Review of Orthopaedics

Review of Orthopaedics

THIRD EDITION

Mark D. Miller, M.D.

WB Carrell Memorial Clinic Associated
Dallas, Texas
Attending Surgeon,
Baylor University Medical Center
Dallas, Texas
Clinical Associate Professor
Uniformed Services University of the Health Sciences
Bethesda, Maryland
Clinical Associate Professor of Orthopaedic Surgery
University of Texas Southwestern Medical Center
Dallas, Texas

Associate Editor:

Mark R. Brinker, M.D.

Director of Acute and Reconstructive Trauma
Director, The Center for Musculoskeletal Research and Outcomes Studies
Fondren Orthopedic Group LLP
Texas Orthopedic Hospital
Houston, Texas
Clinical Associate Professor of Orthopaedic Surgery
Associate Director of Orthopaedic Resident Education
Tulane University School of Medicine
New Orleans, Louisiana
Adjunct Associate Professor of Orthopaedic Surgery
Director of Orthopaedic Basic Science Education
Adjunct Associate Professor, School of Public Health
University of Texas at Houston Medical School
Houston, Texas

W.B. SAUNDERS COMPANY
A Harcourt Health Sciences Company
Philadelphia London New York St. Louis Sydney Toronto

W.B. SAUNDERS COMPANY
A Harcourt Health Sciences Company

The Curtis Center
Independence Square West
Philadelphia, Pennsylvania 19106

Library of Congress Cataloging-in-Publication Data

Review of orthopaedics/[edited by] Mark D. Miller; associate editor, Mark R. Brinker.—3rd ed.

p. cm.

Includes bibliographical references and index.

ISBN 0–7216–8153–0

1. Orthopedics Outlines, syllabi, etc. I. Miller, Mark D. II. Brinker, Mark R. [DNLM: 1. Bone Diseases Outlines. 2. Joint Diseases Outlines. WE 18.2 R454 2000]

RD731.R44 2000 616.7—dc21

DNLM/DLC 99–16737

Editor: Richard H. Lampert
Designer: Marie Gardocky-Clifton
Production Manager: Natalie Ware
Manuscript Editor: Scott Filderman
Illustration Coordinator: Peg Shaw

REVIEW OF ORTHOPAEDICS ISBN 0–7216–8153–0

Printed in the United States of America.

Last digit is the print number: 9 8 7 6 5 4 3 2 1

To my father, an outstanding educator and leader.
I never met a person who didn't admire him.

To my mother, who taught me the value of persistence
and the fact that "Millers don't get B's."

MDM

Contributors

Mark R. Brinker, M.D.
Director of Acute and Reconstructive Trauma; Director, The Center for Musculoskeletal Research and Outcomes Studies, Fondren Orthopedic Group LLP, Texas Orthopedic Hospital, Houston, Texas; Clinical Associate Professor of Orthopaedic Surgery and Associate Director of Orthopaedic Resident Education, Tulane University School of Medicine, New Orleans, Louisiana; Adjunct Associate Professor of Orthopaedic Surgery, Director of Orthopaedic Basic Science Education, and Adjunct Associate Professor, School of Public Health, University of Texas at Houston Medical School, Houston, Texas
Basic Sciences

Tally H. Eddings III, M.D.
Department of Orthopedic Surgery, Duke University, Durham, North Carolina
Adult Trauma

Mark A. Erickson, M.D.
Assistant Professor, Department of Orthopaedic Surgery, University of Colorado Health Sciences Center, Denver, Colorado
Pediatric Orthopaedics

Deborah Anne Frassica, M.D.
Assistant Professor of Oncology, Johns Hopkins University, Baltimore, Maryland
Orthopaedic Pathology

Frank J. Frassica, M.D.
Professor of Orthopaedic Surgery and Oncology, Johns Hopkins University, Baltimore, Maryland
Orthopaedic Pathology

Paul T. Freudigman, M.D.
Director of Orthopaedic Trauma, Baylor University Medical Center, Dallas, Texas
Adult Trauma

Michael E. Goldsmith, M.D.
Clinical Instructor, Georgetown University Medical Center, Washington, D.C.
Spine

Ben A. Gomez, M.D.
Assistant Professor of Orthopaedic Surgery, Wright State University, Dayton, Ohio
Anatomy

Frank Gottschalk, M.D.
Professor of Orthopaedic Surgery, University of Texas Southwestern Medical Center, Dallas, Texas
Rehabilitation: Gait, Amputations, Prosthetics, Orthotics

Kerry G. Jepsen, M.D.
Senior Resident, Department of Orthopaedic Surgery, Wilford Hall USAF Medical Center, Lackland AFB, San Antonio, Texas
Principles of Practice and Statistics

William C. Lauerman, M.D.
Associate Professor of Orthopaedic Surgery and Chief, Division of Spine Surgery, Georgetown University Medical Center, Washington, D.C.
Spine

Edward F. McCarthy, Jr., M.D.
Associate Professor of Pathology and Orthopaedics, Johns Hopkins University, Baltimore, Maryland
Orthopaedic Pathology

Edward J. McPherson, M.D.
Associate Professor of Orthopaedics, University of Southern California, USC Center for Arthritis, Los Angeles, California
Adult Reconstruction

Mark D. Miller, M.D.
WB Carrell Memorial Clinic Associated, Dallas, Texas; Attending Surgeon, Baylor University Medical Center, Dallas, Texas; Clinical Associate Professor, Uniformed Services University of the Health Sciences, Bethesda, Maryland; Clinical Associate Professor of Orthopaedic Surgery, University of Texas Southwestern Medical Center, Dallas, Texas
Sports Medicine; Anatomy

Mark S. Mizel, M.D.
Associate Professor, Department of Orthopaedics and Rehabilitation, University of Miami, Miami, Florida
Disorders of the Foot and Ankle

Richard S. Moore, Jr., M.D.
Associate Professor, Department of Orthopaedics, Duke University, Durham, North Carolina
Adult Trauma

Gregory S. Motley, M.D.
Orthopaedic Surgeon, Nashville, North Carolina
Adult Trauma

Kevin Plancher, M.D.
Director, Plancher Hand and Sports Medicine, Stamford, Connecticut
Principles of Practice and Statistics

Amy Jo Ptaszek, M.D.
Clinical Assistant Professor of Orthopaedic Surgery, University of Texas Health Sciences Center–San Antonio; Chief of Foot and Ankle Surgery, Wilford Hall USAF Medical Center, Lackland AFB, San Antonio, Texas
Disorders of the Foot and Ankle

Damian M. Rispoli, M.D.
Orthopaedic Surgeon, Lakesheath AFB Hospital, England
Principles of Practice and Statistics

Mark Sobel, M.D.
Director, Orthopaedic Foot and Ankle Service, Beth Israel Medical Center–North Division, New York, New York
Disorders of the Foot and Ankle

Raymond M. Stefko, M.D.
Chief, Pediatric Orthopedics, and Assistant Orthopedic Residency Program Director, Wilford Hall USAF Medical Center, Lackland AFB, San Antonio, Texas
Pediatric Orthopaedics

Steven M. Topper, M.D.
Assistant Professor, Orthopaedics and Plastic Surgery, Oregon Health Sciences University, Portland, Oregon; Attending Congenital Hand Surgeon, Shriners Hospital for Children, Portland, Oregon
Hand and Microsurgery

Foreword

The Third Edition of the *Review of Orthopaedics* exhibits an increasing maturity and enhanced focus on a topic that is very much needed and very well done. The goal is to provide a condensed, yet quite comprehensive, overview of the spectrum of orthopaedics. This goal is much needed as demonstrated by the enthusiasm with which the first two editions of this work was accepted. This Third Edition exemplifies Dr. Miller's ongoing commitment to this important challenge. This version is a distinct refinement from the previous two editions. The standardized format allows facility of use as the reader becomes familiar with this layout. The chapters thoroughly review the full spectrum of anatomy, pathology, and treatment options. This edition emphasizes surgical technique more so than before as well as potential pitfalls. The references are also very much up-to-date and relevant. Thus, this continues to provide a very effective and efficient opportunity to review the full spectrum of orthopaedic topics. As such, this volume should prove of value to the medical student, house officer, and practicing orthopaedic surgeon alike. Dr. Miller has, in my judgment, admirably obtained the goal defined in his Preface, that is, to continue to refine and to improve the comprehensive distillation of orthopaedics in a straightforward, simple, and intelligible manner that is easily comprehended, referenced, and applied. Dr. Miller and his colleagues are to be commended for this effort, which has been a singular value to the orthopaedic community, particularly those in training.

BERNARD F. MORREY, M.D.

Preface

Ten years ago, I convinced a skeptical editorial staff at W.B. Saunders Company of the need for a review book in orthopaedics. A decade, several editors, and three editions later, I am proud of the overwhelming success of *Review of Orthopaedics*. This book, and the review course that it fostered, has truly become the orthopaedic resident's best friend. I am honored to make a contribution to the education of a generation of orthopaedic residents and surgeons.

What's new in this edition of *Miller*? First and foremost, I have waged war on typos, omissions, and minor errors. I am indebted to the many individuals who took me seriously when I asked for comments and suggestions—thank you, and please continue to help us make this book, your book, even better in future editions. Second, I am pleased to introduce a new chapter, "Principles of Practice and Statistics," to the third edition. This chapter was developed as a direct result of new challenges (and test questions in a variety of forums) in the practice of orthopaedic surgery. I would be remiss if I did not highlight major revisions as a result of the authors' diligent efforts in the following chapters: "Basic Sciences," "Adult Reconstruction," "Hand," "Rehabilitation," and "Trauma." Although every chapter has been updated and scrutinized, those chapters in particular benefited from the insightful and unselfish contributions of a brilliant group of academic stars.

Welcome to the Third Edition . . . Now, let's get to work!

MARK D. MILLER, M.D.

NOTICE

Medicine is an ever-changing field. Standard safety precautions must be followed, but as new research and clinical experience broaden our knowledge, changes in treatment and drug therapy become necessary or appropriate. Readers are advised to check the product information currently provided by the manufacturer of each drug to be administered to verify the recommended dose, the method and duration of administration, and the contraindications. It is the responsibility of the treating physician, relying on experience and knowledge of the patient, to determine dosages and the best treatment for the patient. Neither the publisher nor the editor assumes any responsibility for any injury and/or damage to persons or property.

THE PUBLISHER

Contents

1

Basic Sciences

Mark R. Brinker

Section 1

Bone

I. **Histology of Bone**

A. Types—Normal bone is lamellar and can be cortical or cancellous. Immature and pathologic bone is woven, is more random with more osteocytes than lamellar bone, has increased turnover, and is weaker and more flexible than lamellar bone. Lamellar bone is stress-oriented; woven bone is not stress-oriented.

1. Cortical Bone (Compact Bone) (Fig. 1–1) (Table 1–1)—Makes up 80% of the skeleton and is composed of tightly packed osteons or haversian systems that are connected by haversian (or Volkmann's) canals. These canals contain arterioles, venules, capillaries, nerves, and possibly lymphatic channels. Interstitial lamellae lie between the osteons. Fibrils frequently connect lamellae but do not cross cement lines (where bone resorption has stopped and new bone formation has begun). Cement lines define the outer border of an osteon. Nutrition is via the intraosseous circulation (canals and canaliculi [cell processes of osteocytes]). Cortical bone is characterized by a slow turnover rate, a relatively high Young's modulus (*E*), and a higher resistance to torsion and bending than cancellous bone.
2. Cancellous Bone (Spongy or Trabecular Bone) (Fig. 1–1)—Less dense and undergoes more remodeling according to lines of stress (Wolff's law). It has a higher turnover rate, has a smaller Young modulus, and is more elastic than cortical bone.

B. Cellular Biology

1. Osteoblasts—Form bone. Derived from undifferentiated mesenchymal cells. These cells have more endoplasmic reticulum, Golgi apparatus, and mitochondria than other cells (to fulfill the cell's role in the synthesis and secretion of matrix). More differentiated, metabolically active cells line bone surfaces and less active cells in "resting regions" or

Table 1–1.

Types of Bone

Microscopic Appearance	Subtypes	Characteristics	Examples
Lamellar	Cortical	Structure is oriented along lines of stress Strong	Femoral shaft
	Cancellous	More elastic than cortical bone	Distal femoral metaphysis
Woven	Immature	Not stress oriented	Embryonic skeleton Fracture callus
	Pathologic	Random organization Increased turnover Weak Flexible	Osteogenic sarcoma Fibrous dysplasia

Modified from Brinker, M.R., and Miller, M.D.: Fundamentals of Orthopaedics. Philadelphia, WB Saunders, 1999, p. 1.

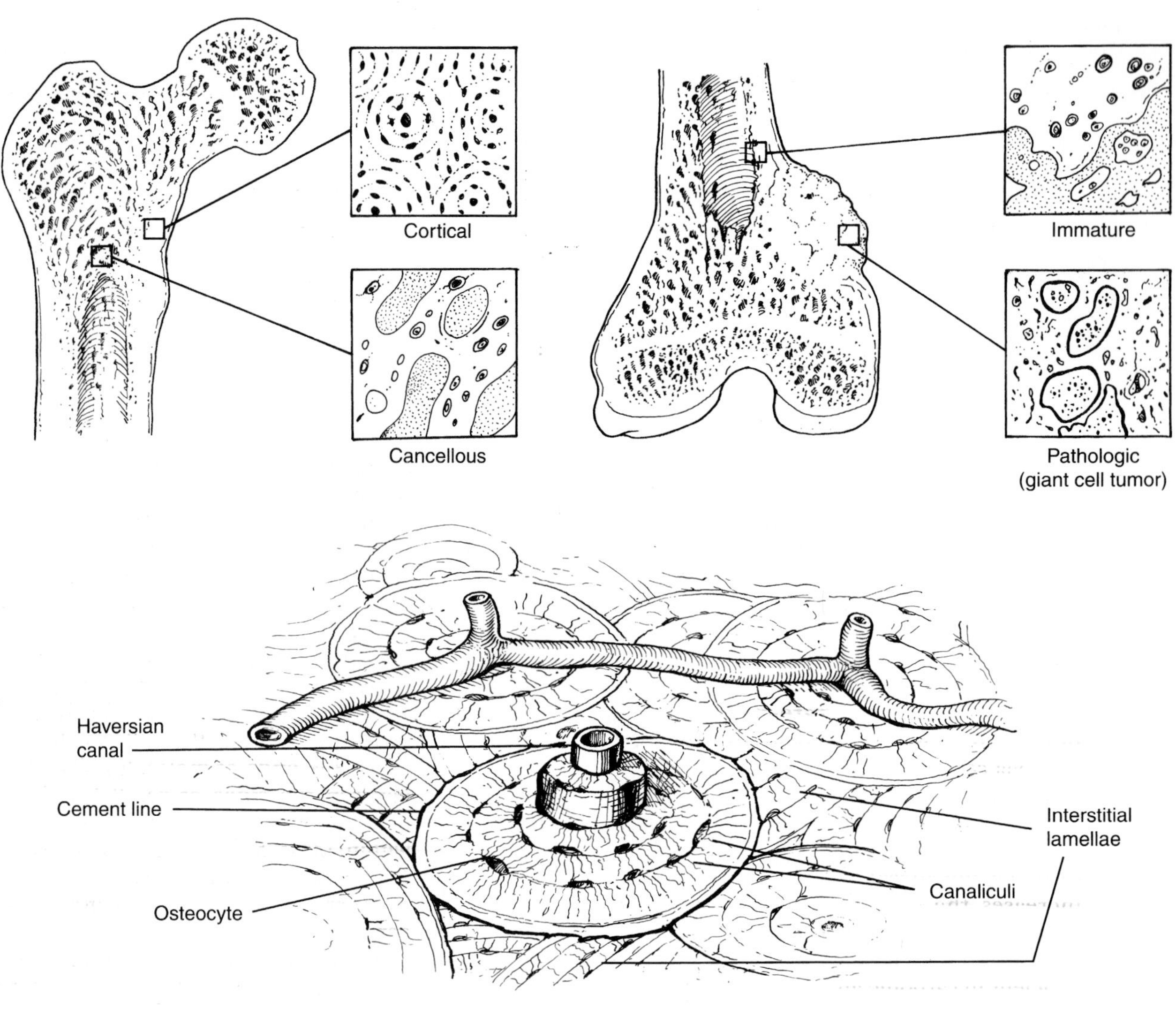

Figure 1–1. Types of bone. *Cortical* bone consists of tightly packed osteons. *Cancellous* bone consists of a meshwork of trabeculae. In *immature* bone, there is unmineralized osteoid lining the immature trabeculae. In *pathologic bone,* atypical osteoblasts and architectural disorganization are seen. (From Brinker, M.R., and Miller, M.D.: Fundamentals of Orthopaedics. Philadelphia, WB Saunders, 1999, p. 2.)

entrapped cells maintain the ionic milieu of bone. Disruption of the lining cell layer activates these cells. Osteoblast differentiation in vivo is effected by the interleukins, platelet-derived growth factor (PDGF), and insulin-derived growth factor (IDGF). Osteoblasts show high alkaline phosphatase activity, produce type I collagen, respond to parathyroid hormone (PTH), and produce osteocalcin (stimulated by 1,25-dihydroxyvitamin D). Osteoblasts have receptor-effector interactions for: (1) PTH; (2) 1,25-dihydroxyvitamin D; (3) glucocorticoids; (4) prostaglandins; and (5) estrogen (Table 1–2). Certain antiseptic agents as an irrigation solution have been shown to be toxic to cultured osteoblasts. These include hydrogen peroxide and povidone-iodine (Betadine) solution and scrub. Bacitracin is generally believed to be less toxic on osteoblasts.

2. Osteocytes (see Fig. 1–1)—Make up 90% of the cells in the mature skeleton and serve to maintain bone. These cells represent former osteoblasts that have been trapped within newly formed matrix (which they help preserve). Osteocytes have an increased nucleus/cytoplasm ratio with long interconnecting cytoplasmic processes and are not as active in matrix production as osteoblasts. Osteocytes have an important role in controlling the extracellular concentration of calcium and phosphorus; they are directly stimulated by calcitonin and inhibited by PTH.
3. Osteoclasts—Resorb bone. These multinucleated, irregularly shaped giant cells originate from hematopoietic tissues (**monocyte**

Table 1–2.

Bone Cell Types, Receptor Types, and Effects

Cell Type	Receptor	Effect
Osteoblast	PTH	Releases a secondary messenger (exact mechanism unknown) to stimulate osteoclastic activity. Activates adenylate cyclase.
	1-25 Vitamin D_3	Stimulates matrix and alkaline phosphatase synthesis and production of bone-specific proteins (such as osteocalcin).
	Glucocorticoids	Inhibits the synthesis of DNA, production of collagen, and synthesis of osteoblastic proteins.
	Prostaglandins	Activates adenylate cyclase and stimulates resorption of bone.
	Estrogen	Anabolic (bone production) and anticatabolic (prevents bone resorption) effect on bone. Increases the levels of mRNA for alkaline phosphatase and inhibits the activation of adenylate cyclase.
Osteoclast	Calcitonin	Inhibits the function of osteoclasts (inhibits bone resorption).

progenitors form giant cells by fusion) and possess a ruffled ("brush") border (plasma membrane enfoldings that increase surface area and are important in bone resorption) and a surrounding clear zone. Bone resorption occurs in depressions known as Howship's lacunae and occurs more rapidly than bone formation; bone formation and resorption are linked ("coupled"). **Osteoclasts synthesize tartrate-resistant acid phosphate.** Osteoclasts bind to bone surfaces via cell attachment (anchoring) proteins (**integrins**). The integrin attachment to bone effectively seals the space below the osteoclast. Osteoclasts produce hydrogen ions (via carbonic anhydrase) to lower the pH, which increases the solubility of hydroxyapatite crystals, and the organic matrix is removed by proteolytic digestion. Patients who are deficient in carbonic anhydrase cannot resorb bone by this mechanism. **Osteoclasts have specific receptors for calcitonin** to allow them to directly regulate bone resorption (Table 1–2). **Osteoclasts are responsible for the bone resorption seen in multiple myeloma and metastatic bone disease. Interleukin-1 (IL-1) is a potent stimulator of osteoclastic bone resorption and has been found in the membranes surrounding loose total joint implants. IL-10 suppresses osteoclast formation.**

4. Osteoprogenitor Cells—Become osteoblasts. These local mesenchymal cells line haversian canals, endosteum, and periosteum, awaiting the stimulus to differentiate into osteoblasts.
5. Lining Cells—Narrow, flattened cells that form an "envelope around bone."

C. Matrix—Composed of organic components (40%) and inorganic components (60%).

1. Organic Components—Make up 40% of the dry weight of bone. Organic components include collagen, proteoglycans, noncollagenous matrix proteins (glycoproteins, phospholipids, phosphoproteins), and growth factors and cytokines.

a. Collagen—Responsible for the tensile strength of bone. Makes up 90% of the organic matrix of bone and is composed primarily of type I collagen (the word "bone" contains the word "one" as its terminal three letters, so it is easy to remember that bone is composed primarily of type I collagen). Collagen structure consists of a triple helix of two α_1 and one α_2 chains that are quarter-staggered to produce a collagen fibril. **Hole zones** (gaps) exist within the collagen fibril between the **ends** of molecules. **Pores** exist between the **sides** of parallel molecules. Mineral deposition (calcification) occurs within these hole zones and pores (Fig. 1–2). Cross-linking decreases solubility and increases the tensile strength of collagen.

b. Proteoglycans—Partially responsible for the compressive strength of bone, they inhibit mineralization. Composed of glycosaminoglycan (GAG)-protein complexes (discussed later in Section 2: Joints).

c. Matrix Proteins (Noncollagenous)—Promote mineralization and bone formation. Matrix proteins include osteocalcin (bone γ-carboxyglutamic acid–containing protein [bone Gla protein]), osteonectin (SPARC), osteopontin, and others. **Osteocalcin** (produced by osteoblasts) attracts osteoclasts and is directly related to the regulation of bone density. Osteocalcin is the most abundant noncollagenous matrix protein of bone and accounts for 10–20% of the noncollagenous protein of bone. The synthesis of osteocalcin is inhibited by PTH and stimulated by 1,25-dihydroxyvitamin D. **Osteocalcin levels can be measured in the serum or urine as a marker of bone turnover.** Osteocalcin levels in urine and serum are elevated in Paget's disease, renal osteodystrophy, and hyperparathyroidism. **Osteonectin** (secreted by platelets and osteoblasts) is postulated to play a role in the regulation

MINERAL ACCRETION: *BIOLOGICAL CONSIDERATIONS*
HETEROGENEITY WITHIN A COLLAGEN FIBRIL

PROGRESSIVELY INCREASING MINERAL MASS DUE TO:

1. INCREASED NUMBER OF NEW MINERAL PHASE PARTICLES (NUCLEATION)
   a. HETEROGENEOUS NUCLEATION BY MATRIX IN COLLAGEN HOLES (? PORES)
   b. 2° CRYSTAL INDUCED NUCLEATION IN HOLES AND PORES
2. INITIAL GROWTH OF PARTICLES TO ~ 400Å x 15–30Å x 50–75Å

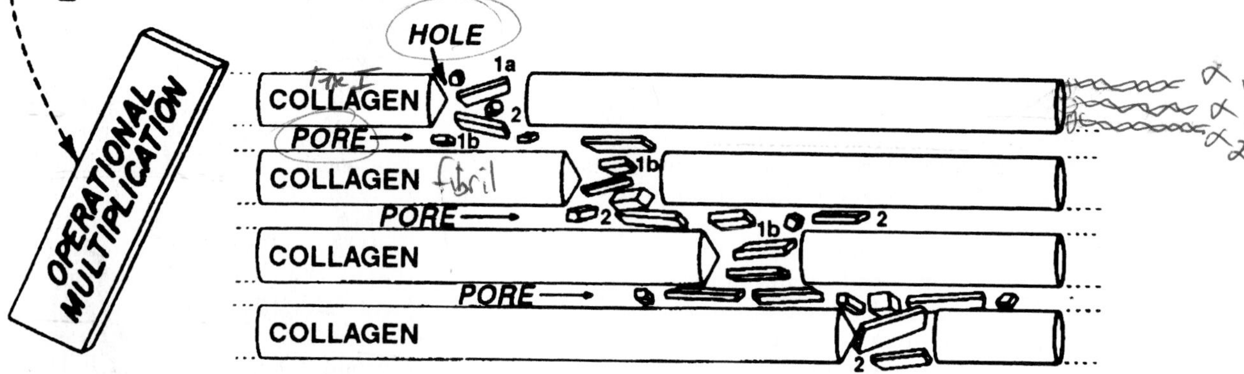

Figure 1–2. Mineral accretion. (From Simon, S.R., ed.: Orthopaedic Basic Science, 2nd ed., p. 139. Rosemont, IL, American Academy of Orthopaedic Surgeons, 1994.)

of calcium or the organization of mineral within the matrix. **Osteopontin** is a cell-binding protein (similar to an integrin).

d. Growth Factors and Cytokines—Present in small amounts in bone matrix. They include (1) transforming growth factor-beta (TGF-β); (2) insulin-like growth factor (IGF); (3) interleukins (IL-1, IL-6); and (4) bone morphogenic proteins (BMP_{1-6}). These proteins aid in bone cell differentiation, activation, growth, and turnover.

2. Inorganic (Mineral) Components—Make up 60% of the dry weight of bone.
   a. Calcium Hydroxyapatite [$Ca_{10}(PO_4)_6(OH)_2$]—Responsible for the compressive strength of bone. Makes up most of the inorganic matrix and is responsible for mineralization of the matrix. Primary mineralization occurs in gaps (holes and pores) in the collagen; secondary mineralization occurs on the periphery.
   b. Osteocalcium Phosphate (Brushite)—Makes up the remaining inorganic matrix.

D. Bone Remodeling—Affected by mechanical function according to Wolff's law. Removal of external stresses can lead to significant bone loss, but this situation can be reversed to varying degrees upon remobilization.

1. General—Bone remodels in response to stress and responds to piezoelectric charges (compression side is electronegative, stimulating osteoblasts [bone formation]; tension side is electropositive, stimulating osteoclasts [bone resorption]). Both cortical and cancellous bone are continuously being remodeled by osteoclastic and osteoblastic activity (Fig. 1–3). Bone remodeling occurs in small packets of cells known as **basic multicellular units (BMUs).** This bone remodeling is modulated by systemic hormones and local cytokines. Bone remodeling occurs throughout life. **The Hueter-Volkmann law** suggests that mechanical factors can influence longitudinal growth, bone remodeling, and fracture repair; compressive forces inhibit growth and tensile forces stimulate growth. The law is postulated to play a role in the progression of scoliosis and Blount's disease.
2. Cortical Bone—Remodels by osteoclastic tunneling (cutting cones) (Fig. 1–4) followed by layering of osteoblasts and successive deposition of layers of lamellae (after the cement line has been laid down) until the tunnel size has narrowed to the diameter of the osteonal central canal. The head of the cutting cone is made up of osteoclasts, which bore holes through hard cortical bone. Behind the osteoclast front are capillaries, followed by osteoblasts, which lay down osteoid to fill the resorption cavity.
3. Cancellous Bone—Remodels by osteoclastic resorption, followed by osteoblasts, which lay down new bone.

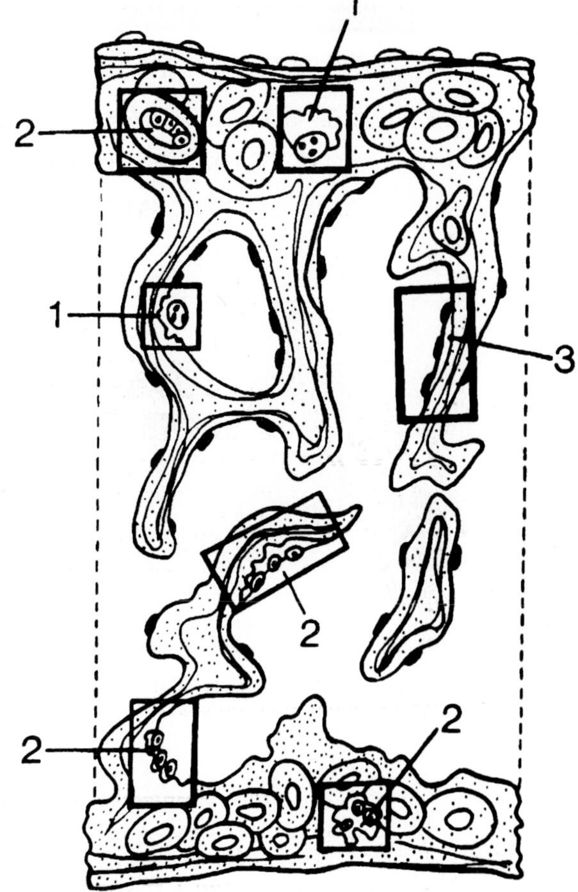

Figure 1–3. Bone remodeling. *1,* Bone resorbed by osteoclastic activity in the cortex and trabeculae. *2,* Osteoblasts form new bone at the site of prior bone resorption. *3,* Osteoblasts become incorporated into bone as osteocytes. (From Simon, S.R., ed.: Orthopaedic Basic Science, 2nd ed., p. 141. Rosemont, IL, American Academy of Orthopaedic Surgeons, 1994.)

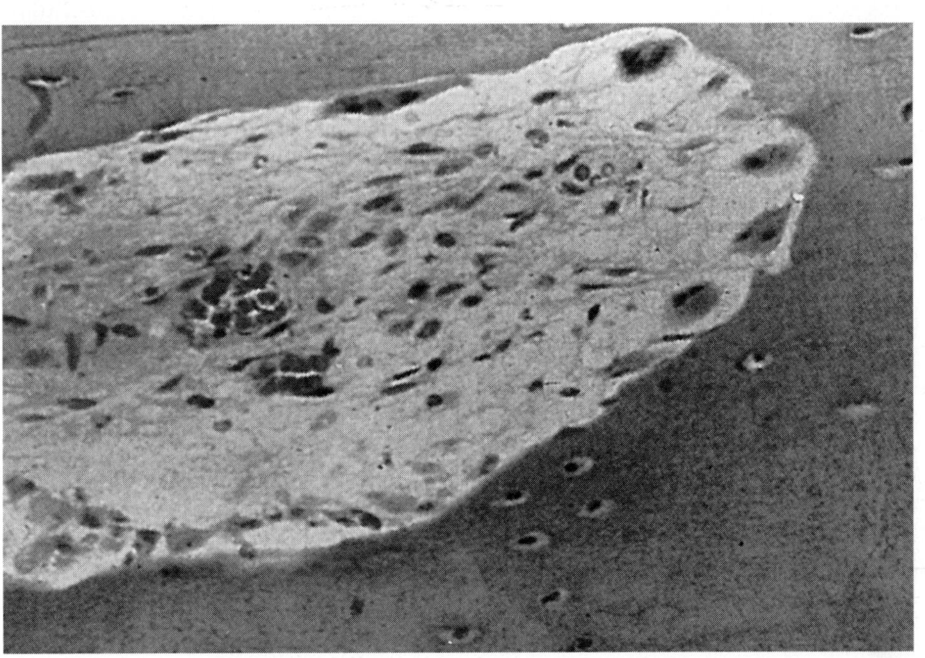

Figure 1–4. Mechanism of cortical bone remodeling via cutting cones. (From Simon, S.R., ed.: Orthopaedic Basic Science, 2nd ed., p. 142. Rosemont, IL, American Academy of Orthopaedic Surgeons, 1994.)

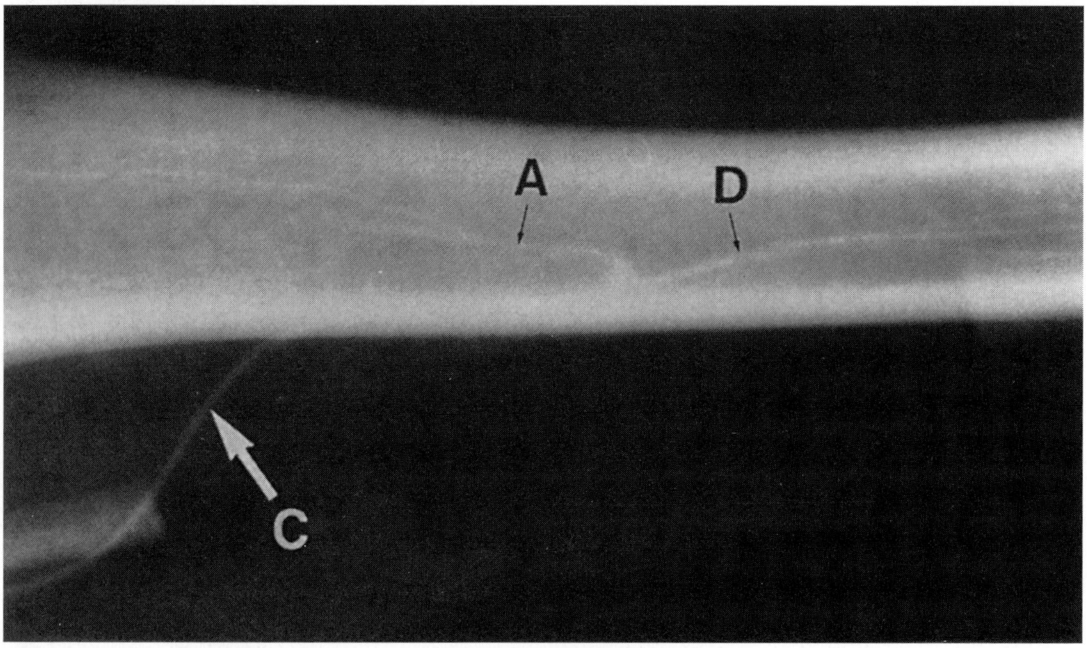

Figure 1–5. Intraoperative arteriogram (canine tibia) demonstrating ascending (*A*) and descending (*D*) branches of the nutrient artery. *C,* Cannula. (From Brinker, M.R., Lipton, H.L., Cook, S.D., and Hyman, A.L.: Pharmacological regulation of the circulation of bone. J. Bone Joint Surg. [Am.] 72:964–975, 1990.)

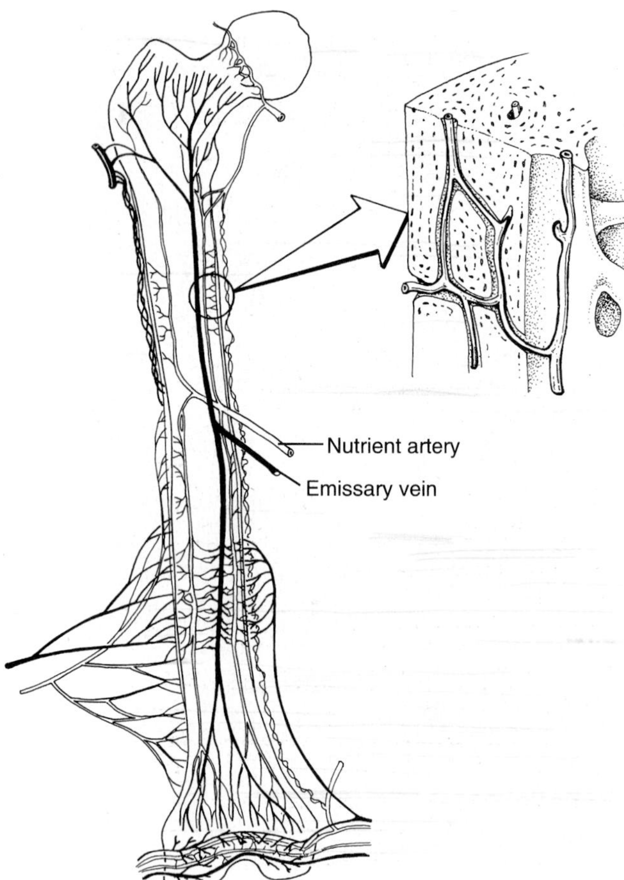

Figure 1–6. Blood supply to bone. (From Brinker, M.R., and Miller, M.D.: Fundamentals of Orthopaedics. Philadelphia, WB Saunders, 1999, p. 4.)

E. Bone Circulation

1. Anatomy—As an organ, bone receives 5–10% of the cardiac output. The long bones receive blood from three sources: (1) nutrient artery system; (2) metaphyseal-epiphyseal system; and (3) periosteal system. Bones with a tenuous blood supply include the scaphoid, talus, femoral head, and odontoid.
    a. Nutrient Artery System—The nutrient artery(s) originate as branches from major arteries of the systemic circulation. The nutrient artery enters the diaphyseal cortex (outer and inner tables) through the nutrient foramen to enter the medullary canal. Once in the medullary canal, the nutrient artery branches into ascending and descending small arteries (Fig. 1–5), which branch into arterioles that penetrate the endosteal cortex to supply at least the inner two-thirds of mature diaphyseal cortex via vessels that traverse the haversian system (Figs. 1–6, 1–7). The nutrient artery system is a **high-pressure** system.
    b. Metaphyseal-Epiphyseal System—Arises from the periarticular vascular plexus (i.e., geniculate arteries).
    c. Periosteal System—Composed primarily of capillaries that supply the outer one-third (at most) of the mature diaphyseal cortex. The periosteal system is a low-pressure system.
2. Physiology
    a. Direction of Flow (Fig. 1–8)
        1. Arterial flow in mature bone is centrifugal (inside to outside), a result of the net effect of the high-pressure nutrient arterial system (endosteal system) and the low-pressure periosteal system.
        2. In the case of a completely displaced fracture with complete disruption of the endosteal (nutrient) system, the pressure head is reversed, the periosteal system predominates, and blood flow is centripetal (outside to inside).
        3. Arterial flow in immature developing bone is centripetal because the periosteum is highly vascularized and is the predominant component of bone blood flow.
        4. Venous flow in mature bone is centripetal; cortical capillaries drain to venous sinusoids, which drain in turn to the emissary venous system.

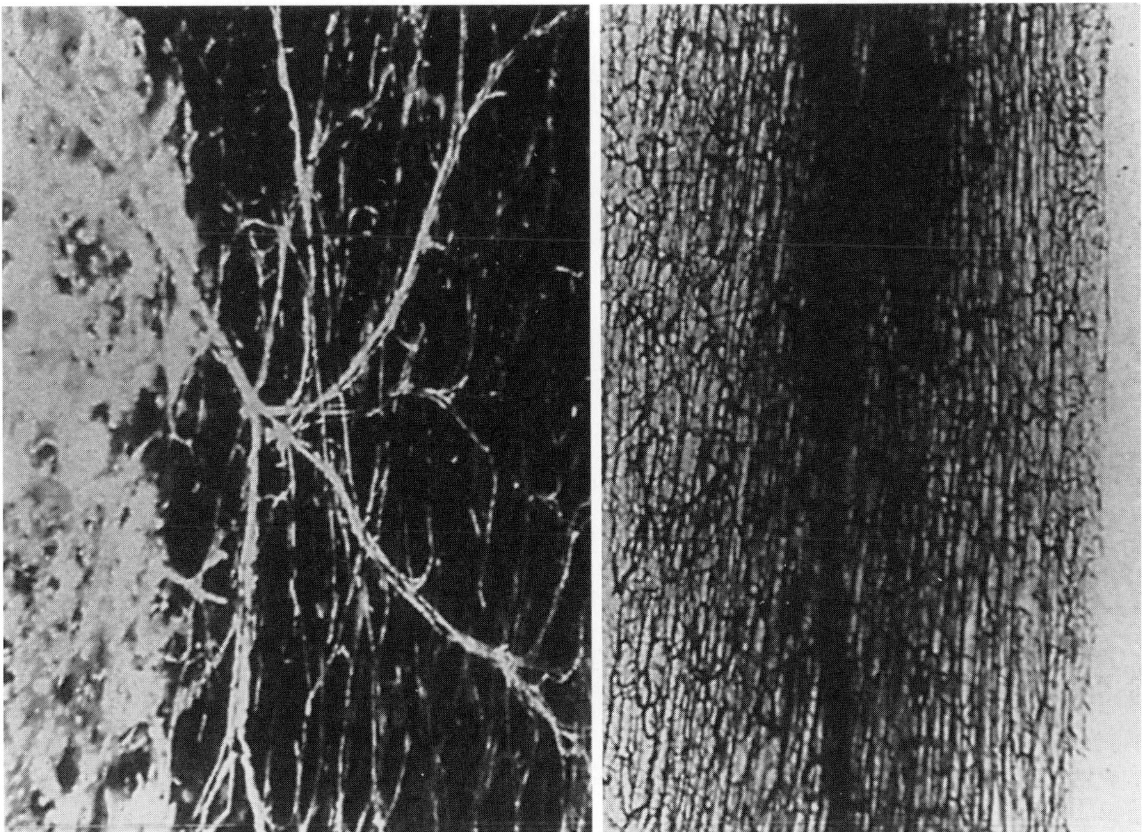

Figure 1–7. Vasculature of cortical bone. (From Simon, S.R., ed.: Orthopaedic Basic Science, 2nd ed., p. 131. Rosemont, IL, American Academy of Orthopaedic Surgeons, 1994.)

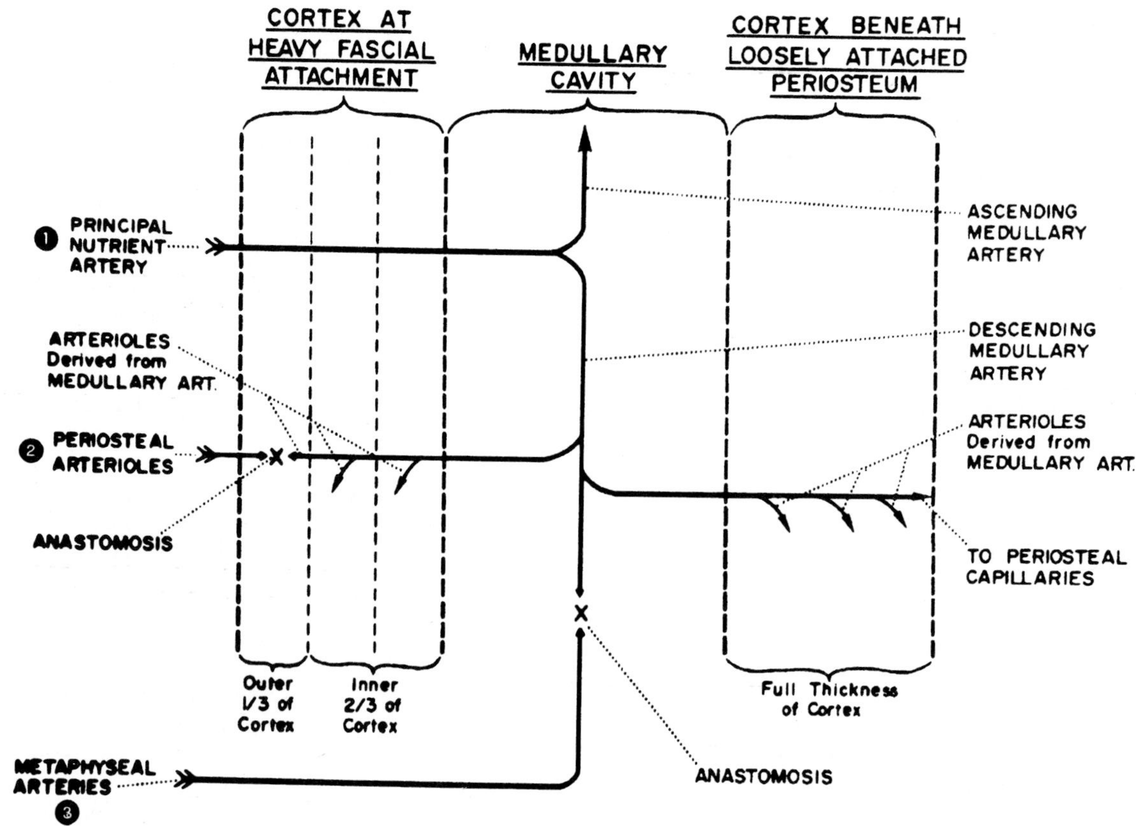

Figure 1–8. Major components of the afferent vascular system of long bone. Components 1, 2, and 3 constitute the total nutrient supply to the diaphysis. Arrows indicate the direction of blood flow. (From Rhinelander, F.W.: Circulation in bone. In Bourne, G., ed.: The Biochemistry and Physiology of Bone, 2nd ed., vol. 2. Orlando, FL, Academic Press, 1972.)

5. Fluid Compartments of Bone

Extravascular	65%
Haversian	6%
Lacunar	6%
RBCs	3%
Other	20%

b. Physiologic States' Effect on Bone Blood Flow
   1. Hypoxia—increases flow
   2. Hypercapnia—increases flow
   3. Sympathectomy—increases flow

3. Fracture Healing—Bone blood flow is responsible for the delivery of nutrients to the site of bony injury. The **initial response** of bone blood flow to a fracture is **decreased flow** secondary to disruption of the vascular anatomy at the fracture site. **Within hours to days, bone blood flow increases** (as part of the **regional acceleratory phenomenon)** and **peaks at approximately 2 weeks.** Blood flow **returns to normal** between **3 and 5 months.** Bone blood flow is the **major determinant** of fracture healing. The major advantage of using unreamed intramedullary (IM) nails is the preservation of the endosteal blood supply. Loose-fitting nails spare cortical perfusion and allow for a more rapid reperfusion when compared with canal filling nails; reaming devascularizes the inner 50–80% of cortex and is the type of canal preparation associated with the greatest delay in revascularization of the endosteal blood supply and the distribution of the nutrient artery.
4. Regulation—Bone blood flow is under the control of metabolic, humoral, and autonomic inputs. The arterial system of bone has great potential for vasoconstriction (from the resting state) and much less potential for vasodilation. The vessels within bone possess a variety of vasoactive receptors (β-adrenergic, muscarinic, thromboxane/prostaglandin) that may be useful in the future for pharmacologic treatment of bone diseases related to aberrant circulation (e.g., osteonecrosis, fracture nonunions).

F. Tissues Surrounding Bone
   1. Periosteum—Connective tissue membrane that covers bone. It is more highly developed in children because of its role in the deposition of cortical bone, which is responsible for growth in bone diameter. The inner layer of periosteum, or cambium, is loose, is more vascular, and contains cells that are capable of becoming osteoblasts (to form bone); these cells are responsible for enlarging the diame-

ter of bone during growth and forming periosteal callus during fracture healing; the outer, fibrous layer is less cellular and is contiguous with joint capsules.

2. Bone Marrow—Source of progenitor cells; controls the inner diameter of bone.
   a. Red Marrow—Hematopoietic (40% water, 40% fat, 20% protein). Red marrow slowly changes to yellow marrow with age, beginning in the appendicular skeleton and later the axial skeleton.
   b. Yellow Marrow—Inactive (15% water, 80% fat, 5% protein).

G. Types of Bone Formation (Table 1–3)

1. **Enchondral Bone Formation/Mineralization**
   a. General Comments—Undifferentiated cells secrete cartilagineous matrix and differentiate into chondrocytes. This matrix mineralizes and is invaded by vascular buds that bring in osteoprogenitor cells. Osteoclasts then resorb calcified cartilage, and osteoblasts form bone. **Remember: Bone replaces the cartilage model; cartilage is not converted to bone. Examples of enchondral bone formation include (1) embryonic long bone formation, (2) longitudinal growth (physis), (3) fracture callus, and (4) the bone formed with the use of demineralized bone matrix.**
   b. Embryonic Long Bone Formation (Figs. 1–9, 1–10)—Formed from mesenchymal anlage, usually at 6 weeks in utero. Enchondral bone formation is responsible for the development of embryonic long bones. Vascular buds invade the mesenchymal model, bringing in osteoprogenitor cells that differentiate into osteoblasts and form the primary centers of ossification at approximately 8 weeks. The cartilage model grows through appositional (width) and interstitial (length) growth. The marrow is formed by resorption of the central portion of the cartilage anlage by invasion of myeloid precursor cells brought in by the capillary buds. Secondary centers of ossification develop at the bone ends, forming epiphyseal centers of ossification (growth plates), which are responsible for longitudinal growth of immature bones. During this developmental stage, there is a rich arterial supply composed of an epiphyseal artery (which terminates in the proliferative zone), metaphyseal arteries, nutrient arteries, and perichondrial arteries (Fig. 1–11).
   c. Physis—Two growth plates exist in immature long bones: (1) a **horizontal** growth plate (the physis); and (2) a **spherical** growth plate that allows growth of the epiphysis. The spherical growth plate has the same arrangement as the physis but is less organized. Acromegaly and spondyloepiphyseal dysplasia affect physeal growth; multiple epiphyseal dysplasia adversely affects growth of the epiphysis. Physeal cartilage is divided into zones based on growth (Fig. 1–11) and function (Figs. 1–12, 1–13).
      1. Reserve Zone—Cells store lipids, glycogen, and proteoglycan aggregates for later growth. Decreased oxygen tension occurs in this zone. **Lysosomal storage diseases (Gaucher's)** and other diseases can affect this zone, which is involved in matrix production.
      2. Proliferative Zone—Longitudinal growth occurs with stacking of chondrocytes (top cell is the dividing

Table 1–3.

Types of Bone Formation

Type of Ossification	Mechanism	Examples of Normal Mechanisms	Examples of Diseases with Abnormal Ossification
Enchondral	Bone replaces a cartilage model	1) Embryonic long bone formation 2) Longitudinal growth (physis) 3) Fracture callus 4) The type of bone formed with the use of demineralized bone matrix	Achondroplasia
Intramembranous	Aggregates of undifferentiated mesenchymal cells differentiate into osteoblasts, which form bone	1) Embryonic flat bone formation 2) Bone formation during distraction osteogenesis 3) Blastema bone	Cleidocranial dysostosis
Appositional	Osteoblasts lay down new bone on existing bone	1) Periosteal bone enlargement (width) 2) The bone formation phase of bone remodeling	Paget's disease Infantile hyperostosis (Caffey's disease) Melorheostosis

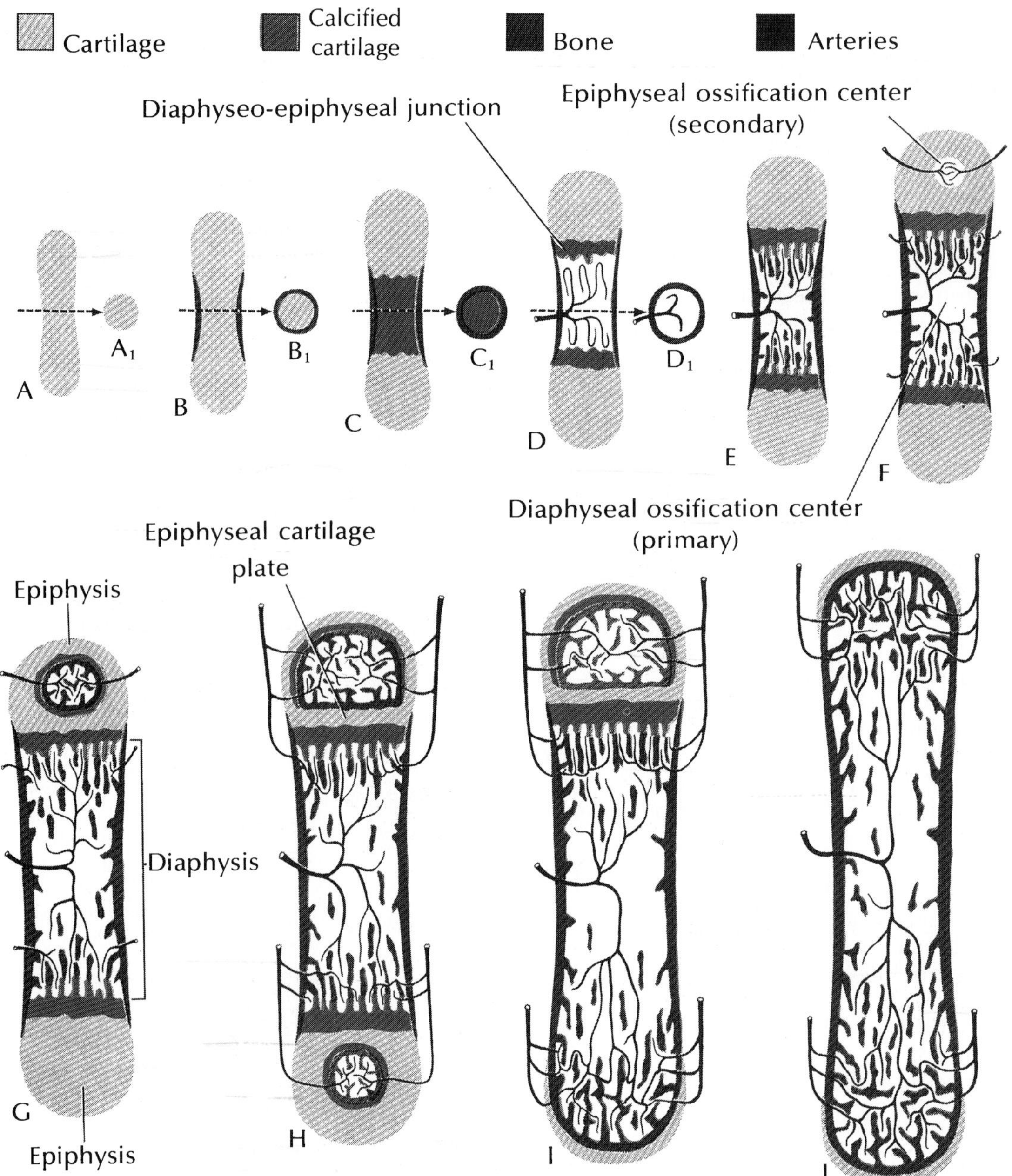

Figure 1–9. Enchondral ossification of long bones. Note that phases *F–J* often occur after birth. (From Moore, K.L.: The Developing Human, p. 346. Philadelphia: WB Saunders, 1982.)

"mother" cell). There is increased oxygen tension and increased proteoglycan in the surrounding matrix, which inhibits calcification. This zone functions in cellular proliferation and matrix production. Defects in this zone (chondrocyte proliferation and column formation) are seen in **achondroplasia** (Fig. 1–13) (does not affect intramembranous bone [width]).

3. Hypertrophic Zone—Sometimes subdivided into three zones: **maturation, degeneration,** and **provisional calcification.** Normal mineralization of matrix occurs in the lower hypertrophic zone. In the hypertrophic zone, cells increase five times in size, accumulate calcium in their mitochondria, and then die (releasing calcium from matrix vesicles). Osteoblasts, which migrate from sinusoidal vessels, use cartilage as a scaffolding for bone formation. Low oxygen tension and decreased proteoglycan aggregates aid in this process. **This zone is widened in rickets** (Fig. 1–13), where little or no provisional calcification occurs. **Enchondromas** also originate in this

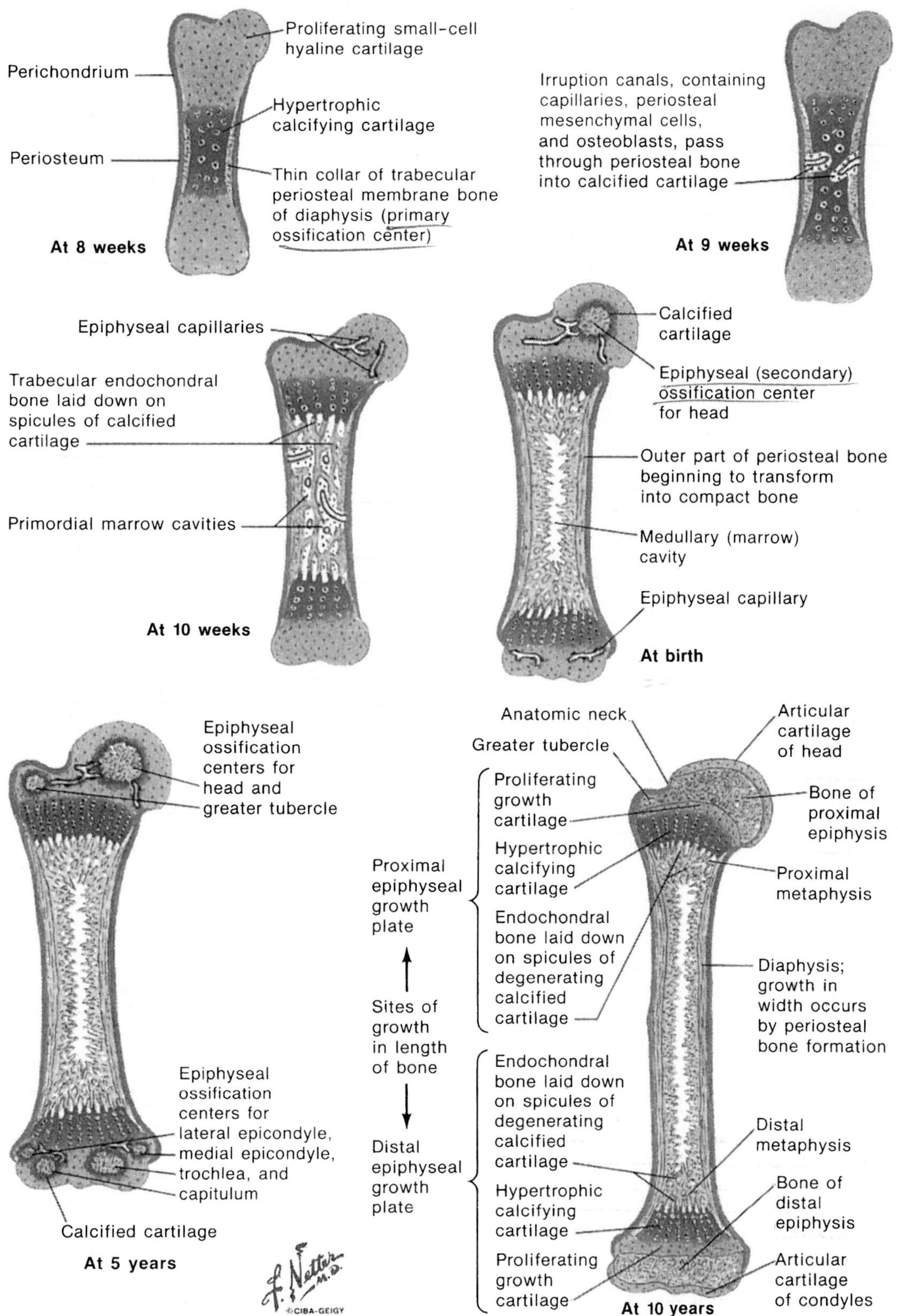

Figure 1–10. Development of a typical long bone: formation of the growth plate and secondary centers of ossification. (From The Ciba Collection of Medical Illustrations, vol. 8, part I, p. 136, 1987. Illustrated by Frank H. Netter. Reprinted by permission.)

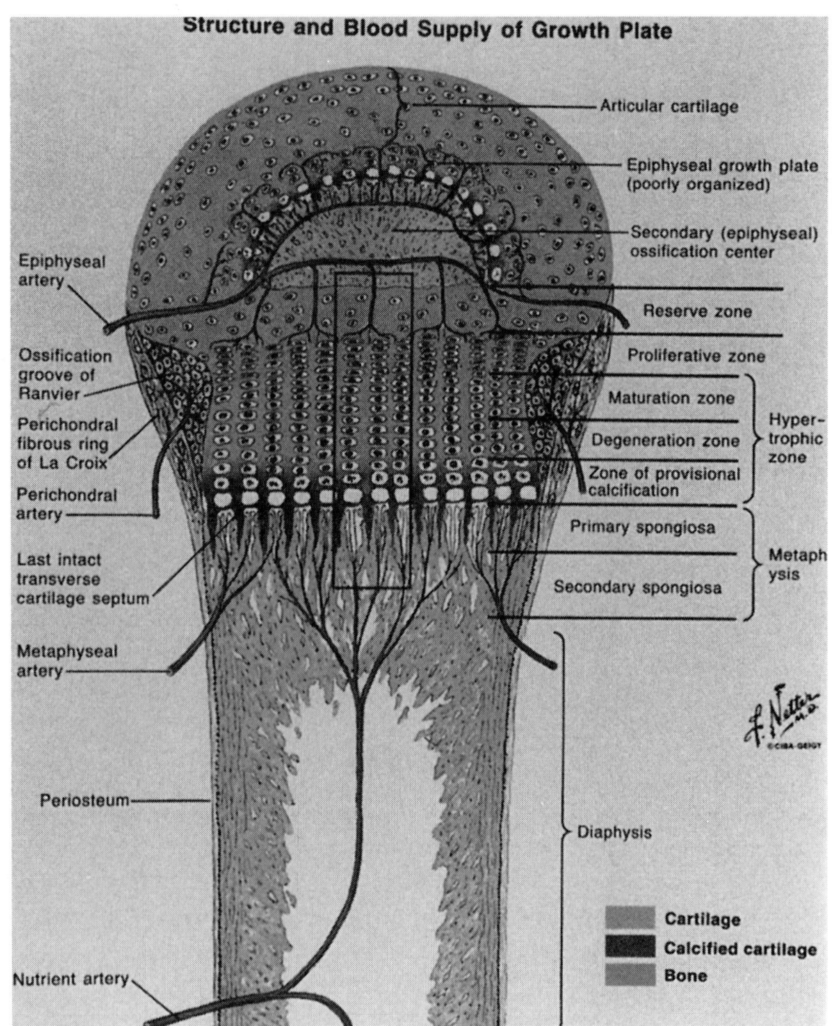

Figure 1–11. Structure and blood supply of a typical growth plate. (From the Ciba Collection of Medical Illustrations, vol. 8, part I, p. 166, 1987. Illustrated by Frank H. Netter. Reprinted by permission.)

zone. **Mucopolysaccharidic diseases** (Fig. 1–13) also affect the zone, leading to chondrocyte degeneration (swollen, abnormal chondrocytes). Physeal fractures are classically believed to occur through the zone of provisional calcification (within the hypertrophic zone), but they probably traverse several zones depending on the type of loading (Fig. 1–14). **The hypertrophic zone is also believed to be involved in slipped capital femoral epiphysis (SCFE). An exception to this is SCFE associated with renal failure; in this case the slippage occurs through the metaphyseal spongiosa.**

d. Metaphysis—Adjacent to the physis, the metaphysis expands with skeletal growth. Osteoblasts from osteoprogenitor cells line up on cartilage bars produced by physeal expansion. Primary spongiosa (calcified cartilage bars) is mineralized to form woven bone and is remodeled to form secondary spongiosa and a "cutback zone" at the metaphysis. Cortical bone is made by remodeling of physeal (enchondral) and intramembranous bone in response to stress along the periphery of the growing long bones.

e. Periphery of the Physis—Composed of two elements.
   1. Groove of Ranvier—Supplies chondrocytes to the periphery of the growth plate for lateral growth (width).
   2. Perichondrial Ring of LaCroix—Dense fibrous tissue anchors and supports the physis.

f. Mineralization—Consists of seeding of collagen hole zones with calcium hydroxyapatite crystals through branching and accretion (crystal growth).

g. Effect of Hormones and Growth Factors on the Growth Plate—Several hormones and growth factors have both direct and indirect effects on the developing growth plate. Some factors are produced and act within the growth plate (paracrine or autocrine), and others are produced at a site distant from the growth plate (endocrine).

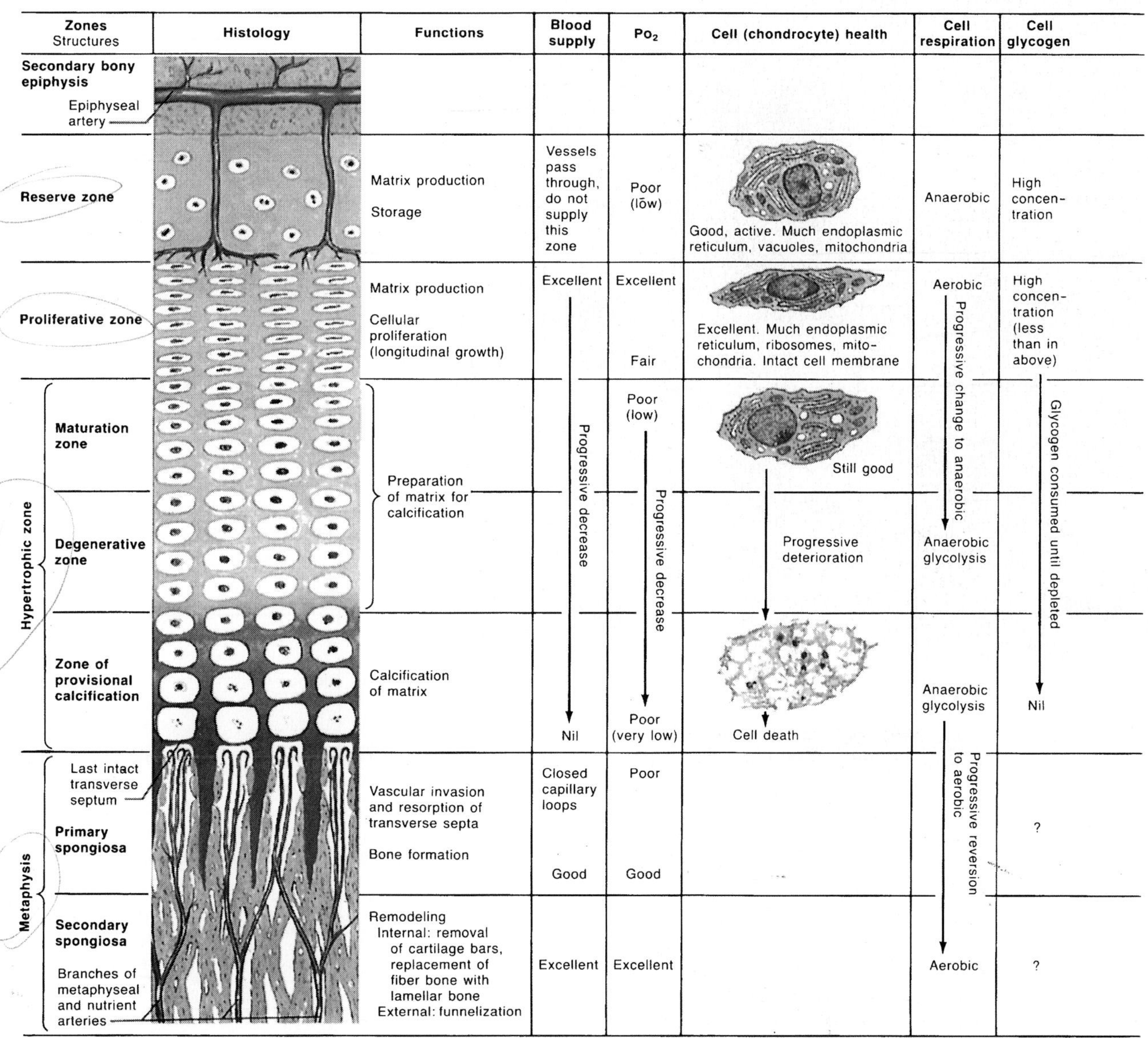

Zones
Structures
Histology
Functions
Blood supply
Po2
Cell (chondrocyte) health
Cell respiration
Cell glycogen
Secondary bony epiphysis
Epiphyseal artery
Reserve zone
Matrix production
Storage
Vessels pass through, do not supply this zone
Poor (lōw)
Good, active. Much endoplasmic reticulum, vacuoles, mitochondria
Anaerobic
High concen-tration
Proliferative zone
Matrix production
Cellular proliferation (longitudinal growth)
Excellent
Excellent
Fair
Excellent. Much endoplasmic reticulum, ribosomes, mito-chondria. Intact cell membrane
Aerobic
High concen-tration (less than in above)
Hypertrophic zone
Maturation zone
Degenerative zone
Preparation of matrix for calcification
Poor (low)
Still good
Progressive deterioration
Progressive change to anaerobic
Anaerobic glycolysis
Glycogen consumed until depleted
Progressive decrease
Progressive decrease
Zone of provisional calcification
Calcification of matrix
Nil
Poor (very low)
Cell death
Anaerobic glycolysis
Nil
Metaphysis
Last intact transverse septum
Primary spongiosa
Vascular invasion and resorption of transverse septa
Bone formation
Closed capillary loops
Good
Poor
Good
Progressive reversion to aerobic
?
Secondary spongiosa
Branches of metaphyseal and nutrient arteries
Remodeling
Internal: removal of cartilage bars, replacement of fiber bone with lamellar bone
External: funnelization
Excellent
Excellent
Aerobic
?

Figure 1–12. Zonal structure, function, and physiology of the growth plate. (From The Ciba Collection of Medical Illustrations, vol. 8, part I, p. 164, 1987. Illustrated by Frank H. Netter. Reprinted by permission.)

Zones Structures	Histology	Functions	Exemplary diseases	Defect (if known)
Secondary bony epiphysis Epiphyseal artery	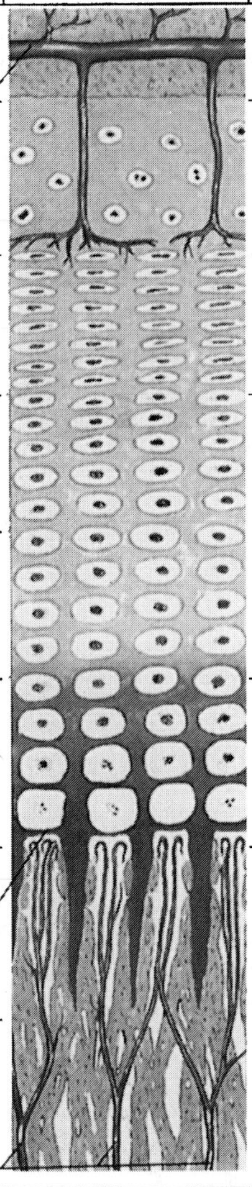			
Reserve zone		Matrix production Storage	Diastrophic dwarfism (also, defects in other zones) Pseudoachondroplasia (also, defects in other zones) Kneist syndrome (also, defects in other zones)	Defective type II collagen synthesis Defective processing and transport of proteoglycans Defective processing of proteoglycans
Proliferative zone		Matrix production Cellular proliferation (longitudinal growth)	Gigantism Achondroplasia Hypochondroplasia Malnutrition, irradiation injury, glucocorticoid excess	Increased cell proliferation (growth hormone increased) Deficiency of cell proliferation Less severe deficiency of cell proliferation Decreased cell proliferation and/or matrix synthesis
Hypertrophic zone: **Maturation zone**; **Degenerative zone**		Preparation of matrix for calcification	Mucopolysaccharidosis (Morquio's syndrome, Hurler's syndrome)	Deficiencies of specific lysosomal acid hydrolases, with lysosomal storage of mucopolysaccharides
Hypertrophic zone: **Zone of provisional calcification**		Calcification of matrix	Rickets, osteomalacia (also, defects in metaphysis)	Insufficiency of Ca^{++} and/or P for normal calcification of matrix
Metaphysis: Last intact transverse septum; **Primary spongiosa**		Vascular invasion and resorption of transverse septa Bone formation	Metaphyseal chondrodysplasia (Jansen and Schmid types) Acute hematogenous osteomyelitis	Extension of hypertrophic cells into metaphysis Flourishing of bacteria due to sluggish circulation, low PO_2, reticuloendothelial deficiency
Metaphysis: **Secondary spongiosa**; Branches of metaphyseal and nutrient arteries		Remodeling Internal: removal of cartilage bars, replacement of fiber bone with lamellar bone External: funnelization	Osteopetrosis Osteogenesis imperfecta Scurvy Metaphyseal dysplasia (Pyle disease)	Abnormality of osteoclasts (internal remodeling) Abnormality of osteoblasts and collagen synthesis Inadequate collagen formation Abnormality of funnelization (external remodeling)

Figure 1–13. Zonal structure and pathologic defects of cellular metabolism. (From The Ciba Collection of Medical Illustrations, vol. 8, part I, p. 165, 1987. Illustrated by Frank H. Netter. Reprinted by permission.)

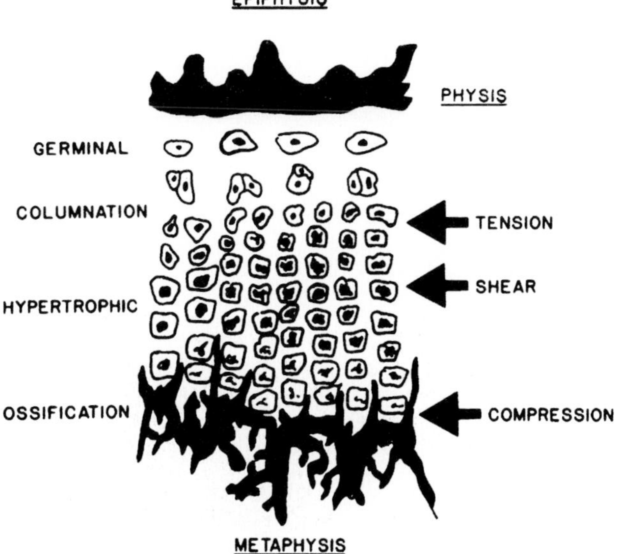

Figure 1–14. Histologic zone of failure varies with the type of loading applied to a specimen. (From Moen, C.T., and Pelker, R.R.: Biomechanical and histological correlations in growth plate failure. J. Pediatr. Orthop. 4:180–184, 1984.)

The actions of hormones and growth factors are via their effect on chondrocytes and matrix mineralization (summarized in Fig. 1–15 and Table 1–4).

2. **Intramembranous Ossification**—Occurs without a cartilage model. Undifferentiated mesenchymal cells aggregate into layers (or membrane). These cells differentiate into osteoblasts and deposit organic matrix that mineralizes to form bone. **Examples of intramembranous bone formation include (1) embryonic flat bone formation (pelvis, clavicle, vault of skull), (2) bone formation during distraction osteogenesis, and (3)**

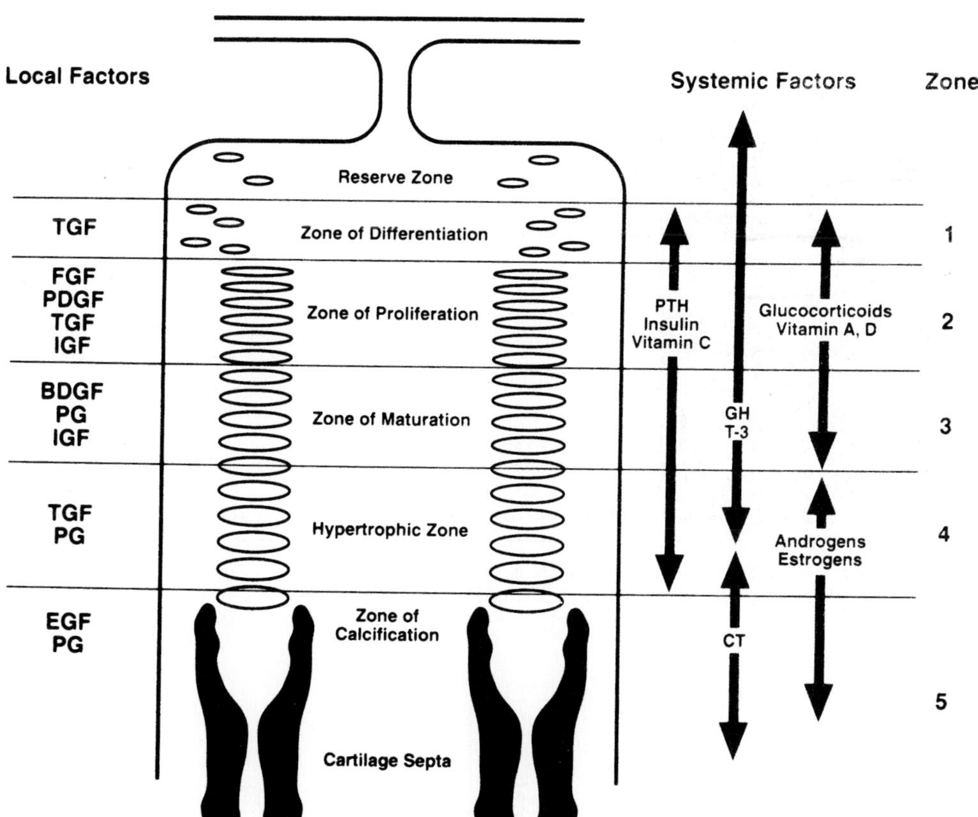

Figure 1–15. Growth plate, demonstrating the proposed sites of action of hormones, growth factors, and vitamins. (From Simon, S.R., ed.: Orthopaedic Basic Science, 2nd ed., p. 197. Rosemont, IL, American Academy of Orthopaedic Surgeons, 1994.)

Table 1–4.

Effects of Hormones and Growth Factors on the Growth Plate

Hormone/ Factor	Systemic/ Local Derivation	Biologic Effect				Zone Primarily Affected
		Proliferation	Macro-Molecule Biosynthesis	Maturation Degradation	Matrix Calcification	
Thyroxine	Systemic (thyroid)	+ (T_3 with IGF-I)	0	+ (T_3 alone)	0	Proliferative zone and upper hypertrophic zone
Parathyroid	Systemic (parathyroid)	+	+ + (Proteoglycan)	0	0	Entire growth plate
Calcitonin	Systemic (thyroid)	0	0	+	+	Hypertrophic zone and metaphysis
Excess corticosteroids	Systemic (adrenals)	–	–	–	0	Entire growth plate
Growth hormone	Systemic (pituitary)	+ (through IGF-I locally)	+ (Slight)	0	0	Proliferative zone
Somatomedins	Systemic Local paracrine (liver, chondrocytes)	+	+ (Slight)	0	0	Proliferative zone
Insulin	Systemic (pancreas)	+ (through IGF-I receptor)	0	0	0	Proliferative zone
1,25-$(OH)_2D_3$	Systemic (liver, kidney)	0	0	+ (Indirect effect serum [Ca] × [PO])		Hypertrophic zone
24,25-$(OH)_2D_3$	Systemic (liver, kidney)	+	+ (Collagen II)	0	0	Proliferative zone and hypertrophic zone

Vitamin A	Systemic (diet)	0	0	−	0	Hypertrophic zone
Vitamin C	Systemic (diet)	0	+ (Collagen)	0	+ (Matrix vesicles)	Proliferative zone and hypertrophic zone
EGF	Local paracrine (endothelial cells)	+	− (Collagen)	0	0	Metaphysis
FGF	Local paracrine (endothelial cells)	+	0	0	0	Proliferative zone
PDGF	Local paracrine (platelets)	+	+ (Noncollagenous proteins)	0	0	Proliferative zone
TGF-β	Local paracrine (platelets, chondrocytes)	±	±	0	0	Proliferative zone and hypertrophic zone
BDGF	Local paracrine (bone matrix)	0	+ (Collagen)	0	0	Upper hypertrophic zone
IL-1	Local paracrine (inflammatory cells, synoviocytes)	0	−	+ + Activates tissue metalloproteinases	0	Entire growth plate
Prostaglandin	Local autocrine	±	+ (Proteoglycan) − (Collagen and alkaline phosphatase)	0	Bone resorption with osteoclasts	Hypertrophic zone and metaphysis

+, increase stimulation; 0, no known effect; −, inhibitory; ±, depending on the local hormonal milieu.

EGF, epidermal growth factor; FGF, fibroblast growth factor; PDGF, platelet-derived growth factor; TGF-β, transforming growth factor-beta; BDGF, bone-derived growth factor; IL-1, interleukin-1; IGF-I, Insulin-like growth factor I.

From Simon, S.R.: Orthopaedic Basic Science, 2nd ed., p. 196. Rosemont, IL, American Academy of Orthopaedic Surgeons, 1994; reprinted by permission.

Table 1–5.

Biologic and Mechanical Factors Influencing Fracture Healing

Biologic Factors	Mechanical Factors
Patient age	Soft-tissue attachments to bone
Comorbid medical conditions	Stability (extent of immobilization)
Functional level	Anatomic location
Nutritional status	Level of energy imparted
Nerve function	Extent of bone loss
Vascular injury	
Hormones	
Growth factors	
Health of the soft-tissue envelope	
Sterility (in open fractures)	
Cigarette smoke	
Local pathologic conditions	
Level of energy imparted	
Type of bone affected	
Extent of bone loss	

blastema bone (occurs in young children with amputations).

3. **Appositional Ossification**—Osteoblasts align themselves on the existing bone surface and lay down new bone. **Examples of appositional ossification include (1) periosteal bone enlargement (width) and (2) the bone formation phase of bone remodeling.**

II. **Bone Injury and Repair**

A. **Fracture Repair**—The response of bone to injury can be thought of as a continuum of processes, beginning with **inflammation,** proceeding through **repair** (soft callus followed by hard callus), and finally ending in **remodeling.** Fracture healing may be influenced by a variety of biologic and mechanical factors (Table 1–5).

1. Stages of Fracture Repair

a. Inflammation—Bleeding from the fracture site and surrounding soft tissues creates a hematoma (and fibrin clot), which provides a source of hematopoietic cells capable of secreting growth factors. Subsequently fibroblasts, mesenchymal cells, and osteoprogenitor cells are present at the fracture site, and granulation tissue forms around the fracture ends. Osteoblasts, from surrounding osteogenic precursor cells, fibroblasts, or both proliferate.

b. Repair—Primary callus response occurs within 2 weeks. If the bone ends are not in continuity, **bridging (soft) callus** occurs. The soft callus later is replaced, via the process of enchondral ossification, by woven bone (hard callus). Another type of callus, **medullary callus,** supplements the bridging callus, although it forms more slowly and occurs later (Fig. 1–16). The amount of callus formation is indirectly proportional to the amount of immobilization of the fracture. Primary cortical healing, which resembles normal remodeling, occurs with rigid immobilization and anatomic (or near-anatomic) reduction. Fracture healing varies with the method of treatment (Table 1–6). With closed treatment, "enchondral healing" with periosteal bridging callus occurs. With rigidly fixed fractures (compression plate), direct osteonal or primary bone healing occurs without visible callus. The initial histologic change observed in hypertrophic nonunions treated with plate

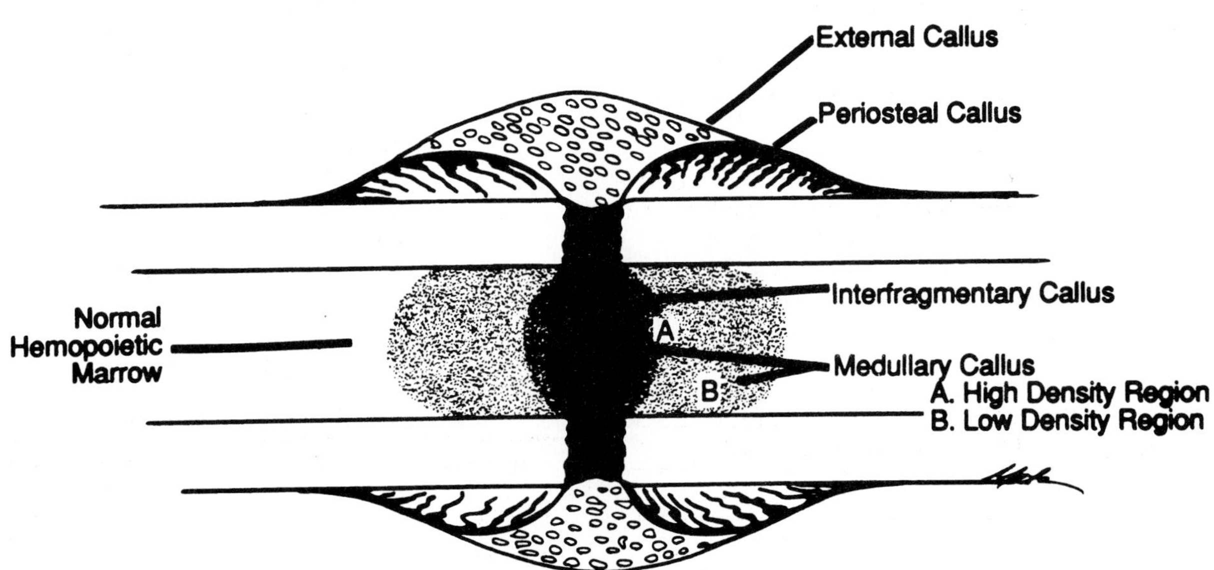

Figure 1–16. Histology of typical fracture healing. (From Brighton, C.T., and Hunt, R.M.: Early histological and ultrastructural changes in medullary fracture callus. J. Bone Joint Surg. [Am.] 73:832–847, 1991.)

Table 1–6.

Type of Fracture Healing Based on Type of Stabilization

Type of Immobilization	Predominant Type of Healing	Comments
Cast (closed treatment)	Periosteal bridging callus	Enchondral ossification
Compression plate	Primary cortical healing (remodeling)	Cutting cone–type remodeling
Intramedullary nail	Early—periosteal bridging callus Late—medullary callus	Enchondral ossification
External fixator	Dependent on extent of rigidity Less rigid—periosteal bridging callus More rigid—primary cortical healing	
Inadequate	Hypertrophic nonunion	Failed endochondral ossification Type II collagen predominates

stabilization is fibrocartilage mineralization.

c. Remodeling—This process begins during the middle of the repair phase and continues long after the fracture has clinically healed (up to 7 years). Remodeling allows the bone to assume its normal configuration and shape based on the stresses to which it is exposed (Wolff's law). Throughout the process, woven bone formed during the repair phase is replaced with lamellar bone. Fracture healing is complete when there is repopulation of the marrow space.

2. Biochemistry of Fracture Healing—Four biochemical steps of fracture healing have been described (Table 1–7).
3. Growth Factors of Bone
   a. Bone Morphogenic Protein (BMP)—Osteoinductive; induces metaplasia of mesenchymal cells into osteoblasts. **The target cell for BMP is the undifferentiated perivascular mesenchymal cell.** BMP stimulates bone formation.
   b. Transforming Growth Factor-Beta (TGF-β)—Induces mesenchymal cells to produce type II collagen and proteoglycans. Also induces osteoblasts to synthesize collagen. TGF-β is found in fracture hematomas and is believed to **regulate cartilage and bone formation in fracture callus.** Coating porous implants with TGF-β enhances bone ingrowth.
   c. Insulin-Like Growth Factor II (IGF-II)—Stimulates type I collagen, cellular proliferation, cartilage matrix synthesis, and bone formation.
   d. Platelet-Derived Growth Factor (PDGF)—Released from platelets; attracts inflammatory cells to the fracture site (chemotactic).
4. Hormonal Effects on Fracture Healing (Table 1–8)
5. Ultrasound and Fracture Healing
   a. Clinical studies show that low-intensity pulsed ultrasound accelerates fracture healing and increases the mechanical strength of callus, including torque and stiffness.
   b. The postulated mechanism of action is that the cells responsible for fracture healing respond favorably to the mechanical energy transmitted by the ultrasound signal.
6. Effect of Radiation on Bone
   a. Long-term changes of bone injury after high-dose irradiation are the result of changes in the haversian system and a decrease in overall cellularity.
   b. Immediate postoperative irradiation has an adverse effect on the incorporation of anterior spinal interbody strut grafts (a delay in postoperative irradiation of 3 weeks eliminates these adverse effects).
   c. High-dose irradiation (90 kGy—the dose needed for viral inactivation) of allograft bone significantly reduces its structural integrity.
7. Electricity and Fracture Healing

Table 1–7.

Biochemical Steps of Fracture Healing

Step	Collagen Type
Mesenchymal	I, II, (III, V)
Chondroid	II, IX
Chondroid-osteoid	I, II, X
Osteogenic	I

Table 1–8.

Endocrine Effects on Fracture Healing

Hormone	Effect	Mechanism
Cortisone	–	Decreased callus proliferation
Calcitonin	+?	Unknown
TH/PTH	+	Bone remodeling
Growth hormone	+	Increased callus volume

TH/PTH, thyroid hormone/parathyroid hormone.

a. Definitions
   1. Stress-Generated Potentials—Serve as signals that modulate cellular activity. Piezoelectric effect and streaming potentials are examples of stress-generated potentials.
   2. Piezoelectric Effect—Charges in tissues are displaced secondary to mechanical forces.
   3. Streaming Potentials—Occur when electrically charged fluid is forced over a tissue (cell membrane) with a fixed charge.
   4. Transmembrane Potentials—Generated by cellular metabolism.

b. Fracture Healing—Electrical properties of cartilage and bone depend on their charged molecules. Devices intended to stimulate fracture repair by altering a variety of cellular activities have been introduced.

c. Types of Electrical Stimulation
   1. Direct Current (DC)—Stimulates an inflammatory-like response (stage I).
   2. Alternating Current (AC)—"Capacity coupled generators." Affects cyclic AMP, collagen synthesis, and calcification during the repair stage.
   3. Pulsed Electromagnetic Fields (PEMFs)—Initiate calcification of fibrocartilage (cannot induce calcification of fibrous tissue).

B. Bone Grafting—Bone grafts have four important properties (Table 1–9).
   1. Graft Properties
      a. Osteoconductive matrix—acts as a scaffold or framework into which bone growth occurs.
      b. Osteoconductive factors—growth factors such as BMP and TGF-β that promote bone formation.
      c. Osteogenic cells—include primitive mesenchymal cells, osteoblasts, and osteocytes.
      d. Structural integrity
   2. Overview of Bone Grafts—Commonly, autografts (from same person) or allografts (from another person) are used. Cancellous bone is commonly used for grafting nonunions or cavitary defects because it is quickly remodeled and incorporated (via creeping substitution). Cortical bone is slower to turn over than cancellous bone and is used for structural defects. **Osteoarticular (osteochondral) allografts** are being used with increasing frequency for tumor surgery. These grafts are immunogenic (cartilage is vulnerable to inflammatory mediators of immune response [cytotoxic injury from antibodies and lymphocytes]); the articular cartilage is preserved with glycerol or dimethyl sulfoxide (DMSO) treatment; **cryogenically preserved grafts leave few viable chondrocytes.** Tissue-matched fresh osteochondral grafts produce minimal immunogenic effect and incorporate well. Vascularized bone grafts, though technically difficult, allow more rapid union with preservation of most cells. Vascularized grafts are best employed for irradiated tissues or when large tissue defects exist. (However, there may be donor site morbidity with the vascularized grafts [i.e., fibula].) Nonvascular bone grafts are used more commonly than vascularized grafts. Allograft bone can be (1) fresh (increased antigenicity); (2) fresh frozen—less immunogenic than fresh, preserves bone morphogenic protein (BMP); (3) freeze-dried (lyophilized)—loses structural integrity and depletes BMP, **least immunogenic and purely osteoconductive and lowest likelihood of viral transmission,** commonly known as "croutons"; and (4) in bone matrix gelatin (BMG—digested source of BMP).

Table 1–9.

Types of Bone Grafts and Bone Graft Properties

Graft	Osteoconduction	Osteoinduction	Osteogenic Cells	Structural Integrity	Other Properties
Autograft					
Cancellous	Excellent	Good	Excellent	Poor	Rapid incorporation
Cortical	Fair	Fair	Fair	Excellent	Slow incorporation
Allograft	Fair	Fair	None	Good	**Fresh** has the highest immunogenicity **Freeze-dried** is the least immunogenic but has the least structural integrity (weakest) **Fresh frozen** preserves BMP
Ceramics	Fair	None	None	Fair	
Demineralized bone matrix	Fair	Good	None	Poor	
Bone marrow	Poor	Poor	Good	Poor	

BMP, bone morphogenic protein.
Modified from Brinker, M.R., and Miller, M.D.: Fundamentals of Orthopaedics. Philadelphia, WB Saunders, 1999, p. 7.

Table 1–10.

Stages of Graft Healing

Stage	Activity
1—Inflammation	Chemotaxis stimulated by necrotic debris
2—Osteoblast differentiation	From precursors
3—Osteoinduction	Osteoblast and osteoclast function
4—Osteoconduction	New bone forming over scaffold
5—Remodeling	Process continues for years

Demineralized bone matrix (Grafton) is both osteoconductive and osteoinductive. Bone marrow cells of a bone allograft incite the greatest immunogenic response compared with other constituents. Five stages of graft healing have been recognized (Urist) (Table 1–10).

3. **Specific Bone Graft Types**
   a. Cortical Bone Grafts—Incorporate through slow remodeling of existing haversian systems via a process of resorption (which weakens the graft) followed by deposition of the new bone (restoring its strength). Resorption is confined to the osteon borders, and the interstitial lamellae are preserved.
   b. Cancellous Grafts—Revascularized more quickly; osteoblasts lay down new bone on old trabeculae, which are later remodeled (“creeping substitution”). All allografts must be harvested with sterile technique, and donors must be screened for potential transmissible diseases. The major factors influencing bone graft incorporation are shown in Figure 1–17.
   c. Synthetic Bone Grafts—Composed of calcium, silicon, or aluminum.
      1. Silicate-Based Grafts—Incorporate the element silicon (Si) in the form of silicate (silicon dioxide).
         a. Bioactive Glasses
         b. Glass-Ionomer Cement
      2. Calcium Phosphate-Based Grafts—Capable of osseoconduction and osseointegration. **These materials biodegrade at a very slow rate.** Many are prepared as ceramics (apatite crystals are heated to fuse the crystals [sintered]).
         a. Tricalcium Phosphate
         b. Hydroxyapatite (example: Collagraft Bone Graft Matrix [Zimmer, Inc., Warsaw, IN]; purified bovine dermal fibrillar collagen plus ceramic hydroxyapatite granules and tricalcium phosphate granules.
      3. Calcium Sulfate—Osteoconductive (example: OsteoSet [Wright Medical Technology Inc., Arlington, TN]).
      4. Calcium Carbonate (chemically unaltered marine coral)—Is resorbed and replaced by bone (osteoconductive) (example: Biocora [Inoteb, France]).
      5. Corralline Hydroxyapatite—Calcium carbonate skeleton is converted to calcium phosphate via a thermoexchange process (example: Interpore 200 and 500 [Interpore Orthopaedics, Irvine, CA]).
      6. Other Materials
         a. Aluminum Oxide—Alumina ceramic bonds to bone in response to stress and strain between implant and bone.

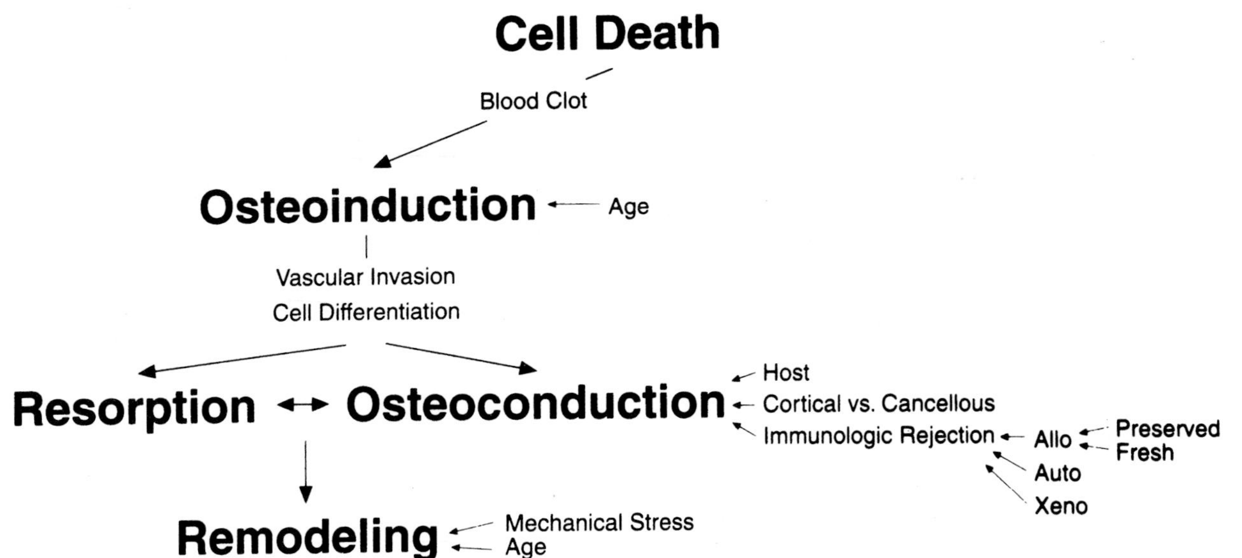

Figure 1–17. Major factors influencing bone graft incorporation. (From Simon, S.R., ed.: Orthopaedic Basic Science, 2nd ed., p. 284. Rosemont, IL, American Academy of Orthopaedic Surgeons, 1994.)

b. Hard Tissue—Replacement polymer.

C. Distraction Osteogenesis (Fig. 1–18)
1. Definition—The use of distraction to stimulate formation of bone
2. Clinical applications
   a. Limb lengthening
   b. Hypertrophic nonunions
   c. Deformity correction (via differential lengthening)
   d. Segmental bone loss (via bone transport)
3. Biology
   a. Under optimal stable conditions, **bone is formed via intramembranous ossification.**
   b. In an unstable environment, bone forms via enchondral ossification or, in an extremely unstable environment, a pseudoarthrosis may occur.
   c. Histologic Phases
      1. Latency phase (5–7 days)
      2. Distraction phase (1 mm per day, approximately 1 inch per month)
      3. Consolidation phase (typically twice as long as the distraction phase)
4. Conditions that Promote Optimal Bone Formation During Distraction Osteogenesis
   a. Low-energy corticotomy/osteotomy

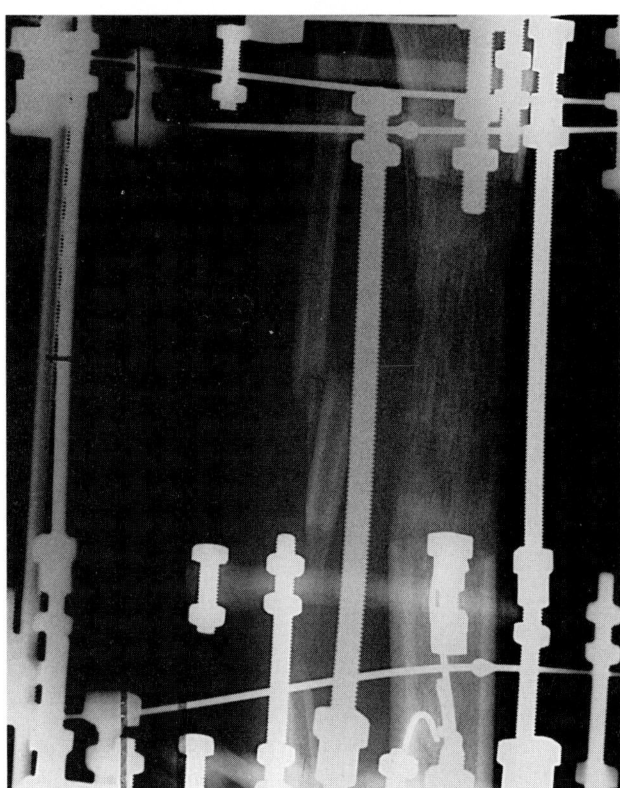

Figure 1–18. Radiograph of a patient who has undergone bone transport for a large distal tibial segmental defect. This AP radiograph of the proximal tibia shows early regeneration of distraction osteogenesis; bone formation is via intramembranous ossification.

   b. Minimal soft-tissue stripping at the corticotomy site (preserve blood supply)
   c. Stable external fixation to eliminate torsion, shear, and bending moments
   d. Latency period (no lengthening) of 5–7 days
   e. Distraction at 1/4 mm 3 to 4 times per day (0.75–1.0 mm per day)
   f. Neutral fixation interval (no distraction) during consolidation
   g. Normal physiologic use of the extremity, including weight-bearing

D. Heterotopic Ossification (HO)—Ectopic bone forms in the soft tissues, most commonly in response to an injury or a surgical dissection. Myositis ossificans (MO) is a form of HO that occurs specifically when the ossification is in muscle. Patients with traumatic brain injuries are particularly prone to HO, and recurrence after operative resection is likely if the neurologic compromise is severe. When resecting HO that has formed after THA (resection should be delayed for a minimum of 6 months after THA), radiation is a useful adjuvant therapy to prevent the recurrence of HO; **irradiation (usually in doses of 700 rad) prevents proliferation and differentiation of primordial mesenchymal cells into osteoprogenitor cells that can form osteoblastic tissue.** Oral diphosphonate inhibits mineralization of osteoid but does not prevent the formation of osteoid matrix; when the oral diphosphonate therapy is discontinued, mineralization with formation of HO may occur. The incidence of HO for THA in patients with Paget's disease is high (approximately 50%).

III. Conditions of Bone Mineralization, Bone Mineral Density, and Bone Viability

A. Normal Bone Metabolism
1. Calcium—Bone serves as a reservoir for more than 99% of the body's calcium. Calcium is also important in muscle and nerve function, the clotting mechanism, and many other areas. Plasma calcium (less than 1% of total body calcium) is about equally free and bound (usually to albumin). It is absorbed from the gut (duodenum) by active transport (ATP and calcium-binding protein required), which is regulated by 1,25-$(OH)_2$-vitamin D_3 and by passive diffusion (jejunum). It is 98% reabsorbed by the kidney (60% in the proximal tubule). The dietary requirement of **elemental calcium** is approximately 600 mg/day for children, increasing to about 1300 mg/day for adolescents and young adults (growth spurt [age 10–25 years]). The requirement for adult men and women (age 25–65 years) is 750 mg/day. Pregnant women require 1500 mg/day, and **lactating women require 2000 mg/day. Postmenopausal women and patients with a healing long bone fracture require 1500 mg/day.** Most

people have a positive calcium balance during their first three decades of life and a negative balance after the fourth decade. About 400 mg of calcium is released from bone daily. Calcium may be excreted in stool. **The primary homeostatic regulators of serum calcium are PTH and 1,25 $(OH)_2$ Vit D.**

2. Phosphate—In addition to being a key component of bone mineral, phosphate has an important role in enzyme systems and molecular interactions (metabolite and buffer). Approximately 85% of the body's phosphate stores are in bone. Plasma phosphate is mostly in the unbound form and is reabsorbed by the kidney (in the proximal tubule). Dietary intake of phosphate is usually adequate; the daily requirement is 1000–1500 mg/day. Phosphate may be excreted in urine.
3. Parathyroid Hormone (PTH)—An 84-amino-acid peptide synthesized in and secreted from the chief cells of the (four) parathyroid glands. PTH helps regulate plasma calcium. PTH directly activates osteoblasts and modulates renal phosphate filtration. Decreased calcium levels in the extracellular fluid stimulate release of PTH, which acts at the intestine, kidney, and bone (Table 1–11). PTH may also have a role in bone loss in the elderly. **PTH-related protein and its receptor have been implicated in metaphyseal dysplasia.**
4. Vitamin D—Naturally occurring steroid that is activated by UV irradiation from sunlight or utilized from dietary intake (Fig. 1–19). It is hydroxylated to the 25-(OH)-vitamin D_3 form in the liver and is hydroxylated a second time in the kidney. Conversion to the 1,25-$(OH)_2$-vitamin D_3 form activates the hormone, whereas conversion to the 24,25-$(OH)_2$-vitamin D form inactivates it (Fig. 1–20). The active form works at the intestine, kidney, and bone (see Table 1–11). Phenytoin (Dilantin) causes impaired metabolism of vitamin D.
5. Calcitonin—A 32-amino-acid peptide hormone made by the clear cells in the parafollicles of the thyroid gland; this hormone also has a limited role in calcium regulation. Increased calcium levels in the extracellular milieu cause secretion of calcitonin. Like PTH, calcitonin secretion is controlled by a β_2 receptor. **The main biologic effect of calcitonin is to inhibit osteoclastic bone resorption (osteoclasts have calcitonin receptors). Calcitonin acts to decrease serum calcium levels.** Calcitonin may also have a physiologic role in fracture healing and the treatment of osteoporosis.

Table 1–11.

Regulation of Calcium and Phosphate Metabolism

Parameter	Parathyroid Hormone (PTH) (Peptide)	1,25-$(OH)_2$D (Steroid)	Calcitonin (Peptide)
Origin	Chief cells of parathyroid glands	Proximal tubule of kidney	Parafollicular cells of thyroid gland
Factors stimulating production	Decreases serum Ca^{2+}	Elevated PTH Decreased serum Ca^{2+} Decreased serum P_i	Elevated serum Ca^{2+}
Factors inhibiting production	Elevated serum Ca^{2+} Elevated 1,25$(OH)_2$D	Decreased PTH Elevated serum Ca^{2+} Elevated serum P_i	Decreased serum Ca^{2+}
Effect on end-organs for hormone action			
Intestine	No direct effect Acts indirectly on bowel by stimulating production of 1,25-$(OH)_2$D in kidney	Strongly stimulates intestinal absorption of Ca^{2+} and P_i	?
Kidney	Stimulates 25-(OH)D-1α-OH_{ase} in mitochondria of proximal tubular cells to convert 25-(OH)D to 1,25-$(OH)_2$D Increases fractional resorption of filtered Ca^{2+} Promotes urinary excretion of P_i	?	?
Bone	Stimulates osteoclastic resorption of bone Stimulates recruitment of preosteoclasts	Strongly stimulates osteoclastic resorption of bone	Inhibits osteoclastic resorption of bone ? Role in normal human physiology
Net effect on Ca^{2+} and P_i concentrations in extracellular fluid and serum	Increased serum Ca^{2+} Decreased serum P_i	Increased serum Ca^{2+} Increased serum P_i	Decreased serum Ca^{2+} (transient)

1,25-$(OH)_2$D, 1,25-dihydroxyvitamin D; PTH, parathyroid hormone; 25-(OH)D, 25-hydroxyvitamin D.

Adapted from an original figure by Frank H. Netter. From The Ciba Collection of Medical Illustrations, vol. 8, part I, p. 179.

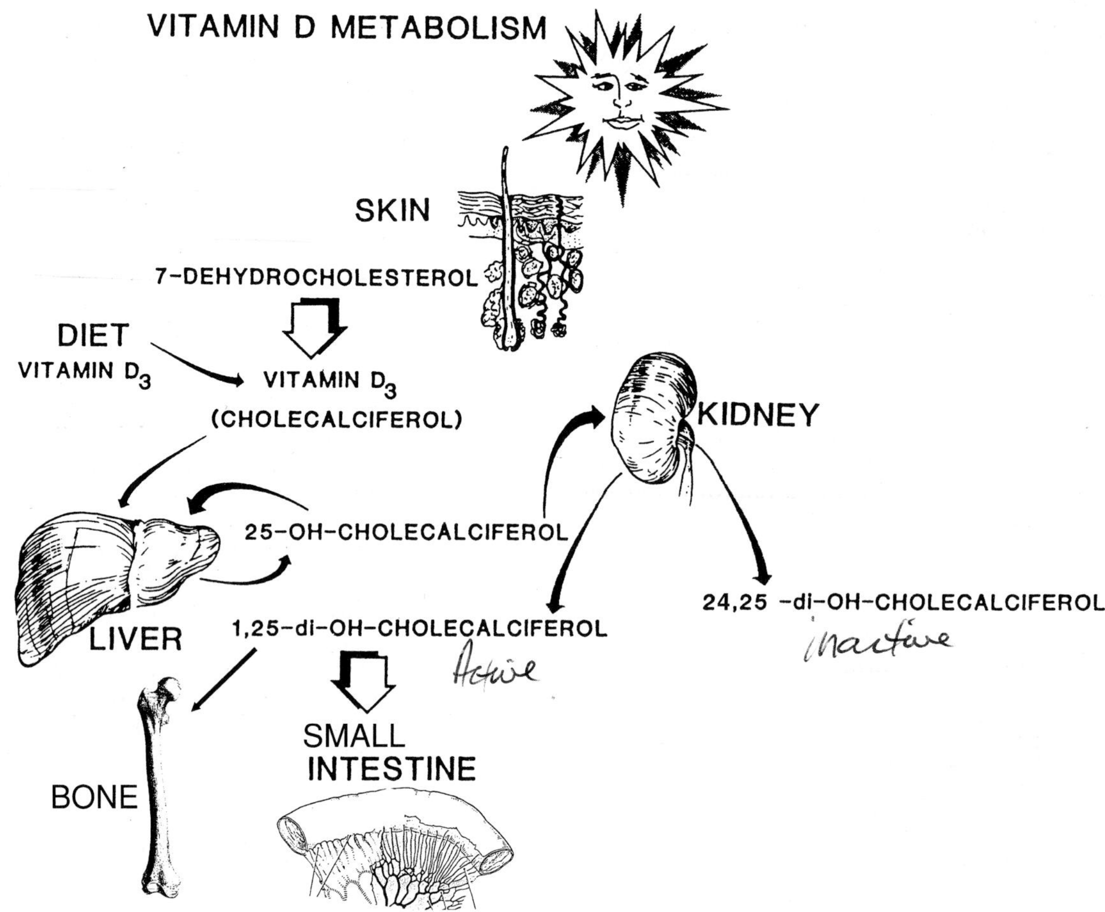

Figure 1–19. Vitamin D metabolism. (Modified from Orthopaedic Science Syllabus, p. 11. Park Ridge, IL, American Academy of Orthopaedic Surgeons, 1986.)

6. Other Hormones—The following hormones also have an effect on bone metabolism.
   a. Estrogen—**Prevents bone loss by inhibiting bone resorption** (a decrease in urinary pyridoline cross-links is observed). **However, because bone formation and resorption are coupled, estrogen therapy also decreases bone formation (see discussion of Bone Loss, which follows).** Supplementation is helpful in postmenopausal women but only if it is started within the first 5–10 years after the onset of menopause. The risk of endometrial cancer for patients taking estrogen is reduced when it is combined with cyclic progestin therapy.
   b. Corticosteroids—**Increase bone loss** (decrease gut absorption by decreasing binding proteins and decrease bone formation [cancellous bone more affected than cortical bone] through inhibition of collagen synthesis). Adverse effects may be reduced with alternate-day therapy.
   c. Thyroid Hormones—Affect bone resorption more than bone formation, **leading to osteoporosis** (large [thyroid-suppressive] doses of thyroxine can lead to osteoporosis).
   d. Growth Hormone—**Causes a positive calcium balance** by increasing gut ab-

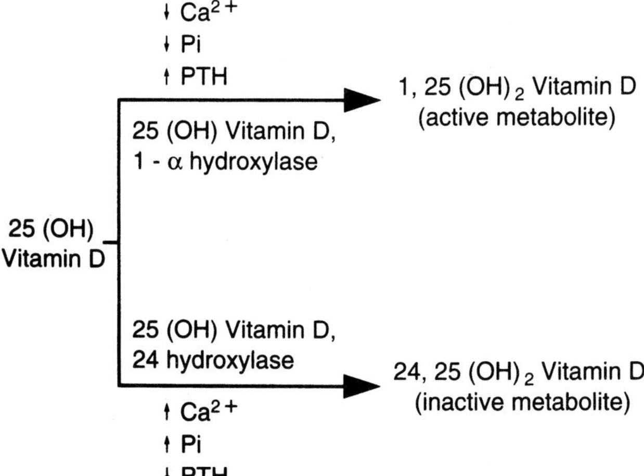

Figure 1–20. Vitamin D metabolism in the renal tubular cell. (From Simon, S.R., ed.: Orthopaedic Basic Science, 2nd ed., p. 165. Rosemont, IL, American Academy of Orthopaedic Surgeons, 1994.)

sorption of calcium more than its increase in urinary excretion. Insulin and somatomedins participate in this effect.

e. Growth Factors—TGF-β, PDGF, and mono/lymphokines have a role in bone and cartilage repair (discussed elsewhere within this chapter).

7. Interaction—Calcium and phosphate metabolism is affected by an elaborate interplay of hormones and even the levels of the metabolites themselves. Feedback mechanisms play an important role in the regulation of plasma levels of calcium and phosphate. It is now believed that peak bone mass usually occurs between 16 and 25 years of age and is greater in men and African Americans. After this peak, bone loss occurs at a rate of 0.3–0.5% per year (2–3% per year for untreated women during the sixth through tenth years after menopause).

8. Bone Loss—Occurs at the onset of menopause, when there is both accelerated bone formation and resorption. **Markers of bone resorption include urinary hydroxyproline and pyridoline cross-links (when there is bone resorption, both of these are elevated). Serum alkaline phosphatase is a marker for bone formation (elevated when bone formation is increased). Estrogen therapy for osteoporosis results in a decrease in urinary pyridoline (decreased bone resorption) and a decrease in serum alkaline phosphatase (decreased bone formation).**

B. Conditions of Bone Mineralization—Include hypercalcemic disorders, hypocalcemic disorders, and hypophosphatasia (Tables 1–12, 1–13, and 1–14).

1. Hypercalcemia—Can present as polyuria, kidney stones, excessive bony resorption ± fibrotic tissue replacement (osteitis fibrosa cystica), CNS effects (confusion, stupor, weakness), and GI effects (constipation).

a. Primary Hyperparathyroidism—Caused by overproduction of PTH, usually as a result of a parathyroid adenoma (which generally affects only one parathyroid gland). Excessive PTH causes a net **increase in plasma calcium** (from all three sources) and a **decrease in plasma phosphate** (due to enhanced urinary excretion). It results in **increased osteoclastic resorption** and failure of repair attempts (poor mineralization due to low phosphate). Diagnosis is based on signs and symptoms of hypercalcemia (described earlier) and characteristic laboratory results (increased serum calcium, PTH, urinary phosphate; decreased serum phosphate). Bony changes include osteopenia, osteitis fibrosa cystica (fibrous replacement of marrow), **"brown tumors"** (increased giant cells, extravasation of RBCs, hemosiderin staining, fibrous tissue hemosiderin), and chondrocalcinosis. Radiographs may demonstrate deformed, osteopenic bones, fractures, "shaggy" trabeculae, areas of radiolucency (phalanges,

Table 1–12.

Overview of Clinical and Radiographic Aspects of Metabolic Bone Diseases

Disease	Etiology	Clinical Findings	Radiographic Findings
Hypercalcemia			
Hyperparathyroidism	PTH overproduction—adenoma	Kidney stone, hyperreflexia	Osteopenia, osteitis fibrosa cystica
Familial syndromes	PTH overproduction—MEN/renal	Endocrine/renal abnormalities	Osteopenia
Hypocalcemia			
Hypoparathyroidism	PTH underproduction—idiopathic	Neuromuscular irritability, eye	Calcified basal ganglia
PHP/Albright's	PTH receptor abnormality	Short MC/MT, obesity	Brachydactyly, exostosis
Renal osteodystrophy	CRF—↓ phosphate excretion	Renal abnormalities	"Rugger jersey" spine
Rickets (osteomalacia)			
Vit. D–deficient	↓ Vit. D diet; malabsorption	Bone deformities, hypotonia	"Rachitic rosary," wide growth plates, fxs
Vit. D–dependent (types I and II)	(see Table 1–13)	Total baldness	Poor mineralization
Vit. D–resistant (hypophosphatemic)	↓ Renal tubular phosphate resorption	Bone deformities, hypotonia	Poor mineralization
Hypophosphatasia	↓ Alkaline phosphatase	Bone deformities, hypotonia	Poor mineralization
Osteopenia			
Osteoporosis	↓ Estrogen—↓ bone mass	Kyphosis, fx	Compression vertebral fx, hip fx
Scurvy	Vit. C deficiency—defective collagen	Fatigue, bleeding, effusions	Thin cortices, corner sign
Osteodense			
Paget's disease	Osteoclastic abn.—↑ bone turnover	Deformities, pain, CHF, fxs	Coarse trabeculae, "picture frame" vertebrae
Osteopetrosis	Osteoclastic abn.—unclear	Hepatosplenomegaly, anemia	Bone within bone

↓, decreased; ↑, increased; Def., defective; abn., abnormality; PTH, parathyroid hormone; MC, metacarpal; MT, metatarsal; CRF, chronic renal failure; CHF, congestive heart failure; fxs, fractures; PHP, pseudohypoparathyroidism; MEN, multiple endocrine neoplasia.

Table 1–13.

Laboratory Findings and Clinical Data Regarding Patients with the Various Metabolic Bone Diseases

Disorder	Serum Ca	Serum Phos	Alk Phos	PTH	25 (OH) Vit D	1,25-$(OH)_2$ Vit D	Urinary Calcium	Other Findings/ Possible Findings	Treatment	Comments
Primary hyperparathyroidism	↑	N or ↓	N or ↑	↑	N	N or ↑	↑	Active turnover seen on bone biopsy with peritrabecular fibrosis **Brown tumors**	Surgical excision of parathyroid edema Treat hypercalcemia (see text)	Most commonly due to parathyroid adenoma. Because PTH stimulates conversion of the inactive form to the active form [1,25 (OH_2) Vit D] in the kidney, ↑ production of PTH leads to ↑ levels of 1,25 $(OH)_2$ Vit D
Malignancy with bony metastases	↑	N or ↑	N or ↑	N or ↓	N	N or ↓	↑	Destructive lesions in bone	Treat cancer and hypercalcemia (see text)	↑ Calcium levels may lead to ↓ PTH production via feedback mechanism. ↓ 1,25 $(OH)_2$ Vit D levels are due to ↓ PTH (which is responsible for conversion of the inactive to the active form of Vit D in the kidney). Multiple myeloma will display an abnormal urinary and serum protein electrophoresis
Hyperthyroidism	↑	N	N	N or ↓	N	N	↑	↑ Free thyroxin index ↓ thyroid-stimulating hormone Tachycardia, tremors		↑ Calcium levels due to ↑ bone turnover (hypermetabolic state)
Vitamin D intoxication	↑	N or ↑	N or ↑	N or ↓	↑↑↑	N	↑			History of excessive Vit D intake Dietary vitamin D is converted to 25(OH) Vit D in the liver This results in very high concentrations of 25(OH) Vit D that cross-react with intestinal Vit D receptors to ↑ resorption of calcium to cause hypercalcemia
Hypoparathyroidism	↓	↑	N	↓	N	↓	↓	Basal ganglia calcification Hypocalcemic findings		↓ PTH production most commonly follows surgical ablation of the thyroid (with the parathyroid) gland ↓ PTH leads to ↓ serum calcium and ↑ serum phosphate (due to ↓ urinary excretion of phosphate) Because PTH stimulates conversion from the inactive to the active form of Vit D (in the kidney), 1,25 $(OH)_2$ Vit D is also ↓
Pseudohypoparathyroidism	↓	↑	N	N or ↑	N	↓	↓	Hypocalcemic findings		PTH has no effect at the target cells (in the kidney, bone, and intestine) due to a PTH receptor abnormality. This leads to a ↓ in the active form of Vit D. Therefore, serum calcium levels are ↓ due to: 1) the lack of effect of PTH on bone 2) ↓ levels of 1,25 $(OH)_2$ Vit D
Renal osteodystrophy (high-turnover bone disease of renal disease [secondary hyperparathyroidism])	↓ (or N)	↑↑↑	↑	↑↑↑	N	↓	—	Findings of secondary hyperparathyroidism "Rugger jersey" spine Osteitis fibrosa Amyloidosis	1) Correct underlying renal abnormality 2) Maintain normal serum phosphorous and calcium 3) Dietary phosphate restriction 4) Phosphate binding antacid (calcium carbonate) 5) Administration of the active form of Vit D—1,25 $(OH)_2$ Vit D (calcitriol)	↓ Renal phosphorous excretion leads to hyperphosphatemia Phosphorous retention leads to ↓ serum calcium and ↑↑↑ PTH (which can lead to secondary hyperparathyroidism) Elevated BUN and creatinine Associated with long-term hemodialysis

Renal osteodystrophy (low-turnover bone disease of renal disease [aluminum toxicity])	↑ (or N)	N or ↑	↑	N (or mildly elevated)	N	↓	—	"Rugger jersey" spine Osteitis fibrosa Amyloidosis Osteomalacia may be seen		PTH levels are ↓ because of: 1) Frequent episodes of hypercalcemia 2) Direct inhibitory effect of aluminum on PTH **No secondary hyperparathyroidism is present** Elevated BUN and creatinine Associated with long-term hemodialysis
Nutritional rickets—vitamin D deficiency	↓ or N	↓	↑	↑	↓	↓	↓	Osteomalacia, hypotonia Muscle weakness, tetany Bowing deformities of the long bones Rachitic rosary	Oral administration of Vit D (1500–5000 IU/day)	With ↓ vitamin D intake, intestinal calcium and phosphate absorption are reduced leading to hypocalcemia. ↓ Serum calcium stimulates ↑ PTH (secondary hyperparathyroidism) that leads to bone resorption and to ↑ serum calcium (toward or to normal levels) Sources of vitamin D include: 1) Sunlight 2) Fish liver foods 3) Fortified milk
Nutritional rickets—calcium deficiency	↓ or N	↓	↑	↑	N	↑ (or N)	↓	Similar clinical findings as vitamin D deficiency	Oral administration of calcium (700 mg/day)	Hypocalcemia leads to secondary hyperparathyroidism. ↑ PTH leads to enhanced renal conversion of 25(OH) Vit D to $1,25(OH)_2$ Vit D
Nutritional rickets—phosphate deficiency	N	↓	↑	**N**	N	↑ ↑ ↑	N	No changes of secondary hyperparathyroidism are seen	Oral supplementation of phosphate	Neither secondary hyperparathyroidism nor Vit D deficiency is present ↓ Serum phosphate leads to ↑ renal production of $1,25(OH)_2$ Vit D
Hereditary vitamin D–dependent rickets type I ("pseudovitamin D deficiency")	↓	↓	↑	↑	N (or ↑)	↓ ↓ ↓	↓	Osteomalacia Clinical findings similar (but more severe) than nutritional rickets—vitamin D deficiency	Oral administration of physiologic doses (1–2 μg/day) of $1,25(OH)_2$ Vit D	There is a defect in renal 25(OH) Vit D 1 α hydroxylase. This enzymatic defect inhibits conversion from the inactive form [25(OH) Vit D] to the active form [$1,25(OH)_2$ Vit D] of vitamin D in the kidney
Heredity vitamin D–dependent rickets type II ("hereditary resistance to $1,25(OH)_2$ Vit D")	↓	↓	↑	↑	N (or ↑)	↑ ↑ ↑	↓	Osteomalacia Alopecia Clinical findings similar (but more severe) than nutritional rickets—vitamin D deficiency	Long-term (3–6 months) daily administration of high-dose vitamin D analogue [$1,25(OH)_2$ Vit D or 1 α (OH) Vit D] plus 3 g/day of elemental calcium	There is an intracellular receptor defect for $1,25(OH)_2$ Vit D Patients with this disorder have the highest $1,25(OH)_2$ Vit D levels observed in humans; this ↑ ↑ ↑ level of $1,25(OH)_2$ Vit D distinguishes hereditary vitamin D–dependent rickets type II from type I (the level of $1,25(OH)_2$ Vit D is ↓ ↓ ↓)
Hypophosphatemic rickets (vitamin D–resistant rickets) ("phosphate diabetes") (Albright's syndrome is an example of a hypophosphatemic syndrome)	N	↓ ↓ ↓	↑	N	N	N	N	Osteomalacia No changes of secondary hyperparathyroidism Classic triad: 1) Hypophasphatemia 2) Lower limb deformities 3) Stunted growth rate	Oral administration of elemental phosphate (1–3 g/day) plus high-dose vitamin D (20,000–70,000 IU/day). Vitamin D administration is needed to counterbalance the hypocalcemic effect of phosphate administration, which otherwise could lead to severe secondary hyperparathyroidism	There is an inborn error in phosphate transport (probably located in the proximal nephron). This leads to failure of reabsorption of phosphate in the kidney and "spilling" of phosphate (phosphate diabetes) in the urine While the absolute levels of $1,25(OH)_2$ Vit D are normal, they are inappropriately low considering the degree of phosphaturia [production of $1,25(OH)_2$ Vit D is normally stimulated by ↓ serum phosphorous (see Table 1–11)] **This is the most commonly encountered form of rickets**
Hypophosphatasia	↑	↑	↓ ↓ ↓	N	N	N	↑	Osteomalacia Early loss of teeth	There is no established medical therapy	There is an inborn error in the tissue-nonspecific (kidney, bone, liver) isoenzyme of alkaline phosphatase Elevated urinary phosphoethanolamine is diagnostic

Table 1–14.

Differential Diagnosis of the Metabolic Bone Diseases Based on Blood Chemistries

↑ Calcium	↓ Calcium	Normal Calcium	↑ Phosphorus	↓ Phosphorus	Normal Phosphorus
Primary hyperparathyroidism Hyperthyroidism Vitamin D intoxication Malignancy without bony metastasis Malignancy with bony metastasis Multiple myeloma Lymphoma Sarcoidosis Milk-alkali syndrome Severe generalized immobilization Multiple endocrine neoplasias Addison's disease Steroid administration Peptic ulcer disease Hypophosphatasia	Hypoparathyroidism Pseudohypoparathyroidism Renal osteodystrophy (high-turnover bone disease) Nutritional rickets—vitamin D deficiency Nutritional rickets—calcium deficiency Hereditary vitamin D–dependent rickets (types I and II)	Osteoporosis Pseudohypoparathyroidism Nutritional rickets—vitamin D deficiency Nutritional rickets—calcium deficiency Nutritional rickets—phosphate deficiency Hypophosphatemic rickets	Malignancy with bony metastasis Multiple myeloma Lymphoma Vitamin D intoxication Hypoparathyroidism Pseudohypoparathyroidism Renal osteodystrophy Hypophosphatasia Sarcoidosis Milk-alkali syndrome Severe generalized immobilization	Primary hyperparathyroidism Malignancy without bony metastasis Nutritional rickets—vitamin D deficiency Nutritional rickets—calcium deficiency Nutritional rickets—phosphate deficiency Hereditary vitamin D–dependent rickets (types I and II) Hypophosphatemic rickets	Osteoporosis Primary hyperparathyroidism Malignancy with bony metastasis Multiple myeloma Lymphoma Hyperthyroidism Vitamin D intoxication Renal osteodystrophy (*only* low-turnover bone disease) Sarcoidosis Milk-alkali syndrome Severe generalized immobilization

distal clavicle, skull), and calcification of the soft tissues. Histologic changes include osteoblasts and osteoclasts active on both sides of trabeculae (as seen in Paget's disease), areas of destruction, and wide osteoid seams. Surgical parathyroidectomy is curative.

b. Other Causes of Hypercalcemia
   1. Familial Syndromes—Hypercalcemia can result from pituitary adenomas associated with multiple endocrine neoplasia (MEN) types I and II and from familial hypocalciuric hypercalcemia (which is caused by poor renal clearance of calcium).
   2. Other causes of hypercalcemia—Include malignancy (most common), PTH-related protein secretion (lung carcinoma) and lytic bone metastases and lesions (such as multiple myeloma), hyperthyroidism, vitamin D intoxication, prolonged immobilization, Addison's disease, steroid administration, peptic ulcer disease (milk-alkali syndrome), kidney disease, sarcoidosis, and hypophosphatasia. Hypercalcemia related to malignancy can be life-threatening. Initial treatment should include hydration with normal saline (reverses dehydration). Hypercalcemia of malignancy can occur in the absence of extensive bone metastasis; hypercalcemia of malignancy most commonly results from the release of systemic growth factors and cytokines that stimulate osteoclastic bone resorption (at bony sites not involved in the tumor process).

c. Treatment of Hypercalcemia
   1. Hydration (saline diuresis)
   2. Loop diuretics
   3. Dialysis (for severe cases)
   4. Mobilization (prevents further bone resorption)
   5. Specific drug therapy (bisphosphonates, mithramycin, calcitonin, and galium nitrate)

2. Hypocalcemia—Low plasma calcium can result from low PTH or vitamin D_3. Hypocalcemia leads to increased neuromuscular irritability (tetany, seizures, Chvostek's sign), cataracts, fungal infections of the nails, EKG changes (prolonged QT interval), and other signs and symptoms. The body's response to hypocalcemia is shown in Figure 1–21.
   a. Hypoparathyroidism—Decreased PTH causes diminished plasma calcium and increased plasma phosphate (urinary excretion not enhanced because of lack of PTH). Common findings include fungal infections of the nails, hair loss, and blotchy skin due to pigment loss (vitiligo). Skull radiographs may show basal ganglia calcification. **Iatrogenic hypoparathyroidism most commonly follows thyroidectomy.**
   b. Pseudohypoparathyroidism (PHP)—A rare genetic disorder caused by a lack of effect of PTH at the target cells. PTH level is normal or even high, but PTH action at the cellular level is blocked by an abnormality at the receptor, by the cAMP system, or by a lack of required cofactors (e.g., Mg^{2+}). **Albright hereditary osteodystrophy,** a form of PHP, is associated with short first, fourth, and

Table 1–14. *Continued*

Differential Diagnosis of the Metabolic Bone Diseases Based on Blood Chemistries

↑ PTH	↓ PTH	Normal PTH	↑ $1,25(OH)_2$ Vit D	↓ $1,25(OH)_2$ Vit D	Normal $1,25(OH)_2$ Vit D
Primary hyperparathyroidism Pseudohypoparathyroidism Renal osteodystrophy Nutritional rickets—vitamin D deficiency Nutritional rickets—calcium deficiency Hereditary vitamin D–dependent rickets (types I and II)	Malignancy with bony metastasis Malignancy without bony metastasis Multiple myeloma Lymphoma Hyperthyroidism Vitamin D intoxication Hypoparathyroidism Sarcoidosis Milk-alkali syndrome Severe generalized immobilization	Osteoporosis Malignancy with bony metastasis Multiple myeloma Lymphoma Vitamin D intoxication Pseudohypoparathyroidism Renal osteodystrophy (*only* low-turnover bone disease) Nutritional rickets—phosphate deficiency Hypophosphatemic rickets Hypophosphatasia Sarcoidosis Hyperthyroidism Milk-alkali syndrome Severe generalized immobilization	Primary hyperparathyroidism Nutritional rickets—calcium deficiency Nutritional rickets—phosphate deficiency Hereditary vitamin D–dependent rickets type II Sarcoidosis	Malignancy with bony metastasis Malignancy without bony metastasis Multiple myeloma Lymphoma Hypoparathyroidism Pseudohypoparathyroidism Renal osteodystrophy Nutritional rickets—vitamin D deficiency Hereditary vitamin D–dependent rickets type I	Osteoporosis Primary hyperparathyroidism Malignancy with bony metastasis Multiple myeloma Lymphoma Hyperthyroidism Vitamin D intoxication Nutritional rickets—calcium deficiency Hypophosphatemic rickets Hypophosphatasia

fifth MCs and MTs, brachydactyly, exostoses, obesity, and diminished intelligence. Pseudopseudohypoparathyroidism (pseudo-PHP) is a normocalcemic disorder that is phenotypically similar to PHP. However, in pseudo-PHP there is a normal response to PTH.

c. Renal Osteodystrophy (Fig. 1–22)—A spectrum of disorders of bone mineral metabolism in patients with chronic renal disease. Renal disease (impaired renal function) leads to the body's inability to excrete certain endogenous and exogenous substances and compromises mineral homeostatis, which leads to abnormalities of bone mineral metabolism. Renal bone diseases are subdivided into high-turnover disease (due to chronically elevated serum PTH) and low-turnover disease (excess deposition of aluminum into bone or normal or reduced serum PTH).

1. High-turnover bone disease of renal disease–sustained increased secretion of PTH can lead to **secondary hyperparathyroidism.** Factors contributing to sustained increased secretion of PTH (and ultimately hyperplasia of the chief cells of the parathyroid gland [secondary hyperparathyroidism]) include:
   a. Diminished renal phosphorous excretion—chronic renal failure leads to an inability to excrete phosphate. Phosphorous retention promotes the secretion of PTH by three mechanisms: (1) hyperphos-

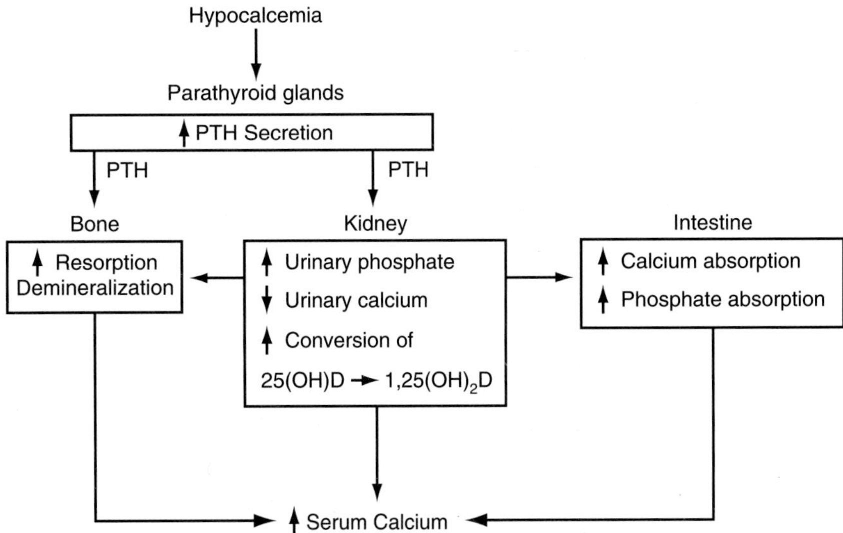

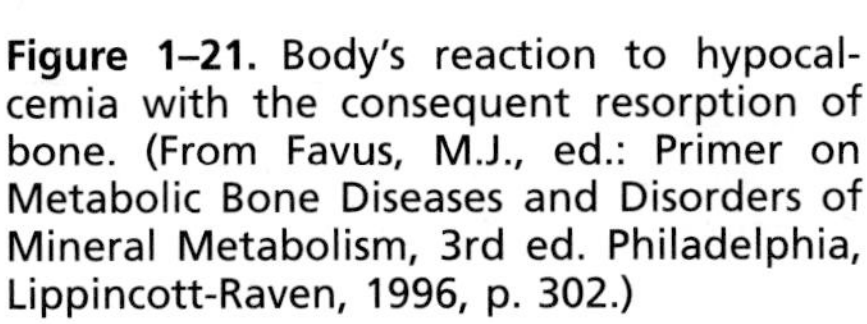

Figure 1–21. Body's reaction to hypocalcemia with the consequent resorption of bone. (From Favus, M.J., ed.: Primer on Metabolic Bone Diseases and Disorders of Mineral Metabolism, 3rd ed. Philadelphia, Lippincott-Raven, 1996, p. 302.)

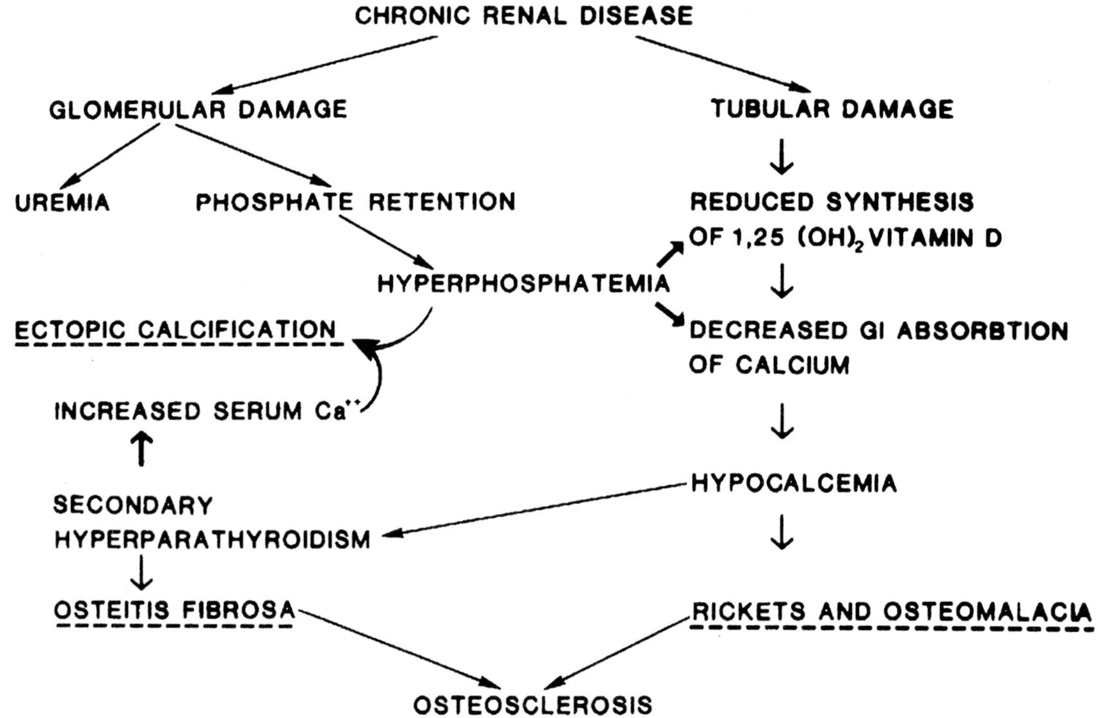

Figure 1–22. Pathogenesis of bone changes in renal osteodystrophy. (From Simon, S.R., ed.: Orthopaedic Basic Science, 2nd ed., p. 171. Rosemont, IL, American Academy of Orthopaedic Surgeons, 1994.)

phatemia leads to lowered serum calcium directly, and thereby stimulates PTH; (2) phosphorous impairs renal 1α hydroxylase activity, therefore impairing production of 1,25 $(OH)_2$ Vit D; (3) phosphorous retention may directly increase the synthesis of PTH. Increased secretion of PTH can lead to secondary hyperparathyroidism.

b. Hypocalcemia
c. Impaired renal calcitriol [1,25 $(OH)_2$ Vit D_2]
d. Alterations in the control of PTH gene transcription secretion
e. Skeletal resistance to the actions of PTH

2. Low-turnover bone disease of renal disease (adynamic lesion of bone and osteomalacia)—**these patients do not have secondary hyperparathyroidism,** and the serum levels of PTH are normal or mildly elevated. Bone formation and turnover are reduced. Aluminum toxicity—aluminum negatively affects bone mineral metabolism in several ways:
   a. Impairs differentiation of precursor cells to osteoblasts.
   b. Impairs proliferation of osteoblasts.
   c. Impairs the release of PTH from the parathyroid gland.
   d. Disrupts the mineralization process. Depending on the severity of involvement, the low-turnover lesion may represent an adynamic lesion or osteomalacia.
   e. Adynamic lesion—accounts for the majority of cases of low-turnover bone disease in patients with chronic renal failure.
   f. Osteomalacia—in addition to slowed bone formation and turnover, there is a defect in the mineralization of newly formed bone. In renal osteodystrophy, radiographs may demonstrate a "rugger jersey" spine, like that in childhood osteopetrosis, and soft-tissue calcification. **An additional complication of chronic dialysis is the accumulation of beta-2 microglobulin, which leads to amyloidosis. Amyloidosis may be associated with carpal tunnel syndrome, arthropathy, and pathologic fractures.** The material in amyloidosis stains pink

with Congo red. Laboratory tests in renal osteodystrophy show an abnormal glomerular filtration rate (GFR); increased alkaline phosphatase, BUN, and creatinine; and decreased venous bicarbonate. Treatment should be directed at relieving the urologic obstruction or kidney disease.

d. Rickets (Osteomalacia in Adults)—**Failure of mineralization** leading to changes in the physis (increased width and disorientation) and bone (cortical thinning, bowing). The causes of rickets and osteomalacia are summarized in Table 1–15.

1. Nutritional Rickets (see Table 1–13)
   a. Vitamin D Deficiency Rickets—Almost eliminated after addition of vitamin D to milk in the United States; the disease is still seen in Asian immigrants, patients with dietary peculiarities, premature infants, and those with malabsorption (sprue) or chronic parenteral nutrition. Decreased intestinal absorption of calcium and phosphate leads to secondary hyperparathyroidism (PTH continues to be produced because of low plasma calcium). **Laboratory studies** show **low normal calcium** (maintained by high PTH), **low phosphate** (excreted because of the effect of PTH), **increased PTH,** and **low levels of vitamin D.** Enlargement of the costochondral junction (**"rachitic rosary"**), bony deformities (**bowing of the knees,** "codfish" vertebrae), retarded bone growth (defect in the hypertrophic zone with widened osteoid seams and physeal cupping), muscle hypotonia, dental disease, pathologic fractures (Looser's zones [pseudofracture on the compression side of bone]), **milkman's fracture** [pseudofracture in adults]), a waddling gait, and other problems may result. Affected children are commonly below the fifth percentile for height. Treatment with vitamin D (5000 IU daily) resolves most deformities. Characteristic radiographic changes seen in rickets include physeal widening, physeal cupping, and coxa vara.
   b. Calcium Deficiency Rickets (Fig. 1–23)
   c. Phosphate Deficiency Rickets
2. Hereditary Vitamin D–Dependent Rickets—This rare disorder can be subdivided in two types: vitamin D–dependent rickets type I, and vitamin D–dependent rickets type II. The disorders' features are similar to those of nutritional rickets–vitamin D deficiency, except they **may be worse** and patients may have total baldness.
   a. Vitamin D–Dependent Rickets Type I—**The defect is in renal 25(OH) Vit D 1 α-hydroxylase.** Therefore, there is inhibition of

Table 1–15.

Causes of Rickets and Osteomalacia

NUTRITIONAL DEFICIENCY
- Vitamin D deficiency
- Dietary chelators (rare) of calcium
  - Phytates
  - Oxalates (spinach)
- Phosphorus deficiency (unusual)
  - Antacid (aluminum-containing) abuse leading to severe dietary phosphate binding

GASTROINTESTINAL ABSORPTION DEFECTS
- Postgastrectomy (rare today)
- Biliary disease (interference with absorption of fat-soluble vitamin D)
- Enteric absorption defects
  - Short bowel syndrome
  - Rapid-transit (gluten-sensitive enteropathy) syndromes
  - Inflammatory bowel disease
    - Crohn's disease
    - Celiac disease

RENAL TUBULAR DEFECTS (RENAL PHOSPHATE LEAK)
- X-linked dominant hypophosphatemic vitamin D–resistant rickets (VDRR) or osteomalacia
- Classic Albright's syndrome or Fanconi's syndrome type I
- Fanconi's syndrome type II
- Phosphaturia and glycosuria
- Fanconi's syndrome type III
- Phosphaturia, glycosuria, aminoaciduria
- Vitamin D–dependent rickets (or osteomalacia) type I (a genetic or acquired deficiency of renal tubular 25-hydroxyvitamin D 1-alpha hydroxylase enzyme that prevents conversion of 25-hydroxy-vitamin D to the active polar metabolite 1,25-dihydroxy-vitamin D)
- Vitamin D–dependent rickets (or osteomalacia) type II (this entity represents enteric end-organ insensitivity to 1,25-dihydroxy-vitamin D and is probably caused by an abnormality in the 1,25-dihydroxy-vitamin D nuclear receptor)
- Renal tubular acidosis
  - Acquired—associated with many systemic diseases
  - Genetic
    - Debre-De Toni-Fanconi syndrome
    - Lignac-Fanconi syndrome (cysteinosis)
    - Lowe's syndrome

RENAL OSTEODYSTROPHY

MISCELLANEOUS CAUSES
- Soft-tissue tumors secreting putative factors
  - Fibrous dysplasia
  - Neurofibromatosis
  - Other soft-tissue and vascular mesenchymal tumors
- Anticonvulsant medication (induction of the hepatic P450 microsomal enzyme system by some anticonvulsants—phenytoin, phenobarbital, mysoline—causes increased degradation of vitamin D metabolites)
- Heavy metal intoxication
- Hypophosphatasia
- High-dose diphosphonates
- Sodium fluoride

Adapted from Simon, S.R.: Orthopaedic Basic Science, 2nd ed., p. 169. Rosemont, IL, American Academy of Orthopaedic Surgeons, 1994.

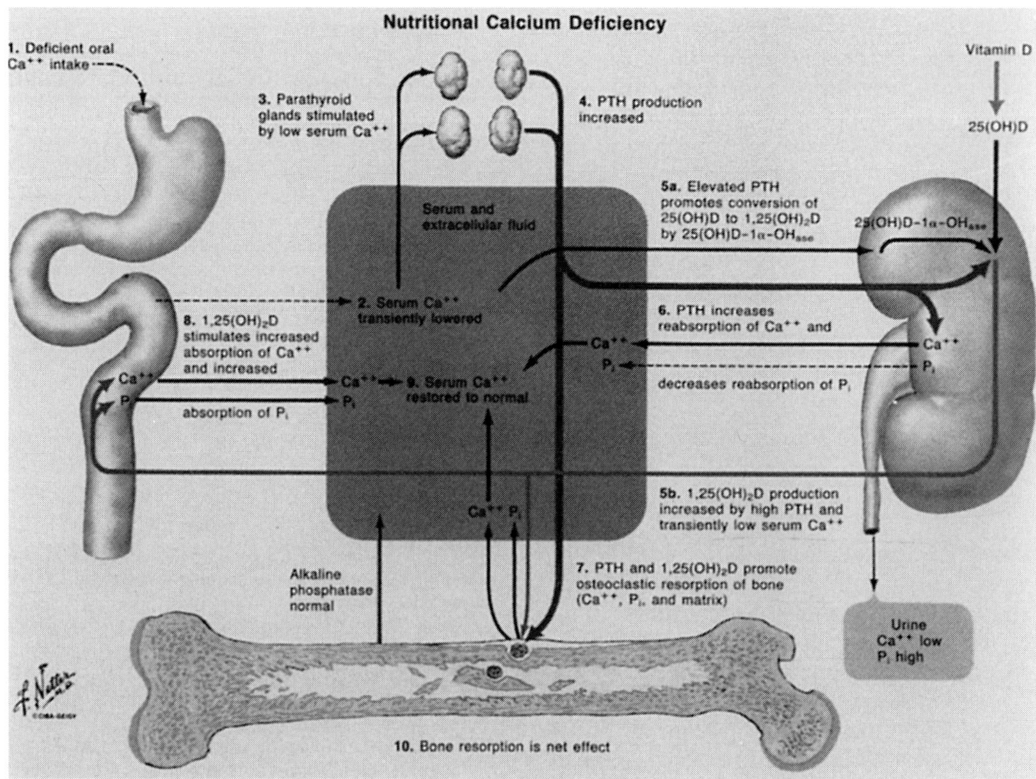

Figure 1–23. Nutritional calcium deficiency. (From The Ciba Collection of Medical Illustrations, vol. 8, part I, p. 184, 1987. Illustrated by Frank H. Netter. Reprinted by permission.)

conversion of the inactive form of vitamin D to the active form of vitamin D. The inheritance pattern is autosomal recessive (AR). The gene responsible is on chromosome 12q14.

b. Vitamin D–Dependent Rickets Type II—**The defect is in an intracellular receptor for 1, 25(OH)$_2$ Vit D.**

3. Familial Hypophosphatemic Rickets (Vitamin D–Resistant Rickets; a.k.a. "Phosphate Diabetes")—**X-linked dominant disorder that is a result of impaired renal tubular reabsorption of phosphate. This is the most commonly encountered form of rickets.** Affected patients have a normal GFR and an impaired vitamin D$_3$ response. Phosphate replacement (1–3 g daily) with high-dose vitamin D$_3$ can correct the effects of the disorder, which are similar to those of the other forms of rickets.

3. Hypophosphatasia—AR disorder caused by an inborn error in the tissue-nonspecific isoenzyme of alkaline phosphatase that leads to **low levels of alkaline phosphatase,** which is required for the synthesis of inorganic phosphate, important in bone matrix formation. **Features are similar to those of rickets,** and treatment may include phosphate therapy. **Increased urinary phosphoethanolamine is diagnostic.**

C. Conditions of Bone Mineral Density—Bone mass is regulated by the relative rates of deposition and withdrawal (Fig. 1–24).

1. Osteopenia

a. Osteoporosis—Age-related **decrease in bone mass** usually associated with loss of estrogen in postmenopausal women (Fig. 1–25). Osteoporosis is responsible for more than 1 million fractures per year (vertebral body most common). The lifetime risk of fracture in white women after 50 years of age is approximately 75%; the risk of hip fracture is 15–20%. **Osteoporosis is a quantitative, not a qualitative, defect in bone.** Sedentary, thin **Caucasian women of northern European descent,** particularly **smokers,** heavy **drinkers,** and patients on **phenytoin (impairs vitamin D metabolism),** with low-calcium and low-vitamin D diets **who breast-fed their infants,** are at greatest risk. **Cancellous bone is most markedly affected.** Clinical features include kyphosis and vertebral fractures (compression fractures of T11–L1 [creating an anterior wedge-shaped defect or resulting in a centrally depressed "codfish" vertebrae]), hip fractures, and distal radius fractures. Two

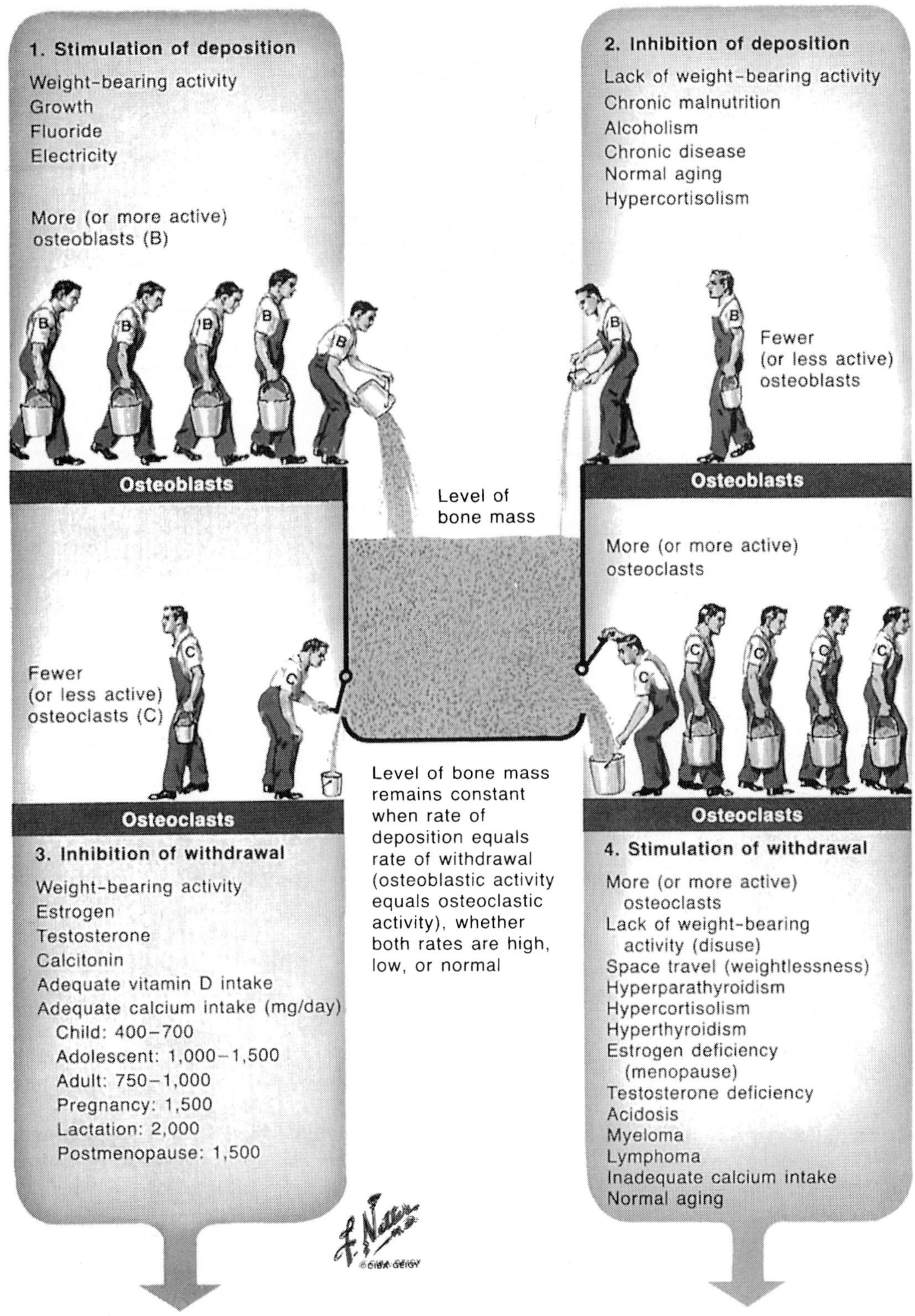

Figure 1–24. Four mechanisms of bone mass regulation. (From The Ciba Collection of Medical Illustrations, vol. 8, part I, p. 181, 1987. Illustrated by Frank H. Netter. Reprinted by permission.)

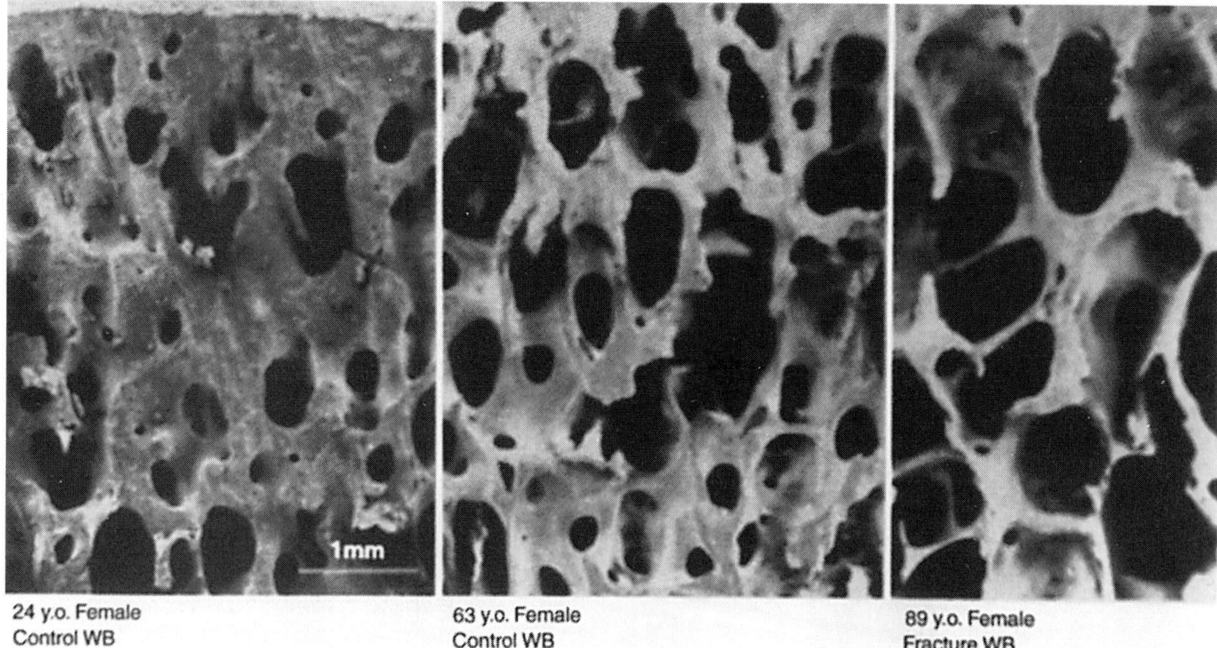

Figure 1–25. Age-related changes in density and architecture of human trabecular bone from the lumbar spine. (Reprinted from Keaveney, T.M., and Hayes, W.C.: Mechanical properties of cortical and trabecular bone. Bone 7:285–344, 1993, with permission from Elsevier Science.)

types of osteoporosis have been characterized: type I (postmenopausal) and type II (age-related).

1. Type I Osteoporosis (Postmenopausal)—Affects trabecular bone primarily; vertebral and distal radius fractures are common.
2. Type II Osteoporosis (Age-Related)—Seen in patients older than 75 years; affects both trabecular and cortical bone; is related to poor calcium absorption; hip and pelvic fractures are common.

Laboratory studies, including urinary calcium and hydroxyproline and serum alkaline phosphatase, are helpful for evaluating osteopenic conditions. **Results of these laboratory studies are usually unremarkable in osteoporosis;** but hyperthyroidism (osteoporosis is reversible), hyperparathyroidism, Cushing's syndrome, hematologic disorders, and malignancy should be ruled out. **Plain radiographs are usually not helpful unless bone loss is >30%.** Special studies used for the work-up of osteoporosis include single-photon (appendicular) and double-photon (axial) absorptiometry, quantitative CT, and dual-energy x-ray absorptiometry (DEXA). **DEXA is most accurate with less radiation.** Biopsy (after tetracycline labeling) may be used to evaluate the severity of osteoporosis and to identify osteomalacia. Histologic changes in osteoporosis are thinning of trabeculae, decreased size of osteons, and enlargement of haversian and marrow spaces. Physical activity, calcium supplements (more effective in type II [age-related] osteoporosis), **estrogen-progesterone therapy (in type I [postmenopausal] osteoporosis) works best when initiated within 6 years of menopause),** and fluoride (inhibits bone resorption, but bone is more brittle) have a role in the treatment of osteoporosis. Bisphosphonates bind to bone resorption surfaces and inhibit osteoclastic membrane ruffling without destroying the cells. Other drugs, such as intramuscular calcitonin, may also be helpful but are expensive and may cause hypersensitivity reactions. The future of bone augmentation with PTH, growth factors, prostaglandin inhibitors, and other modes of therapy remains to be determined. **An overview of recommended treatments for osteoporosis is shown in Figure 1–26.** The best prophylaxis for patients at risk for osteoporosis comprises: (1) diet with adequate calcium intake; (2) weight-bearing exercise program; and (3) estrogen therapy evaluation at menopause.

3. Idiopathic Transient Osteoporosis of the Hip—Uncommon; diagnosis of exclusion; most common during the third trimester of pregnancy in women but can also occur in men. Presents with groin pain, limited ROM, and localized osteopenia (without a history of

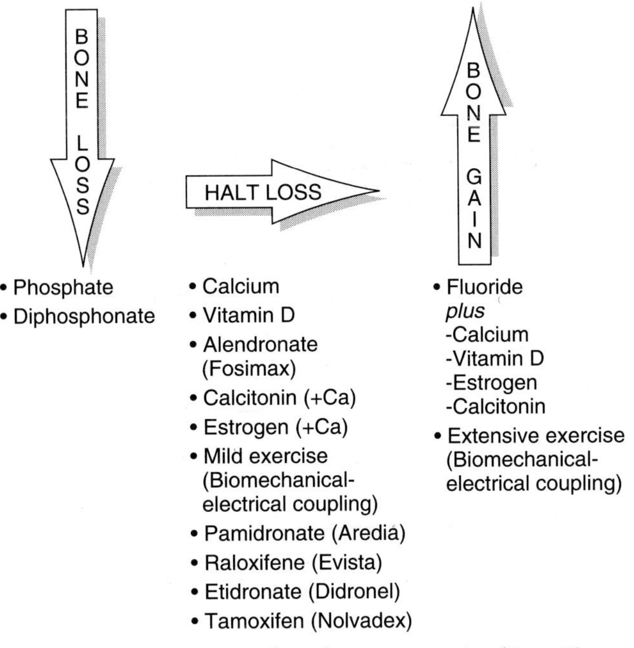

Figure 1–26. Treatment options for osteoporosis. (From Simon, S.R., ed.: Orthopaedic Basic Science, 2nd ed., p. 174. Rosemont, IL, American Academy of Orthopaedic Surgeons, 1994.)

trauma). Treatment includes limited weight-bearing and analgesics. The disease is generally self-limited and tends to resolve spontaneously after 6–8 months (this distinguishes transient osteoporosis from osteonecrosis, in which the symptoms are progressive and do not resolve spontaneously). Stress fractures may occur.

4. Bone Loss Related to Spinal Cord Injury—With paraplegia and quadraplegia, bone mineral loss occurs throughout the skeleton (except the skull) for approximately 16 months and levels off at two-thirds of the original bone mass (high risk of fracture). Bone loss occurs to the greatest extent in the lower extremities.

b. Osteomalacia—Discussed with rickets. **Defect in mineralization** results in a large amount of **unmineralized osteoid (qualitative defect).** Osteomalacia is caused by vitamin D–deficient diets, GI disorders, renal osteodystrophy, and certain drugs (aluminum-containing phosphate-binding antacids [aluminum deposition in bone prevents mineralization], and phenytoin [Dilantin]). **Like osteoporosis, osteomalacia is also associated with chronic alcoholism.** It is commonly associated with Looser's zones (microscopic stress fractures), other fractures, biconcave vertebral bodies, and a trefoil pelvis seen on plain radiographs. Biopsy (transiliac) is required for diagnosis (histologically, widened osteoid seams are seen). Femoral neck fractures are common in patients with osteomalacia. Treatment usually includes large doses of vitamin D. Osteoporosis and osteomalacia are compared in Figure 1–27.

c. Scurvy—**Vitamin C (ascorbic acid) deficiency produces a decrease in chondroitin sulfate synthesis, which leads to defective collagen growth and repair and impaired intracellular hydroxylation of collagen peptides.** Clinical features include fatigue, gum bleeding, ecchymosis, joint effusions, and iron deficiency. Radiographic changes may include thin cortices and trabeculae and metaphyseal clefts (corner sign). Laboratory studies are normal. Histologic changes include replacement of primary trabeculae with granulation tissue, areas of hemorrhage, and widening of the zone of provisional calcification in the physis. **The greatest effect on bone formation occurs in the metaphysis.**

d. Marrow Packing Disorders—Myeloma, leukemia, and other disorders can cause osteopenia (see Chapter 8, Orthopaedic Pathology).

e. Osteogeneis Imperfecta (see Chapter 2, Pediatric Orthopaedics)—**Caused by abnormal collagen synthesis (failure of normal collagen cross-linking). Abnormality is primarily due to a mutation in the genes that are responsible for the production of type I collagen.**

2. Increased Osteodensity

a. Osteopetrosis (Marble Bone Disease)—A group of bone disorders that lead to increased sclerosis and obliteration of the medullary canal due to **decreased osteoclast (and chondroclast) function** (a failure of bone resorption). The number of osteoclasts may be increased, decreased, or normal. The disorder may result from an abnormality of the immune system (thymic defect). Histologically, osteoclasts lack the normal ruffled border and clear zone. The marrow spaces become filled with **necrotic calcified cartilage,** and cartilage may be trapped within osteoid. Empty lacunae and plugging of haversian canals are also seen. The most severe infantile AR "malignant" form leads to a "bone within a bone" appearance on radiographs, hepatosplenomegaly, and aplastic anemia. Bone marrow transplantation (of osteoclast precursors) can be life-saving during childhood. High doses of calcitriol ± steroids may also be helpful. The autosomal dominant (AD) "tarda" (benign) form **(Albers-Schönberg disease)** demonstrates generalized

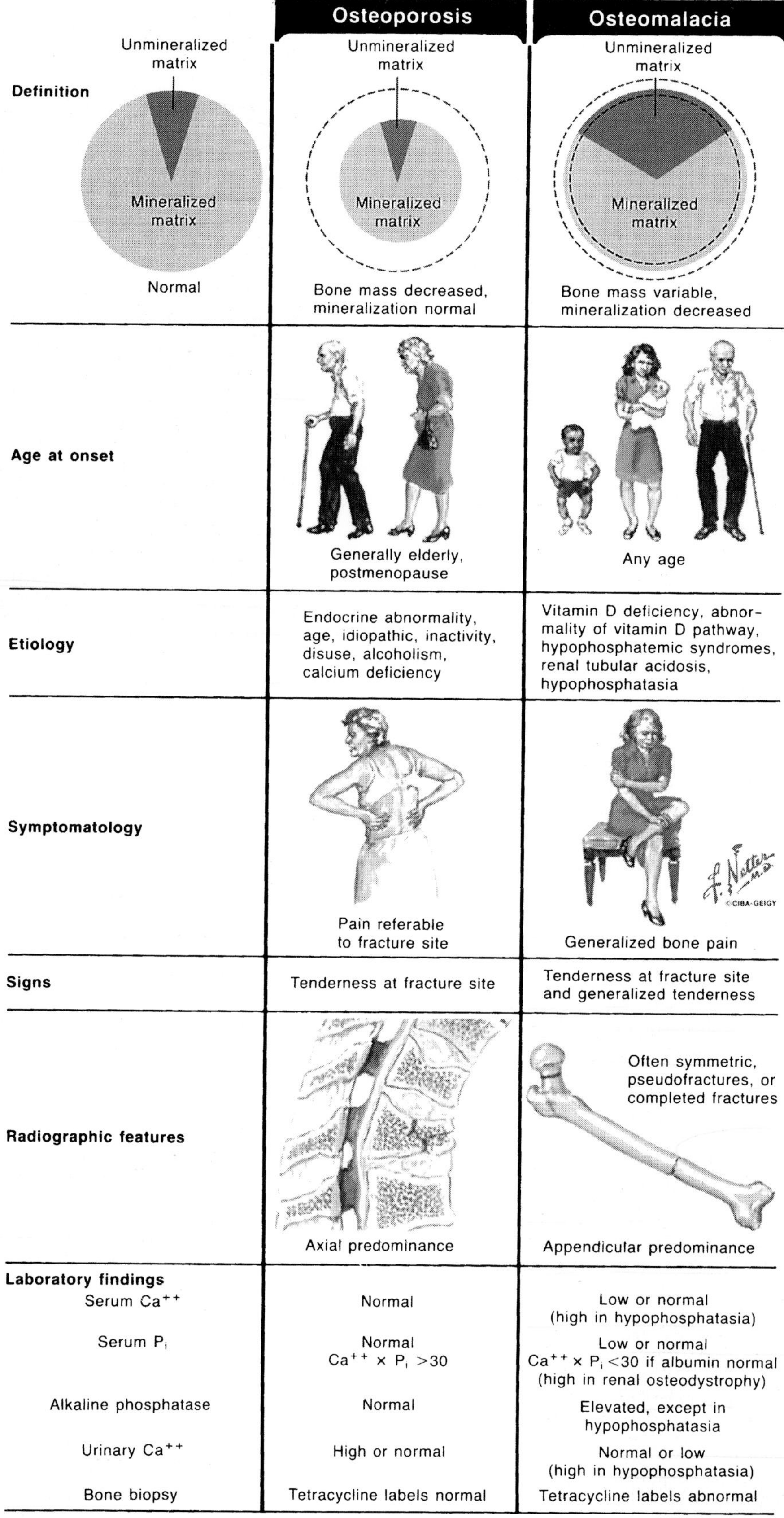

Comparison of Osteoporosis and Osteomalacia

	Osteoporosis	Osteomalacia
Definition (Normal: Unmineralized matrix / Mineralized matrix)	Unmineralized matrix / Mineralized matrix Bone mass decreased, mineralization normal	Unmineralized matrix / Mineralized matrix Bone mass variable, mineralization decreased
Age at onset	Generally elderly, postmenopause	Any age
Etiology	Endocrine abnormality, age, idiopathic, inactivity, disuse, alcoholism, calcium deficiency	Vitamin D deficiency, abnormality of vitamin D pathway, hypophosphatemic syndromes, renal tubular acidosis, hypophosphatasia
Symptomatology	Pain referable to fracture site	Generalized bone pain
Signs	Tenderness at fracture site	Tenderness at fracture site and generalized tenderness
Radiographic features	Axial predominance	Often symmetric, pseudofractures, or completed fractures Appendicular predominance
Laboratory findings		
Serum Ca^{++}	Normal	Low or normal (high in hypophosphatasia)
Serum P_i	Normal $Ca^{++} \times P_i > 30$	Low or normal $Ca^{++} \times P_i < 30$ if albumin normal (high in renal osteodystrophy)
Alkaline phosphatase	Normal	Elevated, except in hypophosphatasia
Urinary Ca^{++}	High or normal	Normal or low (high in hypophosphatasia)
Bone biopsy	Tetracycline labels normal	Tetracycline labels abnormal

Figure 1–27. Osteoporosis versus osteomalacia. (From The Ciba Collection of Medical Illustrations, vol. 8, part I, p. 228, 1987. Illustrated by Frank H. Netter. Reprinted by permission.)

osteosclerosis (including the typical **"rugger jersey" spine**), usually without other anomalies (Figs. 1–28, 1–29). The AR form is more severe (malignant form) and can lead to death during infancy. Pathologic fractures through abnormal (brittle) bone are common.

b. Osteopoikilosis ("Spotted Bone Disease")—Islands of deep cortical bone appear within the medullary cavity and the cancellous bone of the long bones (especially in the hands and feet). These areas are usually asymptomatic, and there is no known incidence of malignant degeneration.

3. Conditions that can display both decreased and increased osteodensity (depending on the phase of the disease)
   a. Paget's Disease—Discussed in Chapter 8, Orthopaedic Pathology **(elevated serum alkaline phosphatase and urinary hydroxyproline are seen)**
      1. Active Phase
         a. Lytic Phase—Intense osteoclastic bone resorption
         b. Mixed Phase
         c. Sclerotic Phase—Osteoblastic bone formation predominates
      2. Inactive Phase

D. Conditions of Bone Viability
   1. Osteonecrosis—Osteonecrosis (ON) represents death of bony tissue (usually adjacent to a joint surface) from causes other than infection. It is usually caused by loss of blood supply due to trauma or another etiology (e.g., after a slipped capital femoral epiphysis). **Recent studies suggest that idiopathic ON of the femoral head and Legg-Calvé-Perthes disease occur in patients with coagulation abnormalities** (deficiency of antithrombin factors protein C and protein S and increased levels of lipoprotein (a)). Osteonecrosis commonly affects the hip joint, leading to eventual collapse and flattening of the femoral head. The condition is associated with steroid and heavy alcohol use; it is also associated with blood dyscrasias (e.g., sickle cell disease), dysbaric (Caisson's disease), excessive radiation therapy, and Gaucher's disease.
      a. Etiology—Theories regarding the etiology of ON vary (Fig. 1–30). It may be related to enlargement of space-occupying marrow fat cells, which leads to ischemia of adjacent tissues. Vascular insults and other factors may also be significant. Idiopathic ON (Chandler's disease) is diagnosed when no other cause can be identified. Idiopathic, alcohol, and dysbaric ON are associated with multiple insults. ON may arise secondary to an underlying hemoglobinopathy (such as sickle cell disease) or a marrow disorder (such as hemochromatosis). The inci-

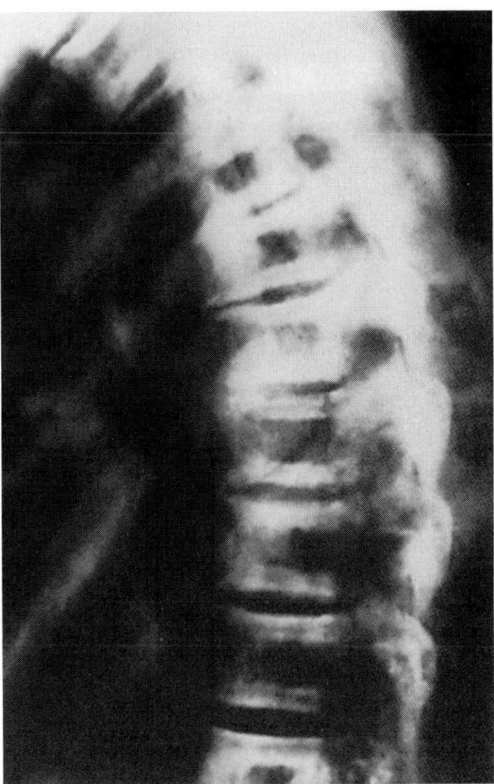

Figure 1–29. Typical "rugger jersey" spine seen in osteopetrosis. (From Tachdijian, M.O.: Pediatric Orthopaedics, 2nd ed., p. 797. Philadelphia, WB Saunders, 1990.)

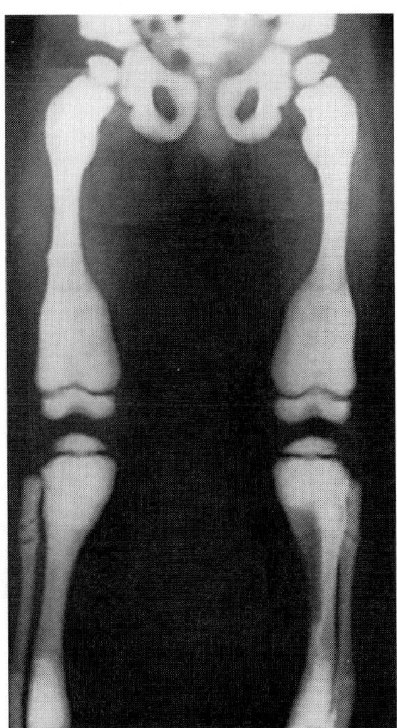

Figure 1–28. Typical "marble bone" appearance of osteopetrosis. (From Tachdijian, M.O.: Pediatric Orthopaedics, 2nd ed., p. 795. Philadelphia: WB Saunders, 1990.)

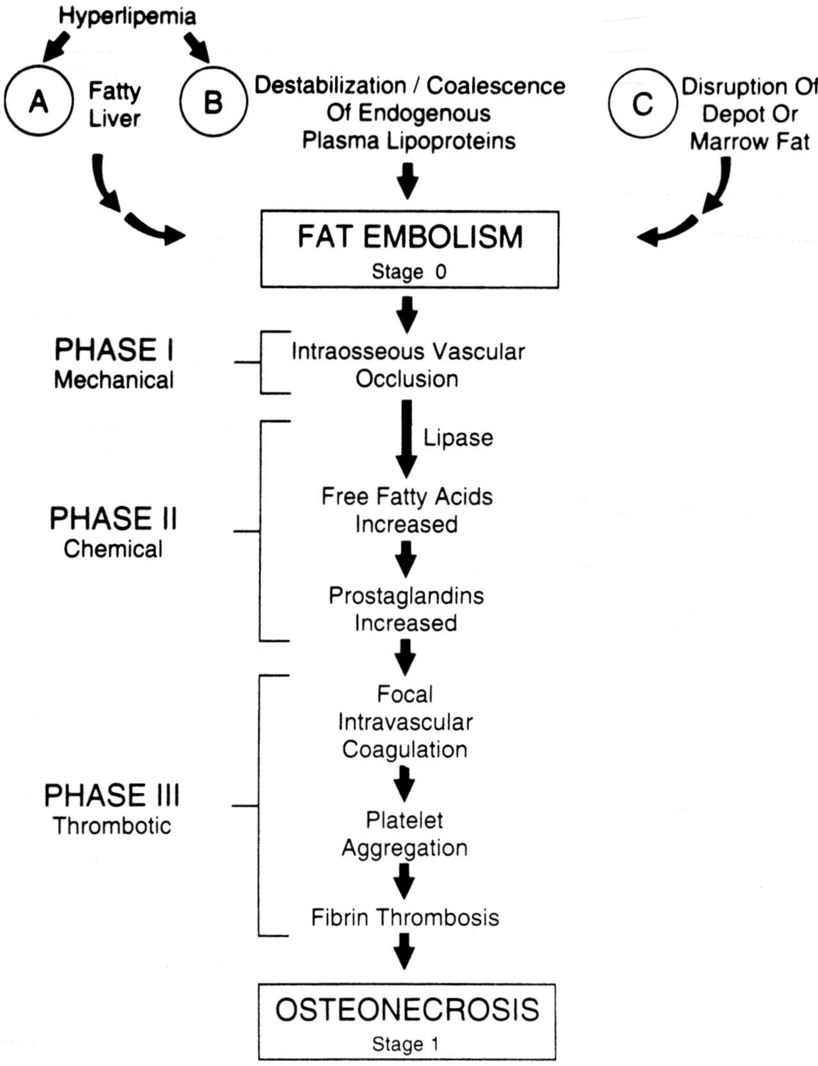

Figure 1–30. Possible mechanisms of intraosseous fat embolism leading to focal intravascular coagulation and osteonecrosis. (From Jones, J.P., Jr.: Fat embolism and osteonecrosis. Orthop Clin North Am 16:595–633, 1985.)

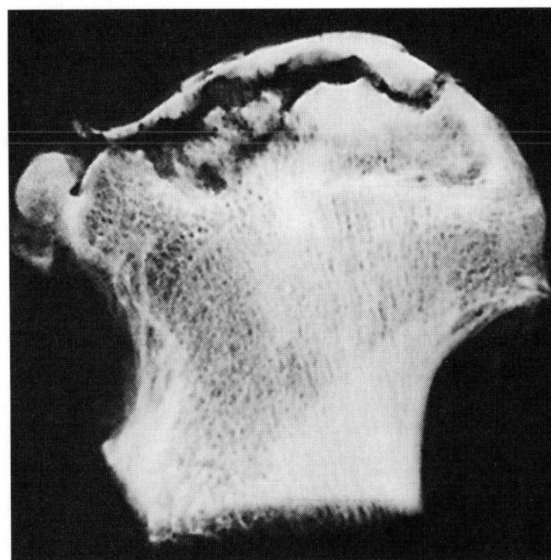

Figure 1–31. Fine-grain radiograph demonstrating space between the articular surface and subchondral bone: "crescent sign" of osteonecrosis. (From Steinberg, M.E.: The Hip and Its Disorders, p. 630. Philadelphia, WB Saunders, 1991.)

dence of ON of the femoral head in renal transplant patients has been reduced by the use of cyclosporine.

b. Pathologic Changes—Grossly necrotic bone, fibrous tissue, and subchondral collapse may be seen (Figs. 1–31, 1–32). Histologically, early changes involve autolysis of osteocytes (14–21 days) and necrotic marrow, followed by inflammation with invasion of buds of primitive mesenchymal tissue and capillaries. Later, **new woven bone is laid down on top of dead trabecular bone.** This stage is followed by resorption of the dead trabeculae and remodeling during a process of **"creeping substitution."** It is during this process that the bone is weakest, and **collapse (crescent sign, seen on radiographs)** and fragmentation can occur.

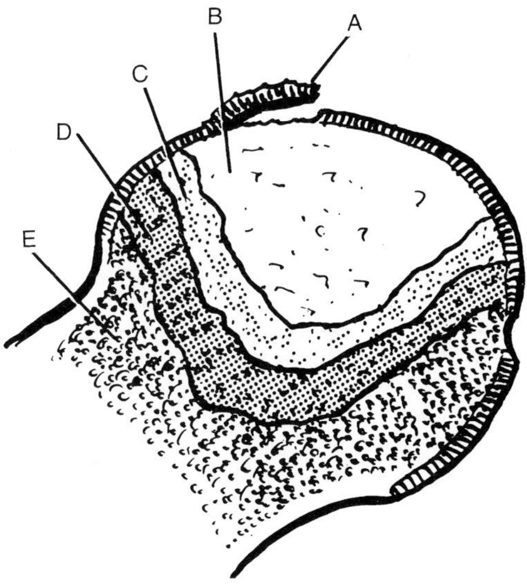

Figure 1–32. Pathology of avascular necrosis. *A,* Articular cartilage. *B,* Necrotic bone. *C,* Reactive fibrous tissue. *D,* Hypertrophic bone. *E,* Normal trabeculae. (From Steinberg, M.E.: The Hip and Its Disorders, p. 630. Philadelphia, WB Saunders, 1991.)

Table 1–16.

Common Osteochondroses

Disorder	Site	Age (Years)
Van Neck's disease	Ischipubic synchrondrosis	4–11
Legg-Calvé-Perthes disease	Femoral head	4–8
Osgood-Schlatter disease	Tibial tuberosity	11–15
Sinding-Larsen-Johansson syndrome	Inferior patella	10–14
Blount's disease (infant)	Proximal tibial epiphysis	1–3
Blount's disease (adolescent)	Proximal tibial epiphysis	8–15
Sever's disease	Calcaneus	9–11
Köhler's disease	Tarsal navicular	3–7
Freiberg's infarction	Metatarsal head	13–18
Scheuermann's disease	Discovertebral junction	13–17
Panner's disease	Capitellum of humerus	5–10
Thiemann's disease	Phalanges of hand	11–19
Kienböck's disease	Carpal lunate	20–40

c. Evaluation—Careful history-taking (risk factors) and physical examination (e.g., decreased ROM, limp) should precede additional studies. Evaluation of other joints (especially the contralateral hip) is important in order to identify the disease process early. The process is bilateral in the hip in 50% of cases of idiopathic ON and up to 80% of steroid-induced ON. MRI **(earliest positive study)** and bone scanning are helpful for making an early diagnosis. Femoral head pressure measurement is possible but invasive. Pressure >30 mm Hg or increased >10 mm Hg with injection of 5 mL of saline (stress test) is considered abnormal (but these values have varied widely from one investigation to another).

d. Treatment—Replacement arthroplasty of the hip is associated with increased loosening. Nontraumatic ON of the distal femoral condyle and proximal humerus may improve spontaneously without surgical correction. The precise role of core decompression remains unresolved, but results are best for early hip disease (Ficat stage I).

2. Osteochondroses—Can occur at traction apophyses in children and may or may not be associated with trauma, inflammation of the joint capsule, or vascular insult/secondary thrombosis. The pathology is similar to that described for ON in the adult. Table 1–16 shows the common osteochondroses (*know them!*). Most are discussed separately in the chapters covering the respective sites of disease.

Section 2
Joints

I. **Articular Tissues**

A. Cartilage—There are several types of cartilage. **Growth plate (physeal) cartilage** has been previously discussed; fibrocartilage is important for tendon and ligament insertion into bone (and for healing of articular cartilage); **elastic cartilage** is seen in tissues such as the trachea; **fibroelastic cartilage** makes up menisci; and finally, **articular cartilage** is critical to the function of joints and is the focus of this section. Articular cartilage functions in decreasing friction and in load distribution. Classically, mature articular cartilage has been described as avascular, aneural, and alymphatic. Chondrocytes receive nutrients and oxygen from synovial fluid via diffusion through the cartilage matrix. The pH of cartilage is 7.4; changes in pH can disrupt the structure of cartilage. **Unlike mature articular cartilage, immature articular cartilage has a stem cell population.** Animal models (rabbit knee) suggest that autologous osteochondral progenitor cells can be isolated (from bone marrow) and grown in vitro. These cells do not appear to lose their ability to differentiate into cartilage or bone and therefore may be clinically useful for repairing articular cartilage defects (and subchondral bone). Animal models (rabbit) also suggest that TGF-β can induce chondrogenesis in periosteal explants cultured in agarose gel.

1. Articular Cartilage Composition

a. Water (65–80% of wet weight)—Allows for deformation of the cartilage surface in response to stress by shifting in and out of cartilage. Water is not distributed homogeneously throughout cartilage (65% at the deep zone, 80% at the surface). Water content increases (90%) in osteoarthritis (Table 1–17). Water is also responsible for nutrition and lubrication. Increased water content leads to increased permeability, decreased strength, and decreased Young's modulus (*E*).

b. Collagen (10–20% of wet weight; >50% of dry weight) (Fig. 1–33)—Type II collagen accounts for approximately 90–95% of the total collagen content of articular cartilage and allows for a cartilaginous framework and **tensile strength.** Increased amounts of glycine, proline, hydroxyproline, and hydrogen bonding are responsible for its unique characteristics. Hydroxyproline is unique to collagen and can be measured in the urine to assess bone turnover. Small amounts of types V, VI, IX, X, and XI collagen are present in the matrix of articular cartilage. An overview of collagen types for all tissues is shown in Table 1–18. Collagen type VI is a minor component of normal articular cartilage, but its content increases significantly in early osteoarthritis. **Collagen type X is produced only by hypertrophic**

Table 1–17.

Biochemical Changes of Articular Cartilage

	Aging	Osteoarthritis (OA)
Water content (hydration; permeability)	↓	↑
Collagen	Content remains relatively unchanged	Becomes disorderly (breakdown of matrix framework) Content ↓ in severe OA Relative concentration ↑ (due to loss of proteoglycans)
Proteoglycan content (concentration)	↓ (also the length of the protein core and GAG chains decreases)	↓
Proteoglycan synthesis		↑
Proteoglycan degradation	↓	↑ ↑ ↑
Chondroitin sulfate concentration (includes both chondroitin 4 and 6–sulfate)	↓	↑
Chondroitin 4–sulfate concentration	↓	↑
Keratin sulfate concentration	↑	↓
Chondrocyte size	↑	
Chondrocyte number	↓	
Modulus of elasticity	↑	↓

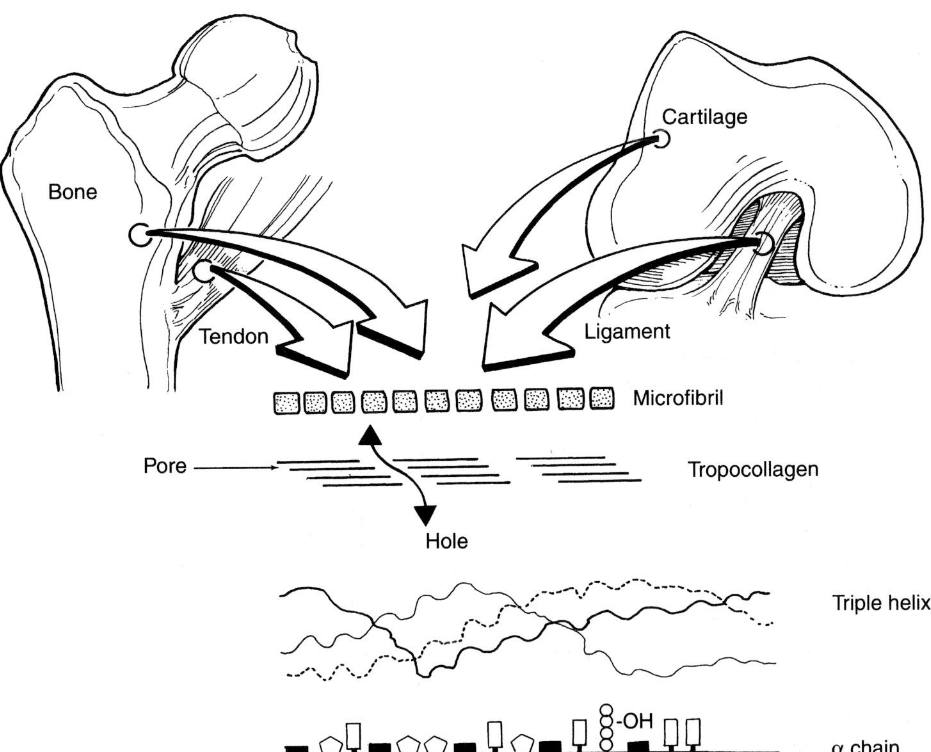

Figure 1–33. Microstructure of collagen. Collagen is composed of microfibrils that are quarter-staggered arrangements of tropocollagen. Note hole and pore regions for mineral deposition (for calcification). Tropocollagen, in turn, is made up of a triple helix of α chains of polypeptides. (From Brinker, M.R., and Miller, M.D.: Fundamentals of Orthopaedics. Philadelphia, WB Saunders, 1999, p. 3.)

chondrocytes during enchondral ossification (growth plate, fracture callus, HO formation). Type X collagen is associated with calcification of cartilage; a genetic defect in type X collagen is responsible for Schmid's metaphyseal chondrodysplasia; the hypertrophic physeal zone is the zone primarily affected by the type X collagen defect. Collagen type XI is an adhesive that holds the collagen latticework together.

c. Proteoglycans (10–15% of wet weight)—Protein polysaccharides responsible for the **compressive strength** of cartilage. Proteoglycans are produced by chondrocytes, are secreted into the extracellular matrix, and are composed of subunits known as **glycosaminoglycans** (GAGs, disaccharide polymers). **These GAGs include two subtypes of chondroitin sulfate (the most prevalent GAG in cartilage) and keratin sulfate. The concentration of chondroitin-4-sulfate decreases with age, that of chondroitin-6-sulfate remains essentially constant, and that of keratin sulfate increases with age.** GAGs are bound to a protein core by sugar bonds to form a proteoglycan aggrecan molecule. Link proteins stabilize aggrecan molecules to hyaluronic acid to form a proteoglycan aggregate. Proteoglycans have a half-life of 3 months, are responsible for the porous structure of cartilage, and serve to trap and hold water **(regulate matrix hydration).** A proteoglycan aggregate and an aggrecan molecule are represented in Figure 1–34.

d. Chondrocytes (5% of wet weight)—Active in protein synthesis and possess a double effusion barrier; produce collagen, proteoglycans, and some enzymes for cartilage metabolism; less active in the calcified zone. Deeper zones of cartilage have

Table 1–18.

Types of Collagen

Type	Location
I	Bone Tendon Meniscus Annulus of intervertebral disc Skin
II	Articular cartilage Nucleus pulposus of intervertebral disc
III	Skin Blood vessels
IV	Basement membrane (basal lamina)
V	Articular cartilage (in small amounts)
VI	Articular cartilage (in small amounts) Tethers the chondrocyte to its pericellular matrix
VII	Basement membrane (epithelial)
VIII	Basement membrane (epithelial)
IX	Articular cartilage (in small amounts)
X	Hypertrophic cartilage Associated with calcification of cartilage (matrix mineralization)
XI	Articular cartilage (in small amounts) (acts as an adhesive)
XII	Tendon
XIII	Endothelial cells

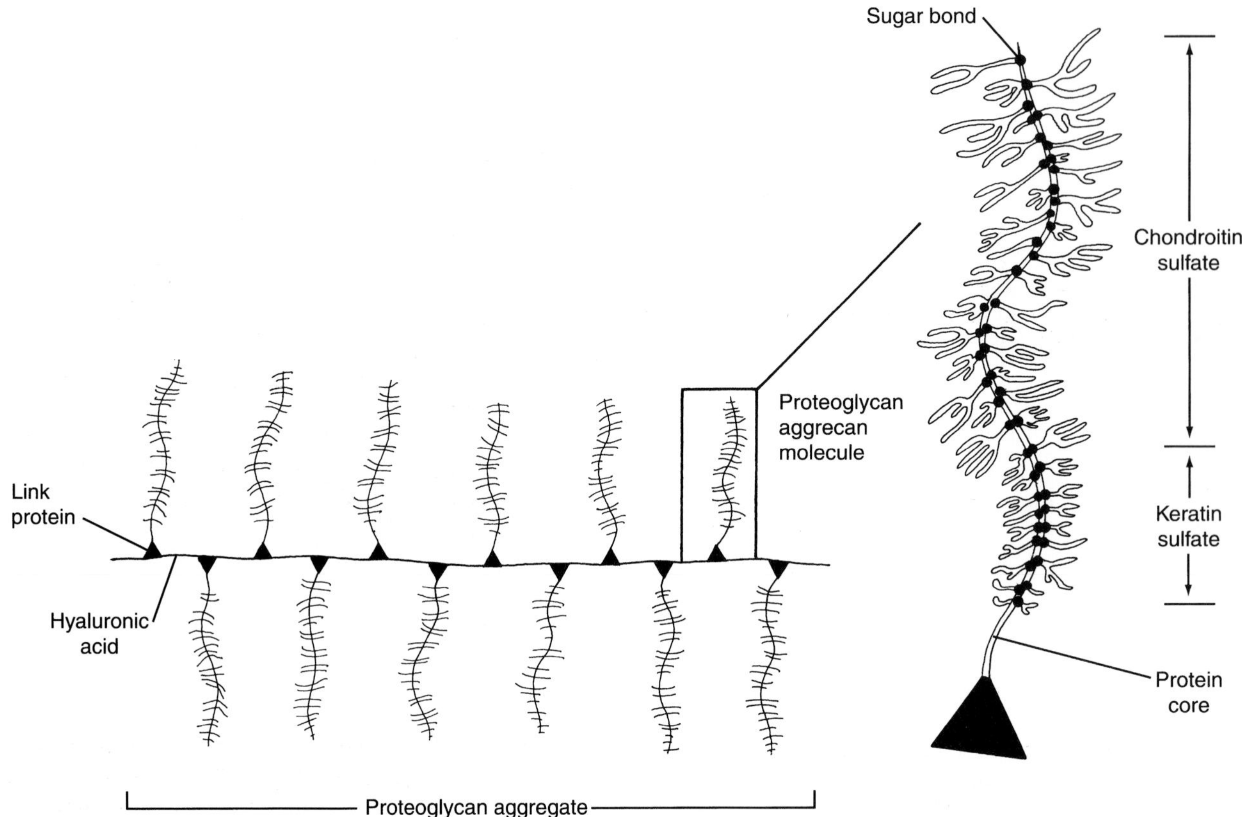

Figure 1–34. Proteoglycan aggregate and aggrecan molecule. (From Brinker, M.R., and Miller, M.D.: Fundamentals of Orthopaedics. Philadelphia, WB Saunders, 1999, p. 9.)

chondrocytes with decreased rough endoplasmic reticulum (RER) and increased intraplasmic filaments (degenerative products). Chondroblasts, which are derived from undifferentiated mesenchymal cells (stimulated by motion), are later trapped in lacunae to become chondrocytes.

e. Other Matrix Components
  1. Adhesives (fibronectin, chondronectin, anchorin CII)—Involved in interactions between chondrocytes and fibrils. Fibronectin may be associated with osteoarthritis.
  2. Lipids—Unknown function.

2. Articular Cartilage Layers—The various layers of articular cartilage are described in Table 1–19 and are illustrated in Figure 1–35. **The tangential zone has a high concentration of collagen fibers** arranged at right angles to each other (and parallel to the articular surface). The zone of calcified cartilage forms a transitional zone of intermediate stiffness between articular cartilage and subchondral bone.

3. Articular Cartilage Metabolism
  a. Collagen Synthesis—The events and sites involved in collagen synthesis are shown in Figure 1–36.
  b. Collagen Catabolism—Little is known of the exact mechanism. Enzymatic processes have been proposed such that metalloproteinase collagenase cleaves the triple helix. Mechanical factors may also play a role.
  c. Proteoglycan Synthesis (Fig. 1–37)—A se-

Table 1–19.

Articular Cartilage Layers

Layer	Width (μm)	Characteristic	Orientation	Function
Gliding zone (superficial)	40	↓ Metabolic activity	Tangential	vs. Shear
Transitional zone (middle)	500	↑ Metabolic activity	Oblique	vs. Compression
Radial zone (deep)	1000	↑ Collagen size	Vertical	vs. Compression
Tidemark	5	Undulating barrier	Tangential	vs. Shear
Calcified zone	300	Hydroxyapatite crystals		Anchor

↑, increased; ↓, decreased.

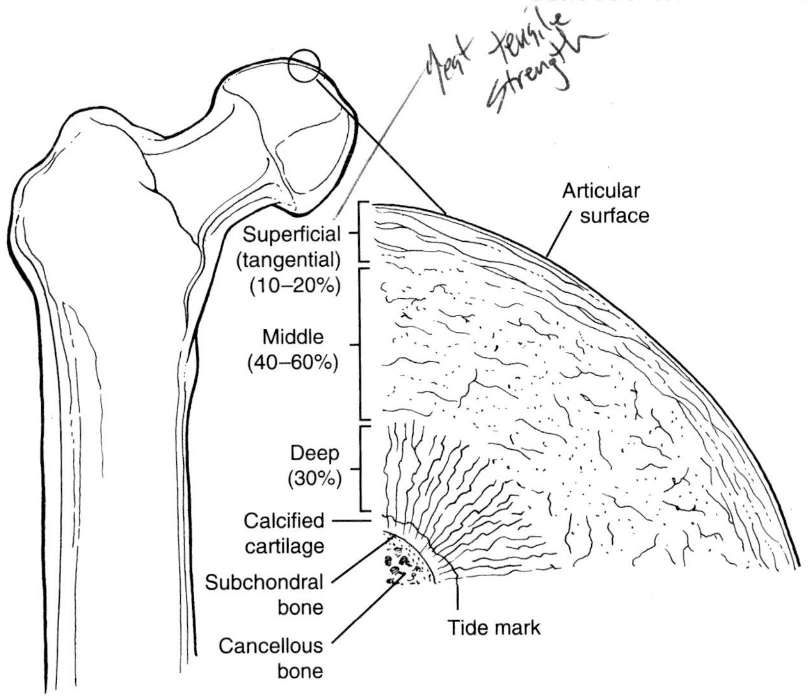

Superficial (tangential) (10–20%)
Middle (40–60%)
Deep (30%)
Calcified cartilage
Subchondral bone
Cancellous bone
Articular surface
Tide mark

Figure 1–35. Articular cartilage layers. (From Brinker, M.R., and Miller, M.D.: Fundamentals of Orthopaedics. Philadelphia, WB Saunders, 1999, p. 9.)

ries of molecular events beginning with proteoglycan gene expression and transcription of messenger RNA and concluding with proteoglycan aggregate formation in the extracellular matrix.

d. Proteoglycan Catabolism (Fig. 1–38)

4. Articular Cartilage Growth Factors—Regulate cartilage synthesis; may have a role in osteoarthritis.

a. Platelet-Derived Growth Factor (PDGF)—May play a role in the healing of cartilage lacerations (and perhaps osteoarthritis).

b. Transforming Growth Factor-Beta (TGF-β)—**Stimulates proteoglycan synthesis while suppressing synthesis of type II collagen.** Stimulates the formation of plasminogen activator inhibitor-1 and tissue inhibitor of metalloproteinase (TIMP), which prevent the degradative action of plasmin and stromelysin.

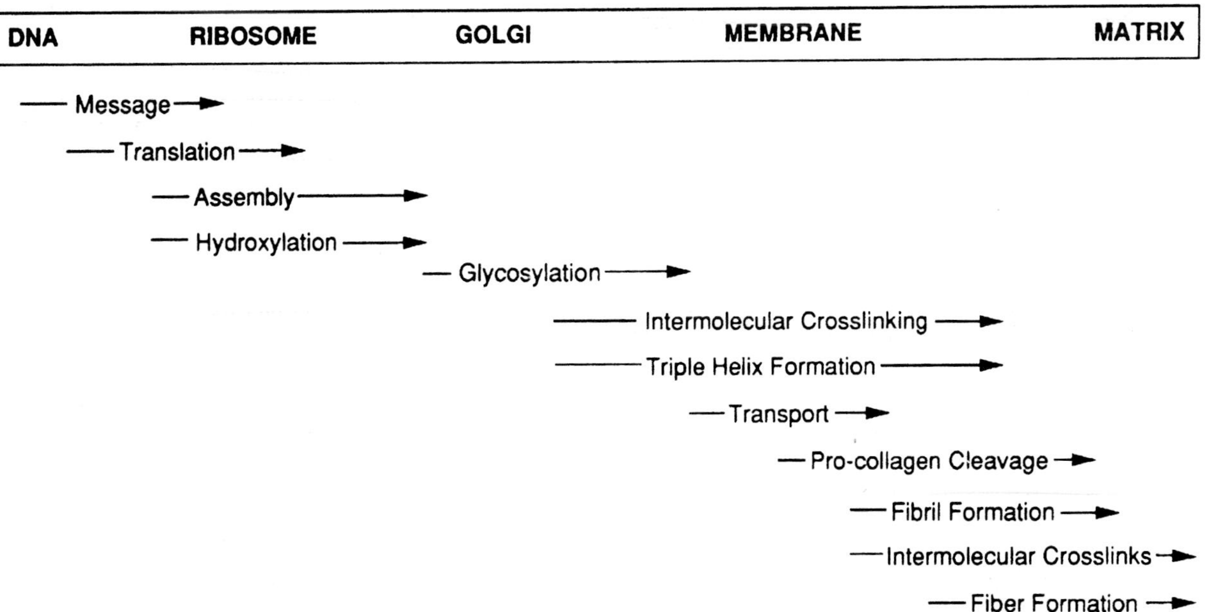

Figure 1–36. Collagen synthesis is accomplished at various intracellular sites. (From Mankin, H.J., and Brandt, K.D.: Biochemistry and metabolism of articular cartilage in osteoarthritis. In Moskowitz, R.W., Howell, D.S., Goldberg, V.M., et al., eds.: Osteoarthritis: Diagnosis and Medical/Surgical Management, 2nd ed., p. 124. Philadelphia, WB Saunders, 1992.)

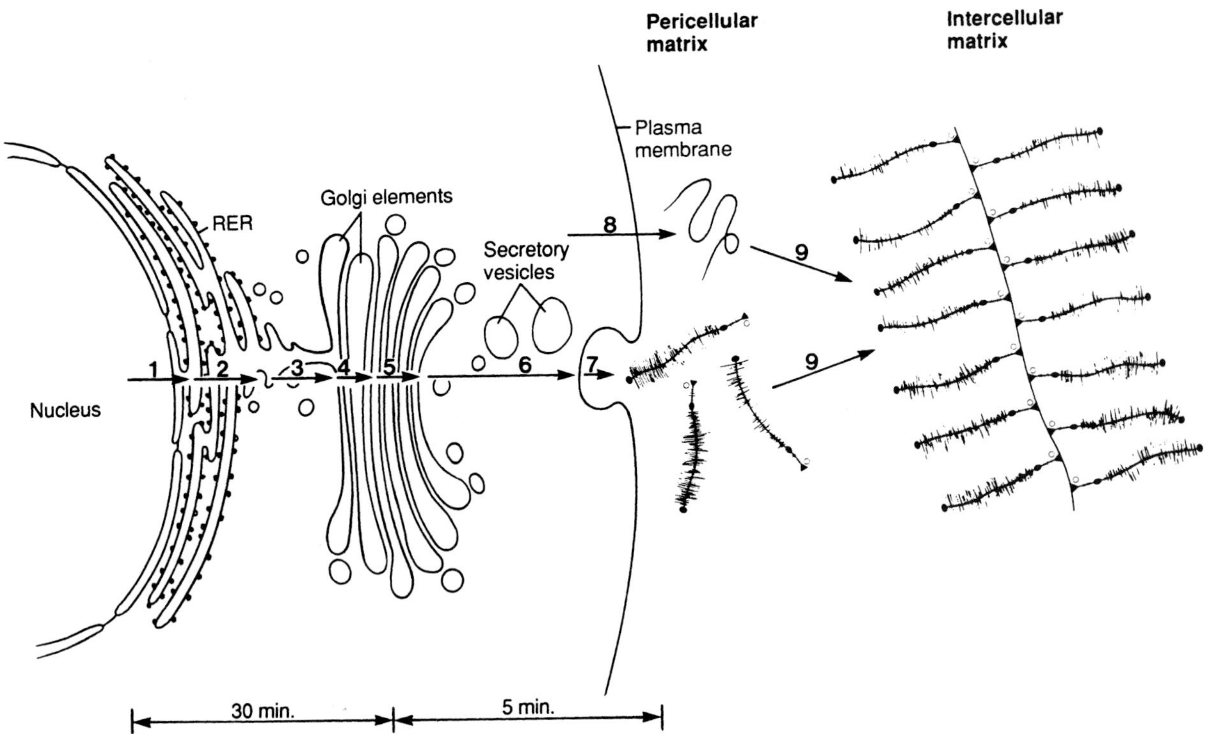

Figure 1–37. Synthesis and secretion of proteoglycan aggrecan molecules and link protein by a chondrocyte. *1,* Transcription of aggrecan and link protein genes to mRNA. *2,* Translation of mRNA to form protein core. *3,* Transportation. *4, 5, cis* and medial *trans* Golgi compartments, respectively, where glycosaminoglycan chains are added to the protein core. *6,* Transportation to the secretory vesicles. *7,* Release into the extracellular matrix. *8, 9,* Hyaluronate from the plasma membrane binds with the aggrecan and link proteins to form aggregates in the extracellular matrix. RER, rough endoplasmic reticulum. (From Simon, S.R., ed.: Orthopaedic Basic Science, 2nd ed., p. 13. Rosemont, IL, American Academy of Orthopaedic Surgeons, 1994.)

c. Fibroblast Growth Factor (Basic) (b-FGF)—Stimulates DNA synthesis in adult articular chondrocytes; may play a role in the cartilage repair process.

d. Insulin-Like Growth Factor-I (IGF-I)—Previously known as somatomedin C. Stimulates DNA and cartilage matrix synthesis in adult articular cartilage and immature cartilage of the growth plate.

5. Lubrication and Wear Mechanisms of Articular Cartilage (Figs. 1–39, 1–40, 1–41)

a. General Comments—The primary mechanism responsible for lubrication of articular cartilage (low coefficient of friction) during dynamic function is **elastohydrodynamic lubrication.** The coefficient of friction for human joints (such as the knee and hip) is in the range of 0.002–0.04. Factors that decrease the coefficient of friction of articular cartilage include: fluid film formation, elastic deformation of articular cartilage, synovial fluid, and efflux of fluid from the cartilage. Factors that increase the coefficient of friction include: fibrillation of articular cartilage. Almost all joints, during range of motion, undergo both rolling and sliding. Pure rolling occurs when the instant center of rotation is at the rolling surfaces; pure sliding occurs with pure translation (without an instant center of rotation).

b. Specific Types of Lubrication (Figs. 1–39 and 1–40)

1. **Elastohydrodynamic Lubrication—The predominant mechanism during dynamic joint function.** Deformation of articular surfaces and thin films of the joint lubricants separate the surfaces (the coefficient of friction is primarily due to the properties of the lubricant, not the surfaces). Coefficient of friction is generally low.
2. **Boundary Lubrication** (Slippery Surfaces)—The bearing surface is largely nondeformable, and therefore the lubricant only partially separates the surfaces.
3. **Boosted Lubrication** (Fluid Entrapment)—Describes the concentration of lubricating fluid in pools trapped by regions of bearing surfaces that are making contact. Coefficient of friction is generally higher for boosted than elastohydrodynamic.
4. **Hydrodynamic Lubrication**—Fluid separates the surfaces under load.
5. **Weeping Lubrication**—Fluid shifts to loaded areas.

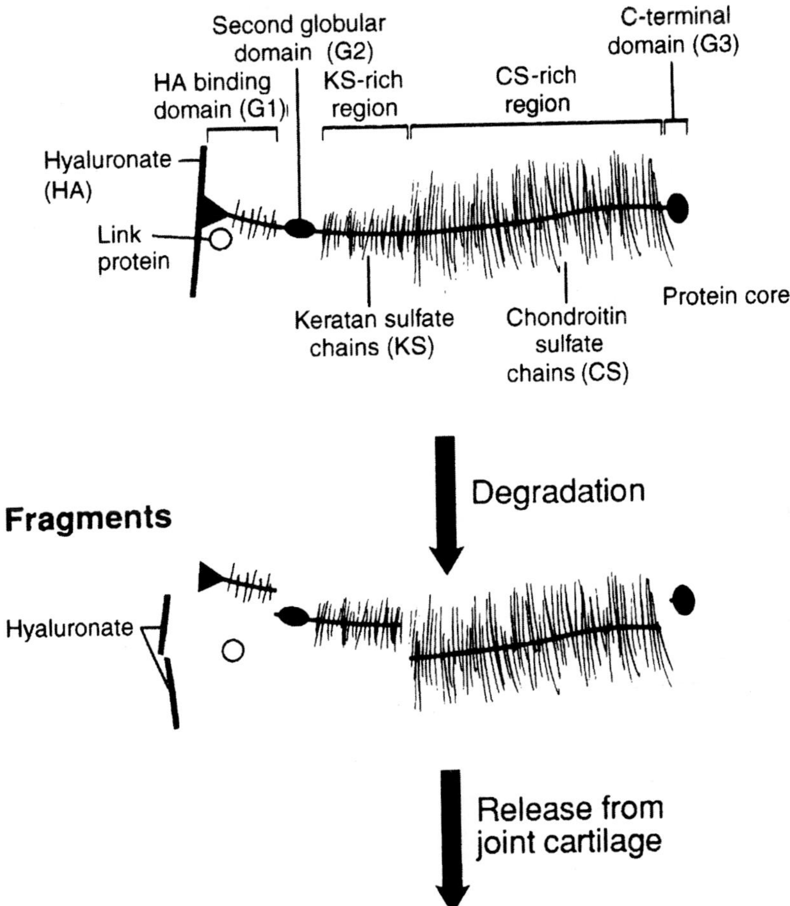

Figure 1–38. Proteoglycan degradation in articular cartilage. Cleavage of the G1 and G2 domains make the fragments nonaggregating. (Modified from Simon, S.R., ed.: Orthopaedic Basic Science, 2nd ed., p. 14. Rosemont, IL, American Academy of Orthopaedic Surgeons, 1994.)

6. Articular Cartilage Aging (and Other Special Circumstances) (see Table 1–17)—With aging, chondrocytes become larger, acquire increased lysosomal enzymes, and no longer reproduce (so cartilage becomes relatively hypocellular). **Cartilage has increased stiffness and decreased solubility with aging.** With aging, cartilage proteoglycans decrease in mass and size (decreased length of the chondroitin sulfate chains) and change in proportion (decreased concentration of chondroitin sulfate and **increased concentration of keratin sulfate).** Protein content increases with aging, and **water content decreases.** These changes decrease the elasticity of cartilage. Moderate impact to a joint without fracture results in decreased proteoglycan concentration and increased tissue hydration.
7. Articular Cartilage Healing—**Deep lacerations** extending below the tidemark that penetrate the underlying subchondral bone may heal with fibrocartilage. **The fibrocartilage is produced by undifferentiated marrow mesenchymal stem cells** that differentiate into cells capable of producing fibrocartilage (this is the theory behind abrasion chon-

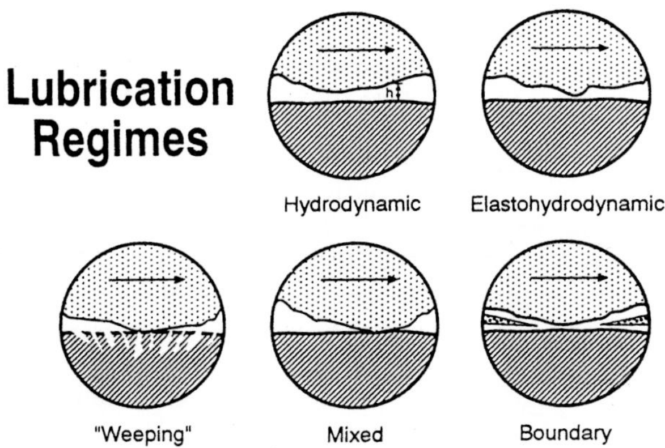

Figure 1–39. Types of lubrication. (From Simon, S.R., ed.: Orthopaedic Basic Science, 2nd ed., p. 465. Rosemont, IL, American Academy of Orthopaedic Surgeons, 1994.)

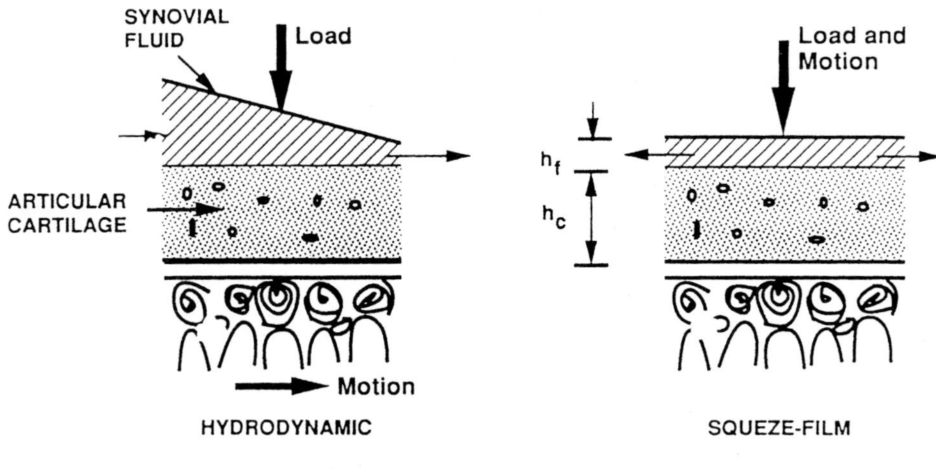

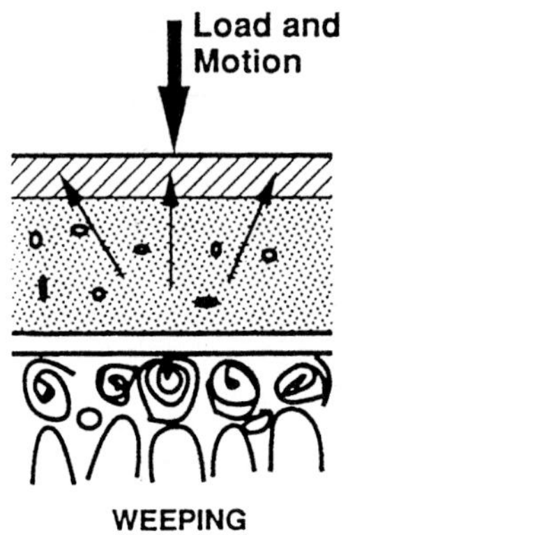

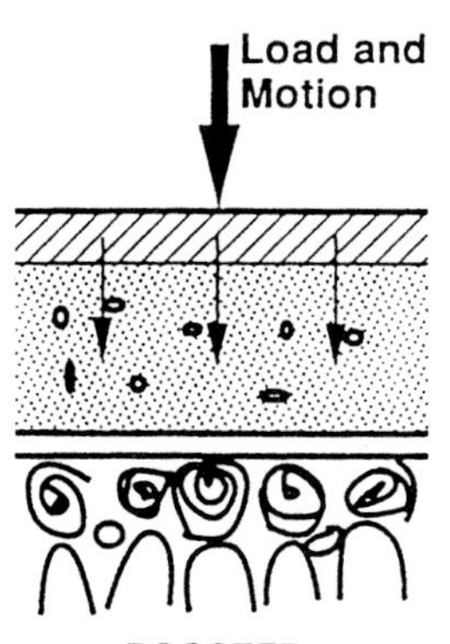

Figure 1–40. Fluid film lubrication models include Hydrodynamic, Squeeze-Film, Weeping, and Boosted. (From Mow, V.C., and Soslowsky, L.J.: Friction, lubrication, and wear of diarthrodial joints. In Basic Orthopaedic Biomechanics, Mow, V.C., and Hayes, W.C., eds., pp. 245–292. New York, Raven Press, 1991.)

droplasty). Remember, fibrocartilage is not as durable as hyaline cartilage. Blunt trauma may induce changes in cartilage similar to those seen with osteoarthritis. **Superficial articular cartilage** lacerations that do not cross the tidemark cause chondrocytes to proliferate but do not heal. Continuous passive motion is believed to have a beneficial effect on cartilage healing; immobilization of a joint leads to atrophy or cartilage degeneration. In experimental animals, 4 weeks of joint disuse (knee immobilization) results in a decrease in the ratio of proteoglycan to collagen, which returns to normal after 8 weeks of joint mobilization. Joint instability (transection of the ACL) leads to an initial decrease in the ratio of proteoglycan to collagen (at 4 weeks), but a late (12 weeks) elevation in the ratio of proteoglycan to collagen and an increase in hydration. Joint instability leads to a marked decrease in hyaluronan, whereas disuse does not.

Wear Mechanisms
Adhesion
Abrasion
Transfer
Fatigue
Third Body

Figure 1–41. Wear mechanisms. (From Simon, S.R., ed.: Orthopaedic Basic Science, 2nd ed., p. 466. Rosemont, IL, American Academy of Orthopaedic Surgeons, 1994.)

B. Synovium—Synovium mediates the exchange of nutrients between blood and joint (synovial) fluid. Synovial tissue is composed of vascularized connective tissue that lacks a basement membrane. Two cell types are present in synovium: **type A cells**, which are important in **phagocytosis**; and **type B cells (fibroblast-like cells),** which produce synovial fluid (broth). Other undifferentiated cells have a reparative role. A third type of cell, type C, may exist as an intermediate cell type. **Synovial fluid** is made up of hyaluronic acid, lubricin (a lubricating glycoprotein), proteinase, collagenases, and prostaglandins. Synovial fluid is an ultrafiltrate (dialysate) of blood plasma added to fluid produced by the synovial membrane; it contains no RBCs, clotting factors,

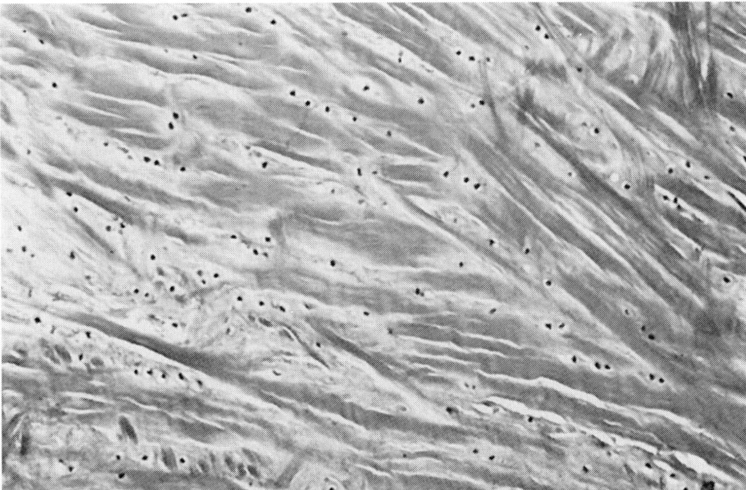
Figure 1–42. Histology of menisci.

or hemoglobin. It **lubricates articular cartilage and provides nourishment through diffusion. Synovial fluid exhibits non-newtonian flow characteristics** (the viscosity coefficient μ is not a constant; the fluid is not linearly viscous), and its **viscosity increases as the shear rate decreases. Lubricin, a glycoprotein,** is the key lubricating component of synovial fluid. **Hyaluronan molecules** in the knee become entangled and behave like an elastic solid during high-strain activities (running, jumping). Analysis of synovial fluid in disease processes is important and is discussed later in this section under Arthroses.

C. Meniscus—Functions to deepen the articular surface of a variety of synovial joints (acromioclavicular [AC], sternoclavicular [SC], glenohumeral, hip, knee) and thereby broaden the contact area to distribute the load such as on the tibial plateau. The meniscus of the knee is the focus of this section. **After total meniscetomy of the knee, 20% of patients have significant arthritic lesions, and 70% have x-ray changes at 3 years' follow-up; all patients experience arthrosis by 20 years. The severity of degenerative changes is proportional to the amount of meniscus exised.**

1. Anatomy (Knee Meniscus)—Triangular semilunar structure. Peripheral border is attached to the joint capsule. Medial meniscus is semicircular; lateral meniscus is circular.
2. Histology—Meniscus is composed of **fibroelastic cartilage** (Fig. 1–42). There is an interlacing network of collagen fibers, proteoglycans, glycoproteins, and cellular elements (Table 1–20).

Table 1–20.

Histologic Features of Meniscus

EXTRACELLULAR MATRIX
Collagen—**primarily type I collagen** (55–65% of dry weight)
Also types II, III, V, and VI (5–10% of dry weight)
Superficial layer—mesh-like fibers oriented primarily radially
Surface layer—(deep to superficial layer) irregularly aligned collagen bundles
Middle layer—(deep) parallel circumferential fibers
Elastin (0.6% of dry weight)
Proteoglycans } (1–3% of dry weight)
Glycoproteins }
Adhesive glycoproteins (fibronectin, thrombospondin)
CELLULAR COMPONENTS—synthesize and maintain extracellular matrix
—anaerobic metabolism (few mitochondria)
Chondrocytes } **Fibrochondrocytes:**
Fibroblasts }
Fusiform cells
Found in superficial layer
Resemble fibroblasts and chondrocytes
Found in lacunae
Contain abundant endoplasmic reticulum (ER) and Golgi
Ovoid cells
Found in surface and middle layer
Contain abundant ER and Golgi

Table 1–21.

Comparison of Common Arthritides

Arthritis	Age	Sex	SYM?	Joints	Physical Exam
Noninflammatory					
Osteoarthritis	Old	M > F	Asym	Hip, knee, CMC	↓ ROM, crepitus
Neuropathic	Old	M > F	Asym	Foot, ankle, LE	Effusion, unstable
ARF	Child	M = F	Asym	Mig; lg joints	Red tender joint, rash
Ochronosis	Adult	M = F	Asym	Lg joints/spine	↓ ROM, locking
Inflammatory					
Rheumatoid	Young	F > M	Sym	Hands, feet	Ulnar dev, claw toes
SLE	Young	F > M	Sym	PIP, MCP, knee	Red swollen joint, rash
JRA	Child	F > M	Sym	Knee, multiple	Swollen joint, normal color
Relapsing polychondritis	Old	M = F	Sym	All joints	Eye, ear involved
Spondyloarthropathies					
AS	Young	M > F	Sym	SI, spine, hip	Rigid spine, "chin on chest"
Reiter's syndrome	Young	M > F	Asym	Wt-bearing	Urethral D/C, conjunctivitis
Psoriatic	Young	M = F	Asym	DIP, small joints	Rash, sausage digit, pitting
Entereopathic	Young	M > F	Asym	Wt-bearing	Synovitis, GI manifestations
Crystal Deposition Disease					
Gout	Young	M > F	Asym	Great toe, LE	Tophi, red, swollen
Chondrocalcinosis	Old	M = F	Asym	Knee, LE	Acute swelling
Infectious					
Pyogenic	Any	M = F	Asym	Any joint	Red, hot, swollen
Tuberculous	Old	M > F	Asym	Spine, LE	Indolent, swelling
Lyme disease	Young	M = F	Asym	Any joint	Acute effusion
Fungal	Any	M > F	Asym	Any joint	Indolent
Hemorrhagic					
Hemophilia	Young	M	Asym	Knee, UE (elbow, shoulder)	↓ ROM, swelling
Sickle cell	Young	M = F	Asym	Hip, any bone	Pain, ↓ ROM
PVNS	Young	M = F	Asym	Knee, LE	Pain, synovitis

ARF, acute rheumatic fever; SLE, systemic lupus erythematosus; JRA, juvenile rheumatoid arthritis; AS, ankylosing spondylitis; PVNS, pigmented villonodular synovitis; Asym, asymmetric; Sym, symmetric; CMC, carpometacarpal; LE, lower extremity; Mig, migratory; Lg, large; PIP, proximal interphalangeal; MCP, metacarpophalangeal; SI, sacroiliac; DIP, distal interphalangeal; UE, upper extremity; ↓ ROM, decreased range of motion; D/C, discharge; GI, gastrointestinal; ASO, antistreptolysin O; ESR, erythrocyte sedimentation rate; CRP, C-reactive protein; RF, rheumatoid factor; ANA, antinuclear antibody; alk. phos, alkaline phosphatase; CPK, creatine phosphokinase; HLA, human leukocyte antigen; Birefr., birefringent; WBC, white blood cells; PPD, purified protein derivative; AFB, acid fast bacilli; ELISA, enzyme linked immunosorbent assay; PTT, partial thromboplastin time; resorp., resorption; arth, arthritis; MT, metatarsal; DIP, distal interphalangeal; Art, articular; fibrocart, fibrocartilage; Eryth. marg, erythema marginatum; Pericard., pericardial; Pulm, pulmonary; Eryth., erythema; ECM, erythema chronicum migrans; Neuro., neurologic; NSAID, nonsteroidal anti-inflammatory drugs; TJA, total joint arthroplasty; Tx, treat/treatment; reconstr. surg., reconstructive surgery; RA, rheumatoid arthritis; ASA, acetylsalicylic acid; PT, physical therapy; I&D, incise and drain; IV, intravenous; 5-FU, 5-flucytosine.

3. Innervation and Blood Supply (Knee Meniscus)—The peripheral two-thirds of the menisci is innervated by type I and type II nerve endings (concentrated in the anterior and posterior horns with few fibers in the meniscal body). **Menisci obtain blood supply from the geniculate arteries.** Vessels branch to form a circumferentially arranged plexus that supplies the **peripheral 25% of the meniscus;** the remaining portion of the meniscus receives its nutrition via diffusion. Peripheral meniscal tears in the vascularized region ("red zone") can heal via fibrovascular scar formation; more central tears in the avascular region ("white zone") cannot. **The cell responsible for healing a meniscal tear is the fibrochondrocyte. Peripheral meniscal tears with a rim width <4 mm have the best healing characteristics.**

II. **Arthroses**

A. Introduction—Arthroses can be classified into four basic groups based on their common characteristics. The arthritides are summarized in Table 1–21.

1. **Noninflammatory Arthritides**—Include osteoarthritis, neuropathic arthropathy, acute rheumatic fever, and a variety of other entities (osteonecrosis, osteochondritis dissecans, osteochondromatosis).
2. **Inflammatory Arthritides**—Include a wide range of rheumatologic disorders: rheumatoid arthritis, systemic lupus erythematosus, the spondyloarthropathies, and crystalline arthropathies. These disorders may be associated with an HLA complex region.
3. **Infectious Arthritides**—Include pyogenic arthritis, tuberculous arthritis, fungal arthritis, and Lyme disease.

Table 1–21. *Continued*

Comparison of Common Arthritides

Lab Tests	Radiography	Systemic	Treatment
Nonspecific	Asym. narrowing, eburnation, cysts, osteophytes	None	NSAID, arthrodesis, osteotomy, TJA
For underlying disease	Destruction/heterotopic bone	None	Brace, TJA contraindicated
ASO titer	Usually normal	Eryth. marg. nodules, carditis	Symptomatic
Urine homogentisic acid	Destruction, disc calcification	Spondylosis	Supportive
ESR, CRP, RF	Sym. narrow, periart. resorp.	Pericard. & pulm. disease	Pyramid Tx. synovitis, reconstr. surg.
ANA	Less destruction	Cardiac, renal, pancytopenia	Drug therapy like RA
RF/ANA	Juxta-art. late, osteopenia	Iridocyclitis, rash	ASA; 75% remission
ESR	Normal	Ear, cardiac	Supportive, dapsone?
ESR, alk. phos., CPK, HLA-B27	SI arth., bamboo spine	Uveitis	PT, NSAID, osteotomy
ESR, WBC, HLA-B27	MT head erosion, periostitis	Urethritis, conjunctivitis, ulcer	PT, NSAID, sulfa?
ESR, HLA-B27	DIP—pencil in cup	Rash, conjunctivitis	Drug therapy as for RA
ESR, HLA-B27	Normal	Eryth. nodosum, pyoderma	Tx bowel disease, symptomatic
Uric acid; − Birefr. crystals	Soft tissue swell, erosions	Tophi, renal stones	Colchicine, indomethacin
+ Birefr. rod-shaped crystals	Art, fibrocart. calcified	Ochronosis, hyperparathyroidism, hypothyroidism	Symptomatic, avoid surgery
WBC, ESR, bacteria	Joint narrowing (late)	Fever, chills, infection	I&D, IV antibiotics
PPD, AFB, cultures	Both sides, cysts	Lung, multiorgan	Antibiotics ± I&D
Culture, ELISA	Usually normal	ECM rash, neuro., cardiac	Penicillin, tetracycline
Special studies/cultures	Minimal changes	Immunocompromised	5-FU, amphotericin
PTT, factor VIII	Squared-off patella	Soft tissue bleeding	Support, synovectomy, TJA (unless + inhibitor)
Sickle prep.	Osteonecrosis	Infarcts, osteonecrosis	
Aspirate, biopsy	Juxtacortical erosion	None	Surgical excision

4. **Hemorrhagic Arthritides**—Include hemophilic arthropathy, sickle cell joint destruction, and pigmented villonodular synovitis.

B. Joint Fluid Analysis (Table 1–22)

1. Noninflammatory Arthritides—200 WBCs with 25% PMNs; glucose and protein equal serum values; normal viscosity (high), straw color, firm mucin clot.
2. Inflammatory Arthritides—2000–75,000 WBCs with up to 50% PMNs; moderately decreased glucose (25 mg/dL lower than serum glucose); low viscosity, yellow-green, friable mucin clot. **Synovial fluid complement** is decreased in rheumatoid arthritis and normal in ankylosing spondylitis.
3. Infectious Arthritides—More than 80,000 WBCs with more than 75% PMNs, a positive Gram stain (also positive cultures later), low glucose (25 mg/dL lower than serum glucose), opaque fluid, increased synovial lactate.

C. Noninflammatory Arthritides

1. Osteoarthritis (Degenerative Joint Disease)

Table 1–22.

Joint Fluid Analysis

Types of Arthritis	White Blood Cells	Polymorphonuclear Leukocytes (%)	Other Characteristics
Noninflammatory	200	25	Joint aspirate glucose and protein equal to serum values
Inflammatory	2000–75,000	50	↓ Joint aspirate glucose
Infectious	>80,000	>75	Thick cloudy fluid + Gram stain + Cultures ↓ Joint aspirate glucose, ↑ joint aspirate protein

From Brinker, M.R., and Miller, M.D.: Fundamentals of Orthopaedics. Philadelphia, WB Saunders, 1999, p. 26.

(see Table 1–21)—Although it is the **most common form** of arthritis, little is known about this disease.

a. Etiology—On a cellular level, osteoarthritis (OA) may be a result of a failed attempt of chondrocytes to repair damaged cartilage. Osteoarthritic cartilage is characterized by **increased water content** (in contrast with the decreased water content seen with aging) (see Table 1–17), **alterations in proteoglycans** (shorter chains and increased chondroitin/keratin sulfate ratio), **collagen abnormalities** (disrupted by collagenase), and **binding of proteoglycans to hyaluronic acid** (caused by the action of proteolytic enzymes from increased prostaglandin E [PGE] and decreased numbers of link proteins). Levels of cathepsins B and D and the **metalloproteinases** (collagenase, gelatinase, stromelysin) **are increased in OA cartilage. Interleukin-1** (IL-1) enhances enzyme synthesis and may have a **catabolic effect** leading to cartilage degeneration; GAGs and polysulfuric acid may have a protective effect. **A comparison of the biochemical changes seen in articular cartilage with aging and osteoarthritis is shown in Table 1–17.** The cascade of enzymes involved in the degradation of articular cartilage is shown in Figure 1–43. Cartilage degeneration is encouraged by shear stress and is prevented with normal compressive forces. Excessive stresses and inadequate chondrocyte response lead to degeneration. Genetic predisposition may be an important factor in OA. **Postmenopausal arthritis of the medial clavicle** is seen in elderly women on the dominant extremity side and is not associated with any systemic arthritis. Treatment is with nonsteroidal anti-inflammatory drugs (NSAIDs). **Rapidly destructive OA** occurs most commonly in the hip and may mimic septic arthritis, rheumatoid arthritis, seronegative arthritis, neuropathic arthritis, or ON. In the hip, the femoral head may be so flattened that is appears to have "sheared off."

b. General Characteristics—From a larger perspective, OA can be primary (from an intrinsic defect) or secondary (from trauma, infection, or congenital disorders). Changes that occur in OA begin with deterioration and loss of the bearing surface, followed by the development of osteophytes and breakdown of the osteochondral junction. Later, disintegration of the cartilage with subchondral microfractures exposes the bony surface. **Subchondral cysts** (which arise secondary to microfracture and may contain an amorphous gelatinous material) and **osteophytes,** which are part of this process, along with **"joint space narrowing"** and eburnation of bone

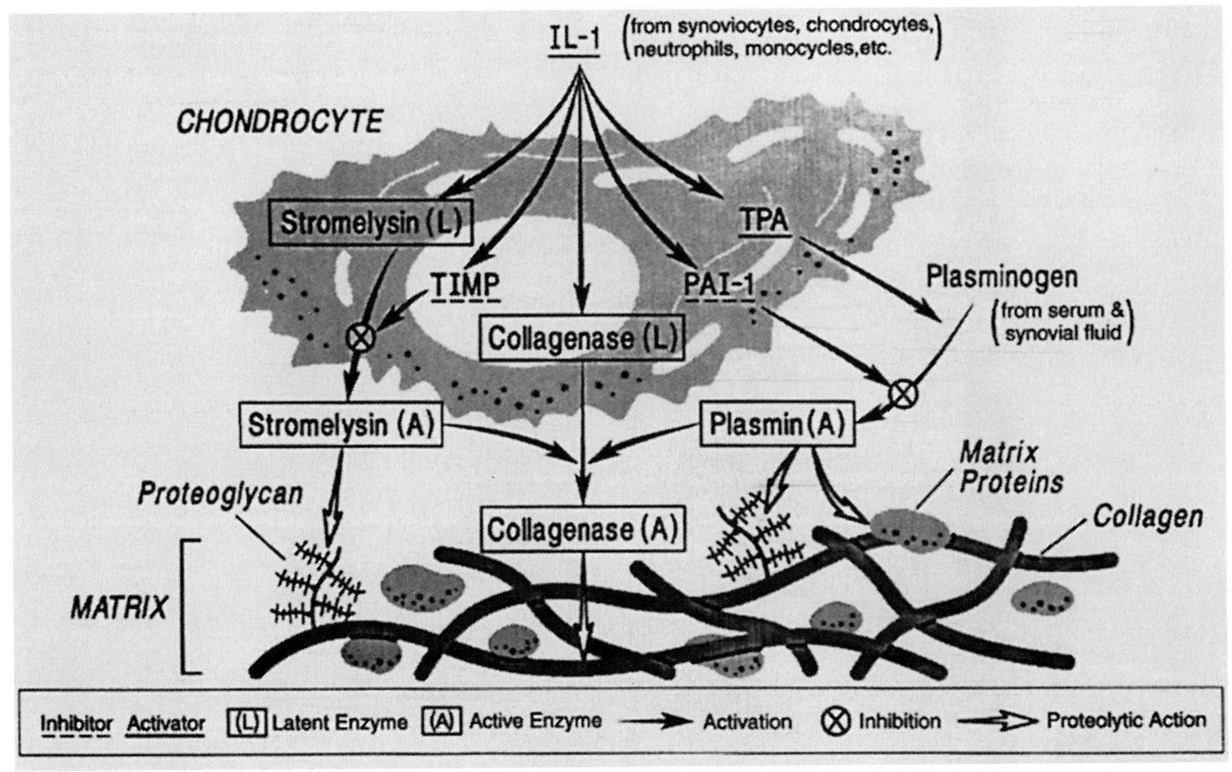

Figure 1–43. Enzyme cascade of interleukin-1-stimulated degradation of articular cartilage. (From Simon, S.R., ed.: Orthopaedic Basic Science, 2nd ed., p. 40. Rosemont, IL. American Academy of Orthopaedic Surgeons, 1994.)

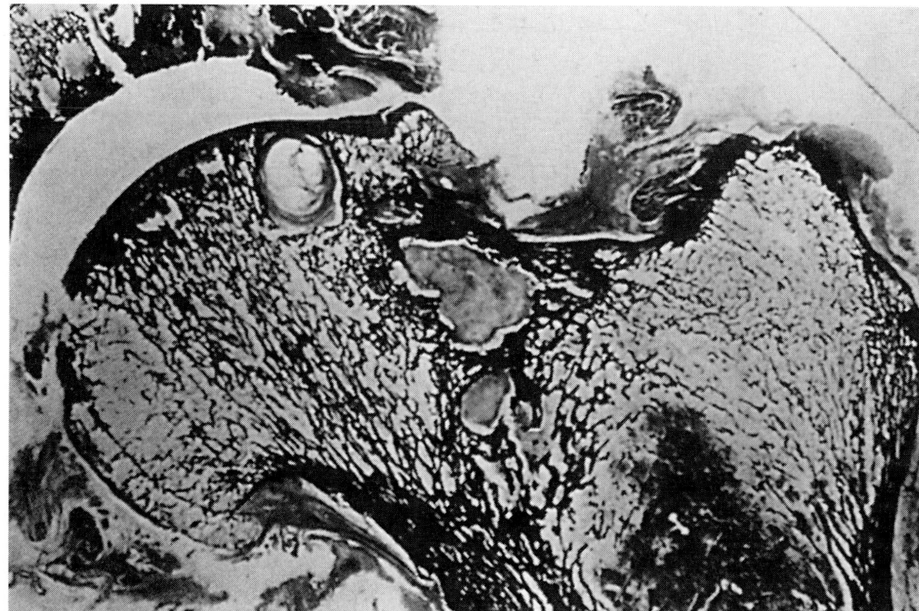

Figure 1–44. Macro section of an osteoarthric human femoral head demonstrating subarticular cysts, sclerotic bone formation, and ,an inferior femoral head osteophyte. (From Simon, S.R., ed.: Orthopaedic Basic Science, 2nd ed., p. 35. Rosemont, IL, American Academy of Orthopaedic Surgeons, 1994.)

are demonstrated on radiographs. Microscopic changes include loss of superficial chondrocytes, **chondrocyte cloning** (>1 chondrocyte per lacuna), replication and breakdown of the tidemark, fissuring, cartilage destruction with eburnation of subchondral "pagetoid" bone, and other changes (Figs. 1–44, 1–45). Notable features on physical examination include decreased ROM and crepitus. **The knee is the most common joint affected in OA.** Treatment begins with supportive measures (e.g., activity modification, cane) and includes NSAIDs (misoprostol [Cytotec] may lower GI complications via a prostaglandin effect). A variety of surgical procedures ranging from arthroscopic débridement to total joint arthroplasties (TJAs) may be useful in advanced cases that are resistant to nonoperative treatment.

c. Radiographic Characteristics—Osteophytes and "joint space" narrowing. Subchondral cysts from microfractures/bone repair.
   1. Hand—DIP, PIP, CMC
   2. Hip—Superolateral involvement
   3. Knee—Asymmetric involvement

2. Neuropathic Arthropathy (Charcot's Joint)

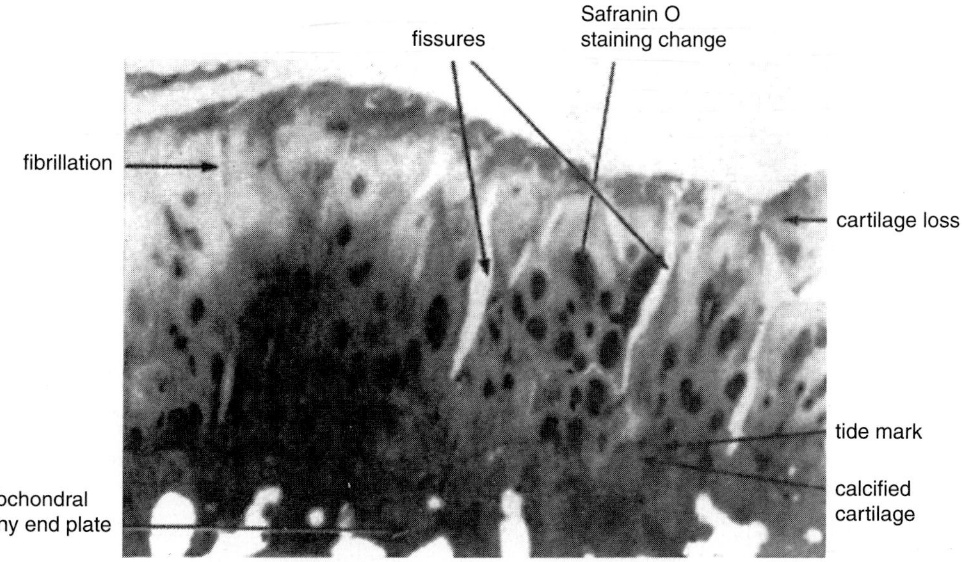

Figure 1–45. Low-power micrograph of osteoarthritis demonstrating fibrillation, fissures, and cartilage loss. (From Simon, S.R., ed.: Orthopaedic Basic Science, 2nd ed., p. 34. Rosemont, IL, American Academy of Orthopaedic Surgeons, 1994.)

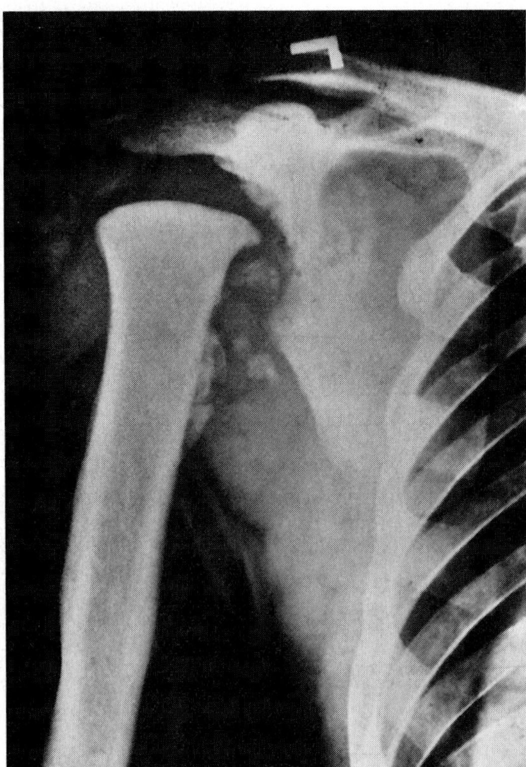

Figure 1–46. AP radiograph of a shoulder showing severe destructive changes characteristic of neuropathic arthropathy. (From Weissman, B.N.W., and Sledge, C.B.: Orthopedic Radiology. Philadelphia, WB Saunders, 1986, p. 238.)

(see Table 1–21 and Fig. 1–46)—An extreme form of OA caused by a disturbance in the sensory innervation of a joint. Causes include diabetes (foot), tabes dorsalis (lower extremity), **syringomyelia (the most common cause of upper-extremity neuropathic arthropathy** [most commonly in the shoulder and elbow]), Hansen's disease (the second most common cause of neuropathic joints in the upper extremity), myelomeningocele (ankle and foot), congenital insensitivity to pain (ankle and foot), and other neurologic problems. A Charcot joint develops in 25% of patients with syringomyelia (80% of them involve the upper extremity). Typically seen in an older patient with an unstable, painless, swollen joint, who may present with a hemarthrosis. Radiographs show advanced (severe) destructive changes on both sides of the joint, scattered "chunks" of bone embedded in fibrous tissue, joint distention by fluid, and heterotopic ossification. **It may be very difficult, based on physical examination and plain radiographs, to differentiate Charcot's arthropathy and osteomyelitis.** Symptoms common to the two conditions include swelling, warmth, erythema, minimal pain, and a variable white blood cell count and ESR. Both conditions are common in diabetic patients. **Whereas the technetium bone scan may look similar (both will be "hot") for osteomyelitis and Charcot's arthropathy, an indium leukocyte scan will be hot (positive) for osteomyelitis and "cold" (negative) for Charcot's arthropathy.** Treatment of Charcot's arthropathy is focused on limitation of activity and appropriate bracing or casting **(the best indicator for discontinuation of a total contact cast is that the skin temperature of the involved side is similar to that of the uninvolved side).** A Charcot joint is usually a contraindication for total joint arthroplasty and the use of other orthopaedic hardware.

3. Acute Rheumatic Fever (see Table 1–21) (Sometimes Included in the Inflammatory Group)—Formerly the most common cause of childhood arthritis, acute rheumatic fever has rarely been seen since the advent of antibiotics. Arthritis and arthralgias can follow **untreated group A β-hemolytic strep infections** and can present with acute onset of red, tender, extremely painful joint effusions. Systemic manifestations include carditis, erythema marginatum (painless macules with red margins usually involving the abdomen but never seen on the face), subcutaneous nodules (extensor surfaces of the upper extremities), and chorea. The arthritis is **migratory** and typically involves **multiple large joints.** Diagnosis is based on the **Jones criteria** (preceding strep infection with two major criteria [carditis, polyarthritis, chorea, erythema marginatum, subcutaneous nodules] or one major and two minor criteria [fever, arthralgia, prior rheumatic fever, elevated ESR, prolonged PR interval on EKG]). **Antistreptolysin O titers are elevated in 80% of affected patients.** Treatment includes penicillin and salicylates.
4. Ochronosis (see Table 1–21)—Degenerative arthritis resulting from **alkaptonuria,** a rare inborn defect of the **homogentisic acid oxidase enzyme system** (tyrosine and phenylalanine catabolism). **Excess homogentisic acid is deposited in the joints** and then polymerizes (turns black) and leads to early degenerative changes. Homogentisic acid can also deposit in other tissues (e.g., the heart valves). These patients may also present with **black urine. Ochronotic spondylitis** (Fig. 1–47), which usually occurs during the fourth decade of life, includes progressive degenerative changes and **disc space narrowing and calcification.**
5. Secondary Pulmonary Hypertrophic Osteoarthropathy—A clinical diagnosis. Involves a lung tumor mass, joint pain and stiffness, periostitis of the long bones, and clubbing of the fingers.

D. Inflammatory Arthritides—An overview of commonly confused laboratory findings in inflammatory arthritic conditions is shown in Tables

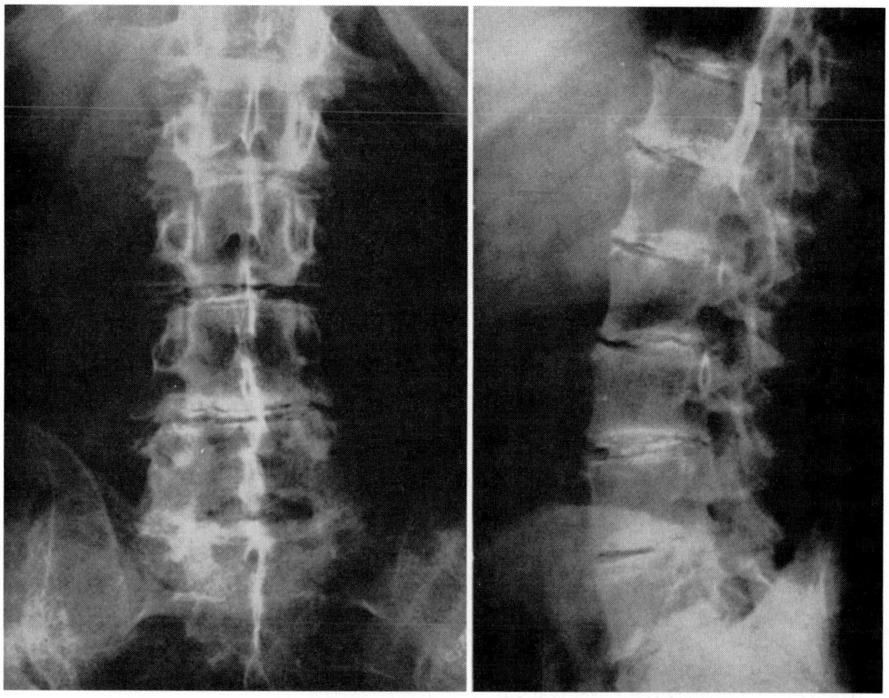

Figure 1–47. Ochronosis. Irregular calcification and narrowing of the intervertebral discs are present. Radiolucent streaks, evident anteriorly between the vertebral bodies, are not uncommon. There is only minimal lipping of the vertebral bodies. (Courtesy of Samuel Fisher, M.D.)

1–23 and 1–24. As a general rule, inflammatory arthritides produce radiographic evidence of destruction on both sides of a joint.

1. Rheumatoid Arthritis (RA) (see Table 1–21)—The most common form of inflammatory arthritis, RA affects 3% of women and 1% of men. Several of the following diagnostic criteria, developed by the American Rheumatism Association, are required: morning stiffness, swelling, nodules, positive laboratory tests, and radiographic findings.
   a. Etiology—Unclear, but probably related to a cell-mediated immune response (T cell) that incites an inflammatory response initially against soft tissues and later against cartilage (chondrolysis) and bone (periarticular bone resorption). **The primary cellular mediator of tissue destruction in RA is mononuclear cells.** RA may be associated with an infectious etiology or an HLA locus **(HLA-DR4 and -DW4).** Lymphokines and other inflammatory mediators initiate a destructive cascade that leads to joint destruction. RA cartilage is sensitive to PMN degradation and IL-1 effects (phospholipase A_2, PGE_2, and plasminogen activators). **Class II molecules** are involved in antigen–T-lymphocyte interaction.
   b. General Characteristics—Usually an insidious onset of morning stiffness and polyarthritis. Most commonly the hands (ulnar deviation and subluxation of the MCPs) and the feet (MTPs, claw toes, and hallux valgus) are affected early, but involvement of the knees, elbows, shoulders, ankles, and

Table 1–23.

Commonly Confused Laboratory Findings in Inflammatory Arthritic Conditions

Finding	May Be Positive for	Usually Negative for
Rheumatoid factor (RF)	Rheumatoid arthritis Sjögren's syndrome Sarcoid Systemic lupus erythematosus	Ankylosing spondylitis Gout Psoriatic arthritis Reiter's syndrome
HLA-B27*	Ankylosing spondylitis Reiter's syndrome Psoriatic arthritis Enteropathic arthritis	
Antinuclear antibody (ANA)	Systemic lupus erythematosus Sjögren's syndrome Scleroderma	

*Approximately 6% of all whites are HLA-B27–positive.

Modified from Brinker, M.R., and Miller, M.D.: Fundamentals of Orthopaedics. Philadelphia, WB Saunders, 1999, p. 27.

Table 1–24.

Associations Between Human Leukocyte Antigen Alleles and Susceptibility to Some Rheumatic Diseases

Disease	HLA Marker	Frequency (%) in Patients (Whites)	Frequency (%) in Controls (Whites)	Relative Risk
Ankylosing spondylitis	B27	90	9	87
Reiter's syndrome	B27	79	9	37
Psoriatic arthritis	B27	48	9	10
Inflammatory bowel disease with spondylitis	B27	52	9	10
Adult rheumatoid arthritis	DR4	70	30	6
Polyarticular juvenile rheumatoid arthritis	DR4	75	30	7
Pauciarticular juvenile rheumatoid arthritis	DR8	30	5	5
	DR5	50	20	4.5
	DR2.1	55	20	4
Systemic lupus erythematosus	DR2	46	22	3.5
	DR3	50	25	3
Sjögren syndrome	DR3	70	25	6

From Nepom, B.S., and Nepom, G.T.: Immunogenetics and the rheumatic diseases. In McCarty, D.J., ed.: Arthritis and Allied Conditions: A Textbook of Rheumatology, 12th ed. Philadelphia, Lea & Febiger, 1993.

cervical spine is also common. **Subcutaneous nodules** are seen in 20% of RA patients (over their lifetime) and are strongly associated with positive serum rheumatoid factor (RF). Synovium and soft tissues are affected first; only later are joints significantly involved. Pannus ingrowth denudes articular cartilage and leads to chondrocyte death. **Laboratory findings** include **elevated ESR and C-reactive protein and a positive RF titer (immunoglobulin M, IgM)** in approximately 80% of patients. Joint fluid assays can also demonstrate RF, decreased complement levels, and other helpful findings. **Systemic manifestations** can include rheumatoid vasculitis, pericarditis, and pulmonary disease (pleurisy, nodules, fibrosis). Popliteal cysts in rheumatoid patients (confirmed by ultrasonography) can mimic thrombophlebitis. Felty's syndrome is RA with splenomegaly and leukopenia. Still's disease is acute-onset JRA with fever, rash, and splenomegaly. Sjögren's syndrome is an autoimmune exocrinopathy often associated with RA. Symptoms include **decreased salivary and lacrimal gland secretion** (keratoconjunctivitis sicca complex) and lymphoid proliferation. **Treatment** of RA is aimed at controlling synovitis and pain, maintaining joint function, and preventing deformities. A multidisciplinary approach involving therapeutic drugs, physical therapy, and sometimes surgery is necessary to achieve these goals. A "pyramid" approach to drug therapy for rheumatoid patients involves beginning with NSAIDs and slowly progressing to antimalarials, remittive agents (methotrexate, suphasalazine, gold, and penicillamine), steroids, cytotoxic drugs, and finally experimental drugs. This pyramidal approach has been challenged in recent years, and a more aggressive approach (beginning with remittive agents) has been advocated. Surgery includes synovectomy (indicated only if aggressive drug therapy fails), soft-tissue realignment procedures (usually not favored because the deformity progresses), and various reconstructive procedures (RA patients are at increased risk for infection after TJA). Chemical and radiation synovectomy can be successful if it is done early. **Operative synovectomy** (open or arthroscropic), especially in the knee, **decreases the pain and swelling associated with the synovitis but does not prevent radiographic progression or the future need for TKA, nor does it improve joint ROM.** After all forms of synovectomy, the synovium initially regenerates normally, but with time it degenerates back to rheumatoid synovial tissue. Evaluation of the cervical spine with preoperative radiographs is important.

c. Radiographic Characteristics (Fig. 1–48)—Include **periarticular erosions** and **osteopenia.** Areas commonly affected are the hand, wrist, and C-spine. In the hand and wrist the MCPs, PIPs, and carpal bones are commonly involved. In the knee, osteoporosis and erosions may be seen in all three compartments. **Protrusio acetabuli** (medial displacement of the acetabulum beyond the radiographic teardrop with medial migration of the femoral head into the pelvis) is common in RA and can also be seen with ankylosing spondylitis, Paget's disease, metabolic bone diseases, Marfan's syndrome, Otto's pelvis, and other conditions.

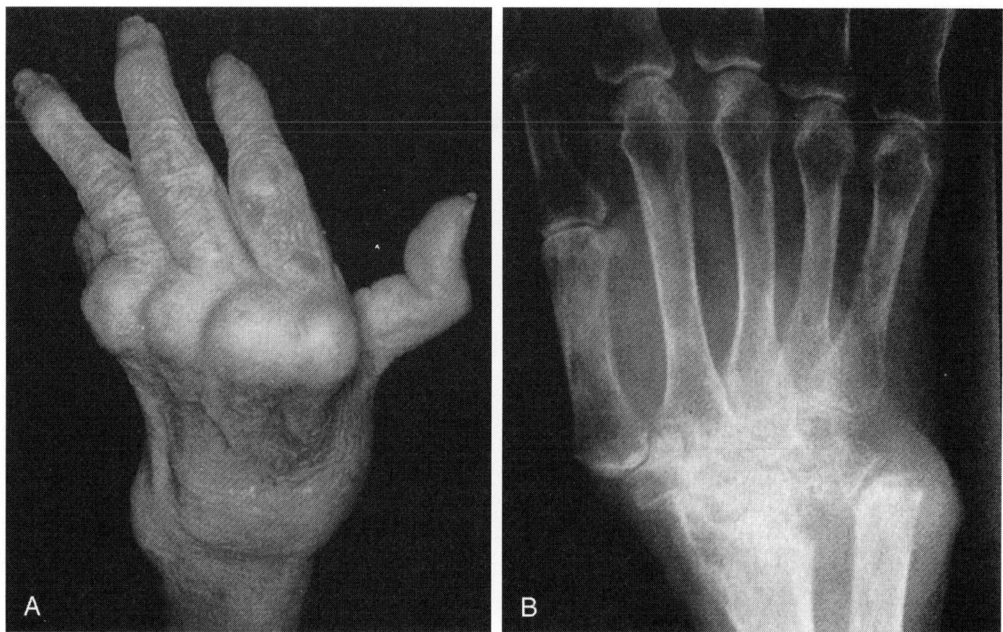

Figure 1–48. *A,* Clinical photograph of the hand of a patient with advanced rheumatoid arthritis. Note ulnar drift of the metacarpophalangeal (MCP) joints caused by the ulnar shift of the extensor tendons, dislocations of the MCP joints, and thumb deformities. *B,* AP radiograph of the hand and wrist of a patient with rheumatoid arthritis. Note severe erosive destruction of the distal radioulnar joint and diffuse osteopenia. (From Bogumil, G.P.: The hand. In Wiesel, S.W., and Delahay, J.N: Essentials of Orthopaedic Surgery, 2nd ed. Philadelphia, WB Saunders, 1997, p. 263.)

2. Systemic Lupus Erythematosus (SLE) (see Tables 1–21, 1–23, and 1–24)—Chronic inflammatory disease of unknown origin usually affecting women (especially African Americans). Probably immune complex–related. Manifestations include **fever, butterfly malar rash,** pancytopenia, pericarditis, nephritis, and polyarthritis. **Joint involvement is the most common feature,** affecting more than 75% of SLE patients. Arthritis typically presents as acute, red, tender swelling of the PIPs, MCPs, and carpus as well as the knees and other joints. **SLE is typically not as destructive as RA.** Treatment for SLE arthritis usually includes the same medications described for RA. Mortality in SLE is usually related to renal disease. Differential diagnosis of SLE includes polymyositis and dermatomyositis, which also present with symmetric weakness ± a characteristic "heliotropic" rash of the upper eyelids. SLE patients are typically positive for antinuclear antibody (ANA) and HLA-DR3 and may be positive for RF.
3. Polymyalgia Rheumatica—A common disease of the elderly. Aching and stiffness of the shoulder and pelvic girdle, associated with malaise, headaches, and anorexia, are common symptoms. Physical examination is usually unremarkable. Laboratory studies are notable for a **markedly elevated ESR,** anemia, increased alkaline phosphatase, and increased immune complexes. **This disorder may be associated with temporal arteritis,** which requires a biopsy for definitive diagnosis; temporal arteritis requires timely treatment with high-dose steroids and if left untreated may result in total blindness. Polymyalgia rheumatica is usually treated symptomatically, with steroid use for refractory cases.
4. Juvenile Rheumatoid Arthritis (JRA) (see Tables 1–21 and 1–24)—JRA is also discussed in Chapter 2, Pediatric Orthopaedics. Three major types of JRA are recognized: systemic (20%), polyarticular (50%), and pauciarticular (30%). **Seronegative** denotes RF-negative, **seropositive** denotes RF-positive. **Pauciarticular** denotes four or fewer joints are involved, **polyarticular** denotes five or more joints are involved. **Early-onset** denotes onset of disease before the teens, **late-onset** denotes onset of disease as a teenager or later. **Seronegative polyarticular JRA** is characterized by five or more joints being involved and is seen more frequently in girls. **Seropositive polyarticular JRA** also involves five or more joints, is seen more frequently in girls, exhibits a **positive RF** and **destructive degenerative joint disease (DJD),** and **frequently develops into adult RA. Early-onset pauciarticular JRA** involves four or fewer joints, is seen more frequently in girls, and is associated with **iridiocyclitis** in 50% of cases (particularly those with a positive ANA). **Late-onset pauciarticular JRA** involves four or fewer joints and is seen in **boys** more commonly than girls. JRA may also be associated with

an HLA locus (HLA-DR2, HLA-DR4, HLA-DR5, HLA-DR8, and HLA-B27 in boys). Treatment of JRA includes high-dose aspirin, only occasionally gold or remittive agents (refractory polyarticular), and frequent ophthalmologic examinations (with a slit lamp) for asymptomatic ocular involvement. **The most common joint affected in JRA is the knee** (66%), followed by the ankle (25%), finger/wrist (33%), and hip and C-spine (3%).

5. Relapsing Polychondritis (see Table 1–21)—Rare disorder associated with episodic **inflammation, diffuse self-limited arthritis,** and progressive cartilage destruction ± systemic vasculitis. The disorder typically involves the **ears (thickening of the auricle);** also seen are inflammatory eye disorders, tracheal involvement, hearing disorders, and sometimes cardiac involvement. It may be an autoimmune disorder (type II collagen affected). Treatment is supportive, although dapsone may have a role in the future.
6. Spondyloarthropathies/Enthesopathies (Occur at Ligament Insertions into Bone)—Characterized by a **positive HLA-B27** (sixth chromosome, "D" locus) and a **negative RF** titer.
   a. Ankylosing Spondylitis (AS) (see Tables 1–21, 1–23, and 1–24)—Bilateral sacroiliitis ± acute anterior uveitis in an HLA-B27–positive man is diagnostic of this disease. There is insidious onset of back and hip pain during the third to fourth decade of life. The disease progresses for approximately 20 years **(progressive spinal flexion deformities).** Radiographic changes (Fig. 1–49) in the spine include **squaring of the vertebrae, vertical syndesmophytes,** obliteration of sacroiliac (SI) joints, and "whiskering" of the enthesis. Ascending ankylosis of the spine usually begins in the thoracolumbar (TL) spine, often causing the entire spine to become rigid. Spinal manifestations include the "chin on chest" deformity (which may require corrective osteotomy of the cervicothoracic junction), **difficult cervical spine fractures (associated with epidural hemorrhage [high mortality rate]) that are best diagnosed via CT scan (75% rate of neurologic involvement),** and severe kyphotic deformities (corrected via a posterior closing wedge osteotomy). Spondylodiscitis may develop in the late stage of AS. Lower spinal deformities with hip flexion deformities and pain (plus **morning stiffness)** are often helped with bilateral total hip arthroplasty (THA). Protrusio acetabuli is associated with AS and requires special THA techniques. The need for prophylaxis for heterotopic bone formation has been questioned in patients with AS undergoing routine primary, noncemented THA. Initial treatment with physical therapy (PT) and NSAIDs (phenylbutazone is best but can cause bone marrow depression) may be helpful. AS is often associated with heart disease and pulmonary fibrosis. Other extraskeletal manifestations include: iritis; aortitis, colitis, arachnoiditis, amyloidosis, and sarcoidosis. Pulmonary involvement (restriction of chest excursion [<2 cm]), hip involvement, and young age at onset of disease are prognostic indicators of poor outcomes in patients with AS.

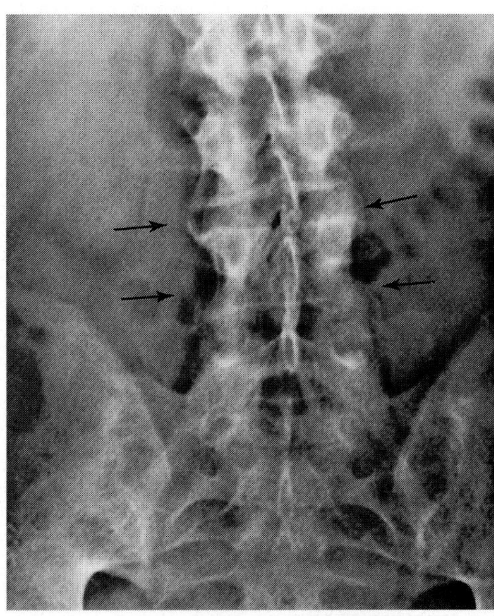

Figure 1–49. AP radiograph of the lumbar spine and sacroiliac joints demonstrating marginal syndesmophytes (*arrows*) typical in ankylosing spondylitis. Note bilateral involvement of the sacroiliac joints. (From Bullough, P.G., and Vigorita, V.J.: Atlas of Orthopaedic Pathology. Philadelphia, Gower Medical Publishing, 1984, p. 8.11, by permission of Mosby.)

   b. Reiter's Syndrome (see Tables 1–21, 1–23, and 1–24) (Fig. 1–50)—Classic presentation is a young man with the triad: **conjunctivitis, urethritis, and oligoarticular arthritis** ("can't see, pee, or bend the knee"). Painless **oral ulcers, penile lesions,** and **pustular lesions** on the extremities, **palms,** and **soles (keratoderma blennorrhagicum),** as well as plantar heel pain, are also common. The arthritis usually has an abrupt onset of asymmetric swelling and pain in the weight-bearing joints. Recurrence is common and can lead to erosions of the MT heads and calcaneal periostitis. Approximately **80–90% of patients with Reiter's syndrome are HLA-B27–positive,** and 60% with chronic disease have **sacroiliitis.** Treatment includes NSAIDs, PT, and possibly sulfa drugs in the future.
   c. Psoriatic Arthropathy (see Tables 1–21, 1–23, and 1–24)—Affects approximately 5–

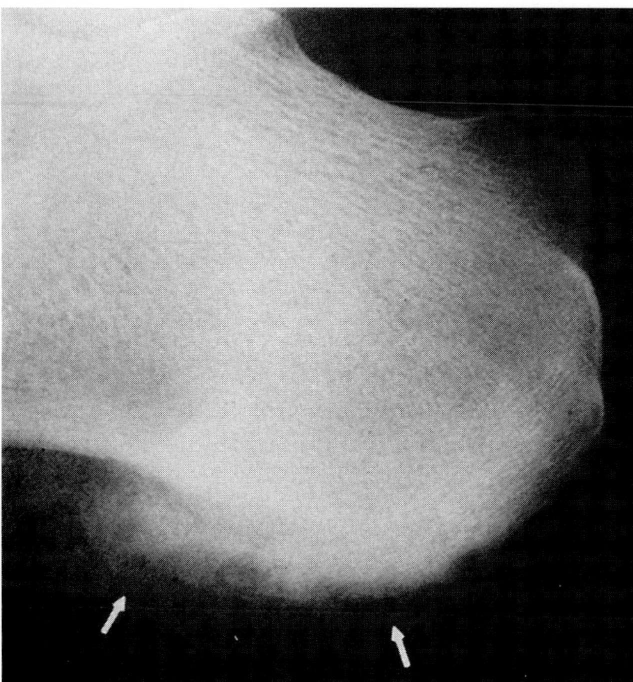

Figure 1–50. Lateral radiograph of the calcaneus of a patient with Reiter's syndrome shows fluffy perosteal calcifications (*arrows*).

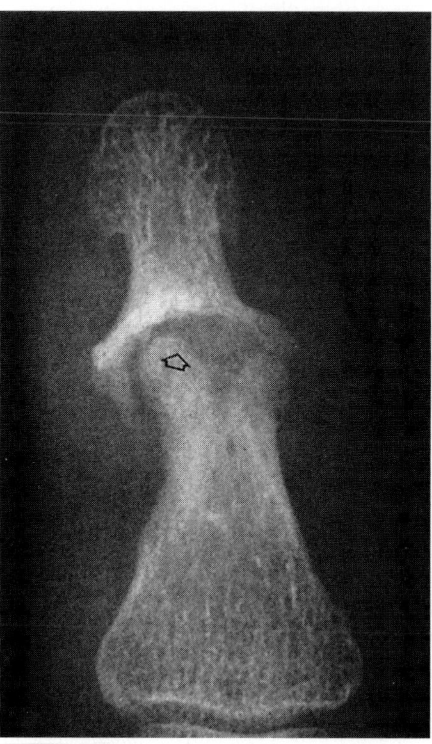

Figure 1–51. AP radiograph of the distal interphalangeal joint of the foot in a patient with psoriatic arthritis shows the classic "pencil and cup" deformity.

10% of patients with psoriasis. Many HLA loci may be involved, but HLA-B27 is found in 50% of patients with psoriatic arthritis. Many forms exist; most patients have the oligoarticular form, which (asymmetrically) affects the small joints of the hands and feet. **Nail pitting** (also fragmentation and discoloration), **"sausage" digits, and "pencil in cup" deformity (with DIP involvement)** are characteristic (Fig. 1–51). Treatment is similar to that for RA.

d. Enteropathic Arthritis (see Tables 1–21, 1–23, and 1–24)—Approximately 10–20% of Crohn's disease and ulcerative colitis patients experience peripheral joint arthritis, and 5% or more experience axial disease. The arthritis is nondeforming and occurs more commonly in the large, weight-bearing joints. It usually presents as an acute monarticular synovitis that may precede any bowel symptoms. Enteropathic arthritis is HLA-B27–positive in approximately half of all affected persons and is associated with AS in 10–15% of cases.

7. Crystal Deposition Disease

a. Gout (see Table 1–21 and Fig. 1–52)—Disorder of nucleic acid metabolism causing hyperuricemia, which leads to monosodium urate (MSU) crystal deposition in joints. Inflammatory mediators (proteases, chemotactic factors, prostaglandins, leukotriene B_4, and free oxygen radicals) are activated by the crystals **(inhibited by colchicine).** Crystals also activate platelets,

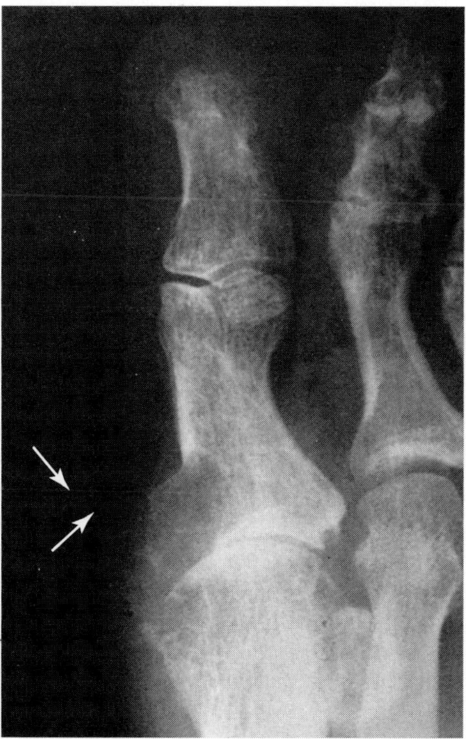

Figure 1–52. AP radiograph of the great toe of a patient with gout. Note soft-tissue swelling and "punched out" periarticular erosions (*arrow*) and sclerotic overhangings bordering the joint. (From Bullough, P.G., and Vigorita, V.J.: Atlas of Orthopaedic Pathology. Philadelphia, Gower Medical Publishing, 1984, p. 5.4.)

phagocytosis **(inhibited by phenylbutazone and indomethacin [Indocin]),** IL-1, and the complement system. Local polypeptides may inhibit the crystal inflammatory response via a glycoprotein "coating." Recurrent attacks of arthritis, especially in men 40–60 years of age (usually in the lower extremity, **especially the great toe [podagra]),** crystal deposition as **tophi** (ear helix, eyelid, olecranon, Achilles; usually seen in the chronic form), and renal disease/stones (2% Ca^{2+} versus normal 0.2%) are characteristic. The kidneys are the second most commonly affected organ. **Gout may be precipitated by chemotherapy for myeloproliferative disorders. Radiographs may show soft-tissue changes and "punched-out" periarticular erosions with sclerotic overhanging borders** (see Fig. 1–52). An elevated serum uric acid level is not diagnostic of gout; the demonstration of MSU crystals is mandatory for the diagnosis. Demonstration of **thin, tapered intracellular crystals that are strongly negatively birefringent** (Fig. 1–53) in joint aspirate is essential for the diagnosis. **Initial treatment with indomethacin** (75 mg tid) is indicated, followed by a rheumatology consultation (patients with GI symptoms or a history of peptic ulcer disease should receive intravenous colchicine for acute attacks). **Allopurinol** is used to lower serum uric acid levels in hyperuricemic patients with chronic gout and is given prior to chemotherapy for myeloproliferative disorders. **Allopurinol is a xanthine oxidase inhibitor** (xanthine oxidase is needed for the conversion of hypoxanthine to xanthine, and xanthine to uric acid). Colchicine can be used for **prophylaxis after recurrent attacks.**

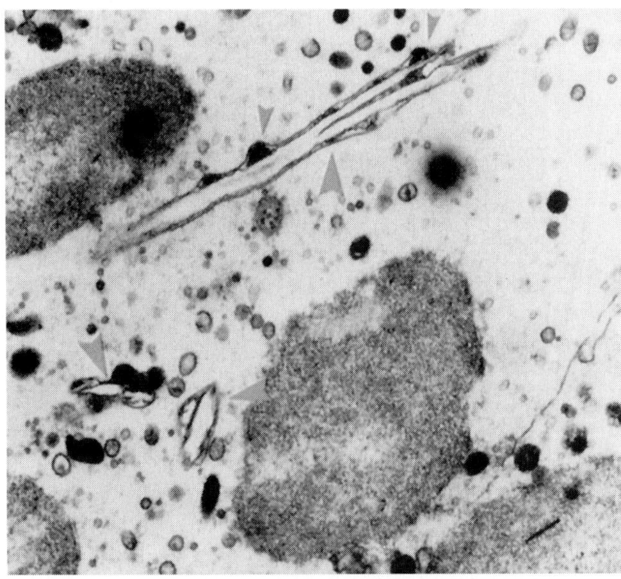

Figure 1–53. A neutrophil has phagocytosed a number of MSU crystals (*large arrows*). Although the crystals have almost completely dissolved, the outlines of the vacuoles remain, one still needle-shaped. Lysosomes discharge their contents directly into the phagosomes (*small arrows*). (Magnification, ×22,000; original magnification, ×31,250.) (From Krey, P.R., and Lazaro, D.M.: Analysis of Synovial Fluid. Summit, NJ, Ciba-Geigy, 1992.)

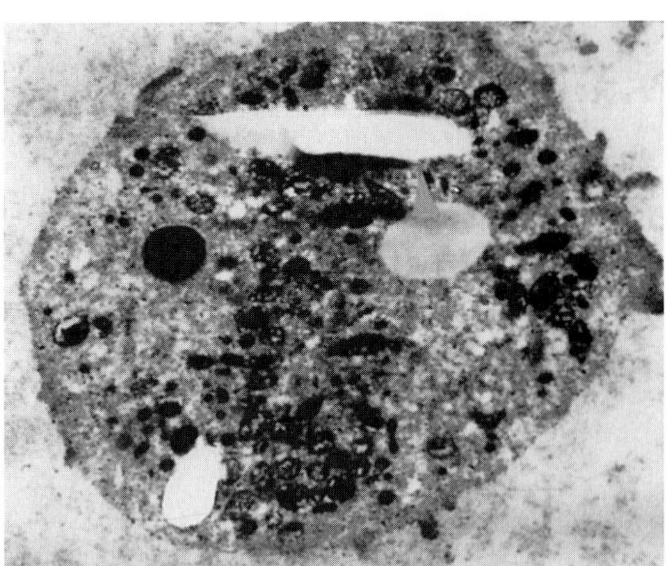

Figure 1–54. A synovial fluid leukocyte showing the outline of a phagocytosed CPPD crystal that has dissolved (*arrow*). (Magnification, ×14,000; original magnification, ×17,000.) (From Krey, P.R., and Lazaro, D.M.: Analysis of Synovial Fluid. Summit, NJ, Ciba-Geigy, 1992.)

b. Chondrocalcinosis (see Table 1–21)—caused by several disorders, including (1) **calcium pyrophosphate (dihydrate crystal) deposition disease (CPPD—a.k.a. pseudogout),** (2) ochronosis, (3) hyperparathyroidism, (4) hypothyroidism, and (5) hemochromatosis. **CPPD** (a common cause of chondrocalcinosis) is a disorder of pyrophosphate metabolism that occurs in older patients and occasionally causes acute attacks (usually in the lower extremities, especially the **knee),** which can be mistaken for septic arthritis. **Short, blunt, rhomboid-shaped crystals that are weakly positively birefringent** (Fig. 1–54) are seen in neutrophilic leukocytes after aspiration of the knee of a person with CPPD. **Chondrocalcinosis of knee menisci is often related to a previous knee injury.** Radiographs show fine linear calcification in hyaline cartilage and more diffuse calcification of **menisci** (Fig. 1–55) **and other fibrocartilage** (acetabular labrum, triangular fibrocartilage complex). NSAIDs are often helpful. Intra-articular yttrium-90 injections have also been successful in chronic cases.

c. Calcium Hydroxyapatite Crystal Deposition Disease—Also associated with chon-

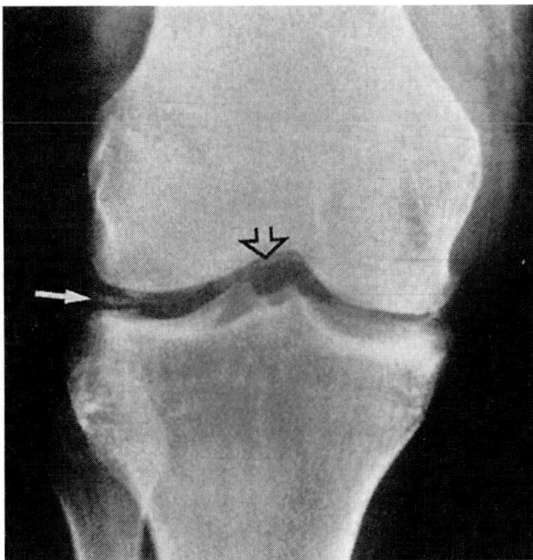

Figure 1–55. AP radiograph demonstrating calcium pyrophosphate deposition disease (pseudogout) in the meniscus of the knee. Note calcification within the (fibrocartilage) meniscus (*closed arrow*) and articular involvement with fine linear calcification of hyaline cartilage (*open arrow*). (From Weissman, B.N.W., and Sledge, C.B.: Orthopaedic Radiology, p. 549. Philadelphia, WB Saunders, 1986).

drocalcinosis and DJD. It is a **destructive arthropathy** commonly seen in the knee and shoulder. The **"Milwaukee shoulder"** is basic calcium phosphate deposition in the shoulder along with cuff tear arthropathy. Calcium hydroxyappatite crystals are too small to see with light microscopy, and treatment of the arthropathy is generally supportive.

d. Birefringence
   1. Positive—The long axis of the crystal is parallel to the compensator (of the microscope) and the crystal is blue.
   2. Negative—The long axis of the crystal is parallel to the compensator and the crystal is yellow. (*Note:* when the long axis of the crystal is perpendicular to the compensator, the rules of color are reversed.)
   3. Weak—Dull crystal
   4. Strong—Bright, shiny crystal

E. Infectious Arthritides
   1. Pyogenic Arthritis (see Table 1–21)—Results from hematogenous spread or by extension of osteomyelitis. Commonly occurs in children and is discussed in detail in Chapter 2, Pediatric Orthopaedics. In adult patients, pyogenic arthritis occurs more commonly in persons who are at risk, including IV drug abusers (especially the SC and SI joints); sexually active young adults (gonococcal infection [intracellular diplococci], especially if seen with skin papules); diabetics (feet and lower extremities); and RA patients. It is also seen after trauma (fight bites, open injuries) or surgery (iatrogenic). Histology may demonstrate synovial hyperplasia, numerous PMNs, and cartilage destruction. Destruction of cartilage can be direct (proteolytic enzymes) or indirect (caused by pressure and lack of nutrition). Treatment includes I&D(s) and up to several weeks of antibiotics.
   2. Tuberculous Arthritis (see Table 1–21)—The chronic granulomatous infection caused by *Mycobacterium tuberculosis* usually involves joints by **hematogenous spread.** The spine and lower extremities are most often involved, typically in Mexicans and Asians. It is monarticular in 80% of cases. Radiographically, tuberculous arthritis causes changes on both sides of the joint. Diagnosis is helped with a **positive PPD,** demonstration of **acid-fast bacilli** and **"rice bodies" (fibrin globules) in the synovial fluid,** positive cultures (may take several weeks), and characteristic radiographs (subchondral osteoporosis, cystic changes, notch-like bony destruction at the edge of the joint, and joint space narrowing with osteolytic changes on both sides of the joint). Histology may demonstrate **characteristic granulomas with Langhans' giant cells** (peripheral nuclei). Treatment includes I&D and long-term antibiotics (isoniazid, rifampin, pyrazinamide, and pyridoxine).
   3. Fungal Arthritis (see Table 1–21)—More common in neonates, **AIDS patients,** and drug users. Pathogens include *Candida albicans.* KOH preparations of synovial fluid are helpful because cultures require prolonged incubation. Arthritis can be treated with 5-flucytosine. Blastomycosis, coccal infections, and other fungal infections often require treatment with amphotericin (this treatment is sometimes administered intraarticularly with fewer side effects).
   4. Lyme Disease (see Table 1–21)—Acute, self-limited joint effusions (especially in the shoulder and knee) that recur at frequent intervals. It is caused by the **spirochete *Borrelia burgdorferi*** (*Borrelia garinii* in Europe), which is transmitted by **tick bites** *(Ioxodes)* endemic in half of the United States. Transmission of *B. burgdorferi* occurs in approximately 10% of bites by infected ticks. Sometimes called the "great mimicker." Systemic signs may include a characteristic "bull's-eye" rash **(erythema chronicum migrans)** and neurologic (Bell's palsy is common) or cardiac symptoms. The disease occurs in three stages (I—rash, II—neurologic symptoms, III—arthritis). **Immune complexes and cryoglobulins accumulate in the synovial fluid** of affected persons. Diagnosis is confirmed by ELISA testing, which should be sought in endemic areas after a Gram stain and joint cultures of an infectious aspirate show no organisms. **Treatment** is with doxycycline, amoxicillin,

cefuroxime, clarithromycin, or ceftriaxone (for carditis).

F. Hemorrhagic Effusions

1. Hemophilic Arthropathy (see Table 1–21)—**X-linked recessive disorder, factor VIII deficiency** (hemophilia A—classic) or factor IX deficiency (hemophilia B—Christmas disease) associated with repeated hemarthrosis due to minor trauma, leading to synovitis, cartilage destruction (enzymatic processes), and joint deformity. Severity of disease is related to the degree of factor deficiency (mild, 5–25% levels; moderate, 1–5% levels; severe, 0–1% levels). Repeated episodes of hemarthrosis lead to replacement of the normal joint capsule with dense scar tissue. **The knee is most commonly involved,** followed by the elbow, ankle, shoulder, and spine. Joint swelling, decreased ROM, and pain are characteristic. **A joint aspirate should be obtained to rule out a concomitant infection.** Radiographs later in the disease process may demonstrate a **"squared off" patella (Jordan's sign** [also seen in JRA]), widening of the intercondylar notch, and enlarged femoral condyles that appear to "fall off" the tibia. Ultrasonography can be used to diagnose and follow intramuscular bleeding episodes. **Iliacus hematomas can cause femoral nerve palsies.** Management includes correction of factor levels, splints, compressive dressings, bracing, and analgesics. Occasionally, steroids are helpful. Surgical management includes synovectomy (for recurrent hemarthroses and synovial hypertrophy refractory to conservative treatment), TJA (for end-stage arthropathy), or arthrodesis (especially for the ankle). **Synovectomy** has been shown to reduce the incidence of recurrent hemarthroses (less pain and swelling). **Synoviorthesis** (destruction of synovial tissue by intra-articular injection of a radioactive agent) with colloidal ^{32}P chromic phosphate may be useful for the treatment of chronic hemophilic synovitis that is resistant to conventional treatment. **Factor levels** should be maintained near 100% during the first postoperative week and at 50–75% during the second week. There is a high incidence of HIV positivity in hemophiliacs (up to 90%). **The presence of an inhibitor that represents an IgG antibody to the clotting factor protein (that causes the patient to**

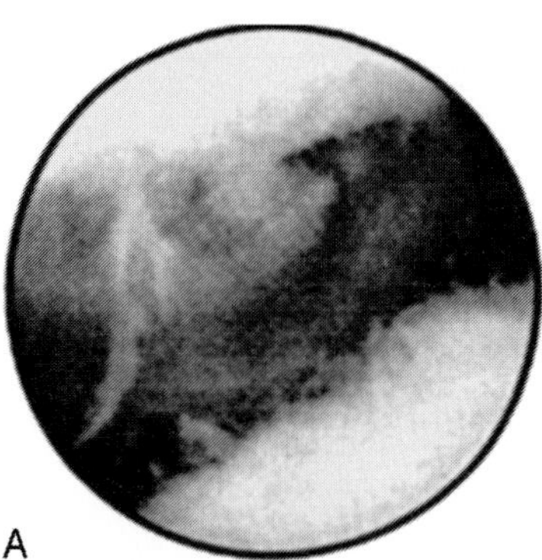

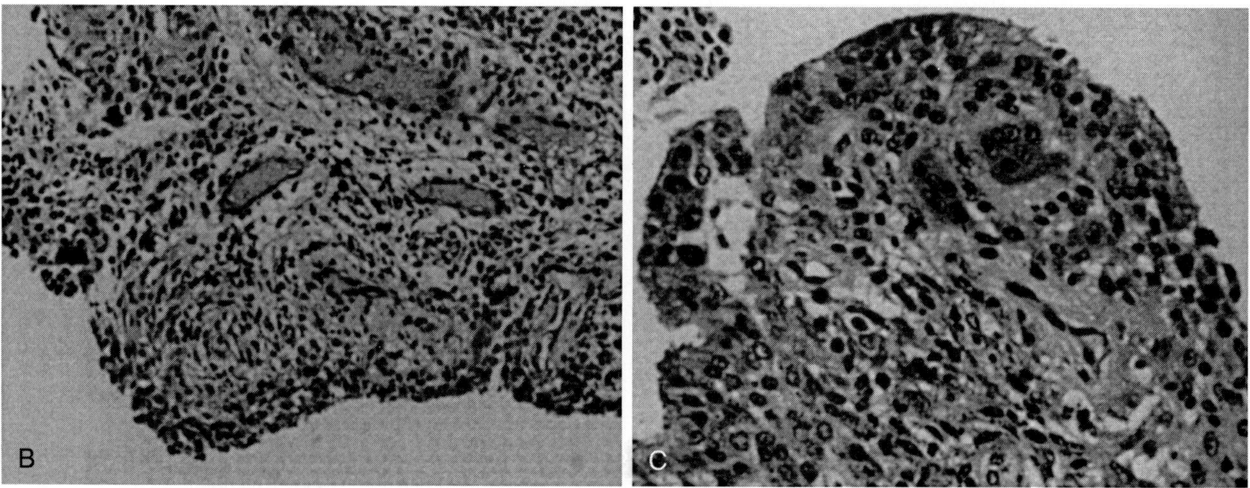

Figure 1–56. Localized pigmented villonodular synovitis. *A,* Arthroscopic view localized to the medial knee joint. *B,* Histologic picture shows vascular channels, giant cells, and blood pigments (hematoxylin and eosin stain, ×100). *C,* Giant cells in synovial villus (hematoxylin and eosin stain, ×400).

have no response to factor replacement therapy) is a relative contraindication to any elective surgical procedure. Inhibitor is present in 5–25% of patients and can develop at any time. New monoclonal recombinant factor VIII products are prone to induce inhibitors. When an inhibitor to factor VIII develops, other strategies to provide hemostasis must be used.

2. Sickle Cell Disease—Hemoglobin SS is found in 1% of North American blacks and leads to local infarction due to capillary stasis. Bony infarcts and ischemic necrosis may occur in multiple bones in sickle cell disease (thalassemia does not produce infarcts or ischemic necrosis). Dactylitis with MC/MT periosteal new bone formation may also be seen. Osteomyelitis is not uncommon in patients with sickle cell disease **(*Salmonella* is the most characteristic organism, and *Staphylococcus* is the most common).** The ESR is usually falsely low. ON (especially of the femoral head, which leads to joint destruction and may require THA) is common in sickle cell patients. Results of TJA are poor owing to ongoing negative bone remodeling. *Salmonella* spread can come from a gallbladder infection.

3. Pigmented Villonodular Synovitis (PVNS) (see Table 1–21) (Fig. 1–56)—Synovial disease with **exuberant proliferation of villi and nodules.** The synovium is frequently rust-colored or brown because of extensive **hemosiderin deposits.** Pain, swelling, synovitis, and a **rust-colored or bloody effusion** are common. **The knee is the most frequent site of PVNS,** with occasional involvement of the hip and ankle. Radiographs show well-defined juxtacortical erosions with sclerotic margins. Histologic features include pigmented synovial histiocytes, foam cells (lipid-laden histiocytes), and multinucleated giant cells. Treatment is surgical excision **(total synovectomy)** of the affected synovium. Microscopic residual disease may be treated with intra-articular dysprosium (a radioisotope).

Section 3

Neuromuscular and Connective Tissues

I. **Skeletal Muscle and Athletics**
   A. Noncontractile Elements (Fig. 1–57)
      1. Muscle Body—Epimysium surrounds individual muscle bundles; **perimysium** surrounds muscle fascicles; and **endomysium** surrounds individual fibers.
      2. Myotendon Junction—**The weak link in the muscle, often the site of tears,** especially with eccentric contractions. Sarcolemma filaments interdigitate with the basement membrane (type IV collagen) and tendon tissue (type I collagen). Involution of muscle cells in this region gives maximum surface area for attachment. Linking proteins and specialized membrane proteins are also present.
      3. Sarcoplasmic Reticulum—Stores calcium in intracellular membrane-bound channels, including T-tubules (which go to each myofibril) and cisternae (small storage areas) (Fig. 1–58).
   B. Contractile Elements (Fig. 1–57)—Derived from myoblasts. Each muscle is composed of several muscle **fascicles,** which in turn contain muscle **fibers** (the basic unit of contraction); fibers are composed of **myofibrils** (1–3 μm in diameter and 1–2 cm long); a myofibril is a

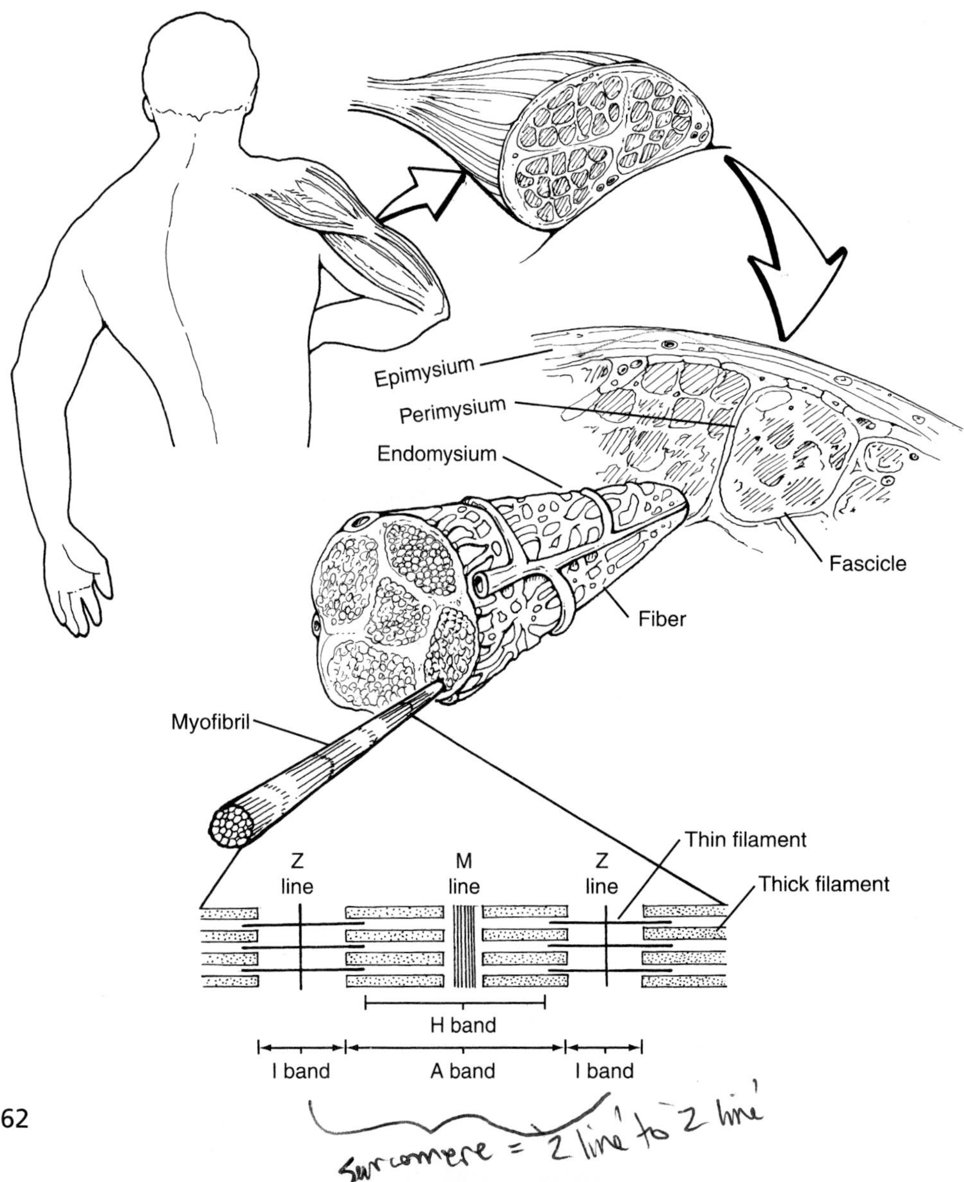

Figure 1–57. Skeletal muscle architecture. (From Brinker, M.R., and Miller, M.D.: Fundamentals of Orthopaedics. Philadelphia, WB Saunders, 1999, p. 10.)

Sarcomere = Z line to Z line

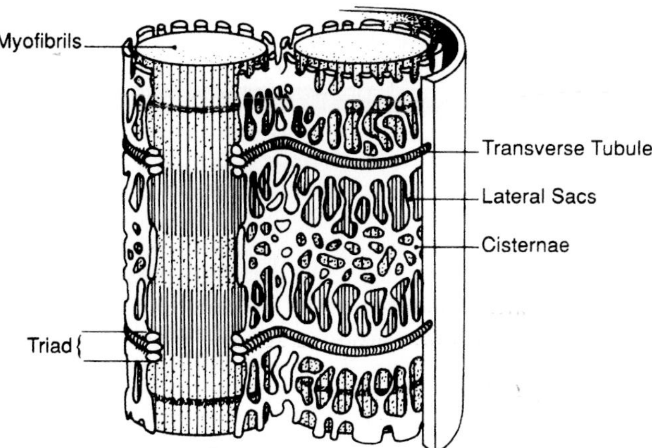

Figure 1–58. Sarcoplasmic reticulum. Action potentials travel down the transverse tubules, causing calcium release from the outer vesicles. (From Simon, S.R., ed.: Orthopaedic Basic Science, 2nd ed., p. 94. Rosemont, IL, American Academy of Orthopaedic Surgeons, 1994.)

collection of **sarcomeres.** A muscle fiber is an elongated cell. Fibers are most commonly arranged in parallel bundles but can run oblique to one another, as in a bipennate muscle. The architectural arrangement of muscle fibers is specific for the specific function required.

1. Sarcomere—Composed of thick and thin filaments in an intricate arrangement that allows the fibers to slide past each other. Thick filaments are composed of **myosin,** and thin filaments are composed of **actin.**

Table 1–25.

Sarcomere

A band	Contains actin and myosin
I band	Contains actin only
H band	Contains myosin only
M line	Interconnecting site of the thick filaments
Z line	Anchors the thin filaments

From Brinker, M.R., and Miller, M.D.: Fundamentals of Orthopaedics. Philadelphia, WB Saunders, 1999, p. 11.

The sarcomere is arranged into bands and lines, as shown in Figure 1–57 and detailed in Table 1–25. The **H band** contains only thick (myosin) filaments, and the **I band is composed solely of thin (actin) filaments.** Thin filaments are attached to the **Z line** and extend across I bands, partially into the A band. Each sarcomere is bounded by two adjacent Z lines.

C. Action—Stimulus for a muscle contraction originates in the cell body of a nerve and is carried toward the neuromuscular junction via an electrical impulse that is propagated down the entire length of the axon (from the spinal cord to skeletal muscle). Once the impulse reaches the **motor end plate** (a specialized synapse formed between muscle and nerve) (Fig. 1–59), acetylcholine (stored in presynaptic vesicles) is released. Acetylcholine then diffuses across the **synaptic cleft** (50 nm) to bind a specific receptor on the muscle membrane (myasthenia gravis

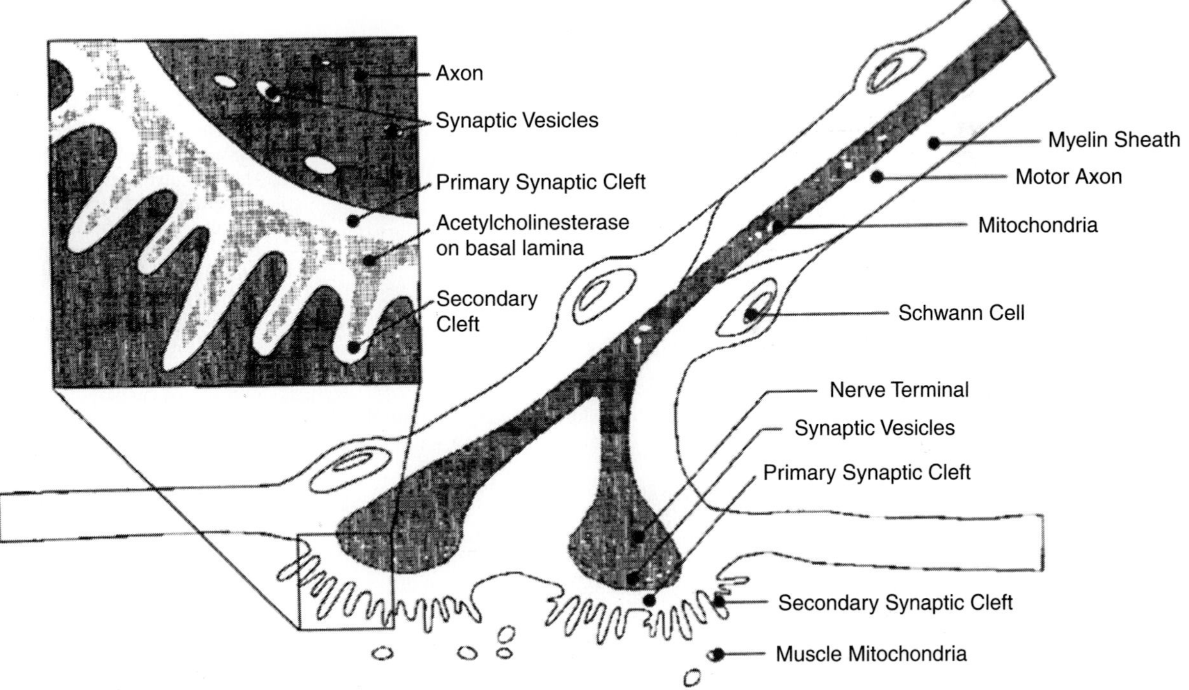

Figure 1–59. Motor end plate. (From Simon, S.R., ed.: Orthopaedic Basic Science, 2nd ed., p. 93. Rosemont, IL, American Academy of Orthopaedic Surgeons, 1994.)

Table 1–26.

Agents that Affect Neuromuscular Impulse Transmission

Agent	Site of Action	Mechanism	Effect
Nondepolarizing drugs (curare, pancuronium, vecuronium)	Neuromuscular junction	Competitively binds to acetylcholine receptor to block impulse transmission	Paralytic agent (long term)
Depolarizing drugs (succinylcholine)	Neuromuscular junction	Binds to acetylcholine receptor to cause temporary depolarization of muscle membrane	Paralytic agent (short term)
Anticholinesterases (neostigmine, edrophonium)	Autonomic ganglia	Prevents breakdown of acetylcholine to enhance its effect	Reverses effect of nondepolarizing drugs; muscarinic effects (bronchospasm, bronchorrhea, bradycardia)

is a shortage of acetylcholine receptors). This binding triggers depolarization of the sarcoplasmic reticulum, releasing calcium. Calcium binds to troponin (on the thin filaments), causing them to change the position of tropomycin (also on the thin filaments) and exposing the actin filament. Actin-myosin cross-bridges form; and with the breakdown of ATP, the thick and thin filaments slide past one another, contracting the muscle. Table 1–26 shows the effects of some

Table 1–27.

Types of Muscle Contractions

Type of Muscle Contraction	Definition	Example	Phases
Isotonic	**Muscle tension is constant through the range of motion.** Muscle length changes through the range of motion. This is a measure of dynamic strength.	Biceps curls using free weights.	**Concentric Contraction**—The muscle shortens during the contraction. Tension within the muscle is proportional to the externally applied load. An example of an isotonic concentric contraction is the "curl" (elbow moving toward increasing flexion) portion of a biceps curl. **Eccentric Contraction**—The muscle lengthens during the contraction (internal force is less than external force). **Eccentric contractions have the greatest potential for high muscle tension and muscle injury.** An example of an isotonic eccentric contraction is "the negative" (elbow moving toward increasing extension) portion of a biceps curl.
Isometric	Muscle tension is generated but the length of the muscle remains unchanged. This is a measure of static strength.	Pushing against an immovable object (such as a wall).	
Isokinetic	Muscle tension is generated as the muscle maximally contracts at a constant velocity over a full range of motion. Isokinetic exercises are best for maximizing strength and are a measure of dynamic strength.	Isokinetic exercises require special equipment, such as a cybex machine.	Concentric Eccentric

Table 1–28.

Characteristics of Human Skeletal Muscle Fiber Types

Characteristic	Type I	Type IIA	Type IIB
Other names	Red, slow twitch (ST) Slow oxidative (SO)	White, fast twitch (FT) Fast oxidative glycolytic (FOG)	Fast glycolytic (FG)
Speed of contraction	Slow	Fast	Fast
Strength of contraction	Low	High	High
Fatigability	Fatigue-resistant	Fatigable	Most fatigable
Aerobic capacity	High	Medium	Low
Anaerobic capacity	Low	Medium	High
Motor unit size	Small	Larger	Largest
Capillary density	High	High	Low

From Simon, S.R.: Orthopaedic Basic Science, 2nd ed., p. 100. Rosemont, IL, American Academy of Orthopaedic Surgeons, 1994.

commonly used agents that affect impulse transmission.

D. Types of Muscle Contractions—Table 1–27

E. Types of Muscle Fibers—Include fast and slow twitch; compose individual motor units (motor nerve and fibers innervated). Table 1–28 shows the characteristics of type I and type II muscle fibers.

1. Slow Twitch (ST) (Type I; Oxidative ["Red"]) Fibers—**Aerobic** and therefore have **more mitochondria,** enzymes, and triglycerides (energy source) than type II fibers. They have low concentrations of glycogen and glycolytic enzymes (ATPase). A helpful way to remember: **"slow red ox"** (slow-twitch fibers are slower, are typically more vascularized [red], and undergo aerobic oxidation). Type I fibers specialize in **endurance activities.** Slow-twitch fibers are the first lost without rehabilitation.
2. Fast Twitch (FT) (Type II; Glycolytic ["White"]) Fibers—Contract more quickly, and their motor units are larger and stronger than ST fibers' (increased ATPase). However, they do it at the expense of efficiency and are **anaerobic.** These fibers develop a large amount of force per cross-sectional area, with high contraction speeds and quick relaxation times. Type II fibers are well suited for high-intensity, short-duration activities (sprinting) and fatigue rapidly. These fibers have low intramuscular triglycerine stores. Type IIA and IIB fibers are associated with sprinting (ATP-CP system). Subtypes of type II fibers are based on myosin heavy chains.

F. Energetics—Three energy systems may be used to generate muscle activity. Which of these three systems is used depends on the duration and intensity of the muscular activity required (Fig. 1–60).

1. **Adenosine Triphosphate—Creatine Phosphate (ATP-CP) System (also known as the Phosphagen System)**
   a. The phosphagen system meets the metabolic requirements for intense muscle activities that last up to 20 seconds such as **sprinting a 100 to 200 meter dash.**
   b. This system uses stored carbohydrates from within the muscle fiber itself (and converts these stored carbohydrates to energy).
   c. **This system does not use oxygen and does not produce lactate;** it is therefore alactive anaerobic activity.
   d. The energy from this system is derived from the high-energy phosphate bonds during hydrolysis

$$ATP \rightarrow ADP + P + Energy$$
$$ADP \rightarrow AMP + P + Energy$$

2. **Lactic Anaerobic System (also known as Lactic Acid Metabolism)** (Fig. 1–61)

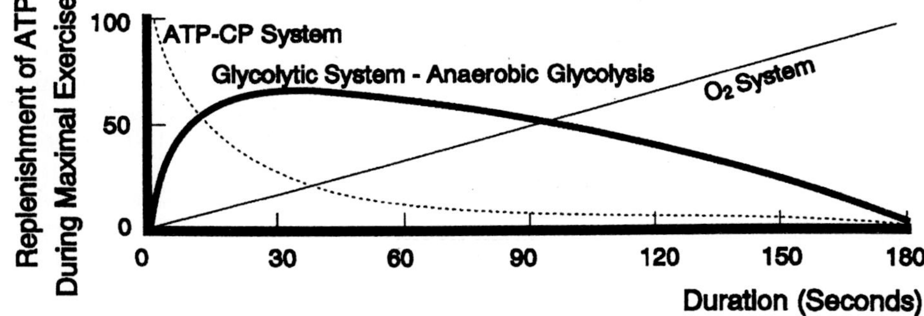

Figure 1–60. Energy sources for muscle activity. (From Simon, S.R., ed.: Orthopaedic Basic Science, 2nd ed., p. 102. Rosemont, IL, American Academy of Orthopaedic Surgeons, 1994.)

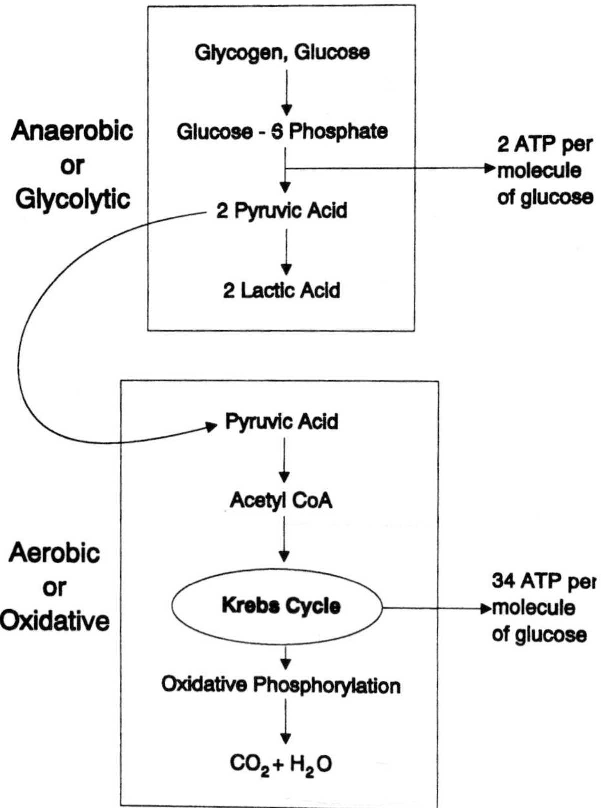

Figure 1–61. ATP production via anaerobic and aerobic breakdown of carbohydrates: Glycolysis and anaerobic metabolism occurs in the cytoplasm; oxidative phosphorylation occurs in the mitochondria. (From Simon, S.R., ed.: Orthopaedic Basic Science, 2nd ed., p. 104. Rosemont, IL, American Academy of Orthopaedic Surgeons, 1994.)

a. The lactic anaerobic system meets the metabolic requirements for episodes of intense muscle activities that last for 20–120 seconds such as a **400 meter sprint.**

b. Anerobic metabolism involves the hydrolysis of glucose molecules to ultimately produce lactic acid plus enough energy to convert two molecules of ADP to ATP.

3. **Aerobic System** (Figs. 1–61 and 1–62)

a. When oxygen is available, the aerobic system is responsible for the replenishment of ATP through oxidative phosphorylation and the Krebs cycle. This system uses glucose or fatty acids to produce ATP.

b. The aerobic system meets the metabolic requirements for **episodes of longer duration and lower-intensity muscle activities.**

G. Athletes and Training—The distribution of FT versus ST fibers is genetically determined; however, different types of training can selectively improve these fibers. **Endurance athletes typically have a higher percentage of ST fibers,** whereas athletes participating in "strength"-type sports (and sprinters) have more FT fibers. **Training for endurance sports** consists of decreased tension and increased repetitions, which helps increase the efficiency of the ST fibers and increase the number of mitochondria, capillary density, and oxidative capacity. **Training for strength** consists of increased tension and decreased repetitions, which leads to an increased number of myofibrils/fibers and **hypertrophy (increased cross-sectional area) of FT (type II) fibers.** The most reliable parameter to estimate the potential for contractile force of skeletal muscle is the cross-sectional area of the muscle. Both endurance and strength training slow the increase of lactate in response to exercise. **Isokinetic exercises produce more strength gains than do isometric exercises.** Isotonic exercises produce a uniform increase in strength throughout the ROM of a joint. Oxygen consumption (VO_2) is an important consideration in athletic training. **Plyometric exercises** consist of a muscle stretching cycle followed closely by a rapid shortening cycle. The stretching leads to storage of elastic energy, which adds to the force generated by a concentric muscle contraction. **Plyometrics are the most efficient method of conditioning for improvement in power. Closed chain rehabilitation exercise** is defined as extremity loading with the most distal part of the extremity stabilized or not moving; it places less stress on the anterior cruciate ligament (ACL) and allows for physiologic co-contraction of the musculature around the knee, which minimizes joint shear forces. **Weight reduction** with fluid and food restriction (wrestlers, boxers, and jockeys trying to "make weight") is associated with reduced cardiac output, increased heart rate, smaller stroke volumes, lower oxygen consumption, decreased renal blood flow, and electrolyte loss. **Anabolic (androgenic) steroids** cause increased muscle strength (due to increased protein synthesis and an increase in aggressive behavior that promotes increased weight training), increased body weight, testicular atrophy, reduction in testosterone and gonadotropic hormones, oligospermia, azoospermia, gynecomastia, hypertension, striae, cystic acne, alopecia (irreversible), liver tumors, increased LDL, decreased HDL, and abnormal liver isoenzymes (LDH). Anabolic steroids do not increase aerobic power or capacity for muscular exercise. Athletes who use pure testosteone extract to enhance performance have both anabolic and androgenic effects. The anabolic effects include muscle development, increased muscle mass, and erythropoiesis. Doping control (drug testing) for anabolic steroids is tested by the International Olympic Committee using urine sampling. **Aerobic conditioning (cardiorespiratory fitness)** in a healthy adult is recommended 3–5 days per week for 20–60 minutes per session (training at 60–90% of maximum heart rate). Long-distance runs increase aerobic capacity and endurance but decrease

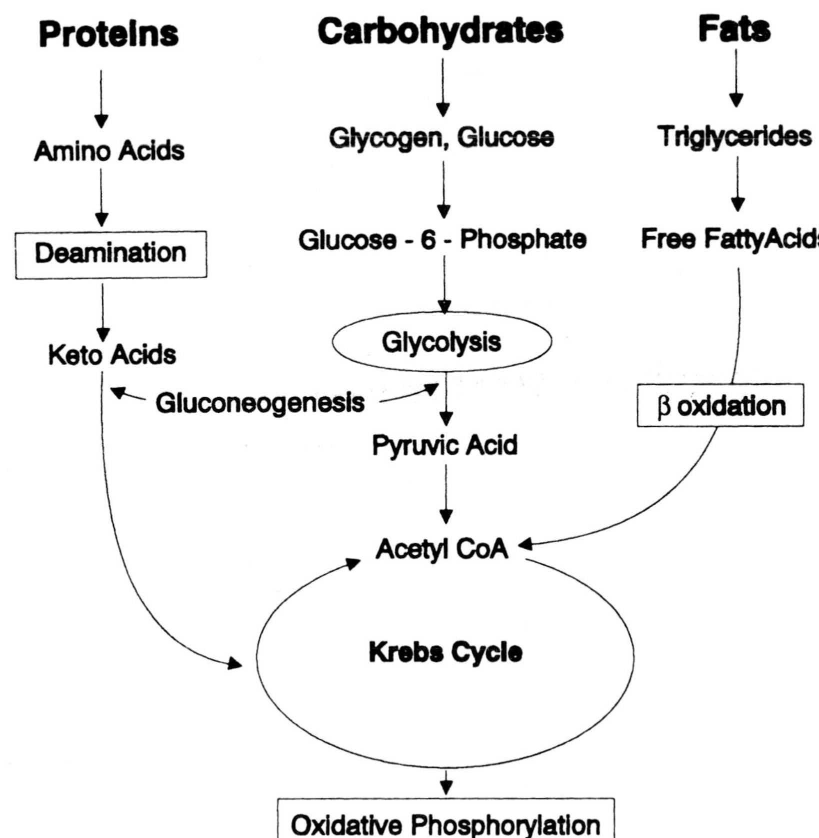

Figure 1–62. Aerobic system for ATP (energy) production of skeletal muscle. (From Simon, S.R., ed.: Orthopaedic Basic Science, 2nd ed., p. 103. Rosemont, IL, American Academy of Orthopaedic Surgeons, 1994.)

flexibility and optimum explosive strength. Aerobic conditioning has proved effective in lowering the incidence of back injury in workers and in helping the elderly to remain ambulatory. A significant decline in aerobic fitness occurs after just 2 weeks of no training ("detraining"). A syncopal episode in a young athlete can suggest a serious underlying cardiac abnormality (and a risk of sudden death); a timely medical evaluation is mandatory prior to returning to athletics. The most common cause of **sudden death** in young athletes is hypertrophic obstructive cardiomyopathy. Abdominal injuries in athletes most commonly affect the kidney. Wraparound polycarbonate glasses should be worn to protect the eyes in racquet sports. **Carbohydrate loading** involves increasing carbohydrates 3 days prior to an event (marathon) and decreasing physical activity. The best **fluid replacement** regimen for a competitive athlete is to replace enough water to maintain prepractice weight and maintain a normal diet. Fluid carbohydrate and electrolyte replacement is most effective when the osmolality of the replacement fluid is <10% (glucose polymers minimize osmolality); fluid absorption by the gut is enhanced by solutions of low osmolality. Treatment of heat cramps includes passive stretching, cooling, and fluid/electrolyte replacement.

H. Female Athletes—Three common problems in young female athletes are **amenorrhea, osteoporosis,** and **anorexia.** Amenorrhea results from a decrease in the percentage of body fat, increased training, hormonal changes, competitive running before menarche, and changes in the hypothalamic-pituitary axis. Exercise-induced secondary amenorrhea leads to premature bone demineralization. Initial management includes increasing weight, decreasing exercise, and possibly administration of cyclic estrogens or progesterones.

I. Muscle Injury—As noted earlier, most **muscle strains** (the most common sports injury) occur at the myotendinous junction. These injuries occur most commonly in muscles that cross two joints (hamstring, gastrocnemius), with increased type II fibers. Initially there is inflammation and later fibrosis. Muscle activation (via stretching) allows twice the energy absorption prior to failure; "bouncing" types of stretching are deleterious. **Muscle soreness** may result from eccentric muscle contractions and may be associated with changes in the I band of the sarcomere. **Tears in muscle occur most commonly at the myotendinous junction and are most commonly the result of a rapid (high-velocity) eccentric contraction; eccentric contractions develop the highest forces that can be seen in skeletal muscle.** Muscle tears typically heal with dense scarring. Surgical repair of clean lacerations in the midbelly of skeletal muscle usually results in minimal regeneration of muscle fibers distally, scar formation at the laceration, and recovery of about one-half of muscle strength. Denervation causes muscle atrophy and increased sensitivity to acetylcholine, causing spontaneous fibrillations at 2–4 weeks after damage to the motor axon. Spasticity is related to increased muscle activity with increasingly rapid stretch. Muscle strength gains during the first 10 days of rehabilitation after injury are due to improved neural firing patterns. Strength gains seen in the later phases of rehabilitation are due to increases in ROM, muscle fiber size, muscle repair, and tendon repair. Trunk extensors are stronger than trunk flexors.

J. Immobilization—Causes changes in the number of sarcomeres at the musculotendinous junction and acceleration of granulation tissue response in the injured muscle. Immobilization in lengthened positions decreases contractures and increases strength. Atrophy can result from disuse or altered nervous system recruitment. Electrical stimulation can help offset these effects.

II. **Nervous System**

A. Organization

1. Central Nervous System (CNS)—**Stroke** patients may continue to improve up to 6 months after their vascular event. **Traumatic brain injury** patients may improve for up to 18 months. **Spinal cord injury patients who present less than 8 hours after their injury have the best chance for optimizing their neurologic outcome if given methylprednisone. Patients presenting less than 3 hours from the time of injury should receive an initial bolus of 30 mg/kg followed by an infusion of 5.4 mg/kg/hr for 24 hours. Patients presenting between 3 and 8 hours from the time of injury should receive an initial bolus of 30 mg/kg followed by an infusion of 5.4 mg/kg/hr for 48 hours.** **Concussion** (Table 1–29) is a jarring injury to the brain that results in disturbance (to some degree) of cerebral function. Grade I injuries are mild, and the athlete may return to play if he or she becomes asymptomatic. Grade II injuries are moderate and are characterized by retrograde amnesia (which persists for several minutes after the injury) despite the resolution of confusion and disorientation. A first-time grade II concussion allows return to play after a week without symptoms. Long periods without play (months) are required for a third-time grade I concussion, a second grade II, or a grade III (severe) concussion. Folic acid, as a dietary supplement, can decrease the chance of having a child with myelomeningocele.

2. Peripheral Nervous System (PNS) (Fig. 1–63)
   a. Nerves—Bundles of axons enclosed in a connective tissue sheath
   b. Nerve fiber—Axon plus surrounding Schwann cell sheath
      1. Myelinated Fibers—An axon is considered myelinated once it reaches a diameter of 1–2 μm. One myelinated axon is associated with one Schwann cell. Conduction velocity is faster than in unmyelinated fibers.
      2. Unmyelinated fibers—One Schwann cell surrounds several axons. Conduction velocity is relatively slow.

3. Nerve Fibers
   a. Afferents—Transmit information from sensory receptors to the CNS.
   b. Somatic Afferents—Afferent fibers originate in receptors in muscle, skin, and the sensory organs of the head (vision, hearing, taste, smell).
   c. Visceral Afferents—Afferent fibers originate in viscera.
   d. Efferents—Transmit information from the CNS to the periphery. Motor efferents are those that innervate skeletal muscle fibers.
   e. Somatic Nerves—Innervate skin, skeletal muscle, and joints.
   f. Autonomic Nerves (Splanchnics)—Innervate viscera.

B. Histology and Signal Generation

1. Neuron (Fig. 1–63)—Composed of four re-

Table 1–29.

Concussion

Severity	Characteristics	Treatment
Grade I (mild)	No loss of consciousness No retrograde amnesia	Return to play as soon as aymptomatic (Long-term suspension of play for a third-time grade I concussion)
Grade II (moderate)	Loss of consciousness <5 minutes Retrograde amnesia (there is always some permanent loss of memory regarding the injury itself) Confusion and disorientation resolve rapidly	*First episode*—Return to play after asymptomatic for 1 week *Repeat episode*—Long-term suspension of play
Grade III (severe)	Prolonged unconsciousness Permanent retrograde amnesia Confusion and disorientation persist	Long-term suspension of play

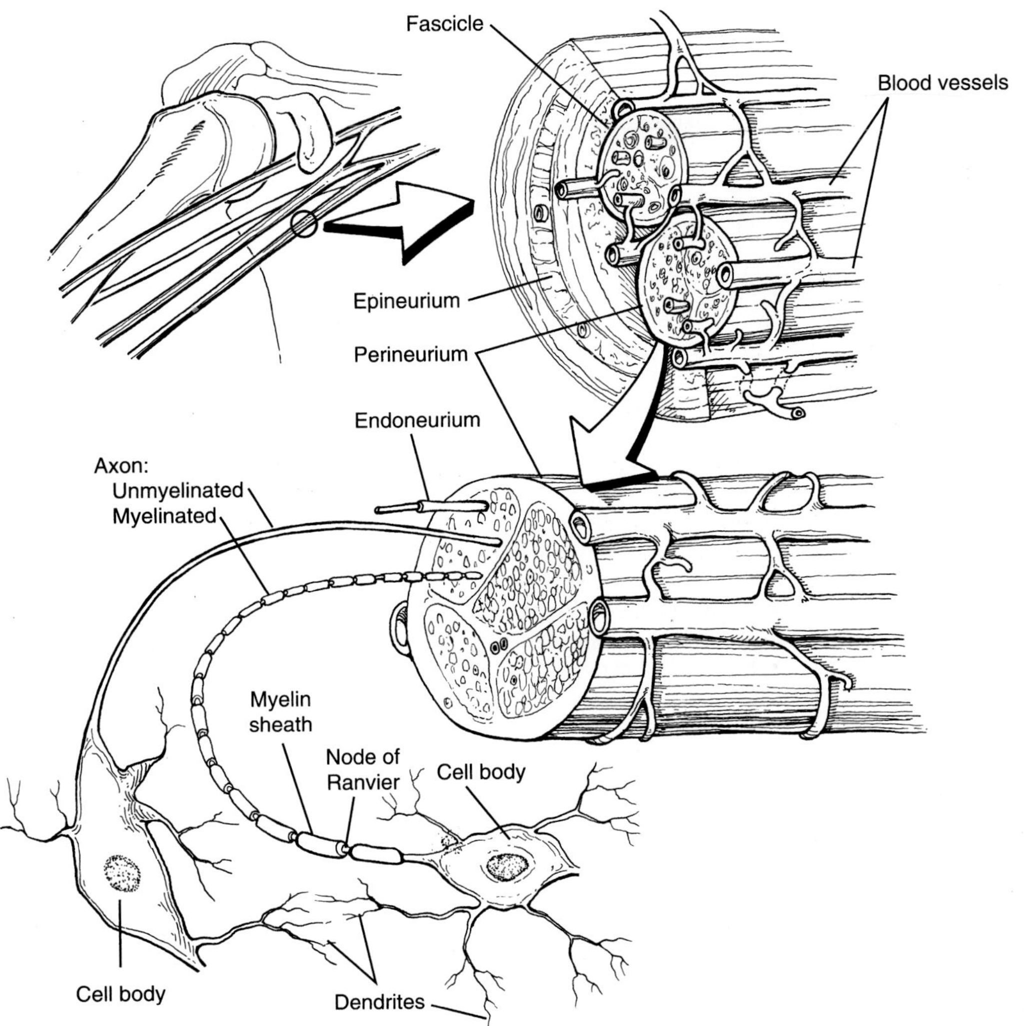

Figure 1–63. Nerve architecture. (From Brinker, M.R., and Miller, M.D.: Fundamentals of Orthopaedics. Philadelphia, WB Saunders, 1999, p. 13.)

gions: cell body, axon, dendrites, and presynaptic terminal.

a. Cell Body—The neurons' metabolic center; accounts for less than 10% of the size of the neuron; gives rise to a single axon.
b. Axon—Primary conducting vehicle of the neuron; conveys electrical signals (over long distances) via action potentials.
c. Dendrites—Thin processes that branch from the cell body to receive input (synaptic) from surrounding nerve cells.
d. Presynaptic Terminals—Transmit information from one neuron to another (to the cell body or dendrites of the "receiving" neuron).

2. Glial Cells (Fig. 1–64)—Three basic types have been described: Schwann cells, oligodendrocytes, and astrocytes.
   a. Schwann cells—**Responsible for myelinating peripheral nerve axons** (forms an elongated double-membrane structure). Loss of the myelin sheath (demyelination) causes disruption in the conduction of action potentials along the axon. Myelin is composed of lipid (70%) and protein (30%).
   b. Oligodendrocytes—Found only in the CNS; responsible for the formation of myelin.
   c. Astrocytes—Most common of the glial cells. Found only in the CNS. Astrocytes have many functions but serve primarily as a supporting structure of the brain.
3. Resting and Action Potentials
   a. Resting Potential—Results from unequal distribution of ions on either side of the neuronal cell membrane (lipid bilayer). The four most plentiful ions about the cell membrane are Na^+, K^+, Cl^-, and a group of other organic ions (A^-). The resting potential of a neuron is −50 to −80 mV (inside the cell is negative relative to outside the cell) (Fig. 1–65).
   b. Action Potential—Transmits signals rapidly via electrical impulses to other neurons or effector organs (e.g., muscle). De-

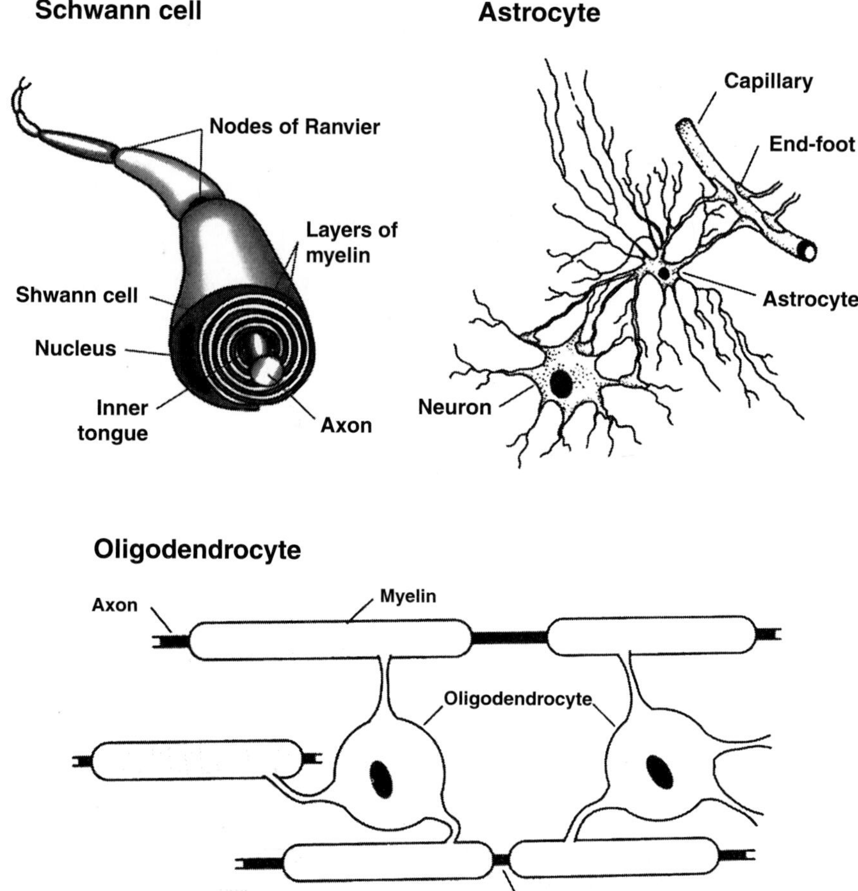

Figure 1–64. Glial cells include the Schwann cell, astrocytes, and oligodendrocytes. (From Simon, S.R., ed.: Orthopaedic Basic Science, 2nd ed., p. 320. Rosemont, IL, American Academy of Orthopaedic Surgeons, 1994.)

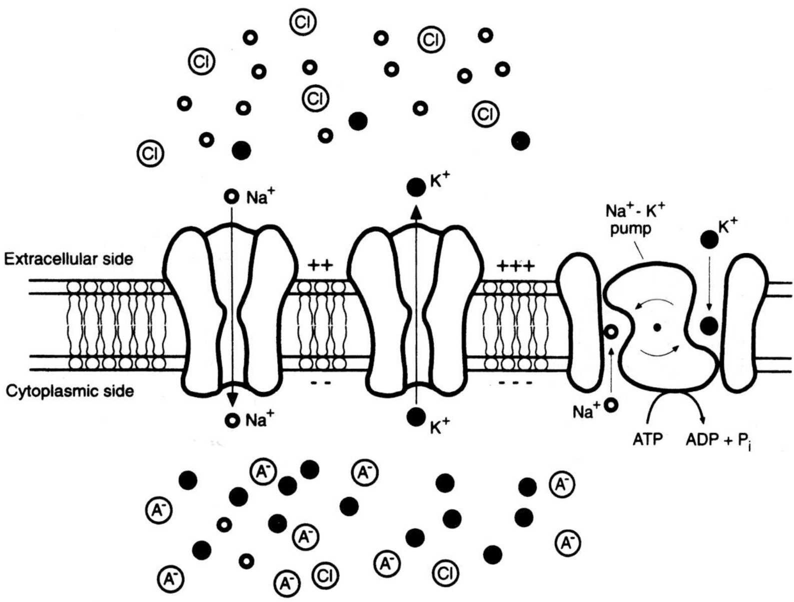

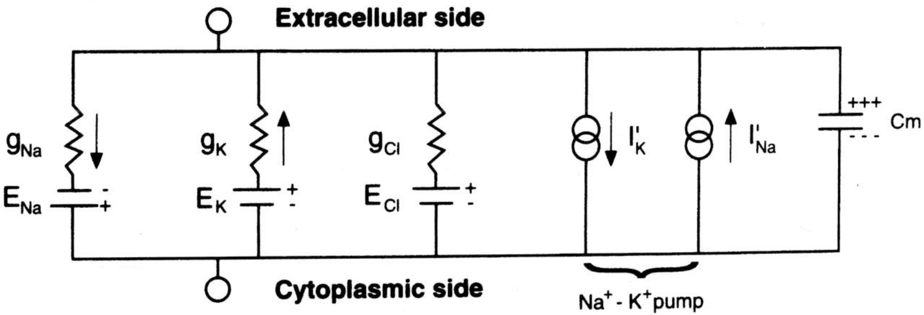

Figure 1–65. Electrolyte transport across cell walls. *Top,* Passive fluxes of Na^+ and K^+ into and out of the cell are balanced by the energy-dependent sodium-potassium pump. *Bottom,* Electrical circuit model of a neuron at rest. (From Simon, S.R., ed.: Orthopaedic Basic Science, 2nd ed., p. 332. Rosemont, IL, American Academy of Orthopaedic Surgeons, 1994.)

depolarization and the action potential result from an increase in cell membrane permeability to Na^+ in response to a stimulus. This process is related to gated ion channels (Fig. 1–66), which are of three types: voltage-gated channels, mechanical gated channels, and chemical-transmitter gated channels. Action potentials propagate via both passive current flow and active membrane changes (Fig. 1–67).

C. Sensory System—Receives messages from the environment and other parts of the body via transmission from **sensory receptors** (located peripherally) to the CNS. The four attributes of a stimulus are quality, intensity, duration, and location. Sensory receptor types include photoreceptors (vision), mechanoreceptors (hearing, balance, mechanical stimuli), thermoreceptors (temperature), chemoreceptors (taste, smell), and nociceptors (pain). Neurogenic pain (and inflammatory) mediators are identifiable within the dorsal root ganglion of the lumbar spine. The pain associated with an osteoid osteoma comes from prostaglandins secreted by the tumor itself.

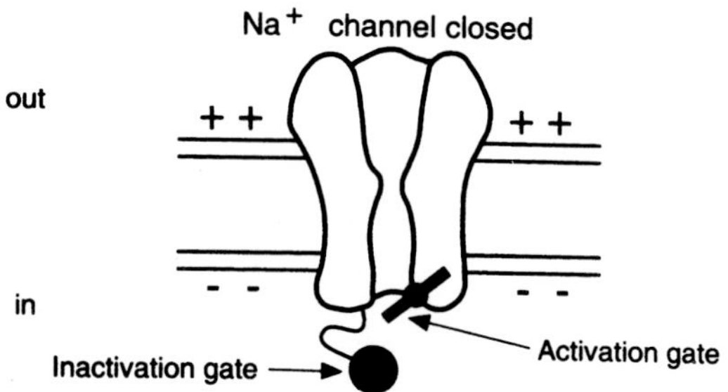

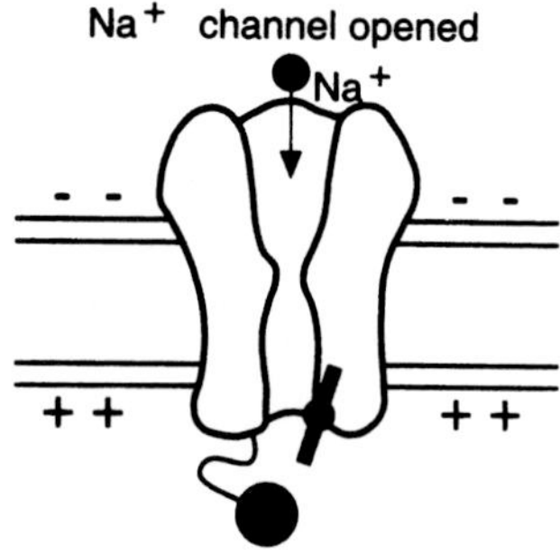

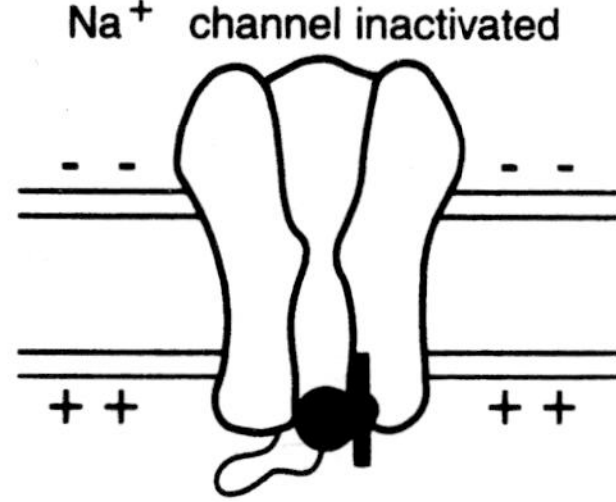

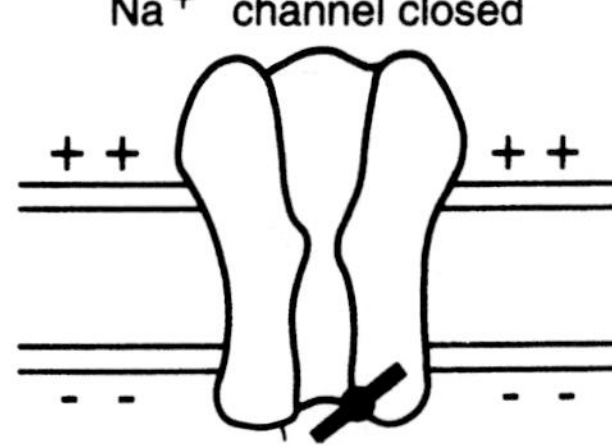

Figure 1–66. Gated sodium channel response during an action potential. *Top to bottom:* rest, depolarization, maintenance of depolarization, repolarization. (From Kandel, E.R., Schwartz, J.H., and Jessel, T.M.: Principles of Neural Science, 3rd ed., p. 14. Norwalk, CT, Appleton & Lange, 1991.)

1. Somatosensory System—Conveys three modalities: mechanical, pain, and thermal. Each of these three somatic modalities is mediated by a specific type of sensory receptor (Table 1–30). Somatosensory input from each of these three modalities is transmitted to the spinal cord (or brainstem) via the **dorsal root ganglion** (Fig. 1–68).

D. Motor System–Organized into four areas: spinal cord, brainstem, motor cortex, and premotor cortical areas (basal ganglia and cerebellum).

1. Spinal Cord (Fig. 1–68)—Contains white matter (peripheral) and gray matter (central).
   a. White Matter—Ascending and descending fiber tracts of myelinated and unmyelinated axons.
   b. Gray Matter—Contains neuronal cell bodies, glial cells, dendrites, and axons (myelinated and unmyelinated). Three types of neurons are found in spinal cord gray matter.
      1. Motoneurons (α and γ)—Axons exit the CNS via ventral roots.
      2. Interneurons—Axons remain in the spinal cord.
      3. Tract Cells—Send axons that ascend to supraspinal centers.
   c. Spinal Cord Reflexes (Table 1–31)—A reflex is a "stereotyped response" to a specific sensory stimulus. **The pathway of a reflex involves a sensory organ (receptor), an interneuron, and a motoneuron.**
      1. Monosynaptic Reflex—Only one synapse is involved (between receptor and effector).
      2. Polysynaptic Reflex—Involves one or more interneurons. **Most human reflexes are polysynaptic.**
2. Motor Unit—Composed of an α-motoneuron and the muscle fibers it innervates. Motor units are of four types based on the physiologic demands of the motor unit: type S (slow, fatigue-resistant); type FR (fast, fatigue-resistant); type FI (fast, fatigue-intermediate); and type FF (fast-fatigue). Table 1–32 shows an overview of the motor unit subtypes.
3. Upper and Lower Motoneurons

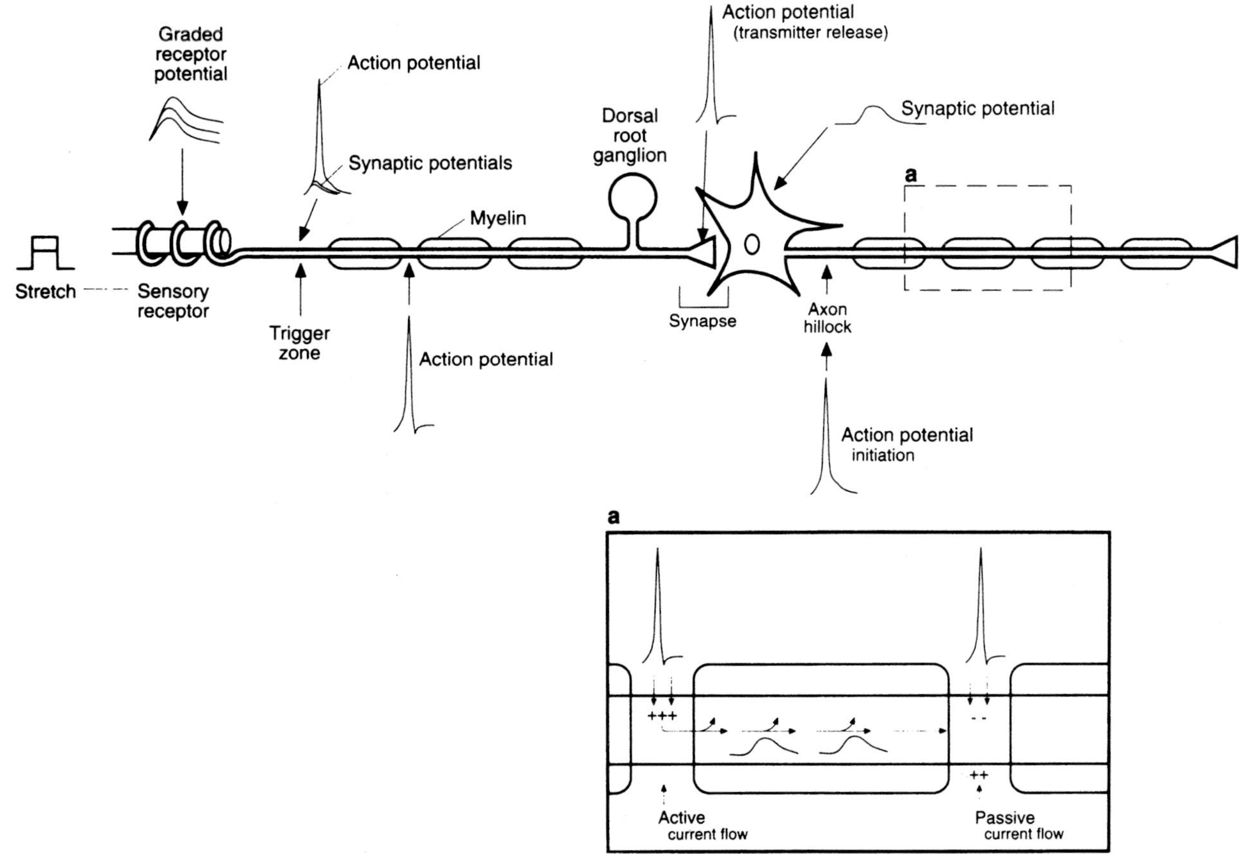

Figure 1–67. Action potential is propagated to the terminal region, where it triggers the release of transmitter, which initiates a synaptic potential in the motoneuron. Action potential propagation results from the spread of local passive depolarizing currents between the nodes of Ranvier (*inset*). At the nodes, voltage-gated channels open, producing an action potential. (From Simon, S.R., ed.: Orthopaedic Basic Science, 2nd ed., p. 337. Rosemont, IL, American Academy of Orthopaedic Surgeons, 1994.)

Table 1–30.

Receptor Types

Receptor Type	Fiber Type	Quality
Nociceptors		
Mechanical	Aδ	Sharp, pricking pain
Thermal and mechanothermal	Aγ	Sharp, pricking pain
Thermal and mechanothermal	C	Slow, burning pain
Polymodal	C	Slow, burning pain
Cutaneous and subcutaneous mechanoreceptors		
Meissner's corpuscle	Aβ	Touch
Pacini's corpuscle	Aβ	Flutter
Ruffini's corpuscle	Aβ	Vibration
Merkel's receptor	Aβ	Steady skin indentation
Hair-guard, hair-tylotrich	Aβ	Steady skin indentation
Hair-down	Aβ	Flutter
Muscle and skeletal mechanoreceptors		
Muscle spindle primary	Aα	Limb proprioception
Muscle spindle secondary	Aβ	Limb proprioception
Golgi tendon organ	Aα	Limb proprioception
Joint capsule mechanoreceptor	Aβ	Limb proprioception

From Kandel, E.R., Schwartz, J.H., and Jessel, T.M., eds: Principles of Neural Science, 3rd ed., p. 342. Norwalk, CT, Appleton & Lange, 1991.

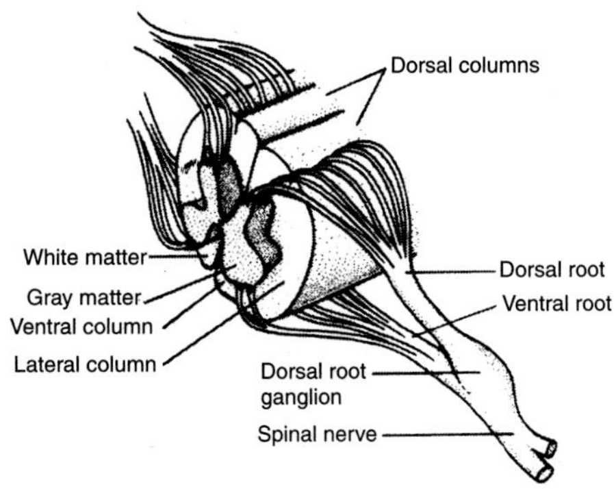

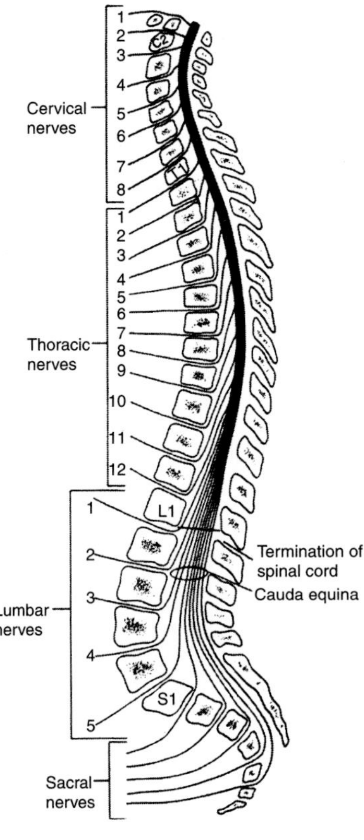

Figure 1–68. Spinal cord anatomy. *Left,* Each spinal nerve has a doral (sensory) and a ventral (motor) root. Dorsal roots are branches from dorsal root ganglia cells; ventral roots are motor axons from cells in the ventral horn. *Right,* Note that the spinal cord terminates at the L1 vertebra. The dorsal and ventral roots of the lumbar and sacral nerves are collectively called the cauda equina. (From Kandel, E.R., Schwartz, J.H., and Jessell, T.M.: Principles of Neural Science, 3rd ed., pp. 285–286. Norwalk, CT, Appleton & Lange, 1991.)

a. Upper Motoneurons—Located in the descending pathways of the cortex, brainstem, and spinal cord.
b. Lower Motoneurons—Located in the ventral gray matter of the spinal cord.
c. Motoneuron Lesions—**A synopsis of findings in patients with upper and lower motoneuron lesions is shown in Table 1–33. Spasticity** is a common finding in patients with an **upper motoneuron lesion.**

E. Peripheral Nerve
1. Morphology (see Fig. 1–63)—The peripheral nerve is a highly organized structure composed of nerve fibers, blood vessels, and connective tissues. Axons, coated with a fibrous tissue called **endoneurium,** are grouped into nerve bundles called **fascicles** that in turn are covered with connective tissue called **perineurium.** Peripheral nerves are composed of one (mono-), a few (oligo-), or several (poly-) fascicles and surrounding areolar connective tissue **(epineurium)** enclosed within an epineural sheath.
2. Nerve Fibers (Axons) (2–25 μm in Diameter)—Three types of nerve fiber are shown in Table 1–34.
3. Conduction—As has been previously discussed, myelinated axons conduct action potentials rapidly, facilitated by gaps between Schwann cells known as **nodes of Ranvier.**
4. Blood Supply
   a. Extrinsic—Vessels run in loose connective tissue surrounding the nerve trunk.
   b. Intrinsic—Vascular plexuses in the epineurium, perineurium, and endoneurium

Table 1–31.

Summary of Spinal Reflexes

Segmental Reflex	Receptor Organ	Afferent Fiber
Phasic stretch reflex	Muscle spindle (primary endings)	Type Ia (large myelinated)
Tonic stretch reflex	Muscle spindle (secondary endings)	Type II (intermediate myelinated)
Clasp-knife response	Muscle spindle (secondary endings)	Type II (intermediate myelinated)
Flexion withdrawal reflex	Nociceptors (free nerve endings), touch and pressure receptors	Flexor-reflex afferents: small unmyelinated cutaneous afferents (A-delta, C and muscle afferents, group III)
Autogenic inhibition	Golgi tendon organ	Type 1b (large myelinated)

From Simon, S.R.: Orthopaedic Basic Science, 2nd ed., p. 350. Rosemont, IL, American Academy of Orthopaedic Surgeons, 1994.

Table 1–32.

General Characteristics of Motor Unit Types

Parameter	Motor Unit Types FF	FR	S
Muscle unit physiology[a]			
Contraction time	Fastest	Slightly slower	Slowest
Sag	Present	Present	Absent
Maximum tension	Largest	Smaller	Smallest
Fatigue index	<0.25	<0.75–1.00	0.7–1.0
Muscle unit anatomy[b]			
Innervation ratio	2.9	2.1	1.0
Fiber cross-sectional area	1.3	0.98	1.0
Specific tension	1.4	1.2	1.0
Muscle unit metabolism			
Fiber type	FG	FOG	SO
Myosin heavy chain	IIB	IIA	I
Glycogen	High	High	Low
Hexokinase	Low	Intermediate	High
Glycolytic enzymes	High	High	Low
Oxidative enzymes	Low	High	High
Cytochrome c	Low	High	High
Capillary supply	Sparse	Rich	Very rich
Motoneuron			
Cell body size	Largest	Slightly smaller	Smallest
Conduction velocity	Fastest	Slighly slower	Slowest
After-hyperpolarization duration	Shortest	Slightly shorter	Longest
Input resistance	Lowest	Slightly higher	Highest

FF, fast fatigable; FR, fast fatigue-resistant; S, fatigue-resistant; FG, fast glycolytic; FOG, fast oxidative glycolytic; SO, slow oxidative.
[a]Data relative to the FF unit.
[b]Data relative to the slow unit.
From Simon, S.R.: Orthopaedic Basic Science, 2nd ed., p. 344. Rosemont, IL, American Academy of Orthopaedic Surgeons, 1994; reprinted by permission.

(with interconnections between these three plexuses).

F. Injury to the Nervous System—**Peripheral nerve injury** leads to death of the distal axons and **wallerian degeneration** (of myelin), which extends distal to the somatosensory receptor. Proximal axonal budding occurs (after a 1-month delay) and leads to regeneration at the rate of about 1 mm/day (possibly 3–5 mm/day in children). Pain is the first modality to return. **Nerve injury may be characterized as one of three types (Table 1–35).** Cortical evoked potential testing is the most sensitive method of predicting neural compression. Mechanical deformation of a compressed peripheral nerve is greatest in superficial regions and in zones between compressed and uncompressed segments. **Nerve stretching** also can affect function: 8% elongation diminishes microcirculation to the nerve, and 15% elongation disrupts axons. Nerve regeneration is influenced by contact guidance (attraction of regenerating nerve to the basal lamina of the Schwann cell), neurotrophism (factors enhancing growth), and neurotropism (preferential attraction toward nerves rather than other tissues). **"Stingers"** (or "burners") refer to neuropraxia from a stretch injury to the brachial plexus; they are seen most commonly in football players. Time needed for re-

Table 1–33.

Findings in Upper and Lower Motoneuron Lesions

Findings	Upper Motoneuron Lesions	Lower Motoneuron Lesions
Strength	Decreased	Decreased
Tone	Increased	Decreased
Deep tendon reflexes	Increased	Decreased
Superficial tendon reflexes	Decreased	Decreased
Babinski's sign	Present	Absent
Clonus	Present	Absent
Fasciculations	Absent	Present
Atrophy	Absent	Present

From Simon, S.R.: Orthopaedic Basic Science, 2nd ed., p. 354. Rosemont, IL, American Academy of Orthopaedic Surgeons, 1994.

Table 1–34.

Types of Nerve Fibers

Type	Diameter (μm)	Myelination	Speed	Examples
A	10–20	Heavy	Fast	Touch
B	<3	Intermediate	Medium	ANS
C	<1.3	None	Slow	Pain

ANS, autonomic nervous system.

Table 1–35.

Types of Nerve Injuries

Injury	Pathophysiology	Prognosis
Neuropraxia	Reversible conduction block characterized by local ischemia and selective demyelination of the axon sheath	Good
Axonotmesis	More severe injury with disruption of the axon and myelin sheath but leaving the epineurium intact	Fair
Neurotmesis	Complete nerve division with disruption of the endoneurium	Poor

covery from a stinger is variable as are residual sequela (such as permanent muscle atrophy). Neurologic studies (EMG/NCS) may be useful to document the extent of the injury in patients with muscle atrophy or motor weakness. **Cauda equina** syndrome is discussed in detail in Chapter 7, Spine. A double-level cauda equina nerve root compression (even at low pressures) results in a dramatic reduction in impulse conduction and blood flow as compared with a single-level cauda equina compression. The nucleus pulposus induces an inflammatory response when in contact with the nerve roots. The inflammatory response includes leukotaxis, increased vascular permeability, and decreased nerve conduction velocities.

G. Nerve Repair—Several methods are available. Younger patients have a better chance of recovery than do older patients after an operative repair of a nerve transection.

1. Direct Muscular Neurotization—Inserts the proximal stump of the nerve into the affected muscle belly. Results in less than normal function but is indicated in selected cases.
2. Epineural Repair—Primary repair of the outer connective tissue layer of the nerve at the site of injury after resecting the proximal neuroma and distal glioma. Care is taken to

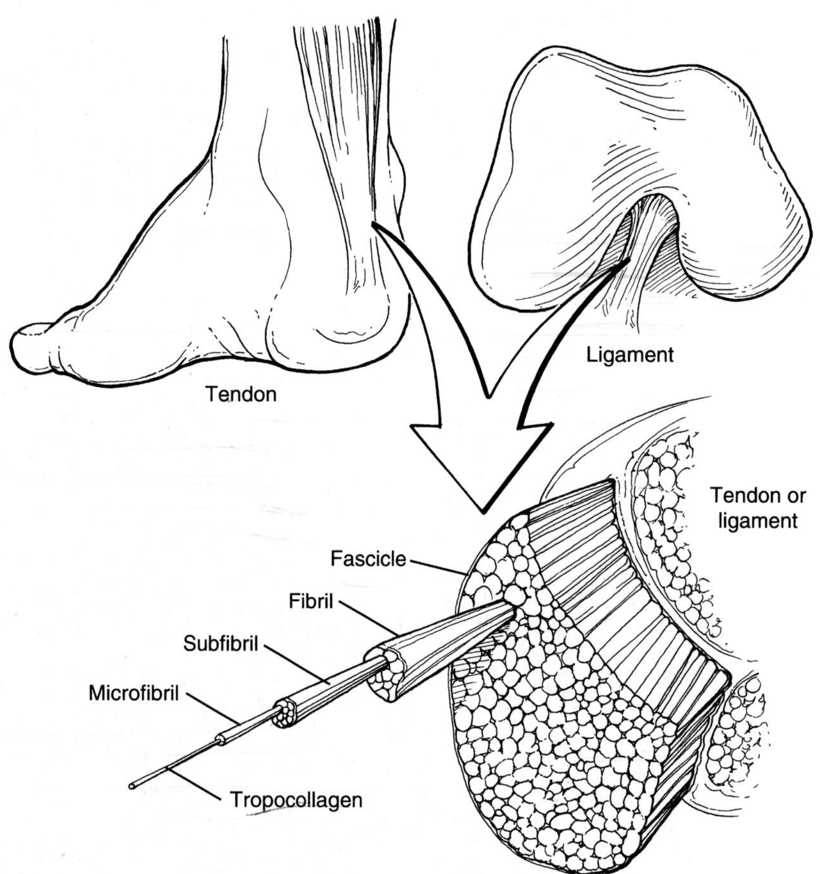

Figure 1–69. Tendon and ligament architecture. (From Brinker, M.R., and Miller, M.D.: Fundamentals of Orthopaedics. Philadelphia, WB Saunders, 1999, p. 15.)

ensure proper rotation and lack of tension on the repair.

3. Grouped Fascicular Repair—Primary repair is also performed after resection of the neuroma and glioma, but individual fascicles are reapproximated under microscopic control. Used for large nerves, but no significant improvement in results over epineural repair has been demonstrated.

III. Connective Tissues

A. Tendons (Fig. 1–69)—Dense, regularly arranged tissues that attach muscle to bone. Tendons are composed of fascicles (groups of collagen bundles), separated by **endotenon** and surrounded by **epitenon.** Tendons consist of fibroblasts (predominant cell type) arranged in parallel rows (Fig. 1–70) in fascicles (composed of fibrils) with surrounding loose areolar tissue (peritenon). Fibroblasts produce mostly type I collagen (85% of the dry weight of tendon). **Insertion of tendon into bone is by way of four transitional tissues (for force dissipation): tendon, fibrocartilage, mineralized fibrocartilage (Sharpey's fibers), and bone.** Two types of tendons exist: (1) paratenon-covered tendons and (2) sheathed tendons. Paratenon-covered tendons are also known as vascular tendons because many vessels supply a rich capillary system (Fig. 1–71). With a sheathed tendon, a mesotenon (vincula) carries a vessel that supplies only one segment of the tendon; avascular areas receive nutrition via diffusion from vascularized segments (Fig. 1–72). Because of these differences in vascular supply, paratenon-covered ten-

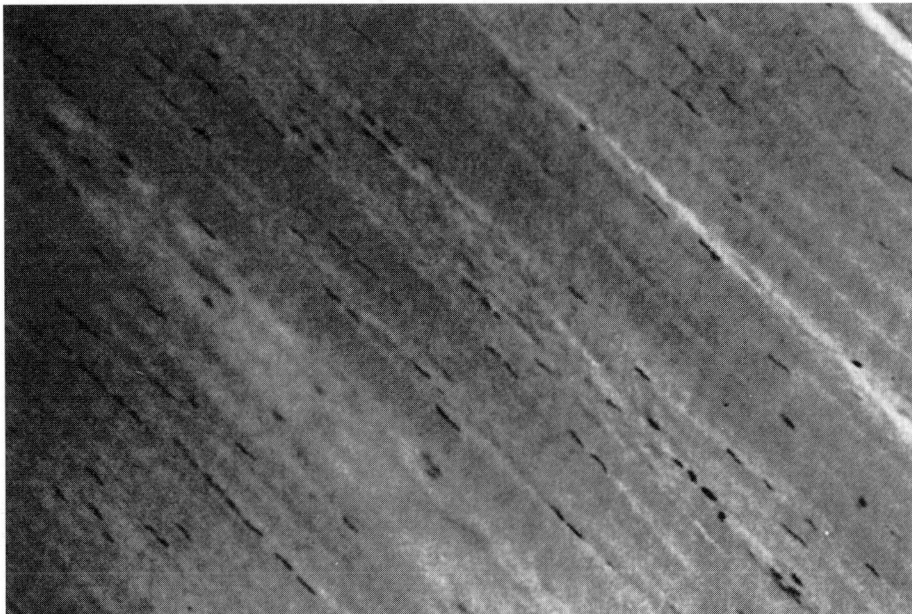

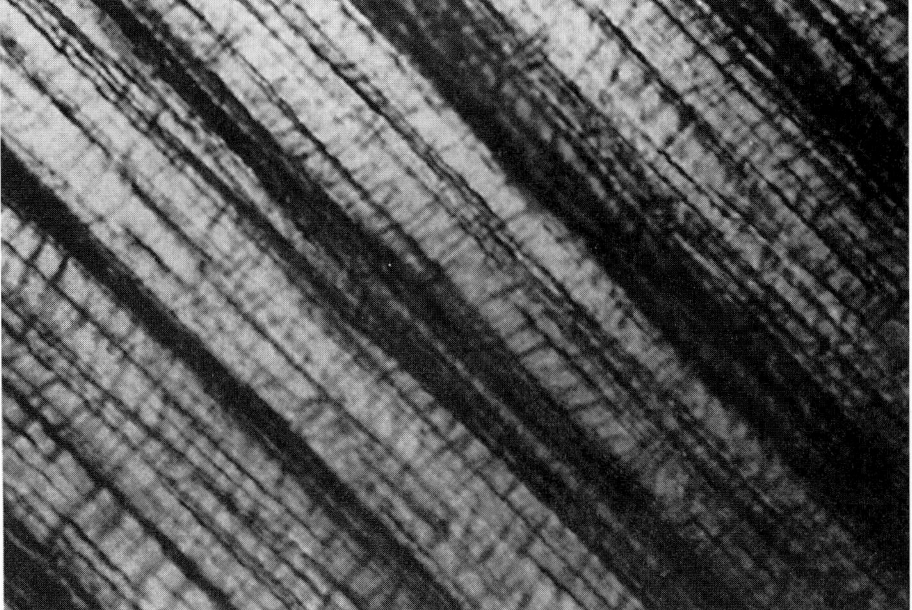

Figure 1–70. *Top,* Photomicrograph of a flexor tendon with parallel rows of fibroblasts and collagen bundles. *Bottom,* Polarized light photograph of the same section illustrating parallel, longitudinally arranged collagen bundles. (From Simon, S.R., ed.: Orthopaedic Basic Science, 2nd ed., p. 49. Rosemont, IL, American Academy of Orthopaedic Surgeons, 1994.)

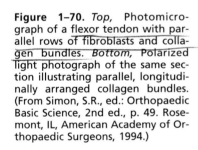

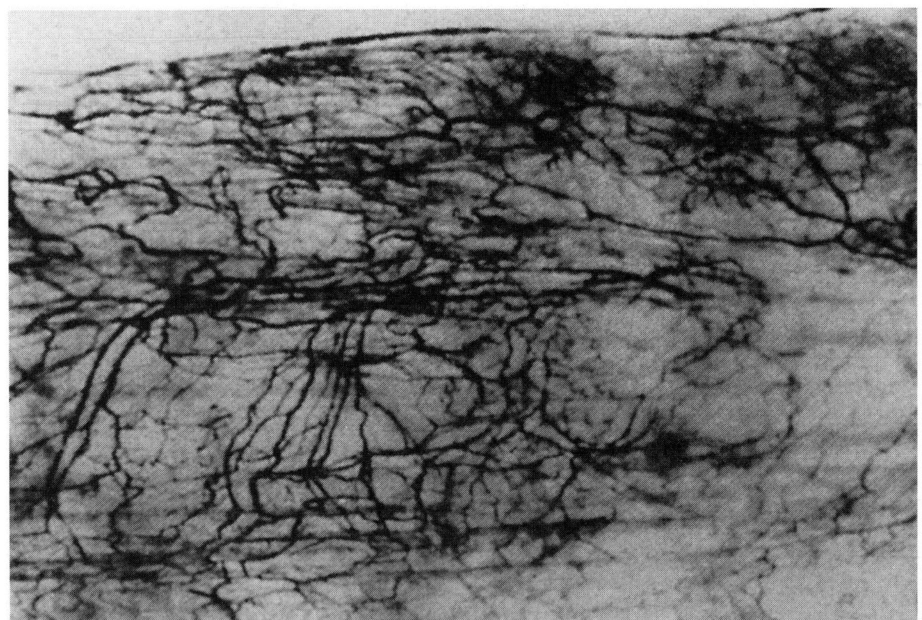

Figure 1–71. India ink injection of rabbit calcaneal tendon (Spalteholz technique) demonstrating the vasculature of the paratenon. (From Simon, S.R., ed.: Orthopaedic Basic Science, 2nd ed., p. 50. Rosemont, IL, American Academy of Orthopaedic Surgeons, 1994.)

dons heal better than sheathed tendons. Tendinous structures tend to orient themselves along stress lines. Tendinous healing in response to injury is initiated by fibroblasts that originate in the epitenon and macrophages that initiate healing and remodeling. Treatment of injuries affects the repair process. Tendon healing occurs in large part through intrinsic capabilities. Tendon repairs are **weakest at 7–10 days;** they regain most of their original strength at 21–28 days and achieve **maximum strength at 6 months.** Early mobilization allows increased ROM but results in decreased tendon repair strength. Immobilization leads to increased strength in the tendon substance at the expense of ROM. However, immobilization tends to decrease the strength at the tendon-bone interface. Bony avulsions of tendon insertions heal more rapidly than midsubstance tendon tears. Animal experiments (goats) have demonstrated no significant benefit from the creation of a trough (to expose the tendon to cancellous bone) for a tendon repair as compared to direct tendon repair to cortical bone.

B. Ligaments (see Fig. 1–69)—Composed of type I collagen (70% of the dry weight of ligament), these structures have a role in stability of joints. Their ultrastructure is similar to that of tendons, but the fibers are more variable and have a **higher elastin content. Unlike tendons, ligaments have a "uniform microvascularity," which receives its supply at the insertion site.** They also possess mechanoreceptors and free nerve endings that may play a role in stabilizing joints. Collagen sliding plays an important role in changes in ligament length (during growth and contracture). **Ligament insertion into bone** represents a transition from one material to another and can be classified into two types: **indirect insertion** (more common) and **direct insertion.** With an indirect insertion, the superficial fibers of the ligament insert at acute angles into the periosteum. Direct insertions display superficial and deep fibers; the deep fibers attach to bone at 90 degree angles, and the **transition from ligament to bone occurs in four phases: ligament, fibrocartilage, mineralized fibrocartilage, and bone.** Healing (in three phases, as in bone) is benefited from normal stress and strain across the joint. **Early ligament healing is with type III collagen that is later converted to type I collagen.** Immobilization adversely affects the strength (elastic modulus decreases) of an intact ligament and of a ligament repair. In animal studies (rabbit), the breaking strength of the MCL was reduced dramatically (reduced 66%) after 9 weeks of cast immobilization. There is a slow reversal of the negative effects of immobilization on ligaments after remobilization. The mechanical properties of a ligament return toward normal much more rapidly than those of an insertion site. Exercise causes an increase in the mechanical and structural properties of a ligament. **The most common mechanism of ligament failure is rupture of sequential series of collagen fiber bundles** distributed throughout the body of the ligament and not localized to one specific area. **Ligaments do not plastically deform** ("they break, not bend"). **Midsubstance ligament tears are common in adults; avulsion injuries are more common in children.** Local injection of corticosteroids at the site of an injured ligament has been shown to be detrimental to the healing process. **Avulsion of ligaments typically occurs between the unmineralized and mineralized fibrocartilage layers.** The most common site of failure during the immediate

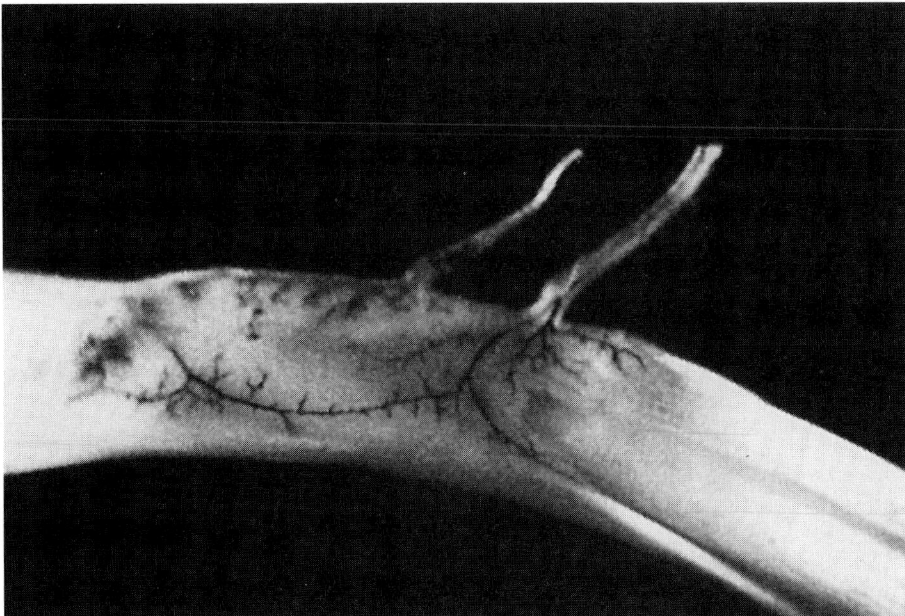

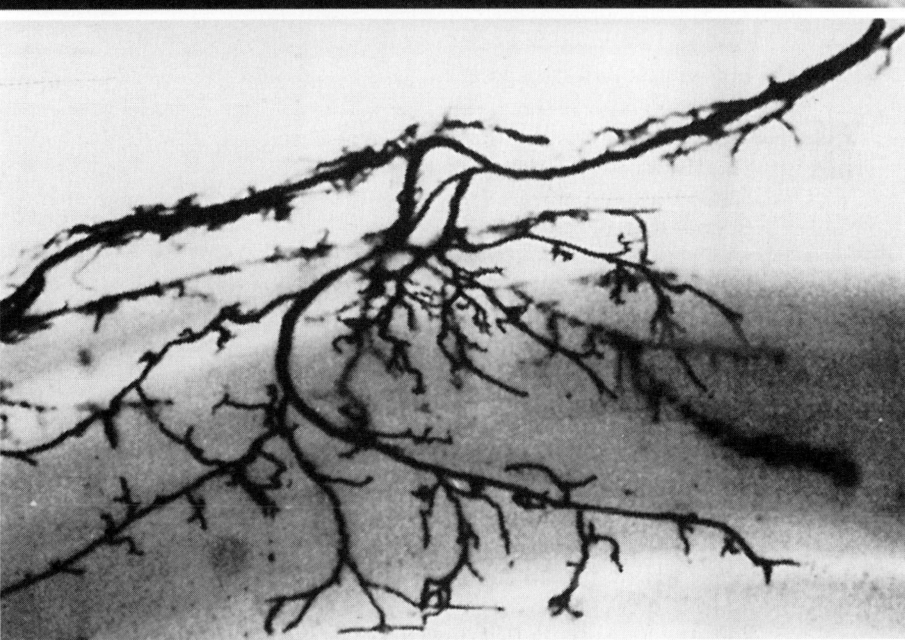

Figure 1–72. *Top,* India ink specimens demonstrating the vascular supply of the flexor tendons via vincula. *Bottom,* Close-up of the specimen. (From Simon, S.R., ed.: Orthopaedic Basic Science, 2nd ed., p. 51. Rosemont, IL, American Academy of Orthopaedic Surgeons, 1994.)

postoperative period of a bone-patellar tendon-bone ACL reconstruction is the fixation site. **The major blood supply of the cruciate ligaments is the middle genicular artery.** Most patients with Marfan's syndrome have abnormalities of fibrillin (a structural protein of ligaments).

C. Intervertebral Discs—Allow motion and stability of the spine. Composed of two components: the central nucleus pulposus (a hydrated gel with compressibility; high GAG/low collagen) and a surrounding annulus fibrosis (allows for extensibility and increased tensile strength; high collagen/low GAG). Composed of 85% water, proteoglycans, and **collagen types I and II** (type I in the annulus; type II in the nucleus pulposus). The aging disc shows decreased water content, decreased proteoglycan content, size, and concentration (however, the concentration of keratin sulfate increases with age), and increased collagen. Nerve fibers are present in the superficial layer of the annulus. Various neuropeptides, which are believed to be involved in sensory transmission, nociceptive transmission, neurogenic inflammation, and skeletal metabolism, have been described and include: substance P, calcitonin gene–related peptide (GCRP), vasoactive intestinal peptide (VIP), and the c-flanking peptide of neuropeptide Y (CPON). Cigarette smoking is a predisposing factor to degenerative disc disease.

D. Soft-Tissue Healing

1. Four phases of soft-tissue healing have been described.

a. Hemostasis—Primary platelet plug is formed within 5 minutes. Secondary clotting (via the coagulation cascade) uses fibrin and occurs within the first 10–15 minutes of injury. Fibronectin, a large glycoprotein, binds fibrin and cells and acts as a chemotactic factor. Platelets release factors that activate the next phase of healing.
b. Inflammation—Involves débridement of injured/necrotic tissue utilizing macrophages and occurs within the first week after injury. It has three stages: (1) activation (immediate); (2) amplification (48–72 hours); and (3) débridement (using bacteria, phagocytosis, and matrix [biochemical] means). Prostaglandins help to mediate the inflammatory response.
c. Organogenesis—Occurs at 7–21 days and consists of tissue modeling. Mesenchymal precursors differentiate into myofibroblasts. Angiogenesis occurs. Further differentiation leads to the final stage of healing.
d. Remodeling (of Individual Tissue Lines)—Begins shortly after repair and continues for up to 18 months. Realignment and cross-linking of collagen fibers allows increased tensile strength.

2. Growth Factors—Require activation, are redundant, and function with feedback loop mechanisms.
   a. Chemotactic Factors—Attract cells. The factors include prostaglandins (PMNs), prostanoids (PMNs), complement (PMNs and macrophages), PDGF (macrophages and fibroblasts), and angiokines (endothelial cells).
   b. Competence Factors—Activate dormant (G_0) cells. Include PDGF and prostaglandins.
   c. Progression Factors—Allow cell growth. Induce epidermal growth factor, IL-1, and somatomedins.
   d. Inductive Factors—Stimulate differentiation. Include angiokines, bone morphogenic protein, and specific tissue growth factors.
   e. Transforming Factors—Cause dedifferentiation and proliferation.
   f. Permissive Factors—Enhancing factors; include fibronectin and osteonectin.

E. Soft-Tissue Implants
   1. Introduction—Usually used around the knee (ACL); implants can be allografts, autografts, and synthetics.
   2. Allografts—Have no donor-site morbidity but incite an immune response and may transmit infection. The immunogenic response can be reduced with treatment (freeze-drying), but it decreases strength (deep freezing without drying does not significantly affect strength). If not harvested under sterile conditions, treatment with cold ethylene oxide gas may have adverse affects **(graft failure)**, particularly if >3 M rad irradiation is used in conjunction (2 M rad with ethylene oxide does not appear to significantly decrease the mechanical properties). Allograft ligaments exhibit slower, less predictable histologic recovery than autografts.
   3. Synthetic Ligaments—Unlike autografts or allografts, these structures have no initial period of weakness. However, they suffer from wear (debris) and are associated with **sterile joint effusions** with increased levels of neutral proteinases **(collagenase** and gelatinase) and chondrocyte activation factor (IL-1).

F. Miscellaneous
   Platelet-derived growth factor, transforming growth factor-β, and epidermal growth factor have been associated with fibroblastic proliferation in Dupuytren's contracture. A defect in the metabolism of fibrillin (a component of the elastic fiber system) has been demonstrated in some patients with adolescent idiopathic scoliosis.

Section 4

Cellular and Molecular Biology, Immunology, and Genetics of Orthopaedics

The fields of molecular biology, immunology, and genetics, are rapidly expanding. Recent advancements have been made in these areas, specifically in the field of musculoskeletal science. It is the intent of this section on Cellular and Molecular Biology, Immunology, and Genetics of Orthopaedics to serve as an introduction to the basic concepts of these fields.

I. **Cellular and Molecular Biology**

A. Chromosomes—Humans have 23 pairs (46) of chromosomes. Chromosomes are located in the nucleus of every cell in the body. Each chromosome contains at least 150,000 **genes.** Although every cell has 46 chromosomes, the genes located on these chromosomes are regulated so a relatively small number of genes are expressed for any given cell. In this way the regulation of **gene expression** determines the unique biologic qualities of each cell. Chromosomes contain both deoxyribonucleic acid (DNA) and ribonucleic acid (RNA).

B. DNA—Located within the chromosome (in the cell nucleus), DNA is responsible for regulating cellular functions via **protein synthesis.** DNA has been classically described as a double helix (double-stranded) that contains **two sugar molecules** (each strand of DNA represents one sugar molecule), each of which has one of four nitrogenous bases (adenine, guanine, cytosine, thymine) (Fig. 1–73). The nitrogenous bases from one strand are linked to those of the other strand via hydrogen bonds. (In DNA, adenine is always linked to thymine, and guanine is always linked to cytosine.) DNA is important for three cellular processes: (1) DNA replication; (2) transcription of messenger RNA (mRNA); (3) regulation of cell division and the production of mRNA. All nuclear DNA is housed in the 23 chromosome pairs.

C. Nucleotide—Made up of the sugar molecule strand plus a nitrogen base. The nucleotide sequence in one strand of DNA determines the complimentary nucleotide sequence in the other (adenine to thymine, guanine to cytosine). The genetic message is grouped into three-letter words known as **codons.** The codon specifies one of the possible 20 amino acids that are the building blocks of all proteins (Fig. 1–74).

D. Gene—Portion of DNA that codes for a specific enzyme ("one gene equals on enzyme").

E. Transcription (Fig. 1–75)—In order to produce a specific protein (to regulate cellular functions), the DNA of the gene that is coding for that specific protein must be transcribed to an mRNA (via RNA polymerase).

F. Translation (Fig. 1–75)—Process by which mRNA builds proteins from amino acids.

G. Protein Coding and Regulation—**A codon** is a sequence of three nucleotides in a strand of DNA or RNA that provides the genetic code information for a specific amino acid (Fig. 1–76). Between functional coding sequences are large noncoding sequences known as **regulating DNA.** The **gene promoter** is an important portion of the regulatory DNA and is required for the initiation of transcription. **Consensus**

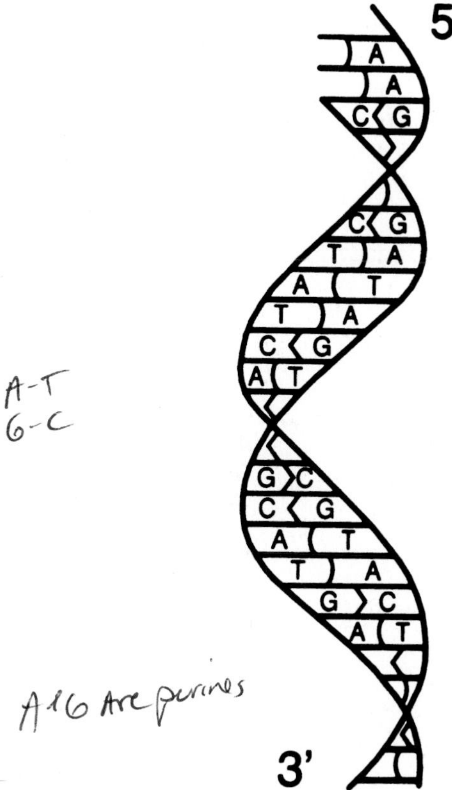

Figure 1–73. DNA structure. The two deoxyribose strands are connected by a pair of nucleotides (which form the rung of the ladder) connected by hydrogen bonds. A, adenine; T, thymine; C, cytosine; G, guanine. (From Simon, S.R., ed.: Orthopaedic Basic Science, 2nd ed., p. 221. Rosemont, IL, American Academy of Orthopaedic Surgeons, 1994.)

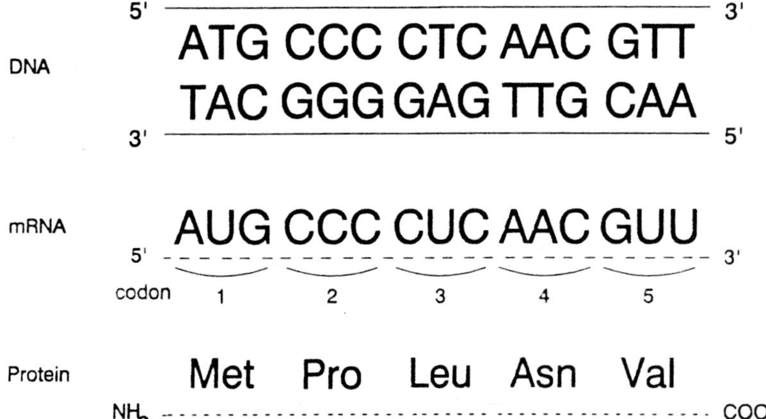

Figure 1–74. A genetic message begins as a double-stranded DNA molecule, which serves as the template for messenger RNA. The mRNA, in groups of three nucleotides to a codon, directs the order of amino acids in protein. (From Ross, D.W., ed.: Introduction to Molecular Medicine, 2nd ed., p. 4. New York, Springer-Verlag, 1996.)

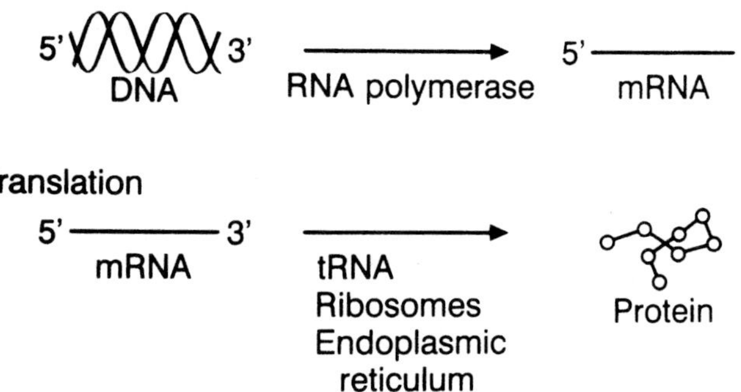

Figure 1–75. DNA information is transcribed into RNA in the nucleus. mRNA is then transported to the cytoplasm where translation into proteins occurs in the endoplasmic reticulum. DNA, deoxyribonucleic acid; RNA, ribonucleic acid; mRNA, messenger RNA; tRNA, transfer RNA. (From Simon, S.R., ed.: Orthopaedic Basic Science, 2nd ed., p. 222. Rosemont, IL, American Academy of Orthopaedic Surgeons, 1994.)

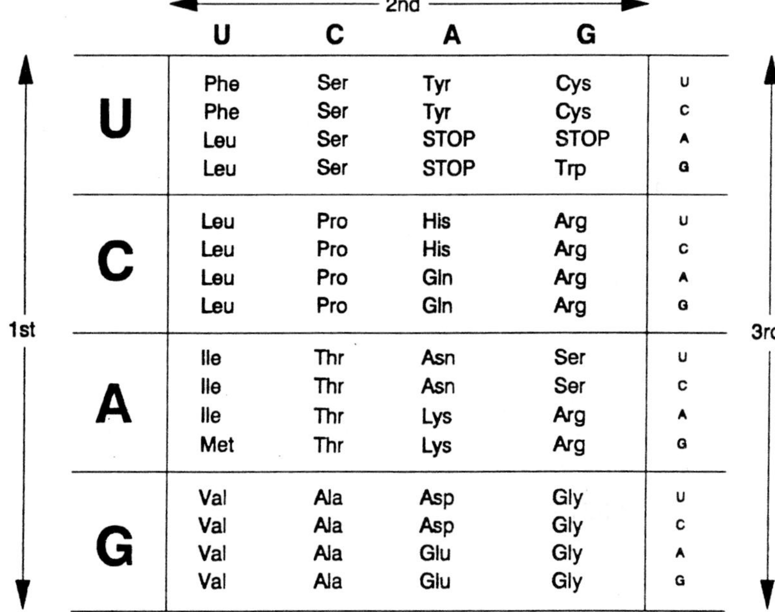

1st	U	C	A	G	3rd
U	Phe	Ser	Tyr	Cys	U
	Phe	Ser	Tyr	Cys	C
	Leu	Ser	STOP	STOP	A
	Leu	Ser	STOP	Trp	G
C	Leu	Pro	His	Arg	U
	Leu	Pro	His	Arg	C
	Leu	Pro	Gln	Arg	A
	Leu	Pro	Gln	Arg	G
A	Ile	Thr	Asn	Ser	U
	Ile	Thr	Asn	Ser	C
	Ile	Thr	Lys	Arg	A
	Met	Thr	Lys	Arg	G
G	Val	Ala	Asp	Gly	U
	Val	Ala	Asp	Gly	C
	Val	Ala	Glu	Gly	A
	Val	Ala	Glu	Gly	G

Figure 1–76. The genetic code for translation of the triplet nucleotide codons of mRNA into amino acids in proteins. (From Ross, D.W., ed.: Introduction to Molecular Medicine, 2nd ed., p. 7. New York, Springer-Verlag, 1996.)

sequences (named for a specific nucleotide sequence) serve as binding sites for specific proteins involved in gene regulation. **Gene enhancers** are binding sites for proteins involved in the regulation of transcription. Protein coding and regulation are shown in Figure 1–77.

H. Techniques of Study—Used to study genetic (inherited) disorders.
   1. Restriction Enzymes—Used to cut DNA at a precise, reproducible cleavage location. Fragments of DNA that have been cleaved using restriction enzymes are known as **restriction fragments.**
   2. Agarose Gel Electrophoresis—When exposed to an electrical field, negatively charged DNA is attracted toward the positive pole of the field and moves through the agarose gel in which it has been placed. The gel acts as a "sieve" to the extent that small DNA fragments move more easily (migrate further from the original position) through the gel than large fragments. Agarose gel is commonly used after the use of (and in conjunction with) restriction enzymes.
   3. DNA Ligation—Process of attaching genes removed from human DNA to pieces of nonhuman DNA known as **plasmids.** The purpose of this process is to facilitate the study of specific genes. Two DNA fragments linked together (via the ligation process) form **recombinant DNA.**
   4. Plasmid Vectors—A gene to be studied is ligated into a plasmid (which is then known as a **recombinant plasmid**) and inserted into a bacterium using a process known as **transformation.** The recombinant plasmid then replicates and increases the amount of recombinant DNA inside the bacterium.
   5. Genomic Screening (Fig. 1–78)
   6. Transgenic Animals (Fig. 1–79)—Used to investigate the function of cloned genes. A transgenic animal is produced by inserting a foreign gene **(transgene)** into a single-cell embryo, which then duplicates repeatedly and carries the transgene to every cell in the body.
   7. Southern Hybridization—Technique used to identify a **particular DNA sequence** in an extract of mixed DNA.
   8. Northern Hybridization—Technique used to identify a particular **RNA sequence** in an extract of mixed RNA.
   9. Polymerase Chain Reaction (PCR) Amplification—**Method used to repetitively synthesize (amplify) a specific DNA sequence** in vivo such that the number of DNA copies doubles each cycle. PCR amplification has gained widespread use and has been employed for the prenatal diagnosis of sickle cell disease and screening DNA for gene mutations.

II. **Immunology**
   A. Overview—Immunology is the study of the body's defense mechanisms. Areas of particular relevance to the musculoskeletal system are infection, transplantation, tumors, autoimmune disorders (e.g., rheumatoid arthritis), and bone remodeling. Two types of immune responses have been described: nonspecific and specific.
   B. Nonspecific Immune Response—**Inflammatory reaction** that begins when an antigen is recognized as foreign. This response may arise as a result of a fracture, soft-tissue injury, or foreign body. Histamine is released and results in local vasodilation (exudate) with phagocytic cells that enzymatically digest "offending material." The inflammatory response may be enhanced by ac-

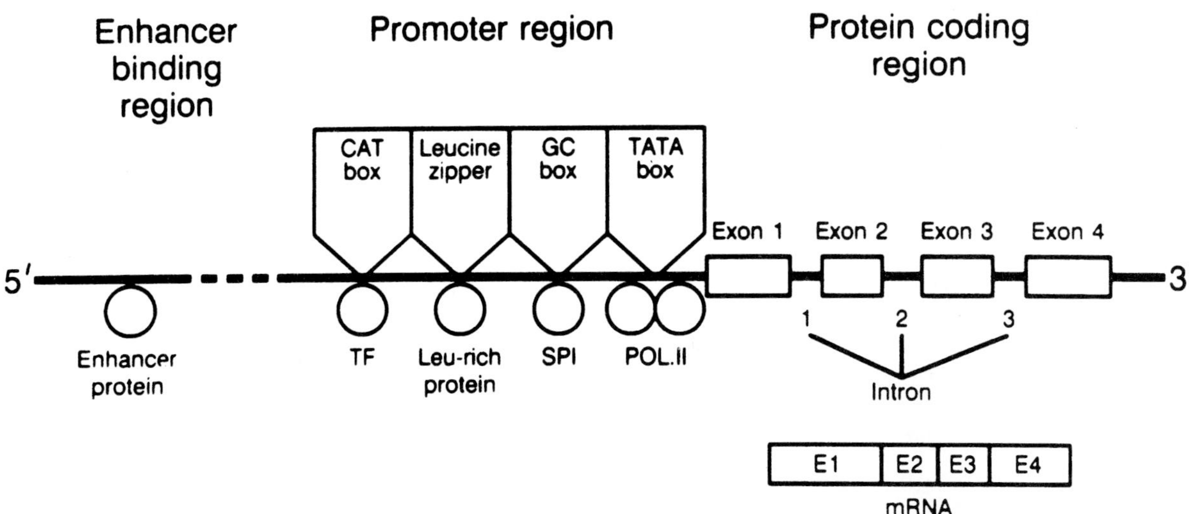

Figure 1–77. Protein coding and regulation. mRNA, messenger ribonucleic acid; TF, transcription factor; POL II, RNA polymerase II; SPI, serum promotor. (From Simon, S.R., ed.: Orthopaedic Basic Science, 2nd ed., p. 223. Rosemont, IL, American Academy of Orthopaedic Surgeons, 1994.)

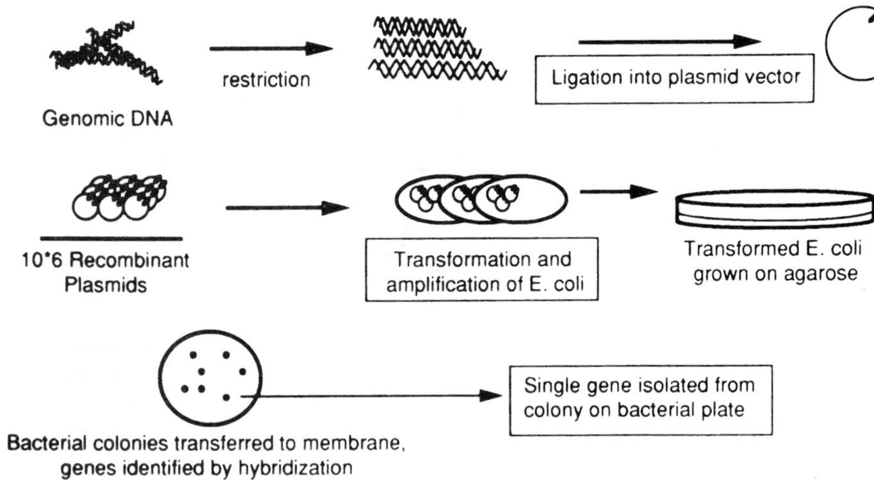

Figure 1–78. Genomic library of recombinant plasmids with fragments of all the DNA in the chromosome. The entire genome, restricted into small fragments, is ligated into plasmid vectors restricted by the same enzymes. These recombinant plasmids transform bacteria, which can be screened to isolate specific genes of interest. (From Simon, S.R., ed.: Orthopaedic Basic Science, 2nd ed., p. 227. Rosemont, IL, American Academy of Orthopaedic Surgeons, 1994.)

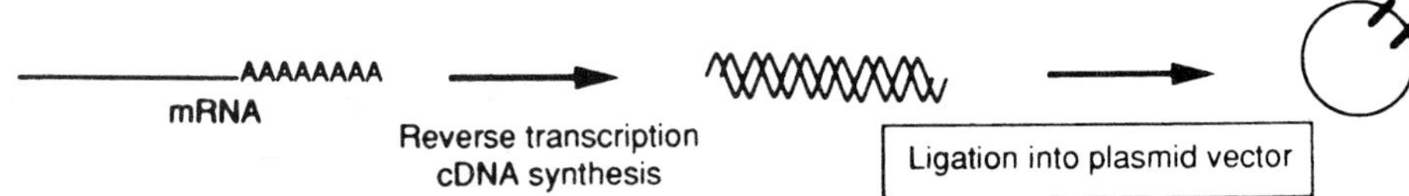

tivation of the complement system or quieted by anti-inflammatory medication.

C. Specific Immune Response (Fig. 1–80)—Includes **cell-mediated** and **humoral antibody-mediated** immune responses. The cells involved in specific immune responses arise from primitive mesenchymal cells from the bone marrow (Fig. 1–81). B lymphocytes mature in the lymph nodes; T lymphocytes originate in the bone marrow and pass through the thymus during fetal development before moving to the lymph nodes and blood. T cells include helper T cells, suppressor T cells, and killer T cells. **Antigens** evoke an immune response. **Macrophages and monocytes** are responsible for processing antigen so it is able to stimulate lym-

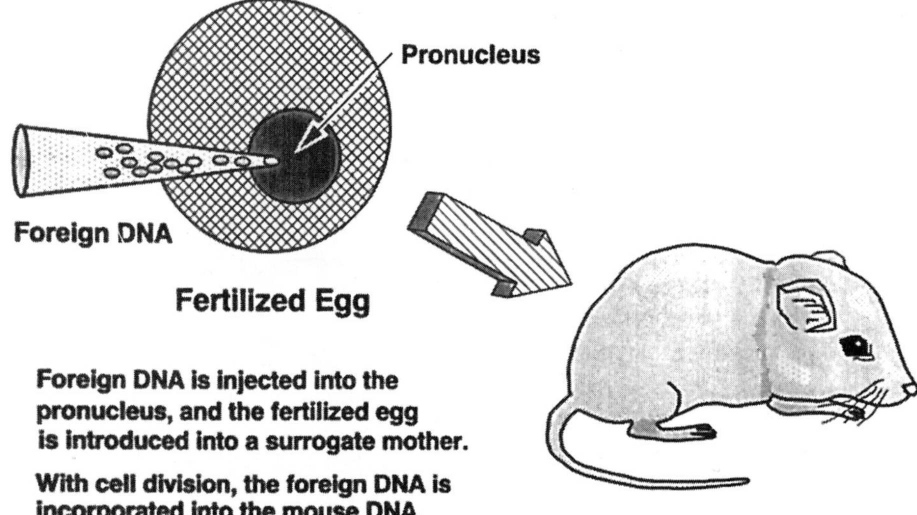

Figure 1–79. Transgenic mice. Recombinant DNA is injected into a fertilized mouse egg. The foreign DNA incorporates into the chromosome with cell division. As the egg develops into an embryo, every cell in the animal contains the foreign DNA. (From Simon, S.R., ed.: Orthopaedic Basic Science, 2nd ed., p. 228. Rosemont, IL, American Academy of Orthopaedic Surgeons, 1994.)

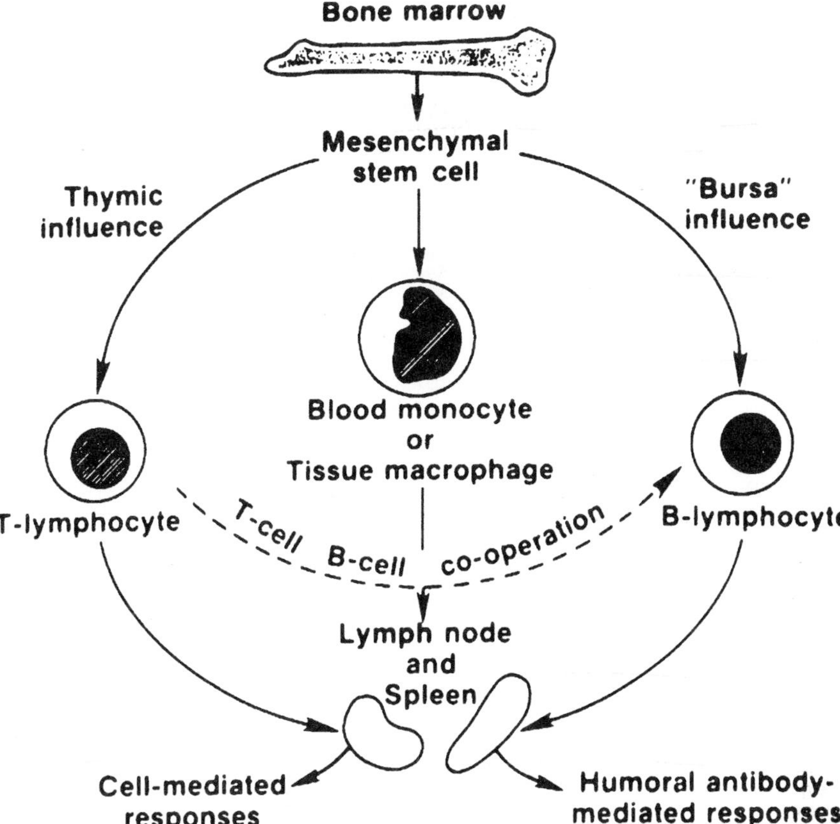

Figure 1–80. Bone marrow primitive mesenchymal cells differentiate into B and T lymphocytes and macrophages and cooperate in cell-mediated and humoral responses. (From Friedlander, G.E.: Immunology. In Albright, J.A., and Brand, R.A., eds.: The Scientific Basis of Orthopaedics, 2nd ed., p. 484. Norwalk, CT, Appleton & Lange, 1987.)

phocytes. Lymphocytes have the unique ability to mount specific reactions to millions of potential antigens. This is possible because lymphocytes are able to rearrange their genes (no other cell can do this) to achieve antigenic diversity (to produce millions of antibodies).

1. **Cell-mediated immune response** (Fig. 1–82)—Involves T lymphocytes. The protein produced by gene rearrangement stays fixed to the surface of T cells to act as a receptor molecule. The T-cell receptor acts indirectly on foreign antigen (it does not bond directly as is seen with B lymphocytes).
2. **Humoral antibody-mediated immune response** (Fig. 1–83)—Involves B lymphocytes. B lymphocytes differentiate into **plasma cells** to produce immunoglobins against specific antigens. B lymphocytes are different from T lymphocytes because **B lymphocytes are associated with immunoglobins and the HLA system.** Immunoglobins are produced by plasma cells in a

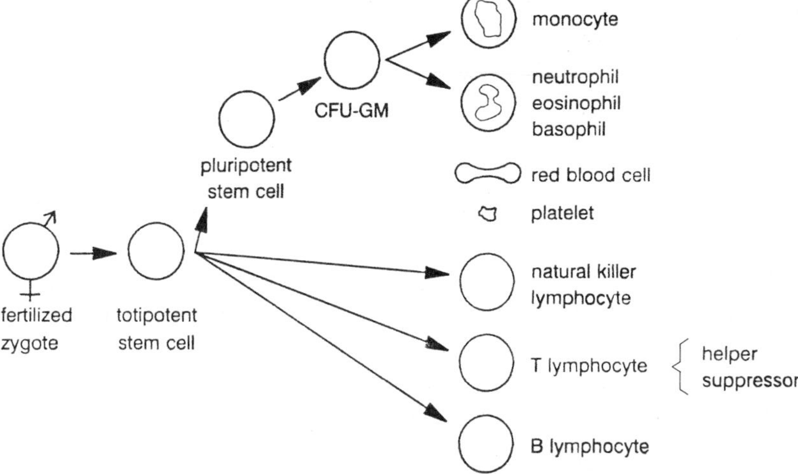

Figure 1–81. Stem cells generate all the cell types of the blood and immune systems by a process of proliferation and differentiation in response to growth signals. CFU-GM = colony-forming unit of the granulocyte/monocyte. (From Ross, D.W., ed.: Introduction to Molecular Medicine, 2nd ed., p. 112. New York, Springer-Verlag, 1996.)

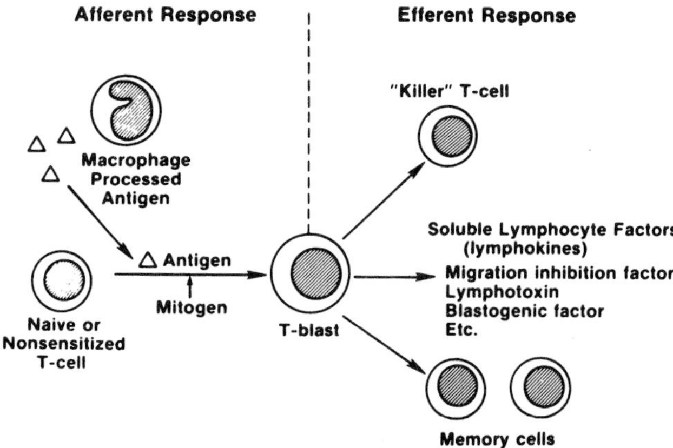

Figure 1–82. The cell-mediated immune response. (From Friedlaender, G.E.: Immunology. In Albright, J.A., and Brand, R.A., eds.: The Scientific Basis of Orthopaedics, 2nd ed. Norwalk, CT, Appleton & Lange, 1987, p. 493.)

"Y" configuration (Fig. 1–84). Five classes of immunoglobulin have been described:
   a. IgA—Mucosal surfaces
   b. IgM—Produced earliest by fetus; largest; rheumatoid factor (RF) is an IgM.
   c. IgG—Most common; arises in response to infection.
   d. IgD—Acts as a receptor.
   e. IgE—Allergic responses

D. Cytokines—Proteins (or glycoproteins) that are cell products secreted in response to a foreign antigen. They are produced by T cells and regulate inflammatory and immune responses. Cytokines have been described in four broad categories.
   1. Interferons
   2. Growth Factors
   3. Colony-Stimulating Factors
   4. Interleukins

E. Complement System (Fig. 1–85)—A group of 25 proteins that act in a "cascading sequence" to amplify an immune response.

F. Immunogenetics—Human leukocyte antigens (HLAs) contribute to the "specificity of immune recognition" and are associated with a variety of rheumatologic diseases. The HLA gene is located on chromosome 6 (short arm); there are six class I loci and 14 class II loci.

G. Transplantation
   1. Allogenic Grafting–Transplantation between nonidentical members of the same species.
   2. Xenografting—Transplantation of tissues across species.
   3. Graft Preparation
      a. Freezing—Cellular response diminished.
      b. Freeze-drying (Lyophilization)—Cellular response nearly undetectable.

H. Oncology (Fig. 1–86)
   1. Cancer is a disease characterized by uncontrolled cell growth. This abnormal cell growth is due to damage to the cell's DNA. The molecular approach to cancer seeks to discover the mechanisms by which normal cells become cancer cells.
   2. Various mechanism may lead to the damage of normal cells, resulting in malignancy. These mechanisms include:
      a. A point mutation in DNA
      b. A gene deletion
      c. A chromosomal translocation (which results in gene rearrangment)
   3. **Oncogenes**—Are growth control genes. Improper expression of an oncogene results in unregulated cell growth as seen in cancer cells.
   4. **Anti-Oncogenes (Tumor Suppressor Genes)**—Suppress growth in damaged cells to inhibit tumors.
   5. Metastases—The sequence of events for primary tumor cells to metastasize to a distant organ are as follows:
      a. Progressive growth of the primary tumor
      b. Neovascularization of the tumor
      c. Basement membrane erosion and invasion. **Matrix metalloproteinases have the capacity to degrade type IV collagen, which is present in the basement membrane** (see Table 1–18). It is therefore believed that matrix metalloproteinases are important for tumor cell metastasis.
      d. Entry of tumor cells into adjacent blood vessels
      e. Detachment of cells from the primary tumor
      f. Embolization of tumor cells into the general circulation
      g. Attachment of tumor cells at a distant site
      h. Invasion into vessel walls; migration into surrounding parenchyma
      i. Progressive tumor growth in the new site
   6. Miscellaneous
      a. **Flow cytometry and cytofluorometry**—A method used to quantify the amount of

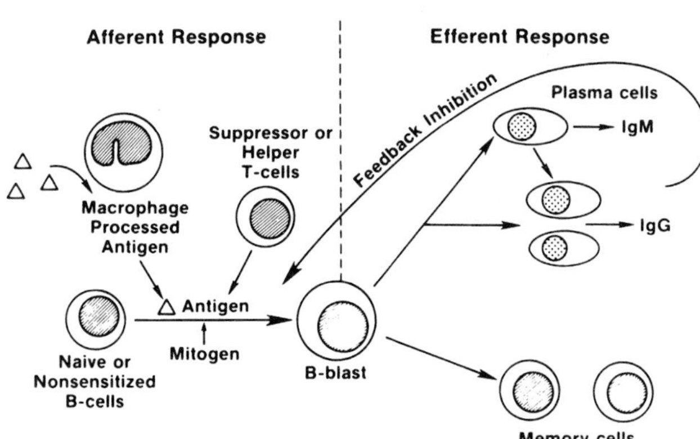

Figure 1–83. The humoral antibody response; activation of B cells and immunoglobin production. (From Friedlaender, G.E.: Immunology. In Albright, J.A., and Brand, R.A., eds.: The Scientific Basis of Orthopaedics, 2nd ed. Norwalk, CT, Appleton & Lange, 1987, p. 492.)

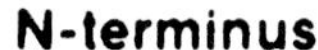

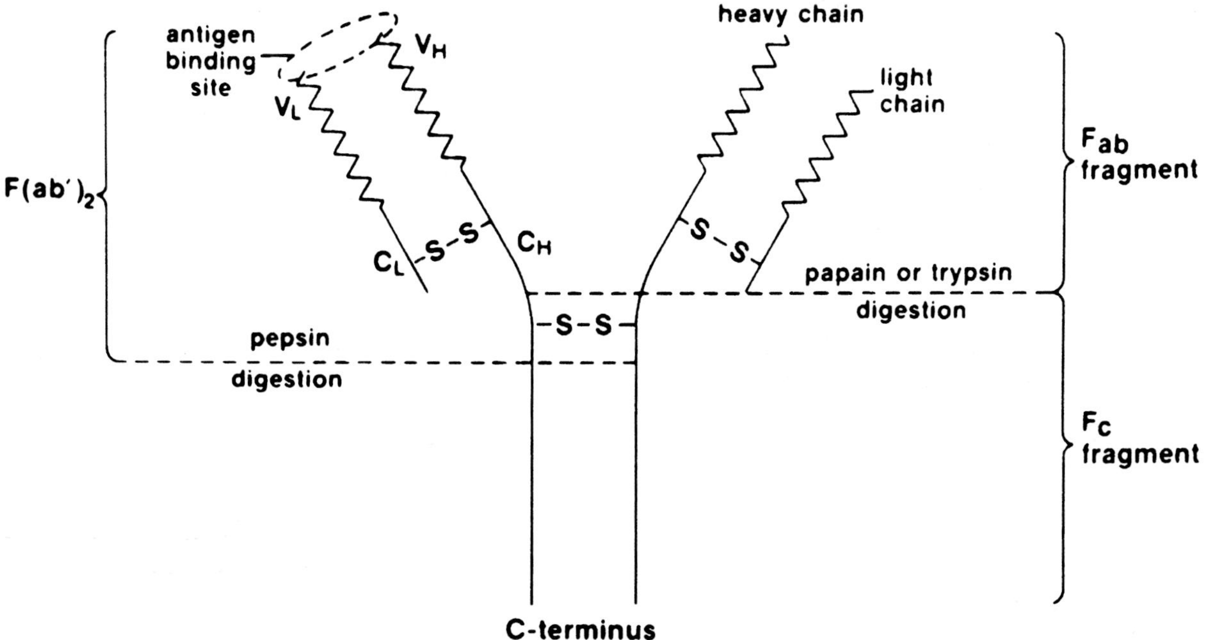

Figure 1–84. Basic subunit structure of the immunoglobulin molecule. (From Friedlander, G.E.: Immunology. In Albright J.A., and Brand, R.A., eds.: The Scientific Basis of Orthopaedics, 2nd ed., p. 486. Norwalk, CT, Appleton & Lange, 1987.)

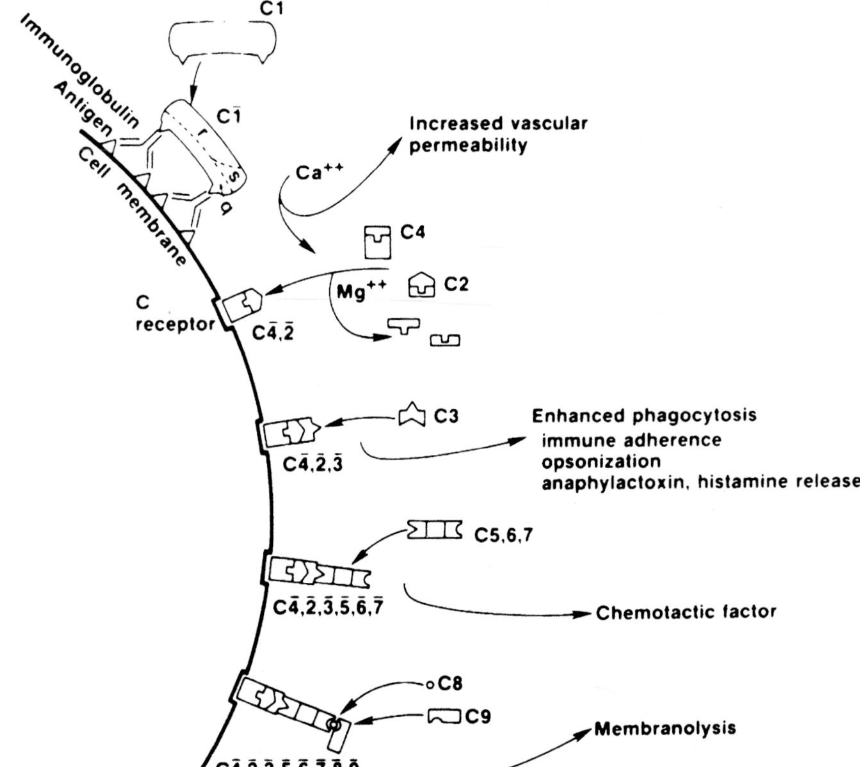

Figure 1–85. Complement cascade. (From Friedlander, G.E.: Immunology. In Albright, J.A., and Brand, R.A., eds.: The Scientific Basis of Orthopaedics, 2nd ed., p. 491. Norwalk, CT, Appleton & Lange, 1987.)

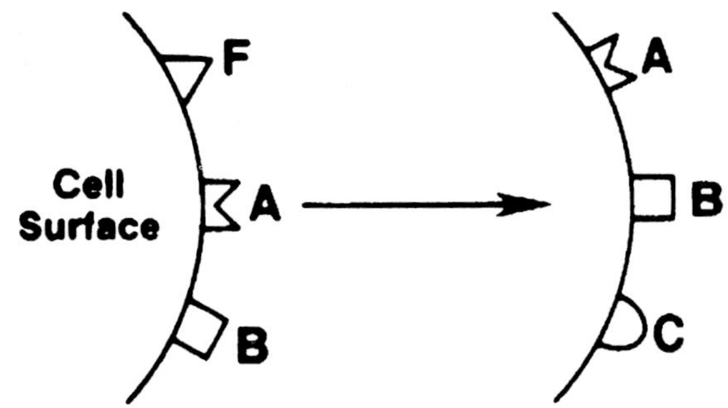

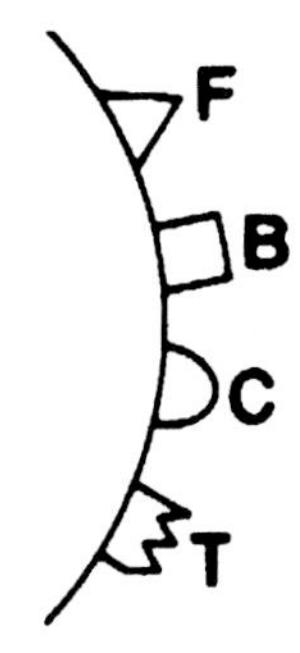

Figure 1–86. Tumor cells have cell-surface antigens common to other normal cells reflecting the tissue of origin (*B, C*). They may also demonstrate antigens normally present only on fetal cells (*F*) and loose antigens common to the cell type of origin (*A*). In addition, they acquire new tumor-associated antigens (*T*). (From Friedlander, G.E.: Immunology. In Albright, J.A., and Brand, R.A., eds.: The Scientific Basis of Orthopaedics, 2nd ed., p. 502. Norwalk, CT, Appleton & Lange, 1987.)

DNA in cells. **This technique is useful for determining the amount of abnormal (aneuploid) DNA in a malignant tumor.**

b. **P-glycoprotein** is a cell-wall pump that functions to eliminate natural toxins (and some chemotherapeutic agents) from the cytoplasm. P-glycoprotein allows both cancer and normal cells to develop resistance to chemotherapeutic agents.

I. **Miscellaneous Topics Related to Specific Immune-Related Orthopaedic Conditions**

1. **Latex allergy** has been reported as an intraoperative complication, particularly in patients with myelomenigocele. Latex allergy in these children is likely due to repetitive mucosal and parenteral exposure to latex (e.g., operations, examinations). **Type I hypersensitivity to latex involves IgE antibodies** that are specific for proteins to the sap from the rubber tree (*Hevea brasiliensis*) used to make gloves. Preoperative prophylaxis (cimetidine and diphenyhydramine) decreases the frequency of potentially catastrophic events (anaphylaxis).
2. The development of rheumatoid arthtitis is related to a reaction between T cells (helper/inducer) and antigen-presenting cell macrophage.
3. The foreign-body response to particulate biomaterials appears to be initiated by macrophages. Lymphocytes do not appear to be essential for this response.
4. Endosteal bone erosion (osteolysis; aggressive granulomatous lesions) surrounding an uninfected femoral stem following THA is associated with monocytes-macrophages.

III. **Genetics**

A. Introduction—Although more than 3000 genetic disorders have been identified, the genes responsible for the disorders have been identified in only a small number of musculoskeletal diseases.

B. Mendelian Inheritance—Mendelian traits are those that follow specific patterns of inheritance controlled by a single gene pair ("monogenic"). **A genetic locus** is a specific position on a chromosome that holds a gene. **An allele** is one of several possible alternative forms of a gene. Because the chromosomes are paired (46 chromosomes; 23 pairs [22 pairs of autosomes and 1 pair of sex chromosomes]) there are two copies (loci) for every gene. An individual is said to be **homozygous** if the two alleles present on each of the chromosomes are identical; the individual is said to be **heterozygous** if the alleles differ. The term **phenotype** refers to the features exhibited by an individual due to genetic makeup; **genotype** refers to the presence or absence of particular genes, not the associated traits expressed. Mendelian traits may be inherited by one of four modes:

1. Autosomal dominant
2. Autosomal recessive
3. X-linked dominant
4. X-linked recessive

A detailed description of these four modes of mendelian inheritance is shown in Table 1–36. The overall incidence of mendelian disorders in humans is approximately 1%. Nonmendelian traits may be inherited via "polygenic" transmission (caused by the action of several genes).

C. Mutations—Genetic disorders arise as a result of alterations (mutations) in the genetic material. These mutations may be passed down from generation to generation and may follow mendelian inheritance or the mutation may represent a new mutation **(sporadic mutation)** that occurs in the sperm or egg of the parents or in the embryo.

D. Chromosomal Abnormalities—A chromosomal abnormality results from a disruption in the normal arrangement or number of chromosomes. Chromosomal abnormalities include:

1. Aneuploidy—An abnormal number of chromosomes
   a. Triploidy—Three copies of chromosomes (69 chromosomes).
   b. Tetraploids—Four copies of chromosomes (92 chromosomes).
   c. Monosomy—One chromosome of one pair is absent (45 chromosomes).

Text continued on page 94

Table 1–36.

Mendelian Inheritance

Inheritance Pattern	Description	Punit Square(s)
Autosomal dominant	Typically represent **structural defects** Heterozygote state (Aa) manifests the condition 50% of the offspring are affected (assuming only one parent is affected) Normal offspring do not transmit the condition There is no gender preference	A a a: Aa aa a: Aa aa
Autosomal recessive	Typically represent **biochemical or enzymatic defects** Homozygote state (aa) manifests the condition Parents are unaffected (they are most commonly heterozygotes) 25% of offspring are affected (assuming each parent is a heterozygote) There is no gender preference	A a A: AA Aa a: Aa aa
X-linked dominant	Heterozygote (X′X or X′Y) manifests the condition Affected females (mating with unaffected males) transmit the X-linked gene to 50% of daughters and 50% of sons	X Y X′: X′X X′Y X: XX XY
	Affected males (mating with unaffected females) transmit the X-linked gene to all daughters and no sons	X′ Y X: X′X XY X: X′X XY
X-linked recessive	Heterozygote (X′Y) male manifests the condition Heterozygote (X′X) female is unaffected Affected male (mating with a normal female) transmits the X-linked gene to all daughters (who are carriers) and no sons	X′ Y X: X′X XY X: X′X XY
	Carrier female (mating with a normal male) transmits the X-linked gene to 50% of daughters (who are carriers) and 50% of sons (who are affected)	X Y X′: X′X X′Y X: XX XY

Table 1–37.

Overview of the Inheritance Patterns of Some Musculoskeletal Related Disorders

Autosomal Dominant	Autosomal Recessive	X-Linked Dominant	X-Linked Recessive
Achondroplasia Spondyloepiphyseal dysplasia (congenita form) Multiple epiphyseal dysplasia Metaphyseal chondrodysplasia (Schmid and Jansen types) Kneist dysplasia Malignant hyperthermia Marfan's syndrome Ehlers-Danlos syndrome Osteogenesis imperfecta (types I and IV) Osteochondromatosis Polydactyly	Metaphyseal chondrodysplasia (McKusick type) Diastrophic dysplasia Laron's dysplasia Sickle cell anemia Hurler's syndrome Osteogenesis imperfecta (types II and III) Hypophosphatasia Hereditary vitamin D–dependent rickets Homocystinuria	Hypophosphatemic rickets	Spondyloepiphyseal dysplasia (tarda form) Hemophilia Hunter's syndrome Duchenne's muscular dystrophy

Table 1–38.

Comprehensive Compilation of Inheritance Pattern, Defect, and Associated Gene of Musculoskeletal-Related Disorders

	Disorder	Inheritance Pattern	Defect	Associated Gene
Dysplasias	Achondroplasia	Autosomal dominant	Defect in the fibroblast growth factor (FGF) receptor 3	FGF receptor 3 gene
	Diastrophic dysplasia	Autosomal recessive	Mutation of a gene coding for a sulfate transport protein	Sulfate-transporter gene (chromosome 5)
	Kniest's dysplasia	Autosomal dominant	Defect in type II collagen	COL 2A1
	Laron's dysplasia (pituitary dwarfism)	Autosomal recessive	Defect in the growth hormone receptor	
	McCune-Albright syndrome (polyostotic fibrous dysplasia, café-au-lait spots, precocious puberty)	Sporadic mutation	Germ line defect in the Gsα protein	Mutation of Gsα subunit of the receptor/adenylate cyclase-coupling G proteins
	Metaphyseal chondrodysplasia (Jansen form)	Autosomal dominant		
	Metaphyseal chondrodysplasia (McKusick form)	Autosomal recessive		
	Metaphyseal chondrodysplasia (Schmid-tarda form)	Autosomal dominant	Defect in type X collagen	COL 10A1
	Multiple epiphyseal dysplasia	Autosomal dominant (most commonly)	Cartilage oligomeric matrix protein	
	Spondyloepiphyseal dysplasia	Autosomal dominant (congenita form) X-Linked recessive (tarda form)	Defect in type II collagen	Linked to X p22.12–p22.31 and COL 2A1
	Achondrogenesis	Autosomal recessive	Fetal cartilage fails to mature	
	Apert syndrome	Sporadic mutation/ Autosomal dominant		
	Chondrodysplasia punctata (Conradi-Hünerman)	Autosomal dominant		
	Chondrodysplasia punctata (rhizomelic form)	Autosomal recessive	Defect in subcellular organelles (perioxisomes)	
	Cleiodocranial dysplasia (dysostosis)	Autosomal dominant		
	Dysplasia epiphysealis hemimelica (Trevor's disease)	??		
	Ellis-van Creveld syndrome (chondroectodermal dysplasia)	Autosomal recessive		
	Fibrodysplasia ossifican progressiva	Sporadic mutation/ Autosomal dominant		
	Geroderma osteodysplastica (Walt Disney dwarfism)	Autosomal recessive		
	Grebe chondrodysplasia	Autosomal recessive		
	Hypochondroplasia	Sporadic mutation/ Autosomal dominant		
	Kabuki make-up syndrome	Sporadic mutation		
	Mesomelic dysplasia (Langer type)	Autosomal recessive		
	Mesomelic dysplasia (Nievergelt type)	Autosomal dominant		
	Mesomelic dysplasia (Reinhardt-Pfeiffer type)	Autosomal dominant		
	Mesomelic dysplasia (Werner type)	Autosomal dominant		
	Metatrophic dysplasia	Autosomal recessive		
	Progressive diaphyseal dysplasia (Camurati-Engelmann disease)	Autosomal dominant		
	Pseudoachondroplastic dysplasia	Autosomal dominant		
	Pycnodysostosis	Autosomal recessive		
	Spondylometaphyseal chondrodysplasia	Autosomal dominant		

Table 1–38. *Continued*

Comprehensive Compilation of Inheritance Pattern, Defect, and Associated Gene of Musculoskeletal-Related Disorders

	Disorder	Inheritance Pattern	Defect	Associated Gene
Dysplasias *(Continued)*	Spondylothoracic dysplasia (Jarco-Levin syndrome)	Autosomal recessive		
	Thanatophoric dwarfism	Autosomal dominant		
	Tooth-and-nail syndrome	Autosomal dominant		
	Treacher Collins syndrome (mandibulo-facial dysotosis)	Autosomal dominant		
Metabolic bone diseases	Hereditary vitamin D–dependent rickets	Autosomal recessive	(See Table 1–13)	
	Hypophosphatasia	Autosomal recessive	(See Table 1–13)	
	Hypophosphatemic rickets (vitamin D–resistant rickets)	X-linked dominant	(See Table 1–13)	
	Osteogenesis imperfecta	Autosomal dominant (types I and IV) Autosomal recessive (types II and III)	Defect in type I collagen (abnormal cross-linking)	COL 1A1, COL 1A2
	Albright hereditary osteodystrophy (pseudohypoparathyroidism)	Uncertain	Parathyroid hormone has no effect at the target cells (in the kidney, bone, and intestine)	
	Infantile cortical hyperostosis (Caffey's disease)	???		
	Ochronosis (alkaptonuria)	Autosomal recessive	Defect in the homogentisic acid oxidase system	
	Osteopetrosis	Autosomal dominant (mild, tarda form) Autosomal recessive (infantile, malignant form)		
Connective tissue disorders	Marfan syndrome	Autosomal dominant	Fibrillin abnormalities (some patients also have type I collagen abnormalities)	Fibrillin gene (chromosome 15)
	Ehlers-Danlos syndrome (there are at least 13 varieties)	Autosomal dominant (most common)	Defects in types I and III collagen have been described for some varieties; lysyl oxidase abnormalities	COL 1A2 (for Ehlers-Danlos type VII)
	Homocystinuria	Autosomal recessive	Deficiency of the enzyme cystathionine β-synthase	
Mucopolysaccharidosis	Hunter's syndrome ("gargoylism")	X-linked recessive		
	Hurler's syndrome	Autosomal recessive	Deficiency of the enzyme alpha-L-iduronidase	
	Maroteaux-Lamy syndrome	Autosomal recessive		
	Morquio's syndrome	Autosomal recessive		
	Sanfilippo's syndrome	Autosomal recessive		
	Scheie's syndrome	Autosomal recessive	Deficiency of the enzyme alpha-L-iduronidase	
Muscular dystrophies	Duchenne's muscular dystrophy	X-linked recessive	Defect on the short arm of the X chromosome	Dystrophin gene
	Becker's dystrophy	X-linked recessive		
	Fascioscapulohumeral dystrophy	Autosomal dominant		
	Limb-girdle dystrophy	Autosomal recessive		
	Steinert's disease (myotonic dystrophy)	Autosomal dominant		
Hematologic disorders	Hemophilia (A and B)	X-linked recessive	Hemophilia A–factor VIII deficiency Hemophilia B–factor IX deficiency	
	Sickle cell anemia	Autosomal recessive	Hemoglobin abnormality (hemoglobin S)	
	Gaucher's disease	Autosomal recessive	Deficient activity of the enzyme β-glucosidase (glucocerebrosidase)	

Table continued on following page

Table 1–38. *Continued*

Comprehensive Compilation of Inheritance Pattern, Defect, and Associated Gene of Musculoskeletal-Related Disorders

	Disorder	Inheritance Pattern	Defect	Associated Gene
Hematologic disorders *(Continued)*	Hemochromatosis	Autosomal recessive		
	Niemann-Pick disease	Autosomal recessive	Accumulation of sphingomyelin in cellular lysosomes	
	Smith-Lemli-Opitz syndrome	Uncertain		
	Thalassemia	Autosomal recessive	Abnormal production of hemoglobin A	
	von Willebrand's disease	Autosomal dominant		
Chromosomal disorders with musculoskeletal abnormalities	Down syndrome		Trisomy of chromosome 21	
	Angelman's syndrome		Chromosome 15 abnormality	
	Clinodactyly		Associated with many genetic anomalies including trisomy of chromosomes 8 and 21	
	Edwards' syndrome		Trisomy of chromosome 18	
	Fragile X syndrome	X-linked trait (does not follow the typical pattern of an X-linked trait)		Xq27-Xq28
	Klinefelter's syndrome (XXY)		Male has an extra X chromosome	
	Langer-Giedion syndrome	Sporadic mutation	Chromosome 8 abnormality	
	Nail-patella syndrome	Autosomal dominant	Chromosome 9 abnormality	
	Patau's syndrome		Trisomy of chromosome 13	
	Turner's syndrome (XO)		Female missing one of the two X chromosomes	
Neurologic disorders	Charcot-Marie-Tooth disease	Autosomal dominant (most common)		
	Congenital insensitivity to pain	Autosomal recessive		
	Dejerine-Sottas disease	Autosomal recessive		
	Friedreich's ataxia	Autosomal recessive		
	Huntington's disease	Autosomal dominant		
	Menkes' syndrome	X-linked recessive	Inability to absorb and use copper	
	Pelizaeus-Merzbacher disease	X-linked recessive	Defect in the gene for proteolipid (a component of myelin)	
	Riley-Day syndrome	Autosomal recessive		
	Spinal muscular atrophy (Werdnig-Hoffman disease and Kugelberg-Welander disease)	Autosomal recessive		
	Sturge-Weber syndrome	Sporadic mutation		
	Tay-Sachs disease	Autosomal recessive	Deficiency in the enzyme hexosaminidase A	
Diseases associated with neoplasias	Ewing's sarcoma			11;22 chromosomal translocation
	Multiple endocrine neoplasia I (MENI)	Autosomal dominant		RET
	MENII	Autosomal dominant		
	MENIII	Autosomal dominant	Chromosome 10 abnormality	
	Neurofibromatosis (von Recklinghausen's disease)	Autosomal dominant		NF1, NF2
Miscellaneous disorders	Malignant hyperthermia	Autosomal dominant		
	Osteochondromatosis	Autosomal dominant		
	Polydactyly	Autosomal dominant (a small number of cases of sporadic gene mutations have been reported)		

Table 1–38. *Continued*

Comprehensive Compilation of Inheritance Pattern, Defect, and Associated Gene of Musculoskeletal-Related Disorders

	Disorder	Inheritance Pattern	Defect	Associated Gene
Miscellaneous disorders *(Continued)*	Captodactyly	Autosomal dominant		
	Cerebro-oculo-facio-skeletal syndrome	Autosomal recessive		
	Congenital contractural arachnodactyly			Fibrillin gene (chromosome 5)
	Distal arthrogryposis syndrome	Autosomal dominant		
	Dupuytren's contracture	Autosomal dominant (with partial sex-limitation)		
	Fabry's disease	X-linked recessive	Deficiency of alpha-galactosidase A	
	Fanconi's pancytopenia	Autosomal recessive		
	Freeman-Sheldon syndrome (craniocarpotarsal dysplasia; whistling face syndrome)	Autosomal dominant Autosomal recessive		
	GM1 gangliosidosis	Autosomal recessive		
	Hereditary anonychia	Autosomal dominant Autosomal recessive		
	Holt-Oram syndrome	Autosomal dominant		
	Humeroradial synostosis	Autosomal dominant Autosomal recessive		
	Klippel-Feil syndrome		Faulty development of spinal segments along the embryonic neural tube	
	Klippel-Trenaunay-Weber syndrome	Sporadic mutation		
	Krabbe's disease	Autosomal recessive	Deficiency of galactocerebroside β-galactosidase	
	Larsen's syndrome	Autosomal dominant Autosomal recessive		
	Lesch-Nyham disease	X-linked trait	Absence of the enzyme hypoxanthine guanine phosphoribosyltransferase	
	Madelung's deformity	Autosomal dominant		
	Mannosidosis	Autosomal recessive	Deficiency of the enzyme alpha-monosidase	
	Maple syrup urine disease	Autosomal recessive	Defective metabolism of the amino acids leucine, isoleucine, and valine	
	Meckel syndrome (Gruber's syndrome)	Autosomal recessive		
	Moebius' syndrome	Autosomal dominant		
	Mucolipidosis (oligosaccharidosis)	Autosomal recessive	A family of enzyme deficiency diseases	
	Multiple exostoses	Autosomal dominant		
	Multiple pterygium syndrome	Autosomal recessive		
	Noonan's syndrome	Sporadic mutation		
	Oral-facial-digital (OFD) syndrome	OFDI—X-linked dominant OFDII (Mohr's syndrome)—autosomal recessive		
	Osler-Weber-Rendu syndrome (hereditary hemorrhagic telangiectasia)	Autosomal dominant		
	Pfeiffer's syndrome (acrocephalosyndactyly)	Sporadic mutation/ autosomal dominant		
	Phenylketonuria	Autosomal recessive	Enzyme deficiency characterized by the inability to convert phenylalanine to tyrosine due to a chromosome 12 abnormality	

Table continued on following page

Table 1–38. *Continued*

Comprehensive Compilation of Inheritance Pattern, Defect, and Associated Gene of Musculoskeletal-Related Disorders

	Disorder	Inheritance Pattern	Defect	Associated Gene
Miscellaneous disorders *(Continued)*	Phytanic acid storage disease	Autosomal recessive		
	Progeria (Hutchinson-Gilford progeria syndrome)	Autosomal dominant		
	Proteus syndrome	Autosomal dominant		
	Prune-belly syndrome	Uncertain	Localized mesodermal defect	
	Radioulnar synostosis	Autosomal dominant		
	Rett's syndrome	Sporadic mutation/X-linked dominant		
	Roberts' syndrome (pseudo thalidomide syndrome)	Sporadic mutation/ autosomal recessive		
	Russell-Silver syndrome	Sporadic mutation (possibly X-linked)		
	Saethre-Chotzen syndrome	Autosomal dominant		
	Sandhoff's disease	Autosomal recessive	Enzyme deficiency of hexosaminidase A and B	
	Schwartz-Jampel syndrome	Autosomal recessive		
	Seckel's syndrome (bird-headed dwarfism)	Autosomal recessive		
	Stickler's syndrome (hereditary progressive arthroopthalmopathy)	Autosomal dominant	Collagen abnormality	
	TAR syndrome (thrombocytopenia–aplasia of radius syndrome)	Autosomal recessive		
	Tarsal coalition	Autosomal dominant		
	Trichorrhinophalangeal syndrome	Autosomal dominant		
	Urea cycle defects	Argininemia—autosomal recessive Argininosuccinic aciduria—autosomal recessive Carbamyl phosphate synthetase deficiency—autosomal recessive Citrullinemia—autosomal recessive Ornathine transcarbamylase deficiency—X-linked	A group of enzyme disorders characterized by high levels of ammonia in the blood and tissues	
	VATER association	Sporadic mutation		
	Werner's syndrome	Autosomal recessive		
	Zygodactyly	Autosomal dominant		

d. Trisomy—One chromosome has an extra third chromosome (47 chromosomes).

2. Deletion—A section of one chromosome (in a chromosome pair) is absent.
3. Duplication—An extra section of one chromosome (in a chromosome pair) is present.
4. Translocation—A portion of one chromosome is exchanged with a portion of another chromosome.
5. Inversion—A broken portion of a chromosome reattaches to the same chromosome in the same location but in a reverse direction.

E. The Genetics of Musculoskeletal Conditions and Conditions Associated with Musculoskeletal Abnormalities—Table 1–37 shows the inheritance pattern of the most commonly tested musculoskeletal (and related) disorders. Table 1–38 is a comprehensive compilation of the genetic defects involved (when known) of disorders that display musculoskeletal manifestations.

Section 5

Orthopaedic Infections and Microbiology

I. **Musculoskeletal Infections**—The following should serve as an overview of orthopaedic infections. Specific infections unique to particular orthopaedic areas are covered in detail in the appropriate chapters that follow. In general, the initial treatment regimen recommendations, which follow, are based on the presumed type of infection based on clinical findings and symptoms. Definitive treatment should be based on final culture results when available. **Glycocalyx** is an exopolysaccharide coating that envelops bacteria. Bacterial adherence to biologic implants is promoted by an inflammatory tissue interface and inhibited by a noninflammatory tissue interface.

A. Soft-Tissue Infections

1. Cellulitis—An infection of the subcutaneous tissues. The infection is generally deeper and has less distinct margins in cellulitis than in erysipelas. Clinical findings include erythema, tenderness, warmth, lymphangitis, and lymphadenopathy. **Group A strep is the most common organism; *S. aureus* is much less common.** Antimicrobial therapy includes the penicillinase-resistant synthetic penicillins (PRSPs) (nafcillin or oxacillin), or cefazolin, or for less severe cases, oral dicloxacillin. Alternative treatment regimens include: erythromycin, first-generation cephalosporins, amoxicillin (Augmentin), azithromycin, and clarithromycin.
2. Erysipelas—An infection of the superficial soft tissues characterized by a progressively enlarging, well-demarcated, red, raised, painful plaque. **In nondiabetic patients, the most common organism is group A strep.** The clinical picture is similar to that of cellulitis but is more superficial and the infection is well demarcated; the treatment regimen is the same as with cellulitis. In diabetic patients with erysipelas, the most common organisms are group A strep, *S. aureus*, enterobacteriaceae, and clostridia (uncommon). Early and mild cases are best treated with a second or third-generation cephalosporin or amoxicillin; severe cases may require imipenem (Primaxin), meropenem, or trovafloxacin. Diabetic patients with erysipelas may require surgical débridement to rule out necrotizing fasciitis and obtain definitive cultures. Septic patients should undergo x-ray evaluation to rule out gas in the soft tissues.
3. Necrotizing Fasciitis ("Flesh-Eating Bacteria")—An aggressive, life-threatening fascial infection that may be associated with an underlying vascular disease (particularly diabetes). Necrotizing fasciitis commonly occurs post surgery or post trauma or after a streptococcal skin infection. Many cases of acute necrotizing fasciitis involve several organisms. **The most commonly isolated organism in necrotizing fasciitis is group A strep.** Clostridia or polymicrobial infections (aerobic plus anaerobic) are also seen. **Extensive surgical débridement (involving the entire length of the overlying cellulitis) and intravenous antibiotics are required emergently.** Initial antibiotic treatment is clindamycin plus penicillin G; alternative initial antibiotic treatment includes ceftriaxone or erythromycin.
4. Gas Gangrene—**An infection of muscle that is commonly found in grossly contaminated traumatic wounds (particularly those that are closed primarily).** The clinical presentation usually includes progressive pain, edema (distant from the wound), and a **foul-smelling serosanguineous discharge. Radiographs typically show widespread gas in the soft tissues.** The gas facilitates rapid spread of the infection. Gas gangrene is classically caused by *Clostridium perfringens* or *Clostridium specticum* or other histotoxic *Clostridium* species (gram-positive anaerobic spore-forming rods that produce exotoxins). The exotoxins create local edema, necrosis of fat and muscle, and thrombosis of local vessels. Symptoms include severe pain, high fevers, chills, tachycardia, confusion, and findings consistent with toxemia. **Surgical (radical) débridement with fasciotomies is the primary treatment;** hyperbaric oxygen may be a useful adjuvant therapy, although its effectiveness remains inconclusive. Initial antibiotic therapy should include clindamycin plus penicillin G. Alternative therapies include ceftriaxone or erythromycin.
5. Toxic Shock Syndrome
   a. Staphylococcal Toxic Shock Syndrome—A severe condition caused by the toxin of *Staphylococcus staph aureus*. In orthopaedics, this infection develops secondary to colonization of surgical/traumatic wounds (even after minor trauma). The patient displays fever and hypotension and has an erythematous macular rash with a serous exudate (gram-positive cocci are present). **The wound may look very benign and**

may be misleading with regard to the seriousness of the underlying condition. Toxic shock syndrome can develop in women in association with tampon use and colonization of the vagina with toxin-producing *S. aureus*. **Remember, toxic shock syndrome is a form of toxemia (from toxins produced by *S. aureus*), not a septicemia.** Treatment of wound infections include irrigation and débridement and IV antibiotics. Initial treatment is with a PRSP (nafcillin or oxacillin); alternative antibiotic treatment includes a first-generation cephalosporin. Patients with toxic shock syndrome may also require **emergent fluid resuscitation.**

b. Streptococcal Toxic Shock Syndrome—This condition is commonly associated with erysipelas or necrotizing fasciitis. The offending organism can be group A, B, C, or G *Streptococcus pyogenes.*

6. Surgical Wound Infection—**The most common offending organism is *S. aureus*.** Group A strep and enterobacteriaceae are also not uncommon. **There has been an increase in the incidence of *Staphalococcus epidermidis* wound infections.** Methacillin-resistant *Staphylococcus* species infections have also increased over the past several years and are best treated with vancomycin (alternatives to vancomycin for methacillin–resistant *S. aureus* include teicoplanin, trimethoprim (Bactrim), doxycycline, minocycline, fusidic acid, fosfomycin, rifampin, and novobiocin). Vancomycin-methacillin-resistant *S. aureus* has also been reported; the treatment for these organisms is currently quinupristin/dalfopristin.
7. Bite injuries—Bite injuries are summarized in Table 1–39.
8. Marine injuries—Marine injuries involve organisms that can cause indolent infections. Cultures may take several weeks to grow on culture media. In the patient with a history of a fishing (or other marine) injury who has an indolent low-grade infection, consider atypical mycobacteria (such as *Mycobacterium marinum*). It is important to culture the specimens at 30°C (86°F).

B. Bone Infections

1. Introduction—Osteomyelitis is an infection of bone and bone marrow that may be caused by direct inoculation of an open traumatic wound or by blood-borne organisms (hematogenous). **It is not possible to predict the microscopic organism that is causing osteomyelitis based on the clinical picture and the age of the patient; therefore, a specific microbiologic diagnosis via deep cultures is essential (organisms isolated from sinus tract drainage typically do not accurately reflect the organisms present deep within the wound and within bone).**
2. Acute Hematogenous Osteomyelitis—Bone and bone marrow infection caused by blood-borne organisms. Children are commonly affected (boys are more commonly affected than

Table 1–39.

Bite Injuries

Source of Bite	Organism(s)	Primary Antimicrobial (or Drug) Regimen
Human	*Strep. viridans* (100%) *Bacteroides* *Staph. epidermidis* *Corynebacterium* *Staph. aureus* *Peptostreptococcus* *Eikenella*	Amoxicillin/clavulanate (Augmentin) [*Eikenella* → cefoxitan or ampicillin]
Dog	*Strep. viridans* *Pasteurella multocida* *Bacteroides* *Fusobacterium*	Pencillin V or ampicillin consider antirabies treatment
Cat	*Pasteurella multocida* *Staph. aureus* Possibly tularemia	Amoxicillin/clavulanate (Augmentin) *or* penicillin V
Rat	*Streptobacillus moniliformis*	Ampicillin antirabies treatment *not* indicated
Pig	Polymicrobic (aerobes and anerobes)	Amoxicillin/clavulanate (Augmentin)
Skunk, raccoon, bat	?	Ampicillin antirabies treatment indicated
Pit viper (snake)	*Pseudomonas* Enterobacteriaceae *Staph. epidermidis* *Clostridium*	Antivenom therapy ceftriaxone tetanus prophylaxis
Brown recluse spider	—	Dapsone
Catfish sting	Toxins (may become secondarily infected)	Amoxicillin/clavulanate (Augmentin)

Adapted from Sanford J.P.: Guide to Antimicrobial Therapy, pp. 30–31. Dallas, Antimicrobial Therapy, Inc., 1994.

girls). In children, the infection is most common in the metaphysis or epiphysis of the long bones and is more common in the lower extremity than the upper extremity. Radiographic changes of acute hematogenous osteomyelitis include soft-tissue swelling (early), bone demineralization (10–14 days), and **sequestra** (dead bone with surrounding granulation tissue) and **involucrum** (periosteal new bone) later. Pain, loss of function of the involved extremity, and a soft-tissue abscess may be present. Patients commonly show an elevated WBC count and an elevated ESR; blood cultures may also be positive. **The most sensitive monitor of the course of infection in children with acute hematogenous osteomyelitis is C-reactive protein.** Nuclear medicine studies may be helpful in equivocal cases. **MRI shows changes in bone and bone marrow before plain films.** Empiric therapy should be started after cultures have been obtained, either by aspiration or surgical drainage when indicated. The indications for operative intervention include: (1) drainage of an abscess, (2) débridement of infected tissues to prevent further destruction, and (3) refractory cases that show no improvement following nonoperative treatment. The treatment of acute osteomyelitis may be summarized as follows: (1) identification of the organism(s), (2) selection of appropriate antibiotics, (3) delivery of antibiotics to the site of infection, and (4) halting tissue destruction. Empiric therapy prior to availability of definitive cultures is based on the patient's age and/or special circumstances.

a. **Newborn (up to 4 Months of Age)**—The most common organisms include *S. aureus*, gram-negative bacilli, and group B streptococcus. Primary empiric therapy includes nafcillin or oxacillin plus a third-generation cephalosporin. Alternative antibiotic therapy includes vancomycin plus a third-generation cephalosporin. Newborns with hematogenous osteomyelitis may be afebrile, and the best predictors of the osteomyelitis are local signs in the extremity, including warmth and others. Almost 70% of newborn patients with hematogenous osteomyelitis have positive blood cultures.
b. **Children of 4 Years of Age or Older**—The most common organisms are *S. aureus*, group A Strep, and coliforms (uncommon). The empiric treatment of choice is nafcillin or oxacillin; alternative regimens include vancomycin or clindamycin. When the Gram stain shows gram-negative organisms, a third-generation cephalosporin should be added. It should be noted that **with recent immunization, *H. influenzae* bone infections of hematogenous osteomyelitis have almost been completely eliminated.**
c. **Adults of 21 Years of Age or Older—The most common organism is *S. aureus*,** but a wide variety of other organisms have been isolated. Initial empiric therapy includes nafcillin or oxacillin or cefazolin; vancomycin can be used as an alternative initial therapy.
d. Sickle Cell Anemia—*Salmonella* is a characteristic organism. The primary treatment is with one of the fluoroquinolones (only in adults); alternative treatment is with a third-generation cephalosporin.
e. Hemodialysis Patients and Intravenous Drug Abusers—*S. aureus*, *S. epidermidis*, and *Pseudomonas aeruginosa* are common organisms. The treatment of choice is one of the PRSPs plus ciprofloxacin; an alternative treatment is vancomycin with ciprofloxacin.

3. Acute Osteomyelitis (After Open Fracture or Open Reduction with Internal Fixation)—Clinical findings may be similar to acute hematogenous osteomyelitis. Treatment includes radical irrigation and débridement with removal of orthopaedic hardware as necessary. Open wounds may require rotational or free flaps. The most common offending organisms are *S. aureus*, *P. aeruginosa*, and coliforms. Empiric therapy prior to definitive cultures is nafcillin with ciprofloxacin; alternative therapy is vancomycin with a third-generation cephalosporin. Patients with acute osteomyelitis and vascular insufficiency and those who are immunocompromised generally show a polymicrobic picture.
4. Chronic Osteomyelitis—May arise as a result of an inappropriately treated acute osteomyelitis, trauma, or soft-tissue spread, especially in the Cierney type C elderly host (Table 1–40), the immunosuppressed, diabetics, and IV drug abusers. Chronic osteomyelitis may be classified anatomically (Fig. 1–87). Skin and soft tissues are often involved and the sinus tract may occasionally develop into squamous cell carcinoma. Periods of quiescence (of the infection) are often followed by acute exacerbations. Nuclear medicine studies are often helpful for determining the activity of the disease. **Operative sampling of deep specimens from multiple foci is the most**

Table 1–40.

Infected Host Types

Type	Description	Risk
A	Normal immune response; nonsmoker	Minimal
B	Local or mild systemic deficiency; smoker	Moderate
C	Major nutritional or systemic disorder	High

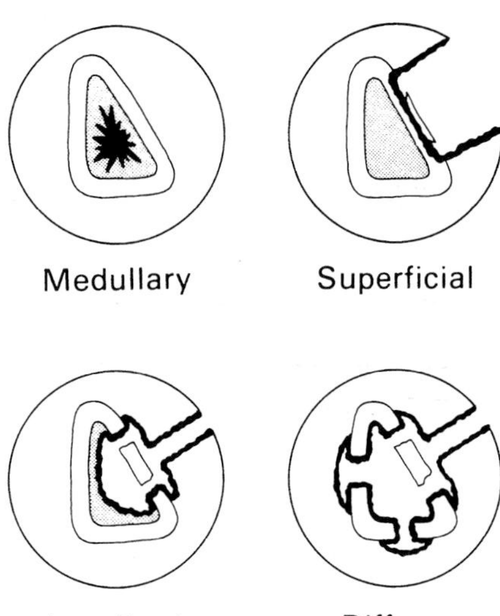

Figure 1–87. Cierney's anatomic classification of adult chronic osteomyelitis. (From Cierney, G., III: Chronic osteomyelitis: Results of treatment. Instr. Course Lect. 39:495, 1990.)

accurate means of identifying the pathologic organisms. A combination of IV antibiotics (based on deep cultures), surgical débridement, bone grafting, and soft-tissue coverage is often required. Unfortunately, amputations are still required in certain cases. *S. aureus*, Enterobacteriaceae, and *P. aeruginosa* are the most frequent offending organisms. **Treatment is based on cultures and sensitivity testing, and empiric therapy is not indicated in chronic osteomyelitis.**

5. Subacute Osteomyelitis—Usually discovered radiologically in a patient with a painful limp and no systemic (and often no local) signs or symptoms. Subacute osteomyelitis may arise secondary to a partially treated acute osteomyelitis or occasionally develops in a fracture hematoma. Unlike in acute osteomyelitis, WBC count and blood cultures are frequently normal. ESR, bone cultures, and radiographs are often useful. Subacute osteomyelitis most commonly affects the femur and tibia; and unlike acute osteomyelitis, it can cross the physis, even in older children. Radiographic changes include **Brodie's abscess** (a localized radiolucency usually seen in the metaphyses of long bones). It is sometimes difficult to differentiate from Ewing's sarcoma. When localized to the epiphysis only, other lesions (e.g., chondroblastoma) must be ruled out. **Epiphyseal osteomyelitis is caused almost exclusively by *S. aureus*.** Treatment of Brodie's abscess in the metaphysis includes surgical curettage. Epiphyseal osteomyelitis requires surgical drainage only if pus is present (48 hours of IV antibiotics followed by 6 weeks of oral antibiotics is curative otherwise).
6. Chronic Sclerosing Osteomyelitis—An unusual infection that primarily involves diaphyseal bones of adolescents. Typified by intense proliferation of the periosteum leading to bony deposition, it may be caused by anaerobic organisms. Insidious onset, dense progressive sclerosis on radiographs, and localized pain and tenderness are common. Malignancy must be ruled out. Surgical and antibiotic therapy are usually not curative.
7. Chronic Multifocal Osteomyelitis—Caused by an infectious agent, it appears in children without systemic symptoms. Normal laboratory values, except for an elevated ESR, are common. Radiographs demonstrate multiple metaphyseal lytic lesions, especially in the medial clavicle, distal tibia, and distal femur. Symptomatic treatment only is recommended because this condition usually resolves spontaneously.
8. Osteomyelitis with Unusual Organisms—Several unusual organisms occur in certain clinical settings (Table 1–41). Radiographs show characteristic features in syphilis (*Treponema pallidum*) (radiolucency in the metaphysis from granulation tissue) and tuberculosis (joint destruction on both sides of a joint). Histology can also be helpful (e.g., tuberculosis with granulomas).

C. Joint Infections
1. Septic Arthritis—Commonly follows hematogenous spread or extension of metaphyseal

Table 1–41.
Unusual Organisms That May Be Found in Osteomyelitis

Organism	Risk Factor(s)	Symptoms/Signs/Findings	Treatment
Serratia marcescens	IV drug abuse	Axial skeleton	Cotrimoxazole
Pseudomonas aeruginosa	IV drug abuse	Nonspecific	Aminoglycoside
Brucella (G−)	Meat handling	Flat bones	Tetracycline/Septra
Salmonella	Sickle cell disease	Asymptomatic	Ampicillin
Anaerobes	Skin contamination	Tissue culture	Clindamycin/cephalosporin
Fungi	Skin contamination	Special study	Amphotericin B
Treponema pallidum	Sexual contact	Nontender swelling	Penicillin
Mycobacteria	TB/leprosy/fishermen	PPD/granuloma/culture at 30°C	PAS, isoniazid

TB, tuberculosis; PPD, purified protein derivative; PAS, *p*-aminosalicylic acid.

osteomyelitis in children. Can also arise as a complication of a diagnostic or therapeutic procedure. Most cases involve infants (hip) and children. **The metaphysis of the proximal femur, proximal humerus, radial neck, and distal fibula are within their respective joint capsules; metaphyseal osteomyelitis can rupture into the joint in these areas. The most common site at which septic arthritis follows acute osteomyelitis is the proximal femur/hip.** RA (tuberculosis most characteristic, *S. aureus* most common) and IV drug abuse (*Pseudomonas* most characteristic) predispose adults. Surgical drainage or daily aspiration is the mainstay of treatment. Open (or arthroscopic) drainage is required for septic hip joints. SI joint sepsis is unusual and is best diagnosed by physical examination (flexion abduction external rotation [FABER] most specific), ESR, bone scan, CT scan, and aspiration. A pannus (much as in inflammatory arthritis) can be seen in tuberculosis infections. Late sequelae of septic arthritis include soft-tissue contractures that can sometimes be treated with soft-tissue procedures (such as a quadricepsplasty). Empiric therapy prior to availability of definitive cultures is based on the patient age and/or special circumstances.

a. **Newborn (up to 3 Months of Age)—The most common organisms include *S. aureus* and group B strep; less common organisms include** Enterobacteriaceae and *N. gonorrhoeae*. Adjacent bony involvement is seen in almost 70% of patients. Blood cultures are commonly positive. Initial treatment is with a PRSP plus a third-generation cephalosporin. Alternative treatment is with a PRSP plus an antipseudomonal aminoglycosidic antibiotic.
b. **Children (3 Months to 14 Years of Age)**—The most common organisms are as follows: *S. aureus*, *Streptococcus pyogenes*, *Streptococcus pneumoniae*, *H. influenzae* **(there has been a marked decrease in the incidence of *H. influenzae* septic arthritis with vaccination),** and gram-negative bacilli. Initial treatment is with a PRSP plus a third-generation cephalosporin; alternative treatment is with vancomycin plus a third-generation cephalosporin.
c. **Acute Monoarticular Septic Arthritis in Sexually Active Adults Ages 15–40 Years**—The most common organisms include *N. gonorrhoeae*, *S. aureus*, streptococci, and aerobic gram-negative bacilli (uncommon). Empiric drug therapy when the Gram stain is negative is ceftriaxone or cefotaxime or ceftizoxime; when the Gram stain shows gram-positive cocci in clusters, the treatment is nafcillin or oxacillin.
d. **Acute Monoarticular Septic Arthritis in Sexually Active Adults Older Than Age 40**—The most common organisms are *N. gonorrhoeae* or *S. aureus* (in persons with RA the most common organisms are *S. aureus*, streptococci, and gram-negative bacilli). Antibiotic treatment is a PRSP plus a third-generation cephalosporin or a PRSP plus ciprofloxacin.
e. **Chronic Monoarticular Septic Arthritis**—The most common organisms are *Brucella*, *Nocardia*, *Mycobacteria*, and fungi.
f. **Polyarticular Septic Arthritis**—The most common organisms are gonococci, *Borrelia burgdorferi*, acute rheumatic fever, or viruses.

2. Septic Bursitis—Most commonly caused by an *S. aureus* infection. Treatment is with a PRSP.
3. Infected Total Joint Arthroplasty—Covered in Chapter 4, Adult Reconstruction, but bears some mention here. Perioperative IV antibiotics are the most effective method for decreasing its incidence, although good operative technique, laminar flow (avoiding obstruction between the air source and the operative wound), and special "space" suits also have a role. The ESR is the most sensitive indicator of infection, but it is nonspecific. Culture of the hip aspirate is sensitive and specific. C-reactive protein may also be helpful. Preoperative skin ulcerations are associated with an increased risk for infecting a TKA. **Acute infections (within 2–3 weeks of arthroplasty) can usually be treated with prosthesis salvage, exchanging only polyethylene components (provided the metallic components are stable).** Synovectomy for an acute TKA infection is also beneficial. **Delayed or chronic TJA infections require implant (and cement) removal.** A staged exchange arthroplasty may later be performed, depending on the virulence of the organism. ***S. epidermidis* is the most common pathogen;** the next most frequent pathogens are *S. aureus* and group B streptococcus. Polymicrobial organisms may form an overlying glycocalyx, making infection control difficult without removing the prosthesis and vigorous débridement. However, according to Cierney, the host is more important than the organism in terms of risk (see Table 1–40). Use of antibiotic-impregnated cement in revision arthroplasties and antibiotic spacers/beads in infected total joints may be helpful. Reimplantation after thorough débridement and use of polymethylmethacrylate (PMMA) with antibiotics has been successful at variable intervals. Some advocate frozen sections at the time of reimplantation to ensure that local tissues have fewer than 5–10 PMNs per high-power field. The most accurate test for infection of a TJA is a tissue culture. Routine

aspiration of all hip joints prior to revision THA results in a high incidence of false-positive cultures; preoperative aspiration of the knee joint prior to revision TKA appears to be a useful study to rule out infection. Most patients who have undergone total joint replacement do not need prophylactic antibiotics when undergoing dental surgery. The most common organism infecting a TJA after a dental procedure is **peptostreptococcus.**

4. Clenched Fist Lacerations (to the Face or Mouth)—Lacerations overlying the joints of the hand (that has struck another person's mouth ["fight bite"]) should be considered a penetrating joint injury. These wounds should be operatively explored, and the patient will need IV antibiotics.

D. Other Infections

1. Tetanus—**A potentially lethal neuroparalytic disease caused by an exotoxin of *Clostridium tetani.*** Prophylaxis against tetanus requires classifying the patient's wound (tetanus prone or nontetanus prone) and a complete history of the patient's immunizations. Tetanus-prone wounds are those that are greater than 6 hours old, have an irregular configuration, have a depth greater than 1 cm or are the result of a projectile injury, crush injury, burn, or frostbite, have devitalized tissue, and are grossly contaminated. Patients with tetanus-prone wounds who have an unknown tetanus status or have received fewer than three immunizations require tetanus and diphtheria toxoids and tetanus immune globulin (human). Patients with tetanus-prone wounds who were fully immunized do not require immune globulin; however, tetanus toxoid should be administered if the wound is severe or more than 24 hours old or if the patient has not received a booster within the past 5 years. The only type of patient with a non–tetanus-prone wound who requires any treatment is one with an unknown immunization history or a history of fewer than three doses of tetanus immunization; these patients require tetanus toxoid. The treatment of established tetanus is primarily to control the patient's muscle spasms with diazepam. Initial antibiotic therapy includes penicillin G or doxycycline; alternative antibiotic therapy includes metronidazole.

2. Rabies—**An acute infection characterized by irritation of the central nervous system that may be followed by paralysis and death. The organism involved in rabies is a neurotropic virus that may be present in the saliva of rabid animals.** In bites of dogs and cats, healthy animals should be observed for 10 days, and there is no need to start anti-rabies treatment. If the dog or cat begins to experience symptoms, human rabies immune globulin with human diploid cell vaccine or rabies vaccine absorbed (inactived) should be started. For bites from dogs and cats that are suspected of being rabid or are known to be rabid, immediately vaccinate the patient. Bites from skunks, raccoons, bats, foxes, and most carnivores should be considered rabid, and the patient should be immunized immediately. Bites from animals that rarely require anti-rabies treatment include the following: mice, rats, chipmunks, gerbils, guinea pigs, hamsters, squirrels, rabbits, and rodents.

3. Puncture Wounds of the Foot—**The most common organism from the puncture of a nail through the sole of a tennis shoe is *Staphylococcus;* the most characteristic organism is *P. aeruginosa.*** *Pseudomonas* infections (gram-negative rod) requires aggressive débridement and appropriate antibiotics (which may often require a two-antibiotic regimen). Initial antibiotic regimen should include ceftazidime or cefepime or tobramycin plus carbenicillin; alternative initial antibiotic regimen might include ciprofloxacin (except in children). The prophylactic antibiotic treatment for a patient presenting with a recent (hours) puncture through the sole of a tennis shoe (without infection) remains controversial. **Osteomyelitis develops in 1–2% of children who sustain a puncture wound through the sole of a tennis shoe.**

4. Diabetic Foot Infections
   a. Limited in Extent (No Osteomyelitis, No Previous History of Foot Infection)—The most common organism is aerobic gram-positive cocci. The antibiotic regimen of choice is clindamycin or a first-generation cephalosporin. Débridement of soft tissues is performed as clinically indicated.
   b. Chronic, Recurrent, Limb-Threatening Diabetic Foot—These infections can be life-threatening and, generally, **cultures show a polymicrobial picture** (including aerobic cocci, aerobic bacilli, and anaerobes). **In early cases or relatively milder cases** of chronic recurrent limb-threatening diabetic foot, the initial antibiotic regimen includes cefoxitin or ciprofloxacin with clindamycin or metronidazole. In cases of **severe chronic recurrent limb-threatening diabetic foot** or when the patient is septic, the antibiotic regimen of choice includes imipenem/cilastatin (Primaxin) or meropenem or timentin or ampicillin/sulbactum (Unasyn) or trovafloxacin or piperacillin—tazobactam or a PRSP with an antipseudomonal aminoglycosidic antibiotic (or aztreonam) with clindamycin. Cultures from diabetic foot

ulcers are unreliable. **Rapid surgical intervention with irrigation and débridement is essential.** Surgical débridement helps differentiate diabetic foot from necrotizing fasciitis or gas gangrene.

5. Paronychia—Infection/inflammation of the paronychial fold on the side of the nail.
   a. Nail Biting and Manicuring—The most common organism is *S. aureus;* anaerobes are also common. The initial antibiotic treatment includes clindamycin; erythromycin is an alternative initial antibiotic treatment.
   b. Dentist, Anesthesiologist, Wrestlers, (Those Who Are in Contact with the Oral Mucosa of Others)—The most common organism is herpes simplex (herpetic whitlow). Patients commonly present with vesicles that contain clear fluid. Gram's stain and routine cultures are negative. The treatment of choice for these patients is acyclovir; there is no need to débride the vesicles.
   c. Dishwashers or Others Who Engage in Activities that Involve Prolonged Immersion in Water—The most common organism is *Candida,* and the treatment is topical clotrimazole.
6. Fungal Infections—Fungi are multicellular organisms with mycelia (branches) that induce a hypersensitivity reaction in tissues, causing chronic granuloma, abscess, and necrosis. Surgical treatment and **amphotericin B** administration are often required. Oral ketoconazole is effective for some limited infections.
7. Human Immunodeficiency Virus (HIV) Infection—Incidence is high in the homosexual male population and is becoming increasingly common in heterosexual patients. Additionally, a large portion of the hemophiliac population is affected. The virus primarily affects the lymphocyte and macrophage cell lines and **decreases the number of T helper cells (formerly known as T4 lymphocytes, now known as CD4 cells). The diagnosis of AIDS requires one of the following two scenarios: (1) an HIV-positive test result plus one of the opportunistic infections (such as pneumocystis), or (2) an HIV-positive test result plus a CD4 count of less than 200 (normal uninfected persons have a CD4 count of 700–1200).** This disease has increased the importance of blood and body fluid handling precautions during trauma management and surgery. The risk of seroconversion from a contaminated needle stick is 0.3%; the risk increases if the exposure involves a larger amount of blood. The risk of seroconversion from mucous membrane exposure is 0.09%. The risk of HIV transmission via a processed musculoskeletal allograft is 1 in 1.5 million; **donor screening is the most important factor in preventing viral transmission. Unfortunately, blood donated for transfusion that tests negative for the HIV antibody may transmit HIV to the blood recipient because there is a delay (in the donor) between infection with HIV and the development of a detectable antibody.** The risk of transmission of HIV via a blood transfusion is 1 in 440,000 to 1 in 600,000 per unit transfused. HIV positivity is not a contraindication to performing required surgical procedures. HIV-positive patients (even those who are asymptomatic) with traumatic orthopaedic injuries (especially open fractures) or those undergoing certain orthopaedic surgical procedures appear to be at increased risk for wound infections as well as non–wound-related complications (e.g., urinary tract infection, pneumonia). Patients with HIV can develop secondary rheumatologic conditions such as Reiter's syndrome. Fetal acquired immunodeficiency syndrome is transmitted across the placenta, and affected children typically have a box-like forehead, wide eyes, a small head, and growth failure.
8. Hepatitis—Three types are commonly recognized.
   a. Hepatitis A—Common in areas with poor sanitation and public health concerns. Not a major problem regarding surgical transmission.
   b. Hepatitis B—Approximately 200,000 people are infected with the hepatitis B virus each year, and there are more than 1 million carriers. Screening and use of a vaccine has reduced the risk of transmission for health care workers. Immune globulin is administered after exposure in nonvaccinated persons. Neither vaccine nor immune globulin administration has been documented as causing HIV transmission.
   c. Hepatitis C (Non-A, Non-B)—The offending virus has been identified (hepatitis C virus). It is the **most common transfusion-associated hepatitis and is also related to IV drug abuse.**
9. Lyme Disease—Discussed in the section on Arthroses. A new Lyme disease vaccine, LYMErix (Recombinant OspA), is available for persons 15–70 years of age.
10. Allograft Infection—May involve up to 20% of allografts; requires aggressive measures to control.
11. Meningococcemia—Can develop in patients with multiple infarcts, such as those with **electrical burns.**
12. Marjolin's Ulcer—Squamous cell carcinoma that develops in patients with chronic drain-

age from sinus tracts. Seen in untreated chronic osteomyelitis.

13. Nutritional Status and Infection—Nutrition is critical to decreasing the incidence of postoperative infection. Malnutrition is common after multiple trauma.
14. Postsplenectomy Patients—Susceptible to streptococcal infections and respond poorly to them.
15. Infections of the Spine (Also Discussed in Chapter 7, Spine)
    a. Discitis—Children present with back pain and may have difficulty walking or sitting. Radiographs may appear normal; bone scans and MRI may show early changes. Initial treatment is immobilization and antibiotics. A biopsy is indicated if the initial treatment fails.
    b. Vertebral Osteomyelitis—Activity-related pain of insidious onset is the most common symptom. Neurologic signs are not usually seen until late in the disease's progression. Weight loss and chills are common. The lumbar spine is the most common site of vertebral osteomyelitis; diabetics are particularly prone to vertebral osteomyelitis. Both a bone scan and MRI are usually diagnostic. Recommended treatment is immobilization and antibiotics. Surgery (I&D and immediate spinal arthrodesis) is needed if: (1) nonoperative treatment fails or (2) there is vertebral collapse with a neurologic deficit.
    c. Epidural Abscess—Onset of symptoms may be rapid. There is often a history of recent trauma. There is generally markedly limited ROM to the lumbar spine and a positive straight leg raising test (indicating a process that is associated with inflammation of the dura or nerve root sleeves). Bone scans are typically negative. MRI and contrast CT are excellent methods of imaging an epidural abscess. Because antibiotics are generally ineffective with an abscess, surgical drainage is necessary.
    d. Postoperative Spinal Infections—Early diagnosis is difficult; clinical findings are often vague, and there are no excellent diagnostic tests. Following spinal surgery, both the ESR and C-reactive protein peak at 2–3 days and may remain elevated for as long as 2 weeks. Fever spikes and a rising ESR indicate infection (don't forget the blood cultures). Treatment is IV antibiotics, operative débridement, and retention of spinal implants.
    e. Other Spinal Infections
        1. Pyogenic infections
        2. Tuberculous spondylitis
        3. Coccidioidomycosis spondylitis

II. **Antibiotics**

A. Introduction—Antibiotics in orthopaedics may be used for (1) prophylactic treatment to prevent postoperative sepsis (for clean surgical cases, proper administration is 1 hour preoperatively and continued for 24 hours postoperatively), (2) providing initial care after an open traumatic wound, and (3) treatment of established infections. Perioperative use of first-generation cephalosporins is efficacious in cases requiring insertion of hardware. Type I and II open fractures require a first-generation cephalosporin; type IIIA open fractures require a first-generation cephalosporin plus an aminoglycoside; penicillin is added for grossly contaminated (type IIIB) open fractures. Overall, *S. aureus* remains the leading cause of osteomyelitis and nongonococcal septic arthritis. In general, the virulence of *S. epidermidis* infections is closely related to orthopaedic hardware. **Clindamycin achieves the highest antibiotic concentrations in bone;** the concentration in bone nearly equals that of serum concentrations after IV administration. **Clindamycin is bacteriostatic.**

B. Antibiotic-Resistant Bacteria—Two types of antibiotic resistance exist.
    1. Intrinsic Resistance—Inherent features of a cell that prevent antibiotics from acting on the cell (such as the absence of a metabolic pathway or enzyme).
    2. Acquired Resistance—A new resistant strain emerges from a population that was previously sensitive (acquired resistance is mediated by plasmids [extrachromosomal genetic elements] and transopsons).

C. Spectrum of Antimicrobial Agents (Table 1–42)

D. Antibiotic Indications and Side Effects (Table 1–43)

E. Mechanism of Action of Antibiotics (Table 1–44)

F. Other Forms of Antibiotic Delivery
    1. Antibiotic Beads or Spacers—PMMA impregnated with antibiotics (usually an aminoglycoside); useful when treating infections with TJA or for osteomyelitis with bony defects. Antibiotic powder is mixed with cement powder; the type of antibiotic to be used is guided by the microorganism present, and dosage depends on the specific antibiotic selected and type of PMMA used. Antibiotics that have been used with PMMA for infection are tobramycin, gentamicin, cefazolin (Ancef) and other cephalosporins, oxacillin, cloxacillin, methicillin, lincomycin, clindamycin, colistin, fucidin, neomycin, kanamycin, and ampicillin. Chloramphenicol and tetracycline appear to be inactivated during polymerization. Antibiotics are eluted from PMMA beads with an exponential decline in elution over a 2-week period and then cease to be present in significant levels locally by 6–8 weeks. Local tis-

Table 1–42.

Overview of Antimicrobial Agents

Penicillins
- *Natural*
  - Penicillin G
  - Penicillin-VK
- *Penicillinase Resistant (PRSP)*
  - Methicillin (Staphcillin, Celbenin)
  - Nafcillin (Unipen, Nafcil)
  - Oxacillin (Prostaphlin, Bactocill)
  - Cloxacillin (Tegopen, Cloxapen)
  - Dicloxacillin (Dynapen, Pathocil)
  - Flucloxacillin (Floxapen, Ladropen, Staphcil)
- *Aminopenicillins*
  - Ampicillin (Omnipen, Polycillin)
  - Amoxacillin (Amoxil)
  - Bacampicillin (Spectrobid)
  - Amoxicillin/clavulanate (Augmentin)
  - Ampicillin/sulbactam (Unasyn)
- *Antipseudomonal Agents*
  - Indanyl carbenicillin (Geocillin)
  - Ticarcillin (Ticar)
  - Ticarcillin/clavulanate (Timentin)
  - Mezlocillin (Mezlin)
  - Piperacillin (Pipracil)
  - Piperacillin/tazobactam (Zosyn)

Cephalosporins
- *First Generation*
  - Cephalothin (Keflin, Seffin)
  - Cefazolin (Ancef, Kefzol)
  - Cephapirin (Cefadyl)
  - Cephradine (Velosef)
  - Cephalexin (Keflex, Keftab)
  - Cefadroxil (Duricef, Ultracef)
- *Second Generation*
  - Cefaclor (Ceclor)
  - Cefamandole (Mandol)
  - Cefoxitin (Mefoxin)
  - Cefuroxime (Zinacef, Kefurox)
  - Cefuroxime axetil (Ceftin)
  - Cefmetazole (Zefazone)
  - Cefotetan (Cefotan)
  - Cefprozil (Cefzil)
  - Cefonicid (Monocid)
  - Loracarbef (Lorabid)
  - Ceftibuten (Cedax)
- *Third Generation*
  - Cefetamet pivoxil (R. 15-8075)
  - Cefoperazone (Cefobid)
  - Cefoperazone (Claforan)
  - Ceftizoxime (Cefizox)
  - Ceftriaxone (Rocephin, Nitrocephin)
  - Ceftazidime (Fortaz, Tazicef, Tazidime)
  - Cefixime (Suprax)
  - Cefpodoxime proxetil (Vantin)
- *Fourth Generation*
  - Cefpirome (HR 810)
  - Cefepime (Maxipime)

Carbapenems
- Imipenem + cilastatin (Primaxin)
- Meropenem (Merrem)

Monobactams
- Aztreonam (Azactam)

Aminoglycosides
- Amikacin (Amikin)
- Gentamicin (Garamycin)
- Kanamycin (Kantrex)
- Netilmicin (Netromycin)
- Tobramycin (Nebcin)

Fluoroquinolones
- Norfloxacin (Noroxin)
- Ciprofloxacin (Cipro)
- Ofloxacin (Floxin)
- Enoxacin (Penetrex)
- Lomefloxacin (Maxaquin)
- Pefloxacin
- Grepafloxacin (Raxar)
- Levofloxacin (Levaquin)
- Sparfloxacin (Zagam)
- Trovafloxacin (Trovan)

Macrolides
- Azithromycin (Zithromax)
- Clarithromycin (Biaxin)
- Erythromycin

Other Antibacterial Agents
- Chloramphenicol (Chloromycetin)
- Clindamycin (Cleocin)
- Vancomycin (Vancocin, Vancoled)
- Teicoplanin (Targocid)
- Doxycycline (Vibramycin)
- Minocycline (Minocin)
- Tetracycline (Terramycin)
- Polymyxin B (Aerosporin)
- Fusidic acid (Fucidin)
- Fosfomycin (Monurol)
- Sulfisoxazole (Gantrisin)
- Trimethoprim/sulfamethoxazole (Bactrim, Septra)
- Metronidazole (Flagyl)

Antifungal Agents
- Amphotericin B (Fungizone)
- Fluconazole (Diflucan)
- Flucytosine (Ancobon)
- Ketaconazole (Nizoral)
- Itraconazole (Sporanox)

Antimycobacterial Agents
- Isoniazid [INH (Nydrazid)]
- Rifampin (Rifadin)
- Ethambutol (Myambutol)
- Streptomycin
- Pyrazinamide
- Ethionamide
- Cycloserine (Seromycin)
- Amikacin (Amikin)
- Capreomycin (Capastat)
- Thioacetazone
- Rifabutin (Mycobutin)

Antiparasitic Agents
- Albendazole (Zentel)
- Atovaquone (Mepron)
- Dapsone
- Mefloquine (Lariam)
- Pentamidine (Pentam 300)
- Pyrimethamine (Daraprim)
- Praziquantel (Biltricide)

Antiviral Agents
- Acyclovir (Zovirax)
- Amantadine (Symmetrel)
- Didanosine (Videx)
- Foscarnet (Foscavir)
- Ganciclovir (Cytovene)
- Zalcitabine (Hivid)
- Zidovudine [AZT (Retrovir)]

Adapted from Gilbert, D.N., Moellering, R.C., and Sande, M.A.: The Sanford Guide to Antimicrobial Therapy, 28th ed. Virginia, Antimicrobial Therapy, Inc., 1998, pp. 55–71.

Table 1–43.

Antibiotic Indications and Side Effects

Antibiotics	Organisms	Complications/Other
Aminoglycosides	G−, PM	Auditory (most common) and vestibular toxicity are caused by destruction of the cochlear and vestibular sensory cells from drug accumulation in the perilymph and endolymph; renal toxcity; neuromuscular blockade
Amphotericin	Fungi	Nephrotoxic
Azactam	G−, no anaerobes	
Carbenicillin/ticarcillin/piperacillin	Better against G−	Bleeding diathesis (carbenicillin)
Cephalosporins		
First generation	Prophylaxis (surgical)	Cephazolin is the drug of choice
Second generation	Some G+/G−	
Third generation	G−, fewer G+	Hemolytic anemia (bleeding diathesis [moxalactam])
Chloramphenicol	*H. influenzae*, anaerobes	Bone marrow aplasia
Ciprofloxacin	G−, methicillin-resistant *S. aureus*	Tendon ruptures; cartilage erosion in children; antacids reduce absorption of cipro; theophylline increases serum concentrations of cipro
Clindamycin	G+, anaerobes	Pseudomembranous enterocolitis
Erythromycin	G+ (PCN allergy)	Ototoxic
Imipenem	G+, some G−	Resistances, seizure
Methicillin/oxacillin/nafcillin	Penicillinase-resistant	Same as penicillin; nephritis (methicillin); subcut. skin slough (nafcillin)
Penicillin	Strep, G+	Hypersensitivity/resistance; hemolytic
Polymyxin/nystatin	GU	Nephrotoxic
Sulfonamides	GU	Hemolytic anemia
Tetracycline	G+ (PCN allergy)	Stains teeth/bone (up to age 8)
Vancomycin	Methicillin-resistance *S. aureus*, *C. difficile*	Ototoxic; erythema with rapid IV delivery

G+, gram positive; G−, gram negative; GU, genitourinary; PM, polymicrobial; PCN, penicillin; subcut, subcutaneous.

sue concentrations of antibiotic are much higher than can be achieved with systemic administration and do not seem to cause problems in doses that are typically used. Extremely high local concentrations of antibiotics can decrease cellular replication or even result in cell death. Increased surface area of PMMA (e.g., with oval beads) enhances elution of antibiotics. Beads are inserted only after thorough débridement. Because PMMA itself is associated with a foreign body reaction, the beads should always be removed. Antibiotic powder in doses of 2 g per 40 g of powdered PMMA (simplex P) does not appreciably affect the compressive strength of PMMA. Much higher concentrations (4–5 g of antibiotic powder per 40 g of PMMA) significantly reduce the compressive strength (important in cemented joint arthroplasties). Antibiotic-impregnated cement spacers, after

Table 1–44.

Mechanism of Action of Antibiotics

Class of Antibiotic	Examples	Mechanism of Action
Beta-lactam antibiotics	Penicillin Cephalosporins	Inhibits bacterial peptidoglycan synthesis (the mechanism is via binding to the penicillin-binding proteins on the surface of the bacterial cell membrane)
Aminoglycosides	Gentamicin Tobramycin	Inhibits protein synthesis (the mechanism is via binding to cytoplasmic ribosomal RNA)
Clindamycin and macrolides	Clindamycin Erythromycin Clarithromycin Azithromycin	Inhibit the dissociation of peptidyl-tRNA from ribosomes during translocation (the mechanism is via binding to 50S-ribosomal subunits)
Tetracyclines		Inhibit protein synthesis (on 70S- and 80S-ribosomes)
Glycopeptides	Vancomycin Teicoplanin	Interfere with the insertion of glycan subunits into the cell wall
Rifampin		Inhibits RNA synthesis in bacteria
Quinolones	Ciprofloxacin Levofloxacin Ofloxacin	Inhibit DNA gyrase

removal of an infected TKA, help to prevent soft-tissue contracture.

2. Osmotic Pump—Method for delivering high concentrations of antibiotics locally. Used mainly for osteomyelitis.
3. Home IV Therapy—Cost-effective alternative for patients requiring long-term IV antibiotics. This treatment is facilitated by the use of a Hickman or Broviac indwelling catheter.
4. Immersion Solution—Contaminated bone from an open fracture may be sterilized (100% effective) by immersion in chlorhexidine gluconate scrub and an antibiotic solution.

Section 6

Perioperative Problems

I. **Pulmonary Problems**

A. General Considerations—Pulmonary function tests and blood gas measurements are often helpful for evaluating baseline status. Thoracic and abdominal surgery can significantly affect these values.

B. Blood Gas Evaluation—The following is a simple working formula and is useful for evaluating blood gases:

$$pO_2 = 7\ (FiO_2) - pCO_2$$

where pO_2 is the **anticipated or normal pO_2** for a given FiO_2 in a normal person, FiO_2 is the percentage of inspired oxygen, and pCO_2 is the value obtained by the blood gas assay.

Example: A 63-year-old man has acute onset of shortness of breath 12 hours after a THA. When you arrive at his bed, he is wearing a face mask with an inspired oxygen (FiO_2) of 60%. Using our working formula the anticipated, or normal, pO_2 for a normal person would be:

$$pO_2 = 7\ (60) - pCO_2 = 420 - pCO_2$$

Now let us assume that a blood gas assay (blood obtained 15 minutes after placing the patient on 60% oxygen) reveals the following **observed values:**

$$pO_2 = 120$$

$$pCO_2 = 60$$

With a pCO_2 of 60, the anticipated (or normal) pO_2 would be

$$pO_2 = 420 - 60 = 360$$

Therefore, for the patient on 60% oxygen with a pCO_2 of 60, we would anticipate a pO_2 of 360 if all were normal. Because the observed pO_2 is only 120, there is obviously a problem with this patient's pulmonary status. To quantify the extent of the patient's problem we must next calculate the **Aa gradient:**

Aa gradient = (anticipated or normal pO_2 [for a given FiO_2]) − (observed pO_2)

Continuing with the example:

$$\text{Aa gradient} = (360) - (120) = 240$$

Finally, the **percent physiologic shunt** may be calculated as follows:

Percent physiologic shunt = Aa gradient/20

Continuing with the example:

$$\text{Percent physiologic shunt} = 240/20 = 12\%$$

C. Thromboembolism—A common problem in orthopaedic patients, especially in those with procedures about the hip. **Risk of thromboembolism is increased with a history of thromboembolism, obesity, malignancy, aging, congestive heart failure (CHF), birth control pill use, varicose veins, smoking, use of general anesthetics** (in contrast with continuous epidural anesthesia, which some authors believe has a lower incidence of thromboemboli), **increased blood viscosity, immobilization, paralysis, and pregnancy.**

1. Deep Venous Thrombosis (DVT)—Clinical suspicion is more helpful than the physical examination findings (pain, swelling, Homan's sign) for DVT. Useful studies include **venography (the "gold standard"),** which is 97% accurate (70% for iliac veins), ^{125}I-labeled fibrinogen (operative site artifact causes false positives), impedence plethysmography (poor sensitivity), duplex ultrasonography (B-mode)—90% accurate for DVT proximal to the trifurcation vessels, and Doppler imaging (immediate bedside tool, often best for the first study). Prophylaxis is the most important factor in decreasing morbidity and mortality, and the methods commonly used are listed in Table 1–45. Because DVT is relatively uncommon after elective spinal surgery, only mechanical prophylaxis (such as compression stockings) is recommended. **The anticoagulation effects of warfarin (Coumadin) are via inhibition of hepatic enzymes, vitamin K epoxide, and perhaps vitamin K reductase. This inhibition results in decreased carboxylation of the vitamin K–dependent proteins: factors II (prothrombin), VII (the first to be affected), IX, and X. Warfarin does not act by directly binding vitamin K or the clotting factors. The anticoagulation effects of warfarin can be reversed with vitamin K or more rapidly with fresh frozen plasma.** Rifampin is an antagonist to warfarin. The diagnosis of DVT postoperatively requires initiation of heparin therapy (followed by later conversion to long-term [3 months] warfarin therapy). **Low-dose warfarin given to a patient with a DVT acts by interfering with the metab-**

Table 1–45.

Thromboembolism Prophylaxis

Method	Effect	Advantages	Disadvantages
Heparin			
Intravenous	Coagulation cascade—antithrombin III inhibitor	Reversible, effective	Control, embolization
Subcutaneous	Antithrombin III inhibitor	Reversible	No effect in extremity surgery
Coumadin*	Coagulation cascade—vitamin K	Most effective, oral	3–5 days to full effect, control
Aspirin	Inhibits platelet aggregation	Easy, no monitoring	Limited efficacy
Dextran	Dilutional	Effective	Fluid overload, bleeding
Pneumatic compression (and foot pumps)	Mechanical	Inexpensive, no bleeding	Bulky
Enoxaparin (Lovenox), a low-molecular-weight heparin	Inhibits clotting—forms complexes between antithrombin III and factors IIa and Xa	Fixed dose, no monitoring	Bleeding

*See text for details.

olism of factors II (prothrombin), VII, IX, and X. Treatment is recommended for all thigh DVTs; however, treatment of DVTs occurring below the popliteal fossa is controversial. **Preoperative identification of a DVT in a patient with lower-extremity or pelvic trauma is an indication for placement of a vena cava filter. Virchow's triad** of factors involved in venous thrombosis are stasis, hypercoagulability, and intimal injury. Thromboembolism formation is summarized in Figure 1–88.

2. Pulmonary Embolism—Pulmonary embolism (PE) should be suspected in postoperative patients with acute onset of pleuritic pain, **tachypnea (90%),** and tachycardia (60%). Initial work-up includes an EKG (right bundle branch block [RBBB], right axis deviation [RAD] in 25%; may also show ST depression or T wave inversion in lead III), a chest radio-

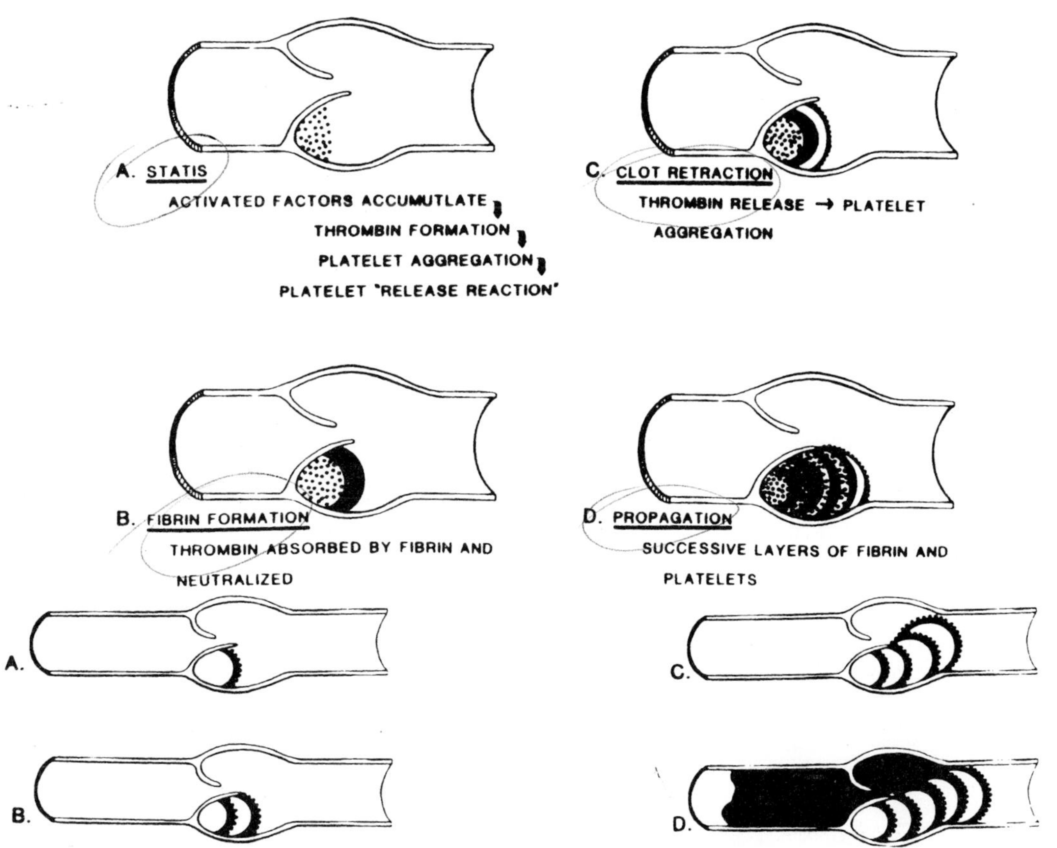

Figure 1–88. Venous thromboembolus formation. (From Simon, S.R., ed.: Orthopaedic Basic Science, 2nd ed., p. 492. Rosemont, IL, American Academy of Orthopaedic Surgeons, 1994.)

Table 1–46.

Frequency of Deep Vein Thrombosis and Fatal Pulmonary Embolism (Diagnosed by Venography)

Unprotected Patients	Frequency (%) DVT	Fatal PE
Elective hip arthroplasty	70	2
Elective knee arthroplasty	80	1
Open meniscectomy	20	?
Hip fracture	60	3.5
Spinal fracture with paralysis	100	~1
Polytrauma patients	35	?
Pelvic/acetabular fracture	20	?

From Simon, S.R.: Orthopaedic Basic Science, 2nd ed., p. 489. Rosemont, IL, American Academy of Orthopaedic Surgeons, 1994.

graph (hyperlucency rare), and ABGs (normal PO_2 does not exclude PE). Nuclear medicine ventilation-perfusion (V/Q) scan may be helpful, but pulmonary angiography (the "gold standard") is required to make the diagnosis if there is any question. Heparin therapy (continuous IV infusion) is initiated for the patient with a proved PE and is monitored by the partial thromboplastin time (PTT). More aggressive therapy (thrombolytic agents, vena cava filter, and other surgical measures) is required in select cases. Seven to ten days of heparin therapy is followed by 3 months of oral warfarin (monitored by the prothrombin time [PT]). Approximately 700,000 people in the United States have an asymptomatic PE each year, of which 200,000 are fatal. The most important factor for survival is early diagnosis with prompt therapy initiation. The incidence of DVT and fatal PE in unprotected patients is summarized in Table 1–46.

3. Coagulation (Fig. 1–89)—A cascading sequence of enzymatic reactions that begins with prothrombin-converting activity and concludes with the formation of a **fibrin** clot (as fibrinogen is converted to fibrin). Two interconnecting pathways have been described.
   a. Intrinsic Pathway—Monitored by PTT. Pathway is activated when factor XII makes contact with the collagen of damaged vessels.
   b. Extrinsic Pathway—Monitored by PT. Pathway is activated by release of thromboplastin into the circulation secondary to cellular injury.
   c. The **bleeding time test measures platelet function.** The **fibrinolytic system** is

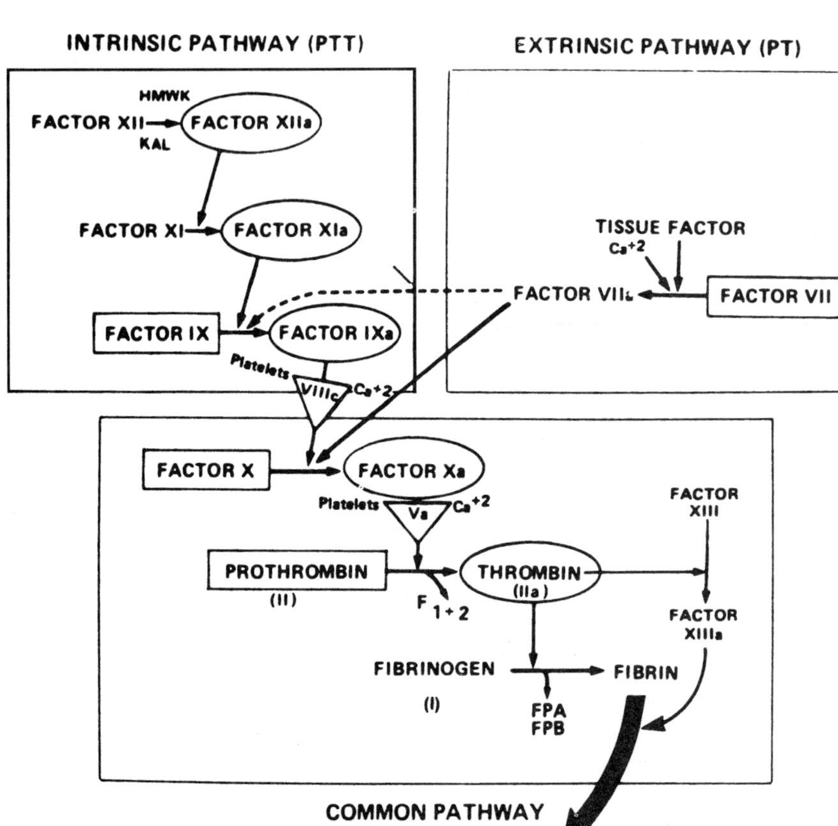

Figure 1–89. Coagulation cascade. (From Stead, R.B.: Regulation of hemostasis. In Goldhaber, S.Z., ed.: Pulmonary Embolism and Deep Venous Thromboembolism, p. 32. Philadelphia, WB Saunders, 1985.)

responsible for dissolving clots. Plasminogen is converted to plasmin (with the help of tissue activators, factor XIIa, and thrombin); plasmin dissolves fibrin clot.

D. Adult Respiratory Distress Syndrome (ARDS)—Acute respiratory failure secondary to pulmonary edema after such events as trauma, shock, or infection. Causes of ARDS include pulmonary infection, sepsis, fat embolism, microembolism, aspiration, fluid overload, atelectasis, oxygen toxicity, pulmonary contusion, and head injury. Tachypnea, dyspnea, hypoxemia, and decreased lung compliance are manifestations of ARDS. **The clinical diagnosis of ARDS after a long-bone fracture is best made using ABGs.** Normal supportive care is often unsuccessful, and a 50% mortality rate is not uncommon. Fluid overload, aspiration, and microscopic emboli may contribute to the development of ARDS. Activation of the complement system leads to further progression. Ventilation with PEEP is important; steroids have not been proven to be efficacious. Early stabilization of long-bone fractures (particularly the femur) decreases the risk of pulmonary complications.

E. Fat Embolism (Fig. 1–90)—Usually seen 24–72 hours after trauma (3–4% of patients with long-bone fractures). It is fatal in 10–15% of cases. **The incidence of clinically significant fat embolism is decreased by early skeletal stabilization.** Onset may be heralded by tachypnea, pulmonary edema, tachycardia, hypoxemia, mental status changes, **confusion,** CNS depression, and **petechiae.** May be caused by bone marrow fat **(mechanical theory),** chylomicron changes as a result of stress **(metabolic theory),** or both. Metabolism to free fatty acids, initiation of the clotting cascade, pulmonary capillary leakage, bronchoconstriction, and alveolar collapse result in a **ventillation-perfusion deficit** (hypoxemia) consistent with ARDS. Treatment includes mechanical ventilation with **high levels of PEEP.** Steroids do not appear to have a prophylactic role. Prevention with early fracture stabilization is key. Over-reaming the femoral canal can decrease the incidence of fat embolism (embolization of marrow contents) during TKA.

F. Pneumonia—Aspiration pneumonia can occur in patients with decreased mentation, supine positioning, and decreased GI motility. Simple preventive measures such as raising the head of the bed and the use of antacids and metoclopramide (Reglan) can help to avoid problems. Appropriate IV antibiotics and pulmonary toilet are required to treat an established pneumonia.

G. Pulmonary Complications of Orthopaedic Disorders—Scoliosis of significant magnitude can cause pulmonary dysfunction. Spontaneous pneumothorax is common in patients with Marfan's syndrome.

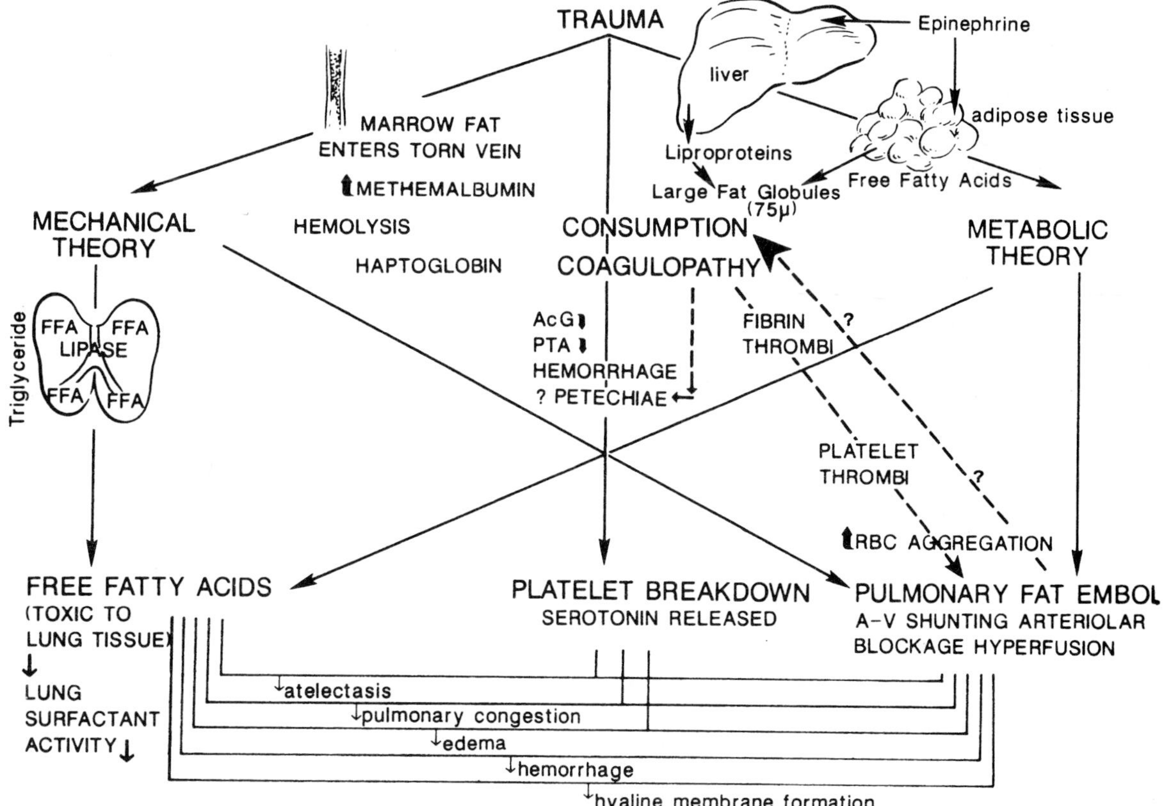

Figure 1–90. Pathological events of fat embolism syndrome. (From Simon, S.R., ed.: Orthopaedic Basic Science, 2nd ed., p. 502. Rosemont, IL, American Academy of Orthopaedic Surgeons, 1994.)

II. **Other Medical Problems (Nonpulmonary)**

A. Nutrition—Adequate nutrition should be ensured prior to elective surgery. Malnutrition may be present in 50% of patients on a surgical ward. Several indicators exist (e.g., anergy panels, albumin levels, transferrin level); **arm muscle circumference measurement is the best indicator of nutritional status.** Wound dehiscence and infection, pneumonia, and sepsis can result from poor nutrition. Lack of enteral feeding can lead to **atrophy of the intestinal mucosae, leading in turn to bacterial translocation.** Nutritional requirements are significantly elevated as a result of stress. Full enteral or parenteral nutrition (nitrogen 200 mg/kg per day) should be provided for patients who cannot tolerate normal intake. Early elemental feeding through a jejunostomy tube can decrease complications in the multiple trauma patient. **Enteral protein supplements have proved effective in patients at risk of developing multiple organ system failure.** The metabolic changes of starvation and stress are compared in Table 1–47.

B. Myocardial Infarction (MI)—Acute chest pain, radiation, and EKG changes are classic and warrant monitoring in an appropriate critical care environment where cardiac enzymes and the EKG can be monitored on a continuing basis. Risk factors of MI include increased age, smoking, elevated cholesterol, hypertension, aortic stenosis, a history of coronary artery disease, and a variety of other factors.

C. GI Complications—Can range from ileus (treated with nasogastric suction [NG tube] and antacids) to upper GI bleeding. Postoperative ileus is common in diabetics with neuropathy. Upper GI bleeding is more likely in patients with a history of ulcers, NSAID use, and smoking. Treatment includes lavage, antacids, and H_2-blockers. Vasopressin (left gastric artery) may be required for more serious cases. Ogilvie's syndrome, which includes cecal distention, can follow total joint replacement surgery. If the cecum is >10 cm on an abdominal flat plate radiograph, it must be decompressed (usually can be done colonoscopically).

D. Decubitus Ulcers—Associated with advanced age, critical illness, and neurologic impairment. Common sites include the sacrum, heels, and buttocks, which may be a source of infection and increased morbidity. Prevention with constant changing of position, special mattresses, and treatment of systemic illness and malnutrition is essential. Once established, débridement and sometimes soft-tissue flaps are required for treatment.

E. Urinary Tract Infection (UTI)—Most common nosocomial infection (6–8%). Causes increased risk for joint sepsis after TJA (but may not be from direct seeding). Established UTIs should be adequately treated preoperatively. Perioperative catheterization (removed 24 hours postoperatively) may reduce the rate of postoperative UTI.

F. Prostatic Hypertrophy—Causes postoperative urinary retention. If the history, physical examination (prostate), and urine flow studies (<17 mL/sec peak flow rate) are suggestive, urologic referral should be accomplished preoperatively.

G. Acute Tubular Necrosis—Can cause renal failure in trauma patients. Alkalization of urine is important during the early treatment of this disorder.

H. Genitourinary (GU) Injury—NSAIDs can affect the kidney, and appropriate screening laboratories are required at regular intervals. Retrograde urethrogram best evaluates lower GU injuries with displaced anterior pelvic fractures.

I. Shock—Capillary blood flow is insufficient for the perfusion of vital tissues and organs. There are four types of shock:

1. Hypovolemic Shock—"Volume loss": decreased cardiac output (CO), increased peripheral vascular resistance (PVR), venous constriction
2. Cardiogenic Shock—"Ineffective pumping":

Table 1–47.

Metabolic Changes of Starvation and Stress

Metabolic Activity	Starvation: Early	Starvation: Late	Stress: Hypermetabolism	Stress: Multisystem
Energy expenditure	↓	↓↓	↑↑	Organ failure
Mediator activation	None	None	++	++
Metabolic responsiveness	Intact	Intact	Abnormal	Abnormal
Primary fuel	CHO	KB	"Mixed" (no KB)	"Mixed" (no KB)
Hepatic gluconeogenesis	↓	↓	↑	↑ or ↓
Hepatic protein synthesis	↓	↓	↑	↑ or ↓
Whole-body protein catabolism	Sl. ↑	Sl. ↑	↑↑	↑↑↑
Urinary nitrogen excretion	Sl. ↑	Sl. ↑	↑↑	↑↑↑
Malnutrition	Slow	Slow	Rapid	Rapid

CHO, carbohydrate; Sl., slight; KB, ketone bodies.
Adapted from Simon, S.R.: Orthopaedic Basic Science, 2nd ed., p. 510. Rosemont, IL, American Academy of Orthopaedic Surgeons, 1994.

decreased CO, increased PVR, venous dilation

3. Vasogenic Shock (PE or pericardial tamponade)—Arteriolar constriction, venous dilation
4. Neurogenic Shock/Septic Shock—"Blood pooling": arteriolar, capillary, and venous dilation

The preferred initial fluid for hypovolemic shock is Ringer's lactate. For patients in shock with a suboptimal response to Ringer's lactate, add blood transfusion; massive blood replacement requires concomitant fresh frozen plasma and platelets. **The best indicator of adequate fluid resuscitation is urine output.** Patients with inadequate fluid resuscitation show metabolic acidosis on ABGs.

J. Compartment Syndrome—Covered in detail in Chapter 10, Trauma. This subject matter is always tested heavily. Questions regarding compartment syndrome of the foot and thigh seem to be "popular."

K. Frostbite
1. Superficial—Treat with general rewarming of the entire body plus immersion of the hands or feet in a warm water bath (106°F, 41.1°C).
2. Deep—Débridement is often necessary.

L. **Wound Healing—Adequate healing following surgery is promoted by:**
1. **Transcutaneous oxygen tension > 30 mm Hg**
2. **Ischemic index (such as the ankle/brachial systolic index) ≥0.45**
3. Albumin >3.0 g/dL
4. Total lymphocyte count of 1500/mm^3

III. **Intraoperative Considerations**

A. Anesthesia—Regional anesthesia may (there is disagreement in the literature) allow quicker recovery, decreased blood loss, and fewer postoperative complications, including reduced blood loss and incidence of DVT/PE in THA patients. Controlled hypotension during surgery helps with blood loss and is a widely accepted technique, especially with THA and spinal arthrodesis (nitroprusside, nitroglycerine, and isoflurane are all effective). Patient positioning on a kneeling frame for spinal surgery decreases: (1) intra-abdominal pressure, (2) pressure on the inferior vena cava, (3) pressure on the vertebral venous system, and (4) blood loss. Transient intraoperative decreases in BP with PMMA insertion are well known. The use of the fiberoptic bronchoscope has benefited surgery on RA patients and others with C-spine abnormalities. The use of local anesthetics for arthroscopy has also gained popularity. **Malignant hyperthermia,** an autosomal dominant, hypermetabolic disorder of skeletal muscle, can be triggered by the use of various anesthetics (especially halothane and succinylcholine) in susceptible patients (e.g., neuromuscular disorders). The disorder involves impaired function of the sarcoplasmic reticulum and calcium homeostasis. Patients with Duchenne's muscular dystrophy, arthrogryposis, and osteogenesis imperfecta are especially at risk. Cell membrane defects affect calcium transport, leading to muscle rigidity and hypermetabolism. Masseter muscle spasm, increased temperature, rigidity, and acidosis are the hallmarks of the disease. Early diagnosis and treatment with **dantrolene sodium (blocks calcium release by stabilizing the sarcoplasmic reticulum while permitting uptake of calcium and thus decreasing the intracellular concentration of calcium),** balancing of electrolytes, increasing urinary output, respiratory support, and cooling are essential. The **most accurate method for diagnosing malignant hyperthermia is muscle biopsy** (in vitro muscle fiber testing).

B. Spinal Cord Monitoring—Usually involves testing the posterior column, but monitoring of other areas is under investigation. Electrical monitoring includes the use of somatosensory cortical evoked potentials (SCEPs) to record summed input from stimulation of peripheral areas. Somatosensory spinal evoked potentials (SSEPs) are more invasive but can be more sensitive. Preoperative recordings are compared with readings (especially latency and amplitude) at critical times during the procedure. The wake-up test is still the standard for monitoring and relies on the lightening of anesthesia and the patient moving selected extremities upon command.

C. Tourniquet—Injuries usually involve the area directly underneath the tourniquet and include nerve and muscle damage. Careful application, wide cuffs, lower pressures (200 mm Hg in the upper extremity and 250 Hg mm in the lower extremity [or 100–150 mm Hg above systolic BP for the lower extremity]), and double cuffs help avoid these problems. Equilibrium can be reestablished within 5 minutes after 90 minutes of tourniquet application but requires 15 minutes after the use of a tourniquet for 3 hours. EMG abnormalities have been reported in 70% of patients after routine surgery using a tourniquet.

IV. **Other Problems**

A. Pain Control—Acute pain implies the presence of potential tissue damage, whereas chronic pain (3–6 months) does not. Nociceptors transduce stimuli through substances, allowing transmission along peripheral nerves (type A and C fibers) to the dorsal column, spinothalamic tract, and thalamus. Modulation is via brainstem centers and endogenous opiates. Postoperative pain control can be targeted at any step. Local prostaglandin inhibitors and long-acting local anesthetics target transduction of pain. Perispinal opiates affect modulation, and systemic opiates affect perception and modulation of pain.
1. Local Anesthetics—Result in a transient and reversible loss of sensation that is confined to

Section 7
Imaging and Special Studies

I. **Nuclear Medicine**

A. Bone Scan—**Technetium-99m phosphate complexes reflect increased blood flow and metabolism and are absorbed onto the hydroxyapatite crystals of bone in areas of infection, trauma, neoplasia, etc.** Whole-body views and more detailed (pin-hole) views can be obtained. It is particularly useful for the diagnosis of subtle fractures; avascular necrosis (hypoperfused [diminished blood flow] early, increased uptake during the reparative phase); osteomyelitis (especially when a triple-phase study is performed or in conjunction with a gallium or indium scan); and THA and TKA loosening (especially femoral components; a technetium scan can be used in conjunction with a gallium scan to rule out concurrent infection). Three-phase (or even four-phase) studies may be helpful for evaluating diseases such as reflex sympathetic dystrophy and osteomyelitis. The three phases of a triple phase bone scan are as follows: ***First phase*** **(blood flow, immediate)**—this phase displays blood flow through the arterial system. ***Second phase*** **(blood pool, 30 minutes)**—this phase displays equilibrium of tracer throughout the intravascular volume. ***Third phase*** **(delayed, 4 hours)**—this phase displays the sites at which the tracer accumulates. Delayed-phase scans may be negative in pediatric septic arthritis. Triple-phase bone scan is the most reliable test for assessing whether a nondisplaced scaphoid fracture exists. A technetium scan is a useful means of evaluating for osteochondritis dessicans of the talus.

B. Gallium Scan—**Gallium-67 citrate localizes in sites of inflammation and neoplasia, probably because of exudation of labeled serum proteins.** Delayed imaging (usually 24–48 hours or more) is required. Frequently used in conjunction with a bone scan—a "double tracer" technique. Gallium is less dependent on vascular flow than technetium and may identify foci that would otherwise be missed. It is difficult to differentiate cellulitis from osteomyelitis on a gallium scan.

C. Indium Scan—**Indium-111–labeled WBCs (leukocytes) accumulate in areas of inflammation and do not collect in areas of neoplasia.** Useful for evaluation of **acute infections** (such as osteomyelitis) and possibly TJA infections.

D. Technetium-Labeled WBC Scan—Similar to indium scan.

E. Radiolabeled Monoclonal Antibodies—May have a role in identifying primary malignancies and metastatic disease.

F. Other Studies

1. Bone Mineral Analysis—Single-photon absorptiometry (usually of the distal radius and cortical bone; has limited utility), dual-photon absorptiometry (vertebral bodies and femoral neck). (For further details see section on Measurement of Bone Density.)
2. Deep Venous Thrombosis/Pulmonary Embolism (DVT/PE) Scan—Radioactive iodine-labeled fibrinogen accumulates in clot and shows up on scanning. Its limitations include inaccuracy in areas of surgical wounds. Radioisotope scanning of the lungs may also help in evaluating regional pulmonary blood flow, but it too is limited at present.
3. Single-Photon Emission Computed Tomography (SPECT)—Uses scintigraphy and CT to evaluate overlapping structures. Femoral head ON, patellofemoral syndrome, and the healing of spondylolytic defects have been evaluated with this technique.

II. **Arthrography**

A. Shoulder—Can be used with a single- or double-contrast technique (better detail). Used for the following studies.

1. Rotator Cuff Tear Diagnosis—Extravasation of contrast through the tear into the subacromial bursa.
2. Adhesive Capsulitis—Diagnosed by demonstrating diminished joint capsule size and loss of the normal axillary fold. May have a role in therapy also by distending the capsule.
3. Recurrent Dislocations—Arthrography may demonstrate a distended capsule or disruption of the glenoid labrum. Can be used in conjunction with tomograms or CT (computed arthrotomography) to better demonstrate capsular or labral pathology.
4. Other Uses—Include diagnosis of bicipital tendon abnormalities, articular pathology, and impingement syndrome.

B. Elbow—Especially when used with tomography, elbow arthrography can be helpful for diagnosing articular cartilage defects/loose bodies and osteochondral fractures.

C. Wrist—Most useful for evaluation of the posttraumatic wrist to demonstrate ligamentous disruption. Digital subtraction techniques are helpful in this area. Demonstration of communication between compartments is used to determine pathology; however, communication is common in asymptomatic patients in the over-40 age group. If a communication is observed at the radius-carpus and midcarpal joint, an S-L or L-T ligament tear should be suspected. Communication at the radius-carpus and distal radius-ulna suggests a TFCC tear.

D. Hip—Different indications in children and adults.
   1. Infants and Children—Arthrography is useful for diagnosing the "septic" hip (obtain aspirate and assess joint damage), congenital dysplasia of the hip (degree of joint incongruity—interposed limbus), and Legg-Calvé-Perthes disease (severity of deformity).
   2. Adolescents and Adults—Used to evaluate arthritis (cartilage destruction and loose bodies), osteochondral fractures, chondrolysis, and THA loosening. Digital subtraction arthrography can be useful in patients with suspected loose THAs.

E. Knee—Can be a useful screening tool in patients with an equivocal history or findings. Accurate for diagnosing most meniscal tears (except tears in the posterior horn of the lateral meniscus) and demonstrates discoid lateral menisci well. Evaluation of cruciate ligaments is less accurate. Abnormalities of articular cartilage, evaluation of loose bodies (air contrast only is recommended), and pathologic synovial tissue (PVNS, popliteal cysts, synovial chondromatosis, plicas) can be demonstrated as well.

F. Ankle—Helpful for evaluating torn ligaments acutely and assessing chronic osseous and osteocartilaginous abnormalities.

G. Spine—May be useful in conjunction with therapeutic injections (of anesthetics and steroids) into facet joints.

III. **Magnetic Resonance Imaging (MRI)**

A. Introduction—Excellent study to evaluate the soft tissues and bone marrow. Used frequently to evaluate ON, neoplasms, infection, and trauma. Allows both axial and sagittal representations. It is contraindicated in patients with pacemakers, cerebral aneurysm clips, or shrapnel or hardware in certain locations.

B. Basic Principles of MRI (Tables 1–48 and 1–49)—MRI uses radiofrequency (Rf) pulses on tissues in a magnetic field and displays images in any plane desired without the use of ionizing radiation. MRI aligns nuclei with odd numbers of protons/neutrons (with a normally random spin) parallel to a magnetic field. Most magnets used have a strength of about 0.5–1.5 Tesla (1 Tesla is 10,000 Gauss). Radiofrequency pulses cause deflection of these particles' nuclear magnetic moments, resulting in an image. The use of surface coils decreases the signal-to-noise ratio. Body coils are used for large joints, smaller coils are available for other studies. Sequences have been developed to demonstrate the differences in T_1 and T_2 relaxation between tissues. **T_1 images are weighted toward fat; T_2 images are weighted toward water.** Typically, T_1-weighted images have TR (time to repetition) values <1000, and T_2 images have TR values >1000. Some tissues appear differently

Table 1–48.

Magnetic Resonance Imaging Terminology

Term	Explanation
T_1	Time constant of exponential growth of magnetism; T_1 measures how rapidly a tissue gains magnetism (see Table 1–49)
T_2	Time constant of exponential decay of signal following an excitation pulse; a tissue with a long T_2 (such as water) maintains its signal (is bright on T_2-weighted image) (see Table 1–49)
T_2*	Similar to T_2 but includes the effects of magnetic field homogeneity
TR	Time to repetition; the time between successive excitation pulses; short TR is less than 80, long TR is greater than 80
TE	Time to echo; the time that an echo is formed by the refocusing pulse; short TE is less than 1000, long TE is greater than 1000
NEX	Number of excitations; higher NEX results in decreased noise with better images
FOV	Field of view
Spin echo	A commonly used pulse sequence in MRI
FSE	Fast spin echo; a type of pulse sequence
GRE	Gradient-recalled echo; a type of pulse sequence

Table 1–49.

Magnetic Resonance Imaging Signal Intensities

Tissue	Appearance on T_1-Weighted Image	Appearance on T_2-Weighted Image
Cortical bone	Dark	Dark
Osteomyelitis	Dark	Bright
Ligaments	Dark	Dark
Fibrocartilage	Dark	Dark
Hyaline cartilage	Gray	Gray
Meniscus	Dark	Dark
Meniscal tear	Bright	Gray
Yellow bone marrow (fatty-appendicular)	Bright	Gray
Red bone marrow (hematopoietic-axial)	Gray	Gray
Marrow edema	Dark	Bright
Fat	Bright	Gray
Normal fluid	Dark	Bright
Abnormal fluid (pus)	Gray	Bright
Acute blood collection	Gray	Dark
Chronic blood collection	Bright	Bright
Muscle	Gray	Gray
Tendon	Dark	Dark
Intervertebral disc (central)	Gray	Bright
Intervertebral disc (peripheral)	Dark	Gray

Modified from Brinker, M.R., and Miller, M.D.: Fundamentals of Orthopaedics. Philadelphia, WB Saunders, 1999, p. 24.

on T_1- and T_2-weighted scans. Water, CSF, acute hemorrhage, and soft-tissue tumors appear dark on T_1 studies and bright on T_2 studies. Other tissues remain basically the same intensity on both images. Cortical bone, rapidly flowing blood, and fibrous tissue are all dark; muscle and hyaline cartilage are gray; and fatty tissue, nerves, slowly flowing (venous) blood, and bone marrow are bright. **T_1 images best demonstrate anatomic structure (high signal-to-noise ratio), whereas T_2 images are most useful for contrasting normal and abnormal tissues.**

C. Specific Applications of MRI
   1. Osteonecrosis—**MRI is the most sensitive method for early detection of ON** (detects early marrow necrosis and ingrowth of vascularized mesenchymal tissue). MRI is highly specific (98%) and reliable for estimating the age and extent of disease. T_1 images demonstrate diseased marrow as dark. MRI allows direct assessment of overlying cartilage.
   2. Infection and Trauma—MRI has excellent sensitivity to increases in free water and demonstrates areas of infection and fresh hemorrhage (dark on T_1 and bright on T_2 studies). **MRI is an excellent (accurate and sensitive) method of evaluating for occult fractures (particularly in the elderly hip).**
   3. Neoplasms—MRI has many applications in the study of primary and metastatic bone tumors. Primary tumors, particularly soft-tissue components (extraosseous and marrow), are well demonstrated on MRI. Although nuclear medicine studies remain the procedure of choice for seeking metastatic foci in bone, MRI has a role in evaluating for skip lesions and spinal metastases. Benign bony tumors are typically bright on T_1 images and dark on T_2 images. Malignant bony lesions are often bright on T_2 images. Differential diagnosis, however, is best made based on plain films.
   4. Spine—Disc disease is well demonstrated on T_2 images. Degenerated discs lose their water content and become dark on T_2-weighted studies; herniated discs (and their extent) are well shown. **Recurrent disc herniation is best diagnosed via MRI scan with gadolinium** and can be differentiated from scar based on the following characteristics: On T_1 image: scar, decreased signal; free fragment, increased signal; extruded disc, decreased signal; on T_2 image: scar, increased signal; free fragment, increased signal; extruded disc, decreased signal. Gadolinium-DTPA can also be used to differentiate scar from disc; it enhances edematous structures in T_1 images. MRI is the best (most sensitive) study for diagnosing early discitis (decreased signal on T_1 and increased signal on T_2). **Recent studies have shown the following regarding MRI findings of the spine in asymptomatic persons:** (1) 28% of subjects over 40 years of age have an abnormality of the cervical spine on MRI, (2) 20–30% of subjects under 40 years of age show evidence of a lumbar disk herniation on MRI, (3) 93% of subjects over 60 years of age show evidence of degeneration or bulging of one or more lumbar disks on MRI.
   5. Bone Marrow Changes—Best demonstrated by MRI (but nonspecific). Five groups of disorders have been described and are shown in Table 1–50.
   6. Knee MRI—Arthrography with MRI can be accomplished with instillation of saline, creating an iatrogenic effusion. This technique can improve joint definition. Knee derangements are well demonstrated on MRI. ACL rupture is correctly diagnosed in 95% of cases. Meniscal pathology has been classified into four groups of myxoid changes (Lotysch) (Table 1–51). **MRI is the best radiologic test to demonstrate a posterior cruciate ligament (PCL) rupture** (physical examination is probably the best test, overall).
   7. Shoulder MRI
      a. Rotator Cuff Tears—Results are improving with use (sensitivity and specificity are about 90%). Grade 0 tears show a normal signal, and grade 1, 2, and 3 tears show an increased signal. The morphology of

Table 1–50.

Imaging Bone Marrow Disorders

Disorder	Pathology	Examples	MRI Changes
Reconversion	Yellow → red	Anemia, metastasis	↓ T_1 image
Marrow infiltration		Tumor, infection	↓ T_1 image
Myeloid depletion		Anemia, chemotherapy	↓ T_1 image
Marrow edema		Trauma, RSD	↓ T_1, ↑ T_2 image
Marrow ischemia		Osteonecrosis	↓ T_1 image

RSD, reflex sympathetic dystrophy; ↑, increased; ↓, decreased.

Table 1–51.

MRI Changes of Meniscal Pathology

Group	Characteristics
I	Globular areas of hyperintense signal
II	Linear hyperintense signal
III	Linear hyperintense signal that communicates with the meniscal surface (tears)
IV	Vertical longitudinal tear/truncation

grade 0 and 1 tears is normal; grade 2 tears show abnormal morphology; and grade 3 tears show discontinuity.

b. Capsular/Labral Tears—MRI is equal to CT arthrography in the presence of an effusion.

8. MRI Spectroscopy—May help with the measurement of metabolic changes (especially ischemic changes).

IV. **Other Imaging Studies**

A. Computed Tomography (CT)—Continues to be important for evaluating many orthopaedic areas. Hounsfield units are used to identify tissue types (−100 = air, −100 to 0 = fat, 0 = water, 100 = soft tissue, 1000 = bone). **CT demonstrates bony anatomy better than any other study.** It also shows herniated nucleus pulposis better than myelography alone and may be helpful in differentiating recurrent disc herniation from scar (like MRI). IV contrast material is administered and taken up in scar tissue but not disc material. CT is used frequently in conjunction with contrast (e.g., arthrogram CT, myelogram CT). Sagittal and three-dimensional reconstruction techniques may expand its indications. Cine-CT (and MRI) may be helpful for evaluating many joint disorders. CT digital radiography (CT scannogram) can be used for accurate demonstration of leg-length discrepancy with minimal radiation exposure. CT best demonstrates joint incongruity following closed reduction of a dislocated hip. **CT scanning is useful for measuring the cross-sectional dural area in the work-up of cervical spinal stenosis; spinal stenosis is present if this area is less than 100 mm². CT is also important for evaluating injuries involving the subtalar joint and for diagnosing tarsal coalitions;** talocalcaneal tarsal coalitions are also well visualized via plain radiographs on the axial (Harris) view. Dynamic CT scan is the test of choice for patients with atlantoaxial rotatory subluxation (Grisel's syndrome is spontaneous atlantoaxial subluxation occuring in conjunction with inflammation of the soft tissues of the neck [such as pharyngitis]).

B. Ultrasonography—Has been used successfully in several areas of orthopaedics.

1. Shoulder—May be useful for diagnosing rotator cuff tears.
2. Hip—Has been shown to be effective in the diagnosis and follow-up of developmental hip dysplasia and to identify iliopsoas bursitis in adults.
3. Knee—Used to assess articular cartilage thickness and identify intra-articular fluid.
4. Other Areas—Helpful for evaluating: soft-tissue masses, hematoma, tendon rupture, abscesses, foreign body location, intraspinal disorders in infants, and the aorta (in patients who are an increased risk for aortic dilation or rupture [such as Marfan's syndrome]).
5. Fractures—Ultrasound may have a role in assessing the progression of fracture healing.

C. Guided Biopsies—Aspiration and core biopsy (using a trephine needle) is helpful in the work-up of musculoskeletal lesions; it is commonly used in conjunction with CT.

D. Myelography—Still useful for evaluating cervical radiculopathy, subarachnoid cysts, and the failed back syndrome. **It is the procedure of choice for extramedullary intradural pathology.** It can be used in conjunction with other studies, such as CT.

E. Discography—Although its use is controversial, it is helpful for evaluating symptomatic disc degeneration. Reproduction of pain with injection and characteristic changes on discograms help identify pathologic discs. It is commonly used in conjunction with CT.

F. Measurement of Bone Density (Noninvasive Methods)—Several methods are available for measuring bone density and assessing the risk of fracture.

1. Single Photon Absorptiometry—The basic principle of this technique is that the density of the cortical bone being tested is inversely proportional to the quantity of photons passing through it. The radioisotope ^{125}I emits a single-energy beam of photons that passes through bone. A sodium iodide scintillation counter detects the transmitted photons. When the bone is denser, there is greater attenuation of the photon beam and fewer photons pass through to the scintillation counter. The best use of single photon absorptiometry is the appendicular skeleton (radius-diaphysis or distal metaphysis); the test cannot be reliably used for the axial skeleton (because of alterations caused by the depth of the soft tissues).
2. Dual Photon Absorptiometry—Like single-photon absorptiometry, dual-photon absorptiometry is an isotope-based means of measuring bone density. Dual-photon absorptiometry, however, allows for measurement of the axial skeleton and the femoral neck (the method accounts for the attenuation of the signal, which is caused by the soft tissues overlying the spine and the hip).
3. Quantitative Computed Tomography—Allows preferential measurement of trabecular bone density (the bone that is at greatest risk for early metabolic changes). The technique involves the simultaneous scanning of phantoms of known density in order to create a standard calibration curve. Precision is excellent; accuracy is within 5–10%. The radiation dose with this technique is higher than that of DEXA.
4. Dual-Energy X-Ray Absorptiometry (DEXA)—**The most reliable method of predicting fracture risk. This method is**

Table 1–52.

Nerve Conduction Study Results

Condition	Latency	Conduction Velocity	Evoked Response
Normal study	Normal	Upper extremities: >45 m/sec Lower extremities: >40 m/sec	Biphasic
Axonal neuropathy	Increased	Normal or slightly decreased	Prolonged, ↓ amplitude
Demyelinating neuropathy	Normal	Decreased (10–50%)	Normal or prolonged, with ↓ amplitude
Anterior horn cell disease	Normal	Normal (rarely decreased)	Normal or polyphasic with prolonged duration and ↓ amplitude
Myopathy	Normal	Normal	↓ Amplitude, may be normal
Neuropraxia			
Proximal to lesion	Absent	Absent	Absent
Distal to lesion	Normal	Normal	Normal
Axonotmesis			
Proximal to lesion	Absent	Absent	Absent
Distal to lesion	Absent	Absent	Normal
Neurotmesis			
Proximal to lesion	Absent	Absent	Absent
Distal to lesion	Absent	Absent	Absent

Modified from Jahss, M.H.: Disorders of the Foot. Philadelphia, WB Saunders, 1982.

the most accurate with a lower radiation dose than quantitative CT.

G. Thermography—Maps body surface temperatures. Thermography has low specificity and is not recommended for clinical evaluation of disorders of the spine.

V. **Electrodiagnostic Studies**

A. Nerve Conduction Studies—Allow evaluation of peripheral nerves and their sensory and motor responses anywhere along their course. Nerve impulses are stimulated and recorded by electronic surface electrodes, allowing calculation of a conduction velocity. Latency (the time between the onset of the stimulus and the response) and the amplitude of the response are measured. Late responses (F and H) allow evaluation of proximal lesions (impulse travels to the spinal cord and returns). Somatosensory evoked potentials can be used to study brachial plexus injuries and for spinal cord monitoring.

B. Electromyography (EMG)—Uses intramuscular needle electrodes to evaluate muscle units. Most studies are done to evaluate for denervation, which demonstrates fibrillations (earliest sign usually at 4 weeks), sharp waves, and an abnormal recruitment pattern.

C. Interpretation—For peripheral nerve entrapment syndromes, distal motor and sensory latencies >3.5 m/sec, nerve conduction velocities of <50 m/sec, and changes over a distinct interval are considered abnormal (Tables 1–52 and 1–53).

Table 1–53.

Electromyographic Findings

Condition	Insertional Activity	Activity at Rest	Minimal Contraction	Interference
Normal study	Normal	Silent	Biphasic and triphasic potentials	Complete
Axonal neuropathy	Increased	Fibrillations and positive sharp waves	Biphasic and triphasic potentials	Incomplete
Demyelinating neuropathy	Normal	Silent (occasional activity)	Biphasic and triphasic potentials	Incomplete
Anterior horn cell disease	Increased	Fibrillations, positive sharp waves, fasciculations	Large polyphasic potentials	Incomplete
Myopathy	Increased	Silent or increased spontaneous activity	Small polyphasic potentials	Early
Neuropraxia	Normal	Silent	None	None
Axonotmesis	Increased	Fibrillations and positive sharp waves	None	None
Neurotmesis	Increased	Fibrillations and positive sharp waves	None	None

Modified from Jahss, M.H.: Disorders of the Foot. Philadelphia, WB Saunders, 1982.

Section 8

Biomaterials and Biomechanics

I. **Basic Concepts**

A. Definitions

1. Biomechanics—Science of the action of forces, internal or external, on the living body.
2. Statics—Study of the action of forces on bodies at rest (in equilibrium).
3. Dynamics—Study of the motion of bodies and forces that produce the motion. There are three subtypes.
   a. Kinematics—Study of motion in terms of displacement, velocity, and acceleration without reference to the cause of the motion.
   b. Kinetics—Relates the action of forces on bodies to their resulting action.
   c. Kinesiology—Study of human movement/motion.

B. Principal Quantities

1. Basic Quantities—Described by the International System of Units (SI) or the metric system.
   a. Length—Meter (m)
   b. Mass—Amount of matter (kilogram [kg])
   c. Time—Second (sec)
2. Derived Quantities (derived from basic quantities)
   a. Velocity—Time rate of change of displacement (m/sec).
   b. Acceleration—Time rate of change of velocity (m/sec^2).
   c. Force—Action of one body on another (kg · m/s^2[N]).

C. Newton's Laws

1. First Law: Inertia—If a zero net external force acts on a body, the body will remain at rest or move uniformly. This law allows us to do static analysis with the equation $\Sigma F = 0$ (the sum of the external forces applied to a body equals zero).
2. Second Law: Acceleration—The acceleration (a) of an object of mass m is directly proportional to the force (F) applied to the object. Helps in dynamic analysis.
3. Third Law: Reactions—For every action there is an equal and opposite reaction. Leads to free body analysis.

D. Scalar and Vector Quantities

1. Scalar Quantities—Have magnitude but no direction. Examples include volume, time, mass, and speed (not velocity).
2. Vector Quantities—Have magnitude and direction. Examples include force and velocity. Vectors have four characteristics: (1) magnitude (length of the vector); (2) direction (head of the vector); (3) point of application (tail of the vector); and (4) line of action (orientation of the vector). Vectors can be added, subtracted, and split into components (resolved) for analysis. The resultant of two vectors follows the principle of "parallelogram of forces."

E. Free Body Analysis—Uses forces, moments, and free body diagrams to analyze the action of forces on bodies. **Know how to solve these problems!**

1. Forces—A push or a pull causing external (acceleration) and internal (strain) effects. Forces can be split into their components (usually in the x and y directions) for easier analysis. Some elementary knowledge of trigonometry is helpful ($F_x = F \cos \theta$, $F_y = F \sin \theta$). Also, remember the following simple approximations:

$$\sin 30° = \cos 60° \cong 0.5$$
$$\sin 45° = \cos 45° \cong 0.7$$
$$\sin 60° = \cos 30° \cong 0.9$$

   Representation of forces acting at a point is often an idealized situation and actually is an integration of a distributed load over its applied area. The **resultant force** is represented as a single force equivalent to a system of forces acting on a body. The **equilibrant force** is of equal magnitude and opposite to the resultant force.
2. Moment (M)—The rotational effect of a force on a body about a point. Any force acting at a distance from a point can produce a moment. The moment (or "torque") equals the force multiplied by the perpendicular distance from a specified point (moment arm): $M = F \times d$. **Mass moment of inertia is resistance to rotation.**
3. Free Body Diagram (FBD)—Sketch of a body or portion thereof isolated from all other bodies and showing all forces acting on it. Weights of objects act through the center of gravity (CG). **The CG for the human body is just anterior to S2.**
4. Free Body Analysis—Can proceed after all forces are represented on the FBD; using the concept of equilibrium (the sum of the forces equal zero, and the sum of the moments equal

zero) [$\Sigma F = 0$ and $\Sigma M = 0$], solve for unknowns. Assumes no change in motion, deformation, or friction. The following steps are used in the analysis.

a. Identify the system (objective, knowns, assumptions).
b. Select a coordinate system.
c. Isolate free bodies—FBD.
d. Apply Newton's laws ($\Sigma F = 0$; $\Sigma M = 0$).
e. Solve for unknowns.

5. Example—Calculate the biceps force necessary to suspend the weight of the forearm (20 N) with the elbow flexed to 90 degrees; assume the biceps insertion is 5 cm distal to the elbow, and the CG of the forearm is 15 cm distal to the elbow (Fig. 1–91). (*Answer:* 60 N.) Also solve for the joint force (J) (Fig. 1–91). (*Answer:* −40 N.)

F. Other Important Basic Concepts

1. Work—Force acts on the body to cause displacement. Work (*W*) = force (only components parallel to the displacement) × distance. Units: N·m [joules].
2. Energy—Ability to perform work (also joules). According to the law of conservation of energy, energy is neither created nor destroyed; it is transferred from one condition to another.
   a. Potential Energy—Stored energy; the ability of a body to do work as a result of its position or configuration (strain energy).
   b. Kinetic Energy—Energy of an object due to its motion ($KE = 1/2\ mv^2$).
3. Friction (f)—Resistance between two bodies when one slides over the other. Oriented opposite to the applied force. When the applied force is >f, motion begins.
4. Piezoelectricity—Electrical charge from deformation of crystalline structures when forces are applied. **Concave (compression) side = electronegative; convex (tension) side = electropositive.**

II. **Biomaterials**

A. Strength of Materials

1. Definition—Branch of mechanics that deals with relations between externally applied loads and the resulting internal effects and deformations induced in the body subjected to these loads.
   a. Loads—Forces that act on a body (compression, tension, shear, torsion).
   b. Deformations—Temporary (elastic) or permanent (plastic) change in the shape of a body. Changes in load produce changes in deformation.
2. Stress—Intensity of internal force: **Stress = force/area.** Used to analyze the internal resistance of a body to a load. Helps in selection of materials. Normal stresses (compressive or tensile) are perpendicular to the surface on which they act. Shear stresses are parallel to the surface on which they act. Stress has the units N/m² (pascals [Pa]).
3. Strain—Relative measure of the deformation (six components) of a body as a result of loading. **Strain = change in length/original length of an object.** It can also be normal or shear. Strain is a proportion and therefore has no units.

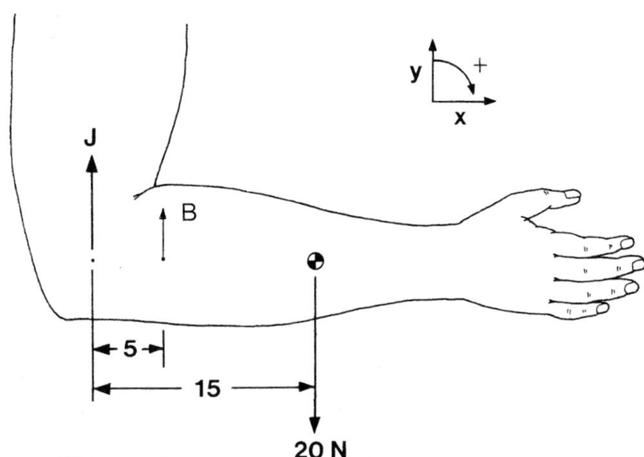

Figure 1–91. Free body diagram (see text for explanation).

Solution: $\sum M_J = 0$
$-B(.05) \quad 20(.15) = 0$
$.05\ B = 3$
$B = 60N$

$\sum F_y = 0$
$+J + B - 20 = 0$
$J = +20 - B$
$J = -40N$

4. Hooke's Law—Basically, stress is proportional to strain up to a limit (the proportional limit).
5. Young's Modulus (of Elasticity, *E*)—Measure of the stiffness of a material or its ability to resist deformation: E = stress/strain (in the elastic range of the stress-strain curve it is the slope). **Modulus of elasticity is the critical factor in load-sharing capacity. A linearly perfect elastic material** has a straight stress-strain curve to the point of failure (the modulus is calculated by dividing the stress at failure (the ultimate stress) by the strain at failure (the ultimate strain).
6. Stress-Strain Curve—Derived by axially loading a body and plotting stress versus strain (Fig. 1–92).
   a. Yield Point (Proportional Limit)—Transition point from the elastic to the plastic range. Usually 0.2% strain in most metals.
   b. Ultimate Strength—Maximum strength obtained by the material.
   c. Breaking Point—Point where the material fractures.
   d. **Plastic Deformation—Change in length after removing the load (before the breaking point) in the plastic range.**
   e. **Strain Energy—The capacity of a material (such as bone) to absorb energy. On a stress-strain curve it is illustrated as the area under the curve.** Total strain energy = recoverable strain energy (resilience) + dissipated strain energy. A measure of the toughness of a material.

B. Materials and Structures
1. Material—Related to a substance or element. Defined by mechanical properties (force, stress, strain) and rheologic properties (elasticity [ability to regain original shape], plasticity [permanent deformation], viscosity [resistance to flow or shear stress], and strength).
   a. **Brittle Materials** (e.g., PMMA)—Exhibit a linear stress-strain curve up to the point of failure. Brittle materials undergo only **fully recoverable (elastic) deformation** prior to failure and have little or no capacity to undergo permanent (plastic) deformation prior to failure.
   b. **Ductile Materials** (e.g., Metal)—Undergo a large amount of plastic deformation prior to failure. Ductility is a measure of post-yield deformation.
   c. **Viscoelastic Materials** (e.g., Bone and Ligaments)—**Exhibit stress-strain behavior that is time-rate dependent** (varies with the material); **the materials deformation depends on the load and its rate of application. The modulus of a viscoelastic material increases as the strain rate increases. The faster a load is applied, the more elastic a viscoelastic material behaves. Viscoelastic behavior is a function of the internal friction of a material.**
   d. **Isotropic Materials—Possess the same mechanical properties in all directions (e.g., a golf ball).**
   e. **Anisotropic Materials—Have mechanical properties that vary with the orientation of loading (e.g., bone).**
   f. Homogeneous Materials—Have a uniform structure or composition throughout.
2. Structure—Related to both the material and the shape of an object and its loading characteristics. A load deformation curve can be constructed similar to a stress-strain curve. The slope of the curve in the elastic range is referred to as the rigidity of the structure. **Bending rigidity of a rectangular structure** is proportional to the base multiplied by the height cubed ($bh^3/12$). **Bending rigidity of a cylinder** is related to the fourth power of the radius. Bending rigidity is closely related to the area moment of inertia (*I*, resistance to bending), which is a function of the width and thickness of the structure, and the polar moment of inertia (*J*), which represents the resistance to torsion (twisting). For more information, see section on Intramedullary Nails. **Deflection associated with bending** is proportional to the applied force (F) divided by the elastic modulus (E) of the material being bent multiplied by the area moment of inertia (I).

$$\text{Deflection} \propto \frac{F}{(E)\,(I)}$$

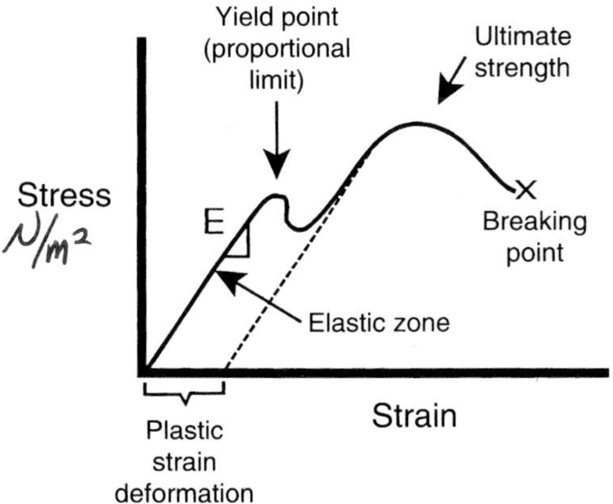

Figure 1–92. Stress-strain curve. (Modified from Miller, M.D.: Review of Orthopaedics, 2nd ed. Philadelphia, WB Saunders, 1996, p. 102.)

C. Orthopaedic Materials
1. Metals—Demonstrate stress-strain curves as discussed earlier. Other important concepts follow.
   a. Fatigue Failure—Occurs with repetitive loading cycles at stress below the ultimate

Table 1–54.

Types of Corrosion

Corrosion	Description
Galvanic	Dissimilar metals[a]; electrochemical destruction
Crevice	Occurs in fatigue cracks with low O_2 tension
Stress	Occurs in areas with high stress gradients
Fretting	From small movements abrading outside layer
Other	Includes inclusion, intergranular, and others

[a]Metals such as 316L stainless steel and Co-Cr-Mo produce galvanic corrosion.

tensile strength. Fatigue failure depends on the magnitude of the stress and number of cycles. If the stress is less than a predetermined amount of stress, called the **endurance limit (the maximum stress under which the material will not fail regardless of how many loading cycles are applied),** the material may be loaded cyclically an infinite number of times (>10^6 cycles) without breaking. Above the endurance limit, the fatigue life of a material is expressed by the stress (*S*) versus the number of loading cycles (*n*), or the *S-n* curve.

b. **Creep (a.k.a. Cold Flow)—Progressive deformation of metals (or other materials [such as polyethylene]) in response to a constant applied force over an extended period of time.** If sudden stress followed by constant loading causes a material to continue to deform, it demonstrates creep. This process can produce a permanent deformity and may affect mechanical function (such as in a TJA).

c. Corrosion—Chemical dissolving of metals as may occur in the high-saline environment of the body. Several types of corrosion may occur (Table 1–54). **316L stainless steel is the most likely metal to undergo pitting and crevice corrosion. The risk of galvanic corrosion is highest between 316L stainless steel and cobalt-chromium (Co-Cr) alloy.** Modular components of THA have direct contact between either similar or dissimilar metals (at the modular junctions) and thereby have corrosion products (metal oxides, metal chlorides, and others). Corrosion can be decreased by using similar metals (e.g., with plates and screws of similar metals), with proper design of implants, and with passivation (a thin layer that effectively separates the metal from the solution [e.g., stainless steel coated by chromium oxide]).

d. Types of Metals—Implants used in orthopaedics are typically made of 316L (L = low carbon) **stainless steel** (iron, chromium, and nickel), "supermetal" alloys **(e.g., cobalt-chromium-molybdenum** [65% Co, 35% Cr, 5% Mo] made with a special forging process), and **titanium alloy** (Ti-6Al-4V). Each possesses a **different stiffness (*E*)** (Fig. 1–93). Problems associated with certain metals include wear, stress shielding (increased in metals with a higher *E*), and ion release (Co-Cr causes macrophage proliferation and synovial degeneration). **Titanium has poor resistance to wear (notch sensitivity);** particulates may incite a histiocytic response; there is an uncertain association between titanium and neoplasms. Polishing, passivation, and ion implantation improve the fatigue properties of titanium alloy. **Titanium is an extremely biocompatible material; it rapidly forms an adherent oxide coating (self-passivation) that covers the surface of titanium (a nonreactive ceramic coating). Another**

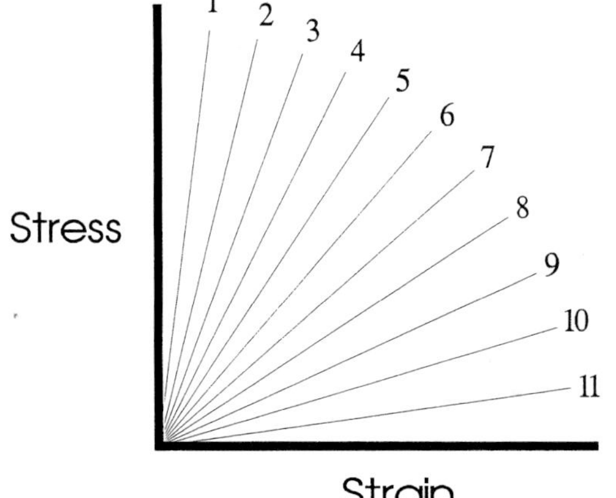

Figure 1–93. Comparison of Young's modulus (relative values, not to scale) for various orthopaedic materials.

advantage of titanium is its relatively low *E* and high yield strength. Cobalt-chrome alloy generates less metal debris (in THA) than does titanium alloy. Problems with orthoses fabrication: stainless steel is heavy and aluminum has a low endurance limit.

2. Nonmetals—Include polyethylene, PMMA (bone cement), silicone, and ceramics.
   a. Polyethylene—Ultra-high-molecular-weight polyethylene (UHMWPE) polymer consists of long chains of carbons used in weight-bearing components of TJAs such as acetabular cups and tibial trays. These materials have wear characteristics superior to those of high-density polyethylene (HDP); they are tough, ductile, resilient, and resistant to wear, and they exhibit low friction. Polyethylenes are viscoelastic and susceptible to abrasion. **Wear damage to a UHMWPE articulating surface is most often caused by third body inclusions. UHMWPE is also thermoplastic and may be altered by temperature or high-dose radiation.** The degradation of polyethylene following gamma irradiation is related to free radical formation. Polyethylenes are weaker than bone in tension and have a low *E.* Wear debris is associated with a histiocytic osteolytic response. Wear is increased with thinner (<6 mm), flatter, carbon fiber-reinforced polyethylene. Metal backing may help minimize plastic deformation of HDP (and loosening) but decreases its effective thickness (wear). Catastrophic wear of polyethylene tibial inserts is associated with varus knee alignment, thin inserts (<6 mm), flat nonconforming inserts, and heat treatments of the insert. **Polyethylene wear debris is the main factor affecting longevity of THAs.**
   b. Polymethylmethacrylate (PMMA; Bone Cement)—Used for fixation (as a grout, not an adhesive) and load distribution for implants. PMMA reaches its ultimate strength within 24 hours. PMMA can also be used as an internal splint for patients with poor bone stock; it should be thought of as a temporary internal splint until the bone heals (if the bone fails to heal, the PMMA will ultimately fail). **PMMA has poor tensile and shear strength. PMMA is strongest in compression (however, it is not as strong as bone in compression), and has a low *E.*** Reduction in the number of voids (porosity) with insertion (vacuum mixing, centrifugation, good technique) increases cement strength and decreases cracking. **PMMA functions by mechanically interlocking with bone. Insertion can lead to a precipitous drop in blood pressure.** Wear particles can incite a macrophage response that leads to loosening of a prosthesis. **Cement failure is often caused by microfracture and fragmentation of cement.**
   c. Silicones—Polymers used for replacement in non-weight-bearing joints. Their poor strength and wear capability are responsible for frequent synovitis with extended use.
   d. Ceramics—Broad class of materials that contain metallic and nonmetallic elements bonded ionically in a highly oxidized state. Include biostable (inert) materials such as Al_2O_3 and bioactive (degradable) substances such as bioglass. **Ceramics typically are brittle (no elastic deformation), have a high *modulus (E)*, a high compressive strength, a low tensile strength, a low yield strain, and poor crack resistance characteristics (low fracture toughness [low resistance to fracture]).** However, ceramics do have the best wear characteristics with polyethylene. Ceramics have a low oxidation rate. Their high conductiveness to tissue bonding is due to **high surface wetability and high surface tension,** which is also responsible for less friction and **diminished wear** ("smooth surface"). Additionally, small grain size allows for an ultrasmooth finish and less friction. Calcium phosphates (e.g., hydroxyapatite) may have application as a coating (plasma sprayed) to allow increased strength of attachment and promote bone healing.
   e. Other Materials—Such as polylactic acid-coated carbon, which serves as a biodegradable scaffolding, and new polymer composites, some with carbon fiber reinforcement, are still investigational. Fabrication of these newer devices involves assembling "piles" of carbon fibers impregnated with matrix polymer (polysulfone or polyetheretherketone). Difficulties with abrasion and impact resistance, radiolucency, and manufacturing are still present.
3. Biomaterials—Possess certain unique characteristics including viscoelasticity (time-dependent stress-strain behavior), creep, and stress relaxation (internal stresses decrease with time). They also are capable of self-adaptation and repair; characteristics change with aging and sampling.
4. Comparison of Common Orthopaedic Materials—Young's modulus of elasticity (*E*) for various orthopaedic materials are compared in Figure 1–93.

D. Orthopaedic Structures
   1. Bone
      a. Mechanical Properties—Bone is a com-

posite of collagen and hydroxyapatite. Collagen has a low *E*, good tensile strength, and poor compressive strength. Calcium apatite is a stiff, brittle material with good compressive strength. The combination is an **anisotropic** material that resists many forces; **bone is strongest in compression, weakest in shear, and intermediate in tension. The mineral content of cortical bone is the main determinant of the elastic modulus of cortical bone.** Cancellous bone is 25% as dense, 10% as stiff, and 500% as ductile as cortical bone. Bone is a dynamic material because of its ability to self-repair, to change with aging (becomes stiffer and less ductile), and to change with prolonged immobilization (becomes weaker). **With aging, there is a decline in the material properties of bone. In an attempt to offset the loss in material properties, bone remodels its geometry such that the inner and outer cortical diameters increase (is bone amazing or what!). The increased diameter of bone increases the area moment of inertia and results in a decrease in the bending stresses on bone.** Stress concentration effects, which occur at points of defects within the bone or implant-bone interface (stress risers), reduce the overall strength of bone to loading. Stress shielding by implants results in osteoporosis of adjacent bone due to lack of normal physiologic stresses. This situation occurs commonly under plates and at the femoral calcar in high-riding total hip arthroplasties. A hole of 20–30% of the bone diameter, regardless of whether it is filled with a screw, reduces overall strength up to 50%, which does not return to normal until 9–12 months after screw removal. Cortical defects can reduce strength 70% or more (less with oval defects, as compared with rectangular defects, due to a smaller stress riser). Bone is anisotropic and viscoelastic. Cortical bone is excellent versus torque; cancellous bone is good versus compressive and shear forces.

b. Fracture—Type is based on mechanism of injury.
   1. **Tension**—By muscle pull, typically transverse, perpendicular to the load and bone axis.
   2. **Compression**—By axial loading of cancellous bone; results in a crush type of fracture.
   3. **Shear**—Commonly around joints; the load is parallel to the bone surface, and the fracture is parallel to the load.
   4. **Bending**—By eccentric loading or direct blows. **The fracture begins on the tension side of the bone and continues transversely/obliquely, eventually bifurcating to produce a butterfly fragment** (with high-velocity bending there will be a comminuted butterfly fracture).
   5. **Torsion—Shear and tensile stresses result in a spiral fracture.** Because torsional stresses are proportional to the distance from the neutral axis to the periphery of a cylinder, **a long bone under torsion experiences the greatest stresses on the outer (periosteal) surface.**

c. **Comminution—A function of the amount of energy transmitted to bone.**

2. Ligaments and Tendons—These structures can sustain 5–10% tensile strain before failure (versus bone, 1–4%). Tension rupture of fibers and shear failure between fibers occurs commonly. Most ligaments can undergo plastic strain to the point at which they cannot function effectively but are still in continuity. Soft-tissue implants include stents, ligament augmentation devices, and scaffoldings. **Tendons** are strong in tension only; *E* is only 10% that of bone but increases with slower loading. Fibers are oriented parallel to each other. Tendons demonstrate stress relaxation and creep. **Ligament** fibers can be oriented parallel if they are required to resist major joint stress or more randomly if they must resist forces from different directions. Stiffness = force/strain, as depicted on a force deformation graph (similar to *E* but does not consider the cross-sectional area). The bone-ligament complex is softer (less stiff—decreased *E*) and has a lower yield point and tensile strength with prolonged immobilization. Bone resorption at the tendon insertion site also occurs.
   a. Stents—Internal splint devices. These include the Proplast Tendon Transfer Stabilizer using synthetic polymers, Goretex prosthetic ligaments, Xenotech (bovine tendon), and polyester implants. All are limited by not allowing adequate collagen ingrowth and therefore eventually fail. Synthetic ligaments produce wear particles that increase levels of proteinases, collagenase, gelatinase, and chondrocyte activation factor.
   b. Ligament Augmentation Devices (LADs)—Such as the Kennedy LAD (polypropylene yarn) and Dacron. LADs do allow some fibrous ingrowth, but their use is limited.
   c. Biodegradable Tissue Scaffoldings—Allow immediate stability and long-term replacement with host tissue. Carbon fiber and polylactic acid (PLA)-coated carbon fiber devices have been used with limited suc-

cess (slow ingrowth is improved with PLA coating).

3. Articular Cartilage—The ultimate tensile strength of cartilage is only 5% that of bone, and *E* is 0.1% that of bone; nevertheless, because of its highly viscoelastic properties, it is well suited for compressive loading. Deformation and shift of water to and from cartilage are largely responsible.
4. Metal Implants
   a. **Screws**—Characterized by pitch (distance between threads), **lead** (distance advanced in one revolution), **root diameter** (minimal/inner diameter α tensile strength), and **outer diameter** (determines holding power [pullout strength]). **To maximize pullout strength, a screw should have a large outer diameter, a small root diameter, and a fine pitch.** Pullout strength of a pedicle screw is most affected by the degree of osteoporosis.
   b. **Plates**—Strength is related to the material and the moment of inertia. **The rigidity (bending stiffness) of a plate is proportional to the thickness (t) to the third power (t^3). Therefore, doubling the thickness of a plate will increase its bending stiffness eight-fold. Plates are most effective when placed on the tension side of a fracture. Plates are load-bearing devices.** Types of plates include static compression (best in the upper extremity; can be stressed for compression), dynamic compression (e.g., tension band plate), neutralization (resists torsion), and buttress (protects bone graft). Stress concentration at open screw holes can lead to implant failure. **Screw holes that remain after removal of a plate and screws represent a stress riser and a site at risk for refracture.** Blade plates provide increased resistance to torsional deformation in subtrochanteric fractures.
   c. **Intramedullary (IM) Nails**—Require a high polar moment of inertia to maximize torsional rigidity and strength. **In characterizing the mechanical characteristics of an IM nail, we describe the torsional rigidity and the bending rigidity. Torsional rigidity** is the amount of torque needed to produce torsional (rotational) deformation (a unit angle of torsional deformation). **Torsional rigidity of an IM nail** (cylinder) depends on both material properties (shear modulus) and structural properties (polar moment of inertia). **Bending rigidity** is the amount of force required to produce a unit amount of deflection. **Bending rigidity of an IM nail** also depends on both material properties (elastic modulus) and structural properties (area moment of inertia). **Bending rigidity of an IM nail is related to the fourth power of the nail's radius.** Reaming allows increased torsional resistance owing to the increased contact area and allows use of a larger nail with increased rigidity and strength. IM nails are better at resisting bending than rotational forces. Unslotted nails allow stronger fixation and a smaller diameter (at the expense of flexibility). **The greatest mechanical advantage of closed section IM nails over slotted nails is increased torsional stiffness.** During IM nail insertion for a femoral shaft fracture, the hoop stresses are lowest for a slotted nail with a thin wall made of titanium alloy. Posterior starting points for femoral nails decrease hoop stresses and iatrogenic comminution of fractures. Implant failure occurs more frequently with smaller-diameter, unreamed IM nails. **IM nails are load-sharing devices.**
   d. External Fixators
      1. **Conventional External Fixators—The stability of fixation of a fracture treated with external fixation is most improved (the most important factor) by allowing the fracture ends to come into contact. Other factors of the external fixator that may be used to enhance stability (rigidity) are:**
         a. **Larger diameter pins (the second most important factor);** the bending rigidity of each pin is proportional to the fourth power of the pin diameter.
         b. **Additional pins.**
         c. **Decreased bone-rod distance;** the bending stiffness of each pin is proportional to the third power of the bone-rod distance.
         d. **Pins in different planes** (pins separated by more than 45 degrees).
         e. **Increased mass of the rods or stacked rods** (a second rod in the same plane provides increased resistance to bending moments in the sagital plane).
         f. **Rods in different planes.**
         g. **Increased Spacing Between Pins**—Placement of the central pins closer to the fracture site and the peripheral pins further from the fracture site (near-near, far-far). For tibial shaft fractures, when comparing the results of external fixation alone with external fixation with additional lag screws, the use of lag screws is associated with a higher refracture rate.
      2. **Circular (Ilizarov) External Fixators**—Circular rings are connected to thin

wires (usually 1.8 mm in diameter) that are fixed to the rings under tension (usually between 90 and 130 kg). Half-pins may also be used but offer better purchase in diaphyseal (not metaphyseal) bone. The optimal orientation of the implants on the ring is 90 degrees to each other to maximize stability (90 degrees is not always possible because of anatomic constraints [such as neurovascular structures]). The bending stiffness of the frame is independent of the loading direction because the frame is circular. At least two implants (wires or half-pins) should be used on each ring. The most stable construct when using two implants on a ring is an olive wire and a half-pin at 90 degrees to each other. When two wires are used on a ring, one wire should be positioned superior to the ring and one should be positioned inferior to the ring (two tensioned wires on the same side of a ring can cause the ring to deform). Factors that enhance stability of circular external fixators include:

a. Larger diameter wires (and half-pins).
b. Decreased ring diameter.
c. The use of olive wires.
d. Additional wires and/or half-pins.
e. Wires (and/or half-pins) crossing at 90 degrees.
f. Increased wire tension (up to 130 kg).
g. Placement of the two central rings close to the fracture site.
h. Decreased spacing between adjacent rings.
i. Increased number of rings.

e. Total Hip Arthroplasty (THA)—Design has evolved to help reduce biomechanical constraints. Femoral components are designed for use with and without cement. Stem length is directly related to rigidity. Minimum compressive and tensile stresses in adjacent structures result from a design with a broad medial surface, a broader lateral surface, and a large moment of inertia. Femoral component design must account for rotational forces. Rotational torque in retroversion is the force most responsible for the initiation of loosening in cemented femoral stems; these rotational torques are increased in femoral stems with a higher offset. **The femoral component should be in neutral or slight valgus to decrease the moment arm, cement stress, and abductor length. Increasing femoral component offset moves the abductor attachment away from the joint center and increases the abductor moment arm; this reduces the abductor force required in normal gait and thus reduces the resultant hip joint reactive force. Unfortunately, increased offset also increases the bending moment on the implant (increased strain), and there is also increased strain on the medial cement mantle. Femoral head size should be a compromise between small (22 mm) components, which decrease friction and torque and polyethlyene volumetric wear but also decrease ROM and stability, and large (36 mm) components that increase friction and torque and polyethylene volumetric wear but also increase ROM and stability.** A 26- or 28-mm head seems to be the ideal size in most instances. The volumetric wear of polyethlyene in hip surface replacement arthroplasty is 4–10 times that of a THA using a 28 mm head; volumetric wear of polyethylene is the most important factor for the relatively poor survivorship of surface replacement hip arthroplasty. Metal backing of acetabular components decreases the stress in cement and cancellous bone. Use of different metal alloys and titanium (with *E* closer to cortical bone) is being investigated. **Polyethylene on titanium makes a poor bearing surface because of excessive wear. The use of titanium on weight-bearing surfaces (poor resistance to wear, notch sensitivity) may lead to fretting, wear debris, and blackening of the soft tissues.** Histiocyte injection of submicron polyethylene debris has been associated with wear synovitis in TJA. UHMWPE serves as a "shock absorber" and should be at least 6 mm thick to prevent creep. Wear rate of UHMWPE in the acetabulum is about 0.1 mm/year. The lowest coefficient of friction is a ceramic femoral head on a ceramic acetabulum. Other new concepts include computer design of THA stems, modularity (increased corrosion at modular metallic junction sites [such as the junction of the head and stem]), custom designs, and more flexible stems. Forging of components appears to be superior to casting.

f. Total Knee Arthroplasty (TKA)—Design has evolved significantly after original design errors that did not take kinematics of the human knee into consideration (i.e., original hinge design). An appropriate compromise between total contact designs with excess stability (and less motion) but less wear and a low-contact design with less stability and increased wear is being approached. Metal alloys are typically used. **Cemented cruciate-substituting**

TKA designs are associated with low polyethylene wear rates and minimal osteolysis (due to the high degree of conformity of the tibiofemoral articulation).

g. Compression Hip Screws—Demonstrate loading characteristics superior to blade plates. Higher-angled plates are subjected to lower bending loads but may be more difficult to insert. Sliding of the screw is proportional to the screw/side plate angle and the length of the screw in the barrel.

5. Implant Fixation—Three basic forms exist: interference fit, interlocking, and biologic.
   a. Interference Fit—Mechanical or press fit components rely on the formation of a fibrous tissue interface. Loosening can occur if stability is not maintained and high-*E* substances are used (leading to increased bone resorption/remodeling).
   b. Interlocking Fit—PMMA (a grout with a low *E*) allows a gradual transfer of stresses to bone (microinterlocking of cement within cancellous bone). Microinterlock may not be achievable when doing a cemented revision of a previously cemented TKA. Aseptic loosening can occur over time. Careful technique with limiting of porosities and gaps and using a 3–5 mm cement thickness yields the best results. Other improvements include low-viscosity cement, better bone bed preparation, plugging and pressurization, and better (vacuum) cement mixing.
   c. Biologic Fit—Tissue ingrowth makes use of fiber-metal composites, void metal composites, or microbeads to create **pore sizes of 100–400 μm (ideally 100–250 μm).** Mechanical stability is required for ingrowth, which is most typically limited to 10–30% of the surface area. Problems include fiber/bead loosening, increased cost, proximal bone resorption (monocyte/macrophage-mediated), corrosion, and decreased implant fatigue strength. Bone ingrowth in the tibial component of an uncemented TKA occurs adjacent to fixation pegs and screws. Bone ingrowth of uncemented TJA components depends on the avoidance of micromotion (may be seen on follow-up radiographs as radiodense reactive lines about the prosthesis) at the bone-implant interface. Canal filling (maximal endosteal contact) of more fully coated femoral stems is an important factor for bone ingrowth.
6. Bone-Implant Unit—The integrated unit is a composite structure that has shared properties. The more accurately the bone cross-section is reconstructed with metallic support, the better the loading characteristics. Plates should act as tension bands. Materials with increased *E* may result in bone resorption, whereas materials with decreased *E* may result in implant failure. **Placement of the implant initiates a race between bone healing and implant failure.**

III. **Biomechanics**

A. Joint Biomechanics: General

1. Degrees of Freedom—Joint motion is described based on rotation and translation in the *x*, *y*, and *z* directions. Therefore **six positions, or degrees of freedom,** are used to describe motion. Fortunately, translations are usually relatively insignificant and can be safely ignored for most joints.
2. Joint Reaction Force (R)—Force generated within a joint in response to external forces (both intrinsic and extrinsic). **Muscle contractions about a joint are the major contributory factor to the joint reaction force.** Values (of R) correlate with the predisposition to degenerative changes. Joint contact pressure (stress) in joints can be minimized by decreasing joint force and increasing contact area.
3. Coupled Forces—Certain joints move in such a way that rotation about one axis is accompanied by an obligatory rotation about another axis, and these movements are coupled. For example, lateral bending of the spine is accompanied by axial rotation, and these movements/forces are coupled.
4. Joint Congruence—Relates to the fit of two articular surfaces and is a necessary condition for joint motion. It can be evaluated radiographically. Movement out of a position of congruity causes increased stress in cartilage by allowing less contact area for distribution of the joint reaction force, predisposing the joint to degeneration.
5. **Instant Center of Rotation**—Point at which a joint rotates. **In joints such as the knee, the location of the instant center changes during the arc of motion (due to joint translation),** following a curved path. The instant center normally lies on a line perpendicular to the tangent of the joint surface at all points of contact. If the instant center lies on the joint surface, a pure rolling motion occurs. Pure sliding motion occurs with no angular change in position and therefore has no instant center.
6. Friction and Lubrication—Resistance between two bodies when one slides over the other. It is not a function of the contact area. Lubrication decreases the coefficient of friction between surfaces. Articular surfaces lubricated with synovial fluid have a coefficient of friction 10 times less than the best synthetic systems. **The coefficient of friction of human joints is 0.002–0.04. The coefficient of friction for joint arthroplasty (metal on UHMWP) is 0.05–0.15 (not as**

Table 1–55.

Hip Biomechanics: Range of Motion

Motion	Average Range (Degrees)	Functional Range (Degrees)
Flexion	115	90 (120 squat)
Extension	30	
Abduction	50	20
Adduction	30	
Internal rotation	45	0
External rotation	45	20

good as human joints). Elastohydrodynamic lubrication is the primary mechanism responsible for lubrication of articular cartilage during dynamic function.

B. Hip Biomechanics
   1. Kinematics
      a. Range of Motion (Table 1–55)
      b. Instant Center—Simultaneous motion in all three planes for this ball-and-socket joint makes analysis impossible.
   2. Kinetics—**The joint reaction force (*R*) in the hip can reach three to six times body weight (*W*) and is primarily due to contraction of muscles crossing the hip.** This phenomenon can be demonstrated with the free body diagram (FBD) in Figure 1–94. If $A = 5$ and $B = 12.5$, using standard FBD analysis:

$$\Sigma M = 0 \text{ (the sum of the moments} = 0)$$
$$-5\ M_y + 12.5\ W = 0$$
$$M_y = 2.5\ W$$
$$\Sigma F_y = 0 \text{ (the sum of the forces} = 0)$$
$$-M_y - W + R_y = 0$$
$$R_y = 3.5\ W$$
$$R = R_y/(\cos 30 \text{ degrees})$$
$$R = \text{(approx.) } 4\ W$$

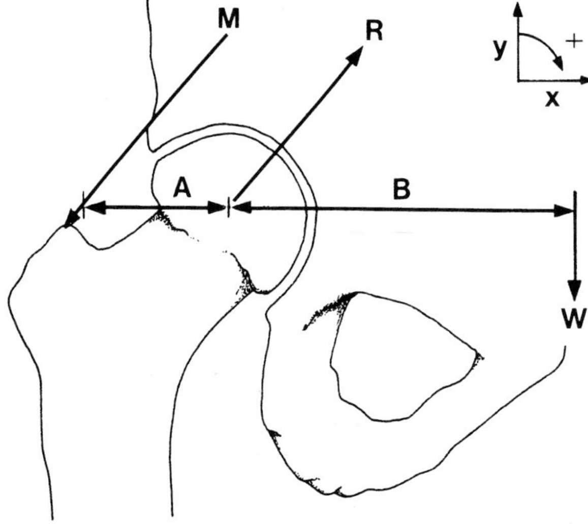

Figure 1–94. Free body diagram (see text for explanation).

One can see that an increase in the ratio of *A/B* (e.g., with medialization of the acetabulum or with a long-neck prosthesis, or with lateralization of the greater trochanter) decreases the joint reaction force. If $A = 7.5$ and $B = 10$, *R* would equal approximately 2.3 *W*. **The joint reaction force (*R*) and abductor moment are both reduced by shifting the body weight over the hip (Trendelenburg gait). A cane in the contralateral hand produces an additional moment and can reduce the joint reaction force up to 60%!** Energy expenditure is 264% of normal with a resection arthroplasty of the hip (such as after a THA infection). The hip and trunk generate approximately 50% (the largest component) of the force generated during a tennis serve.
   3. Other Considerations
      a. Stability—Largely based on the intrinsic stability of the deep-seated "ball-and-socket" design.
      b. Sourcil—Condensation of subchondral bone under the superomedial acetabulum. At this point *R* is maximal (Pauwels).
      c. Gothic Arch—Remodeled bone supporting the acetabular roof with the sourcil at its base (Bombelli).
      d. Neck-Shaft Angle—Varus angulation results in a decreased *R* and increased shear across the neck. **Varus also leads to shortening of the lower extremity and alters the muscle tension resting length of the hip abductors, which may cause a persistent limp.** Valgus angulation creates an increased *R* and decreased shear. Neutral or valgus is better for a THA because PMMA resists shear poorly.
      e. Arthrodesis—**The position for hip arthrodesis should be 25–30 degrees of flexion and 0 degrees of abduction and rotation (ER is better than IR). If the hip is fused in an abducted position, the patient will lurch over the affected lower extremity with an excessive trunk shift, which will later result in lower back pain.** Hip arthrodesis increases oxygen consumption, decreases gait efficiency (to approximately 50% of normal), and increases transpelvic rotation of the contralateral hip.

C. Knee Biomechanics
   1. Kinematics
      a. Range of Motion—ROM of the knee is from 10 degrees of extension (recurvatum) to about 130 degrees of flexion. Functional ROM is from near full extension to about 90 degrees of flexion (117 degrees is required for squatting and lifting). Flexion to approximately 110 degrees is required to arise from a chair after TKA. Rotation varies with flexion. At full extension there

is minimal rotation. At 90 degrees of flexion, 45 degrees of external rotation and 30 degrees of internal rotation are possible. Abduction/adduction is essentially 0 degrees (a few degrees of passive motion is possible at 30 degrees of flexion). Motion about the knee is a complex series of movements about a changing instant center of rotation (i.e., polycentric rotation). There is 0.5 cm of excursion of the medial meniscus and 1.1 cm of excursion of the lateral meniscus during a 0- to 120-degree arc of knee motion.

b. Joint Motion—The instant center of rotation, when plotted, describes a J-shaped curve about the femoral condyle. The instant center of rotation moves posteriorly as the knee goes from extension into flexion. Flexion and extension of the knee involve both **rolling and sliding** motions. The femur internally rotates (external tibial rotation) during the last 15 degrees of extension **("screw home" mechanism** related to the size and convexity of the medial femoral condyle [MFC] and the musculature). **Posterior rollback of the femur on the tibia during knee flexion increases maximum knee flexion.** Normal femoral rollback is compromised when the PCL is sacrificed, as in some TKAs. The axis of rotation of the intact knee is in the MFC. The patellofemoral joint is a sliding articulation (patella slides 7 cm caudally with full flexion), with an instant center near the posterior cortex above the condyles.

2. Kinetics—Extension is via the quadriceps mechanism, through the patellar apparatus; the hamstring muscles are primarily responsible for flexion of the knee.

a. Knee Stabilizers—Although bony contours have a role in knee stability, it is the ligaments and muscles of the knee that play the major role (Table 1–56). The ACL typically is subjected to peak loads of 170 N during walking and up to 500 N with running. The ultimate strength of the ACL in young patients is about 1750 N. The ACL fails by serial tearing at 10–15% elongation. Cadaver studies have shown that sectioning the PCL leads to increased contact pressures in the medial compartment and across the patellofemoral joint.

b. Joint Forces

1. Tibiofemoral Joint—Joint surfaces in the knee are subjected to a loading force equal to **three times body weight during level walking** and up to **four times body weight with walking stairs.** Menisci help with load transmission (bear one-third to one-half of body weight), and removal of these structures increases contact stresses (up to four times load transfer to bone). The quadriceps muscle produces maximal anterior directed force on the tibia at knee flexion of 0–60 degrees.

2. Patellofemoral Joint—The patella aids in knee extension by increasing the lever arm and in stress distribution. This joint has the thickest cartilage in the entire body because it must bear the greatest load—ranging from ½ *W* with normal walking to seven times *W* with squatting and jogging. Loads are proportional to the quadriceps force/knee flexion ratio. **While descending stairs, the compressive force between the patella and the trochlea of the femur reaches 2–3 times body weight. After patellectomy, the length of the moment arm is decreased by the width of the patella (30% reduction) and the power of extension is decreased by 30%.** During TKA the following enhance patella tracking: external rotation of the femoral component, lateral placement of the femoral and tibial components, medial placement of the patellar component, and avoidance of malrotation of the tibial component (avoid internal rotation).

c. Axes of the Lower Extremity (Fig. 1–95)

1. Mechanical Axis of the Lower Extremity—From the center of the femoral head to the center of the ankle. The mechanical axis of a normal lower extremity passes just medial to the medial tibial spine.

2. Vertical Axis—From the center of gravity to the ground.

3. Anatomic Axes—Along the shafts of the femur and tibia. There is a normal valgus angle where these two axes intersect at the knee.

4. Mechanical Axis of the Femur—From the center of the femoral head to the center of the knee.

Table 1–56.

Knee Stabilizers

Direction	Structures
Medial	Superficial MCL (1°), joint capsule, med. meniscus, ACL/PCL
Lateral	Joint capsule, IT band, LCL (mid), lat. meniscus, ACL/PCL (90°)
Anterior	ACL (1°), joint capsule
Posterior	PCL (1°), joint capsule; PCL tightens with IR
Rotatory	Combinations—MCL checks ER; ACL checks IR

IR, internal rotation; ER, external rotation; MCL, medial collateral ligament complex; LCL, lateral collateral ligament complex; IT, iliotibial; ACL, anterior cruciate ligament; PCL, posterior cruciate ligament.

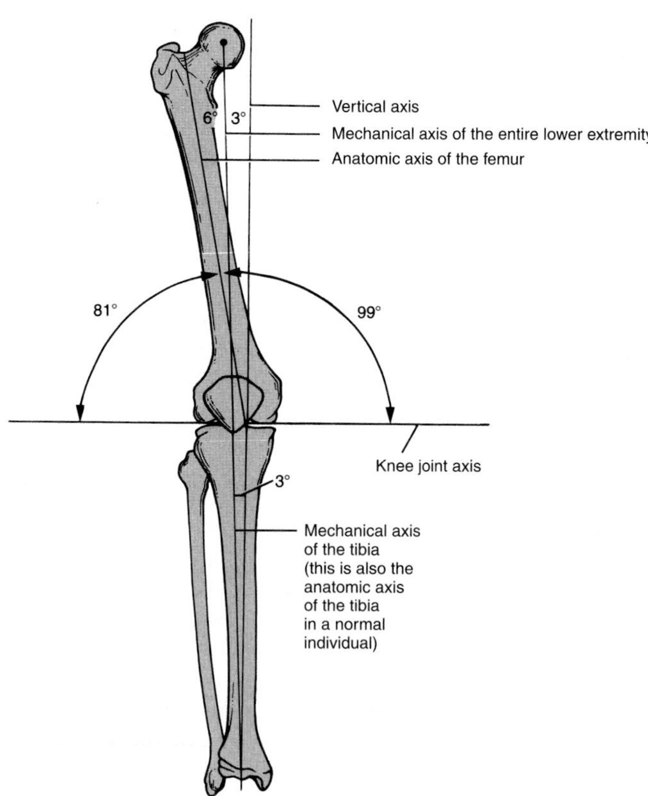

Figure 1–95. Axes of the lower extremity. (Modified from Helfet, D.L.: Fractures of the distal femur. In Browner, B.D., Jupiter, J.B., Levine, A.M., et al., eds.: Skeletal Trauma. Philadelphia, WB Saunders, 1992, p. 1645.)

5. Mechanical Axis of the Tibia—From the center of the tibial plateau to the center of the ankle.
6. Relationships—The mechanical axis of the lower extremity is in 3 degrees of valgus from the vertical axis. The anatomic axis of the femur is in 6 degrees of valgus from the mechanical axis (9 degrees versus the vertical axis). The anatomic axis of the tibia is in 2–3 degrees of varus from the mechanical axis.

d. Arthrodesis—**The position for knee arthrodesis should be 0–7 degrees of valgus and 10–15 degrees of flexion.**

D. Ankle and Foot Biomechanics

1. Ankle

a. Kinematics—Instant center of rotation is within the talus, and the lateral and posterior points are at the tips of the malleoli; they change slightly with movement. The talus is described as forming a cone with the body and trochlea wider anteriorly and laterally. Therefore, the talus and fibula must externally rotate slightly with dorsiflexion. Ankle dorsiflexion and abduction are coupled movements in the ankle. Average ankle ROM is 25 degrees of dorsiflexion, 35 degrees of plantar flexion, and 5 degrees of rotation.

b. Kinetics—The tibial/talar articulation is the major weight-bearing surface of the ankle, supporting compressive forces up to five times body weight on level surfaces and shear (backward-to-forward) forces up to body weight. A large weight-bearing surface area allows for decreased stress (force/area) at this joint. The fibula/talar joint transmits about one-sixth of the force. The highest net muscle moment at the ankle occurs during the terminal stance phase of gait.

c. Other Considerations—Stability is based on the shape of the articulation (mortise that is maintained by the talar shape) and ligamentous support. The greatest stability is in dorsiflexion. During weight-bearing (loaded), the tibial and talar articular surfaces contribute most to joint stability. A windlass action has been described in the ankle, where full dorsiflexion is limited by the plantar aponeurosis, and further tension on the aponeurosis (e.g., with toe dorsiflexion) causes the arch to rise. **A syndesmosis screw limits external rotation of the ankle. Arthrodesis of the ankle should be performed in neutral dorsiflexion, 5–10 degrees of external rotation, and 5 degrees of hindfoot valgus** (anticipate a loss of 70% of the sagittal plane motion of the foot).

2. Subtalar Joint (Talus-Calcaneus-Navicular)—The axis of rotation is 42 degrees in the sagittal plane and 16 degrees in the transverse plane. Described as functioning like an oblique hinge; its motions are also coupled with dorsiflexion, abduction, and eversion in

Table 1–57.
Arches of the Foot

Arch	Components	Keystone	Ligament Support	Muscle Support
Medial longitudinal	Calcaneus, talus, navicular, 3 cuneiforms, 1st–3rd metatarsals	Talus head	Spring (calcaneonavicular)	Tibialis post., flexor digitorum longus, flexor hallucis longus, adductor hallucis
Lateral longitudinal	Calcaneus, cuboid, 4th and 5th metatarsals		Plantar aponeurosis	Abductor digiti minimi, flexor digitorum brevis
Transverse	3 Cuneiforms, cuboid, metatarsal bases			Peroneus longus, tibialis post., adductor hallucis (oblique)

one direction (pronation) and plantar flexion, adduction, and inversion (supination) in the other. Average ROM of pronation is 5 degrees; supination is 20 degrees. Functional ROM is approximately 6 degrees.

3. Transverse Tarsal Joint (Talus-Navicular, Calcaneal-Cuboid)—Motion is based on foot position with two axes of rotation (talonavicular and calcaneocuboid). With eversion of the foot (as during the early stance phase), the two joints are parallel and ROM is permitted. With foot inversion (late stance), external rotation of the lower extremity causes the joints to no longer be parallel, and motion is limited.
4. Foot—Transmits about 1.2 times body weight with walking and three times body weight with running. It is composed of three arches (Table 1–57). The second MT (Lisfranc) joint is "key-like" and stabilizes the second MT, allowing it to carry the most load with gait (the first MT bears the most load while standing). The expected life span of a Plastazote shoe insert in an active adult is less than 1 month (it fatigues rapidly in both compression and shear). Therefore, in a shoe insert, Plastazote should be supported with other materials such as Spenco or PPT.

E. Spine Biomechanics

1. Kinematics—ROM varies with anatomic segment (Table 1–58). Analysis is based on the functional unit **(motion segment = two vertebrae and their intervening soft tissues). Six degrees of freedom exist about all three axes. Coupled motion** (simultaneous rotation, lateral bending, and flexion or extension) is also demonstrated, especially with axial rotation and lateral bending. The instant center of rotation lies within the disc. The normal sagital alignment of the lumbar spine (55–60 degrees of lordosis) exists because of the disc spaces (not the vertebrae); most of the lordosis is between L4 and S1. Loss of disc space height can cause a significant loss of the normal lumbar lordosis. Iatrogenic flat back syndrome of the lumbar spine is the result of a distraction force.
2. Supporting Structures—Anterior supporting structures include the anterior longitudinal ligament, the posterior longitudinal ligament, and the vertebral disc. Posterior supporting structures include the intertransverse ligaments, capsular ligaments and facets, and ligamentum flavum (yellow ligament). The halo vest is the most effective device for controlling cervical motion (because of pin purchase in the skull).
   a. Apophyseal Joints—Resist torsion during axial loading, and the attached capsular ligaments resist flexion. They guide the motion of the motion segment. Direction of motion is determined by the orientation of the facets of the apophyseal joint, which varies with each level. **In the C-spine the facets are oriented 45 degrees to the transverse plane and parallel to the frontal plane. In the T-spine the facets are oriented 60 degrees to the trans-**

Table 1–58.
Range of Motion of Spinal Segments

Level	Flexion/Extension (Degrees)	Lateral Bending (Degrees)	Rotation (Degrees)	Instant Center
Occiput–C1	13	8	0	Skull, 2–3 cm above dens
C1–C2	10	0	45	Waist of odontoid
C2–C7	10–15	8–10	10	Vertebral body below
T-spine	5	6	8	Vertebra below/disc centrum
L-spine	15–20	2–5	3–6	Disc annulus

verse plane and 20 degrees to the frontal plane. In the L-spine the facets are oriented 90 degrees to the transverse plane and 45 degrees to the frontal plane (i.e., they progressively tilt up [transverse plane] and in [frontal plane]). **Cervical facetectomy of greater than 50% causes a significant loss of stability in flexion and torsion. Torsional load resistance in the lumbar spine has a 40% contribution from the facets and a 40% contribution by the disk; the remaining 20% resistance to torsional load is contributed by the ligamentous structures.**

3. Kinetics
   a. Disc—**Behaves viscoelastically and demonstrates creep (deforms with time) and hysteresis (absorbs energy with repeated axial loads and later decreases in function).** Compressive stresses are highest in the nucleus pulposus, and tensile stresses are highest in the annulus fibrosus. Stiffness of the disc increases with increasing compressive load. With higher loads, increased deformation and faster creep can be expected. Repeated torsional loading may separate the nucleus pulposus from the annulus and end-plate and may force nuclear material out through an annular tear (produced by shear forces). Loads are increased with bending and torsional stresses. **After subtotal discectomy, extension is the most stable loading mode. Disc pressures are lowest in the lying supine position on a flat surface. When carrying loads, disc pressures are lowest when the load is carried close to the body.**
   b. Vertebrae—Strength is related to the bone mineral content and size of the vertebrae (increased in the lumbar spine). Fatigue loading may lead to pars fractures. Compression fractures occur at the end-plate. Decreased vertebral body stiffness in osteoporosis is caused by loss of horizontal trabeculae. Increasing implant stiffness for an implant-augmented spinal arthrodesis results in an increased probability of a successful fusion but an increased likelihood of decreased bone mineral content of the bridged vertebrae.

F. Shoulder Biomechanics
1. Kinematics—The scapular plane is 30 degrees anterior to the coronal plane and is the preferred reference for ROM. Abduction of the shoulder requires external rotation of the humerus to prevent greater tuberosity impingement. With internal rotation contractures, patients cannot abduct past 120 degrees. Abduction is a result of glenohumeral motion (120 degrees) and scapulothoracic motion (60 degrees) in a 2:1 ratio. **Deceleration is the most violent phase of pitching; the rotator cuff is the principal decelerator and is susceptible to tensile failure from eccentric loading.** Movement at the acromioclavicular (AC) joint is responsible for the early part of scapulothoracic motion, and sternoclavicular (SC) movement is responsible for the later portion, with clavicular rotation along the long axis. Surface joint motion in the glenohumeral joint is a combination of rotation, rolling, and translation.
2. Kinetics (Table 1–59)—The zero position (Saha)—165 degrees of abduction in the scapular plane—minimizes deforming forces about the shoulder. This position is ideal for reducing shoulder dislocations (or "fractures with traction"). Free-body analysis of the deltoid force (Fig. 1–96) reveals the following:

$$\Sigma M_0 = 0$$
$$3D - 0.05\,W(30) = 0$$
$$D = 0.5\,W$$

3. Stability—Limited about the glenohumeral joint. The humeral head has a surface area larger than the glenoid (48 × 45 versus 35 × 25). Bony stability is limited and relies only on inclination (125 degrees) and retroversion (25 degrees) of the humeral head and slight retrotilt of the glenoid. **The inferior glenohumeral ligament (superior band) is the most important static stabilizer about the shoulder.** The superior and middle glenohumeral ligaments are secondary stabilizers to anterior humeral translation. **Infe-**

Table 1–59.

Shoulder Biomechanics: Muscle Forces

Motion	Muscle Forces	Comments
Glenohumeral		
Abduction	Deltoid, supraspinatus	Cuff depresses head
Adduction	Latissimus dorsi, pectoralis major, teres major	
Forward flexion	Pectoralis major, deltoid (ant.), biceps	
Extension	Latissimus dorsi	
IR	Subscapularis, teres major	
ER	Infraspinatus, teres minor, deltoid (post.)	
Scapular		
Rotation	Upper trapezius, levator scapulae (ant.), serratus ant., lower trapezius	Works through a force couple
Adduction	Trapezius, rhomboid, latissimus dorsi	
Abduction	Serratus ant., pectoralis minor	

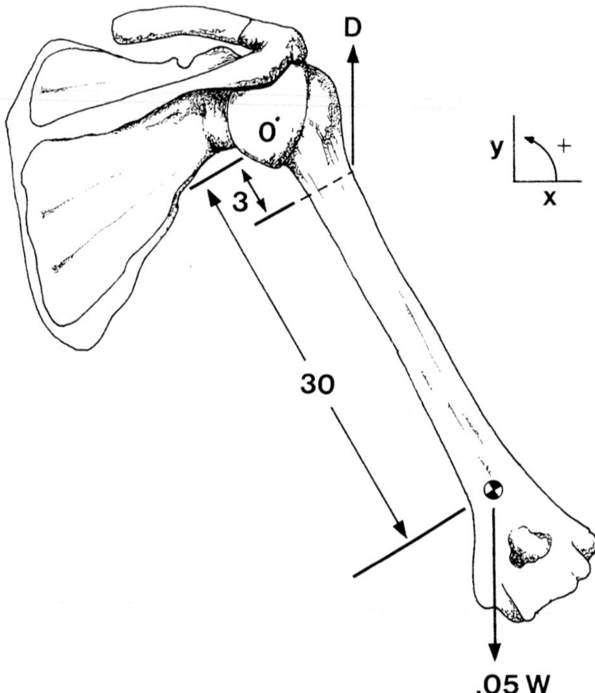

Figure 1–96. Free body diagram (see text for explanation).

rior subluxation of the humeral head is prevented by the shoulder's negative intra-articular pressure. The rotator cuff muscles provide a dynamic contribution to shoulder stability. Stress on the posterior shoulder capsule is greatest during follow-through of throwing. **The position for arthrodesis of the shoulder is 30 degrees of true abduction, 20 degrees of forward flexion, and 40 degrees of internal rotation (avoid excessive external rotation).**

4. Other Joints—The AC joint allows scapular rotation (through the conoid and trapezoid ligaments) and scapular motion (through the AC joint itself). The SC joint allows clavicular protraction/retraction in a transverse plane (through the coracoclavicular ligament), clavicular elevation and depression in the frontal plane (also through the coracoclavicular ligament), and clavicular rotation around the longitudinal axis.

G. Elbow Biomechanics

1. Introduction—The elbow serves three functions: (1) as a component joint of the lever arm when positioning the hand; (2) as a fulcrum for the forearm lever; and (3) as a weight-bearing joint in patients using crutches. During throwing, the elbow functions primarily as a positioner and a means of transferring energy from the shoulder and trunk. Most activities of daily living can be performed with an elbow range of motion of 30–130 degrees of flexion, 50 degrees of supination, and 50 degrees of pronation.
2. Kinematics—Motion about the elbow includes flexion and extension (0–150 degrees with **functional ROM 30–130 degrees;** the axis of rotation is the center of the trochlea) and pronation (P) and supination (S): P = 80 degrees and S = 85 degrees with a **functional P and S of 50 degrees each;** the axis is a line from the capitellum through the radial head and to the distal ulna (defines a cone). The normal carrying angle (valgus angle at the elbow) is 7 degrees for males and 13 degrees for females. This angle decreases with flexion.
3. Kinetics—The forces that act about the elbow have short lever arms and are relatively inefficient, resulting in large joint reaction forces that subject the elbow to degenerative changes. Flexion is primarily by the brachialis and biceps, extension by the triceps, pronation by the pronators (teres and quadratus), and supination by the biceps and supinator. Static loads approach, and dynamic loads exceed, body weight. The FBD in Figure 1–97 demonstrates the inefficiency of elbow flexion.

$$\Sigma M_0 = 0$$
$$-5B + 15W = 0$$
$$B = 3W$$

Because the biceps inserts so close to the joint, it is relatively inefficient and must support three times the weight of the arm and any objects it holds.

4. Stability—Provided partially by articular congruity. **The greatest stability of the elbow comes from the medial side, where the medial collateral ligament (MCL) is the most important stabilizer (especially the anterior oblique fibers).** The MCL stabilizes the elbow to both valgus and distrac-

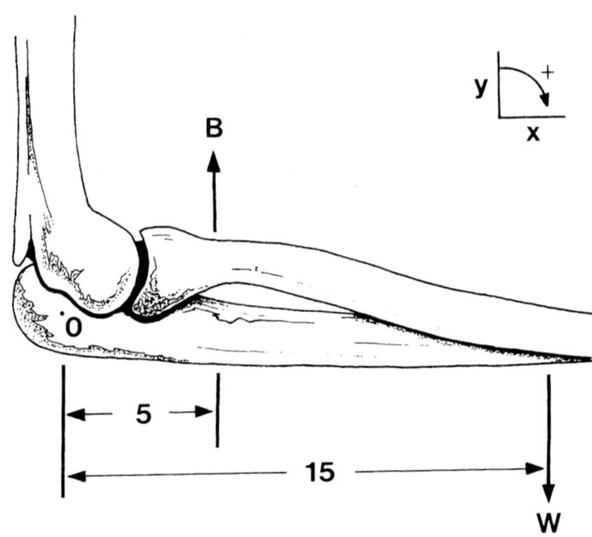

Figure 1–97. Free body diagram (see text for explanation).

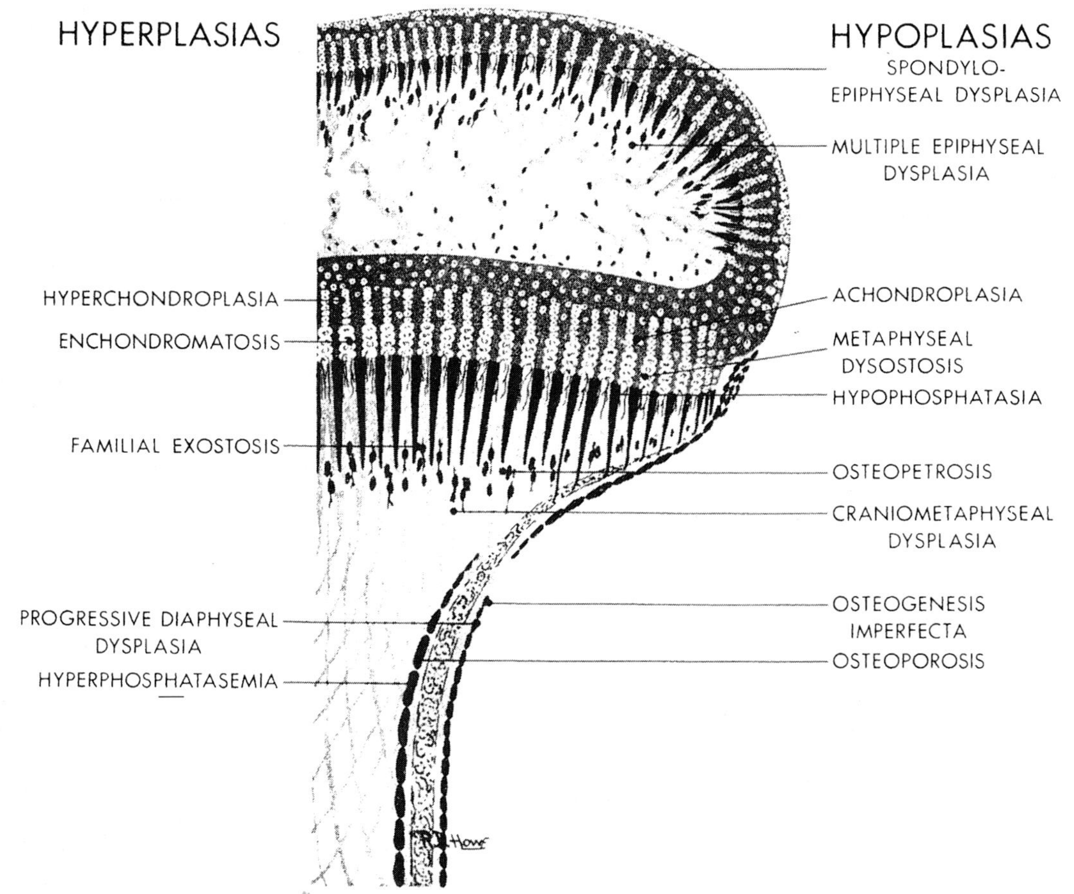

Figure 2–5. Location of abnormalities leading to dysplasias. (From Rubin, P.: Dynamic Classification of Bone Dysplasias. Chicago, Year Book Medical Publishers, 1964.)

tolerated, with a low rate of complications. The patients still have the other underlying problems, however, and limb-lengthening procedures remain controversial in achondroplastic patients.

4. Pseudoachondroplasia—Although considered separately in some classifications, this disorder is clinically similar to achondroplasia. The inheritance pattern is autosomal-dominant. In contrast to achondroplasia, the affected children have normal facies. Radiographs demonstrate metaphyseal flaring and delayed epiphyseal ossification. Orthopaedic manifestations of the disorder include cervical instability, scoliosis with increased lumbar lordosis; significant lower extremity bowing; and hip, knee, and elbow flexion contractures with precocious osteoarthritis.

C. Spondyloepiphyseal Dysplasia—Two forms are generally recognized and must be differentiated from multiple epiphyseal dysplasia (MED). MED and spondyloepiphyseal dysplasia involve epiphyseal development in upper and lower extremities. The distinguishing feature of spondyloepiphyseal dysplasia is the added typical spine involvement.

1. Congenita Form—Short-trunked dwarfism associated with primary involvement of the vertebra (beaking) and epiphyseal centers (affects the proliferative zone), clinical heterogenicity, and AD inheritance. The clinical and radiographic differences are frequently age-related and not distinguishable at birth. Delayed appearance of the epiphysis, flattened facies, platyspondyly, scoliosis, odontoid hypoplasia, coxa vara, and genu valgum are common. Patients should also be screened for associated retinal detachment and myopia.
2. Tarda Form—These patients typically have a variable inheritance pattern and late (age 8–10) manifestations of the disorder, which affects primarily the spine and large joints. Hips may be dislocated, and affected children are often susceptible to premature osteoarthritis (osteotomies may be helpful) and scoliosis (treated like idiopathic scoliosis).

D. Chondrodysplasia Punctata—Characterized by multiple punctate calcifications seen on radiographs during infancy. The AD form (Conradi-Hunermann) has a wide variation of clinical expression. The severe autosomal-recessive (AR) rhizomelic form is usually fatal during the first year of life. Cataracts, asym-

Table 2–1.

Rubin's Classification of Bone Dysplasias

- I. Epiphyseal dysplasias
  - A. Epiphyseal hypoplasias
    - 1. Failure of articular cartilage: spondyloepiphyseal dysplasia
    - 2. Failure of ossification of center: multiple epiphyseal dysplasia
  - B. Epiphyseal hyperplasia
    - 1. Excess of articular cartilage: dysplasia epiphysealis hemimelia
- II. Physeal dysplasia
  - A. Cartilage hypoplasia
    - 1. Failure of proliferating cartilage: achondroplasia
    - 2. Failure of hypertrophic cartilage: metaphyseal dysostosis; cartilage-hair hypoplasia
  - B. Cartilage hyperplasias
    - 1. Excess of proliferating cartilage: hyperchondroplasia (Marfan syndrome)
    - 2. Excess of hypertrophic cartilage: enchondromatosis
- III. Metaphyseal dysplasias
  - A. Metaphyseal hypoplasias
    - 1. Failure to form primary spongiosa: hypophosphatasia
    - 2. Failure to absorb primary spongiosa: osteopetrosis
    - 3. Failure to absorb secondary spongiosa: craniometaphyseal dysplasia
  - B. Metaphyseal hyperplasia
    - 1. Excessive spongiosa: multiple exostoses
- IV. Diaphyseal dysplasias
  - A. Diaphyseal hypoplasias
    - 1. Failure of periosteal bone formation: osteogenesis imperfecta
    - 2. Failure of endosteal bone formation: idiopathic osteoporosis, congenita and tarda
  - B. Diaphyseal hyperplasias
    - 1. Excessive periosteal bone formation: progressive diaphyseal dysplasia (Engelmann's disease)
    - 2. Excessive endosteal bone formation: hyperphosphatasemia (including juvenile Paget's disease and van Buchem's disease)

Adapted from Rubin, P.: Dynamic Classification of Bone Dysplasias. Chicago, Year Book Medical Publishers, 1964.

metric limb shortening that may require surgical correction, and spinal deformities are common.

E. Kniest's Syndrome—AD, short-trunked, disproportionate dwarfism with joint stiffness/contractures, scoliosis, kyphosis, dumbbell-shaped femora, and hypoplastic pelvis and spine. May be related to an abnormality of cartilage proteoglycan metabolism, and physes may have a characteristic "Swiss cheese" appearance histologically. Radiographs show osteopenia and platyspondyly or hypoplasia. Respiratory problems and cleft palate are common. Associated retinal detachment and myopia require an ophthalmology consult. Early therapy for joint contractures is required. Reconstructive procedures may be required for early hip degenerative arthritis. Otitis media and hearing loss are frequent.

F. Metaphyseal Chondrodysplasia—Heterogeneous group of disorders characterized by metaphyseal changes of tubular bones with normal epiphyses. The physis (proliferative and hypertrophic zones) histologically appears to be more affected than the metaphysis; therefore, the term metaphyseal dysostoses has fallen out of favor. The epiphyses are normal. Several types are recognized, including the following:

1. Jansen's (rare)—most severe form; AD, retarded, markedly short-limbed dwarf with wide eyes, monkey-like stance, and hypercalcemia. Striking bulbous metaphyseal expansion of long bones is a distinctive radiographic finding.
2. Schmid's—More common, less severe form. AD, short-limbed dwarf not diagnosed until patient is older, with stunting of growth and bowing of legs due to *coxa vara* and genu varum. Predominantly involves the proximal femur. Metaphyseal lesions heal with bed rest but recur with weight bearing. Often confused with rickets, but laboratory test results are normal.
3. McKusick's—AR, cartilage-Hair dysplasia (hypoplasia of cartilage and small diameter of hair) is seen most commonly among the Amish population and in Finland. Fine, brittle, thin hair is a notable feature. Atlantoaxial instability is common (*odontoid hypoplasia*) and requires flexion-extension lateral radiographs for proper evaluation. Ankle deformity develops due to fibular overgrowth distally. These patients may have abnormal immunologic competence (susceptible to severe reaction from chickenpox).

G. MED—Short-limbed disproportionate dwarfism that often does not manifest until age 5–14. Must differentiate from spondyloepiphyseal dysplasia. A mild form (Ribbing's) and a more severe form (Fairbank's) exist. MED is characterized by irregular, delayed ossification at multiple epiphyses. Short, stunted metacarpals/metatarsals, irregular proximal femora, abnormal ossification (tibial "slant sign" and flattened femoral condyles), valgus knees (consider early osteotomy), waddling gait, and early hip arthritis are common. The proximal femoral involvement can be confused with Perthes'; MED is bilateral and symmetric, has early acetabular changes, and does not have metaphyseal cysts.

H. Dysplasia Epiphysealis Hemimelica (Trevor's Disease)—Essentially an epiphyseal osteochondroma. Most commonly seen at the knee. Partial excision of the prominent overgrowth (if symptomatic) and later osteotomies may be required. Recurrence is a common complication.

I. Progressive Diaphyseal Dysplasia (Camurati-Engelmann Disease)—AD; affected children are often "late walkers" (because of associated muscle weakness), with symmetric cortical thickening of long bones. Radiographs demonstrate widened, fusiform diaphyses with increased bone formation and sclerosis. The tibia, femur, and humerus are most often affected (in that order), affecting only the diaphyseal portion of bone. Symptomatic treatment includes salicylates, nonsteroidal anti-inflammatory drugs, and steroids for refractory cases. Watch for leg-length inequality.

J. Mucopolysaccharidosis—In contrast to the above conditions, these forms of dwarfism are easily differentiated, based on the presence of complex sugars found in the urine. They produce a *proportionate* dwarfism caused by accumulation of mucopolysaccharides due to a hydrolase enzyme deficiency. Mucopolysaccharides consist of glycosaminoglycans attached to a link protein with a hyaluronic acid core (see Chapter 1, Basic Sciences). Four main types include Hurler's, Hunter's, Sanfilippo's, and Morquio's syndromes (Table 2–2). **Morquio's syndrome (AR)** is the most common form and presents by age 18 months to 2 years with waddling gait, knock-knees, thoracic kyphosis, cloudy corneas, and *normal intelligence*. Bony changes include a thickening skull; wide ribs; anterior beaking of vertebrae; wide, flat pelvis; coxa vara with unossified femoral heads, and bullet-shaped metacarpals. C1–C2 instability (due to odontoid hypoplasia) can be seen with Morquio syndrome presenting with myelopathy and requires decompression and cervical fusion. Morquio syndrome is associated with urinary excretion of *keratan sulfate*. **Hurler's syndrome (AR)** is the most severe form and is associated with urinary excretion of *dermatan/heparan sulfate*. **Hunter's syndrome (sex-linked recessive)** is associated with urinary excretion of *dermatan/heparan sulfate*. **Sanfilippo's syndrome (AR)** is associated with urinary excretion of *heparan sulfate*. Hunter's, Hurler's, and Sanfilippo's syndromes are associated with *mental retardation*.

K. Diastrophic Dysplasia—AR; severe, short-limbed dwarfism associated with a disorder of *type II collagen* in the physis. This "*twisted*" dwarf classically has a cleft palate, severe joint contractures (especially hip and knees), cauliflower ears, hitchhiker thumb, rigid club feet, midthoracic kyphoscoliosis, cervical kyphosis (often severe, requiring immediate treatment), thoracolumbar kyphoscoliosis, spina bifida occulta, and atlantoaxial instability due to odontoid hypoplasia. Surgical release of club foot deformities, osteotomies for contractures, and spinal fusion are often required.

L. Cleidocranial Dysplasia (Dysostosis)—AD, proportionate dwarfism that affects bones formed by intramembranous ossification. Patients present with dwarfism and aplasia of portions of or the entire clavicle. Usually unilateral, often the lateral part of the clavicle is missing, and there are delayed skull suture closure, frontal bossing, coxa vara (consider intertrochanteric valgus osteotomy if neck-shaft angle is <100 degrees), delayed ossification of the pubis, and wormian-type bone.

M. Dysplasias Associated with Benign Bone Growths—Include multiple hereditary exostosis (osteochondromatosis), fibrous dysplasia, Ollier's disease (enchondromatosis), and Maffucci's syndrome (enchondromatosis and hemangiomas). These entities are discussed in Chapter 8, Orthopaedic Pathology.

N. Dysplasia Summary—The various types of dysplasia are summarized in Table 2–3.

III. **Chromosomal and Teratologic Disorders**

A. Down's Syndrome (Trisomy 21)—*Most common chromosomal abnormality*; its incidence increases with maternal age. Usually associated with ligamentous laxity, hypotonia, mental retardation, *heart disease* (50%), endocrine disorders (hypothyroidism and diabetes), and premature aging. Orthopaedic problems include metatarsus primus varus, pes planus, spinal abnormalities (**atlantoaxial instability**, scoliosis, spondylolisthesis), hip instability (*open reduction ± osteotomy* usually required), slipped capital femoral epiphysis, patellar dislocation, and symptomatic planovalgus feet. Atlantoaxial instability may be subtle in its presentation, but commonly presents as a loss or change in motor milestones. Atlantoaxial instability is evaluated with flexion-extension radiographs of the C-spine. Asymptomatic children with instability should avoid contact sports, diving, and gymnastics. Atlantoaxial fusion has a high complication rate and is usually reserved for patients with progressive instability, atlanto-dens interval >10 mm, or neurologic symp-

Table 2–2.

Main Types of Mucopolysaccharidosis

Syndrome	Inheritance	Intelligence	Cornea	Urinary Excretion	Other
I Hurler's	AR	MR	Cloudy	Dermatan/heparan sulfate	Worst prognosis
II Hunter's	XR	MR	Clear	Dermatan/heparan sulfate	
III Sanfilippo's	AR	MR	Clear	Heparan sulfate	Normal until 2 years old
IV Morquio's	AR	Normal	Cloudy	Keratan sulfate	Most common

AR, autosomal-recessive; XR, sex-linked recessive; MR, mental retardation.

Table 2–3.

Types of Dysplasia

Dysplasia	Type	Inheritance	Zone	Clinical Findings	Radiographic Features
Achondroplasia	Dis	AD/SM	Epi	Facies, spine abnormalities	Stenosis, leg bowing
SED (congenita)	Dis	AD	Epi	Cleft palate, lordosis	Platyspondyly
SED (pseudoachondroplastic)	Dis	AD/AR	Epi	Normal facies	Fragmented epiphysis
SED (tarda)	Dis	XR	Epi	Kyphosis, hip pain	Hip dysplasia, thick vertebrae
Chondrodysplasia punctata	Dis	AD	Phy	Flat facies	Stippled epiphyses
Kniest's syndrome	Dis	AD	Phy	Retinal detachment, scoliosis	Dumbbell femora
Metaphyseal chondrodysplasia	Dis	AD/AR	Met	Wide eyes, leg bowing	Bowed legs
Multiple epiphyseal	Dis	AD	Epi	Late—waddling gait	Irregular epiphyseal ossification
Dysplasia epiphysealis hemimelia	Dis	—	Met	Bowed legs	Hemienlarged epiphysis
Diaphyseal	Dis	AD	Dia	Delayed walking	Symmetric cortical thickening
Mucopolysaccharidosis	Pro	AD/XR	Hyp	Cornea, urinary sugars, AAI	Thick bone, bullet metacarpals
Diastrophic	Pro	AR	Phy	Palate, ear, thumb	Kyphoscoliosis
Cleidocranial dysostosis	Pro	AR	Met	Absent clavicles	Delayed physeal closure

Dis, disproportionate; Pro, proportionate; AD, autosomal-dominant; AR, autosomal-recessive; SM, spontaneous mutation; XR, sex-linked recessive; Epi, epiphyseal; Phy, physeal; Met, metaphyseal; Dia, diaphyseal; Hyp, hypophyseal; SED, spondyloepiphyseal dysplasia; AAI, atlantoaxial instability.

toms. Preoperative cardiac evaluation is essential.

B. Turner's Syndrome—45,XO females with short stature, sexual infantilism, web neck, and cubitus valgus. Hormonal therapy can exacerbate scoliosis. Renal anomalies (usually minor) are present in two-thirds of patients, and cardiac anomalies are present in one-third. Genu valgum and shortening of the fourth and fifth metacarpals usually require no treatment. *Malignant hyperthermia* is common with anesthetic use.

C. Noonan's Syndrome—Short stature, web neck, and cubitus valgus deformities in boys with normal sexual genotypes. Increased risk for *malignant hyperthermia* with anesthetics.

D. Prader-Willi Syndrome—Chromosome 15 abnormality, causing a floppy, hypotonic infant who becomes an intellectually impaired, obese adult with an insatiable appetite. Growth retardation, hip dysplasia, hypoplastic genitalia, and scoliosis are common.

E. Menkes' Syndrome—Sex-linked recessive disorder of copper transport that affects bone growth and causes characteristic "kinky" hair. May be differentiated from occipital horn syndrome (which also affects copper transport) by the characteristic bony projections from the occiput of the skull in that disorder.

F. Rett's Syndrome—*Progressive impairment* and stereotaxic abnormal hand movements characterize this disorder. It is seen in *girls* at 6–18 months of age, who present with developmental delay much like that seen with cerebral palsy. Affected children typically have *scoliosis* with a C-shaped curve unresponsive to bracing. Anterior diskectomy and interbody fusion combined with posterior fusion and instrumentation are indicated for curves >40 degrees. The posterior fusion should include segmental fixation from the upper thoracic spine to the pelvis inferiorly (Luque-Galveston). Spasticity results in joint contractures, which are treated as in cerebral palsy patients.

G. Teratogens

1. Fetal Alcohol Syndrome—*Maternal alcoholism* can cause growth disturbances, central nervous system dysfunction, dysmorphic facies, hip dislocation, C-spine vertebral and upper extremity congenital fusions, congenital scoliosis, and myelodysplasia.
2. Maternal Diabetes—May lead to heart defects, **sacral agenesis**, and anencephaly. Careful management of pregnant diabetics is essential.
3. Other Teratogens—Includes drugs (e.g., aminopterin, phenytoin, thalidomide), trace metals, maternal conditions, infections, and intrauterine factors; may also lead to orthopaedic manifestations in affected children.

IV. **Hematopoietic Disorders**

A. Gaucher's Disease—Aberrant AR lysosomal storage disease (also known as familial splenic anemia) characterized by accumulation of *cerebroside* in cells of the reticuloendothelial system. Cause is a deficiency of the enzyme *beta-glucocerebrosidase*. Commonly seen in children of Ashkenazic Jewish descent, it is associated with osteopenia, metaphyseal enlargement (failure of remodeling), *femoral head necrosis* (may be confused with Perthes' or MED), "moth-eaten" trabeculae, patchy sclerosis, and "Erlenmeyer's flask" distal femora. Affected patients may complain of bone pain and occasionally experience a "bone crisis" (similar to sickle cell anemia). Bleeding abnormalities are also common. *Hepatosplenomegaly* is a characteristic finding. Histologic examination demonstrates characteristic lipid-laden histiocytes (Gaucher's cells). Treatment is basically supportive; new enzyme therapy is available but is extremely expensive.

B. Niemann-Pick Disease—AR disorder. It is caused by an accumulation of phospholipid (*sphingomyelin*) in reticuloendothelial system cells, which occurs as a result of a deficiency in the enzyme sphingomyelinase. Seen commonly in Eastern European Jews. Marrow expansion and cortical thinning are common in long bones; coxa valga is also seen.

C. Sickle Cell Anemia—Sickle cell disease (affects 1% of African-Americans) is more severe but less common than sickle cell trait (8% prevalence). Crises usually begin at age 2–3 and may lead to characteristic *bone infarctions.* Growth retardation/skeletal immaturity, *osteonecrosis* of femoral and humeral heads, *osteomyelitis (often in diaphysis)*, and septic arthritis are commonly seen in this disorder. *Salmonella* is more commonly seen in children with sickle cell disease. Despite this tendency, *Staphylococcus aureus* is still the most common cause of osteomyelitis in sickle cell patients. Dactylitis (acute hand/foot swelling) is also common. Aspiration and culture are necessary to differentiate infarction from osteomyelitis. Radiographs commonly show osteoporosis and cortical thinning. Preoperative oxygenation and exchange transfusion are helpful for affected patients requiring surgery. Hydroxyurea, a cancer chemotherapeutic agent, has produced dramatic relief of pain when used for bone crises.

D. Thalassemia—It is similar to sickle cell anemia in presentation. Most commonly seen in people of Mediterranean descent. Common symptoms include bone pain and leg ulceration. Radiographs show osteopenia and distorted trabeculae.

E. Hemophilia—X-linked recessive disorder with decreased factor VIII (hemophilia A), abnormal factor VIII with platelet dysfunction (von Willebrand's disease), or factor IX (hemophilia B—Christmas disease); associated with bleeding episodes and skeletal/joint sequelae. Can be mild (5–25% of factor present), moderate (1–5% available), or severe (<1% of factor present).

Hemarthrosis presents with painful swelling and decreased range of motion of affected joints. Deep intramuscular bleeding is also common and can lead to the formation of a *pseudotumor* (blood cyst), which can occur in soft tissue or bone. Ultrasonography can help diagnose bleeding into muscles (most commonly in the lower extremity). Intramuscular hematomas can lead to compression of adjacent nerves (e.g., an *iliacus hematoma may cause femoral nerve paralysis* and may mimic a bleed into the hip joint). Factor levels should be elevated to at least 25% after major bleeding episodes. Radiographic findings in hemophilia include *squaring* of the patellas and condyles, epiphyseal overgrowth with leg-length discrepancy, and generalized osteopenia with resulting fractures, commonly around the knee. Fractures heal in normal time with proper clotting. Cartilage atrophy due to enzymatic matrix degeneration is frequent. Treatment includes fracture management, contracture release, osteotomies, open synovectomy, arthroscopic synovectomy (better motion, shorter hospitalization), radiation synovectomy (useful in patients with antibody inhibitors and poor medical management), and total joint arthroplasty. Treatment of hemophilia has become more complex due to the risk of human immunodeficiency virus (HIV) transmission in factor VIII replacement. Mild to moderate hemophilia A can be treated with desmopressin. Factor VIII levels should be increased for prophylaxis in the following situations: vigorous physical therapy (20%), treatment of hematoma (30%), acute hemarthrosis or soft-tissue surgery (>50%), and skeletal surgery (approach 100% preoperatively and maintain >50% for 10 days postoperatively). Tourniquets can be used, vessels should be ligated rather than cauterized, and rigid fixation of fractures decrease postoperative bleeding. **Antibody inhibitors** are present in 4–20% of hemophiliacs and **are a relative contraindication to surgery.** Large levels of factor VIII, or Autoplex (activated prothrombin), are required to offset these inhibitors. Inhibitor levels of <10 Bethesda units are treatable with high-dose factor VIII. If levels are >10 Bethesda units, more sophisticated treatment (factors IX, VII) is required. Because of the amount of blood component therapy required to treat this disorder, a large percentage of hemophiliacs are *HIV-positive.* The incidence of HIV positivity in the older hemophiliac population (before donor screening and the more recent component treatment) approaches 100%.

F. Leukemia—**The most common malignancy of childhood**. Causes demineralization of bones and septic arthritic and occasionally lytic lesions. One-fourth to one-third of children present with musculoskeletal complaints (back, pelvic, leg pains). Radiolucent "leukemia" lines may be seen in the metaphyses of affected bones in older children. Management of leukemia includes chemotherapy.

G. Acquired Immunodeficiency Syndrome—Caused by HIV. Children born with acquired immunodeficiency syndrome are becoming more common in neonatal units, and supportive care is indicated. Protection for surgeons with patients at risk (e.g., intravenous [IV] drug abusers, homosexuals, hemophiliacs) is essential (see Chapter 1, Basic Sciences).

V. **Metabolic Disease/Arthritides** (see Chapter 1, Basic Sciences)

A. Rickets (referred to as osteomalacia in adults)—Decrease in calcium (and sometimes phosphorus), affecting mineralization at the epiphyses of long bones. Classically, brittle bones with **physeal cupping/widening,** bowing of long bones, transverse radiolucent (Looser's) lines, ligamentous laxity, flattening of the skull, enlargement of costal cartilages (rachitic rosary), and dorsal kyphosis (cat back) characterize this disorder. There are several varieties of rickets based on the underlying abnormality (e.g., gastrointestinal, kidney, diet, end organ), which are discussed in detail in Chapter 1. Histologically, **widened osteoid seams** and "Swiss cheese" trabeculae are characteristic in bone; at the growth plate there is gross distortion of the maturation zone (enlarged and distorted) and a poorly defined zone of provisional calcification.

B. Osteogenesis Imperfecta—Defect in **type I collagen** (procollagen to type 1 collagen sequence and abnormal cross-linking) that leads to decreased collagen secretion, bone fragility (brittle "wormian" bone), short stature, scoliosis, tooth defects (dentinogenesis imperfecta), hearing defects, and ligamentous laxity. Four types have been identified (Sillence), although the disorder is probably best considered as a continuum with different inheritance patterns and severity.

Type	Inheritance	Sclerae	Features
I	AD	Blue	Preschool age (tarda), hearing loss (IA = teeth involved; IB = teeth not affected)
II	AR	Blue	Lethal; concertina femur, beaded ribs
III	AR	Normal	Fractures at birth; progressive, short stature
IV	AD	Normal	Milder form, normal hearing (IVA = teeth involved; IVB = teeth not affected)

Radiographs demonstrate thin cortices and generalized osteopenia. Histologically, increased diameters of haversian canals and osteocyte lacunae, increased numbers of cells, and replicated cement lines are noted, which result in the thin cortices seen on radiographs. Fractures are common; the initial healing is normal, but bone typically does not remodel. Fractures occur less frequently with advancing age (usually cease at puberty). Compression fractures (codfish vertebrae) are also common. The goal of treatment is fracture management and long-term rehabilitation. Bracing of the extremities is indicated early to prevent deformity and minimize fractures. *Sofield's osteotomies* ("shish kebab" multiple long-bone osteotomies with either fixed-length Rush's rods or telescoping [Bailey-Dubow] intramedullary rods) are sometimes required for progressive bowing of long bones. Fractures in children younger than age 2 are treated similarly to those in children without osteogenesis imperfecta. After age 2 years, telescoping intramedullary rods (Bailey-DuBow) can be considered. Although synthetic salmon calcitonin and calcium supplements have been suggested to decrease the number of fractures in some osteogenesis imperfecta patients, no medical therapy has been proved unequivocally effective. Scoliosis is common, and bracing is ineffective treatment. Surgery is necessary for scoliosis deformities exceeding 50 degrees.

C. Idiopathic Juvenile Osteoporosis—Rare, self-limited disorder that appears at age 8–14 with osteopenia, growth arrest, and bone and joint pain. Serum calcium and phosphorus levels are normal. Typically, there is spontaneous resolution 2–4 years after onset of puberty. This disorder must be differentiated from other causes of osteopenia (e.g., osteogenesis imperfecta, malignancy, Cushing's disease).

D. Osteopetrosis—Failure of *osteoclastic* and chondroclastic resorption, probably secondary to a defect in the thymus, leading to dense bone *(marble bone)*, "rugger jersey" spine, *marble bone*, and an "Erlenmeyer flask" proximal humerus/distal femur. Mild form is AD; "malignant" form is AR. **Bone marrow transplant** may be helpful for treating the malignant form (see Chapter 1, Basic Sciences).

E. Infantile Cortical Hyperostosis (Caffey's Disease)—Soft-tissue swelling and bony cortical thickening (especially the jaw and ulna) that *follow a febrile illness* in infants 0–9 months old. Radiographs show characteristic periosteal reaction. This disorder may be differentiated from trauma (and child abuse) based on single-bone involvement. A similar presentation may occur in older children (over 6 months) with hypervitaminosis A. Caffey's disease, however, does not produce bleeding gums, fissures at the corners of the mouth, or the liver enzyme abnormalities associated with hypervitaminosis A. Infection, scurvy, and progressive diaphyseal dysplasia may also be in the differential diagnosis for children of all ages. Condition is benign and self-limiting.

F. Connective Tissue Syndrome—A heterogeneous group of disorders with a broad spectrum of features.

1. Marfan's Syndrome—AD disorder of collagen synthesis (possibly the alpha$_1$ subunit) associated with arachnodactyly (long, slender fingers), pectus deformities, scoliosis, cardiac (valvular) abnormalities, and ocular

findings *(superior lens dislocation)*. Other abnormalities may include dural ectasia and meningocele. Joint laxity is treated conservatively. Scoliosis and spondylolisthesis are common. Bracing is ineffective. The presence of kyphosis with scoliosis requires anterior diskectomy and fusion with posterior fusion and instrumentation. Protrusio acetabuli can be treated with early triradiate cartilage epiphysiodesis.

2. Ehlers-Danlos Syndrome—AD disorder with *hyperextensibility* of "cigarette paper" skin, *joint hypermobility* and dislocation, soft-tissue/bone fragility, and soft-tissue calcification. Failure of other supporting connective tissues can lead to vascular and visceral tears as well. Types II and III (of XI) are the most common and least disabling. Treatment consists of physical therapy, orthotics, and *arthrodesis*; soft-tissue procedures fail.
3. Homocystinuria—AR inborn error of *methionine metabolism* (decreased enzyme cystathionine beta-synthase). Accumulation of the intermediate metabolite homocysteine in the production of the amino acid cysteine can lead to osteoporosis, a marfanoid-like habitus (but with stiffening joints), and *inferior lens dislocation*. The diagnosis is made by demonstrating an increased homocysteine in urine (cyanide-nitroprusside test). This disorder is differentiated from Marfan's syndrome based on the direction of lens dislocation and the presence of osteoporosis in homocystinuria. Spontaneous thrombotic episodes can be initiated by minor procedures, anesthesia, and surgery. Central nervous system effects, including mental retardation, are common in this disorder. Early treatment with vitamin B_6 and a decreased methionine diet is often successful.

G. Juvenile Rheumatoid Arthritis (JRA; Juvenile Chronic Arthritis)—Persistent noninfectious arthritis lasting 6 weeks to 3 months after other possible causes have been ruled out. The term juvenile chronic arthritis is gradually being adopted. To confirm the diagnosis, one of the following is required: rash, presence of rheumatoid factor, iridocyclitis, C-spine involvement, pericarditis, tenosynovitis, intermittent fever, or morning stiffness. JRA affects girls more than boys and commonly involves the wrist (flexed and ulnar-deviated) and hand (fingers extended, swollen, radially deviated). C-spine involvement can lead to kyphosis, facet ankylosis, and atlantoaxial subluxation. Lower extremity problems include flexion contractures (hip and knee flexed, ankle dorsiflexed), subluxation, and other deformities (hip protrusio, valgus knees, equinovarus feet). Five types of JRA are usually identified (Schaller) (Table 2–4). Synovial proliferation leads to joint destruction (chondrolysis) and soft-tissue destruction. Radiographs can show rarefaction of juxta-articular bone. In 50% of patients, symptoms resolve without sequelae; 25% are slightly disabled, and 20–25% have crippling arthritis/blindness. Therapy includes night splinting, salicylates and, rarely, synovectomy (for chronic swelling refractory to medical management). Arthrodesis and arthroplasty may be required for severe JRA. Slit-lamp examination is required twice yearly, as progressive **iridocyclitis** can lead to rapid loss of vision if left untreated.

H. Ankylosing Spondylitis—Typically affects adolescent boys with asymmetric lower extremity large-joint arthritis, heel pain and, sometimes, eye symptoms; hip and back pain (cardinal symptom) may develop later. HLA-B27 test is positive in 90–95% of patients with ankylosing spondylitis or Reiter's syndrome but is also positive in 4–8% of all white Americans. Therefore HLA-B27 is not a good screening test for ankylosing spondylitis. *Limitation of chest-wall expansion* is more specific than HLA-B27. Radiographs show bilateral, symmetric sacroiliac erosion, followed by joint space narrowing, later ankylosis, and late vertebral scalloping (bamboo spine). Nonsteroi-

Table 2–4.

Types of Juvenile Rheumatoid Arthritis

Type	Percent	Joints	ANA	RF	Systemic Symptoms and Signs	Progress (%)
Systemic—Still's	25	Many	–	–	Fever, rash, organomegaly	25
Polyarticular/RF –	15	Many	1/3	–	Mild fever	30
Polyarticular/RF +	15	Many	1/3	+	Mild	25
Pauciarticular I (F)	30	Large	+	–	Iridocyclitis[a]	15
Pauciarticular II (M)	15	Large	–	–	HLA-B27 +, spondylitis	15

ANA, antinuclear antibodies; RF, rheumatoid factor; F, female; M, male.
[a]Slitlamp examination is important to identify iridocyclitis, which is seen early in the pauciarticular form.

dal anti-inflammatory drugs and physical therapy are the mainstays of treatment.

I. Acute Rheumatic Fever—*Autoimmune* process that affects children 5–15 years old; it follows an *untreated streptococcal infection* by 2–4 weeks. Can present with *migratory arthritis*, fever, carditis, subcutaneous nodules, and **erythema marginatum** (pink rash on trunk and extremities but not the face ± history of streptococcus infection). The Jones criteria are used for diagnosis (see Chapter 1, Basic Sciences). Treatment includes salicylates, appropriate antibiotics, and cardiology referral.

VI. **Birth Injuries**

A. Brachial Plexus Palsy—Decreasing in severity as a result of better obstetric management but still 2 per 1000 births have an injury associated with stretching or contusion of the brachial plexus. Occurs most commonly with *large babies, shoulder dystocia, forceps delivery, breech position, and prolonged labor.* Three types are commonly recognized.

Type	Roots	Deficit	Prognosis
Erb-Duchenne	C5, 6	Deltoid, cuff, elbow flexors, wrist and hand dorsiflexors; "waiter's tip" deformity	Best
Total plexus	C5–T1	Sensory and motor; flaccid arm	Worst
Klumpke	C8–T1	Wrist flexors, intrinsics; Horner's	Poor

The key to therapy is maintaining passive range of motion and awaiting return of motor function (up to 18 months). As many as 90% or more cases eventually resolve without intervention. However, **lack of biceps function 3 months after injury** carries a poor prognosis and **may be an indication for surgery** (nerve grafting). Late musculoskeletal surgery can improve functional motion. Options include releasing contractures (Fairbanks'), latissimus and teres major transfer to the shoulder external rotators (L'Episcopo's), tendon transfers for elbow flexion (Clarke's pectoral transfer and Steindler's flexorplasty), proximal humerus rotational osteotomy (Wickstrom's), and microsurgical nerve grafting. Reports have shown that release of the subscapularis tendon for internal rotation contracture, if performed by age 2 years, may result in improved active external rotation of the shoulder, with muscle transfer to assist in active external rotation.

B. Congenital Muscular Torticollis—A congenital deformity resulting from contracture of the sternocleidomastoid muscle. It is associated with other "molding disorders," such as *hip dysplasia and metatarsus adductus* (up to 20% association with hip dysplasia). The differential diagnosis includes C-spine anomalies, ophthalmologic disorders that may require the child to tilt the head to see normally, and posterior fossa brain tumors. The cause of congenital muscular torticollis remains uncertain, although most cases follow a difficult labor and delivery. Studies suggest that the muscle abnormality may be the result of an intrauterine compartment syndrome involving the sternocleidomastoid muscle compartment. Fibrosis of the muscle and a palpable mass are noted within the first 4 weeks of life. Most patients (90%) respond to passive stretching within the first year. Surgery (release of the muscle distally or proximally and distally) may be required if torticollis persists beyond the first year in order to prevent development of permanent plagiocephaly. Torticollis may also be associated with congenital atlanto-occipital abnormalities.

C. Congenital Pseudarthrosis of the Clavicle—May be confused with a fracture but involves the middle third of the clavicle; it does not have associated fracture callus and is not painful at birth. It almost always occurs on the **right side**. Surgical repair should be considered for pain and sometimes cosmesis.

VII. **Cerebral Palsy (CP)**

A. Introduction—**Nonprogressive** neuromuscular disorder with onset before age 2 years, resulting from injury to the immature brain. *The cause is most commonly not identifiable* but can include prenatal intrauterine factors, perinatal infections (toxoplasmosis, other infections, rubella, cytomegalovirus infection, and herpes simplex), *prematurity* (most common), anoxic injuries, and meningitis. This *upper motor neuron* disease results in a mixture of muscle weakness and spasticity. Initially, the abnormal muscle forces cause a dynamic deformity at joints. Persistent spasticity can lead to contractures, bony deformity, and ultimately joint subluxation/dislocation.

B. Classification—CP can be classified based on physiology (according to the movement disorder) or anatomy (according to geographic distribution).

1. Physiologic Classification

a. Spasticity—Characterized by increased muscle tone and hyperreflexia with slow, restricted movements because of simultaneous contraction of agonist and antagonists. This form of CP is the *most common* and is most amenable to improvement of musculoskeletal function by operative intervention.

b. Athetosis—Characterized by a constant succession of slow, writhing, involuntary movements, this form of CP is less common and more difficult to treat.

c. Ataxia—Characterized by an inability to coordinate muscles for voluntary movement, resulting in an unbalanced, wide-based gait. Also less amenable to orthopaedic treatment.

d. Mixed—Typically involves a combination of spasticity and athetosis with total body involvement.

2. Anatomic Classification

a. Hemiplegia—Involves the upper and lower extremities on the same side, usually with spasticity. These children often develop early "handedness." All children with hemiplegia are eventually able to walk, regardless of treatment.

b. Diplegia—Patients have more extensive involvement of the lower extremity than the upper extremity. Most diplegic patients eventually walk. IQ may be normal; strabismus is common.

c. Total Involvement—These children have extensive involvement, low IQ, and high mortality rate; they usually are unable to walk.

C. Orthopaedic Assessment—Based on examination and thorough birth and developmental history. A patient's locomotor profile is based on the persistence of primitive reflexes; the presence of two or more usually means the child will be a nonambulator. Commonly tested reflexes include the Moro startle reflex (normally disappears by age 6 months) and the parachute reflex (normally appears by age 12 months). Surgery to improve function is considered for the child over 3 years old with spastic CP and voluntary motor control. Muscle imbalance yields later bony changes; therefore, the general surgical plan is to perform *soft-tissue procedures early* and, if necessary, *bony procedures later*. Surgery is commonly performed on patients who have no potential for walking or independence, particularly to keep the hips located (to avoid painful arthritis) and to maintain spinal stability (scoliosis surgery) to maintain sitting posture. Use of intramuscular botulinum A toxin to temporarily decrease dynamic spasticity is being investigated at several centers in the United States and Europe. *The mechanism of action of botulinum toxin is a postsynaptic blockade at the neuromuscular junction.* The reduction of dynamic tone with use of botulinum toxin may promote normal muscle growth and avoid development of soft-tissue contractures. Selective dorsal root rhizotomy is a neurosurgical procedure designed to decrease lower extremity spasticity. This treatment, indicated only for spastic CP, includes resection of dorsal rootlets not exhibiting a myographic or clinical response on stimulation. It may help reduce spasticity and complement orthopaedic management in spastic diplegic patients. It requires multilevel laminectomy, which may lead to late instability and deformity. Laminoplasty is now recommended rather than laminectomy. Discussion of specific disorders follows. Discussion of hand disorders is included in Chapter 6, Hand.

D. Gait Disorders—Probably the most common problem seen by the orthopaedist. *Hemiplegics* usually present with *toe walking* only. The use of three-dimensional computerized gait analysis with dynamic electromyography and force plate studies have allowed a more scientific approach to preoperative decision-making and postoperative analysis of the results of cerebral palsy surgery. Specific abnormal gait patterns have been identified (Table 2–5), and surgical procedures have been devised to treat these patterns. The use of gait analysis has allowed a more individualized treatment plan for patients with CP. Lengthening of continuously active muscles and transfer of muscles out of phase is often helpful. Timing and indications for surgery require experience and skill because surgeries should often be done in tandem to best correct the problem (e.g., often, heel-cord lengthening alone exacerbates a

Table 2–5.

Common Gait Abnormalities of the Knee in Cerebral Palsy

	Phase					
	Stance			Swing		
Abnormality	IDS	SLS	SDS	I	M	T
Jump knee	(F	V	V	V	V	(F
Crouch knee	(F	(F	(F	V	V	(F
Stiff knee	V	V	V	(F	(F	V
Recurvatum knee	V	(E	(E	V	V	V

IDS, initial double stance; SLS, single limb stance; SDS, second double stance; I, initial swing; M, midswing; T, terminal swing; F, flexion; V, variable; E, extension.

From Sutherland, D.H., and Davids, J.R.: Common gait abnormalities of the knee in cerebral palsy. Clin. Orthop. 288:139–147, 1993.

Table 2–6.

Surgical Options for Gait Disorders

Problem	Diagnosis	Surgical Options
Hip flexion	Contraction (Thomas')	Psoas tenotomy or recession
Spastic hip	Decreased abduction/uncovered head	Adductor release, osteotomy (late)
Hip adduction	Scissoring gait	Adductor release
Femoral anteversion	Prone internal rotation increased	Osteotomy, VDRO, hamstring lengthening
Knee flexion	Contraction, increased popliteal angle	Hamstring lengthening
Knee hypertension	Recurvatum	Rectus femoris lengthening
Stiff leg gait	Electromyography—hamstring, quadriceps continuous, passive knee flexion decreased with hip extension	Distal rectus transfer to hamstrings
Talipes equinus	Toe walking	Achilles lengthening
Talipes varus	Standing position	Split anterior or posterior tibialis transfer (based on EMG findings)
Talipes valgus	Standing position	Peroneal lengthening, Grice's subtalar fusion, calcaneal lengthening osteotomy
Hallux valgus	Examination/radiographs	Osteotomy, metatarsophalangeal fusion

VDRO, varus derotation osteotomy.

crouched gait). In general, surgery is typically performed in the 4- to 5-year age group. A few generalized guidelines are given in Table 2–6.

E. Spinal Disorders—Most commonly involve scoliosis, which can be severe, making proper wheelchair sitting difficult. **The risk for scoliosis is highest in children with total body involvement (spastic quadriplegic).** Surgical indications include curves >45–50 degrees or worsening pelvic obliquity. Two types of curves occur. Group I curves are double curves with thoracic and lumbar components and little pelvic obliquity. Group II curves are larger lumbar or thoracolumbar curves with marked pelvic obliquity (Fig. 2–6). Treatment is tailored to the needs of the patient. Custom-molded seat inserts allow better positioning but do not prevent curve progression. Small curves with no loss of function or large curves in severely involved patients may require observation alone. Group I curves in ambulators are treated as idiopathic scoliosis with posterior fusion and instrumentation. Group I curves in sitters and group II curves require *anterior and posterior fusion with segmental posterior instrumentation from the upper thoracic spine to the pelvis (Luque-Galveston technique)*. The decision about one-stage versus two-stage anterior and posterior fusion is based on the surgeon's skill and speed, blood loss, and the presence of other factors. Kyphosis is also common and may require fusion and instrumentation. It is important to assess *nutritional status* preoperatively and consider Nissen's fundoplication/gastrostomy tube placement before spinal surgery if indicated.

F. Hip Subluxation/Dislocation—Treated initially with a soft-tissue release (adductor/psoas) plus abduction bracing. Later, hip subluxation/dislocation may require femoral and/or acetabular osteotomies (Dega's) to maintain hip stability. The goal is to keep the hip reduced. Spastic dislocation often leads to painful arthritis, which is difficult to treat. This entity is characterized by four stages:

1. **Hip at Risk**—This situation is the only

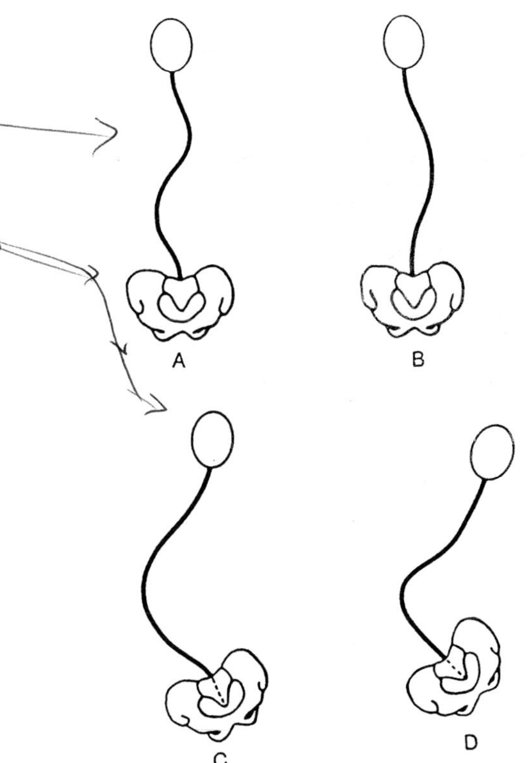

Figure 2–6. Curve patterns of cerebral palsy scoliosis. Group I curves are double curves with thoracic and lumbar components. There is little pelvic obliquity; the curve may be well balanced (*A*); or if the thoracic curve is more significant, there may be some imbalance (*B*). Group II curves are large lumbar or thoracolumbar curves with marked pelvic obliquity. There may be a short fractional curve between the end of the curve and the sacrum (*C*); the curve may continue into the sacrum, with the sacral vertebrae forming part of the curve (*D*). (From Weinstein, S.L.: The Pediatric Spine: Principles and Practice. New York, Raven Press, 1994.)

exception to the general rule of avoiding surgery in CP patients during the first 3 years of life. Characterized by abduction of <45 degrees, with partial uncovering of the femoral head on radiographs. May benefit from *adductor and psoas release*. Neurectomy of the anterior branch of the obturator nerve is now rarely performed because, by converting an upper motor neuron lesion to a lower motor neuron lesion, the muscle is made stiff and fibrotic.

2. **Hip Subluxation**—Best treated with adductor tenotomy in children with abduction of <20 degrees, sometimes with psoas release/recession. *Femoral or pelvic osteotomies* may be considered with femoral coxa valga and acetabular dysplasia.
3. **Spastic Dislocation**—May benefit from *open reduction, femoral shortening, varus derotation osteotomy, and Salter's, Dega's* (Fig. 2–7), *triple or Chiari's osteotomy*. The type of pelvic osteotomy indicated is best determined by obtaining a three-dimensional computed tomography (CT) scan, which will demonstrate the area of acetabular deficiency (anterior, lateral, or posterior) and the congruency of the joint surfaces. *Late dislocations* may best be left out or treated with a *Shanz abduction osteotomy*. In extremely severe cases, a *Girdlestone resection arthroplasty* is performed.
4. Windswept Hips—Characterized by abduction of one hip and adduction of the contralateral hip. Treatment is best directed at attempting to abduct the adducted hip with bracing or tenotomies and releasing the abduction contracture of the contralateral hip.

G. Knee Abnormalities—Usually includes hamstring contractures and decreased range of motion. Hamstring lengthening is often helpful (sometimes increases lumbar lordosis). Distal transfer of an out-of-phase rectus femoris muscle to semitendinosus or gracilis has demonstrated superior results over that of proximal or distal rectus release in improving knee flexion and foot clearance during the early swing phase of gait.

H. Foot and Ankle Abnormalities—Common in CP; gait and dynamic EMG evaluation is often helpful.

1. Equinovalgus Foot—More commonly seen in spastic diplegia. *Caused by spastic peroneals, contracted heel cords, and ligamentous laxity*. Peroneus brevis lengthening is often helpful in correcting moderate valgus. Lateral column-lengthening calcaneal osteotomy is gradually replacing the Grice-Green bone block procedure for correcting hindfoot valgus because it maintains subtalar motion.
2. Equinovarus Foot—More common in

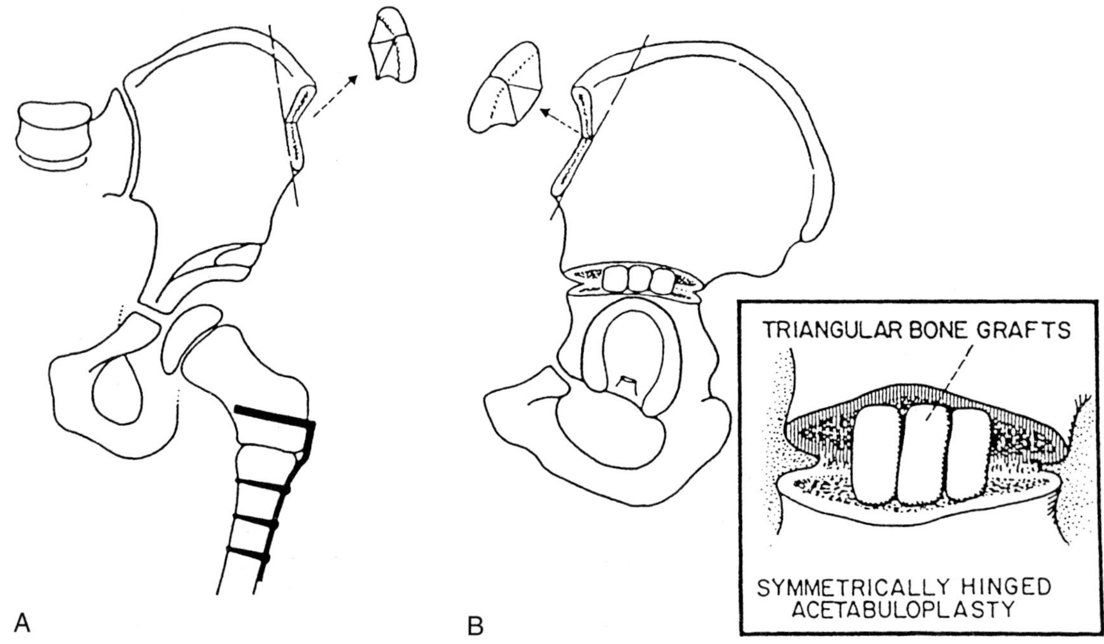

Figure 2–7. Placement of graft for Dega's acetabuloplasty. A bone graft is obtained from the anterosuperior iliac crest and converted to three small triangles, with the base measuring 1 cm (*a*). The grafts are placed in the osteotomy site with the largest placed in the area where maximum improvement of coverage is desired (*b*). The triangular wedges are packed close to each other to prevent collapse, turning, or dislodgment; the result is a symmetric hinging on the triradiate cartilage (*inset*). With the medial wall of the pelvis maintained, the elasticity of the osteotomy keeps the wedges in place. No pins are necessary to maintain the osteotomy. (Adapted from Mubarak, S.J., Valencia, F.G., and Wenger, D.R.: One-stage reconstruction of the spastic hip. J. Bone Joint Surg. [Am.] 74:1352, 1992.)

spastic hemiplegia, *caused by overpull of the posterior or anterior tibialis tendons (or both).* Lengthening of the posterior tibialis is rarely sufficient. Likewise, transfer of an entire muscle (posterior or anterior tibialis) is rarely recommended. **Split muscle transfers are helpful** in certain circumstances, especially **when the affected muscle is spastic during both stance and swing phases** of gait. The split posterior tibialis transfer (rerouting half of the tendon dorsally to the peroneus brevis) is used in cases with spasticity of the muscle, flexible varus foot, and weak peroneals. Complications include decreased foot dorsiflexion. Split anterior tibialis transfer (rerouting half of its tendon laterally to the cuboid) is used in patients with spasticity of the muscle and a flexible varus deformity. Usually the tendon transfer surgery is coupled with an Achilles tendon lengthening to treat the fixed equinous contracture. Most recently, combined split anterior tibial tendon transfer and intramuscular lengthening of the posterior tibial tendon has been recommended for dynamic varus of the hindfoot and adduction of the forefoot during both stance and swing phases of the gait.

VIII. **Neuromuscular Disorders**

A. Arthrogrypotic Syndromes

1. Arthrogryposis Multiplex Congenita (Amyoplasia)—*Nonprogressive* disorder with multiple congenitally rigid joints. It is postulated that *oligohydramnios* may play a role in the etiology. This disorder can be myopathic, neuropathic, or mixed and is associated with a decrease in *anterior horn cells* and other neural elements of the spinal cord. An intrauterine viral infection has been proposed as a possible cause. In some ways arthrogryposis resembles polio, as sensory function is maintained and motor function is lost. Evaluation should include neurologic studies, enzyme tests, and muscle biopsy (at 3–4 months). *Affected patients typically have normal facies, normal intelligence, multiple joint contractures, and no visceral abnormalities.* Upper extremity involvement usually includes adduction and internal rotation of the shoulder, extension of the elbow, and flexion and ulnar deviation of the wrist. Treatment for the elbow deformities consists of passive manipulation and serial casting. Osteotomies are considered after 4 years of age to allow independent eating. One upper extremity should be left in extension at the elbow, for positioning and perineal care, and one elbow in flexion for feeding. *The lower extremity deformities seen in arthrogryposis include teratologic hip dislocations, knee contractures, clubfeet, and vertical talus.* Treatment includes soft-tissue releases (especially hamstrings) for knee contractures and open reduction with femoral shortening for hip dislocation. The foot deformities (clubfoot and vertical talus) are initially treated with a soft-tissue release, but later recurrences may need bone procedures (talectomy). The goal is a stiff, plantigrade foot that enables shoe wear and, possibly, ambulation. Knee contractures should be corrected before hip reduction in order to maintain the reduction. The spine may be involved with characteristic "C-shaped" (neuromuscular) scoliosis. Fractures are also common (25%).
2. Larsen's Syndrome—Similar to arthrogryposis in clinical appearance, but joints are less rigid. The disorder is primarily associated with *multiple joint dislocations* (including bilateral congenital knee dislocations), abnormal (flattened) facies, scoliosis, and *cervical kyphosis.*
3. Distal Arthrogryposis Syndrome—AD disorder that predominantly affects the hands and feet. Ulnarly deviated fingers (at metacarpal joints), metacarpal and proximal interphalangeal flexion contractures, and adducted thumbs with web-space thickening are common. *Clubfoot and vertical talus deformities* are common in the feet.
4. Multiple Pterygium Syndrome—AR disorder characterized by cutaneous flexor surface webs (knee and elbow), congenital vertical talus, and scoliosis.

B. Myelodysplasia (Spina Bifida)

1. Introduction—Disorder of incomplete spinal cord closure or secondary rupture of the developing cord secondary to hydrocephalus. Includes spina bifida occulta (defect in the vertebral arch with confined cord and meninges); meningocele (sac without neural elements protruding through the defect); myelomeningocele (spina bifida; protrusion of the sac with neural elements); and rachischisis (neural elements exposed with no covering). Can be diagnosed in utero (**increased alpha-fetoprotein**). Muscle imbalance and intrauterine positioning frequently lead to hip dislocations, knee hyperextension, and clubfeet. Function is primarily related to the level of the defect and the associated congenital abnormalities. **Sudden changes in function (rapid increase of scoliotic curvature, spasticity, or new neurologic deficit) can be associated with tethered cord, hydrocephalus (most common), or hydromyelia.** Head CT (70% of myelodysplastic patients have hydrocephalus) and myelography or spinal magnetic resonance imaging (MRI) are required. **Fractures are**

Table 2–7.

Characteristics of Myelodysplasia Levels

Level	Hip	Knee	Feet	Orthosis	Ambulation
L1	External rotation/flexed	—	Equinovarus	HKAFO	Nonfunctional
L2	Adduction/flexed	Flexed	Equinovarus	HKAFO	Nonfunctional
L3	Adduction/flexed	Recurvatum	Equinovarus	KAFO	Household
L4	Adduction/flexed	Extended	Cavovarus	AFO	Household plus
L5	Flexed	Limited flexion	Calcaneal valgus	AFO	Community
S1			Foot deformities	Shoes	Near normal

HKAFO, hip-knee-ankle-foot orthosis; KAFO, knee-ankle-foot orthosis; AFO, ankle-foot orthosis.

also common in myelodysplasia, most often about the knee and hip in 3- to 7-year-olds and frequently can be diagnosed only by noting **redness, warmth,** and **swelling.** Fractures are commonly misdiagnosed as infection in these patients. Treatment of fractures is conservative (avoid disuse). Fractures usually heal with abundant callus. The myelodysplasia level is based on the lowest functional level (Table 2–7). *L4 is a key level* because quadriceps can function and allow independent community ambulation.

2. Treatment Principles—Careful observation of patients with myelodysplasia is important. Several myelodysplasia "milestones" have been developed to assess progress.

Age (months)	Function	Treatment
4–6	Head control	Positioning
6–10	Sitting	Supports/orthotics
10–12	Prone mobility	Prone board
12–15	Upright stance	Standing orthosis
15–18	Upright mobility	Trunk/extremity orthosis

Treatment utilizes a team approach to allow maximum function consistent with the patient's level and other abnormalities. Proper use of orthotics is essential in myelodysplasia. Determination of ambulation potential is based on the level of the deficit. Surgery for myelodysplasia focuses on balancing of muscles and correction of deformities. Increased attention has been focused on **latex sensitivity** in myelodysplastic patients; allergic reactions are well described in the literature. Consideration should be given to providing a latex-free environment whenever surgical procedures are performed in spina bifida patients.

3. Hip Problems—Flexion contractures occur commonly in patients with thoracic/high lumbar myelomeningocele due to unopposed hip flexors or in patients who are sitters. Treatment for these patients consists of anterior hip release with tenotomy of the iliopsoas, sartorius, rectus femoris, and tensor fascia lata. For low-lumbar-level patients, the psoas should be preserved for independent ambulation. Hip abduction contracture can cause pelvic obliquity and scoliosis; it is treated with proximal division of the fascia lata and distal iliotibial band release (Ober-Yount procedure). Adduction contractures are treated with adductor myotomy. Hip dislocation occurs frequently in myelodysplastic patients because of paralysis of the hip abductors and extensors with unopposed hip flexors and adductors. **Hip dislocation is most common at the L3/L4 level.** Treatment of hip dislocation is controversial but, in general, containment is considered essential only in patients with a functioning quadriceps. The aim of hip surgery is to maintain range of motion and achieve full hip extension. Containment is a secondary concern. Treatment of hip dislocation is based on the level of the defect: if L2 or higher, leave both hips symmetric; if L4 or lower (and neurologically stable), the dislocation should be reduced. The reduction of a dislocated hip in these patients usually requires (1) correction of muscle imbalance by transfer of the external oblique to augment the hip external rotators; (2) release of soft-tissue contractures; (3) correction of coxa valga with varus derotational osteotomy and acetabular dysplasia with a Pemberton or Shelf acetabuloplasty; and (4) correction of capsular laxity with capsular plication. Stiffness is rarely a problem if all procedures are carried out at one time but may occur after multiple operations. Redislocation may occur no matter what treatment is used to maintain the reduction. Late dislocation at the low lumbar level may be a sign of neurologic decompensation due to a tethered cord, which must be released before reducing the hip.

4. Knee Problems—Usually includes quadriceps weakness (usually treated with knee-ankle-foot orthoses). Flexion deformities

(associated with hip flexion deformities, calcaneovalgus feet, and tethered cord) are not important in wheelchair-bound patients but can be treated with hamstring release and posterior capsular release. Recurvatum (associated with clubfeet and hip dislocation) is rarely a problem and can be treated early with serial casting and knee-ankle-foot orthoses. Tenotomies (quadriceps lengthening) are sometimes required. Valgus deformities are usually not a problem. Sometimes iliotibial band release or late osteotomies are needed.

5. Ankle and Foot Deformities—Objectives are to obtain braceable, plantigrade feet and muscle balance. Affected patients may present with a valgus foot. Total-contact ankle-foot orthoses are often helpful, but clubfoot release, tendon release (anterior tibialis, Achilles), posterior tibialis lengthening, and other procedures may be required. Triple arthrodesis should be avoided in most myelodysplastic patients and is used only for severe deformities with sensate feet. Ankle valgus (resulting from a disparity in fibular versus tibial growth) is addressed by tibial osteotomy or hemiepiphysiodesis (older patients) if the fibula is shortened or Achilles tendon tenodesis to the fibula is performed (patients >8 years).

   Rigid clubfoot, secondary to retained activity or contracture of tibialis posterior and tibialis anterior, is common in L4-level patients. Treatment consists of complete subtalar release via a transverse (Cincinnati) incision, lengthening of tibialis posterior and Achilles tendons, and transfer of tibialis anterior tendon to the dorsal midfoot.

   Secondary hindfoot valgus due to overlengthening of posterior tibial tendon can be treated with a medial displacement calcaneal sliding osteotomy. For severe rotational deformities, distal tibial osteotomy may be required. Subtalar procedures, in general, should be avoided.

6. Spine Problems—Deformity can result from the spine disorder itself, resulting in an upper lumbar kyphosis or other congenital malformation (of hemivertebrae, diastomatomyelia, unsegmented bars) of the spine due to a lack of segmentation or formation. Scoliosis can also occur with severe lordosis as a result of muscular imbalance due to thoracic-level paraplegia. Spinal deformities are often severe and progressive. *Nearly all patients with thoracic-level paraplegia develop scoliosis.* Bracing is generally unsuccessful in treating these spinal deformities. **Rapid curve progression** can be associated with hydrocephalus or a **tethered cord,** which may manifest as lower extremity spasticity (MRI helpful for evaluation). Severe, progressive curves require surgical treatment. This entails anterior and posterior fusion with segmental posterior instrumentation from the upper thoracic spine to the pelvis inferiorly. Segmental Luque's sublaminar wiring with fixation to the pelvis (Galveston's technique) or fixation to the front of the sacrum (Dunn's technique) (Fig. 2–8) may be utilized. Kyphosis in myelodysplasia is a difficult problem. Resection of the kyphosis with local fusion (Lindseth's procedure (Figs. 2–9, 2–10) or fusion to the pelvis is required in severe cases. Infection rates are high due to frequent septicemia and poor skin quality over the lumbar spine.

7. Pelvic Obliquity—Can occur in myelodysplasia as a result of prolonged unilateral hip contractures or scoliosis. Custom seat cushions, thoracolumbosacral orthosis, spinal fusion, and ultimately pelvic osteotomies may be required for treatment.

C. Myopathies (Muscular Dystrophies)—Noninflammatory inherited disorders with progressive muscle weakness. Treatment focuses on physical therapy, orthotics, genetic counseling, and surgery for severe problems (tibi-

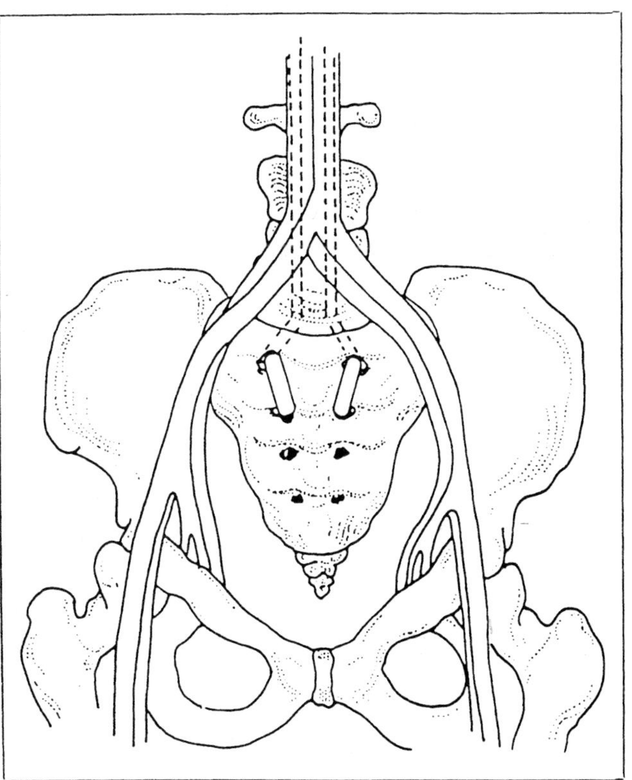

Figure 2–8. Anterior placement of Luque rods through the first sacral foramina. The first sacral foramina are medial to the internal iliac vessels. (From Warner, W.C., and Fackler, C.D.: Comparison of two instrumentation techniques in treatment of lumbar kyphosis in myelodysplasia. J. Pediatr. Orthop. 13:704–708, 1993.)

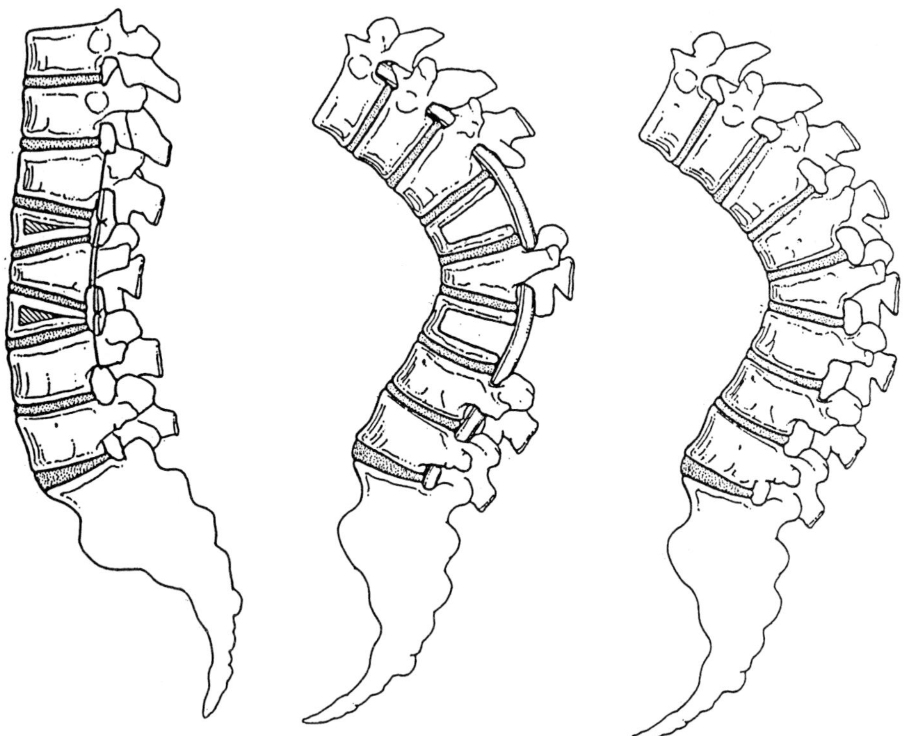

Figure 2–9. *Right to left,* C-shaped kyphosis before removal of the ossific nucleus from its vertebrae. *Center,* Spinous process, lamina pedicle, and ossific nucleus have been removed from the vertebrae above and below the apical vertebrae. Growth plate, disc, and anterior cortex are left intact. *Left,* Deformity is reduced by pushing the apical vertebrae forward and placing tension-band wiring around the pedicles. (From Lindseth, R.E.: Spine deformity in myelomeningocele. Instr. Course Lect. 40:276, 1991.)

alis posterior transfers, release of flexion contractures, and early fusion for neuromuscular scoliosis). *Spinal fusion (often T2 to sacrum) should be done earlier than in idiopathic scoliosis (often at 25 degrees of curvature)* before pulmonary status deteriorates. Several types of muscular dystrophy are classified based on their inheritance pattern.

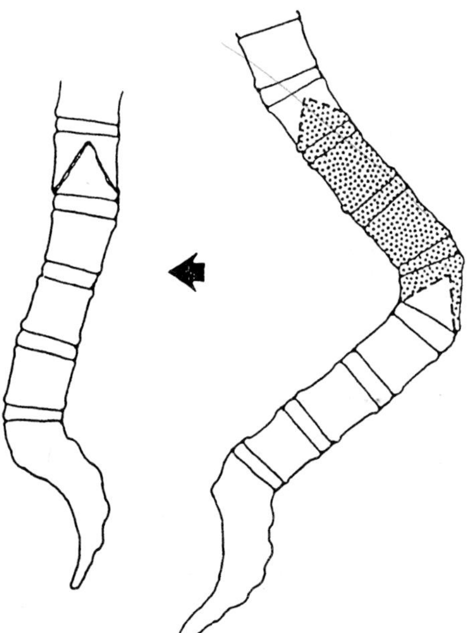

Figure 2–10. Rigid S-shaped kyphosis is corrected by excising the vertebrae between the apex of the kyphosis and the lordosis and fusing the apical vertebrae. (From Lindseth, R.E.: Myelomeningocele. In Morrisey, R.T., ed.: Lovell and Winters' Pediatric Orthopaedics, 3rd ed. Philadelphia, JB Lippincott, 1990, p. 522.)

1. Duchenne's—*Sex-linked recessive* abnormality of young boys, manifested as clumsy walking, decreased motor skills, lumbar lordosis, *calf pseudohypertrophy, positive Gowers' sign* (rises by walking the hands up the legs to compensate for gluteus maximus and quadriceps weakness), **markedly elevated creatine phophokinase (CPK),** and **absent dystrophin protein** on muscle biopsy DNA testing. *Hip extensors are typically the first muscle group affected.* Muscle biopsy sample shows foci of necrosis and connective tissue infiltration. Treatment is based on keeping patients ambulatory as long as possible. Patients lose independent ambulation by age 10, although use of knee-ankle-foot orthoses and release of contractures can extend walking ability for 2–4 years. Patients are usually wheelchair-bound by age 15 years. With no muscle support, scoliosis progresses rapidly between age 13 and 14 years. Patients become bedridden by age 16 due to spinal deformity and are unable to sit for more than 8 hours. Scoliosis should be treated early (25–35 degrees of curvature). Surgical approach includes posterior spinal fusion with segmental instrumentation. These children usually die of cardiorespiratory complications before age 20. Differential diagnosis includes **Becker's** dystrophy (also sex-linked recessive), which is often

seen in 7-year-old, red/green color-blind boys with a similar, but less severe, picture. This diagnosis (Becker's dystrophy) applies to all who live beyond age 22 years without respiratory support; abnormal dystrophin protein is present on muscle biopsy DNA testing.

2. Fascioscapulohumeral—AD disorder typically seen in patients 6–20 years old with facial muscle abnormalities, normal CPK, and winging of the scapula (stabilizes with scapulothoracic fusion).
3. Limb-Girdle—AR disorder; seen in patients 10–30 years old with pelvic or shoulder girdle involvement and increased CPK values.
4. Others—Gowers' (distal involvement, high incidence in Sweden); ocular, oculopharyngeal (high incidence in French Canadians).

D. Myotonic Myopathies—AD disorders with inability of muscles to relax after contractions. There are three basic types.

1. Myotonia Congenita (Thomsen's)—Defect localized to chromosome 7 region, affecting human skeletal muscle chloride channels. Widespread involvement, no weakness, increased hypertrophy. Improves with exercise.
2. Dystrophic Myotonia (Steinert's)—Defect in chromosome 19. Small gonads, heart disease, low IQ, distal/lower extremity involvement, *"dive bomber" EMG.*
3. Paramyotonia Congenita (Eulenburg's)—Defect in chromosome 17 affecting skeletal muscle sodium channels. Myotonic symptoms develop with exposure to cold, especially in the hands (symptoms often respond to quinine or mexiletine).

E. Congenital Myopathies—Nonprogressive AD disorders that present as a "floppy baby." Hypotonia is predominant in the pelvic and shoulder girdles. Muscle biopsy histochemical analysis is required for differentiation of the four types.

F. Polymyositis, Dermatomyositis—Characterized by a febrile illness that may be acute or insidious. Females predominate and typically exhibit photosensitivity and increased CPK and erythrocyte sedimentation rate values. Muscles are tender, brawny, and indurated. Biopsy demonstrates the *pathognomonic inflammatory response.*

G. Hereditary Neuropathies—Disorders associated with multiple central nervous system lesions, including the following:

1. Friedreich's Ataxia—Spinocerebellar degenerative disease with onset before age 10 years. Presents with staggering, wide-based gait; nystagmus; *cardiomyopathy; cavus foot* (treated with plantar release ± metatarsal and calcaneal osteotomies early, and triple arthrodesis later), *and scoliosis* (treated much like idiopathic scoliosis). **Involves motor and sensory defects.** Ataxia limits ambulation by age 30, and death occurs by age 40–50.
2. Charcot-Marie Tooth Disease (Peroneal Muscular Atrophy)—*AD* motor sensory demyelinating neuropathy. Two forms are described: a hypertrophic form (CMT-1), with onset during the second decade of life, and a neuronal form (CMT-2), with onset during the third or fourth decade but with more extensive foot involvement. Orthopaedic manifestations include *pes cavus*, hammer toes with frequent corns/calluses, peroneal weakness, and "stork legs." Low nerve conduction velocities with prolonged distal latencies are noted in peroneal, ulnar, and median nerves. *Intrinsic wasting is noted in hands.* The most severely affected muscles are tibialis anterior, peroneous longus, and peroneous brevis. Treatment includes plantar release, posterior tibial tendon transfer (if hindfoot varus is flexible), triple arthrodesis versus calcaneal and metatarsal osteotomies (if bony deformity is fixed and foot not too short), Jones' procedure for hammer toes, and intrinsic minus procedures for hand deformity. **Involves motor defects much more than sensory defects.**
3. Dejerine-Sottas Disease—AR hypertrophic neuropathy of infancy (CMT-3). Delayed ambulation, pes cavus foot, footdrop, stocking-glove dysesthesia, and spinal deformities are common. Patient confined to wheelchair by third or fourth decade.
4. Riley-Day Syndrome (Dysautonomia)—One of five inherited (AR) sensory and autonomic neuropathies. This disease is found only in patients of *Ashkenazic Jewish ancestry.* Clinical presentation includes dysphagia, alacrima, pneumonia, excessive sweating, postural hypotension, and sensory loss.

H. Myasthenia Gravis—Chronic disease with insidious development of easy muscle fatigability after exercise. Caused by *competitive inhibition of acetylcholine receptors* at the motor end plate by antibodies produced in the thymus gland. Treatment consists of cyclosporin, antiacetylcholinesterase agents, or thymectomy.

I. Anterior Horn Cell Disorders

1. Poliomyelitis—Viral destruction of *anterior horn cells* in the spinal cord and brain stem motor nuclei; all but disappeared in the United States after vaccine was developed. Many surgical procedures still used were developed for treatment of polio. *The hallmark of polio is muscle weakness with normal sensation.*
2. Spinal Muscular Atrophy—AR; loss of

Table 2–8.

Types of Spinal Muscle Atrophy

Type	Onset	Ambulation	Scoliosis First Decade (Degrees)	Survival Age (Years)	Comments
I[a]	Birth	None	60+	0–10	Severe respiratory involvement
II	6 Months	None	50	>35	Has head control
III	1 Year	Orthotics	20	>45	Fusion for scoliosis
IV[b]	Child	Can run	Variable	>55	Lose ambulation by mid-30s

[a]Werdnig-Hoffmann disease.
[b]Kugelberg-Welander disease.

horn cells from the spinal cord. It is the most common diagnosis in girls with progressive weakness. **Werdnig-Hoffman** form—presents at birth, patient has short life span. **Kugelberg-Wellander** form—later onset, patient has long life span. Often associated with *progressive scoliosis* that is best treated surgically like Duchenne's muscular dystrophy curves, except that fusion may be required while patient is still ambulatory (may result in loss of ambulation ability). Patients have symmetric paresis with more involvement of the lower extremity and proximal muscles. Four types of spinal muscle atrophy (Table 2–8) are commonly recognized (Evans and Drennan), but they probably represent the spectrum of a single disease.

J. Acute Idiopathic Postinfectious Polyneuropathy (**Guillain-Barré Syndrome**)—*Symmetric ascending motor paresis caused by demyelination following viral infection.* **Cerebrospinal fluid protein is typically elevated.** Usually self-limited; better prognosis with the acute form.

K. Overgrowth Syndromes

1. Proteus Syndrome—An overgrowth of the hands and feet with bizarre facial disfigurement, scoliosis, genu valgum, hemangiomas, lipomas, and nevi.
2. Klippel-Trenaunay Syndrome—Overgrowth caused by underlying arteriovenous malformations. Associated with cutaneous hemangiomas and varicosities. Severely hypertrophied extremities often require amputation. Selective embolization is a treatment option in selected patients.
3. Hemihypertrophy—Can be caused by various syndromes, but most are idiopathic. Most commonly known cause is *neurofibromatosis.* This disorder is often associated with *renal abnormalities (especially Wilms' tumor).* Management of associated leg-length discrepancy is discussed below.

IX. **Pediatric Spine**

A. Idiopathic Scoliosis

1. Introduction—A lateral deviation and rotational deformity of the spine without an identifiable cause. It may be related to a hormonal, brain-stem, or proprioception disorder. Recent studies have suggested that hormonal factors *(melatonin)* may play a significant role in the cause. Most patients have a positive family history, but there is variable expressivity. The deformity is described as right or left based on the direction of the apical convexity. *Right thoracic curves* are the most common, followed by double major (right thoracic and left lumbar), left lumbar, and right lumbar curves. In adolescents *left thoracic curves* are rare, and *evaluation of the spinal cord by MRI* is suggested to rule out cord abnormalities. Three distinct categories of idiopathic scoliosis have been identified: infantile, juvenile, and adolescent. The adolescent form is the most common. **Risk factors for curve progression include curve magnitudes (>20 degrees), younger age (<12 years), and skeletal immaturity [Risser's stage (0–1)] at presentation** (Table 2–9). About 75% of immature patients with curves of 20–30 degrees will progress at least 5 degrees. Severe curves (>90 degrees) may be associated with cardiopulmonary dysfunction, early death, pain, and a decreased self-image.
2. Diagnosis—Patients are often referred from *school screening* where rotational deformities may be noted on forward flexion testing with a scoliometer. A threshold

Table 2–9.

Incidence of Progression as Related to the Magnitude of the Curve and the Risser Sign

Risser Sign	Percent of Curves That Progressed: 5–19° (Curves)	Percent of Curves That Progressed: 20–29° (Curves)
0, 1	22%	68%
2, 3, 4	1.6%	23%

From Lonstein, J.E., and Carlson, J.M.: The prediction of curve progression in untreated idiopathic scoliosis during growth. J. Bone Joint Surg. [Am.] 66:1067, 1984.

level of 7 degrees is thought to be an acceptable compromise between over-referral and a high false-negative rate. Physical findings include shoulder elevation, waistline asymmetry, trunk shift, limb-length inequality, spinal deformity, and rib rotational deformity (rib hump). Careful neurologic examination for potential spinal cord disorder is important (especially with left thoracic curves). Abnormal neurologic examination results warrant further workup (MRI). Standing posteroanterior and lateral radiographs are obtained, and curves are measured based on the Cobb method (Fig. 2–11). Typically there is *hypokyphosis* of the apical vertebrae in the saggital plane because idiopathic scoliosis is a *lordoscoliotic deformity*. The potential coexistence of spondylolisthesis can also be noted on the lateral x-ray film. Inclusion of the iliac crest on radiographs allows determination of skeletal maturity based on the *Risser sign* (based on ossification of the iliac crest apophysis and graded 0–5). *An MRI scan is obtained for cases with noted structural abnormalities on plain films, excessive kyphosis, juvenile-onset scoliosis (age over 11 years), rapid curve progression, neurologic signs/symptoms, associated syndromes, and left thoracic/thoracolumbar curves.*

3. Treatment—*Based on the maturity of the patient (Risser's stage and presence of menarche), magnitude of the deformity, and curve progression.* Treatment options include *observation, bracing, and surgery.* Exercise and electrical stimulation have not been shown to affect the normal history of curve progression. Bracing may help to halt or slow curve progression but does not reduce the magnitude of the deformity. The Milwaukee brace (cervicothoracolumbosacral orthosis) or Boston underarm brace with Milwaukee superstructure is used for curves with the apex at or above T7. The Boston-type underarm thoracolumbosacral orthosis brace is used for curves with the apex at T8 or below. Patients with thoracic lordosis or hypokyphosis are poor candidates for bracing. *The effectiveness of bracing patients with idiopathic scoliosis is dose-related* (the more the brace is worn each day, the more effective it is). Although the efficacy of full-time wear has been well demonstrated, long-term prospective studies on part-time brace wear are still lacking. Use of the Charleston night-time brace is still under investigation. *The basic options for the surgical treatment of idiopathic scoliosis are anterior spinal fusion (ASF) with instrumentation, posterior spinal fusion (PSF) with instrumentation, or both ASF and PSF.* **The indications for ASF and PSF in idiopathic scoliosis are severe deformities (>75 degrees) and crankshaft prevention (girls <10 years and boys <13 years).** There are multiple comparable "third generation" spinal instrumentation systems available on the market. All of these systems are capable of providing excellent segmental fixation of the spinal column. These systems also allow the surgeon to obtain better correction of the deformities seen in idiopathic scoliosis. The decision between ASF versus PSF is made on a case-by-case basis. *In general, ASF with instrumentation is utilized in thoracolumbar and lumbar curves in order to save lower lumbar fusion levels.* Current research efforts are in progress to extend the use of ASF with instrumentation cranially into the thoracic spine. *The benefits of ASF with instrumentation are saving fusion levels and improved correction. The disadvantages are lumbar kyphosis, thoracic hyperkyphosis, and rod breakage (pseudarthrosis).* **PSF with instrumentation still remains the gold standard for the majority of thoracic and double major curves.** With the newer instrumentation systems, it is generally not necessary to use postoperative bracing or casting. The general treatment guidelines in the chart on the following page apply.

4. Fusion Levels—Successful surgery is based on picking appropriate fusion levels, among other considerations. Several methods have been developed to select the correct levels. The goal is to fuse the spinal levels necessary to establish a well-balanced

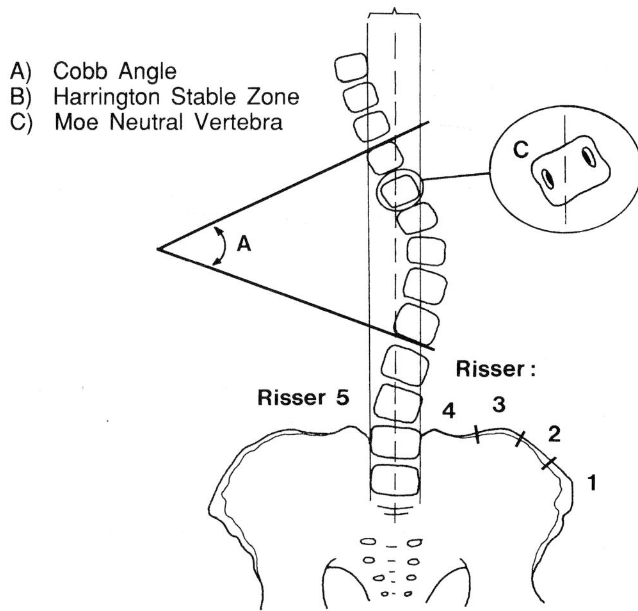

Figure 2–11. Measurements for idiopathic scoliosis. Note Cobb's angle (*A*), Harrington's stable zone (*B*), Moe's neutral vertebra (*C*), and Risser's staging.

Curve (degrees)	Progression (degrees)	Risser	Therapy
0–25	—	Immature	Serial observation
25–30	5–10	Immature	Brace
30–40	—	Immature	Brace
>40	—	Immature	Surgery
>50	—	Mature	Surgery (young adults)

Table 2–11.

Segmental Instrumentation Patterns for Prevention of Coronal Decompensation for Treatment of Thoracic Scoliosis

Group	Criteria for Hook Selection
A	Fused to stable vertebra: one mode of hook orientation on left-sided rod, one rod contour (four hook sites)
B	Fused to one above stable: one mode of hooks, one rod contour (four hook sites)
B-RB	Fused to one above stable: terminal reverse bend and reversal of last two hooks (five hook sites)
C	Fused to stable, with terminal reverse bend between neutral and stable and reverse rod bend (contour) (five hook sites)
D	Fused beyond stable: reverse bend and reversal of hook direction between the stable or neutral vertebra and the distally fused segment (five hook sites)

From Bridwell, K.H., McAllister, J.W., and Betz, R.R.: Coronal decompensation produced by Cotrel-Dubousset "derotation" maneuver for idiopathic right thoracic scoliosis. Spine 16:769–777, 1991.

spine in the coronal and sagittal planes. Harrington recommended fusion one level above and two levels below the end vertebrae if these levels fell within the **stable zone** (within parallel lines drawn vertically up from the lumbosacral facet joints). Moe recommended fusion to the **neutral vertebrae** (without rotation, pedicles symmetric) (see Fig. 2–11). The **stable vertebrae** are defined as the vertebrae that are most closely bisected by the center sacral line (dashed line in Figures 2–11 and 2–12). It is almost never necessary to fuse to the pelvis in adolescent idiopathic scoliosis. Cochran identified a markedly *increased incidence of late, low back pain with fusion to L5 and some increase with fusion to L4*. Therefore, every attempt should be made to stop the fusion at L3 or above. **King and Moe identified five patterns** and treatment options (Table 2–10; see Fig. 2–12). These treatment options were developed in the Harrington instrumentation era. The newer instrumentation systems allow more powerful correction of these deformities. In some instances, the King and Moe fusion levels must be modified to prevent postoperative decompensation. Bridwell noted thoracic decompensation after use of Cotrel-Dubousset instrumentation for right thoracic idiopathic scoliosis. He reviewed his results with five different hook patterns for the King-Moe II, III, and IV curves and recommended stopping the fusion one segment short of the stable vertebra, with all hooks in a distraction mode, or reversal of rod bend and hook on the left side between the neutral and stable vertebra to decrease the incidence of decompensation (Table 2–11; Fig. 2–13). King-Moe type V curves require careful preoperative analysis. If the left shoulder is elevated on presentation, the upper curve must be included in the fusion or the left shoulder will be even more elevated postoperatively. If the shoulders are level and the upper curve is flexible, the lower thoracic curve alone may be fused. If the shoulders are level and the upper thoracic curve is rigid, both the upper and lower curves must be incorporated into the fusion.

5. Complications—The most disastrous complication of spinal surgery is a *neurologic deficit* that was not present preoperatively. Successful surgical intervention is based on careful technique *(intraoperative monitoring [somatosensory evoked potential] is helpful ± Stagnara's wake-up test and clonus tests)*. Apel

Table 2–10.

Patterns of Idiopathic Scoliosis and Treatment Options (After King)

Type	Definition	Flexibility (Flexion-Extension)	Treatment
I	S-shaped thoracolumbar curve; crosses midline	Lumbar < thoracic (or lumbar curve larger)	Fuse lumbar and thoracic vertebrae
II	S-shaped thoracolumbar curve; crosses midline	Lumbar > thoracic (and thoracic curve larger)	Fuse thoracic vertebrae[a]
III	Thoracic curve; lumbar vertebrae do not cross midline	Lumbar vertebrae highly flexible	Fuse thoracic vertebrae
IV	Long thoracic curve	L4 tilts to thoracic curve	Fuse through L4
V	Double thoracic curve	T1 tilts to upper curve	Fuse through T2

[a]Experience with lumbar curves >50 degrees suggests that large lumbar curves should be included in the fusion for rotational correction.

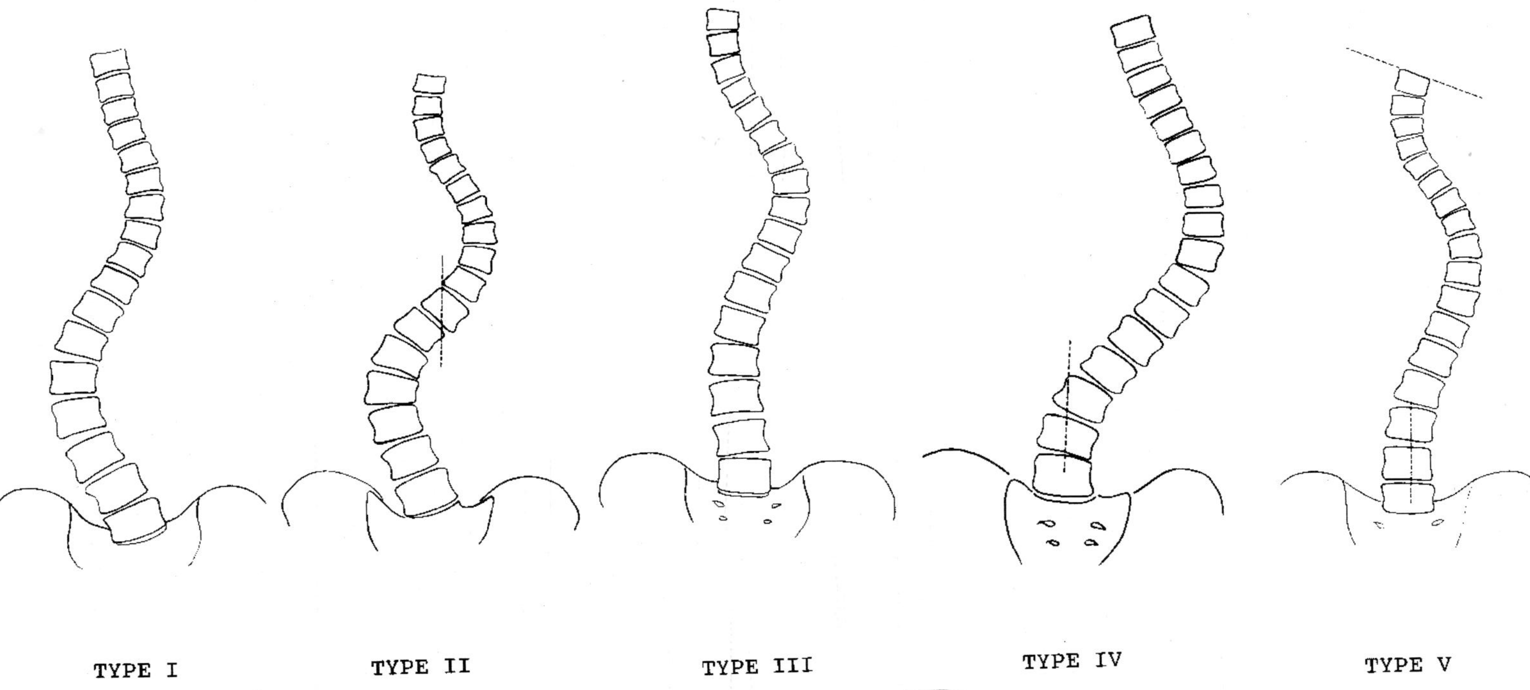

Figure 2–12. Five types of scoliotic curves (I–V). See text for description. (From King, H.A., Moe, J.H., Bradford, D.S., et al.: The selection of fusion levels in thoracic idiopathic scoliosis. J. Bone Joint Surg. [Am.] 65:1302–1313, 1983.)

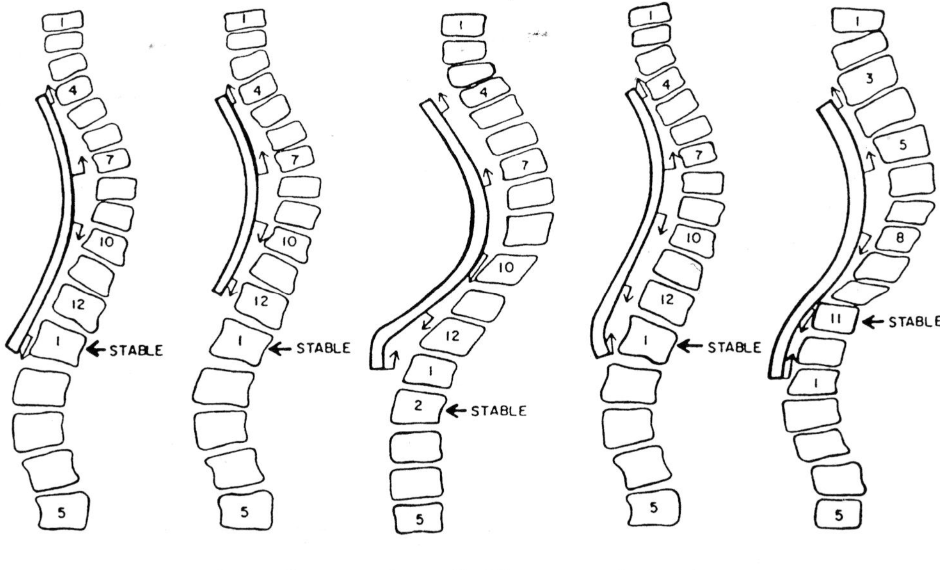

Figure 2–13. Groups A, B, B–RB, C, and D, as described in Table 2–11. See text for further description. (From Bridwell, K.H., McAllister, J.W., Betz, R.R., et al.: Coronal decompensation produced by Cotrel-Dubousset "derotation" maneuver for idiopathic right thoracic scoliosis. Spine 16: 769–777, 1991.)

described the use of somatosensory evoked potential with temporary occlusion of segmental spinal arteries to avoid ischemic neurologic injury during thoracic anterior spinal fusion. It is especially useful in patients with congenital kyphoscoliosis. *Attempting excessive correction or placement of sublaminar wires is associated with an increased risk of neurologic damage.* Minimizing blood loss and the use of autologous blood is important to avoid transfusion-associated problems. *Surgical complications include pseudarthrosis (1–2%), wound infection (1–2%), and implant failure (early hook cutout and late rod breakage).* Late rod breakage frequently signifies failure of fusion. Only an asymptomatic pseudarthrosis (no pain or loss of curve correction) should be observed because the results of the late repair do not differ from those performed earlier. *Use of a compression implant facilitates pseudarthrosis repair.* Creation of a **"flat back syndrome,"** or early fatigability and pain due to loss of lumbar lordosis, can be minimized with rod contouring and effective use of compression and distraction devices. Flat back syndrome is now much *more preventable* with newer instrumentation systems and closer attention to sagittal contour at the time of initial surgery. Treatment of this condition requires revision surgery with posterior closing wedge osteotomies. The results appear to be improved, with maintenance of correction, if anterior release and fusion precede the posterior osteotomies. **The Crankshaft phenomenon** occurs in the setting of continued anterior spinal growth after posterior fusion in skeletally immature patients. It results in increased rotation and deformity of the spine as continued anterior growth causes a spin around the posterior tether (fusion mass). This situation is best avoided by anterior diskectomy and fusion coupled with PSF in immature patients with curves of >50 degrees (Risser's 0–1, girls ≮10 years, boys ≮13 years).

6. Infantile Idiopathic Scoliosis—Presents at age 2 months to 3 years with **left-sided thoracic scoliosis, male predominance, plagiocephaly (skull flattening), and other congenital defects.** Most cases have been reported from Great Britain. The two factors affecting progression most are *curve magnitude and the apical rib-vertebral angle of Mehta.* Most curves less than 25 degrees with rib-vertebral angle of Mehta ≮20 degrees will tend to resolve spontaneously. Therefore, observation is appropriate in these patients. Surgical options for severe curves include instrumentation without fusion (subcutaneous rodding) or ASF/PSF combination. Any severe curve should have MRI preoperatively to rule out any possible spinal cord disease. Treatment is based on the elements in the chart (next page).
7. Juvenile Idiopathic Scoliosis—Scoliosis in 3- to 10-year-olds is similar to adolescent scoliosis in terms of presentation and treatment. *A high risk of curve progression is seen*; 70% require treatment, with 50% needing bracing and 50% requiring surgery. Fusion should be delayed until the onset of the adolescent growth spurt if possible (unless curve magnitude is >50 degrees). The use of spinal instrumentation without fusion (as for infantile scoliosis) may facilitate this delay. In patients with severe deformities

Curve (degrees)	Progression (degrees)	RVAD (degrees)	Treatment
<25	—	<20	Serial observation
25–35	10	20–25	Cast/brace
>35	>10		Neuro/MRI work-up, instrumentation without fusion or combined anterior and posterior fusion

that require surgery, a careful assessment of their skeletal maturity should be done. *Several factors have been identified to assess skeletal maturity: Risser's sign, triradiate cartilage closure, menarchal status, capitellar physis and, most recently, the peak growth velocity.* In patients with multiple risk factors for skeletal immaturity, ASF and PSF with instrumentation should be performed to prevent the occurrence of crankshaft phenomenon.

B. Neuromuscular Scoliosis—Many children with neuromuscular disorders develop scoliosis or other spinal deformities. In general, neuromuscular curves are longer, involve more vertebrae, and are less likely to have compensatory curves than idiopathic scoliosis. Additionally, *neuromuscular curves progress more rapidly and may progress after maturity. These curves may be associated with pelvic obliquity, bony deformities, and cervical involvement—again distinguishing them from idiopathic curves.* Pulmonary complications are also more frequent, including decreased pulmonary function, pneumonia, and atelectasis. For patients who are already wheelchair-bound, curve progression may make them bedridden. Orthotic use is advised until age 10–12 years, at which time corrective fusion is usually performed to provide permanent stability in severe deformities. Underarm (Boston-type) braces are most often used. The surgical treatment of neuromuscular scoliosis often involves the fusion of more levels than for idiopathic curves. Fusion to the pelvis may be required for fixed pelvic obliquity. The *Galveston technique* of pelvic fixation is most commonly used (bending the caudal end of the rods from the lamina of S1 to pass into the posterosuperior iliac spine and between the tables of the ilium just anterior to the sciatic notch). The goal of treatment is stability and truncal balance with a level pelvis. Patients with upper motor neuron disease (CP) are initially treated with a body jacket or seat orthotics but require fusion for curve progression to >50 degrees. *Children with severe involvement require fusion to the sacrum and may require both anterior and posterior procedures.* Posterior fusion alone is associated with higher pseudarthrosis rates and development of the crankshaft phenomenon (delayed bone age is common in neuromuscular patients). Lower motor neuron disease (polio and spinal muscular atrophy) is initially treated with orthotics. If this treatment fails, instrumentation without fusion is carried out in young children (less than 10 years old), with fusion reserved for older children (girls >12 years, boys >14 years). Severe curves require early correction and fusion, usually with Luque's instrumentation. Myopathic disease (muscular dystrophy) often results in rapidly progressive, severe scoliosis and markedly decreased pulmonary function soon after the child is wheelchair-bound. Bracing is not recommended, and fusion (with Luque's instrumentation) is usually done for curves >25 degrees in patients with adequate pulmonary function in order to allow sitting, prolonging their life span.

C. Congenital Spinal Disorders—Due to a developmental defect in the formation of the mesenchymal anlage during the 4th to 6th weeks of development. Three basic types of defect are noted: **failure of segmentation** (typically results in a vertebral bar), **failure of formation** (due to lack of material, may result in hemivertebrae), and **mixed.** Three-dimensional CT is helpful for defining the type (Fig. 2–14) of vertebral anomaly. Spinal MRI scans should be obtained before any surgery to assess for intraspinal anomalies. *Associated anomalies include genitourinary (25%), cardiac (10%), and dysraphism (25%, usually diastomatomyelia—cleft in the spine). Renal ultrasonography is used to rule out associated kidney abnormalities.*

1. Congenital Scoliosis—Most common congenital spinal disorder. **The worst prognosis (most likely to progress) is seen**

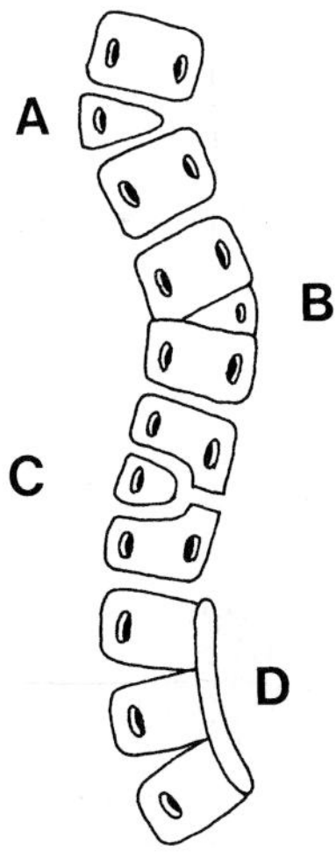

Figure 2–14. Vertebral anomalies leading to congenital scoliosis. *A,* Fully segmented hemivertebra. *B,* Unsegmented hemivertebra. *C,* Incarcerated hemivertebra. *D,* Unilateral unsegmented bar.

with a unilateral unsegmented bar with a contralateral, fully segmented hemivertebra. This deformity should be treated surgically on recognition. The treatment options include ASF and PSF in situ, or convex anterior and posterior hemiepiphysiodesis. The best prognosis is with a block vertebra (bilateral failure of segmentation). A unilateral unsegmented bar is a common disorder and is likely to progress. An incarcerated hemivertebra (within the lateral margins of the vertebrae above and below) has a better prognosis than an unincarcerated (laterally positioned) hemivertebra. A fully segmented hemivertebra is free with normal disc spaces on both sides (higher risk of progression), whereas an unsegmented hemivertebra is fused above and below (lower risk) (see Fig. 2–14). **Unilateral unsegmented bars with contralateral hemivertebrae should be treated operatively when diagnosed;** *other deformities should demonstrate progression before surgical options are considered.* Bracing may be effective for compensatory curves or for smaller, supple curves above a vertebral anomaly, but it is ineffective for controlling congenital curves. Anterior and posterior hemivertebral excision may be indicated for lumbosacral hemivertebrae associated with progressive curves and an oblique take-off (severe truncal imbalance). Isolated hemivertebral excision can destabilize the spine on the convex side and should be accompanied by anterior/posterior arthrodesis with instrumentation to stabilize the adjacent vertebrae. Anterior and posterior convex hemiepiphysiodesis/arthrodesis is safer, but correction of imbalance is less predictable.

Posterior fusion in situ is the gold standard of treatment for most progressive curves. In young patients (girls <10 years, boys <13 years), the crankshaft phenomenon may occur because of continued anterior spinal growth; in these cases anterior/posterior fusion may be required. A summary of treatment recommendations for congenital scoliosis is in the chart at the top of the page.

2. Congenital Kyphosis—May be secondary to failure of formation (type I), failure of segmentation (type II), or mixed abnormalities (type III). **Failure of formation (type I, most common) has the worst prognosis** for progression (95% progress) and neurologic involvement of all spinal deformities. **Type I congenital kyphosis is also the most likely to result in paraplegia (neurofibromatosis is second)**. *The presence of significant congenital kyphosis secondary to failure of formation (type I) is an indication for surgery.* Posterior fusion is favored in young children (<5 years) with curves less than 50 degrees. This is essentially a *posterior (convex) hemiepiphysiodesis.* Combined anterior/posterior fusion is reserved for older children or more severe curves. Anterior vertebrectomy, spinal cord decompression, and anterior fusion followed by posterior fusion are indicated for curves associated with neurologic deficits. A type II congenital kyphosis can be observed to document progression, but progressive curves should be fused posteriorly.

Risk of Progression (Highest to Lowest)	Character of Curve Progression	Treatment Options
Unilateral unsegmented bar with contralateral hemivertebra	Rapid and relentless	Posterior spinal fusion (add anterior fusion for girls <10, boys <12)
Unilateral unsegmented bar	Rapid	Same
Fully segmented hemivertebra	Steady	Anterior spinal fusion Anterior/posterior convex hemiepiphysiodesis (age <5, curve <70°, no kyphosis) Hemivertebra excision
Partially segmented hemivertebra	Less rapid; curve usually <40° at maturity	Observation Hemivertebra excision
Incarcerated hemivertebra	May slowly progress	Observation
Nonsegmented hemivertebra	Little progression	Observation

D. Neurofibromatosis—AD disorder of neural crest origin, often associated with neoplasia and skeletal abnormalities. Two of the following seven findings in the chart are necessary to establish the diagnosis.

Diagnostic Criteria	Requirements
At least six café-au-lait spots	>5 mm (prepubital); >15 mm (mature)
Neurofibromas	Two or more (or one plexiform type)
Axillary/inguinal freckles	Multiple
Osseous lesion	Sphenoid dysplasia, cortical thinning
Optic glioma	Present
Lish nodules	Two or more iris lesions by slit lamp examination
Family history	First-degree relative with neurofibromatosis

The spine is the most common site of skeletal involvement. Careful screening of scoliosis radiographs for vertebral scalloping; enlarged foramina; penciling of transverse processes or ribs; severe apical rotation; short, tight curves; or a paraspinal mass may differentiate this condition from idiopathic scoliosis. Spinal deformity secondary to neurofibromatosis is characteristically kyphoscoliosis in the thoracic region with dystrophic changes, but nondystrophic scoliosis or cervical involvement may also be noted. Nondystrophic scoliosis is treated as appropriate for idiopathic scoliosis, but with dystrophic deformities nonoperative treatment of curves >20 degrees is futile. *Surgical treatment consists of anterior/posterior fusion with instrumentation for patients with progressive dystrophic deformities.* The reported pseudarthrosis rate is intolerably high with PSF alone. If fusion is required in the juvenile age group, anterior and posterior fusion is routinely performed to avoid the crankshaft phenomenon. Neurologic involvement is common in neurofibromatosis and may be caused by the deformity itself: an intraspinal tumor, a soft-tissue mass, or dural ectasia. Therefore, any patient with neurofibromatosis undergoing spinal surgery should have an MRI preoperatively. Because of a high pseudarthrosis rate, some authors recommend routine augmentation of the posterior fusion mass at 6 months postoperatively with repeat iliac crest bone graft. C-spine involvement includes kyphosis or atlantoaxial instability. Posterior fusion with autologous grafting and halo immobilization is recommended for severe C-spine deformity with instability. Isolated kyphosis of the T-spine is treated with anterior decompression of the kyphotic angular cord compression, followed by anterior and posterior fusion.

E. Other Spinal Abnormalities

1. Diastomatomyelia—Fibrous, cartilaginous, or osseous bar creating a longitudinal cleft in the spinal cord. Usually occurs in the lumbar spine and can lead to tethering of the cord with associated neurologic deficits. Intrapedicular widening on plain radiographs is suggestive, and myelo-CT or MRI is necessary to fully define the disorder. A diastomatomyelia must be resected before correction of a spinal deformity, but if otherwise asymptomatic and without neurologic sequelae, it may be simply observed.
2. Sacral Agenesis—Partial or complete absence of the sacrum and lower lumbar spine. **Highly associated with maternal diabetes**, it is often accompanied by gastrointestinal, genitourinary, and cardiovascular abnormalities. Clinically, children have a prominent lower lumbar spine and atrophic lower extremities; they may sit in a "Buddha" position. Motor impairment is at the level of the agenesis, but sensory innervation is largely spared. Management may include amputation or spinal-pelvic fusion.

F. Low Back Pain—In children, complaints of low back pain and especially painful scoliosis should be taken seriously. Acute back pain can be associated with *diskitis* (presents as refusal to sit or walk, increased ESR, and later disc-space narrowing—takes 3 weeks to appear on plain films) or osteomyelitis (systemic illness, leukocytosis). Rang and Wenger discussed the difficulty of differentiating between diskitis and osteomyelitis, and they recommended use of the term infectious spondylitis to describe disc-space infections in children. Occasionally, herniated nucleus pulposus, presenting as sciatica and back pain in older children, occurs and may require operative intervention. *Spondylolysis* is common after athletic injuries, especially activities involving repetitive hyperextension of the lumbosacral spine (gymnastics). Conservative treatment, including avoiding the repetitive activity, is usually adequate. Painful scoliosis often signifies a tumor (e.g., osteoid osteoma) or spinal cord anomaly and should be investigated aggressively. *A bone scan is an excellent screening method for the child or adolescent with back pain.* The use of single photon emission computed tomography scanning has improved detection of occult spondylolysis and osteoid osteoma, and it should be undertaken if plain radiograph results are negative and pain continues for more than 1 month. Further specificity in a still unclear clinical setting may be garnered from CT scanning (spondylolysis, herniated nucleus pulposus) or MRI (infection, herniated nucleus pulposus).

G. Kyphosis

1. Congenital Kyphosis—See Section C, Congenital Spinal Disorders.
2. Scheuermann's Disease—Classic definition is increased thoracic kyphosis (>45 degrees) **with 5 degrees or more anterior wedging at three sequential vertebrae.** Other radiographic findings include disc narrowing, end-plate irregularities, spondylolysis (30–50%), scoliosis (33%), and Schmorl's nodes (Sorenson). Scheuermann's disease is more common in males and typically presents in adolescents with poor posture and occasionally aching pain. Physical examination characteristically shows hyperkyphosis that does not reverse on attempts at hyperextension and tight hamstrings. Neurologic sequelae secondary to disc herniation or extradural spinal cysts are rare but have been reported. Treatment consists of bracing (a modified Milwaukee brace) for a progressive curve in a patient with 1 year or more of skeletal growth

remaining (Risser's 3 or below). Bracing may affect 5–10 degrees of permanent curve correction but is less effective for kyphosis of >75 degrees. For the skeletally mature patient with severe kyphosis (>75 degrees), surgical correction may be indicated. *Posterior fusion with dual rods segmentally attached compression instrumentation is the treatment of choice, preceded by anterior release and interbody fusion for curves of >75 degrees or those not correcting to <55 degrees on hyperextension.* Thorascopic anterior diskectomy and interbody fusion have been used to decrease the morbidity associated with thoracotomy for anterior release and fusion. Lumbar Scheuermann's disease is less common than the thoracic variety but may cause back pain on a mechanical basis (more common in athletes and manual laborers). The pain is usually self-limited. Lumbar Scheuermann's disease also demonstrates irregular vertebral end plates with Schmorl's nodes and decreased disc height, but it is not associated with vertebral wedging.

3. Postural Round Back—Also associated with kyphosis but does not demonstrate vertebral body changes. Forward bending demonstrates kyphosis, but there is no sharp angulation as in Scheuermann's disease. Correction with backward bending and prone hyperextension is typical. Treatment includes a hyperextension exercise program. Occasionally, bracing is required, but surgery is rarely indicated.
4. Other Causes of Kyphosis—Trauma, infections, spondylitis, bone dysplasias (mucopolysaccharidoses, Kniest syndrome, diastrophic dysplasia), and neoplasms. Additionally, *postlaminectomy kyphosis can be severe and requires anterior and posterior fusion early. Performance of total laminectomy in immature patients without stabilization is contraindicated.*

H. Cervical Spine Disorders—Many disorders.

1. Klippel-Feil Syndrome—Multiple abnormal cervical segments due to failure of normal segmentation or formation of cervical somites at 3–8 weeks' gestation. Often associated with congenital scoliosis, renal disease (aplasia 33%), synkinesis (mirror motions), Sprengel's deformity, congenital heart disease, brain-stem abnormalities, or congenital cervical stenosis. *The classic triad of low posterior hairline, short "web" neck, and limited cervical range of motion is seen in fewer than 50% of cases.* Most therapy is conservative, but chronic pain with myelopathy associated with instability may require surgery. Three high-risk fusion patterns are more apt to cause neurologic problems: (1) C2/C3 fusion with occipitalization of the atlas; (2) long fusion with abnormal occipital-cervical junction; and (3) single open cervical interspace. Affected children should avoid collision sports.
2. Atlantoaxial Instability
   a. Anteroposterior Instability—*Associated with Down's syndrome (trisomy 21), JRA, various osteochondrodystrophies, os odontoideum, and other abnormalities.* In patients with Down's syndrome and a normal neurologic examination, simple avoidance of contact sports is appropriate, but with >10 mm of subluxation on flexion-extension films, posterior spinal fusion is indicated (high complication rate). An atlanto-dens interval of >5 mm should be treated with activity restriction in the absence of myelopathy.
   b. Rotatory Atlantoaxial Subluxation—*May present with torticollis; can be caused by retropharyngeal inflammation (Grisel's disease).* It is probably caused by secondary ligamentous laxity and is best *treated with traction and bracing early.* Current diagnosis is by CT scans at the C1–C2 level with the head straightforward, in maximal rotation to the right, and then in maximum rotation to the left (Fig. 2–15). *Late diagnosis may require C1–C2 fusion.* Traumatic atlantoaxial subluxation may present as torticollis, which can be treated initially with a soft collar for up to 1 week. If symptoms persist past this point, cervical traction should be initiated. If discovered late (>1 month), fusion may be required for fixed rotary subluxation. *Rotary subluxation can also be seen in rheumatoid arthritis, ankylosing spondylitis, Down's syndrome, congenital anomalies, and cervical tumors.*
3. Os Odontoideum—Previously thought to be due to the failure of fusion of the base of the odontoid, it appears like a type II odontoid fracture. Evidence suggests that it may represent the residuals of an old traumatic process. Usually seen in place of the normal odontoid process (orthotopic type), but it may fuse to the clivus (dystopic type—more often seen with neurologic compromise). *Treatment is conservative unless instability (>5 mm translation on flexion-extension radiographs) or neurologic symptoms are present, which require a posterior C1-C2 fusion.*
4. Pseudosubluxation of the Cervical Spine—Subluxation of C2 on C3 (and occasionally of C3 on C4) of up to 40% or 4 mm can be normal in children <8 years old because of the orientation of the facets. Rapid resolution of pain, relatively minor trauma,

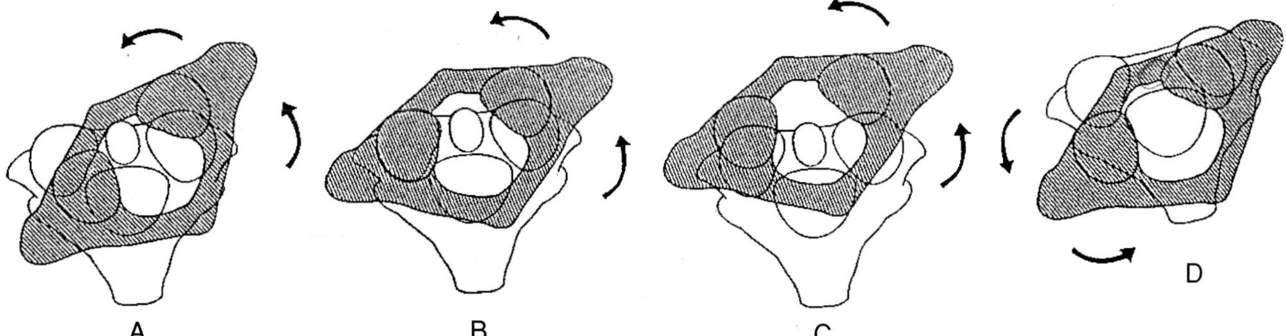

Figure 2–15. Four types of rotary fixation. *(a)* Type I: rotary fixation with no anterior displacement and the odontoid acting as the pivot. *(b)* Type II: rotary fixation with anterior displacement of 3–5 mm, one lateral process acting as the pivot. *(c)* Type III: rotary fixation with anterior displacement of more than 5 mm. *(d)* Type IV: rotary fixation with posterior displacement. (From Fielding, J.W., and Hawkins, R.J.: Atlanto-axial rotatory fixation. J. Bone Joint Surg. [Am.] 59:42, 1977.)

lack of anterior swelling, continued alignment of the posterior interspinous distances and the posterior spinolaminar line (**Schwischuk's line**) on radiographs, and reduction of the subluxation with neck extension help differentiate this entity from more serious disorders.

5. Intervertebral Disc Calcification Syndrome—Pain, decreased range of motion, low-grade fevers, increased ESR, and radiographic disc calcification (within the annulus) without erosion characterize this disorder, which usually involves the C-spine. Conservative treatment is indicated for this self-limited condition.
6. Basilar Impression/Invagination—Bony deformity at the base of the skull causes cephalad migration of the odontoid into the foramen magnum (see Fig. 7–2). Sagittal MRI scan best demonstrates impingement of the dens on the brain stem. Weakness, paresthesias, and hydrocephalus may result. Treatment is often operative and may include transoral resection of the dens, occipital laminectomy, and occipitocervical fusion and wiring.

X. **Upper Extremity Problems** (see Chapter 6, Hand)

A. Sprengel's Deformity—*Undescended scapula often associated with winging, hypoplasia, and omovertebral connections (30%).* It is the most common congenital anomaly of the shoulder in children. Affected scapulae are usually small, relatively wide, and medially rotated. Increased association with Klippel-Feil syndrome, kidney disease, scoliosis, and diastematomyelia. Surgery for cosmetic or functional deformities (decreased abduction) includes distal advancement of the associated muscles and scapula (Woodward) or detachment and movement of the scapula (Schrock, Green). Surgery is best done on the 3- to 8-year-old.

B. Congenital Pseudarthrosis of the Clavicle—*Failure of union of the medial and lateral ossification centers of* ***the right clavicle.*** Cause may be related to pulsations of the underlying subclavian artery. Presents as an enlarging, painless, nontender mass. Radiographs show rounded sclerotic bone at the pseudarthrosis site. *Surgery (open reduction/internal fixation with bone grafting) is indicated for unacceptable cosmetic deformities or with significant functional symptoms (mobility of the fragments and winging of the scapula).* Successful union is predictable (in contrast to congenital pseudarthrosis of the tibia).

C. Deltoid Fibrotic Problems—Short fibrous bands replace the deltoid muscle and cause abduction contractures at the shoulder, with elevation and winging of the scapula when the arms are adducted. Surgical resection of these bands is often required.

XI. **Lower Extremity Problems**

A. Introduction—Lower extremity problems that are best considered as a whole are presented in this section to provide a basis for understanding and comparison.

B. Rotational Problems of the Lower Extremities—Include *femoral anteversion, tibial torsion, and metatarsus adductus.* All of these problems may be a result of intrauterine positioning and commonly present with an *intoeing gait.* These deformities are usually bilateral, and the clinician should be wary of asymmetric findings. Evaluation should include the measurements noted in Table 2–12 and illustrated in Fig. 2–16.

1. Metatarsus Adductus—Forefoot is adducted at the tarsal-metatarsal joint. Usually seen during the first year of life. *May be associated with hip dysplasia (10–15%).* Approximately 85% of cases resolve spontaneously; feet that can be actively corrected to neutral require no treatment. Stretching exercises are used for feet that can be pas-

Table 2–12.

Evaluation of Rotational Problems of the Lower Extremities

Measurement	Technique	Normal Values (Degrees)	Significance
Foot-progression angle	Foot vs. straight line	−5 to +20	Nonspecific rotation
Medial rotation	Prone hip ROM	20–60	>70°, femoral anteversion
Lateral rotation	Prone hip ROM	30–60	<20°, femoral anteversion
Thigh-foot angle	Knee bent, foot up	0–20	<−10°, tibial torsion
Foot lateral border	Convex, medial crease	Straight, flexible	Metatarsus adductus

sively corrected to neutral (heel bisector line lines up with the second metatarsal). Feet that cannot be passively corrected usually respond to serial casting. Metatarsal osteotomies and limited medial release are indicated in resistant cases. The best results with osteotomies are seen when the surgery is performed after 5 years of age. The Heyman-Herndon procedure (complete tarsometatarsal capsulotomy) has fallen into disfavor because of a high incidence of failures at long-term follow-up. Rigidity and heel valgus should be identified and treated with early casting.

2. Tibial Torsion—*The most common cause of intoeing. Usually seen during the second year of life* and can be associated with metatarsus adductus. It is often bilateral and may be secondary to excessive medial ligamentous tightness. Internal rotation of the tibia causes the intoeing gait. This intrauterine "molding" deformity typically resolves spontaneously. Operative correction is rarely necessary except in severe cases, which are addressed with a supramalleolar osteotomy.

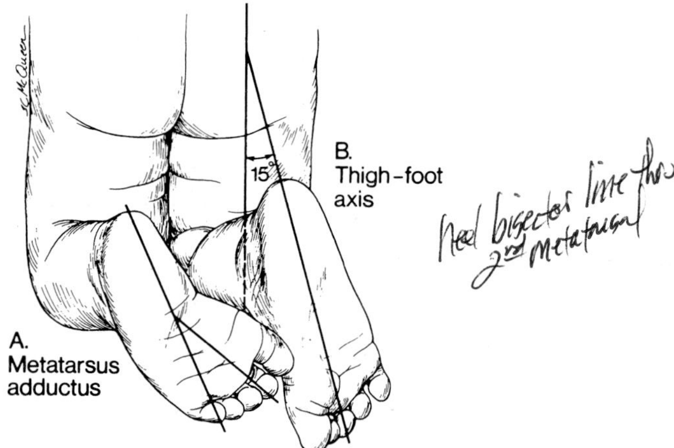

Figure 2–16. *A,* Deviation of the forefoot in metatarsus adductus. *B,* Note also the normal thigh-foot angle (15 degrees); negative thigh-foot angles (<10 degrees) are seen in tibial torsion. (From Fitch, R.D.: Introduction to pediatric orthopedics. In Sabiston, D.C., Jr., ed.: Sabiston's Essentials of Surgery. Philadelphia, WB Saunders, 1987.)

3. Femoral Anteversion—Internal rotation of the femur, *seen in 3- to 6-year-olds*. Increased internal rotation and decreased external rotation are noted on examination of a child with an intoeing gait and whose patellas are internally rotated. Children with this problem classically *sit in a "W" position*. If associated with tibial torsion, femoral anteversion may lead to patellofemoral problems. This disorder usually corrects spontaneously by age 10, but in the older child with less than 10 degrees of external rotation, femoral derotational osteotomy (intertrochanteric is best) may be considered for cosmesis.

XII. **Hip and Femur**

A. Developmental Dysplasia of the Hip (DDH)

1. Introduction—Previously called congenital dysplasia of the hip, this disorder represents abnormal development or dislocation of the hip secondary to capsular laxity and mechanical factors (e.g., intrauterine positioning). **Breech positioning, female sex, and positive family history are risk factors.** Decreased intrauterine space explains the increased incidence of DDH in the first-born child. *Commonly associated with other "packaging problems," such as torticollis (20%) and metatarsus adductus (10%),* it is partially characterized by increased amounts of type III collagen. DDH is seen most commonly in the left hip (67%) in females (85%) with a positive family history (20+%), increased maternal estrogens, and breech births (30–50%). This disorder includes the spectrum of complete dislocation, subluxation, instability, and acetabular dysplasia. The teratologic form is most severe and usually requires early surgery. The teratologic form of DDH is defined as those hips that present with a pseudoacetabulum at or near birth. Teratologic hip dislocations commonly present in association with syndromes such as arthrogryposis or Larsen's syndrome. If left untreated, muscles about the hip become contracted, and the acetabulum becomes more dysplastic and filled with fibrofatty tissue (pulvinar). The capsule becomes redun-

dant, and the head may be trapped by the iliopsoas tendon, causing an "hourglass" constriction. An inverted limbus may block reduction. An abnormal femoral head and "false acetabulum" (pseudoacetabulum) may develop. *Potential obstructions to obtaining a concentric reduction in DDH are iliopsoas tendon, pulvinar, contracted inferomedial hip capsule, and the transverse acetabular ligament.*

2. Diagnosis—Early diagnosis is possible with *Ortolani's test (elevation and abduction of femur relocates a dislocated hip) and Barlow's test (adduction and depression of femur dislocates a dislocatable hip)*. Three phases are commonly recognized: (1) **dislocated** (Ortolani-positive, early; Ortolani-negative, late, when femoral head cannot be reduced); (2) **dislocatable** (Barlow-positive); and (3) **subluxatable** (Barlow-suggestive). *Later diagnosis is made with limitation of hip abduction* in the affected hip as the laxity resolves and stiffness becomes more clinically evident. (*Caution:* Abduction may be decreased symmetrically with bilateral dislocations.) Another sign of dislocation includes a positive *Galeazzi sign*, demonstrated by the clinical appearance of foreshortening of the femur on the affected side. This clinical test is performed with the feet held together and knees flexed (a congenitally short femur can also cause a positive Galeazzi sign). Other clinical findings associated with DDH include asymmetric gluteal folds (less reliable) and a positive Trendelenburg stance. Repeat examination, especially in the infant, is important because a child's irritability can prevent proper evaluation. Radiographs may be helpful in the older child (>3 months), and measurement of the acetabular index (normal <25 degrees), measurement of Perkins' line (normally the ossific nucleus of femoral head is medial to this line), and evaluation of Shenton's line are useful (Fig. 2–17). Later, delayed ossification of the femoral head on the affected side may be seen. Dynamic ultrasonography is also useful for making the diagnosis, especially in young children before ossification of the femoral head (which occurs at age 4–6 months). It is also useful for assessing reduction in a Pavlik harness and diagnosing acetabular dysplasia or capsular laxity; however, it is operator-dependent. Arthrography is helpful after closed reduction to determine concentric reduction.

3. Treatment—Based on achieving and maintaining early "concentric reduction" in order to prevent future degenerative joint disease. Specific therapy is based on the child's age and includes the *Pavlik harness*, which is designed to maintain infants (<6 months) reduced in about 100 degrees of flexion and mild abduction (the "human position" [Salter]). The reduction should be confirmed by radiographs or ultrasound scans after placement in the harness and brace adjustment. The position of the hip should be within the *"safe zone"* of Ramsey (between maximum adduction before redislocation and excessive abduction causing a high risk of avascular necrosis). Impingement of the posterosuperior retinacular branch of the medial femoral circumflex artery has been implicated in osteonecrosis associated with DDH treated in an abduction orthosis. *Pavlik harness treatment is contraindicated in teratologic hip dislocations.* Patients with a narrow safe zone should be considered for an adductor tenotomy. The child is placed in the harness, and radiographs or ultrasound scans are obtained to assess reduction. If unsatisfactory, the harness is adjusted (usually by increasing the amount of flexion), and the study is repeated; *excessive flexion may result in transient femoral nerve palsy.* A stable reduction must be demonstrated in the harness early (within 2–4 weeks). Treatment continues until the hip is reduced and stable. Weaning from the harness is generally done over a period twice as long as the treatment duration. Use of abduction bracing may be considered for residual acetabular dysplasia in a child who is ambulating. Acetabular dysplasia is diagnosed by radiographic parameters (acetabular index >30 degrees). *In children between 6 and 18 months, and younger infants for whom the Pavlik treatment fails, an attempt at closed reduction and spica casting is warranted.* Prereduction traction

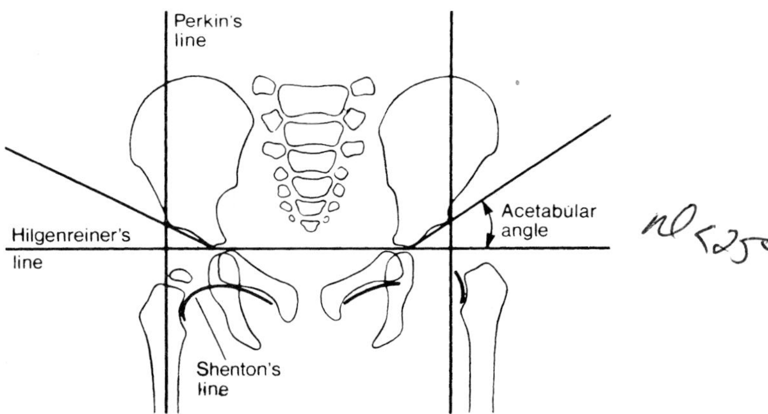

Figure 2–17. Common measurements used to evaluate developmental dysplasia of the hip. Note the delayed ossification, disruption of Shenton's line, and increased acetabular index on the left dislocated hip. (From Fitch, R.D.: Introduction to pediatric orthopaedics. In Sabiston, D.C., Jr., ed.: Sabiston's Essentials of Surgery. Philadelphia, WB Saunders, 1987.)

is controversial. One study has shown that home traction is as safe and efficacious as inpatient traction. Several studies have demonstrated similar rates of osteonecrosis of the femoral head with closed or open reduction with or without preliminary traction. An arthrogram is usually obtained at the time of closed reduction to evaluate the concentricity and stability of the reduction. The arthrogram may show an inverted/obstructive limbus or an hourglass constriction of the capsule, indicating an incomplete/unstable reduction. Alternatively, ultrasonography can be used in the operating room to assess the results of closed reduction. Casting after reduction should be done for at least 4 months, followed by night-time bracing. *Open reduction is reserved for children 12 to 18 months old who fail closed reduction, have an obstructive limbus, or have an unstable safe zone. Open reduction is also the initial treatment for children 18 months and older.* It is usually done through an anterior approach (less risk to the medial femoral circumflex artery) and includes capsulorrhaphy, adductor tenotomy, and perhaps femoral shortening. The major risk associated with both open and closed reductions is osteonecrosis (due to direct vascular injury or impingement versus disruption of the circulation from osteotomies). Failure of open reduction is difficult to treat surgically due to the high complication rate of revision surgery (50% osteonecrosis, 33% pain and stiffness in a recent study). The treatment guidelines in the chart at the top of the page are appropriate.

4. Osteotomies—May be required in toddlers and school-age children. *Osteotomies are indicated for instability, severe acetabular dysplasia, or progressive femoral head subluxation after reduction.* Osteotomies should be done only after congruent reduction, with satisfactory ROM, and after reasonable femoral sphericity is achieved by closed or open methods. *Diagnosis after age 8 years (younger in patients with bilateral DDH) may contraindicate reduction because the acetabulum has little chance to remodel,* although reduction may be indicated in conjunction with salvage procedures. The choice of femoral versus pelvic osteotomy (Fig. 2–18) is sometimes a matter of the surgeon's choice. Some surgeons prefer to perform pelvic osteotomies after age 4 and femoral osteotomies prior to this age. *In general, pelvic osteotomies should be done when severe dysplasia is accompanied by significant radiographic changes on the acetabular side (i.e., increased acetabular index, failure of lateral acetabular ossification), whereas changes on the femoral side (e.g., marked anteversion, coxa valga) are best treated by femoral osteotomies.* Femoral osteotomies rarely correct hip dysplasia successfully after age 5 years. The chart lists common reconstructive osteotomies.

Situation	Findings	Treatment
Newborn		
Dislocated	+ Ortolani's test	Pavlik's harness
Dislocatable	+ Barlow's test	Pavlik's harness
Subluxatable	Barlow's test rides up edge	Supportive/Pavlik's
<6 months old		
Dislocatable/reducible	+ Ortolani's test	Pavlik's harness
Unreducible	− Ortolani's test	Pavlik's harness → traction, closed reduction
>6 months old		
Unreducible	− Ortolani's test	Traction and closed reduction
Failed closed reduction	Medial dye pool >5 mm	Open reduction, psoas tenotomy, capsulorrhaphy, ± femoral shortening osteotomy, ± pelvic osteotomy
>3 years old		
Dislocated	Trendelenburg's gait, leg asymmetry (Allis' test)	Open reduction, psoas tenotomy, capsulorrhaphy, femoral shortening osteotomy, ± pelvic osteotomy

Osteotomy	Procedure	Requirement
Femoral	Intertrochanteric osteotomy (VDRO)	Concentric reduction
Salter's	Innominate osteotomy, open wedge	Concentric reduction
Sutherland's (double)	Salter's + pubic osteotomy	Concentric reduction
Steel's (triple)	Salter's + osteotomy of both rami	Concentric reduction
Dial's	Periacetabular osteotomy	Surgeon's experience
Pemberton's	Through acetabular roof to triradiate cartilage	Concentric reduction
Chiari's	Through ilium above acetabulum (makes new roof)	Salvage procedure for asymmetric incongruity
Shelf's	Slotted lateral acetabular augmentation	Salvage procedure for asymmetric incongruity

The Salter osteotomy may lengthen the affected leg up to 1 cm. *The Pemberton acetabuloplasty is a good choice for residual dysplasia because it reduces acetabular volume* (bends on triradiate cartilage). The Steel (triple) innominate osteotomy is favored for older children because their symphysis pubis does not rotate as well. *Dega-type osteotomies are often favored for paralytic dislocations and patients with posterior acetabular deficiency.* This osteotomy is more versatile

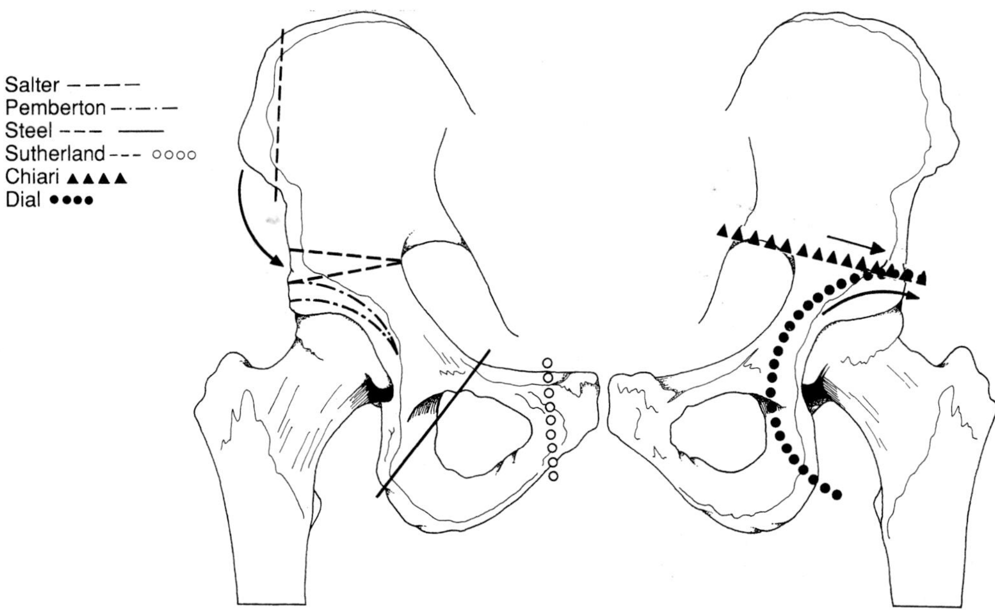

Figure 2–18. Common pelvic osteotomies for treatment of developmental dysplasia of the hip.

and is sometimes used for DDH. The Dial osteotomy is technically difficult and rarely used. *The Chiari osteotomy is recommended for patients with inadequate femoral head coverage and an incongruous joint but is considered a salvage procedure.* The Chiari osteotomy shortens the affected leg and requires periarticular soft-tissue metaplasia for success. Other procedures include the Shelf lateral acetabular augmentation procedure for patients with inadequate lateral coverage or trochanteric advancement in a patient >8 years old with increased trochanteric overgrowth (improves hip abductor biomechanics). *The two pelvic osteotomies that depend on metaplastic tissue (fibrocartilage) for a successful result are the shelf and Chiari osteotomies.*

B. Congenital Coxa Vara—*Decreased neck-shaft angle due to a defect in ossification of the femoral neck.* It is bilateral in one-third to one-half of cases. Coxa vara can be congenital (noted at birth and differentiated from DDH by MRI), developmental (AD, progressive), or acquired (e.g., trauma, Legg-Calvé-Perthes, slipped capital femoral epiphysis). May present with a waddling gait (bilateral) or a painless limp (unilateral). *Radiographs classically demonstrate a triangular ossification defect in the inferomedial femoral neck in developmental coxa vara.* Evaluation of **Hilgenreiner's epiphyseal angle** (the angle between Hilgenreiner's line and a line through the proximal femoral physis) is the key to treatment. *An angle of <45 degrees spontaneously corrects, whereas an angle of >60 degrees (and a neck-shaft angle of <110 degrees) usually requires surgery.* The surgical treatment is a corrective valgus osteotomy of the proximal femur. Proximal femoral (valgus) ± derotation osteotomy (Pauwel) is indicated for a neck-shaft angle <90 degrees, a vertically oriented physeal plate, progressive deformities, or significant gait abnormalities. Concomitant distal/lateral transfer of the greater trochanter may also be indicated to restore more normal hip abductor mechanics.

C. Legg-Calvé-Perthes Disease (Coxa Plana)—Noninflammatory deformity of the proximal femur secondary to a vascular insult, leading to *osteonecrosis of the proximal femoral epiphysis.* Usually seen in boys 4 to 8 years old with delayed skeletal maturation. There is an increase incidence with a positive family history, low birth weight, and abnormal birth presentation. *Symptoms include pain (often knee pain), effusion (from synovitis), and limp. Decreased hip ROM (especially abduction and internal rotation) and a Trendelenburg gait are also common.* **Age is the key to prognosis**. Specifically, the bone age is the best indicator. *Patients presenting with a bone age >6 years have a significantly poorer prognosis.* Bilateral involvement may be seen in 12–15% of cases. However, in bilateral cases the involvement is asymmetric and virtually never simultaneous. *Bilateral involvement may mimic multiple epiphyseal dysplasia.* Differential diagnosis includes septic arthritis, blood dyscrasias, hypothyroidism, and epiphyseal dysplasia. Pathologically, the osteonecrosis is followed by revascularization and resorption via creeping substitution that eventually allows remodeling and fragmentation. Radiographic findings vary with the stage of disease but include cessation of growth of the ossific nucleus, medial joint space widening, and development of a "crescent sign" representing

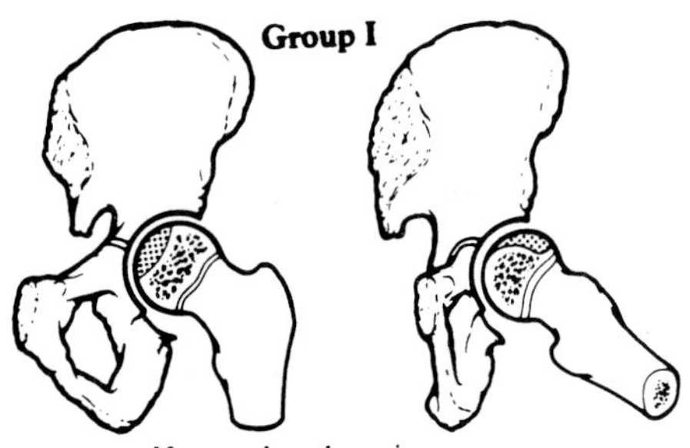

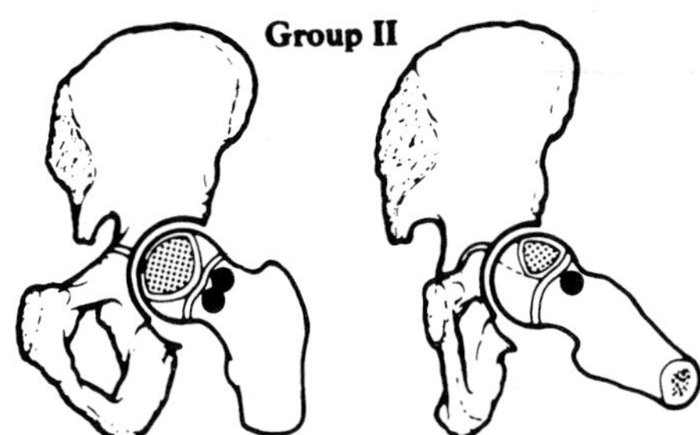

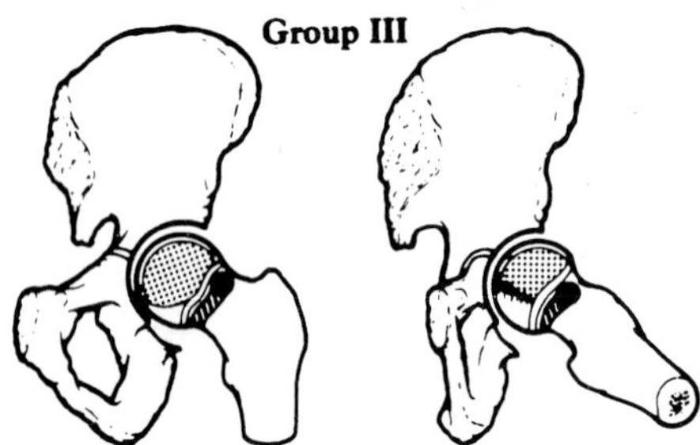

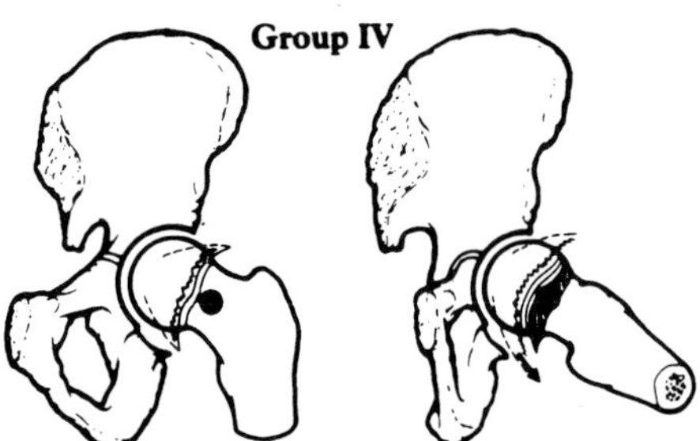

Figure 2–19. Catterall classification of Legg-Calvé-Perthes disease. Note the significant involvement of the lateral margin of the capital femoral epiphysis in groups III and IV (Salter and Thompson "B"). (From Fitch, R.D.: Introduction to pediatric orthopedics. In Sabiston, D.C., Jr., ed.: Sabiston's Essentials of Surgery. Philadelphia, WB Saunders, 1987.)

subchondral fracture. Four radiographic stages (Waldenström's) are usually described based on the appearance of the capital femoral epiphysis.

Stage	Characteristics
Initial	Physeal irregularity, metaphyseal blurring, radiolucencies
Fragmentation	Radiolucencies and radiodensities
Reossification	Normal density returns
Healed	Residual deformity

Catterall has defined four stages based on the amount of femoral involvement (seen as the crescent sign). This grouping has been simplified by Salter and Thompson based on the involvement of the lateral margin of the capital femoral epiphysis (CFE) (Fig. 2–19).

Caterall	Salter and Thompson	Location	Prognosis
I	A	Anterior (seen on lateral view)	Good
II	A	Anterior and partial lateral	Good
III	B	Anterior and lateral margin	Poor
IV	B	Throughout CFE dome	Poor

The crescent sign represents a pathologic subchondral fracture of the resorbing femoral head and is best seen on a frog-leg view of the pelvis. Bone scans and MRI may help identify early involvement but do not correlate with the extent of involvement. Newer, magnified bone scans may help identify the revascularization pattern. These sophisticated studies (bone scan, MRI) are not required for routine cases. *Herring et al. described the lateral pillar classification of femoral head involvement in the fragmentation stage of Perthes' disease* (Fig. 2–20). This radiographic classification is based on the degree of involvement at the lateral pillar of the femoral head. *Group A* has little or no involvement of the lateral pillar and a uniformly good outcome. *Group B* has >50% of lateral pillar height maintained and a good outcome in younger patients (bone age <6 years) but a less fortunate outcome in older patients. *Group C* has <50% of lateral pillar height maintained and a poorer prognosis in all age groups. In group C, essentially all CFEs become aspherical and have a longer duration of fragmentation and reossification stages. This classification has a high correlation for predicting the amount of femoral head deformity at skeletal maturity and is a strong predictor of final outcome. *Maintaining the sphericity of the femoral head is the most important factor in achieving a good result.* Use of circular templates (Mose) is helpful for evaluating this parameter. Early hip degenera-

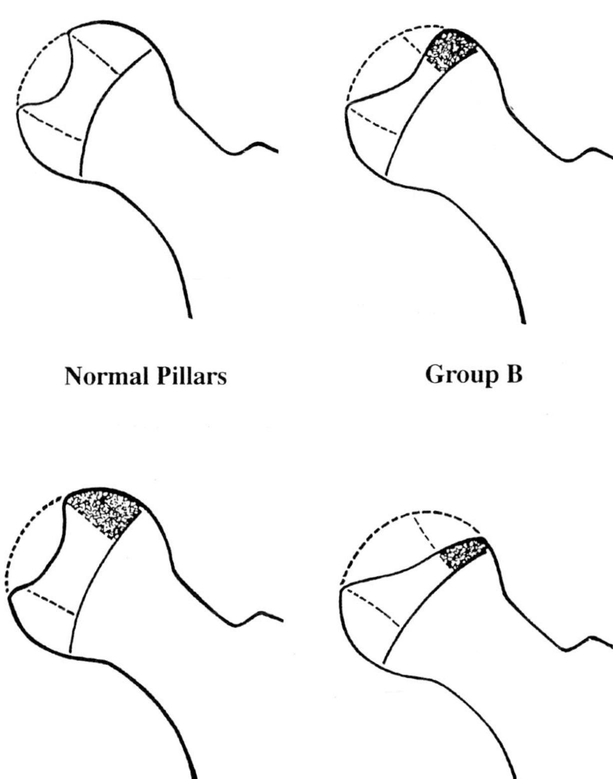

Figure 2–20. Lateral pillar classification of Legg-Calvé-Perthes disease. *Normal pillars,* The pillars were derived by noting the lines of demarcation between the central sequestrum and the remainder of the epiphysis on the anteroposterior radiograph. *Group A,* Normal height of lateral pillar is maintained. *Group B,* More than 50% height of lateral pillar is maintained. *Group C,* Less than 50% height of lateral pillar is maintained. (Adapted from Herring, J.A., Neustadt, J.B., Williams, J.J., et al.: The lateral pillar classification of Legg-Calvé-Perthes disease. J. Pediatr. Orthop. 12:143–150, 1992.)

tive joint disease results from aspherical femoral heads. *Poor prognosis is associated with older children (bone age >6 years), female sex, advanced stages (with lateral margin of the CFE involved), loss of containment, and decreased hip ROM (decreased abduction).* Radiographic findings associated with poor prognosis (*Catterall's "head at risk" signs) include (1) lateral calcification, (2) Gage's sign (V-shaped defect at lateral physis), (3) lateral subluxation, (4) metaphyseal cyst formation, and (5) horizontal growth plate. In general, the goals of treatment are relief of symptoms, restoration of ROM, and containment of the CFE.* Use of outpatient or inpatient traction, anti-inflammatory medications, and partial weight-bearing with crutches for periods of 1–2 days to several weeks is helpful for relieving symptoms. ROM is maintained with traction, muscle releases, exercise, and/or use of a Petrie cast. *Containment of the CFE* by use of traction, muscle releases, abduction bracing, or varus femoral versus pelvic osteotomy is helpful for maintaining CFE sphericity. Herring has described a treatment plan (see bottom of page) based on age and the lateral pillar classification of disease involvement.

Some authors recommend bracing until new bone is seen on the anterolateral portion of the femoral head. Advanced flattening of the femoral head can make it "noncontainable." Because abduction results in hinging and subluxation, bracing at this stage is not effective. Treatment options include Chiari's osteotomy, cheilectomy (of the femoral head prominence), and valgus osteotomy (a technique with some promise). Distal transfer of the greater trochanter is occasionally required to offset overgrowth of the greater trochanter (which is not affected and continues to grow). Overall, the treatment of Perthes' disease is currently quite controversial. *Definitive evidence of the effectiveness of surgical treatment is still lacking.*

D. Slipped Capital Femoral Epiphysis (SCFE)—*Disorder of the proximal femoral epiphysis caused by weakness of the perichondral ring and slippage through the hypertrophic zone of the growth plate.* The femoral head remains in the acetabulum, and the neck displaces anteriorly and externally rotates. *SCFE is seen most commonly in African-American, obese, adolescent boys with a positive family history. Up to 25% of cases are bilateral.* May be associated with hormonal changes in young children, such as hypothy-

Lateral Pillar Classification of Perthes' Disease

Age	Lateral Pillar Classification	Goals of Treatment	Treatment Recommendation
<6 years old	Any	Relief of symptoms	NSAIDs, home traction, avoid weight-bearing
6–8 years old	A	Relief of symptoms	Same as above
	B	Containment	Traction, muscle releases, abduction brace, VDROVs Salter's osteotomy
	C	Containment	Same as type B, but bracing ineffective due to difficulty centering CFE
>9 years old	A	Relief of symptoms	NSAIDs, home traction, avoid weight-bearing
	B	Containment →	(Bracing difficult due to loss of motion and poor compliance),
	C	Containment →	VDRO, Salter's, muscle release, Petrie's cast

roidism, or advanced renal disease. May present with coxalgic, externally rotated gait; decreased internal rotation; thigh atrophy; **and hip, thigh, or knee pain.** Symptoms vary with acuteness of the slip.

Slip	Duration of Symptoms (Weeks)	Symptoms
Acute	<3	Usually no previous symptoms
Chronic	>3	Insidious onset
Acute on chronic		Acute pain with history of chronic hip, thigh, or knee pain

Loder et al. described a new classification of SCFE based on the patients' ability to bear weight at the time of presentation. **Stable slips** are those in which weight-bearing with or without crutches is possible. **Unstable slips** are those in which weight-bearing is not possible because of severe pain. No patients with stable slips developed osteonecrosis, whereas 50% of the patients with unstable slips developed osteonecrosis (in this study of 55 patients, all treated with single pin fixation). Satisfactory results were obtained in 47% of unstable hips and 96% of stable hips. Radiographs show the slip, which is classified based on the percent of slip: grade I, 0–33%; grade II, 33–50%; and grade III, >50%. In mild cases, loss of the lateral overhang of the femoral ossific nucleus *(Klein's line)* and blurring of the proximal femoral metaphysis may be all that is seen on the anteroposterior film. **The recommended treatment is pinning in situ.** Forceful reduction before pinning is not indicated. Pin placement can be done percutaneously with one pin. The pin should be started anteriorly on the femoral neck, ending in the central portion of the femoral head. *Patients presenting at less than 10 years of age should have an endocrine work-up. Prophylactic pinning of the opposite hip is recommended in patients diagnosed with an endocrinopathy (hypothyroidism).* In severe SCFE, the residual proximal femoral deformity may remodel with the patient's remaining growth. Intertrochanteric (Kramer's) or subtrochanteric (Southwick's) osteotomies may be useful in treating the deformities caused by SCFE that fail to remodel. Cuneiform osteotomy at the femoral neck has the potential to correct a higher degree of deformity but remains controversial due to the high reported rates of osteonecrosis (37%) and future osteoarthritis (37%). *Complications associated with SCFE include chondrolysis (narrowed joint space, pain, and decreased motion), osteonecrosis (higher incidence in unstable slips), and degenerative joint disease (pistol grip deformity of the proximal femur).*

E. Proximal Femoral Focal Deficiency (PFFD)—Developmental defect of the proximal femur recognizable at birth. Clinically, patients with PFFD have a short, bulky thigh that is flexed, abducted, and externally rotated. *PFFD can be associated with coxa vara or fibular hemimelia (50%).* Congenital knee ligamentous deficiency and contracture are also common. Treatment must be individualized based on leg-length discrepancy, adequacy of musculature, proximal joint stability, and the presence or absence of foot deformities. The percentage of shortening remains constant during growth. The Aitken classification divides PFFD into four groups (Fig. 2–21). Classes A and B both have a femoral head present, which potentially allows for reconstructive procedures including limb lengthening. Classes C and D do not have a femoral head and present a more difficult treatment dilemma. *Treatment options include amputation, femoral-pelvic fusion (Brown's procedure), Van Ness' rotationplasty, and limb lengthening.*

F. Leg-Length Discrepancy (LLD)—There are many causes of LLD such as congenital disorders (e.g., hemihypertrophy, dysplasias, PFFD, DDH), paralytic disorders (e.g., spasticity, polio), infection (pyogenic disruption of the physis), tumors, and trauma. Long-term problems associated with LLD include inefficient gait, equinus contractures of the ankle, postural scoliosis, and low back pain. The discrepancy must be measured accurately (e.g., with blocks of set height under the affected side, scanogram) and can be tracked with the Green-Anderson or Mosely graph (with serial leg-length films or CT scanograms and bone age determinations). *In general, projected discrepancies at maturity of <2 cm are observed or treated with shoe lifts. Discrepancies of 2–5 cm can be treated with epiphysiodesis of the long side, shortening of the long side (ostectomy), or lengthening. Discrepancies of >5 cm are generally treated with lengthening.* Using standard techniques, lengthening of 1 mm/d is typical. The Ilizarov principles are followed, including metaphyseal corticotomy (preserving the medullary canal and blood supply), followed by gradual distraction. Rarely, one can consider physeal distraction (chondrodiatasis). This procedure must be done near skeletal maturity because the physis almost always closes after this type of limb lengthening. *A gross estimation of LLD can be made using the following assumption of growth per year up to age 16 in boys and age 14 in girls: distal femur, 3/8 in/y (9 mm); proximal tibia, 1/4 in/y (6 mm); and proximal femur 1/8 in/y (3 mm). Use of the Mosely data gives more accurate data.*

G. Lower Extremity Inflammation and Infection (see Chapter 1, Basic Sciences)

1. Transient Synovitis—Most common cause

TYPE		FEMORAL HEAD	ACETABULUM	FEMORAL SEGMENT	RELATIONSHIP AMONG COMPONENTS OF FEMUR AND ACETABULUM AT SKELETAL MATURITY
A		Present	Normal	Short	Bony connection between components of femur Femoral head in acetabulum Subtrochanteric varus angulation, often with pseudarthrosis
B	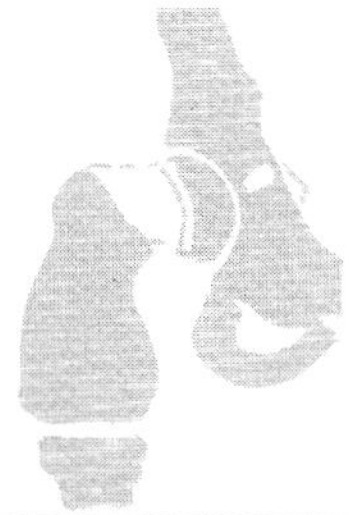	Present	Adequate or moderately dysplastic	Short, usually proximal bony tuft	No osseous connection between head and shaft Femoral head in acetabulum
C	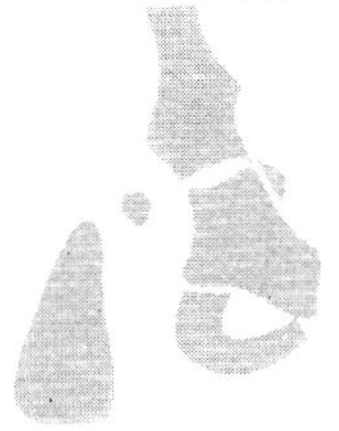	Absent or represented by ossicle	Severely dysplastic	Short, usually proximally tapered	May be osseous connection between shaft and proximal ossicle No articular relation between femur and acetabulum
D	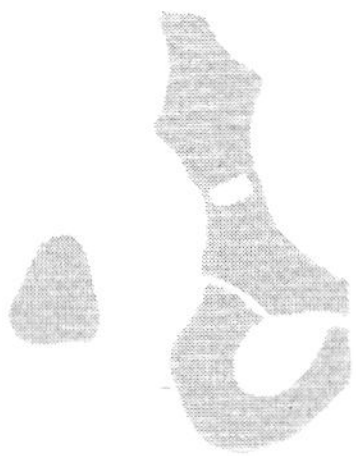	Absent	Absent Obturator foramen enlarged Pelvis squared in bilateral cases	Short, deformed	(none)

Figure 2–21. Aiken's classification of proximal femoral focal deficiency. Note lack of femoral head in types C and D. (From Tachdjian, M.O.: Pediatric Orthopaedics, 2nd ed. Philadelphia, WB Saunders, 1990.)

of painful hips during childhood, but it is *a diagnosis of exclusion. Can be related to viral infection, allergic reaction, or trauma; however, cause is unknown.* Onset can be acute or insidious. Symptoms, which are self-limited, include voluntary limitation of motion and muscle spasm. With transient synovitis, the ESR is usually <20 mm/h. Rule out septic hip with aspiration (especially in children with fever, leukocytosis, or elevated ESR); then observe patient in Buck's traction for 24–48 hours.

2. Osteomyelitis—More common in children because of their rich metaphyseal blood supply and thick periosteum. Most common organism is ***Staphylococcus aureus*** (*except in neonates in whom group B streptococcus is more common*). With the advent of the ***Haemophilus influenzae*** **vaccination,** *H. influenzae* is now a much less common organism in musculoskeletal sepsis. A history of trauma is common in children presenting with osteomyelitis. *Osteomyelitis in children usually begins through hematogenous seeding of a bony metaphysis in the small arterioles that bend just beyond the physis, where blood flow is sluggish and there is poor phagocytosis, creating a bone abscess* (Fig. 2–22). Pus lifts the thick periosteum and puts pressure on the cortex, causing coagulation. Cortical bone may die and become a *sequestrum.* Finally, subperiosteal new bone forms around the dead sequestrum, creating an *involucrum.* Chronic bone abscesses may become surrounded by thick, fibrous tissue and sclerotic bone (*Brodie's abscess*). Clinically, the child presents with a tender, warm, sometimes swollen area over a long-

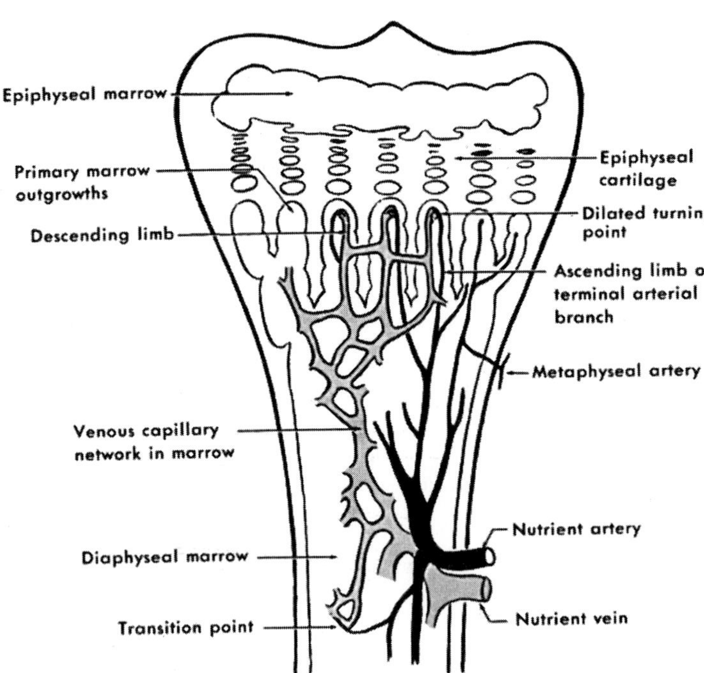

Figure 2–22. Metaphyseal sinusoids where sluggish blood flow increases susceptibility to osteomyelitis. (From Tachdjian, M.O.: Pediatric Orthopaedics, 2nd ed. Philadelphia, WB Saunders, 1990.)

bone metaphysis. Fever may or may not be present. Laboratory tests may be helpful (blood cultures, white blood cell count, ESR, C-reactive protein), and radiologic studies are also useful (radiographs with only soft-tissue edema early, metaphyseal rarefaction late, and bone scans). Definitive diagnosis is made with *aspiration* (50% positive cultures). Intravenous antibiotics are the best initial treatment if osteomyelitis is diagnosed early, prior to radiographic changes or the development of a subperiosteal abscess. Initially, broad-spectrum antibiotics are chosen, followed by antibiotics specific for the organism cultured. *Failure to respond to antibiotics, frank pus on aspiration, or the presence of a sequestered abscess (not accessible to antibiotics) requires operative drainage and débridement.* Specimens should be sent for histology and culture. Some tumors (with necrosis) look like infections. The wound can be closed over a drain. Intravenous antibiotics can be changed to appropriate oral antibiotics after a good response to treatment has been demonstrated (usually at 7–10 days). Antibiotics should be continued until the ESR (or C-reactive protein) returns to normal, usually at 4–6 weeks.

3. Septic Arthritis—Can develop from osteomyelitis (especially in neonates, in whom transphyseal vessels allow proximal spread into the joint) in joints with an intra-articular metaphysis. *The four extremity joints that have an intra-articular metaphysis are the hip, elbow, shoulder, and ankle.* Septic arthritis can also occur as a result of hematogenous spread of infection. Because pus is chondrolytic, septic arthritis in children is an acute surgical emergency. Organisms vary with age.

Age	Common Organisms	Empiric Antibiotics
<12 mo	Staphylococcus group B streptococcus	First generation cephalosporin
6 months–5 years	Staphylococcus, *H. influenzae*	Second or third generation cephalosporin
5–12 years	*S. aureus*	First generation cephalosporin
12–18 years	*S. aureus, N. gonorrhoeae*	Oxacillin/cephalosporin

Septic arthritis presents as a much more acute process than osteomyelitis. Decreased ROM and severe pain with passive motion may be accompanied by systemic symptoms of infection. Radiographs may show widened joint space or even dislocation. *Joint fluid aspirate shows a high white blood cell count (>50,000), glucose level 50 mg/dL less than serum levels, and in patients with gram-positive cocci or gram-negative rods a high lactic acid level.* Ultrasonography can be helpful for identifying the presence of an effusion. Aspiration should be followed by irrigation and débridement in major joints (especially in the hip, culture of synovium is also recommended). Lumbar puncture should be considered in a septic joint caused by *H. influenzae* because of increased incidence of meningitis. Lumbar

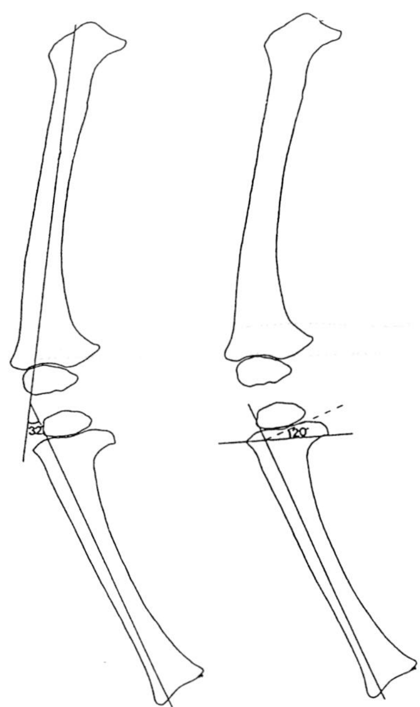

Figure 2–23. Comparison of tibiofemoral angle with Levine and Drennan's metaphyseal-diaphyseal angle in tibia vara. *Tibiofemoral Angle,* Method used to determine the tibiofemoral angle. A line is drawn along the longitudinal axis of the tibia and the femur; the angle between the lines is the tibiofemoral angle (32 degrees). *Metaphyseal-Diaphyseal Angle,* Method used to determine the metaphyseal-diaphyseal angle in the same extremity. A line is drawn perpendicular to the longitudinal axis of the tibia, and another is drawn through the two beaks of the metaphysis to determine the transverse axis of the tibial metaphysis. The metaphyseal-diaphyseal angle (12 degrees) is the angle bisected by the two lines. (Adapted from Levine, A.M., and Drennan, J.C.: Physiological bowing and tibia vara. J. Bone Joint Surg. [Am.] 64:1159, 1982.)

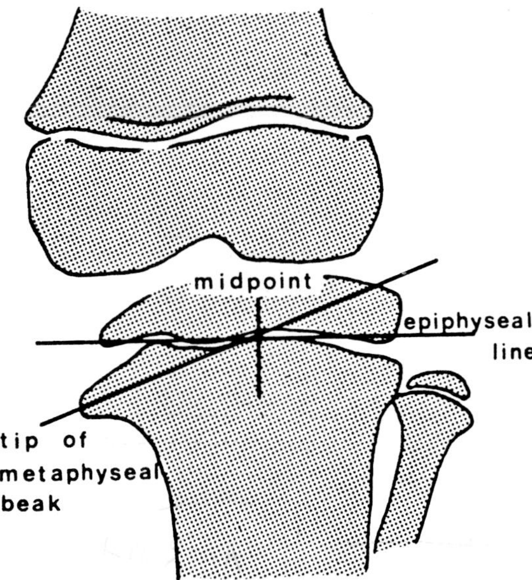

Figure 2–24. Blount's disease and measurement of the epiphyseal-metaphyseal angle. (From Tachdjian, M.O.: Pediatric Orthopaedics, 2nd ed. Philadelphia, WB Saunders, 1990.)

puncture may not be necessary if an antibiotic is selected that is known to cross the blood-brain barrier. Intravenous antibiotics are changed to specific oral antibiotics after a good response to treatment is seen for reliable patients/parents and for those with good drug tolerance. Prognosis is usually good except in patients with a delayed diagnosis. Patients with *Neisseria gonorrhoeae* septic arthritis usually have a preceding migratory polyarthralgia, small red papules, and multiple joint involvement. This organism typically elicits less white blood cell response (less than 50,000) and usually does not require surgical drainage. Large doses of penicillin are required to eliminate this organism.

XIII. **Knee and Leg**

A. Genu Valgum—Normally, genu varum (bowed legs) evolves naturally to genu valgum (knock-knees) by age 2 1/2 years, with a gradual transition to physiologic valgus by age 4 years. Observation of gait is important when evaluating patients to determine if there is a thrust at the onset of weight-bearing.

1. Genu Varum (Bowed Legs)—Normal in children <2 years old. Radiographs in physiologic bowing typically show flaring of the tibia and femur in a symmetric fashion. *Pathologic conditions that can cause genu varum include osteogenesis imperfecta, osteochondromas, trauma, various dysplasias and, most commonly, Blount's disease.* **Blount's disease** (tibia varum) differs from physiologic genu varum because it is caused by a disorder of the posterior medial tibial physis. Affected children are most commonly African-American, obese males. Radiographs may show a *metaphyseal-diaphyseal angle abnormality and metaphyseal beaking.* Drennan's angle of >11 degrees is considered abnormal. This angle is formed between the metaphyseal beaks and is demonstrated in Fig. 2–23. The epiphyseal-metaphyseal angle is also useful (Fig. 2–24). The infantile form of Blount's disease (most common) is usually bilateral and is associated with internal tibial torsion. Adolescent Blount's is less severe and predominantly unilateral. Treatment is based on age and the stage of disease (Langinskiold's I–VI, with VI characterized by a metaphyseal-epiphyseal bony bridge).

Age	Stage	Treatment
<18 mo	I–II	None
18–24 months	I–II	A-frame/Blount's brace (night)
2–3 years	I–II	Modified locked KAFO
3–8 years	III–V	Valgus rotational osteotomy
3–8 years	VI	Resection of bony bridge

2. Genu Valgum (Knock-Knees)—Up to 15 degrees at the knee is common in 2- to 6-year-old children. Patients within this physiologic range do not require treatment. *Pathologic genu valgum may be associated, for example, with renal osteodystrophy (most common cause if bilateral), tumors (e.g., osteochondromas), infections (may stimulate proximal asymmetric tibial growth), or trauma.* Conservative treatment is ineffective in pathologic genu valgum. Consider surgery (at the site of the deformity) in children >10 years old with >10 cm between the medial malleoli or >15–20 degrees of valgus. *Hemiepiphysiodesis or physeal stapling of the medial side is effective before the end of growth for severe deformities.*

B. Tibial Bowing—Three types based on the apex of the curve:

1. Posteromedial—Physiologic bowing usually of the middle and distal thirds of the tibia may be the result of abnormal intrauterine positioning. It is *commonly associated with calcaneovalgus feet and tight anterior structures.* Spontaneous correction is the rule, but follow the patient to evaluate LLD. The most common sequelae of posteromedial bowing is an **average LLD of 3–4 cm,** which may require an age-appropriate epiphysiodesis of the long limb. Tibial osteotomies are not indicated.
2. Anteromedial Tibial Bowing—Typically caused by fibular hemimelia. *A congenital longitudinal deficiency of the fibula is the most common long-bone deficiency.* It is usually *associated with anteromedial bowing, ankle instability, equinovalgus foot (± absent lateral rays), tarsal coalition, and femoral shortening.* Classically, skin dimpling is seen over the tibia. Significant LLD often results from this disorder. The fibular deficiency can be intercalary, which involves the whole bone (absent fibula), or terminal. Fibular hemimelia is frequently associated with femoral abnormalities such as coxa vara and PFFD. Radiographic findings include complete or partial absence of the fibula, ball-and-socket ankle (secondary to tarsal coalitions), and deficient lateral rays in the foot. Treatment varies from a simple shoe lift or bracing to Syme's amputation. *Treatment decisions are based on the degree of foot deformity and the degree of shortening of the limb.* Amputation is usually done to treat limbs with severe shortening and/or a stiff, nonfunctional foot at about 10 months of age. For less severe cases, reconstructive procedures, including lengthening, may be an alternative. This procedure should include resection of the fibular anlage to avoid future foot problems.
3. Anterolateral Tibial Bowing—**Congenital pseudarthrosis of the tibia** is the most common cause of anterolateral bowing. It is often accompanied by *neurofibromatosis* (50%, but only 10% of patients with neurofibromatosis have this disorder). Classification (Boyd's) is based on bowing and the presence of cystic changes, sclerosis, or dysplasia; dysplasia and cystic changes are most common. Initial treatment includes a total contact brace to protect from fractures. Intramedullary fixation with excision of hamartomatous tissue and autogenous bone grafting are options for nonhealing fractures. Vascularized fibular graft or Ilizarov's methods should also be considered if bracing fails. *Osteotomies to correct the anterolateral bowing are contraindicated.* Amputation (Symes') and prosthetic fitting are indicated after two or three failed surgical attempts. Symes' amputation is preferred to below-knee amputation in these patients because the soft tissue available at the heel pad is superior to that in the calf as a weight-bearing stump. The soft tissue in the calf in these patients is often quite scarred and atrophic. The Symes' amputation also alleviates the issue of overgrowth.
4. Other Lower Limb Deficiencies—Include tibial hemimelia, an AD disorder that is a *congenital longitudinal deficiency of the tibia. Tibial hemimelia is the only long-bone deficiency with a known inheritance pattern (AD).* It is much less common than fibular hemimelia and is often associated with other bony abnormalities (especially lobster-claw hand). Clinically, the extremity is shortened and bowed anterolaterally with a prominent fibular head and equinovarus foot, with the sole of the foot facing the perineum. *The treatment for severe deformities with an entirely absent tibia is a knee disarticulation.* Fibular transposition (Brown's)

Category	Age Group	Prognosis	Treatment
I	Birth to adolescence	Excellent	Rest, immobilize
II	Teenage children	Intermediate	Rest, arthroscopic drilling +/− fixation of large defects
III	Adult (20+); closed physis	Poor; fragments/defects	Operative

has been unsuccessful, especially with absent quadriceps function and an absent proximal tibia. When the proximal tibia and quadriceps function are present, the fibula can be transposed to the residual tibia and create a functional below-knee amputation.

C. Osteochondritis Dissecans—An intra-articular lesion, usually of the distal femoral condyle, with disorderly enchondral ossification of epiphyseal growth. Common in 10- to 15-year-olds and can affect many joints, especially the *knee and elbow (capitellum)*. The lesion is thought to be secondary to trauma, ischemia, or abnormal epiphyseal ossification. *The lateral intercondylar portion of the medial femoral condyle is most frequently involved* (seen best on notch view). Classified into three categories based on age at appearance (Pappas) (see chart at bottom of preceding page).

Symptoms include activity-related pain, localized tenderness, stiffness, and swelling ± mechanical symptoms. Radiographs should include the tunnel (notch) view to evaluate the condyles. Differential diagnosis includes anomalous ossification centers. Surgical therapy includes drilling with multiple holes, fixation of large fragments, and bone grafting of large lesions in patients with closed physes. Commonly treated arthroscopically. Poor prognosis is associated with lesions in the lateral femoral condyle and patella. The arthroscopic classification and treatment of osteochondritis dissecans (after Guhl) is shown in the chart at the top of the page.

D. Osgood-Schlatter Disease—An osteochondrosis, or fatigue failure of the tibia tubercle apophysis due to stress from the extensor mechanism in a growing child *(tibial tubercle apophysitis)*. Radiographs may show irregularity and fragmentation of the tibial tubercle. It is usually self-limiting. Late excision of separate ossicles is occasionally required.

Classification	Treatment
Intact lesion	K-wire drilling
Early-separated lesion	In situ pinning
Partially detached lesion	Débridement of base and reduction and pinning
Salvageable loose body	
Unsalvageable loose body	Removal and débridement of base

E. Discoid Meniscus—Abnormal development of the lateral meniscus leads to the formation of a disc-shaped (or hypertrophic), rather than the normal crescent-shaped, meniscus. Typically, radiographs demonstrate widening of the cartilage space on the affected side (up to 11 mm). If symptomatic and torn, discoid meniscus can be arthroscopically débrided.

XIV. **Feet** (Fig. 2–25)

A. Clubfoot (Congenital Talipes Equinovarus)—*Forefoot adductus and supination; hindfoot equinous and varus.* Talar neck deformity (medial and plantar deviation) with medial rotation of the calcaneus and medial displacement of the navicular and cuboid occurs. Clubfoot is more common in males, and half the cases are bilateral. It is associated with *shortened/contracted muscles (intrinsics, tendoachilles, tibialis posterior, flexor hallucis longus, flexor digitorum longus)*, joint capsules, ligaments, and fascia that lead to the associated deformities. *Can be associated with hand anomalies (Streeter's dysplasia), diastrophic dwarfism, arthrogryposis, and myelomeningocele.* Radiographs should include the **dorsiflexion lateral view** (Turco's) in which a talocalcaneal angle of >35 degrees is normal; a smaller angle with a flat talar head is seen with clubfoot. On the AP view a talocalcaneal (Kite's) angle of 20–40 degrees is normal (<20 degrees is seen with clubfoot). The talus–first metatarsal angle is

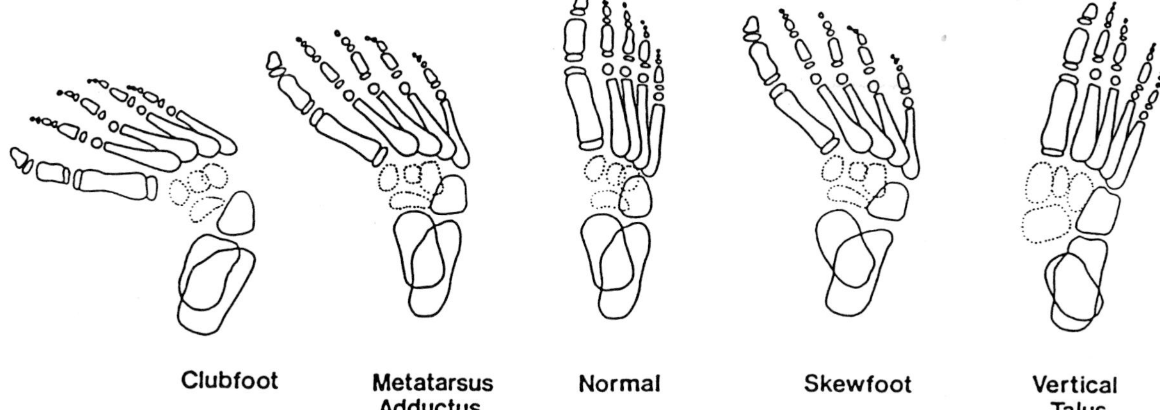

Figure 2–25. Anteroposterior view of common childhood foot disorders. *A,* Varus position of hindfoot and adducted forefoot in clubfoot. *B,* Normal hindfoot and adducted forefoot in metatarsus adductus. *C,* Normal foot. *D,* Valgus hindfoot (with increased talocalcaneal angle) and adducted forefoot in skewfoot. *E,* Increased talocalcaneal angle and lateral deviation of the calcaneus in congenital vertical talus.

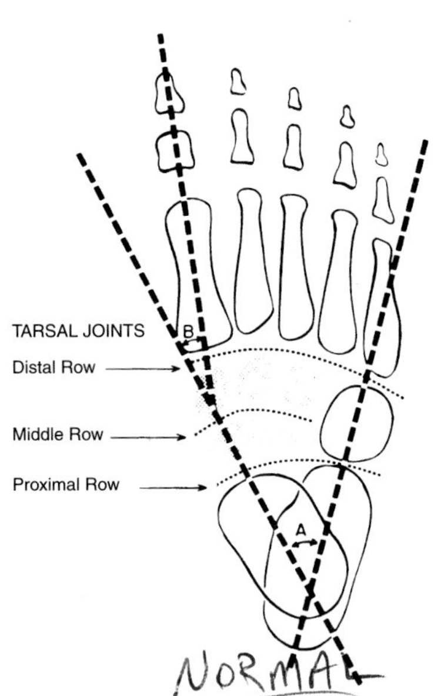

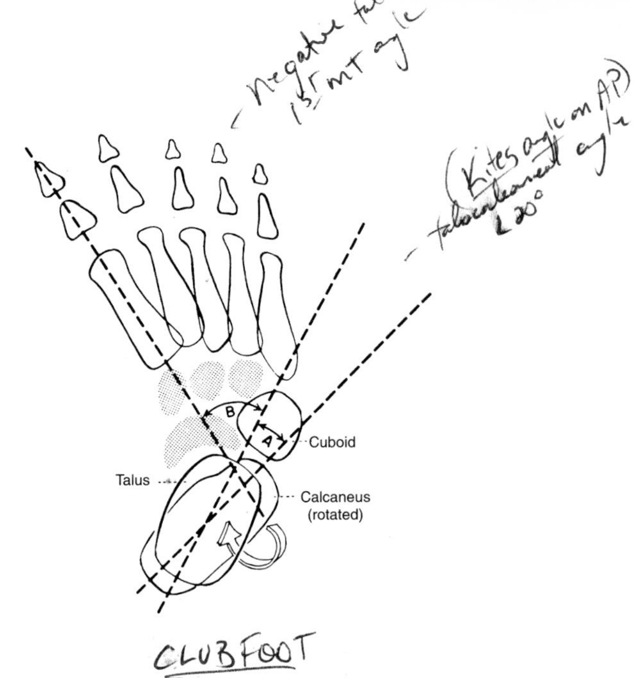

Figure 2–26. Radiographic evaluation of clubfeet. Note the "parallelism" of the talus and calcaneus with a talocalcaneal angle (*A*) of <20 degrees and negative talus–first metatarsal angle (*B*) on the clubfoot side. (From Simmons, G.W.: Analytical radiography of clubfeet. J. Bone Joint Surg. [Br.] 59:485–489, 1974.)

normally 0–20 degrees, a negative talus–first metatarsal angle is seen with clubfoot (Fig. 2–26). "*Parallelism*" of the calcaneus and talus is seen on both views. Only 10–15% of patients with true (rigid, structural) clubfoot respond to serial manipulation and casting. Nevertheless, 3 months of casting is the recommended therapy for children initially. Some cases can be fully corrected with serial casts, although many require corrective surgery. *Surgical soft-tissue release with tendon lengthening is favored in resistant feet, usually at 6–9 months.* The following structures are addressed.

Structure	Procedure
Achilles tendon	Z-lengthening
Calcaneal-fibular ligament	Release
Posterior talofibular ligament	Release
Posterior tibialis tendon	Z-lengthening
Flexor digitorum longus tendon	Z-lengthening
Superficial deltoid	Release
Flexor hallucis longus tendon	Z-lengthening
Tibiotalar, subtalar capsule	Complete release
Talonavicular tibionavicular (pseudo)	Release

The posterior tibial artery must be carefully protected. Often, the dorsalis pedis artery is insufficient. Casting for several months is usually required postoperatively. In older patients (3–10 years old), medial opening or lateral column shortening osteotomy or cuboidal decancellization is recommended. For children who present with refractory clubfoot late (8–10 years old), triple arthrodesis is the only procedure possible for eliminating associated pain and deformity. Triple arthrodesis is contraindicated in patients with insensate feet because it causes a rigid foot that may lead to ulceration. Talectomy may be a better procedure in these patients.

B. Forefoot Adduction (see Fig. 2–19)

1. Metatarsus Adductus (see Section XI: Lower Extremity Problems, Part B: Rotational Problems of the Lower Extremities)—*Adduction of the forefoot is commonly associated with DDH.* A simple clinical grading system has been described by Bleck, which is based on the heel bisector line (Fig. 2–27). Normally, the heel bisector should line up with the second/third toe web space. Four subtypes have been identified (Berg).

Type	Features
Simple MTA	MTA
Complex MTA	MTA + lateral shift of midfoot
Skew foot	MTA + valgus hindfoot
Complex skew foot	MTA, lateral shift, valgus hindfoot

If peroneal muscle stimulation corrects metatarsus adductus, it usually responds to stretching. Otherwise, manipulation and special off-the-shelf orthotics or serial casting may be required. *Surgical options in refractory cases (usually those with a medial skin crease) include abductor hallucis longus recession (for an atavistic first toe), medial capsular release with Evans' calcaneal osteotomy (lateral column shortening), or medial opening cuneiform and lateral closing cuboid osteotomies,* ±

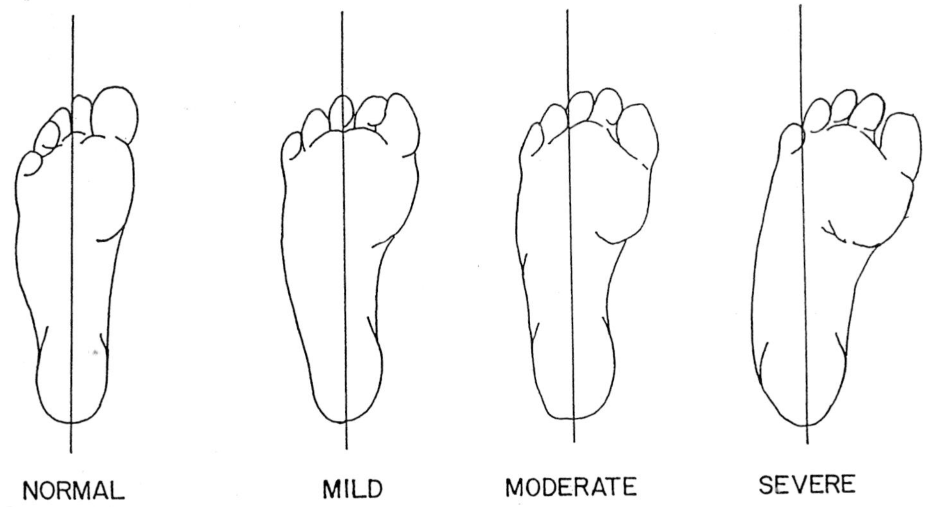

Figure 2–27. Classification of metatarsus adductus. (From Bleck, E.E.: Metatarsus adductus: Classification and relationship to all kinds of treatment. J. Pediatr. Orthop. 3:2–9, 1983.)

metatarsal osteotomies based on the severity of deformity.

2. Medial Deviation of the Talar Neck—Benign disorder of the foot that generally corrects spontaneously.
3. Serpentine ("Z") Foot (Complex Skew Foot)—Associated with residual *tarsometatarsal adductus, talonavicular lateral subluxation, and hindfoot valgus.* Nonoperative treatment is ineffective in correcting the deformity. Surgical treatment of this difficult problem is demanding and may include medial calcaneal sliding osteotomy (for hindfoot valgus), opening wedge cuboid osteotomy and closing wedge cuneiform osteotomy (to correct midfoot lateral subluxation), and metatarsal osteotomies (to correct forefoot adductus). Most cases can be treated symptomatically.

C. Pes Cavus—Cavus deformity of the foot (elevated longitudinal arch) due to fixed plantar flexion of the forefoot. There are four basic types of pes cavus.

Type	Forefoot	Hindfoot	Radiographs
Simple	Balanced	Neutral	Decreased talus-calcaneus angle
Cavorvarus	Plantar flexed	Varus	
Calcaneus	Fixed equinus	Calcaneus	
Equinocavus	Equinus	Equinus	

Pes cavus is commonly associated with neurologic disorders including *polio, CP, Friedreich's ataxia, and Charcot-Marie-Tooth disease.* Full neurologic work-up is mandatory. *Lateral block test (Coleman's)* assesses hindfoot flexibility of the cavovarus foot (a flexible hindfoot corrects to neutral with a lift placed under lateral aspect of foot). Nonoperative management is rarely successful. *Surgical options in supple deformities include plantar release, metatarsal osteotomies, and tendon transfers. If the lateral block test is abnormal (rigid deformity), a calcaneal osteotomy is done.* In the past, triple arthrodesis has been used for rigid deformity in mature patients; the use of calcaneal sliding osteotomy, with multiple metatarsal extension osteotomies, may offer an alternative to subtalar fusion procedures.

D. Pes Calcaneovalgus

1. Congenital Vertical Talus (Convex Pes Valgus)—*Irreducible dorsal dislocation of the navicular on the talus with a fixed equinous hindfoot deformity.* Clinically, the talar head is prominent medially, the sole is convex, the forefoot is abducted and in dorsiflexion, and the hindfoot is in equinovalgus (Persian slipper foot). Patients may demonstrate a "peg-leg" gait (awkward gait with limited forefoot push-off). It is a cause of a rigid flatfoot, *which can be isolated or can occur with chromosomal abnormalities, myeloarthropathies, or neurologic disorders.* **Plantar-flexion lateral radiographs** show that a line along the long axis of the talus passes below the first metatarsal-cuneiform axis (Meary's, tarsal–first metatarsal angle >20 degrees [normal 0–20 degrees dorsal tilt]) (Fig. 2–28). AP radiographs show a talocalcaneal angle of >40 degrees (normal 20–40 degrees). Differential diagnosis includes oblique talus (corrects with plantar flexion), tarsal coalition, and paralytic pes valgus. Three months of corrective casting (foot plantar flexed/inverted) or manipulative stretching is tried initially. *Surgery when the patient is 6–12 months old includes soft-tissue release/lengthening.* Talectomy may be required for resistant cases.
2. Oblique Talus—Talonavicular subluxation that reduces with plantar flexion of foot. Treatment is observation and sometimes a shoe insert University of California, Berke-

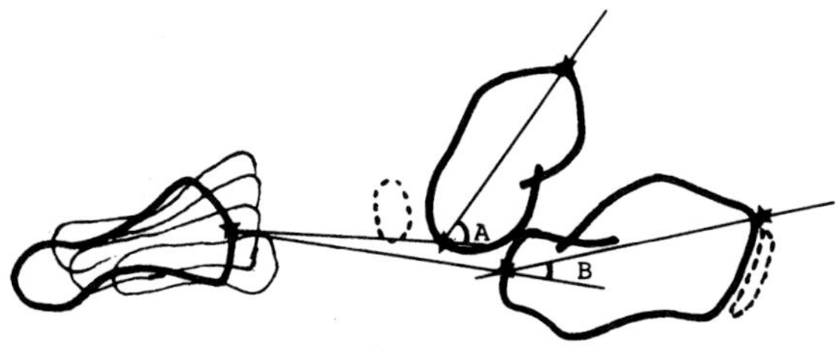

Figure 2–28. Plantar-flexed lateral radiographic features in congenital vertical talus. *A,* Talar axis–metatarsal base angle (normally 3 ± 6 degrees). *B,* Calcaneal axis–metatarsal base angle (normally −9 ± 5 degrees). Both angles are increased in congenital vertical talus. (From Hamanishi, C.: Congenital vertical talus. J. Pediatr. Orthop. 4:319, 1984.)

ley, Laboratory (UCBL). Some patients require pinning of the talonavicular joint in the reduced position and tendoachilles lengthening.

E. Tarsal Coalitions—A disorder of mesenchymal segmentation leading to *fusion of tarsal bones and rigid flatfoot. Most commonly occurs as a talocalcaneal or calcaneonavicular coalition and is the leading cause of peroneal spastic flatfoot.* Symptoms, which appear by age 10–12 years, include calf *pain due to peroneal spasticity, flatfoot, and limited subtalar motion.* Coalitions may be fibrous, cartilaginous, or osseous. *Calcaneonavicular coalition is the most common in children* and is seen on oblique radiographs of the foot (Sloman's). Lateral radiographs may demonstrate an elongated anterior process of the calcaneus *("anteater" sign).* Talocalcaneal coalitions may demonstrate talar beaking on the lateral view (does not denote degenerative joint disease) or an irregular middle facet on Harris' axial view. The best study for identifying and measuring the cross-sectional area of a talocalcaneal coalition is a CT scan. Initial treatment involves immobilization (casting) or orthotics. *Surgery is recommended in resistant cases to resect a symptomatic bar involving <50% of the middle facet in talocalcaneal coalitions. If >50% of the middle facet is involved, then subtalar arthrodesis is preferred. Calcaneonavicular bars usually do well with surgical resection.* Before a patient undergoes resection of a calcaneonavicular coalition, a CT scan should be done to rule out the possibility of a coexisting subtalar coalition. Observation is reasonable for asymptomatic bars in young children. Advanced cases, and cases that fail attempts at resection, often require triple arthrodesis.

F. Calcaneovalgus Foot—Newborn condition associated with intrauterine positioning. It is common in first-born children. Presents with a dorsiflexed hindfoot with eversion and abduction of the hindfoot that is passively correctable to neutral. *Treatment is passive stretching and observation.* Also seen with myelomeningocele at the L5 level due to muscular imbalance between foot dorsiflexors/everters (L4 and L5 roots) and plantar flexors/inverters (S1 and S2 roots).

G. Juvenile Bunions—Often are bilateral and familial. This disorder is less common and usually less severe than the adult form. May be associated with ligamentous laxity and a hypermobile first ray. Usually found in adolescent girls. Wide shoes and arch supports help early. Surgery is indicated in symptomatic patients with an intermetatarsal angle of >10 degrees (metatarsus primus varus) and a hallux valgus angle of >20 degrees. Metatarsus primus varus may require proximal metatarsal osteotomy and distal capsular reefing. Complications include overcorrection and hallux varus. **Recurrence is frequent (>50%),** especially when only soft-tissue procedures are performed. It is best to wait until maturity to reoperate.

H. Köhler's Disease—*Osteonecrosis of the tarsal navicular;* usually presents at about 5 years old. Pain is the typical presenting complaint. Radiographs show sclerosis of the navicular. Symptoms usually resolve spontaneously with decreased activity ± immobilization.

I. Flexible Pes Planus—Foot is flat only when standing and not with toe walking or foot hanging. This is frequently familial and almost always bilateral. Commonly associated with minor lower extremity rotational problems and ligamentous laxity. Symptoms, including aching midfoot or pretibial pain, can occur. Lateral radiographic findings mimic those of vertical talus, but a plantar-flexed lateral view demonstrates that a line along the long axis of the talus passes above the metatarsal-cuneiform axis. Treatment is observation only, with no special shoes. Sometimes, soft arch supports are helpful but not corrective. Thorough evaluation should be completed to rule out tight heel cords and decreased subtalar motion. UCBL heel cups are sometimes indicated for advanced cases with pain (symptomatic treatment only). Calcaneal osteotomy or select fusions may provide pain relief at the expense of inversion/eversion in adolescents with disabling pain refractory to every means of conservative treatment. The radiographic views in the chart may be helpful.

View	Assessment
Standing AP	Talar head coverage, talocalcaneal angle
Standing lateral	Calcaneal/talar equinus, talocalcaneal angle
Oblique	To rule out coalition

J. Habitual Toe Walker—Contracture of the Achilles tendon. Usually responds to serial casting; sometimes requires tendoachilles lengthening.

K. Accessory Navicular—Normal variant seen in up to 12% of the population. Commonly associated with flat feet. Symptoms usually include medial arch pain with overuse. Symptoms usually resolve with activity restriction and/or immobilization. External oblique radiographic views are often helpful for the diagnosis. Most cases resolve spontaneously. Occasionally, excision of the accessory bone is done, which can correct symptoms (but not flatfoot) in most patients.

L. Ball and Socket Ankle—Abnormal formation with a spherical talus (ball) and a cup-shaped tibiofibular articulation (socket). *It usually requires no treatment but should be recognized because of its high association with tarsal coalition (50%), absent lateral rays (50%), fibular deficiency, and leg-length discrepancies.*

M. Congenital Toe Disorders

1. Syndactyly—Fusion of the soft tissues (simple) and sometimes bone (complex) of the toes. Simple syndactyly usually does not require treatment; complex syndactyly is treated as it is in the hand.
2. Polydactyly (Extra Digits)—May be AD and usually involves the lateral ray in patients with a positive family history. Treatment includes ablation of the extra digit and any bony protrusion of the common metatarsal (typically, the border digit is excised, not the best formed digit). The procedure is usually done at age 9–12 months, but some rudimentary digits can be ligated in the newborn nursery.
3. Oligodactyly—Congenital absence of the toes. May be associated with more proximal agenesis (i.e., fibular hemimelia) and tarsal coalition. The disorder usually requires no treatment.
4. Atavistic Great Toe (Congenital Hallux Varus)—Great toe adduction deformity that is often associated with polydactyly. Must be differentiated from metatarsus adductus. Usually, the deformity occurs at the metatarsophalangeal joint and includes a short, thick first metatarsal and a firm band (abductor hallucis longus muscle) that may be responsible for the disorder. Surgery is sometimes required and includes release of the abductor hallucis longus muscle.
5. Overlapping Toe—The fifth toe overlaps the fourth (usually bilaterally) and may cause problems with footwear. Initial treatment includes passive stretching and "buddy" taping. Surgical options include tenotomy, dorsal capsulotomy, and syndactylization to the fourth toe (McFarland).
6. Underlapping Toe (Congenital Curly Toe)—Usually occurs at lateral three toes and is rarely symptomatic. Surgery (flexor tenotomies) is occasionally indicated.

Selected Bibliography

Embryology

Moore, K.L.: The Developing Human. Philadelphia, WB Saunders, 1982.

Bone Dysplasias

Bassett, G.S.: Lower extremity abnormalities in dwarfing conditions. Instr. Course Lect. 39:389–397, 1991.

Bassett, G.S.: Orthopedic aspects of skeletal dysplasias. Instr. Course Lect. 39:381–387, 1991.

Beals, R.K., and Rolfe, B.: Current concepts review: Vater association; a unifying concept of multiple anomalies. J. Bone Joint Surg. [Am.] 71:948–950, 1989.

Bethem, D., Winter, R.B., Lutter, L., et al.: Spinal disorders of dwarfism. J. Bone Joint Surg. [Am] 63:1412–1425, 1981.

Dawe, C., Wynne-Davies, R., and Fulford, G.E.: Clinical variation in dyschondrosteosis: A report on 13 individuals in 8 families. J. Bone Joint Surg. [Br.] 64:377–381, 1982.

Goldberg, M.J.: The Dysmorphic Child: An Orthopedic Perspective. New York, Raven Press, 1987.

Hecht, J.T., Horton, W.A., Reid, C.S., et al.: Growth of the foramen magnum in achondroplasia. Am. J. Med. Genet. 32:528–535, 1989.

Jones, K.L., and Robinson, L.K.: An approach to the child with structural defects. J. Pediatr. Orthop. 3:238–244, 1983.

Kopits, S.E.: Orthopedic complications of dwarfism. Clin. Orthop. 114:153–179, 1976.

McKusick, V.A.: Heritable Disorders of Connective Tissue, 4th ed. St. Louis, CV Mosby, 1972.

Rubin, P.: Dynamic Classification of Bone Dysplasias. Chicago, Year Book Medical Publishers, 1964.

Stanscur, V., Stanscur, R., and Maroteaux, P.: Pathogenic mechanisms in osteochondrodysplasias. J. Bone Joint Surg. [Am.] 66:817–836, 1984.

Swanson, A.B.: A classification for congenital limb malformation. J. Hand Surg. 1:8–22, 1976.

Chromosomal and Teratologic Disorders

Elliot, S., Morton, R.E., and Whitelaw, R.A.J.: Atlantoaxial instability and abnormalities of the odontoid in Down syndrome. Arch. Dis. Child 63:1484–1489, 1988.

Huang, T.J., Lubricky, J.P., and Hammerberg, K.W.: Scoliosis in Rhett syndrome. Orthop. Rev. 23:931–937, 1994.

Loder, R., Lee, C., and Richards, B.: Orthopedic aspects of Rhett syndrome: A multicenter review. J. Pediatr. Orthop. 9:557–562, 1989.

Pueschel, S.M., Herndon, J.H., Gelch, M.M., et al.: Symptomatic atlantoaxial subluxation in persons with Down syndrome. J. Pediatr. Orthop. 4:682–688, 1984.

Rees, D., Jones, M.W., Owen, R., et al.: Scoliosis surgery in the Prader-Willi syndrome. J. Bone Joint Surg. [Br.] 71:685–688, 1989.

Segal, L.S., Drummond, D.S., Zanott, R.M., et al.: Complications of posterior arthrodesis of the cervical spine in patients who have Down syndrome. J. Bone Joint Surg. [Am.] 73:1547–1554, 1991.

Smith, D.W.: Recognizable Pattern of Human Malformation, 2nd ed. Philadelphia, WB Saunders, 1983.

Hematopoietic Disorders

Diggs, L.W.: Bone and joint lesions in sickle-cell disease. Clin. Orthop. 52:119–143, 1967.

Gill, J.C., Thometz, J.C., and Scott, J.P.: Musculoskeletal Problems in Hemophilia in the Child and Adult. New York, Raven Press, 1989.

Triantafylluo, S., Hanks, G., Handal, J.A., et al.: Open and arthroscopic synovectomy in hemophilic arthropathy of the knee. Clin. Orthop. 283:196–204, 1992.

Metabolic Disease/Arthritides

Albright, J.A., and Miller, E.A.: Osteogenesis imperfecta [editorial comment]. Clin. Orthop. 159:2, 1981.

Birch, J.G., and Herring, J.A.: Spinal deformity in Marfan syndrome. J. Pediatr. Orthop. 7:546–552, 1987.

Certner, J.M., and Root, L.: Osteogenesis imperfecta. Orthop. Clin. North Am. 21:151–162, 1990.

Gamble, J.G., Strudwick, W.J., Rinsky, L.A., et al.: Complications of intramedullary rods in osteogenesis imperfecta: Bailey-Dubow rods versus nonelongating rods. J. Pediatr. Orthop. 8:645–649, 1989.

Hensinger, R.N., DeVito, P.D., and Ragsdale, C.G.: Changes in the cervical spine in juvenile rheumatoid arthritis. J. Bone Joint Surg. [Am.] 68:189–199, 1986.

Mankin, H.J.: Rickets, osteomalacia and renal osteodystrophy: An update. Orthop. Clin. North Am. 21:81–96, 1990.

Robelo, I., Peredra, D.A., Silva, L., et al.: Effects of synthetic salmon calcitonin therapy in children with osteogenesis imperfecta. J. Int. Med. Res. 17:401–405, 1989.

Schaller, J.G.: Chronic arthritis in children: Juvenile rheumatoid arthritis. Clin. Orthop. 182:79–89, 1984.

Shapiro, F.: Consequences of an osteogenesis imperfecta diagnosis for survival and ambulation. J. Pediatr. Orthop. 5:456–462, 1985.

Sillence, D.O.: Osteogenesis imperfecta: An expanding panorama of variance. Clin. Orthop. 159:11, 1981.

Sofield, H.A., and Miller, E.A.: Fragmentation realignment and intramedullary rod fixation of deformities of the long bones in children. J. Bone Joint Surg. [Am.] 41:1371, 1959.

Birth Injuries

Canale, S.T., Griffin, T.W., and Hubbard, C.N.: Congenital muscular torticollis: A long-term follow-up. J. Bone Joint Surg. [Am.] 64:810–816, 1982.

Davids, J.R., Wenger, D.R., and Mubarak, S.J.: Congenital muscular torticollis: Sequelae of intrauterine or perinatal compartment syndrome. J. Pediatr. Orthop. 13:141–147, 1993.

Gilbert, A., Brockman, R., and Carlioz, H.: Surgical treatment of brachial plexus birth palsy. Clin. Orthop. 264:39–47, 1991.

Hentze, V.R., and Meyer, R.D.: Brachial plexus microsurgery in children. Microsurgery 12:175–185, 1991.

Jahnke, A.H., Bovill, D.F., McCarroll, H.R., et al.: Persistent brachial plexus birth palsies. J. Pediatr. Orthop. 11:533–537, 1991.

Quinlan, W.R., Brady, P.G., and Regan, B.F.: Congenital pseudarthrosis of the clavicle. Acta Orthop. Scand. 51:489–492, 1980.

Cerebral Palsy

Albright, A.L., Barron, W.B., Fasick, M.P., et al.: Continuous intrathecal baclofen infusion for spasticity of cerebral origin. J.A.M.A. 270:2475–2477, 1993.

Barnes, M.J., and Herring, J.A.: Combined split anterior tibial-tendon transfer and intramuscular lengthening of the posterior tibial tendon. J. Bone Joint Surg. [Am.] 73:734–738, 1991.

Bleck, E.E.: Current concepts review: Management of the lower extremities in children who have cerebral palsy. J. Bone Joint Surg. [Am.] 72:140, 1990.

Bleck, E.E.: Orthopedic Management of Cerebral Palsy. Philadelphia, JB Lippincott, 1987.

Coleman, S.S., and Chestnut, W.J.: A simple test for hindfoot flexibility in the cavovarus foot. Clin. Orthop. 123:60–62, 1977.

Cosgrove, A.P., and Graham, H.K.: Botulinum toxin-A prevents the development of contractures in the hereditary spastic mouse. Dev. Med. Child Neurol. 36:379–385, 1994.

Elmer, E.B., Wenger, D.R., Mubarak, S.J., et al.: Proximal hamstring lengthening in the sitting cerebral palsy patient. J. Pediatr. Orthop. 12:329–336, 1992.

Ferguson, R.L., and Allen, B.L.: Considerations in the treatment of cerebral palsy patients with spinal deformities. Orthop. Clin. North Am. 19:419–425, 1988.

Gage, J.R.: Gait analysis: An essential tool in the treatment of cerebral palsy. Clin. Orthop. 288:126–134, 1993.

Gage, J.R.: The clinical use of kinetics for evaluation of pathologic gait in cerebral palsy. J. Bone Joint Surg. [Am.] 76:622–631, 1994.

Koman, L.A., Mooney, J.F. Goodman, A.: Management of valgus hindfoot deformity in pediatric cerebral palsy patients by medial displacement osteotomy. J. Pediatr. Orthop. 13:180–183, 1993.

Koman, L.A., Mooney, J.F., Smith, B.P., et al.: Management of spasticity in cerebral palsy with botulinum-A toxin: Report of preliminary, randomized, double-blind trial. J. Pediatr. Orthop. 14:299–303, 1994.

Mubarak, S.J., Valencia, F.G., and Wenger, D.R.: One stage correction of the spastic dislocated hip. J. Bone Joint Surg. [Am.] 74:1347–1357, 1994.

Ounpuu, S., Muik, E., Davis, R.B., et al.: Rectus femoris surgery in children with cerebral palsy. Part II. A comparison between the effect of transfer and release of the distal rectus femoris on knee motion. J. Pediatr. Orthop. 13:331–335, 1993.

Rang, M., Silver, R., de la Garza, Jr., et al.: Cerebral palsy. In Lovell, R., and Winter, R., eds: Pediatric Orthopedics, 2nd ed. Philadelphia, JB Lippincott, 1986.

Rang, M., and Wright, J.: What have 30 years of medical progress done for cerebral palsy? Clin. Orthop. 247:55–60, 1989.

Sutherland, D.H., and Davids, J.R.: Common gait abnormalities of the knee in cerebral palsy. Clin. Orthop. 288:139–147, 1993.

Neuromuscular Disorders

Allen, B.L., Jr., and Ferguson, R.L.: The Galveston technique of pelvic fixation with Luque-rod instrumentation of the spine. Spine 9:388–394, 1984.

Beaty, J.H., and Canale, S.T.: Current concepts review: Orthopedic aspects of myelomeningocele. J. Bone Joint Surg. [Am.] 72:626–630, 1990.

Carlson, W.O., Speck, G.J., Vicari, V., et al.: Arthrogryposis multiplex congenita: A long-term follow-up study. Clin. Orthop. 194:115–123, 1985.

Carroll, N.J.: Assessment and management of the lower extremity in myelodysplasia. Orthop. Clin. North Am. 18:709–724, 1987.

Diaz, L.S.: Hip deformities in myelomeningocele. Instr. Course Lect. 40:281–286, 1991.

Drennan, J.C.: Foot deformities in myelomeningocele. Instr. Course Lect. 40:287–291, 1991.

Drummond, D.S., Moreau, M., and Cruess, R.L.: The results and complications of surgery for the paralytic hip and spine in myelomeningocele. J. Bone Joint Surg. [Br.] 62:49–53, 1980.

Emans, J.B.: Current concepts review: Allergy to latex in patients who have myelodysplasia. J. Bone Joint Surg. [Am.] 74:1103–1109, 1992.

Evans, G.A., Drennan, J.C., and Russman, B.S.: Functional classification and orthopedic management of spinal muscular atrophy. J. Bone Joint Surg. [Br.] 63:516–522, 1981.

Hoffer, M.M., Feiwell, E., Perry, R., et al.: Functional ambulation in patients with myelomeningocele. J. Bone Joint Surg. [Am.] 55:137–148, 1973.

Lindseth, R.E.: Spine deformity in myelomeningocele. Instr. Course Lect. 40:273–279, 1991.

Mazur, J.M., Shurtleff, D., Menelaus, M., et al.: Orthopedic management of high-level spina bifida: Early walking compared with early use of a wheelchair. J. Bone Joint Surg. [Am.] 71:56, 1989.

Mendell, J.R., and Sahenk, Z.: Recent advances in diagnosis and classification of Charcot-Marie-Tooth disease. Curr. Opin. Orthop. 4:39–45, 1993.

Shapiro, F., and Bresnan, M.J.: Orthopedic management of childhood neuromuscular disease. Part II. Peripheral neuropathies, Friedreich's ataxia, and arthrogryposis multiplex congenita. J. Bone Joint Surg. [Am.] 64:949–953, 1982.

Shapiro, F., and Specht, L.: Current concepts review: The diagnosis and orthopedic management of inherited muscular disorders of childhood. J. Bone Joint Surg. [Am] 75:439–454, 1993.

Sodergard, J., and Ryoppy, S.: Foot deformities in arthrogryposis multiplex congenita. J. Pediatr. Orthop. 14:768–772, 1994.

Thompson, G.H.: Arthrogryposis multiplex congenita [editorial]. Clin. Orthop. 194:2–3, 1985.

Pediatric Spine

Ali, M.S., and Hooper, G.: Congenital pseudarthrosis of the ulna due to neurofibromatosis. J. Bone Joint Surg. [Br.] 64:600–602, 1982.

Apel, D.M., Marrero, G., King, J., et al.: Avoiding paraplegia during anterior spinal surgery: The role of somatosensory evoked potentials monitoring with temporary occlusion of segmental spinal arteries. Spine 16:S365–S370, 1991.

Bellah, R.D., Summerville, D.A., Treves, S.T., et al.: Low-back pain in adolescent athletes: Detection of stress injury to the pars interarticularis with SPECT. Radiology 180:509–512, 1991.

Bollini, G., Bergion, M., Labriet, C., et al.: Hemivertebrae excision and fusion in children aged less than 5 years. J. Pediatr. Orthop. 1 (part B):95–101, 1993.

Bradford, D.S., Ahmed, K.B., Moe, J.H., et al.: The surgical management of patients with Scheuerman's disease: A review of twenty-four cases managed by combined anterior and posterior spine fusion. J. Bone Joint Surg. [Am.] 62:705–712, 1980.

Bradford, D.S., and Hensinger, R.M., eds.: The Pediatric Spine. New York, Thieme-Stratton, 1985.
Bradford, D.S., Lonstein, J.E., Ogilvie, J.B., et al., eds: Moe's Textbook of Scoliosis and Other Spinal Deformities, 2nd ed. Philadelphia, WB Saunders, 1987.
Bridwell, K.H., McAllister, J.W., Betz, R.R., et al.: Coronal decompensation produced by Cotrel-Dubousset "derotation" maneuver for idiopathic right thoracic scoliosis. Spine 16:769–777, 1991.
Carr, W.A., Moe, J.H., Winter, R.B., et al.: Treatment of idiopathic scoliosis in the Milwaukee brace. J. Bone Joint Surg. [Am.] 62:599–612, 1980.
Crawford, A.H., Jr., and Bagamery, M.: Osseous manifestations of neurofibromatosis in childhood. J. Pediatr. Orthop. 6:72–88, 1986.
Denis, F.: Cotrel-Dubousset instrumentation in the treatment of idiopathic scoliosis. Orthop. Clin. North Am. 19:291–311, 1988.
Dickson, J.H., Erwin, W.D., and Rossi, D.: Harrington instrumentation and arthrodesis for idiopathic scoliosis: A twenty-one year follow-up. J. Bone Joint Surg. [Am.] 72:678–683, 1990.
Dimeglio, A.: Growth of the spine before age 5 years. J. Pediatr. Orthop. 1 (part B):102–107, 1993.
Engler, G.L.: Preoperative and intraoperative considerations in adolescent idiopathic scoliosis. Instr. Course Lect. 38:137–141, 1989.
Fielding, J.W., and Hawkins, R.J.: Atlantoaxial rotatory fixation. J. Bone Joint Surg. [Am.] 59:37–44, 1977.
Fielding, J.W., Hensinger, R.N., and Hawkins, R.J.: Os odontoideum. J. Bone Joint Surg. [Am.] 62:376–383, 1980.
Fitch, R.D., Turi, M., Bowman, B.E., et al.: Comparison of Cotrel-Dubousset and Harrington rod instrumentation in idiopathic scoliosis. J. Pediatr. Orthop. 10:44–47, 1990.
Keller, R.B.: Nonoperative treatment of adolescent idiopathic scoliosis. Instr. Course Lect. 38:129–135, 1989.
King, H.A., Moe, J.H., Bradford, D.S., et al.: The selection of fusion levels in thoracic idiopathic scoliosis. J. Bone Joint Surg. [Am.] 65:1302–1313, 1983.
Koop, S.E., Winter, R.B., and Lonstein, J.E.: The surgical treatment of instability of the upper part of the cervical spine in children and adolescents. J. Bone Joint Surg. [Am.] 66:403–411, 1984.
Kostuik, J.P.: Current concepts review: Operative treatment of idiopathic scoliosis. J. Bone Joint Surg. [Am.] 72:1108–1112, 1990.
Lenke, L.G., Bridwell, K.H., Baldus, C., et al.: Cotrel-Dubousset instrumentation for idiopathic scoliosis. J. Bone Joint Surg. [Am.] 74:1056–1068, 1992.
Lonstein, J.E.: Adolescent idiopathic scoliosis: Screening and diagnosis. Instr. Course Lect. 38:105–113, 1989.
Lonstein, J.E., Bjorklunk, S., Wanninger, M.H., et al.: Voluntary school screening for scoliosis in Minnesota. J. Bone Joint Surg. [Am.] 64:481–488, 1982.
Lonstein, J.E., and Carlson, J.M.: Prognostication in idiopathic scoliosis. Orthop. Trans. 5:22, 1981.
Lonstein, J.E., and Carlson, J.M.: The prediction of curve progression in untreated idiopathic scoliosis during growth. J. Bone Joint Surg. [Am.] 66:1061–1071, 1984.
Lowe, T.G.: Current concepts review: Scheuermann's disease. J. Bone Joint Surg. [Am.] 72:940–945, 1990.
Luque, E.R.: Segmental spinal instrumentation for correction of scoliosis. Clin. Orthop. 163:192–198, 1982.
McFarland, B.: Congenital deformity of the spine and limbs. In Modern Trends in Orthopedics. New York, PB Hoeber, 1950.
McMaster, M.J., and Ohtsuka, K.: The natural history of congenital scoliosis: A study of two hundred and fifty-one patients. J. Bone Joint Surg. [Am.] 64:1128–1137, 1982.
Mehta, M.H.: The rib-vertebra angle in the early diagnosis between resolving and progressive infantile scoliosis. J. Bone Joint Surg. [Br.] 54:230–243, 1972.
Mielke, C.H., Lonstein, J.E., Denis, F., et al.: Surgical treatment of adolescent idiopathic scoliosis: A comparative analysis. J. Bone Joint Surg. [Am.] 71:1170–1177, 1989.
Miller, J.A.A., Nachemson, A.L., and Schultz, A.B.: Effectiveness of braces in mild idiopathic scoliosis. Spine 9:632–635, 1984.
Montgomery, S., and Hall, J.: Congenital kyphosis: Surgical treatment at Boston Children's Hospital. Orthop. Trans. 5:25, 1981.
Pang, D., and Wilberger, J.E., Jr.: Spinal cord injury without radiographic abnormalities in children. J. Neurosurg. 57:114–129, 1982.
Ring, D., and Wenger, D.R.: Magnetic resonance imaging scans in discitis: Sequential studies in a child who needed operative drainage; a case report. J. Bone Joint Surg. [Am.] 76:596–601, 1994.
Schrock, R.D.: Congenital abnormalities at the cervicothoracic level. Inst. Course Lect. 6:1949.
Scoles, P.V., and Quinn, T.P.: Intervertebral discitis in children and adolescents. Clin. Orthop. 162:31–36, 1982.
Smith, A.D., Koreska, J., and Moseley, C.F.: Progressive scoliosis in Duchenne muscular dystrophy. J. Bone Joint Surg. [Am.] 71:1066–1074, 1989.
Sorenson, K.H.: Scheuermann's Juvenile Kyphosis. Copenhagen, Munksgaard, 1964.
Tolo, V.T.: Surgical treatment of adolescent idiopathic scoliosis. Instr. Course Lect. 38:143–156, 1989.
Tredwell, S.J., Newman, D.E., and Lockitch, G.: Instability of the upper cervical spine in Down syndrome. J. Pediatr. Orthop. 10:602–606, 1990.
Weinstein, S.L.: Adolescent idiopathic scoliosis: Prevalence and natural history. Instr. Course Lect. 38:115–128, 1989.
Weinstein, S.L.: Idiopathic scoliosis: Natural history. Spine 11:780–783, 1986.
Weinstein, S.L., and Ponseti, I.V.: Curve progression in idiopathic scoliosis. J. Bone Joint Surg. [Am.] 65:447–455, 1983.
Winter, R.B.: Congenital spine deformity: "What's the latest and what's the best?" Spine 14:1406–1409, 1989.
Winter, R.B., and Lonstein, J.E.: Adult idiopathic scoliosis treated with Luque or Harrington rods and sublaminar wiring. J. Bone Joint Surg. [Am.] 71:1308–1313, 1989.
Winter, R.B., Lonstein, J.E., Drogt, J., et al.: The effectiveness of bracing in the nonoperative treatment of idiopathic scoliosis. Spine 11:790–791, 1986.
Winter, R.B., Moe, J.H., Bradford, D.S., et al.: Spine deformity in neurofibromatosis: A review of 102 cases. J. Bone Joint Surg. [Am.] 61:677–694, 1979.
Winter, R.B., Moe, J.H., and Lonstein, J.E.: Posterior spinal arthrodesis for congenital scoliosis: An analysis of the cases of two hundred and ninty patients, five to nineteen years old. J. Bone Joint Surg. [Am.] 66:1188–1197, 1984.
Winter, R.B., Moe, J.H., and Lonstein, J.E.: The incidence of Klippel-Feil syndrome in patients with congenital scoliosis and kyphosis. Spine 9:363–366, 1984.
Winter, R.B., Moe, J.H., and Lonstein, J.E.: The surgical treatment of congenital kyphosis: A review of 94 patients age 5 years or older, with 2 years or more follow-up in 77 patients. Spine 10:224–231, 1985.

Upper Extremity Problems

Carson, W.G., Lovell, W.W., and Whitesides, T.E., Jr.: Congenital elevation of the scapula: Surgical correction by the Woodward procedure. J. Bone Joint Surg. [Am.] 62:1199–1207, 1981.
Fitch, R.D.: Introduction to pediatric orthopedics. In Sabiston, D.C., Jr., ed.: Sabiston's Essentials of Surgery. Philadelphia, WB Saunders, 1987.
Green, W.T.: The surgical correction of congenital elevation of the scapula (Sprengel's deformity). J. Bone Joint Surg. [Am.] 149, 1957.
Liebovic, S.J., Erlich, M.G., and Zaleske, D.J.: Sprengel deformity. J. Bone Joint Surg. [Am.] 72:192–197, 1990.
Woodward, J.W.: Congenital elevation of the scapula: Correction by release and transplantation of muscle origins. J. Bone Joint Surg. [Am.] 43:219–228, 1961.

Lower Extremity Problems

Berg, E.F.: A reappraisal of metatarsus adductus and skewfoot. J. Bone Joint Surg. [Am.] 68:1185–1196, 1986.
Bleck, E.E.: Metatarsus adductus: Classification and relationship to outcomes of treatment. J. Pediatr. Orthop. 3:2–9, 1983.
Crawford, A.H., and Gabriel, K.R.: Foot and ankle problems. Orthop. Clin. North Am. 18:649–666, 1987.
Green, W.B.: Metatarsus adductus and skewfoot. Instr. Course Lect. 43:161–178, 1994.
Kling, T.F., and Hensinger, R.N.: Angular and torsional deformities of the lower limbs in children. Clin. Orthop. 176:136–147, 1983.
Staheli, L.T., Clawson, D.K., and Hubbard, D.D.: Medial femoral torsion: Experience with operative treatment. Clin. Orthop. 146:222–225, 1980.
Staheli, L.T., Corbett, M., Wyss, C., et al.: Lower extremity rotational problems in children: Normal values to guide management. J. Bone Joint Surg. [Am.] 67:39–47, 1985.

Hip and Femur

Abraham, E., Garst, J., and Barmada, R.: Treatment of moderate-to-severe slipped capital femoral epiphysis with extracapsular base-of-neck osteotomy. J. Pediatr. Orthop. 13:924–302, 1993.

Beaty, J.H.: Legg-Calvé-Perthes disease: Diagnostic and prognostic techniques. Instr. Course Lect. 38:291–296, 1989.

Berkeley, M.E., Dickson, J.H., Cain, T.E., et al.: Surgical therapy for congenital dislocation of the hip in patients who are 12 to 36 months old. J. Bone Joint Surg. [Am.] 66:412–420, 1984.

Bialik, V., Fishman, J., Katzir, J., et al.: Clinical assessment of hip instability in the newborn by an orthopedic surgeon and a pediatrician. J. Pediatr. Orthop. 6:703–705, 1986.

Bialik, V., Reuveni, A., Pery, M., et al.: Ultrasonography in developmental displacement of the hip: A critical analysis of our results. J. Pediatr. Orthop. 9:154–156, 1989.

Blanco, J.S., Taylor, B., and Johnston, C.E., II: Comparison of single pin vs. multiple pin fixation in treatment of slipped capital femoral epiphysis. J. Pediatr. Orthop. 12:384–389, 1992.

Boal, D.K., and Schwenkter, E.P.: The infant hip: Assessment with real-time ultrasound. Radiology 157:667–672, 1985.

Boyer, D.W., Mickelson, M.R., and Ponseti, I.V.: Slipped capital femoral epiphysis: Long-term follow-up study of 121 patients. J. Bone Joint Surg. [Am.] 63:85–95, 1981.

Canale, S.T.: Problems and complications of slipped capital femoral epiphysis. Instr. Course Lect. 38:281–290, 1989.

Canale, S.T., Harkness, R.M., Thomas, P.A., et al.: Does aspiration of bones and joints affect results of later bone scanning? J. Pediatr. Orthop. 5:23–26, 1985.

Castelein, R.M., and Sauter, A.J.M.: Ultrasound screening for congenital dysplasia of the hip in newborns: Its value. J. Pediatr. Orthop. 8:666–670, 1988.

Catterall, A.: Legg-Calvé-Perthes disease. Instr. Course Lect. 38:297–303, 1989.

Catterall, A.: Legg-Calvé-Perthes syndrome. Clin. Orthop. 158:41–52, 1981.

Chiari, K.: Medial displacement osteotomy of the pelvis. Clin. Orthop. 98:55–71, 1974.

Christensen, F., Soballe, K., Ejsted, R., et al.: The Catterall classification of Perthes disease: An assessment of reliability. J. Bone Joint Surg. [Br.] 68:614–615, 1986.

Clarke, N.M.P., Clegg, J., and Al-Chalabi, A.N.: Ultrasound screening of hips at risk for CDH: Failure to reduce the incidence of late cases. J. Bone Joint Surg. [Br.] 71:9–12, 1989.

Crawford, A.H.: The role of osteotomy in the treatment of slipped capital femoral epiphysis. Instr. Course Lect. 38:273–280, 1989.

Daoud, A., and Saighi-Bouaouina, A.: Treatment of sequestra, pseudarthroses, and defects in the long bones of children who have chronic hematogenous osteomyelitis. J. Bone Joint Surg. [Am.] 71:1448–1468, 1989.

Epps, C.H., Jr.: Current concepts review: Proximal femoral focal deficiency. J. Bone Joint Surg. [Am.] 65:867–870, 1983.

Fabry, F., and Meire, E.: Septic arthritis of the hip in children: Poor results after late and inadequate treatment. J. Pediatr. Orthop. 3:461–466, 1983.

Faciszewski, T., Coleman, S.S., and Biddolpf, G.: Triple innominate osteotomy for acetabular dysplasia. J. Pediatr. Orthop. 13:426–430, 1993.

Faciszewski, T., Keifer, G., and Coleman, S.S.: Pemberton osteotomy for residual acetabular dysplasia in children who have congenital dislocation of the hip. J. Bone Joint Surg. [Am.] 5:643–649, 1993.

Fackler, C.D.: Nonsurgical treatment of Legg-Calvé-Perthes disease. Instr. Course Lect. 38:305–308, 1989.

Gage, J.R., and Winter, R.B.: Avascular necrosis of the capital femoral epiphysis as a complication of closed reduction of congenital dislocation of the hip: A critical review of twenty years' experience at Gillette Children's Hospital. J. Bone Joint Surg. [Am.] 54:373–388, 1972.

Galpin, R.D., Roach, J.W., Wenger, D.R., et al.: One-stage treatment of congenital dislocation of the hip in older children, including femoral shortening. J. Bone Joint Surg. [Am.] 71:734–741, 1989.

Green, N.E., and Edwards, K.: Bone and joint infections in children. Orthop. Clin. North Am. 18:555–576, 1987.

Harke, H.T., and Grissom, L.E.: Performing dynamic ultrasonography of the infant hip. A.J.R. Am. J. Roentgenol. 155:837–844, 1990.

Harris, I.E., Dickens, R., and Menelaus, M.B.: Use of the Pavlik harness for hip displacements: When to abandon treatment. Clin. Orthop. 281:29–33, 1992.

Herndon, W.A., Knaur, S., Sullivan, J.A., et al.: Management of septic arthritis in children. J. Pediatr. Orthop. 6:576–578, 1986.

Herring, J.A.: Current concepts review: The treatment of Legg-Calvé-Perthes disease. J. Bone Joint Surg. [Am.] 76:448–457, 1994.

Herring, J.A., Neustadt, J.B., Williams, J.J., et al.: The lateral pillar classification of Legg-Calvé-Perthes disease. J. Pediatr. Orthop. 12:143–150, 1992.

Iwasaki, K.: Treatment of congenital dislocation of the hip by the Pavlik harness: Mechanisms of reduction and usage. J. Bone Joint Surg. [Am.] 65:760–767, 1983.

Jackson, M.A., and Nelson, J.D.: Etiology and medical management of acute suppurative bone and joint infections in pediatric patients. J. Pediatr. Orthop. 2:313–323, 1982.

Kalamchi, A., and McFarland, R., III: The Pavlik harness: Results in patients over three months of age. J. Pediatr. Orthop. 2:3–8, 1982.

Kershaw, C.J., Ware, H.E., Pattinson, R., et al.: Revision of failed open reduction of congenital dislocated hip. J. Bone Joint Surg. [Br.] 75:744–749, 1993.

Koval, K.J., Lehman, W.B., Rose, D., et al.: Treatment of slipped capital femoral epiphysis with a cannulated screw technique. J. Bone Joint Surg. [Am.] 71:1370–1377, 1989.

Lewin, J.S., Rosenfield, N.H., Hoffer, P.B., et al.: Acute osteomyelitis in children: Combined Tc-99 and gallium-67 imaging. Radiology 158:795–804, 1986.

Loder, R.T., Arbor, A., and Richards, B.S.: Acute slipped capital femoral epiphysis: The importance of physeal stability. J. Bone Joint Surg. [Am.] 75:1134–1140, 1993.

Mausen, J.P.G.M., Rozing, P.M., and Obermann, W.R.: Intertrochanteric corrective osteotomy in slipped capital femoral epiphysis: A long-term follow-up study of 26 patients. Clin. Orthop. 259:100–109, 1990.

McAndrew, M.P., and Weinstein, S.L.: A long-term follow-up of Legg-Calvé-Perthes disease. J. Bone Joint Surg. [Am.] 66:860–869, 1984.

Morrissey, R.T., ed.: Lovell and Winter's Pediatric Orthopedics, 3rd ed. Philadelphia, JB Lippincott, 1990.

Morrissey, R.T.: Principles of in situ fixation in chronic slipped capital epiphysis. Instr. Course Lect. 38:257–262, 1989.

Moseley, C.F.: Assessment and prediction in leg length discrepancy. Instr. Course Lect. 38:325–330, 1989.

Mubarak, S.J., Beck, L.R., and Sutherland, D.H.: Home traction in the management of congenital dislocation of the hips. J. Pediatr. Orthop. 6:721–723, 1986.

Mubarak, S.J., Garfin, S., Vance, R., et al.: Pitfalls in the use of the Pavlik harness for treatment of congenital dysplasia, subluxation, and dislocation of the hip. J. Bone Joint Surg. [Am.] 63:1239–1248, 1981.

Norlin, R., Hammerby, S., and Tkaczuk, H.: The natural history of Perthes disease. Int. Orthop. 15:13–16, 1991.

Paley, D.: Current techniques of limb lengthening. J. Pediatr. Orthop. 8:73–92, 1988.

Pizzutillo, P.D.: Developmental dysplasia of the hip. Instr. Course Lect. 43:179–184, 1994.

Price, C.T.: Metaphyseal and physeal lengthening. Instr. Course Lect. 38:331–336, 1989.

Ramsey, P.L., Lasser, S., and MacEwen, G.D.: Congenital dislocation of the hip: Use of the Pavlik harness in the child during the first 6 months of life. J. Bone Joint Surg. [Am.] 58:1000–1004, 1976.

Rennie, A.M.: The inheritance of slipped upper femoral epiphysis. J. Bone Joint Surg. [Br.] 64:180–184, 1982.

Richardson, E.G., and Rambach, B.E.: Proximal femoral focal deficiency: A clinical appraisal. South. Med. J. 72:166–173, 1979.

Ring, D., and Wenger, D.R.: Magnetic resonance imaging scans in discitis. J. Bone Joint Surg. [Am.] 76:596–601, 1994.

Ritterbusch, J.F., Shantharam, S.S., and Gelinas, C.: Comparison of lateral pillar classification and Catterall classification of Legg-Calvé-Perthes disease. J. Pediatr. Orthop. 13:200–202, 1993.

Salter, R.B., Hansson, G., and Thompson, G.H.: Innominate osteotomy in the management of residual congenital subluxation of the hip in young adults. Clin. Orthop. 182:53–68, 1984.

Simons, G.W.: A comparative evaluation of the current methods for open reduction of the congenitally displaced hip. Orthop. Clin. North Am. 11:161–181, 1980.

Southwick, W.O.: Compression fixation after biplane intertrochanteric

osteotomy for slipped capital femoral epiphysis. J. Bone Joint Surg. [Am.] 55:1218–1224, 1973.
Staheli, L.T., and Chew, D.E.: Slotted acetabular augmentation in childhood and adolescence. J. Pediatr. Orthop. 12:569–580, 1992.
Staheli, L.T., Coleman, S.S., Hensinger, R.N., et al.: Congenital hip dysplasia. Instr. Course Lect. 33:350–363, 1984.
Steele, H.H.: Triple osteotomy of the innominate bone. J. Bone Joint Surg. [Am.] 55:343–350, 1973.
Stromqvist, B., and Sunden, G.: CDH diagnosed at 2 to 12 months of age. J. Pediatr. Orthop. 9:208–212, 1989.
Sutherland, D.H., and Greenfield, R.: Double innominate osteotomy. J. Bone Joint Surg. [Am.] 59:1082–1091, 1977.
Suzuki, S., and Yamamuro, T.: Avascular necrosis in patients treated with Pavlik harness for congenital dislocation of the hip. J. Bone Joint Surg. [Am.] 72:1048–1055, 1990.
Tachdjian, M.O.: Pediatric Orthopedics, 2nd ed. Philadelphia, WB Saunders, 1990.
Tetzlaff, T.R., McCracken, G.H., Jr., and Nelson, J.D.: Oral antibiotic therapy for skeletal infections in children. II. Therapy of osteomyelitis and arthritis. J. Pediatr. 92:485–490, 1978.
Tonnis, D., Storch, K., and Ulbrich, H.: Results of newborn screening for CDH with and without sonography and correlation of risk factors. J. Pediatr. Orthop. 10:145–152, 1990.
Tredwell, S.J., and Davis, L.A.: Prospective study of congenital dislocation of the hip. J. Pediatr. Orthop. 9:386–390, 1989.
Viere, R.G., Birch, J.F., Herring, J.A., et al.: Use of the Pavlik harness in congenital dislocation of the hip: An analysis of failures of treatment. J. Bone Joint Surg. [Am.] 72:238–244, 1990.
Weiner, D.S.: Bone graft epiphysiodesis in the treatment of slipped capital femoral epiphysis. Instr. Course Lect. 38:263–272, 1989.
Wenger, D.R.: Congenital hip dislocation. Instr. Course Lect. 38:343–354, 1989.
Zionts, L.E., and MacEwen, G.D.: Treatment of congenital dislocation of the hip in children between the ages of one and three years. J. Bone Joint Surg. [Am.] 68:829–846, 1986.

Knee and Leg

Brown, F.W., and Pohnert, W.H.: Construction of a knee joint in meromelia tibia (congenital absence of the tibia): A 15-year follow-up study. J. Bone Joint Surg. [Am.] 54:1333, 1972.
Dickhaut, S.C., and DeLee, J.C.: The discoid lateral meniscus syndrome. J. Bone Joint Surg. [Am.] 64:1068–1073, 1982.
Guhl, J.: Osteochondritis dissecans. In Shahriaree, H., ed.: O'Conner's Textbook of Arthroscopic Surgery. Philadelphia, JB Lippincott, 1984.
Hayashi, L.K., Yamaga, H., Ida, K., et al.: Arthroscopic meniscectomy for discoid lateral meniscus in children. J. Bone Joint Surg. [Am.] 70:1495–1499, 1988.
Insall, J.: Current concept review: Patellar pain. J. Bone Joint Surg. [Am.] 64:147–152, 1982.
Jacobsen, S.T., Crawford, A.H., Miller, E.A., et al.: The Syme amputation in patients with congenital pseudarthrosis of the tibia. J. Bone Joint Surg. [Am.] 65:533–537, 1983.
Langenskiold, A.: Tibia vara: Osteochondrosis deformans tibiae: Blount's disease. Clin. Orthop. 158:77–82, 1981.
Letts, M., and Vincent, N.: Congenital longitudinal deficiency of the fibula (fibular hemimelia): Parental refusal of amputation. Clin. Orthop. 287:160–166, 1993.
Morrissey, R.T.: A symposium: Congenital pseudarthrosis. Clin. Orthop. 166:1–61, 1982.
Paterson, D.: Congenital pseudarthrosis of the tibia. Clin. Orthop. 247:44–54, 1989.
Poppas, A.M.: Osteochondrosis dissecans. Clin. Orthop. 158:659–669, 1981.
Roach, J.W., Shindell, R., and Green, N.E.: Late onset pseudarthrosis of the dysplastic tibia. J. Bone Joint Surg. [Am.] 75:1593–1601, 1993.
Schoenecker, P.L., Capelli, A.M., Miller, E.A., et al.: Congenital longitudinal deficiency of the tibia. J. Bone Joint Surg. [Am.] 71:278–287, 1989.
Schoenecker, P.L., Meade, W.C., Pierron, R.L., et al.: Blount's disease: A retrospective review and recommendations for treatment. J. Pediatr. Orthop. 5:181–186, 1985.

Feet

Adelar, R.S., Williams, R.M., and Gould, J.S.: Congenital convex pes valgus: Results of an early comprehensive release and a review of congenital vertical talus at Richmond Crippled Childrens Hospital and the University of Alabama at Birmingham. Foot Ankle 1:62–73, 1980.
Chambers, R.B., Cook, T.M., and Cowell, H.R.: Surgical reconstruction for calcaneonavicular coalition: Evaluation of function and gait. J. Bone Joint Surg. [Am.] 64:829–836, 1982.
Coleman, S.S.: Complex Foot Deformities in Children. Philadelphia, Lea & Febiger, 1983.
Cowell, H.R.: The management of clubfoot [editorial]. J. Bone Joint Surg. [Am.] 67:991–992, 1985.
Crawford, A.H., Marxen, J.L., and Osterfeld, D.L.: The Cincinnati incision: A comprehensive approach for surgical procedures of the foot and ankle in childhood. J. Bone Joint Surg. [Am.] 64:1355–1358, 1982.
Cummings, R.J., and Lovell, W.W.: Current concepts review: Operative treatment of congenital idiopathic clubfoot. J. Bone Joint Surg. [Am.] 70:1108–1112, 1988.
Hamanishi, C.: Congenital vertical talus: Classification with 69 cases and new measurement system. J. Pediatr. Orthop. 4:318–326, 1984.
Jacobs, R.F., Adelman, L., Sack, C.M., et al.: Management of *Pseudomonas* osteochondritis complicating puncture wounds of the foot. Pediatrics 69:432–435, 1982.
Jahss, M.H.: Evaluation of the cavus foot for orthopedic treatment. Clin. Orthop. 181:52–63, 1983.
McHale, K.A., and Lenhart, M.K.: Treatment of residual clubfoot deformity, the "bean-shaped" foot, by opening wedge medial cuneiform osteotomy and closing wedge cuboid osteotomy: Clinical review and cadaver correlations. J. Pediatr. Orthop. 11:374–381, 1991.
McKay, D.W.: New concept of and approach to clubfoot treatment: Section I. Principles and morbid anatomy. J. Pediatr. Orthop. 2:347–356, 1982.
Onley, B.W., and Asher, M.A.: Excision of symptomatic coalition of the middle facet of the talocalcaneal joint. J. Bone Joint Surg. [Am.] 69:539–544, 1987.
Oppenheim, W., Smith, C., and Christe, W.: Congenital vertical talus. Foot Ankle 5:198–204, 1985.
Pentz, A.S., and Weiner, D.S.: Management of metatarsus adductovarus. Foot Ankle 14:241–246, 1993.
Peterson, H.A.: Skewfoot (forefoot adduction with heel valgus). J. Pediatr. Orthop. 6:24–30, 1986.
Simons, G.W.: Analytical radiography of club feet. J. Bone Joint Surg. [Br.] 59:485–489, 1974.
Simons, G.W.: Complete subtalar release in club feet: Part I. A preliminary report. Part II. Comparison with less extensive procedures. J. Bone Joint Surg. [Am.] 67:1044–1065, 1985.
Thometz, J.G., and Simons, G.W.: Deformity of the calcaneocuboid joint in patients who have talipes equinovarus. J. Bone Joint Surg. [Am.] 75:190–195, 1993.
Turco, V.J.: Resistant congenital clubfoot: One-stage posteromedial release with internal fixation: A follow-up report of a 15 year experience. J. Bone Joint Surg. [Am.] 61:805–814, 1979.
Victoria-Diaz, A., and Victoria-Diaz, J.: Pathogenesis of idiopathic clubfoot. Clin. Orthop. 185:14–24, 1984.
Zinman, C., Wolfson, N., and Reis, N.D.: Osteochondritis dissecans of the dome of the talus: Computed tomography scanning in diagnosis and follow-up. J. Bone Joint Surg. [Am.] 70:1017–1019, 1988.

3

Sports Medicine

Mark D. Miller

I. **Knee**

A. Anatomy and Biomechanics—Although a thorough discussion of anatomy is included in Chapter 11, a brief review of knee anatomy is relevant.

1. Ligaments—Four major ligaments and several other supporting ligaments and structures provide stability to the knee joint.
   a. Anterior cruciate ligament (ACL) originates in a broad, irregular, oval-shaped area just anterior to and between the intercondylar eminences of the tibia and inserts in a semicircular area on the posteromedial aspect of the lateral femoral condyle. It is approximately 33 mm long and 11 mm in diameter. The ACL is often said to be composed of two "bundles"—**an anteromedial bundle that is tight in flexion and a posterolateral bundle that is tight in extension.** The blood supply to both cruciate ligaments is via branches of the middle geniculate artery. Mechanoreceptor nerve fibers within the ligament may have a proprioceptive role.
   b. Posterior cruciate ligament (PCL) originates from a broad, crescent-shaped area on the medial femoral condyle and **inserts on the tibia in a sulcus that is below the articular surface.** It is also composed of two bundles—an **anterolateral portion that is tight in flexion and a posteromedial portion that is tight in extension.** Variable meniscofemoral ligaments (Humphry's—anterior; Wrisberg's—posterior) originate from the lateral meniscus and insert into the substance of the PCL.
   c. Medial collateral ligament (MCL) is composed of superficial (tibial collateral ligament) and deep (medial capsular ligament) fibers. The ligament originates from the medial femoral epicondyle and inserts on the proximal tibia. The deep portion of the ligament is intimately associated with the medial meniscus (coronary ligaments).
   d. Lateral collateral ligament (LCL), or fibular collateral ligament, originates on the lateral femoral epicondyle and inserts on the lateral aspect of the fibular head. It is a cord-like structure that **inserts proximal and posterior to the insertion of the popliteus tendon.**
   e. Medial and lateral supporting structures are best considered in layers (Fig. 3–1). Recent research has added to our knowledge of the anatomy of the posterolateral corner of the knee. The popliteus and its attachment to the fibular head **(popliteal fibular ligament)** are key structures in this area.

Medial Structures

Layer	Components
I	Sartorius and fascia
II	Superfical MCL, posterior oblique ligament, semimembranosus
III	Deep MCL, capsule

Lateral Structures

Layer	Components
I	Iliotibial tract, biceps, fascia
II	Patellar retinaculum, patellofemoral ligament, LCL
III	Arcuate ligament, fabellofibular ligament, capsule

2. Menisci are crescent-shaped fibrocartilaginous structures that are triangular in cross-section. Only the **peripheral 20–30% of the menisci are vascularized** (medial and lateral genicular arteries). The medial meniscus is more C-shaped, and the lateral meniscus is more circular in shape (see Fig. 3–1). These structures, which deepen the articular surfaces of the tibial plateau and have a role in stability, lubrication, and nutrition, are connected anteriorly by the transverse ligament.
3. Joint Relationships—The height of the lateral femoral condyle is greater than that of the medial condyle. The alignment of the condyles is also different; the lateral condyle is relatively straight, but the medial condyle is curved (allowing the medial tibial plateau to rotate externally in full extension—the "screw home mechanism"). The lateral condyle can also be identified by its terminal sulcus and groove of the popliteus insertion (Fig. 3–2). The patellofemoral joint is composed of the patella (with variably sized medial and lateral facets) and the femoral trochlea. The patella is restrained in the trochlea by the valgus axis of the quadriceps mecha-

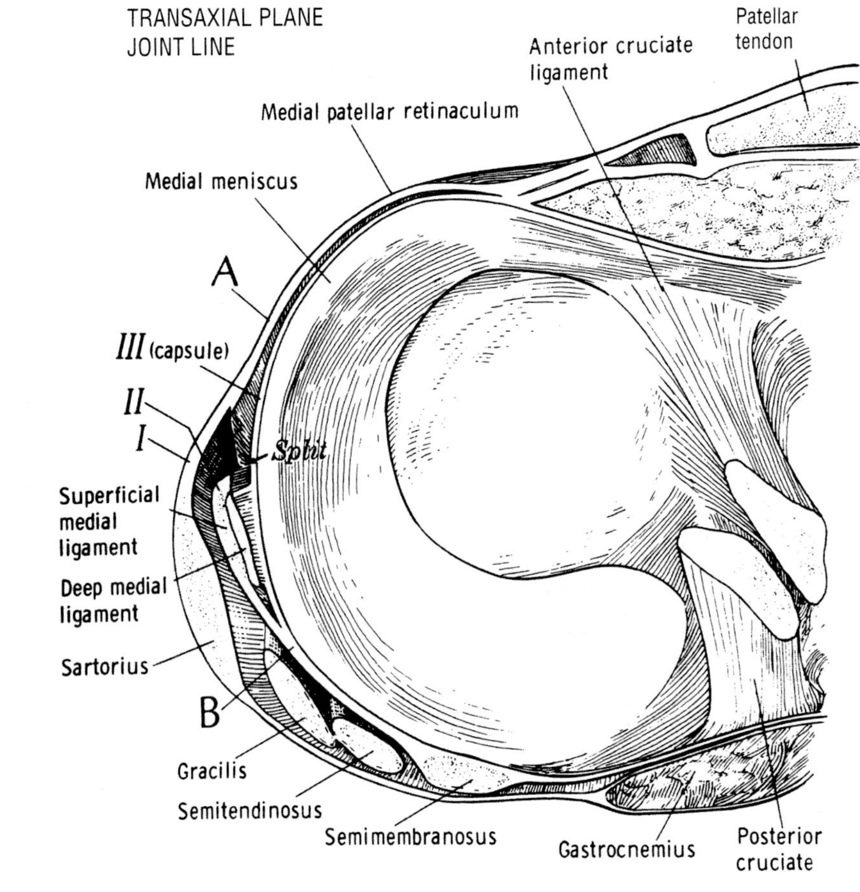

A

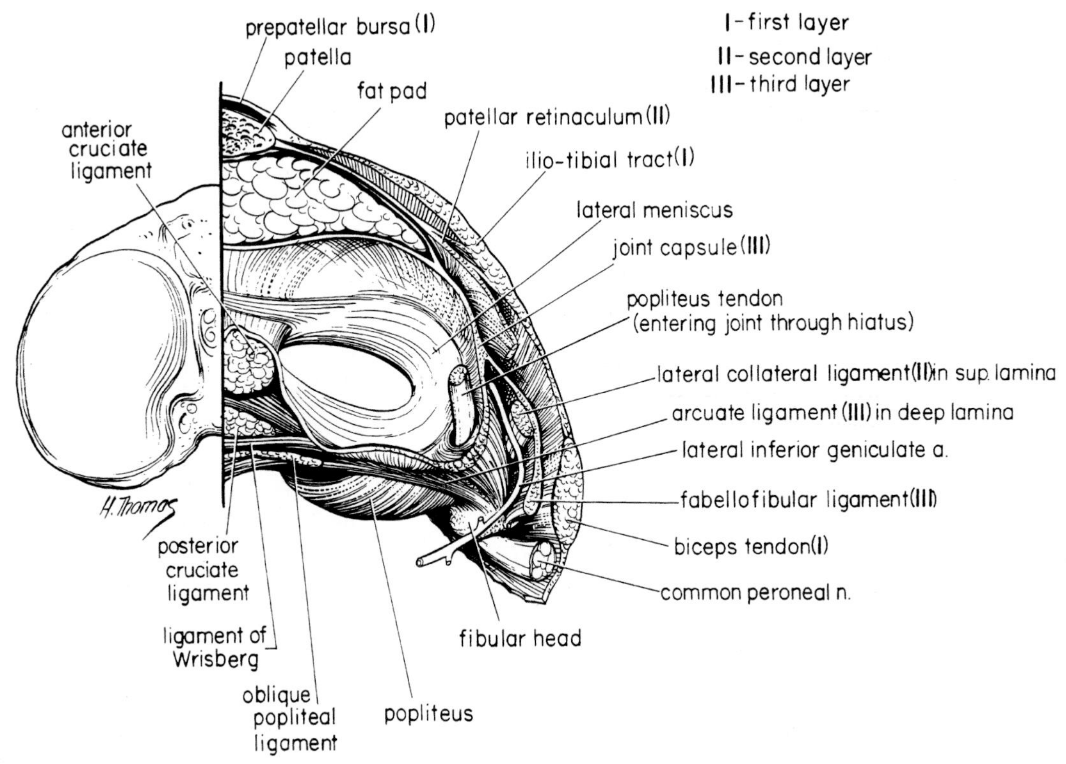

B

Figure 3–1. Medial and lateral supporting structures of the knee. *A,* Medial structures of the knee include the sartorius and its fascia and the patellar retinaculum (layer I), the hamstring tendons and superficial MCL (layer II), and the deep MCL (layer III). (From Warren, L.F., and Marshal, J.L.: The supporting structures and layers of the medial side of the knee. J. Bone Joint Surg. [Am.] 61:56–62, 1979.) *B,* Lateral structures of the knee include the iliotibial tract and biceps (layer I), patellar retinaculum (layer II), and capsule and LCL (layer III). (From Seebacher, J.R., Ingilis, A.E., Marshall, J.L., et al.: The structure of the posterolateral aspect of the knee. J. Bone Joint Surg. [Am.] 64:536–541, 1982.)

Figure 3–2. Relationships of the femoral condyles. *A,* On the lateral projection, the lateral condyle projects more anteriorly and is notched. Anteroposterior *(B)* and posteroanterior *(C)* view demonstrating the difference in size and curvature of the medial femoral condyle. (From Tria, A.J., and Klein, K.S.: An Illustrated Guide to the Knee. New York, Churchill Livingstone, 1992, p. 5.)

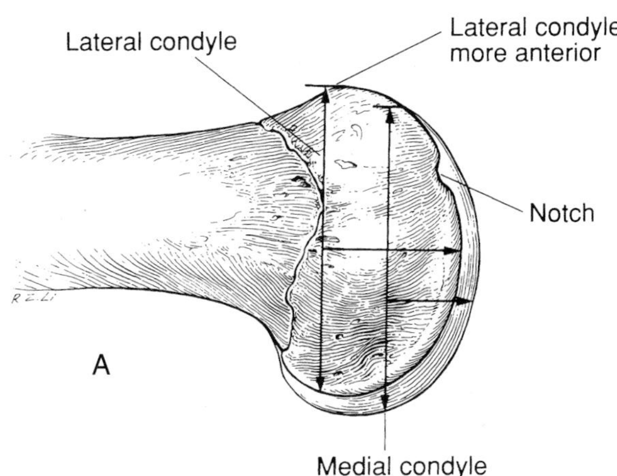

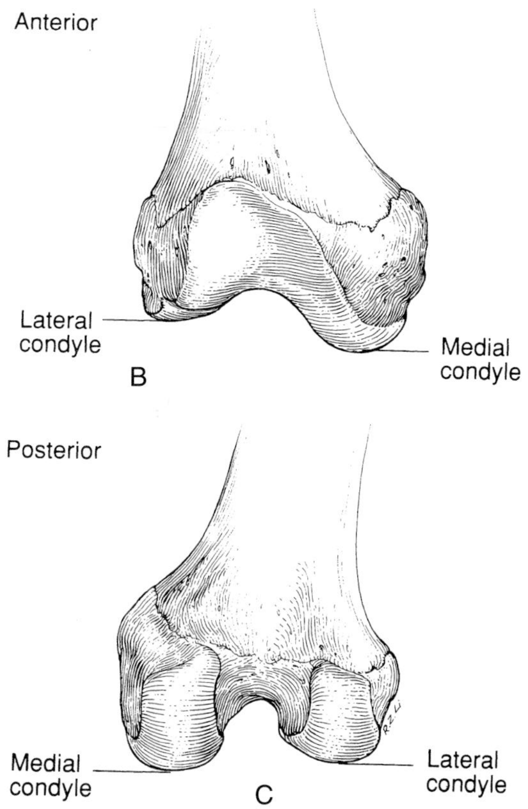

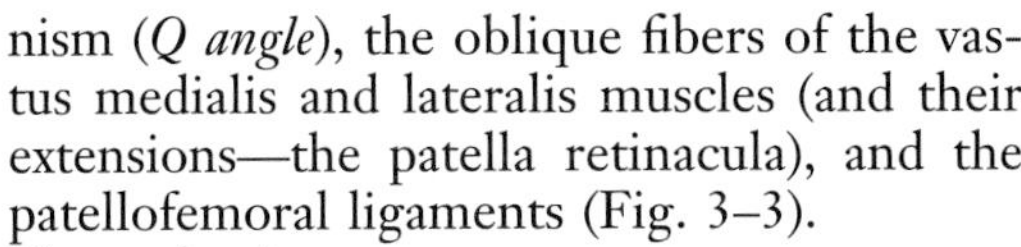
nism (*Q angle*), the oblique fibers of the vastus medialis and lateralis muscles (and their extensions—the patella retinacula), and the patellofemoral ligaments (Fig. 3–3).

4. Biomechanics
   a. Knee ligaments serve primarily as passive restraints to knee motion.

Ligament	Restraint
ACL	Anterior translation of the tibia
PCL	Posterior tibial displacement
MCL	Valgus angulation
LCL	Varus angulation

The tensile strength of the ACL is approximately 2200 N. The tensile strength of a 10-mm patellar tendon graft (young specimen) is more than 2900 N and is about 30% stronger when rotated 90 degrees. However, this strength quickly diminishes in vivo. The concept of ligament "isometry" remains controversial. Reconstructed ligaments should reapproximate normal anatomy and lie within the flexion axis in all positions of knee motion. Other considerations, such as graft impingement and avoiding flexion contractures, are equally important.

   b. Menisci are composed of collagen fibers that are arranged radially and longitudinally (Fig. 3–4). The longitudinal fibers help dissipate the hoop stresses in the menisci, and the combination of fibers allows the meniscus to expand under compressive forces and increase the contact area of the joint. The lateral meniscus has twice the excursion of the medial meniscus during knee range of motion and rotation.

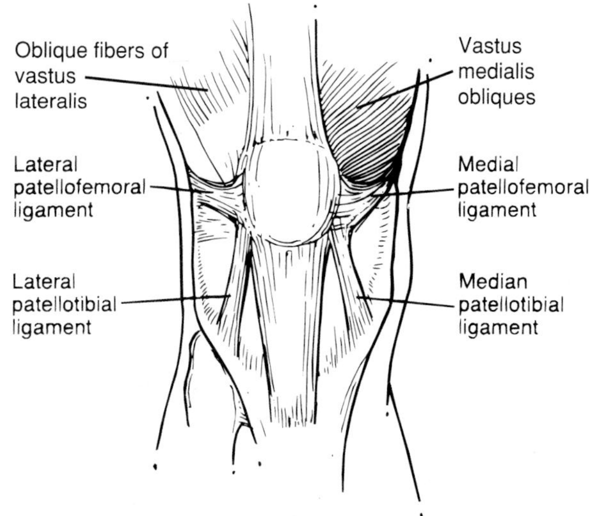

Figure 3–3. Patellar restraints include the patellofemoral and patellotibial ligaments as well as the oblique fibers of the vastus medialis and lateralis. (From Walsh, W.M.: Patellofemoral joint. In DeLee, J.C., and Drez, D., Jr., eds.: Orthopaedic Sports Medicine: Principles and Practice. Philadelphia, WB Saunders, 1994, p. 1168.)

c. The patellofemoral joint must withstand forces that are over three times that of body weight. **The main restraint to lateral displacement of the patella is the medial patellofemoral ligament.**

B. History and Physical Examination

1. History—Several key historical points should be sought:

History	Significance
Pain after sitting/stair climbing	Patellofemoral etiology
Locking/pain with squatting	Meniscal tear
Noncontact injury with "pop"	ACL tear, patellar dislocation
Contact injury with "pop"	Collateral ligament, meniscus, fracture
Acute swelling	ACL, peripheral meniscus tear, osteochondral fx, ± capsule tear
Knee "gives way"	Ligamentous laxity, patellar instability
Anterior force—**dorsiflexed foot**	PCL or patellar injury
Dashboard injury	

2. Physical Examination—The following are key examination points and may be best elicited with an examination under anesthesia (as shown at the bottom of this page).

3. Instrumented Knee Laxity Measurement—KT-1000 and 2000 (MED-metric, San Diego, CA) is the most commonly accepted device for standardized laxity measurement. The manual maximum anterior displacements are the most commonly reported values and are based on side-to-side comparison (>3 mm significant). PCL laxity can also be measured with this device, although it is less accurate.

C. Imaging the Knee—In addition to standard radiographs, certain other findings and views can be helpful (as shown at the top of page 199).

Many of these findings are illustrated in Figure 3–5A. Evaluation of patella height is accomplished by one of three commonly used methods (Fig. 3–5B).

D. Knee Arthroscopy

1. Portals—Standard portals include a superomedial or superolateral inflow portal (made with the knee in extension) and inferomedial and inferolateral portals (made with the knee in flexion) for instruments and the arthroscope, respectively (Fig. 3–6). Accessory portals, sometimes helpful for visualizing the

Examination	Method	Significance
Standing/gait	Observe gait	Based on pathology
Deformity	Observe patient standing	Based on pathology
Effusion	Patella: ballot/milk	Ligament/meniscus injury (acute), arthritis (chronic)
Point of maximum tenderness	Palpate for tenderness	Based on location **(joint line tenderness = meniscus tear)**
Range of motion	Active and passive	Block = meniscus injury (bucket handle), loose body, ACL tear impinging
Patella crepitus	With passive ROM	Patellofemoral pathology
Patella grind	Push patella with quadriceps contraction	Patellofemoral pathology
Patella apprehension	Push patella lat. at 20–30° flexion	**Patella subluxation/dislocation**
Q angle	ASIS-patella-tibial tubercle	Increased with patella malalignment
Flexion Q Angle	ASIS-patella-tibial tubercle	Increased with patella malalignment
J sign	Lateral deviation of the patella in extension	
Ext rotation recurvatum	Pick up great toes; **knee-varus and hyperextension**	
Patella tilt	Tilt up laterally	>15° = Lax <0° = tight lateral constraint
Patella glide	Like apprehension	>50° = Incr. medial const laxity
Active glide	Lat. excursion with quad. contraction	Lat. > prox. excursion = incr. Functional Q angle quadriceps
Quadriceps circumference	10 cm (VMO), 15 cm (quad.)	Atrophy from inactivity
Symmetric extension	Back of knee from ground or prone heel height difference	Contracture, displaced meniscal tear, or other mechanical block
Varus/valgus stress	30°	**MCL/LCL laxity (grade I–III)**
Varus/valgus stress	0°	MCL/LCL and PCL
Apley's	Prone-flexion compression	DJD, meniscal pathology
Lachman	Tibia forward at 30° flexion	**ACL injury (most sensitive)**
Finacetto	Lachman with tibia subluxing beyond post. horns of menisci	ACL injury (severe)
Ant. drawer	Tibia forward at 90° flexion	ACL injury
Int. rotation drawer	Foot int. rotated with drawer	Tighter = (normal), looser = ACL injury
Ext. rotation drawer	Foot ext. rotation with drawer	Loose (normal), looser = ACL/MCL injury
Pivot shift	Flexion with int. rotation and valgus	ACL injury (EUA)
Pivot jerk	Extension with int. rotation and valgus	ACL injury (EUA)
Posterior drawer	Tibia backward at 90° flexion	PCL Injury
Tibia sag.	Flex 90°, observe	PCL
90° quad. Act	Extend flexed knee	PCL
Asymmetric external rotation	"Dial" feet externally at 30° and 90° flexion	**Asymmetric increased external rotation >10°–15° = Posterolateral corner (PLC) injury. If asymmetric at both 30° and 90° = PCL + PLC**
Ext. rotation recurvatum	Pick up great toes	PLC injury
Reversed pivot	Extension with ext. rotation and valgus	PLC injury
Posterolateral drawer	Post. drawer, lat. > med.	PLC injury

View/Sign	Finding	Significance
Lateral-high patella	Patella alta	Patellofemoral pathology
Congruence angle	$\mu = -6° \ SD = 11°$	Patellofemoral pathology
Tooth sign	Irregular ant. patella	Patellofemoral chondrosis
Varus/valgus stress view	Opening	Collateral ligament injury; Salter-Harris fracture
Lateral capsule (Segund) sign	Small tibial avulsion off lateral tibia	ACL tear
Pellegrini-Stieda lesion	Med. femoral condyle avulsion	Chronic MCL injury
Lateral stress view—Stress to anterior tibia with knee 70° flexed	Asymmetric posterior tibial displacement	PCL injury
PA flexion weight-bearing		Early DJD, OCD, notch evaluation
Fairbank's changes	Square condyle, peak eminences, ridging, narrowing	Early DJD (postmeniscectomy)
Square lateral condyle	Thick joint space	Discoid meniscus
Arthrogram	Dye outline	Meniscal tear
MRI	Intra-articular path	Specific for lesion
Bone scan		Stress fractures, early DJD, RSD
CT		Tibial plateau fractures, patellar tilt

posterior horns of the menisci and PCL, include the posteromedial portal (1 cm above the joint line behind the MCL [avoid saphenous nerve branches]) and the posterolateral portal (1 cm above the joint line between the LCL and biceps tendon [avoiding the common peroneal nerve]). The transpatellar portal (1 cm distal to the patella, splitting the patellar tendon fibers) can be used for central viewing or grabbing but should be avoided in patients requiring subsequent autogenous patellar tendon harvesting. Other less commonly used portals include the medial and lateral midpatellar portals; the proximal superomedial portal (4 cm proximal to the patella), which is used for anterior compartment visualization; and the far medial and far lateral portals, which are used for accessory instrument placement (loose body removal).

2. Technique—A systematic examination of the knee should include evaluation of the patellofemoral joint, medial and lateral gutters, medial and lateral compartments, and the notch. The posteromedial corner can best be visualized with a 70 degree arthroscope placed through the notch (modified Gillquist's view).

E. Menisci

1. Meniscal tear is the most common injury to the knee that requires surgery. **The medial meniscus is torn approximately three times more frequently than the lateral meniscus.** Traumatic meniscal tears are common in young patients with sports-related injuries. Degenerative tears usually occur in older patients and can have an insidious onset. Meniscal tears can be classified based on their location in relation to the vascular supply (and healing potential), their position (anterior, middle, or posterior third), and their appearance and orientation (Fig. 3–7).
   a. Partial Meniscectomy—Tears that are not amenable to repair (e.g., peripheral, longitudinal tears), excluding tears that do not require any treatment (e.g., partial-thickness tears, tears <5 mm in length, and tears that cannot be displaced >1–2 mm), are best treated by partial meniscectomy. In general, complex, degenerative, and central/radial tears are resected with minimal normal meniscus being resected. A motorized shaver is helpful for creating a smooth transition zone. The role of lasers or other devices for this purpose is still under investigation. There is some concern with iatrogenic chondral injury caused by lasers.

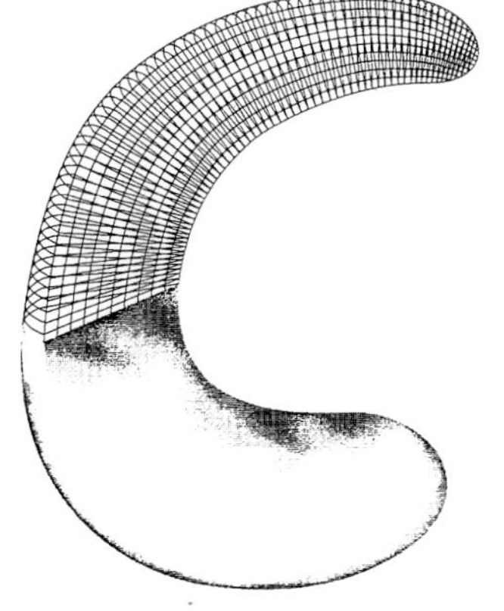

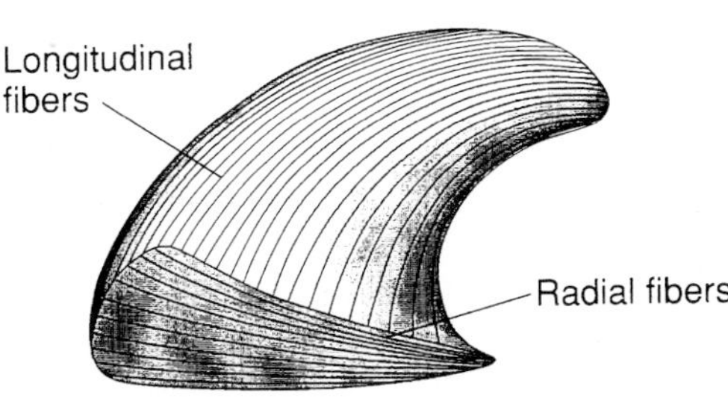

Figure 3–4. Longitudinal and radial fibers of the menisci. (From Tria, A.J., and Klein, K.S.: An Illustrated Guide to the Knee. New York, Churchill Livingstone, 1992, p. 37.)

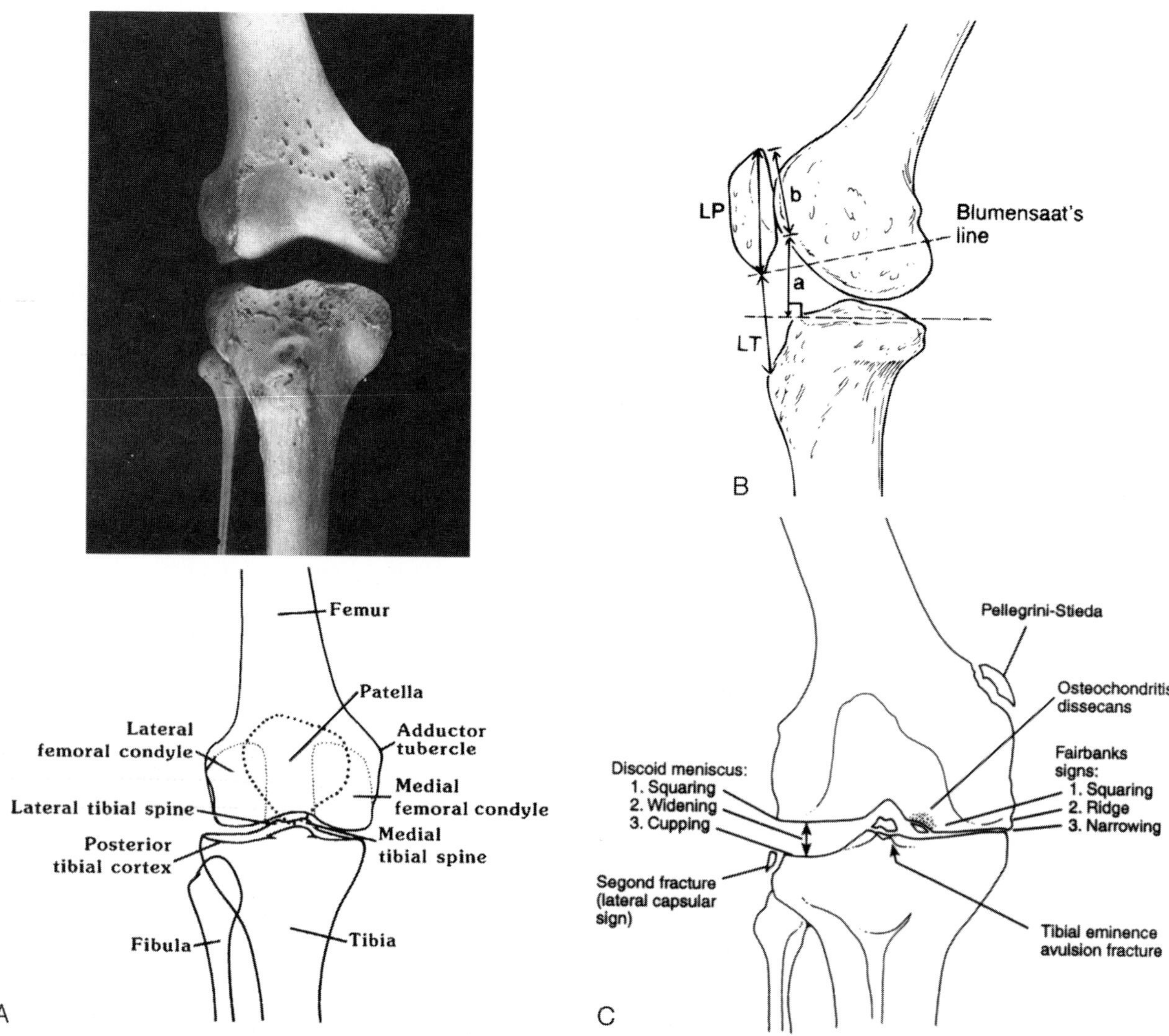

Figure 3–5. *A,* Anterior view and drawing demonstrating the bones of the knee. (From Weissman, B.N.W., and Sledge, C.B.: Orthopedic Radiology. Philadelphia, WB Saunders, 1986, p. 498.) *B,* Three popular methods for evaluating patella alta and baja. (1) **Blumensaat's line**: With the knee flexed 30 degrees, the lower border of the patella should lie on a line extended from the intercondylar notch. (2) **Insall-Salvati index**: Patella tendon length (LT) to patella length (LP) ratio, or index, should be 1.0. An index of >1.2 is alta and <0.8 is baja. (3) **Blackburne-Peel index**: Ratio of the distance from the tibial plateau to the inferior articular surface of the patella (a) to the length of the patella articular surface (b) should be 0.8. An index of >1.0 is alta. (From Harner, C.D., Miller, M.D. and Irrgang, J.J.: Management of the stiff knee after trauma and ligament reconstruction. In Siliski, J.M., ed.: Traumatic Disorders of the Knee. New York, Springer-Verlag, 1994, p. 364.) *C,* Common radiographic abnormalities.

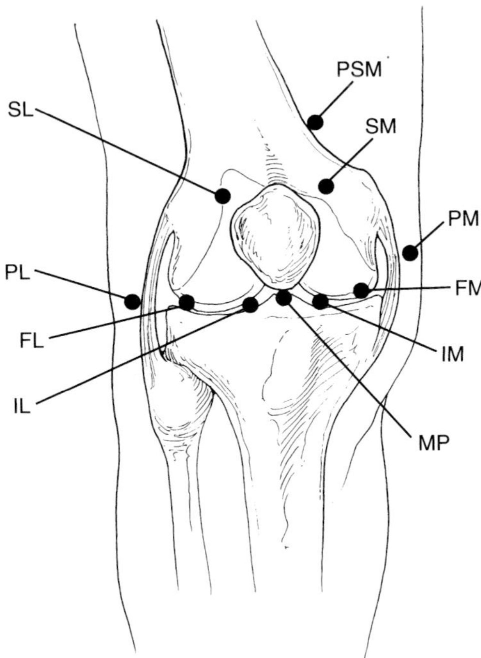

Figure 3–6. Arthroscopic portals. (PSM = proximal superomedial; FM = far medial; IM = inferomedial; MP = midpatellar; IL = inferolateral; FL = far lateral; PL = posterolateral; SL = superolateral) (From Miller, M.D., Osborne J.R., Warner J.J.P., et al.: MRI-Arthroscopy Correlative Atlas. Philadelphia, WB Saunders, 1997, p. 50.)

b. Meniscal Repair—Should be accomplished for all peripheral longitudinal tears, especially in young patients. Augmentation techniques (fibrin clot, vascular access channels, synovial rasping) may extend the indications for repair. Four techniques are commonly used: open, "outside-in," "inside-out," and "all-inside" (Fig. 3–8). Newer techniques for all-inside repairs (arrows, darts, staples, screws, etc.) are currently in early clinical use; however, they are probably not as reliable as vertical mattress sutures. Regardless of the technique used, it is essential to **protect the saphenous nerve branches during medial repairs and the peroneal nerve during lateral repairs** (Fig. 3–9) Results of meniscal repair are good, especially with acute, peripheral tears in young patients undergoing concurrent ACL reconstruction.

2. Meniscal Cysts—Most commonly occur in conjunction **with horizontal cleavage tears of the lateral meniscus** (Fig. 3–10). Operative treatment consisting of arthroscopic partial meniscectomy and decompression through the tear (sometimes including "needling" of the cyst) has been shown to be effective. En bloc excision is no longer favored for most meniscal cysts. Popliteal (Baker's) cysts are also related to meniscal disorder and will usually resolve with treatment. They are classically **located between the semimembranosus and medial head of the gastrocnemius.**

3. Discoid Menisci ("Popping Knee Syndrome")—Can be classified as (1) incomplete, (2) complete, or (3) Wrisberg's variant (Fig. 3–11). Patients may develop mechanical symptoms, or "popping," with the knee in extension. Plain radiographs may demonstrate a widened joint space, squaring of the lateral condyle, cupping of the lateral tibial plateau, and a hypoplastic lateral intercondylar spine. Magnetic resonance imaging (MRI) can be helpful and can also show associated tears. Treatment includes partial meniscectomy (saucerization) for tears, meniscal repair for peripheral detachments (Wrisberg's variant), and **observation for discoid menisci without tears.**

4. Meniscal Transplantation—Remains controversial but may be indicated for young patients who have had near-total meniscectomy (especially lateral meniscectomy) and who have early chondrosis. Indications and techniques are evolving.

F. Osteochondral Lesions

1. Osteochondritis Dissecans—Involves subchondral bone and overlying cartilage separation, most likely as a result of occult trauma. The lesion most often involves the **lateral aspect of the medial femoral condyle**. Children with open growth plates have the best prognosis, and often these lesions can be observed simply. In situ lesions can be treated with retrograde drilling. Detached lesions may require abrasion chondroplasty or newer, more aggressive, techniques.

2. Cartilage Injury—Usually occurs on the medial femoral condyle, often from shearing injuries. Débridement and chondroplasty are currently recommended for symptomatic lesions. Displaced osteochondral fragments can sometimes be replaced and secured with small recessed screws or absorbable pins. Several new treatment options for discrete, isolated, full-thickness cartilage injuries are in early clinical use. These include microfracture, periosteal patches (+/− chondrocyte implantation), and osteochondral transfer (plugs) (Fig. 3–12). Donor site problems and the creation of true articular cartilage at the recipient site are still challenges.

3. Degenerative Joint Disease—Diffuse chondral damage is best treated with reconstructive techniques such as osteotomies and replacements, which are addressed in the chapter that follows.

G. Synovial Lesions

1. Pigmented Villonodular Synovitis—Patients may present with pain and swelling and may have a palpable mass. Synovectomy is effective, but there is a high recurrence rate.

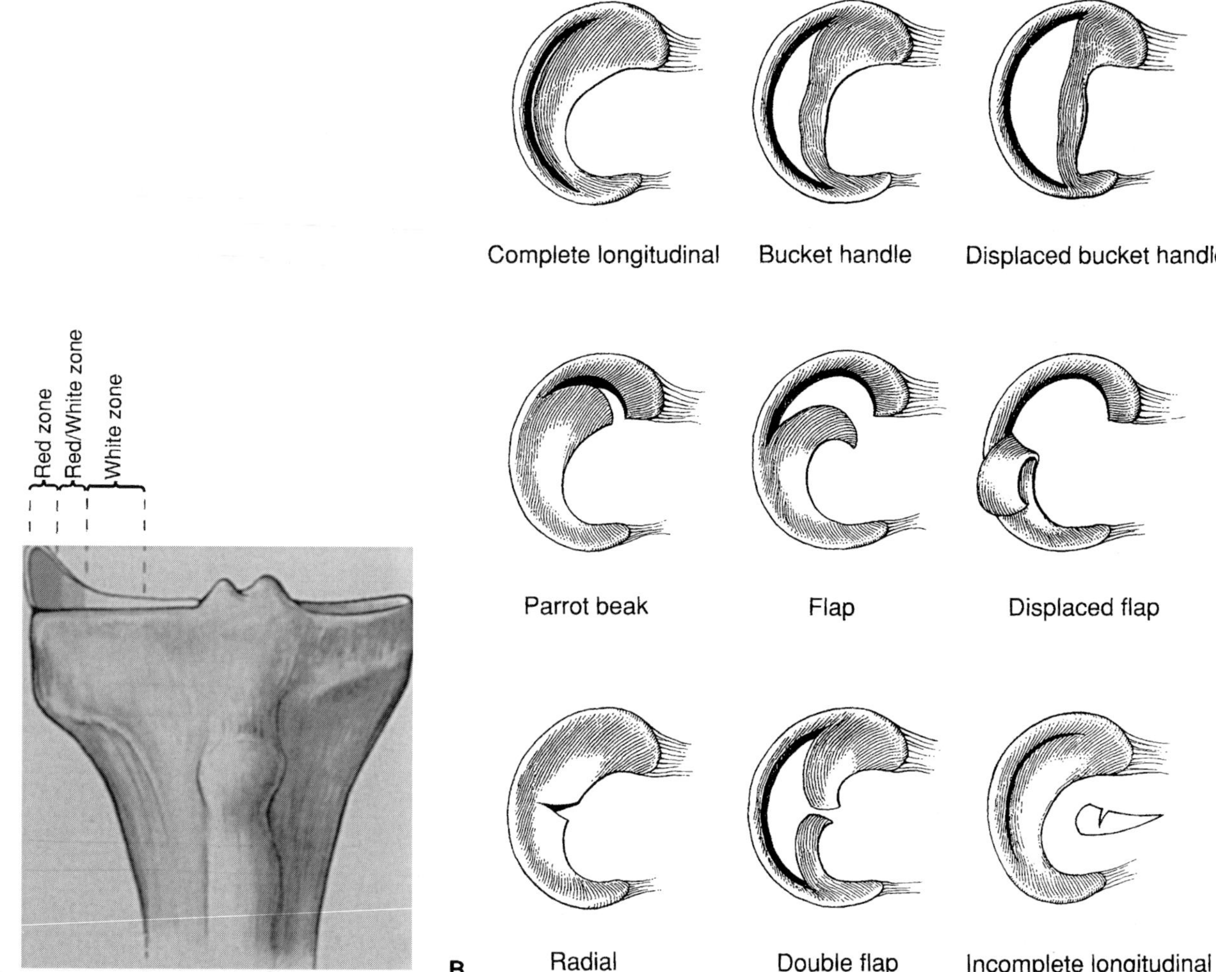

Figure 3–7. Classification of meniscal tears. *A,* Vascular zones. The red-red zone has the highest potential for meniscal healing, and the white-white zone has essentially no potential for healing without enhancement. (Modified from Miller, M.D., Warner, J.J.P., and Harner, C.D.: Meniscal repair. In Fu, F.H., Harner, C.D., and Vince, K.G., eds.: Knee Surgery. Baltimore, Williams & Wilkins, 1994, p. 616.) *B,* Common meniscal tear appearance and orientation. (From Tria, A.J., and Klein, K.S.: An Illustrated Guide to the Knee. New York, Churchill Livingstone, 1992.)

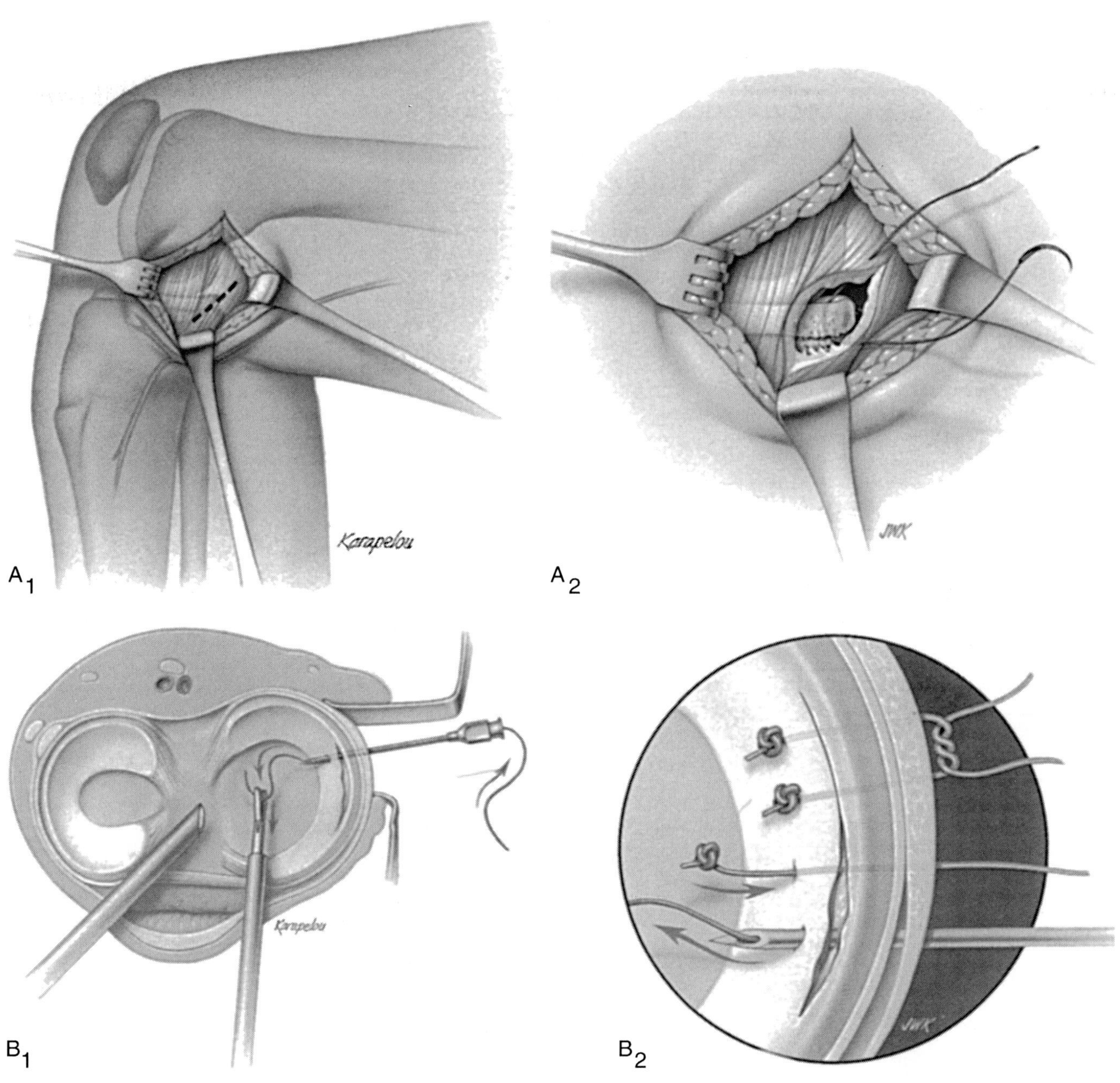

Figure 3–8. Meniscal repair techniques. *A,* Open repair of the medial meniscus (right knee). *B,* "Outside-in" medial meniscal repair (right knee).

Illustration continued on following page

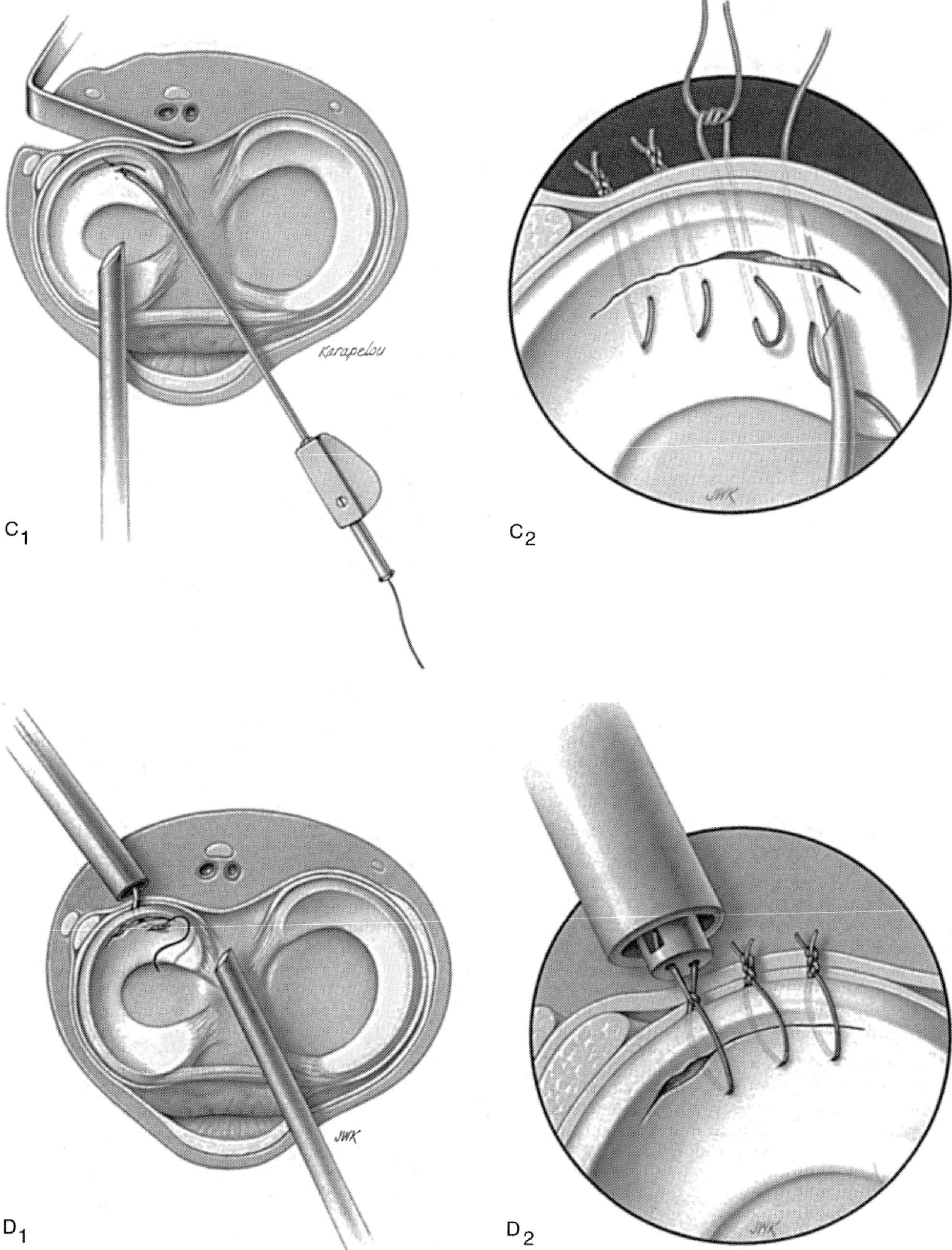

Figure 3–8 *Continued. C,* "Inside-out" lateral meniscal repair (right knee). *D,* "All inside" lateral meniscal repair (right knee). (From Miller, M.D.: Atlas of meniscal repair. Op. Tech. Orthop. 5(1):70–71, 1995.)

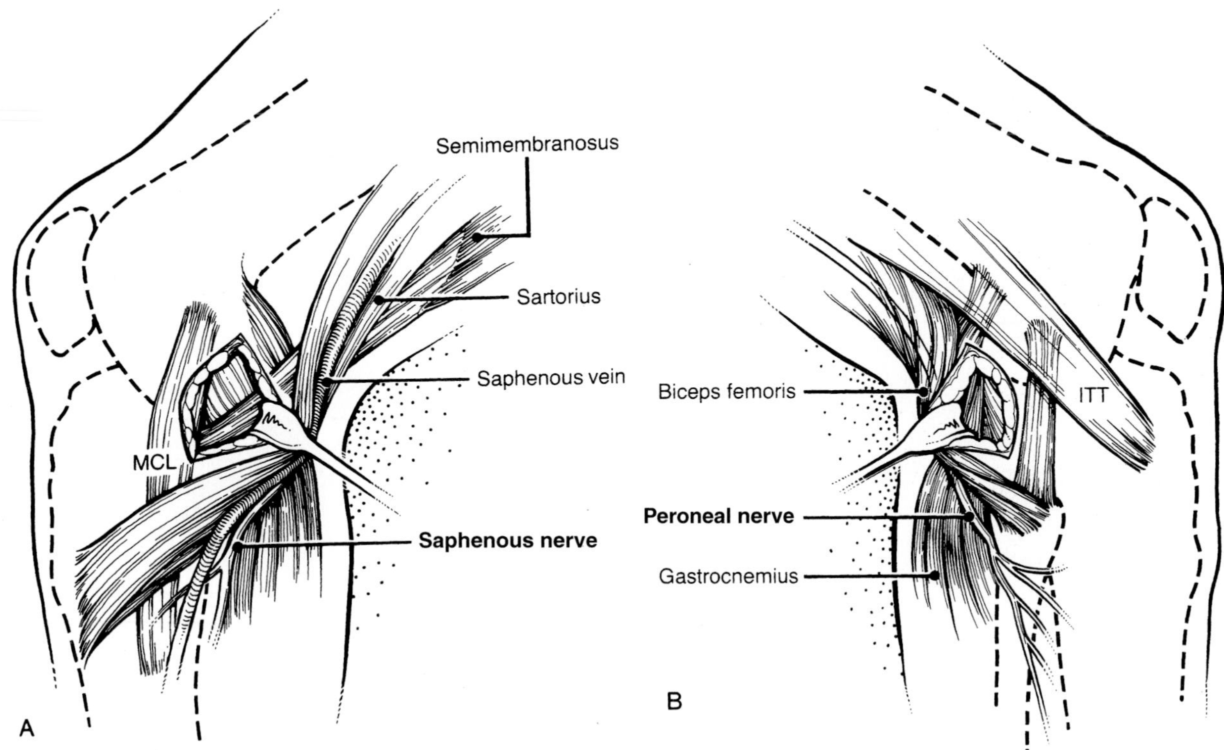

Figure 3–9. Incisions for meniscal repair must be planned to allow for retraction and protection of the saphenous nerve branches during medial meniscal repairs *(A)* and the peroneal nerve during lateral meniscal repairs *(B).* (From Scott, W.N., ed.: Arthroscopy of the Knee: Diagnosis and Treatment. Philadelphia, WB Saunders, 1990.)

Arthroscopic techniques are just as effective as traditional open procedures.

2. Other synovial lesions that respond to synovectomy include (osteo)chondromatosis, pauciarticular juvenile rheumatoid arthritis, and hemophilia. Additional arthroscopic portals are required for complete synovectomy.
3. Plicae—Synovial folds that are embryologic

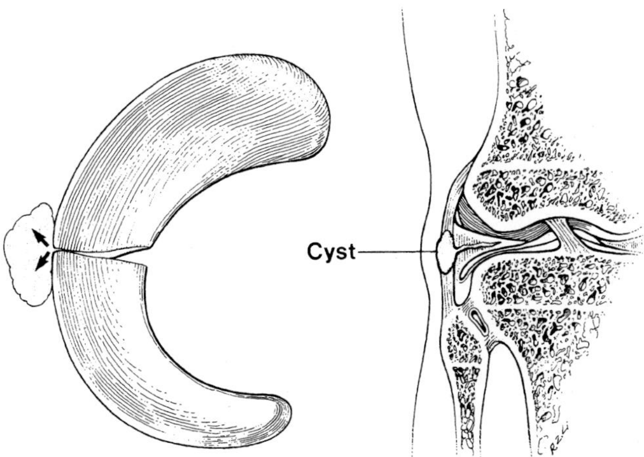

Figure 3–10. Meniscal cysts most commonly involve the lateral meniscus. (From Tria, A.J., and Klein, K.S.: An Illustrated Guide to the Knee. New York, Churchill Livingstone, 1992, p. 101.)

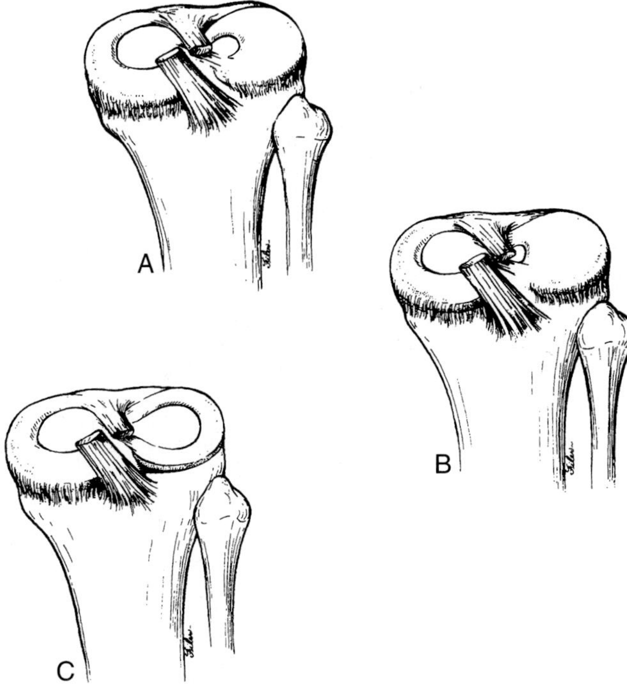

Figure 3–11. Classification of lateral discoid menisci. *A,* Incomplete. *B,* Complete. *C,* Wrisberg's ligament variant. (From Neuschwander, D.C.: Discoid lateral meniscus. In Fu, F.H., Harner, C.D., and Vince, K.G., eds.: Knee Surgery. Baltimore, Williams & Wilkins, 1994, p. 394.)

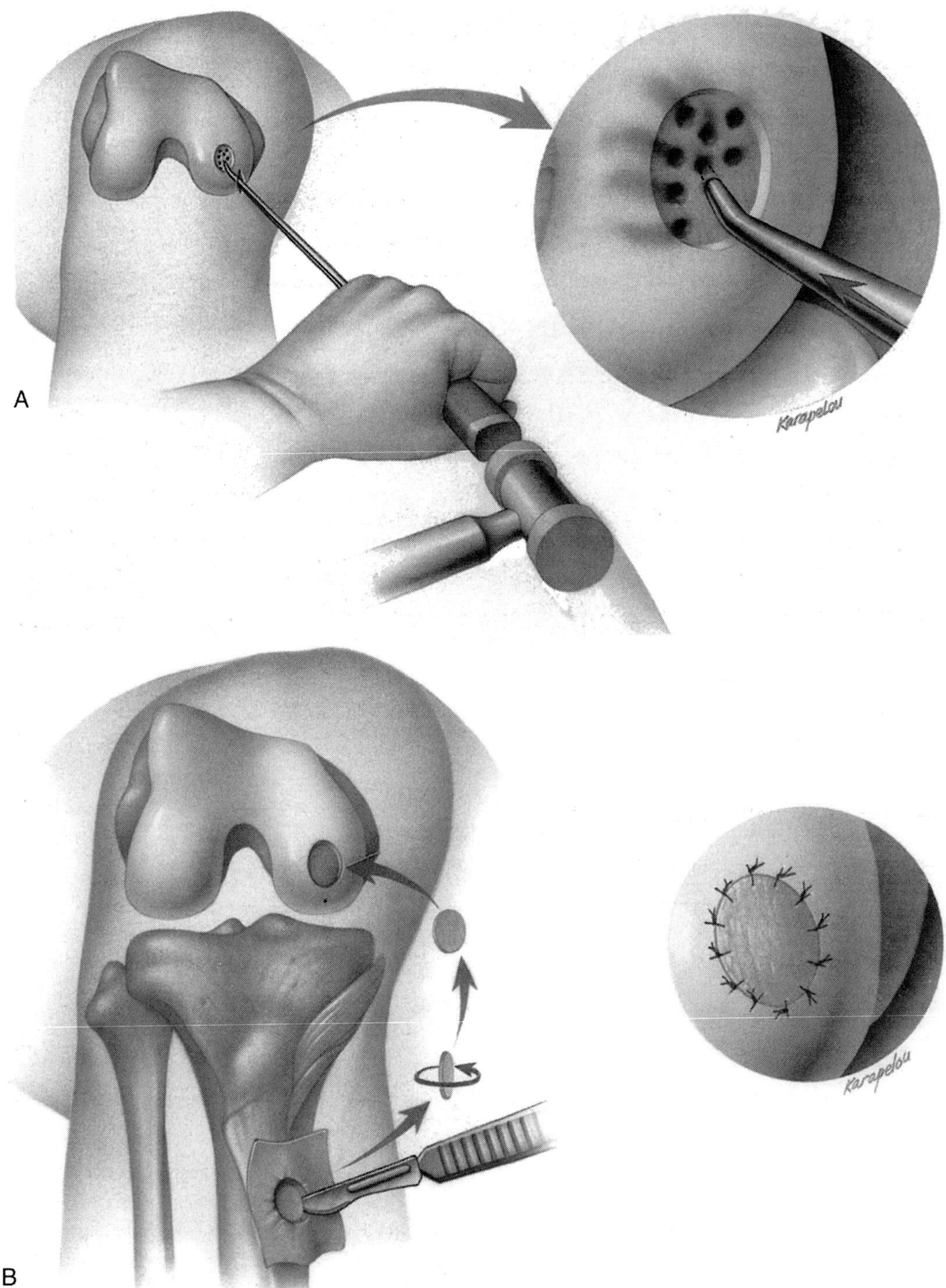

Figure 3–12. Treatment of chondral injuries. *A,* Microfracture. Awls, with various degrees of angulation, are introduced throughout the ipsilateral arthroscopic portal and are used to penetrate the subchondral bone and encourage stem cell production of "cartilage-like" tissue. *B,* Periosteal graft. Periosteum is used as a "patch." The inner cambium layer is rotated so that it is facing outward. The patch is carefully sewn in place, and "cartilage" may grow out from the undifferentiated cambium layer of the graft.

Illustration continued on opposite page

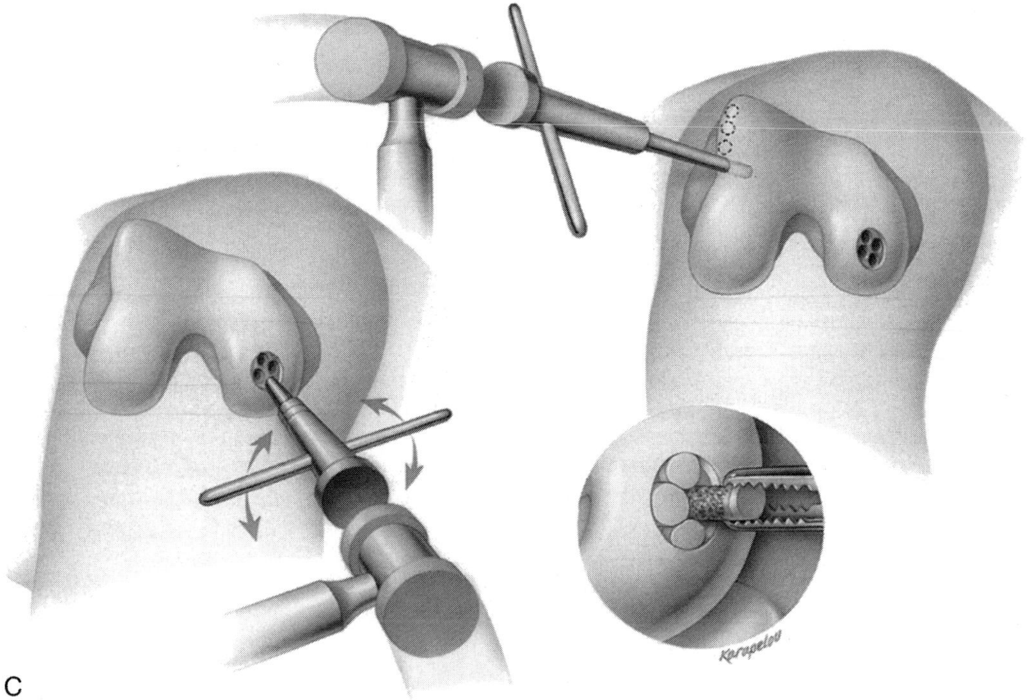

Figure 3–12 *Continued. C,* Osteochondral plugs. Cylindrical "plugs" of exposed bone are removed from the defect. Plugs of normal non-weightbearing cartilage and bone are harvested and placed into the defect. (From Miller MD: Atlas of chondral injury treatment. Op. Tech. Orthop. 7[4]:289–294, 1997.)

remnants. Occasionally, they are pathologic, particularly the medial patellar plica. This plica can cause abrasion of the medial femoral condyle and sometimes responds to arthroscopic excision.

H. Ligamentous Injuries

1. ACL Injury—Controversy continues regarding the development of late arthritis in ACL-deficient versus reconstructed knees. Nevertheless, chronic ACL deficiency is associated with a higher incidence of complex meniscal tears not amenable to repair. Although the arthritis issue remains controversial, ACL-deficient knees have an increased incidence of chondral injury and meniscal tears over time. Bone bruises (trabecular microfractures) occur in over half of acute ACL injuries and are typically located near the sulcus terminalis on the lateral femoral condyle and the posterolateral aspect of the tibia. Although the long-term significance of these injuries is unknown, they may be related to late cartilage injury. Treatment decisions should be individualized based on age, activity level, instability, associated injuries, and other factors (Fig. 3–13). ACL injuries are often the result of noncontact pivoting injuries and are commonly associated with an

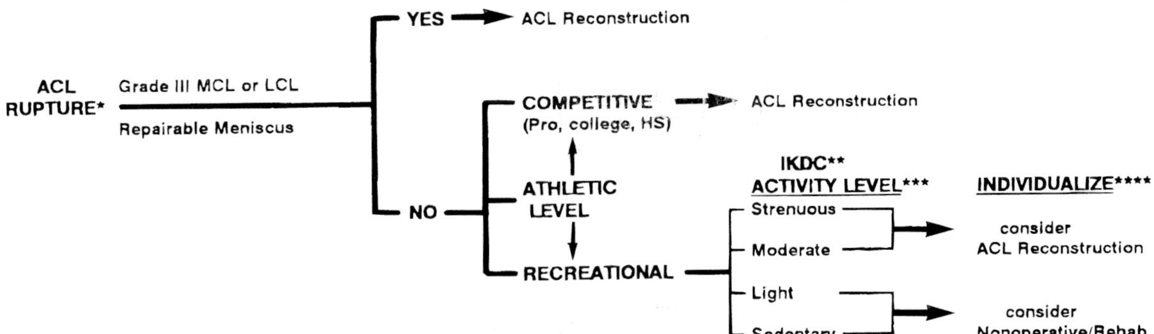

Figure 3–13. Algorithm for the treatment of ACL ruptures. *midsubstance tears; **IKDC (International Knee Documentation Committee); ***activity level; strenuous, jumping/pivoting sports; moderate, heavy manual work, skiing; light manual work, running; sedentary, activities of daily living; ****individualize based on age, arthritis, occupation, activity modification, other medial conditions. (From Spindler, K.P., and Walker, R.N.: General approach to ligament surgery. In Fu, F.H., Harner, C.D., and Vince, K.G., eds.: Knee Surgery. Baltimore, Williams & Wilkins, 1994, p. 652.)

audible "pop" with immediate swelling. The **Lachman test is the most sensitive examination for acute ACL injuries.** Intra-articular reconstruction (usually with bone-patella, tendon-bone, or hamstring autograft) is currently favored for patients who meet the criteria indicated in Figure 3–13. Rehabilitation has evolved, and early motion and weight-bearing are encouraged in most protocols. Closed chain rehabilitation has been emphasized because it allows physiologic co-contraction of the musculature around the knee. Complications most commonly are a result of aberrant tunnel placement (often the femoral tunnel is placed too far anteriorly, limiting flexion) and early surgery (resulting in knee stiffness). **Arthrofibrosis, which can occur more commonly with acute ACL reconstruction**, and aberrant hardware placement (interference screw divergence of >30 degrees [for endoscopic femoral tunnels] and >15 degrees [for tibial tunnels]) can also result in complications. The existence and treatment of "partial" ACL tears is also controversial, although clinical examination and functional stability remain the most important factors.

2. PCL Injury—Treatment is controversial, although reports suggest that nonoperative management may result in late patellar and medial femoral condyle chondrosis. Injuries occur most commonly as a result of a direct blow to the anterior tibia with the knee flexed (the "dashboard injury") or **hyperflexion with a plantar flexed foot** without a blow; hyperextension injuries can also result in PCL rupture. The **key examination is the posterior drawer test** with an absent or posteriorly-directed tibial "step-off." Nonoperative treatment is favored for most isolated PCL injuries. **Bony avulsion fractures can be repaired primarily with good results**, although primary repair of midsubstance PCL (and ACL) injuries has not been successful. **Chronic PCL deficiency can result in late chondrosis of the patellofemoral compartment and/or medial femoral condyle.** PCL reconstruction is recommended for functionally unstable or combined injuries (Fig. 3–14).
3. Collateral Ligament Injury
   a. MCL Injury—Occurs as a result of valgus stress to the knee. Pain and **instability with valgus stress testing at 30 degrees of flexion** (and not in full extension) is diagnostic. Injuries most commonly occur at the femoral insertion of the ligament. **Nonoperative treatment (hinged knee brace)** is highly successful for isolated MCL injuries. Prophylactic bracing may be helpful for football players. Rarely, advancement and reinforcement of the ligament are necessary for chronic injuries that do not respond to conservative treatment. Chronic injuries may have calcification at the medial femoral condyle insertion (Pellegrini-Stieda *sign*). Pellegrini-Stieda *syndrome*, which can occur with chronic MCL injury, usually responds to a brief period of immobilization followed by motion.
   b. LCL Injury—Injury to the LCL ligament is uncommon. Varus instability in 30 degrees of flexion is diagnostic. Isolated LCL injuries should be managed nonoperatively.
4. Posterolateral Corner Injuries—These injuries occur rarely as isolated injuries but more commonly are associated with other ligamentous injuries (especially the PCL). Because of poor results with chronic reconstructions, **acute repair is advocated. Examination for increased external rotation,** external rotation recurvatum test, posterolateral drawer test, and reverse pivot shift test are important. Early anatomic repair is often successful, but these injuries are frequently missed. Procedures recommended for

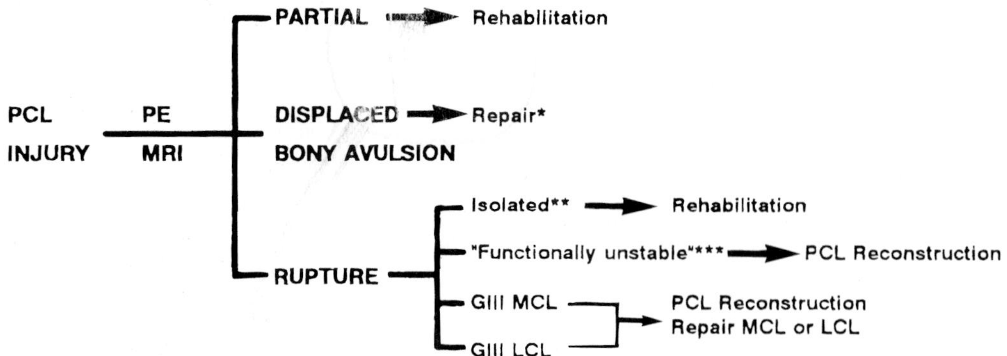

Figure 3–14. Algorithm for treatment of PCL injuries. *with an intact ligament; **without posterolateral injury or combined ligamentous injury; ***failed rehabilitation or unstable/symptomatic with activities of daily living. (From Spindler, K.P., and Walker, R.N.: General approach to ligament surgery. In Fu, F.H., Harner, C.D., and Vince, K.G., eds.: Knee Surgery. Baltimore, Williams & Wilkins, 1994, p. 655.)

chronic injuries include posterolateral corner advancement, popliteus bypass, biceps tenodesis and, more recently, "split" grafts, which are used to reconstruct both the LCL and the popliteus/posterolateral corner (Fig. 3–15).

5. Multiple Ligament Injuries—Combined ligamentous injuries (especially ACL/PCL injuries) can be a result of a knee dislocation, and neurovascular injury must be suspected. **The incidence of vascular injury following anterior knee dislocation is 30 to 50%.** Liberal use of vascular studies is recommended early (Fig. 3–16). Dislocations are classified based on the direction of tibial displacement (Fig. 3–17). Treatment is usually operative. Emergent surgical indications include popliteal artery injury, open dislocations, and irreducible dislocations. Most surgeons recommend delaying surgery 5–12 days to ensure that there is no vascular injury. The use of the arthroscope, especially with a pump, must be limited during these procedures because of the risk of fluid extravasation. Avulsion injuries can be repaired primarily; however, interstitial injuries must be reconstructed.

I. Anterior Knee Pain
  1. Introduction—Anterior knee pain is classified based on etiologic factors (Table 3–1). The term "chondromalacia" should be replaced with a specific diagnosis based on this classification.
  2. Trauma—Includes fractures of the patella (discussed in Chapter 10) and tendon injuries.

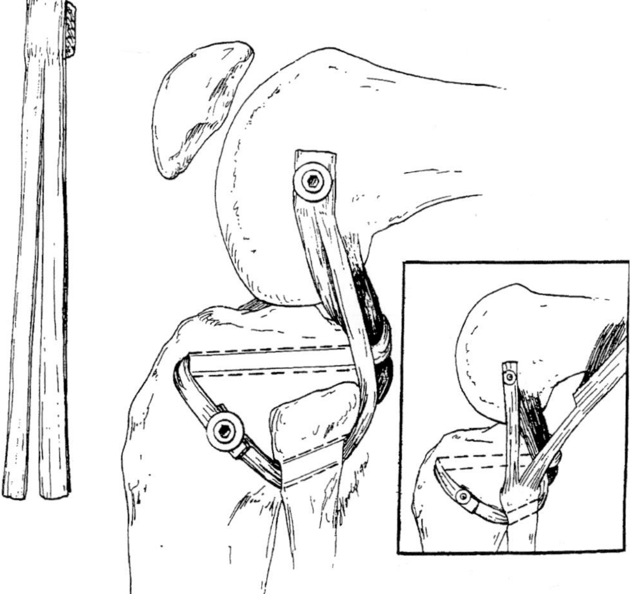

Figure 3–15. Split posterolateral corner graft. (From McKernan, D.J., and Paulos, L.E.: Graft selection. In Fu, F.H., Harner, C.D., and Vince, K.G., eds.: Knee Surgery. Baltimore, Williams & Wilkins, 1994, p. 669.)

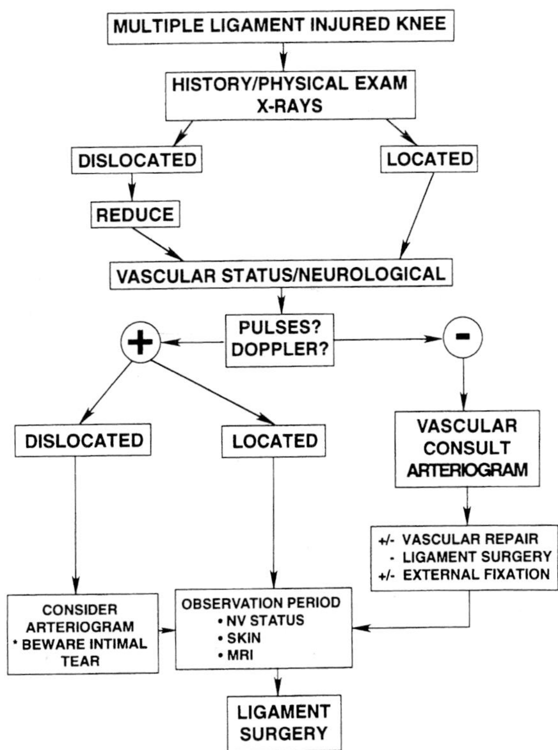

Figure 3–16. Algorithm for the treatment of multiple knee ligament injuries. (From Marks, P.H., and Harner, C.D.: The anterior cruciate ligament in the multiple ligament–injured knee. Clin. Sports Med. 12:825–838, 1993.)

  a. Tendon Ruptures—Quadriceps tendon ruptures are more common than patellar tendon ruptures and occur most commonly in patients over 40 years old with indirect trauma. Patellar tendon ruptures occur in young patients with direct or indirect trauma. Both types of tendon rupture are more common in patients with underlying disorders of the tendon. A palpable defect and inability to extend the knee are diagnostic. Primary repair with temporary stabilization is indicated.
  b. Overuse Injuries
    1. Patellar Tendinitis (Jumper's Knee)—This condition, most common in athletes who participate in sports such as basketball and volleyball, is associated with pain and tenderness near the inferior border of the patella (worse in extension than flexion). Treatment includes nonsteroidal anti-inflammatory drugs (NSAIDs), physical therapy (strengthening and ultrasound), and orthotics (rarely surgery—excision of necrotic tendon fibers).
    2. Quadriceps Tendinitis—Less common but just as painful. Patients may note painful clicking and localized pain. Operative treatment is occasionally necessary.

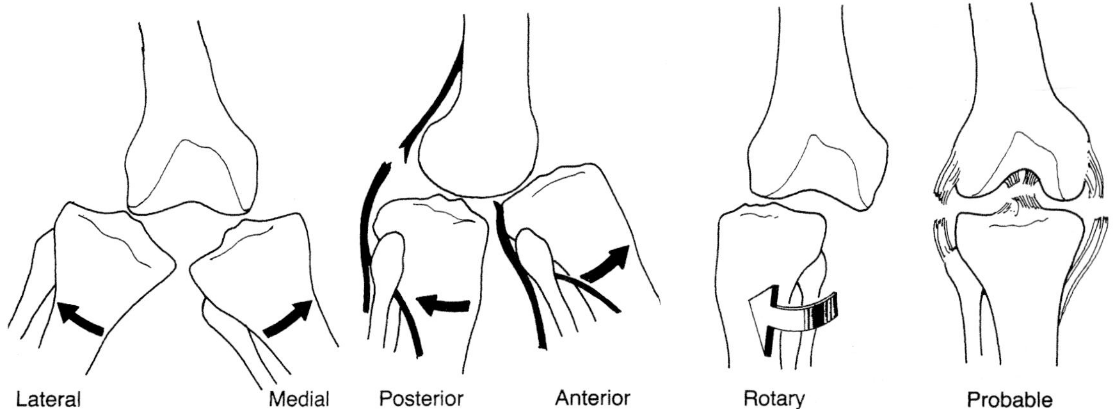

Figure 3–17. Classification of knee dislocations. (From Miller, M.D., Cooper, D.E., and Warner, J.J.P.: Review of Sports Medicine and Arthroscopy. Philadelphia, WB Saunders, 1995, p. 51.)

3. Prepatellar Bursitis (Housemaid's Knee)—It is the most common form of bursitis of the knee and is associated with a history of prolonged kneeling. Supportive treatment (knee pads, occasional steroid injections) and (although rarely) bursal excision are recommended.
4. Iliotibial Band Friction Syndrome—Can occur in runners (especially running hills) and cyclists and is a result of abrasion between the iliotibial band and the lateral femoral condyle. Localized tenderness, worse with the knee flexed 30 degrees, is common. The Ober test (patient lies in a lateral decubitus position and abduction and hyperextension of the hip demonstrate tightness of the iliotibial band) is helpful in making the diagnosis. Rehabilitation is usually successful. Surgical excision of an ellipse of the iliotibial band is occasionally necessary.
5. Semimembranosus Tendinitis—Most common in male athletes in their early thirties, this condition can be diagnosed with nuclear imaging and responds to stretching and strengthening.

c. Late Effects of Trauma
1. Patellofemoral Arthritis—Injury and malalignment can contribute to patellar degenerative joint disease. Lateral release may be beneficial early; however, other procedures may be required for advanced patellar arthritis. Options include anterior or anteromedial transfer of the tibial tubercle, or patellectomy for severe cases.
2. Anterior Fat Pad Syndrome (Hoffa's Disease)—Trauma to the anterior fat pad can lead to fibrous changes and pinching of the fat pad, especially in patients with genu recurvatum. Activity modification, ice, and knee padding can be helpful. Occasionally, arthroscopic excision is beneficial.
3. Reflex Sympathetic Dystrophy—Characterized by **pain out of proportion to physical findings**, reflex sympathetic dystrophy is an exaggerated response to injury. Three stages, progressing from swelling, warmth, and hyperhidrosis to brawny edema and trophic changes and finally to glossy, cool, dry skin and stiffness, are typical. Patellar osteopenia and a "flamingo gait" are also common. Treatment includes nerve stimulation, NSAIDs, and sympathetic or epidural blocks, which can be both diagnostic and therapeutic.

d. Patellofemoral Dysplasia
1. Lateral Patellar Facet Compression Syndrome—This problem is associated with a tight lateral retinaculum and excessive lateral tilt without excessive patellar mobility. Treatment includes activity modification, NSAIDs, and vastus medialis obiquus strengthening. Arthroscopy and **lateral release** are occasionally required. The **best candidates have a neutral or negative tilt and medial patellar glide less than one quadrant with a lateral patellar glide less than three quadrants**. Arthroscopic visualization through a superior portal demonstrates that the patella does not articulate medially by 40 degrees of knee flexion. Lateral release requires care to ensure that **adequate hemostasis** is achieved postoperatively and that the patella can be passively tilted 80 degrees.
2. Patellar Instability—Recurrent subluxation/dislocation of the patella can be characterized by lateral displacement of the patella, a shallow intercondylar sulcus, or patellar incongruence. When

Table 3–1.

Classification of Patellofemoral Disorders

I. Trauma (conditions caused by trauma in the otherwise normal knee)
  A. Acute trauma
    1. Contusion (924.11)
    2. Fracture
      a. Patella (822)
      b. Femoral trochlea (821.2)
      c. Proximal tibial epiphysis (tubercle) (823.0)
    3. Dislocation (rare in the normal knee) (836.3)
    4. Rupture
      a. Quadriceps tendon (843.8)
      b. Patellar tendon (844.8)
  B. Repetitive trauma (overuse syndromes)
    1. Patellar tendinitis ("jumper's knee") (726.64)
    2. Quadriceps tendinitis (726.69)
    3. Peripatellar tendinitis (e.g., anterior knee pain of the adolescent due to hamstring contracture) (726.699)
    4. Prepatellar bursitis ("housemaid's knee") (726.65)
    5. Apophysitis
      a. Osgood-Schlatter disease (732.43)
      b. Sinding-Larsen-Johansson disease (732.42)
  C. Late effects of trauma (905)
    1. Posttraumatic chondromalacia patellae
    2. Posttraumatic patellofemoral arthritis
    3. Anterior fat pad syndrome (posttraumatic fibrosis)
    4. Reflex sympathetic dystrophy of the patella
    5. Patellar osseous dystrophy
    6. Acquired patella infera (719.366)
    7. Acquired quadriceps fibrosis
II. Patellofemoral dysplasia
  A. Lateral patellar compression syndrome (LPCS) (718.365)
    1. Secondary chondromalacia patellae (717.7)
    2. Secondary patellofemoral arthritis (715.289)
  B. Chronic subluxation of the patella (CSP) (718.364)
    1. Secondary chondromalacia patellae (717.7)
    2. Secondary patellofemoral arthritis (715.289)
  C. Recurrent dislocation of the patella (RDP) (718.361)
    1. Associated fractures (822)
      a. Osteochondral (intra-articular)
      b. Avulsion (extra-articular)
    2. Secondary chondromalacia patellae (717.7)
    3. Secondary patellofemoral arthritis (715.289)
  D. Chronic dislocation of the patella (718.362)
    1. Congenital
    2. Acquired
III. Idiopathic chondromalacia patellae (717.7)
IV. Osteochondritis dissecans
  A. Patella (732.704)
  B. Femoral trochlea (732.703)
V. Synovial plicae (727.8916) (anatomic variant made symptomatic by acute or repetitive trauma)
  A. Medial patellar ("shelf") (727.89161)
  B. Suprapatellar (727.89163)
  C. Lateral patellar (727.89165)

Orthopaedic ICD-9-CM Expanded Diagnostic Codes in parentheses.
From Merchant, A.C.: Classification of patellofemoral disorders. Arthroscopy 4:235, 1988.

associated with femoral anteversion, genu valgum, and pronated feet, the symptoms can be exacerbated, especially in adolescents ("miserable malalignment syndrome"). Extensive rehabilitation is often curative. Surgical procedures include proximal and/or distal realignment procedures. Acute, first-time patella dislocations may be best treated with arthroscopic evaluation/débridement and acute repair of the medial patellofemoral ligament (usually at the medial epicondyle).

e. Chondromalacia—Although this term has fallen into disfavor, articular damage and changes to the patella are common. Treatment is usually symptomatic. Débridement procedures are of questionable benefit.

f. Abnormalities of Patellar Height—Patella alta (high-riding patella) and baja (low-riding patella) are determined based on various measurements made on lateral radiographs of the knee (see Fig. 3–5). Patella alta can be associated with patellar instability because the patella may not articulate with the sulcus, which normally constrains the patella. Patella baja is often the result of fat pad and tendon fibrosis and may require proximal transfer of the tubercle for refractory cases.

J. Pediatric Knee Disorders

1. Physeal Injuries—Most commonly involve Salter-Harris II fractures of the distal femoral physis. Pain, swelling, and an inability to ambulate are common. **Stress radiographs may be necessary to make the diagnosis.** Open reduction and internal fixation are indicated for Salter-Harris III and IV fractures and Salter-Harris I and II fractures that cannot be adequately reduced. It is important to counsel the parents that, unlike with other type II fractures, knee physeal injuries may have a worse prognosis.

2. Ligament Injuries—Most ligament injuries are treated like those in adults. Midsubstance ACL injuries in skeletally immature individuals remains a subject of considerable debate. Procedures that do not violate the growth plate are usually recommended for patients who fail nonoperative management. Avulsion fractures of the intercondylar eminence of the tibia are treated with closed treatment; if this treatment fails, arthroscopic reduction and fixation of the fragment are undertaken. Midsubstance injuries may be best addressed with procedures that avoid the physis, especially on the femoral side.

3. Traction Apophysitis—Includes Osgood-Schlatter disease and Sinding-Larsen-Johansson disease; it is usually treated symptomatically. Occasionally, procedures such as ossicle excision are indicated for refractory cases.

II. **Other Lower Extremity Sports Medicine Problems**

A. Nerve Entrapment Syndromes

1. Ilioinguinal Nerve Entrapment—This nerve can be constricted by hypertrophied abdominal muscles as a result of intensive training. Hyperextension of the hip may exacerbate the pain that patients experience, and hyper-

esthesia symptoms are common. Surgical release is occasionally necessary.

2. Obturator Nerve Entrapment—Can lead to chronic medial thigh pain, especially in athletes with well-developed hip adductor muscles (e.g., skaters). Nerve conduction studies are helpful for establishing the diagnosis. Treatment is usually supportive.
3. Lateral Femoral Cutaneous Nerve Entrapment—Can lead to a painful condition termed **meralgia paresthetica.** Tight belts and prolonged hip flexion may exacerbate symptoms. Release of compressive devices, postural exercises, and nonsteroidal anti-inflammatory drugs (NSAIDs) are usually curative.
4. Saphenous Nerve Entrapment—Compressed at Hunter's canal or in the proximal leg, this nerve can cause painful symptoms inferior and medial to the knee.
5. Peroneal Nerve Entrapment—The common peroneal nerve can be compressed behind the fibula or injured by a direct blow to this area. The superficial peroneal nerve can be entrapped about 12 cm proximal to the tip of the lateral malleolus, where it exits the fascia of the anterolateral leg, as a result of inversion injuries. **Fascial defects** can be present as well, contributing to the problem. Compartment release is sometimes indicated. The deep peroneal nerve can be compressed by the inferior extensor retinaculum, leading to **anterior tarsal tunnel syndrome,** sometimes necessitating release of this structure.
6. Tibial Nerve Entrapment—When the tibial nerve is compressed under the flexor retinaculum behind the medial malleolus, it may result in **tarsal tunnel syndrome.** Electromyelography/nerve conduction study evaluation is helpful, and surgical release is sometimes indicated. Distal entrapment of the first branch of the lateral plantar nerve (to the adductor digiti quinti) has also been described.
7. Medial Plantar Nerve Entrapment—Occurs at the point where the flexor digitorum longus and flexor hallucis longus cross (knot of Henry) and is most commonly caused by external compression by orthotics. Commonly called **jogger's foot,** this condition usually responds to conservative measures.

B. Contusions
   1. Iliac Crest Contusions—Direct trauma to this area can occur in contact sports; known commonly as a **hip pointer.** An avulsion of the iliac apophysis should be ruled out in adolescent athletes. Treatment consists of ice, compression, pain control, and placing the affected leg on maximum stretch. Additional padding is indicated after the acute phase.
   2. Groin Contusions—An avulsion fracture of the lesser trochanter must be ruled out before supportive treatment.
   3. Quadriceps Contusions—Can result in hemorrhage and late myositis ossificans. Acute management includes cold compression and **immobilization in flexion.** Close monitoring for compartment syndrome should be accomplished acutely.

C. Muscle Injuries
   1. Hamstring Strain—This common injury is often the result of sudden stretch on the musculotendinous junction during sprinting. These injuries can occur anywhere in the

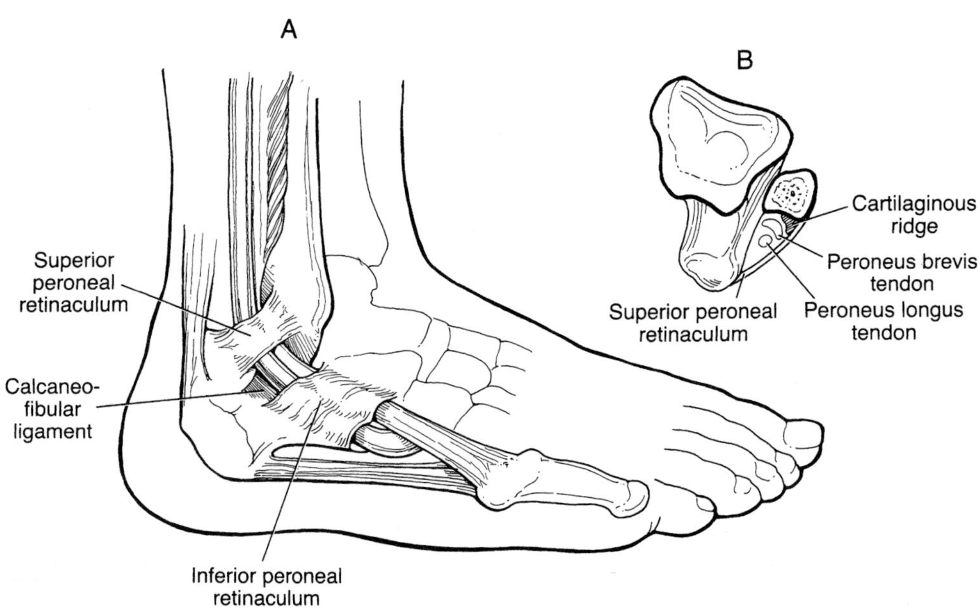

Figure 3–18. Normal relationship of the peroneal tendons. Note the superior and inferior retinacula and the cartilaginous ridge on the posterolateral fibula. *A,* Lateral view. *B,* Superior view. (From Miller, M.D., Cooper, D.E., and Warner, J.J.P.: Review of Sports Medicine and Arthroscopy. Philadelphia, WB Saunders, 1995, p. 82.)

posterior thigh. Treatment is supportive, followed by stretching and strengthening. To prevent recurrence, return to play should be delayed until strength is approximately 90% of the opposite side.

2. Adductor Strain—Common in sports such as soccer, these injuries must be differentiated from subtle hernias.
3. Rectus Femoris Strain—Acute injuries are usually located more distally on the thigh, but chronic injuries are more commonly near the muscle origin. Treatment includes ice and stretching/strengthening.
4. Gastrocnemius-Soleus Strain—Nicknamed **tennis leg** because of its common association with that sport, this injury is probably much more common than rupture of the plantaris tendon. Supportive treatment is indicated.

D. Tendon Injuries

1. Peroneal Tendon Injuries
   a. Subluxation/Dislocation—Violent dorsiflexion of the inverted foot can result in injury of the fibro-osseous peroneal tendon sheath. Diagnosis is confirmed by observing the subluxation or dislocation by means of eversion and dorsiflexion of the foot. Plain radiographs may demonstrate a rim fracture of the lateral aspect of the distal fibula. Treatment of acute injuries includes restoration of the normal anatomy (Fig. 3–18). Chronic reconstruction involves groove-deepening procedures, tissue transfers, or bone block techniques.
   b. Longitudinal Tears of the Peroneal Tendons (Especially Brevis Tendon)—Recognized with increasing frequency. Repair and decompression are generally recommended.
2. Posterior Tibialis Tendon Injury—This injury can occur in older athletes. Débridement of partial ruptures and flexor digitorum longus transfer for chronic injuries are recommended.
3. Achilles Tendon Injuries
   a. Tendinitis—Overuse injury to the Achilles tendon usually responds to rest and physical therapy modalities. Progression to partial rupture may necessitate surgical excision of scar and granulation tissue.
   b. Rupture—Complete rupture of the tendon is caused by maximal plantar flexion with the foot planted. Patients may relate that they felt as if they were "shot." The Thompson test (squeezing the calf results in plantar flexion of the foot normally) is helpful for confirming the diagnosis. Treatment remains controversial; however, recurrence rates can be reduced with primary repair.

E. Chronic/Exertional Compartment Syndrome—Although more commonly encountered with trauma, sports-related compartment syndrome is becoming more frequently diagnosed. Athletes (especially runners and cyclists) may note pain that has a gradual onset during exercise, ultimately restricting their performance. Compartment pressures taken before, during, and after exercise **(pressures >15 mm Hg 15 minutes after exercise, or absolute values above 15 mm Hg while resting or above 30 mm Hg after exercise)** can help establish the diagnosis. The anterior and deep posterior compartments of the leg are most often involved. Fasciotomy is sometimes indicated for refractory cases (Fig. 3–19).

F. Stress Fractures

1. Common Characteristics—A history of overuse with an insidious onset of pain and localized tenderness and swelling are typical. Bone scan can be diagnostic, even with normal plain radiographs. Treatment includes protected weight-bearing, rest, cross-training, analgesics, and therapeutic modalities.
2. Femoral Neck Stress Fractures—Tension, or transverse, fractures are more serious than compression fractures and may require operative stabilization.
3. Femoral Shaft Fractures—Usually respond

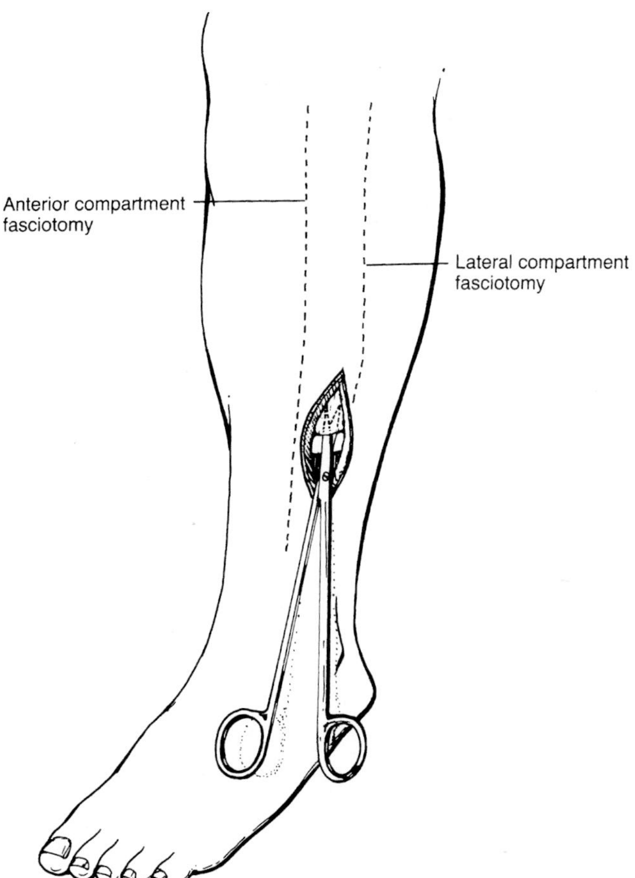

Figure 3–19. Anterior and lateral compartment release. (From DeLee, J.C., and Drez, D., Jr.: Orthopaedic Sports Medicine: Principles and Practice. Philadelphia, WB Saunders, 1994, p. 1618.)

to protected weight-bearing but can progress to complete fractures if unrecognized.

4. Tibial Shaft Fractures—Can be difficult. Persistence of the "dreaded black line" (Fig. 3–20) for more than 6 months, especially with a positive bone scan, can be an indication for bone grafting.
5. Tarsal Navicular Fractures—Can be challenging. Immobilization and **no weight-bearing** are important during the early management of these stress fractures.
6. Jones Fractures—Fractures at the metaphyseal diaphyseal junction of the fifth metatarsal in the athlete can be **treated more aggressively with early open reduction and internal fixation to allow an earlier return to conditioning activities.**

G. Other Hip Disorders

1. Snapping Hip—Condition in which the iliotibial band abruptly catches on the greater trochanter, or by iliopsoas impingement on the hip capsule. The iliotibial condition, more common in females with wide pelves and prominent trochanters, can be exacerbated by running on banked surfaces. The snapping may be reproduced with passive hip flexion from an adducted position. Stretching/strengthening modalities, such as ultrasonography and, occasionally, surgical release, may relieve the snapping. This condition must be differentiated from the less common snapping iliopsoas tendon, which can be diagnosed with extension and internal rotation of the hip from a flexed and externally rotated position. Arthrography and/or bursography may also be helpful in making the diagnosis.
2. Traumatic Avascular Necrosis—Traumatic hip subluxation can disrupt the arterial blood supply to the hip and result in avascular necrosis. Early recognition of these injuries, seen in football players, is essential.
3. Proximal Femoral Fractures—Can occur in athletes, especially cross-country skiers (**skier's hip**). Release bindings may reduce the incidence of these injuries.

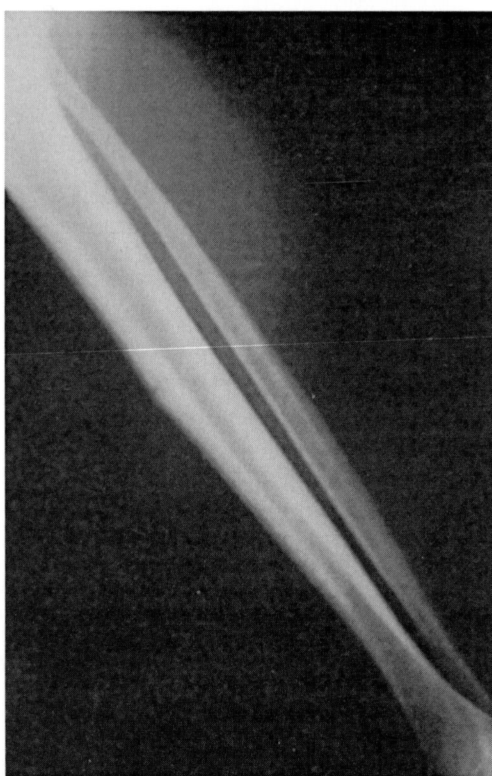

Figure 3–20. Radiograph demonstrating the "dreaded black line" associated with an impending complete fracture of the tibial shaft. (From Miller, M.D., Cooper, D.E., and Warner, J.J.P.: Review of Sports Medicine and Arthroscopy. Philadelphia, WB Saunders, 1995, p. 81.)

H. Other Foot and Ankle Disorders

1. Plantar Fasciitis—Inflammation of the plantar fascia, usually in the central to medial subcalcaneal region, is common in runners. Rest, orthotics, stretching, and NSAIDs are helpful. Occasionally, plantar fasciotomy is necessary, but recovery can be protracted.
2. Os Trigonum—An unfused fractured os trigonum can cause impingement with plantar flexion of the foot, especially in ballet dancers. Treatment may include local anesthetic injection and other supportive measures. Surgical excision of the offending bone is occasionally necessary.
3. Ankle Sprains—These injuries are common in athletes and most often **involve the anterior talofibular ligament.** The Ottawa ankle rules indicate that radiographs are required only in patients with distal (especially posterior) tibia or fibula tenderness, tenderness at the base of the 5th metatarsal or navicular, and an inability to bear weight. Surgical treatment is reserved for recurrent, symptomatic ankle instability with excessive tilt and drawer on examination/stress radiographs that has not responded to orthotics and peroneal strengthening over an extended period. Anatomic procedures (Brostrom's) are usually successful. Involvement of the subtalar joint requires tendon rerouting procedures that include this joint. Patients with "high" ankle sprains involving the syndesmosis require recovery periods almost twice those for common ankle sprains.
4. Turf Toe—Severe dorsiflexion of the MTP joint of the great toe can result in a tender, stiff, swollen toe. Treatment includes motion, ice, and taping. If symptoms persist, a stress fracture of the proximal phalanx should be ruled out with a bone scan.

I. Arthroscopy

1. Hip Arthroscopy—A relatively new procedure; advocates suggest that loose body removal, synovectomy, and labral débridement are indications. Lateral decubitus or, more

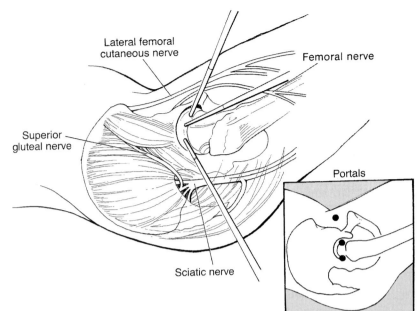

Figure 3–21. Portals for hip arthroscopy include the anterior portal and two portals adjacent to the greater trochanter. (From Miller, M.D., Cooper, D.E., and Warner, J.J.P.: Review of Sports Medicine and Arthroscopy. Philadelphia, WB Saunders, 1995, p. 107.)

recently, supine positioning with approximately 50 pounds of traction with a well-padded perineal post is recommended. Three portals are commonly used for instrumentation—one on each side of the greater trochanter and an additional anterior portal (Fig. 3–21).

2. Ankle Arthroscopy—Indications include treatment of osteochondral injuries of the talus, débridement of post-traumatic synovitis, anterolateral impingement, removal of anterior tibiotalar spurring, and cartilage débridement in conjunction with ankle fusions. Supine positioning with the leg over a well-padded bolster and an external traction device are currently popular. Five portals have been suggested (Fig. 3–22), but most surgeons avoid the posteromedial portal, because of risk to the posterial tibial artery and tibial nerve, and the anterocentral portal, because of risk to the dorsalis pedis and deep peroneal nerve. The "nick and spread" method is advocated for the **anterolateral portal (superficial peroneal nerve) and the anteromedial portal (saphenous vein).** Treatment of osteochondral injuries of the talus, including drilling of the base of these lesions and fixation of replaceable lesions, has been advocated. **Lateral lesions are usually traumatic, shallow, and anterior; medial**

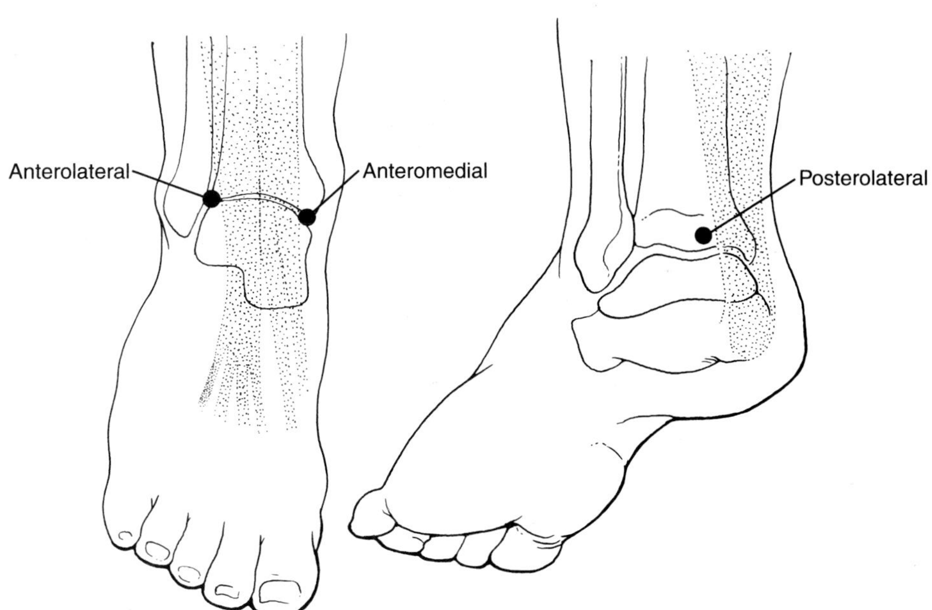

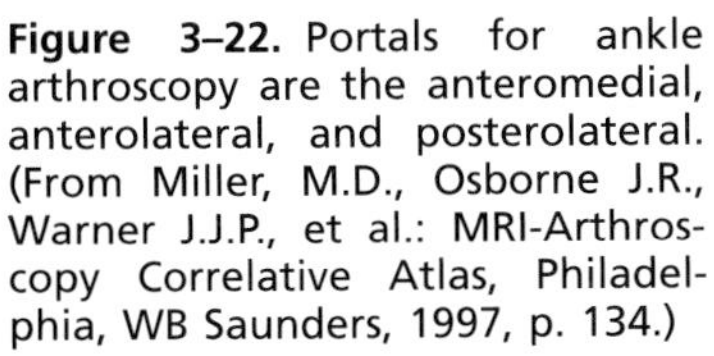
Figure 3–22. Portals for ankle arthroscopy are the anteromedial, anterolateral, and posterolateral. (From Miller, M.D., Osborne J.R., Warner J.J.P., et al.: MRI-Arthroscopy Correlative Atlas, Philadelphia, WB Saunders, 1997, p. 134.)

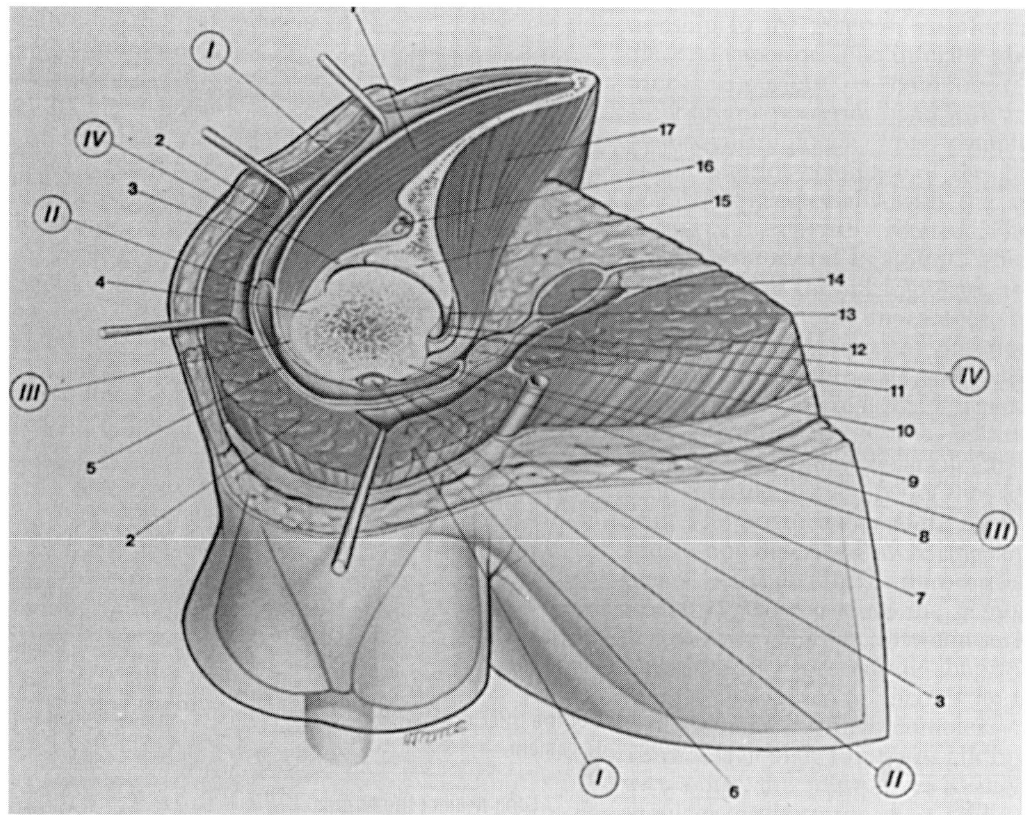

Figure 3–26. Cross-sectional view of the right shoulder at the level of the lesser tuberosity. Note the four layers of the shoulder and their components: I—deltoid (2), pectoralis major (12), cephalic vein (9); II—conjoined tendon (10), pectoralis minor (14), claviopectoral fascia (7); III—subdeltoid bursa (5), rotator cuff muscles (1, 17), glenohumeral capsule (11), greater tuberosity (4), long head of biceps (6), lesser tuberosity (8), fascia (3), synovium (13), glenoid (15). (From Cooper, D.E., O'Brien, S.J., and Warren, R.F.: Supporting layers of the glenohumeral joint: An anatomic study. Clin. Orthop. 289:144–155, 1993.)

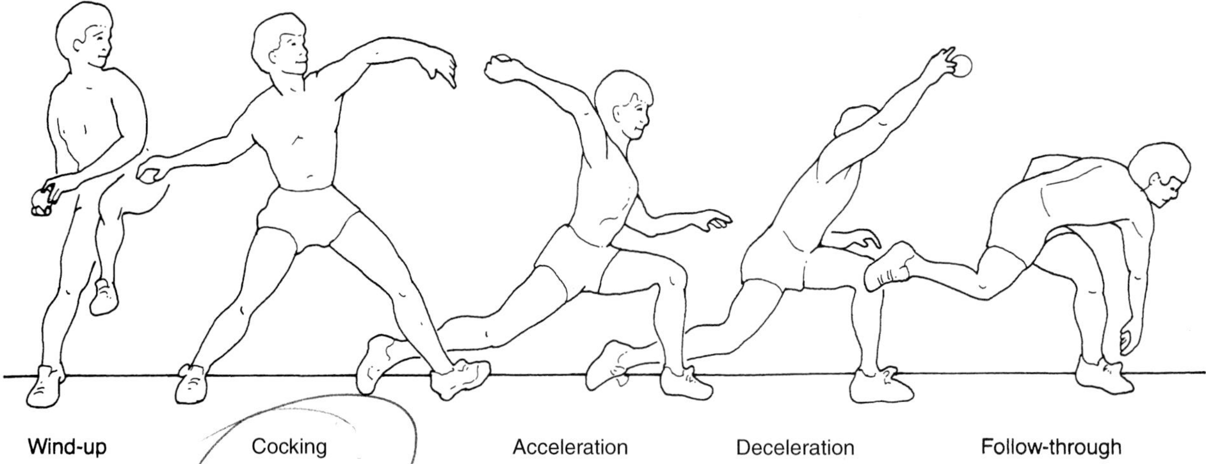

Figure 3–27. The five phases of throwing. (From Miller, M.D., Cooper, D.E., and Warner, J.J.P.: Review of Sports Medicine and Arthroscopy. Philadelphia, WB Saunders, 1995, p. 123.)

Examination	Technique	Significance
Impingement sign	Passive FF >90°	Pain = impingement syndrome
Impingement test	Same after subacromial lidocaine	Relief of pain = impingement syndrome
Hawkins test	Passive FF 90° and int. rotation	Pain = impingement syndrome
Apprehension test	Abd. 90° and ext. rotation	Apprehension = ant. shoulder instability
Relocation test (Fig. 3–28)	Supine apprehension with posterior force	Relief of apprehension = ant. shoulder instability
Posterior apprehension	Forward flexion 90°, internal rotation, posterior force	Apprehension = posterior instability
Sulcus sign	Downward traction on arm	Presence of sulcus below acromion = inferior laxity
Crossed chest adduction test	Passive FF 90° and adduction	Pain = acromioclavicular pathology
AC injection	Same after AC lidocaine injection	Relief of symptoms = acromioclavicular pathology
Bicipital tenderness	Localized tenderness	Bicipital tendinitis
Yergason test	Resisted supination	Pain = bicipital tendinitis
Speed test	Resisted forward elevation of arm	Pain = bicipital tendinitis
Lift-off sign	Arm behind back lifted posteriorly	Inability to accomplish = subscapularis rupture
Wright's test	Ext-Abd-ER arm, neck rotated away	Loss of pulse and reproduction of Sx = thoracic outlet syndrome
Spurling test (Fig. 3–29)	Lat. flexion, rotation and compression of neck	Cervical spine pathology

B. History and Physical Examination

1. History—Age and chief complaint are two important considerations. Instability, acromioclavicular injuries, and distal clavicle osteolysis are more common in young patients. Rotator cuff tears, arthritis, and proximal humeral fractures are more common in older patients. Direct blows are usually responsible for acromioclavicular separations. Instability is related to injury to the abducted, externally rotated arm. Chronic overhead pain and night pain are associated with rotator cuff tears.
2. Physical Examination—Observation and palpation can lead to important diagnostic clues. Evaluation of range of motion (normally 160 degrees forward flexion, 30–60 degrees external rotation, and internal rotation T6) and strength testing are also important. Special testing includes the following examinations (as shown at the top of this page).

C. Imaging the Shoulder—The trauma series of radiographs includes a "true" anteroposterior view (plate is placed parallel to the scapula, about 45 degrees from the plane of the thorax) and an axillary lateral view. Other views that are sometimes helpful include a scapular Y or transscapular view and anteroposterior radiographs in internal and external rotation. Special radiographic views have also been developed for certain other abnormalities. For example, the supraspinatus outlet view is helpful in the evaluation of impingement (Fig. 3–30).

D. Shoulder Arthroscopy

1. Portals—Standard portals include the posterior portal (2 cm distal and medial to posterolateral border of acromion, used for the scope), anterior portals (lateral to the coracoid and below the biceps, used for instrumentation), lateral portal (for acromioplasty), and supraspinatus (Neviaser's) portal for anterior glenoid visualization (rarely used), as demonstrated in Fig. 3–31. The port of Wilmington has recently been described, and may be useful for repair of *S*uperior *L*abral *A*ntero*P*osterior (SLAP) lesion (as shown at the bottom of this page).
2. Technique—Orderly evaluation of the biceps tendon, articular surfaces, rotator cuff, labrum, and glenohumeral ligaments should be accomplished. Subacromial bursoscopy can allow coracoacromial ligament resection, acromioplasty, and distal clavicle resection.

View/Sign	Findings	Significance
Supraspinatus outlet view (Fig. 3–30)	Acromial morphology (types I–III)	Type III (hooked) acromion associated with impingement
30° Caudal tilt view	Subacromial spurring	Area below level of clavicle = impingement area
Zanca 10° cephalic tilt	AC joint pathology	AC DJD, distal clavicle osteolysis
West Point	Anteroinferior glenoid evaluation	Bony Bankart lesion seen with instability
Garth view	Anteroinferior glenoid evaluation	Bony Bankart
Stryker notch	Humeral head evaluation	Hill-Sachs impression fracture with recurrent dislocation episodes
AP int. rot.	Humeral head evaluation	**Hill-Sachs defect**
Hobbs view	Sternoclavicular injury	Anteroposterior dislocations
Serendipity view	Sternoclavicular injury	Ant.-post. dislocation
45° Abduction true AP	Glenohumeral space	Subtle DJD
Arthrography	Rotator cuff injuries	Dye above cuff = tear
CT	Fractures	Classification easier
MRI ± arthro-MRI	Soft tissue evaluation	Labral, cuff, muscle tears

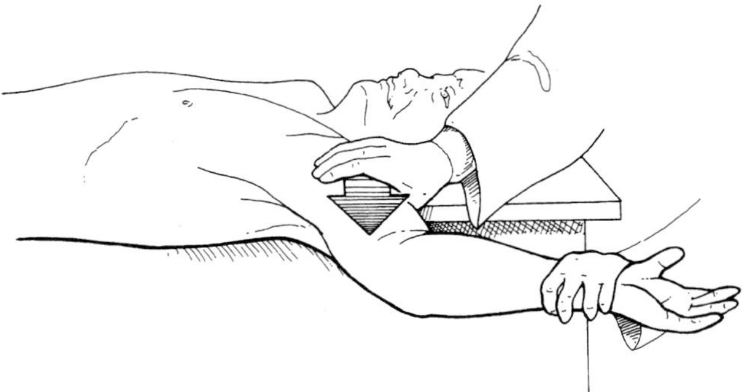

Figure 3–28. Relocation test. Anterior pressure on the proximal arm relocates the humerus and causes relief of apprehension. (From Miller, M.D., Cooper, D.E., and Warner, J.J.P.: Review of Sports Medicine and Arthroscopy. Philadelphia, WB Saunders, 1995, p. 128.)

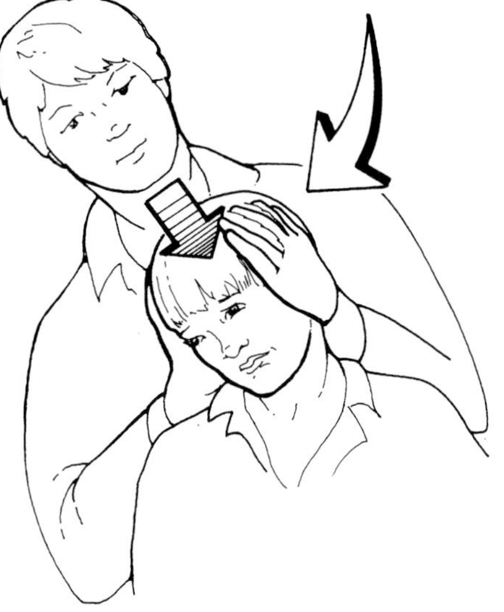

Figure 3–29. Spurling's test. Lateral flexion and rotation with some compression may cause nerve root encroachment and pain on the ipsilateral side in patients with cervical nerve root impingement. (From Miller, M.D., Cooper, D.E., and Warner, J.J.P.: Review of Sports Medicine and Arthroscopy. Philadelphia, WB Saunders, 1995, p. 129.)

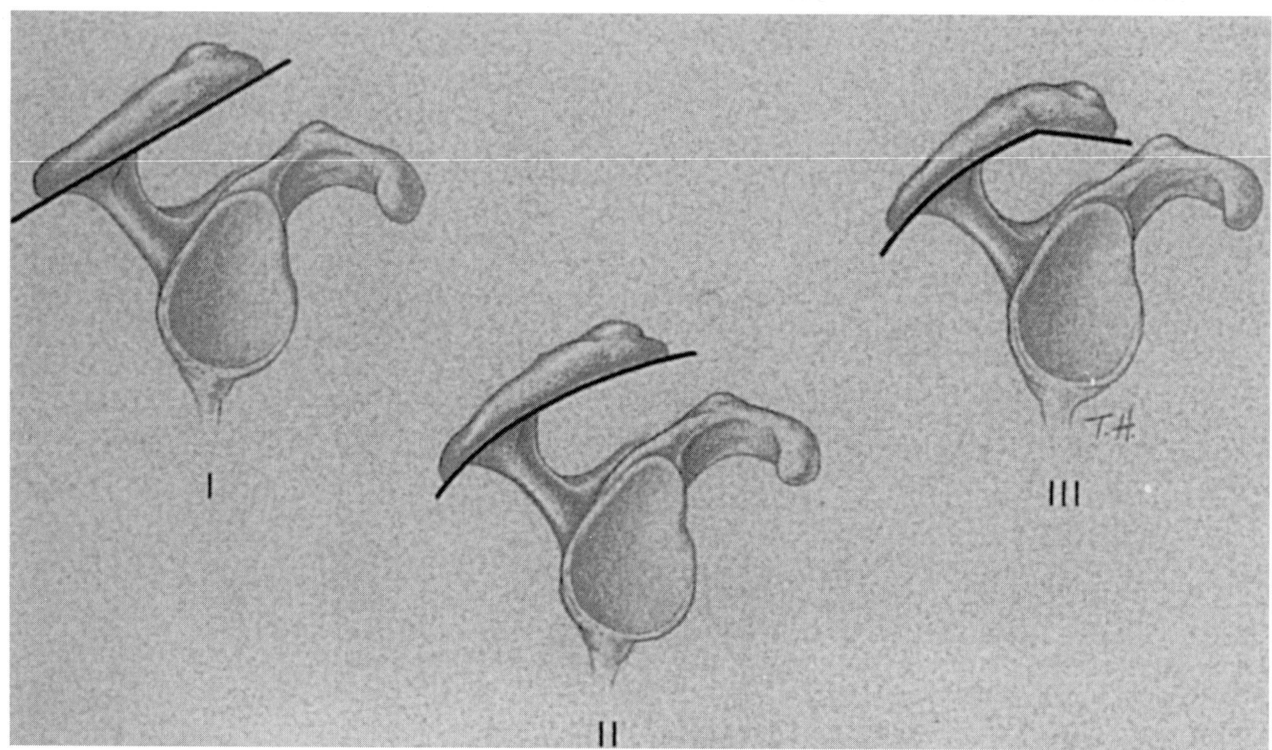

Figure 3–30. Acromion morphology is classified on the basis of the supraspinatus outlet view as originally described by Bigliani. (From Esch, J.C.: Shoulder arthroscopy in the older age group. Op. Tech. Orthop. 1:200, 1991.)

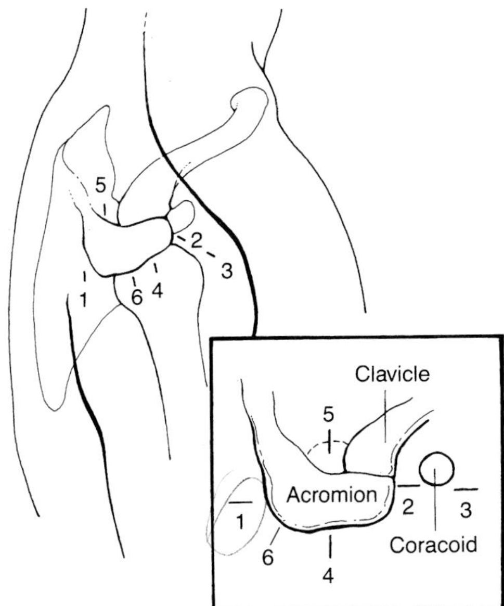

Figure 3–31. Arthroscopic portals of the shoulder. 1, posterior; 2, anterosuperior; 3, anteroinferior; 4, lateral; 5, supraspinatus (Neviaser's); 6, port of Wilmington. (From Miller, M.D., Cooper, D.E., and Warner, J.J.P.: Review of Sports Medicine and Arthroscopy. Philadelphia, WB Saunders, 1995, p. 135.)

E. Shoulder Instability

1. Diagnosis—The shoulder is the most commonly dislocated joint in the body. Anterior dislocations, by far the most common, are often classified based on the mechanism of injury. Diagnosis of instability is based on history, physical examination, and imaging. *T*raumatic *U*nilateral dislocations with a *B*ankart lesion often require *S*urgery (*TUBS*) because they typically occur in young patients and have recurrence rates of up to 80–90% with nonoperative management. *A*traumatic *M*ultidirectional *B*ilateral shoulder dislocation/subluxation often responds to *R*ehabilitation, and sometimes an *I*nferior capsular shift is required (*AMBRI*). **Anterior dislocations may be associated with greater tuberosity fractures; posterior dislocations may have associated lesser tuberosity fractures. Axillary nerve injuries and rotator cuff tears can also occur in conjunction with anterior dislocations, especially in older individuals.**

2. Treatment—Nonoperative management of anterior shoulder instability includes immobilization for 2–4 weeks based on the age of the patient (longer for young patients) followed by an aggressive rotator cuff strengthening program. Arthroscopic Bankart's repair may be effective in young active patients with first-time traumatic shoulder dislocations. Many procedures have been developed for recurrent instability, including the following (as shown at the bottom of this page).

   Complications of open procedures can also include subscapularis overtightening (Z-lengthening required) or rupture (repair +/− pectoralis transfer required) and hardware problems. In addition to these "open" procedures, several techniques for arthroscopic treatment of anterior instability have been developed. These procedures specifically address the Bankart lesion and not the capsule, and they are therefore not indicated for patients with multidirectional instability or multiple recurrences (with capsular stretching). Popular fixation methods include transglenoid suture techniques (Caspari, Morgan, Maki), absorbable tacks (Warren), and suture anchors (Snyder and others). Although the role for arthroscopic treatment of shoulder instability is still unclear, it is perhaps most efficacious for young patients who do not participate in contact sports with first- (or second-) time traumatic dislocations, without systemic laxity.

   Thermal shrinkage procedures have become immensely popular; however, their efficacy has yet to be proved.

3. Posterior Shoulder Instability—Much less common and less amenable to surgical correction. Acute dislocations, in which the patient may present with an internally rotated arm and coracoid and posterior prominence, do well with acute reduction and immobilization. **An axillary lateral radiograph is required to make the diagnosis.** Nonoperative treatment should emphasize external rotator and posterior deltoid strengthening. Surgical management is difficult because the posterior capsule is often very thin; however, posterior capsular shift procedures can be helpful in refractory cases.

Procedure	Essential Features	Complications
Bankart	Reattachment of labrum (and IGHLC) to glenoid	"Gold standard"
Staple capsulorraphy	Capsular reattachment and tightening	Staple migration/articular injury
Putti-Platt	Subscapularis advancement capsular coverage	Decreased external rotation, DJD
Magnuson-Stack	Subscapularis transfer to greater tuberosity	Decreased external rotation
Boyd-Sisk	Transfer of biceps laterally and posteriorly	Nonanatomic, recurrence
Bristow	Coracoid transfer to inferior glenoid	Nonunion, migration, recurrence, missed labral tears
Bone block osteotomy	Anterior bone block	Nonunion, migration, articular injury
Capsular shift	Inferior capsule shifted superiorly—"pants over vest"	Overtightening, "gold standard" for multidirectional instability

Table 3–2.

Stages of Subacromial Impingement Syndrome

Stage	Age (Years)	Pathology	Clinical Course	Treatment
I	<25	Edema and hemorrhage	Reversible	Conservative
II	25–40	Fibrosis and tendinitis	Activity-related pain	Therapy/operative
III	>40	AC spur and cuff tear	Progressive disability	Acromioplasty/repair

F. Impingement Syndrome/Rotator Cuff Disease

1. Diagnosis—Although traditionally considered a disease of the older population, rotator cuff impingement and tears are becoming increasingly common in throwing athletes because of repetitive overuse. Neer identified three stages of subacromial impingement (Table 3–2). Patients typically present with pain during overhead activities and have characteristic physical examination findings and radiographs (see above).
2. Treatment—Nonoperative treatment includes activity modification, modalities such as ultrasonography and iontophoresis, subacromial corticosteroid injection, and rotator cuff strengthening. Surgical treatment includes subacromial decompression (removal of the coracoacromial ligament and subacromial spur) and rotator cuff repair (into a bony trough at the greater tuberosity) if necessary. Arthroscopic subacromial decompression can be as successful as open decompression when correctly performed and may allow earlier rehabilitation because the majority of the deltoid insertion is spared. Arthroscopic or arthroscopically-assisted rotator cuff repair can also be successful for small, easily mobilized tears.
3. Rotator Cuff Arthropathy—This condition is associated with glenohumeral joint degeneration in conjunction with a massive chronic tear of the cuff. Hemiarthroplasty with a large head may be helpful if the anterior deltoid is preserved.
4. Subcoracoid Impingement—This unusual condition is associated with a laterally placed coracoid that can impinge on the proximal humerus with forward flexion and internal rotation. Computed tomography (CT) with the arm in the provocative position and relief with local anesthetic injection in the area can reveal the diagnosis. Treatment may include resection of the lateral aspect of the coracoid process.
5. Internal Impingement—Impingement of the posterior labrum and cuff can occur in throwing athletes with external rotation and anterior translation (secondary impingement). Treatment may include arthroscopic labral débridement/repair.

G. Biceps Tendon Injuries

1. Biceps Tendinitis—Often associated with impingement syndrome, it can also exist as an isolated entity. Tenderness along the bicipital groove, the Speed and Yergason tests (see chart), can help confirm the diagnosis. Treatment of associated impingement syndrome often relieves symptoms. Rarely, tenodesis of the biceps tendon into the proximal humerus using a "keyhole" technique can be helpful in chronic injuries or tears.
2. Biceps Tendon Subluxation—Most often associated with a subscapularis tear, this condition is associated with instability and medial displacement of the tendon out of its groove. Occasionally, the tendon must be relocated into a deepened groove and stabilized operatively.
3. Superior Labral Lesions—SLAP lesions have been classified into seven varieties (Fig. 3–32).

Type	Description	Treatment
I	Biceps fraying, intact anchor on superior labrum	Arthroscopic débridement
II	Detachment of biceps anchor	Reattachment/stabilization
III	Bucket-Handle superior labral tear; biceps intact	Arthroscopic débridement
IV	Bucket-Handle tear of superior labrum into biceps	Repair or tenodesis of tendon based on symptoms and condition of remaining tendon
V	Labral tear + SLAP	Stabilize both
VI	Superior flap tear	Débride
VII	Capsular injury + SLAP	Repair and stabilize

H. Acromioclavicular and Sternoclavicular Injuries

1. Acromioclavicular Separation—This common athletic injury results from a direct fall onto the shoulder. Acromioclavicular separations are classified as shown in Figure 3–33 and in this chart. Treatment of type III injuries is controversial, but most surgeons currently favor nonoperative management. Type IV–VI injuries should be reduced and stabilized with some form of temporary coraco-

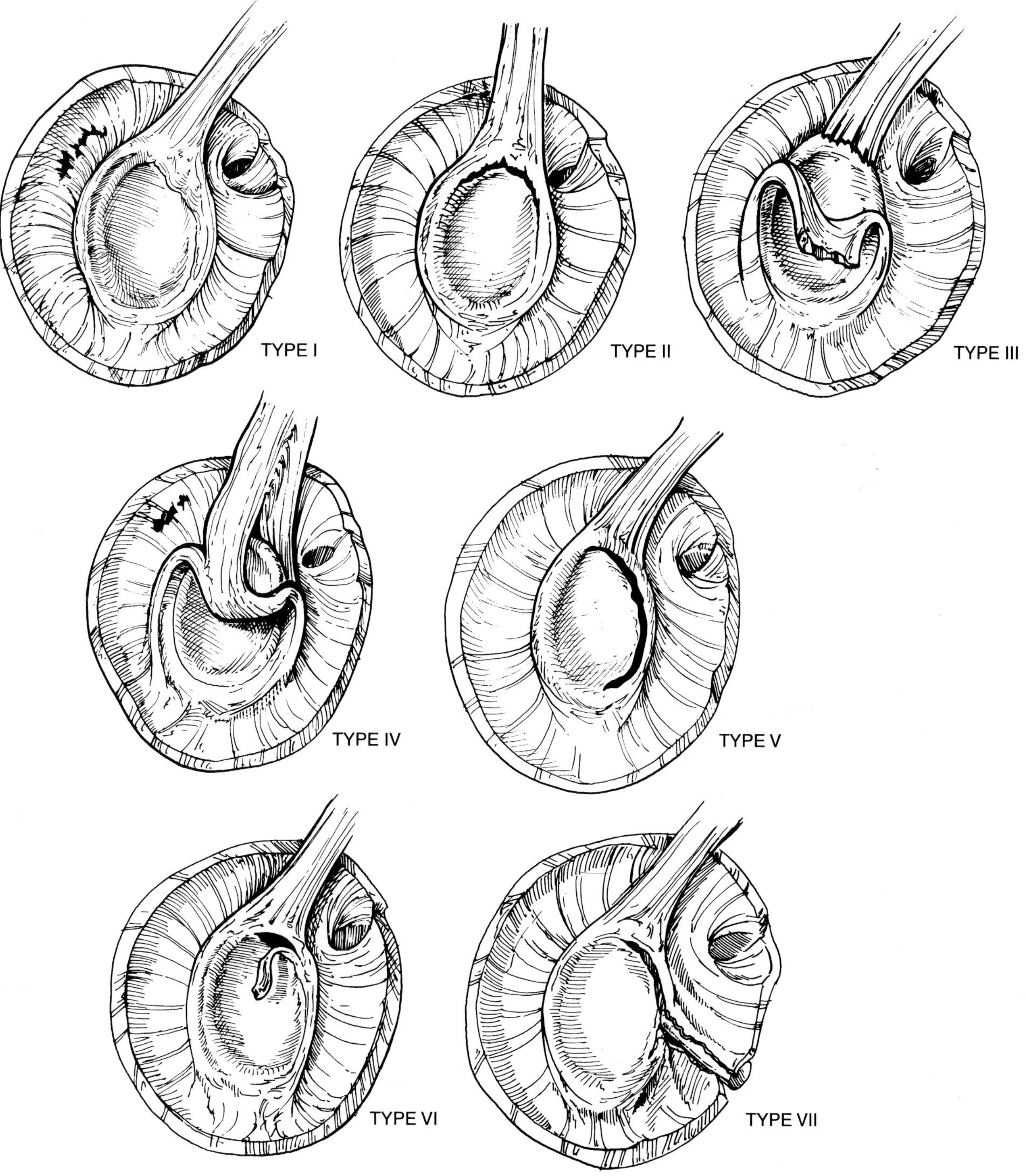

Figure 3–32. Superior labral anterior posterior lesions types I–IV and types V–VII. (From Miller, M.D., Osborne J.R., Warner J.J.P., et al.: MRI-Arthroscopy Correlative Atlas. Philadelphia, WB Saunders, 1997, p. 157.)

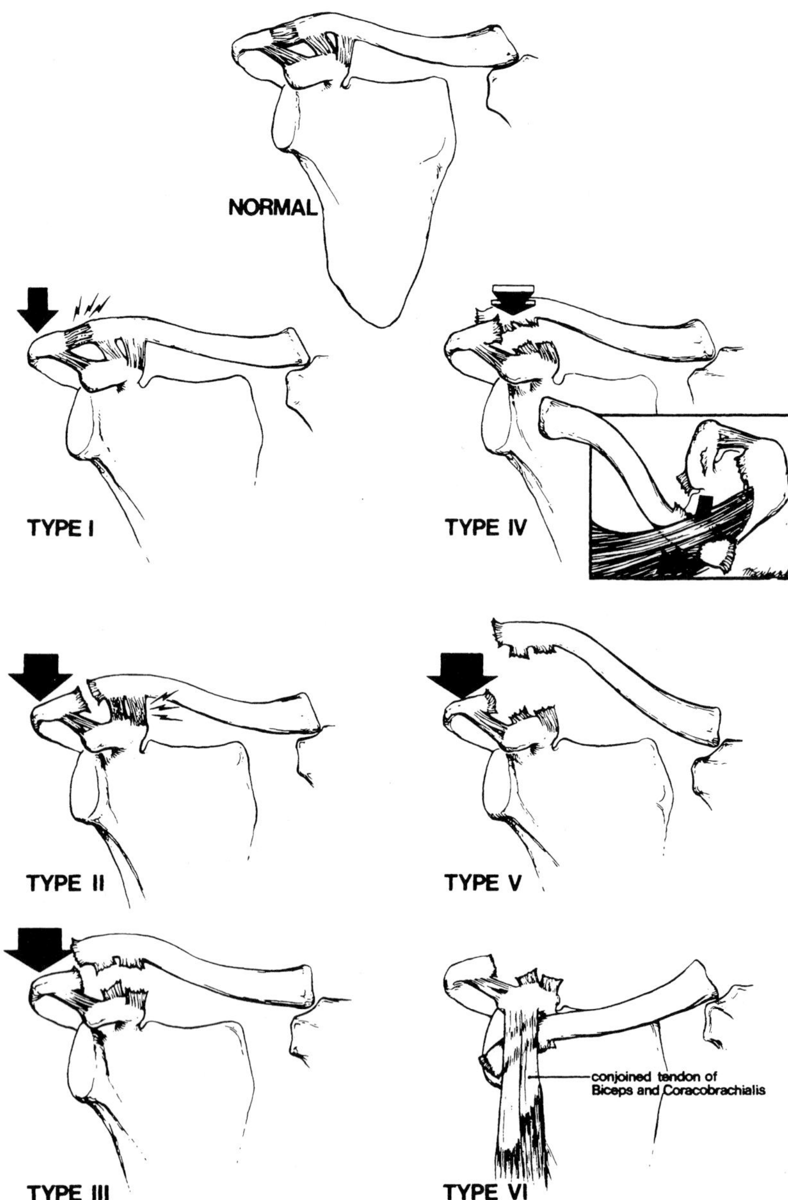

Figure 3–33. Classification of acromioclavicular (AC) separations. Type I injuries involve only an AC sprain. Type II injuries are characterized by complete AC tear but intact coracoclavicular (CC) ligaments. Type III injuries involve both the AC and CC ligaments with a CC distance of 125–200% of the opposite shoulder. Type IV injuries are associated with posterior displacement of the clavicle through the trapezius muscle. Type V injuries involve superior displacement with a CC distance of more than twice the opposite side. This injury is usually associated with rupture of the deltotrapezial fascia, leaving the distal end of the clavicle subcutaneous. Type VI injuries are rare and are defined based on inferior displacement of the clavicle below the coracoid. (From Rockwood, C.A., Jr., and Young, D.C.: Disorders of the acromioclavicular joint. In Rockwood, C.A., Jr., and Matsen, F.A., III, eds.: The Shoulder, 2nd ed. Philadelphia, WB Saunders, 1998, p. 495.)

clavicular fixation. Some type IV acromioclavicular separations can be treated with closed reduction. Chronic injuries may require transfer of the coracoacromial ligament into the resected end of the distal clavicle (modified Weaver-Dunn procedure).

2. Distal Clavicle Osteolysis—Common in **weight lifters, this condition is associated with osteopenia** and cystic changes to the distal clavicle. It often responds to activity modification but occasionally requires distal clavicle resection.
3. Acromioclavicular Degenerative Joint Disease—May be present in conjunction with impingement syndrome. Localized tenderness, pain with crossed-chest adduction, and joint narrowing and osteophytes on radiographs lead to the diagnosis. Treatment may include open or arthroscopic distal clavicle resection (Mumford's procedure).
4. Sternoclavicular (SC) Subluxation/Dislocation—Often caused by motor vehicle accidents or direct trauma, this injury can be best diagnosed by CT. Closed reduction is often successful. Hardware should be avoided.

I. Muscle Ruptures

1. Pectoralis Major—Injury to this muscle is caused by excessive tension on a maximally eccentrically contracted muscle, often in weight lifters. Localized swelling and ecchymosis, a palpable defect, and weakness with adduction and internal rotation are characteristic. Surgical repair to bone is usually necessary.
2. Deltoid—Complete rupture of this muscle is

unusual, and injuries are most often strains or partial tears. Repair to bone is required for complete injury.

3. Triceps—Most often associated with systemic illness or steroid use. Primary repair of avulsions is indicated.
4. **Subscapularis**—Can occur with anterior dislocations or following anterior shoulder surgery. Increased external rotation and a **"lift-off sign"** may be present. Surgical reattachment is indicated. Occasionally, a pectoralis transfer may be required.

J. Calcifying Tendinitis and Adhesive Capsulitis

1. Calcifying Tendinitis—Usually involves the supraspinatus tendon and may be associated with tendon degeneration. Radiographs demonstrate characteristic calcification within the tendon. Physical therapy, modalities such as ultrasonography and iontophoresis, and aspiration are usually successful. Operative treatment (removal of the deposit) is occasionally necessary.
2. Adhesive Capsulitis—Also known (inaccurately) as "frozen shoulder," this disorder is characterized by pain and restricted glenohumeral motion. Arthrography may demonstrate a loss of the normal axillary recess. Three clinical stages and four arthroscopic stages have been defined.

Stage	Characteristics
Clinical:	
Painful	Gradual onset of diffuse pain
Stiff	Decreased ROM; affects activities of daily living
Thawing	Gradual return of motion
Arthroscopic:	
1	Patchy fibrinous synovitis
2	Capsular contraction, fibrinous adhesions, synovitis
3	Increased contraction, resolving synovitis
4	Severe contracton

Treatment includes NSAIDs, passive motion and, occasionally, manipulation under anesthesia. The role of arthroscopy in the treatment of adhesive capsulitis is controversial.

K. Nerve Disorders

1. Brachial Plexus Injury—Minor traction and compression injuries, commonly known by football players as "burners" or "stingers," can be serious if they are recurrent or persist for more than a short time. **If burners occur more than one time, the player should be removed from competition until cervical spine radiographs can be obtained.** More significant injuries, such as root avulsions, can be devastating. There are three grades of nerve injury commonly recognized:

Grade	Description	Pathophysiology
1	Neuropraxia	Selective demyelination of the axon sheath
2	Axonotmesis	Axon and myelin sheath disruption
3	Neurotmesis	Epineurium and endoneurium disruption

2. Thoracic Outlet Syndrome—Compression of the nerves and vessels that pass through the scalene muscles and first rib can result in this disorder. Patients may note pain and ulnar paresthesias. The Wright test, described previously, and neurologic evaluation can be diagnostic. First-rib resection is occasionally required.
3. Long Thoracic Nerve Palsy—Injury to this nerve can result in scapular winging secondary to serratus anterior dysfunction. Bracing and, rarely, pectoralis major transfer are required.
4. Suprascapular Nerve Compression—Ganglia and other lesions can compress the suprascapular nerve, resulting in weakness and atrophy of the supraspinatus and infraspinatus muscles. Neurologic studies and MRI can demonstrate nerve impingement, which usually responds to surgical release. Cysts may be associated with SLAP tears and respond to arthroscopic decompression.

L. Other Shoulder Disorders

1. Glenohumeral Degenerative Joint Disease—Overuse injuries, aberrant hardware, and other conditions can result in arthritis of this joint. Arthroscopic débridement may have a role in the early stages of this disease, but occasionally arthroplasty is required. Progressive pain, decreased range of motion, and inability to perform activities of daily living are reasonable indications for considering prosthetic replacement. Hemiarthroplasty is preferred to total shoulder arthroplasty unless the glenoid is significantly affected because of the problems with glenoid component loosening. The humeral component should be placed in 30–40 degrees of retroversion in most cases. Less retroversion is recommended for prosthetic replacement in fractures and posterior dislocations. **In addition to glenoid loosening, subscapularis rupture is also a complication of shoulder replacement.** Neutral rotation is favored in patients with posterior fracture dislocations. Fusion is rarely indicated, but the position should be 20–30 degrees flexion, 40 degrees abduction, and 25–45 degrees internal rotation.
2. Snapping Scapula—This unusual disorder can be caused by irregularities of the medial scapula or the scapulothoracic bursa. Physical

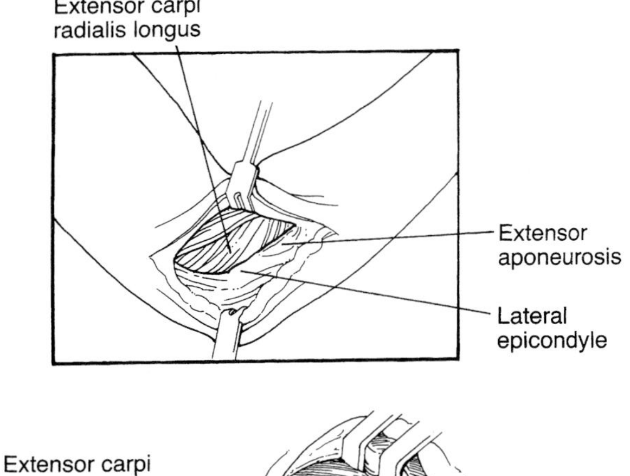

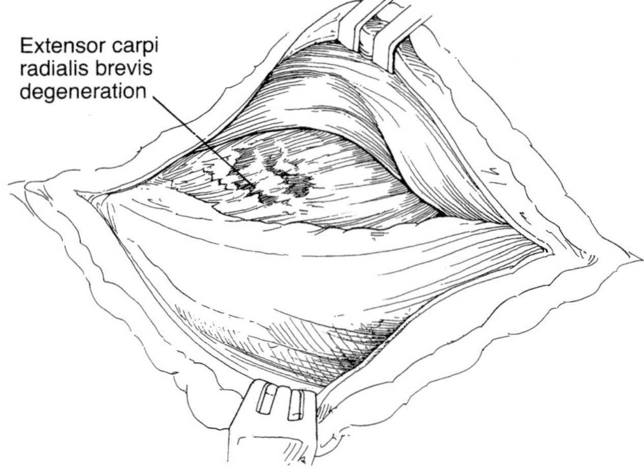

Figure 3–34. Operative exposure for lateral epicondylitis. (From Miller, M.D., Cooper, D.E., and Warner, J.J.P.: Review of Sports Medicine and Arthroscopy. Philadelphia, WB Saunders, 1995, p. 178.)

therapy, local injections, and other nonoperative treatment options are usually successful. Occasionally, resection of the medial border of the scapula is necessary. Arthroscopic bursectomy may also have a role in the treatment of this disorder.

3. Scapular Winging—This can occur as a result of a long thoracic nerve injury (medial winging) or a cranial nerve XI injury (lateral winging). Medial winging usually responds to serratus anterior strengthening, and lateral winging may improve with trapezius strengthening.
4. Reflex Sympathetic Dystrophy—Much as in the knee, this disorder can be a difficult problem. Stellate ganglion blocks may be helpful in the management of this condition.
5. Little Leaguer's Shoulder—This disorder, actually a Salter-Harris type I fracture of the proximal humerus, responds to rest and activity modification. Radiographs may demonstrate widening of the proximal humeral physis.

IV. **Other Upper Extremity Sports Medicine Problems**

A. Tendon Injuries

1. Lateral Epicondylitis (Tennis Elbow)—Degeneration at the extensor muscle group origin, principally in the **extensor carpi radialis brevis**, can be a result of overuse injuries or poor technique in racket sports. Localized tenderness, exacerbated by resisted wrist extension, is common. Therapy that includes stretching, strengthening, ultrasonography, and electrical stimulation can be helpful for this condition. Orthotics that are designed to decentralize the area of stress (tennis elbow strap) are also useful. Equipment modifications (more flexible racket, larger head, larger grip) may also be helpful. Surgical options include release of the common extensor origin and/or débridement of the pathologic tissue (Fig. 3–34).
2. Medial Epicondylitis (Golfer's Elbow)—This condition is less common and more difficult to treat than lateral epicondylitis. The affected area is at the pronator teres–flexor carpi radialis interface. Treatment is similar to that for lateral epicondylitis.
3. Distal Biceps Tendon Avulsion—Acute onset of pain in the antecubital fossa following a sudden force overload with the elbow partially flexed is common. Reattachment of the tendon with a two-incision (Boyd-Anderson) technique or with suture anchors through an anterior incision is favored. It is important not to disrupt the syndesmosis.
4. Distal Triceps Tendon Avulsion—Sudden loss of elbow extension and a palpable defect is the classic history. Early repair is favored for this rare injury.

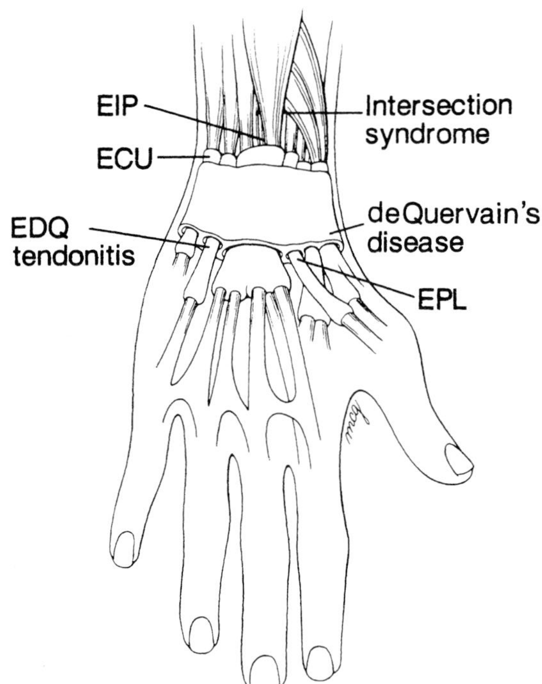

Figure 3–35. Location of common sites of tendinitis about the wrist. EIP, extensor indicis proprius; ECU, extensor carpi ulnaris; EDQ, extensor digiti quinti; EPL, extensor pollicis longus. (From Kiefhaber, T.R., and Stern, P.J.: Upper extremity tendinitis and overuse syndromes in the athlete. Clin. Sports Med. 11:43, 1992.)

5. De Quervain's Disease—Stenosing tenosynovitis of the first dorsal compartment of the wrist can occur with racket sports and in golfers. This site of tendinitis is only one of many in the wrist (Fig. 3–35). The Finkelstein test (ulnar deviation of the wrist with the thumb in the palm) is diagnostic. Treatment includes activity modification, local injection and, occasionally, surgical release.
6. Flexor Carpi Radialis/Ulnaris Tendinitis—Associated with overuse, this condition usually responds to NSAIDs, rest and, rarely, tenolysis.
7. Extensor Carpi Ulnaris—Tendinitis and even subluxation of this tendon can be treated with immobilization with the wrist in pronation. Occasionally, it is necessary to débride or stabilize the tendon in the sixth dorsal compartment.
8. Intersection Syndrome—Irritation and inflammation at the crossing point of the tendons of the first dorsal compartment (abductor pollicis longus and extensor pollicis brevis) and the second dorsal compartment (extensor carpi radialis longus and extensor carpi radialis brevis) can cause pain and crepitus ("squeakers"). Splinting, local injections, and decompression may be indicated.
9. Other Extensor Tendon Tendinitis—Includes the extensor pollicis longus, extensor digiti quinti, and extensor indicis proprius. Usually responds to local measures and, rarely, surgical release.
10. Flexor Digitorum Profundus Avulsion Injuries—Commonly known by the appropriate term "Jersey finger," these injuries require operative repair.
11. Mallet/Baseball Finger—Avulsion of the terminal extensor tendon in the finger can usually be treated with extension splinting of the distal interphalangeal joint for 6+ weeks.

B. Ligamentous Injuries
1. Ulnar (Medial) Collateral Ligament of the Elbow—Injury to this ligament is usually the result of a valgus stress. The all-important **anterior band of this ligament** is commonly involved, especially in baseball pitchers. The diagnosis is based on clinical examination findings (Fig. 3–36) and sometimes MRI. Reconstruction using a palmaris longus tendon graft (Fig. 3–37) is occasionally required for chronic injuries. Repair of acute injuries is usually less successful.
2. Lateral Collateral Ligament Injuries of the Elbow—This injury has only recently been characterized. Patients may complain of recurrent clicking or locking while extending the elbow. Clinically, posterolateral rotatory subluxation can be demonstrated by the lat-

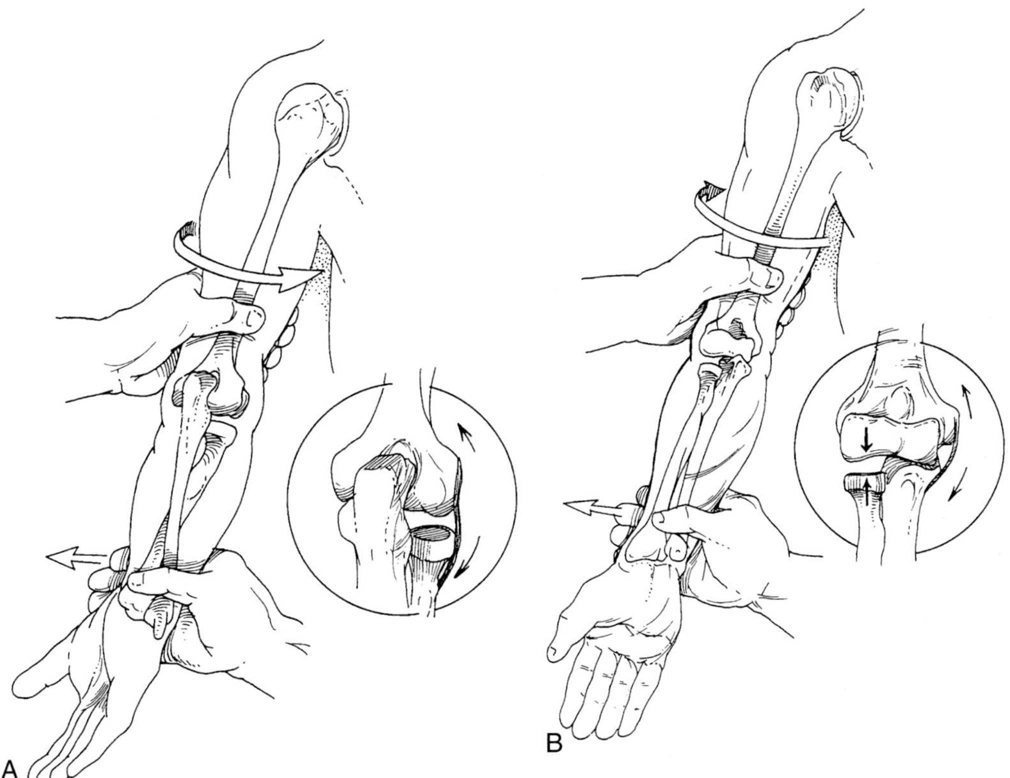

Figure 3–36. Varus *(A)* and valgus *(B)* instability testing of the elbow. Note the position and rotation of the arm. (From Morrey, B.F.: The Elbow and Its Disorders, 2nd ed. Philadelphia, WB Saunders, 1994, p. 83.)

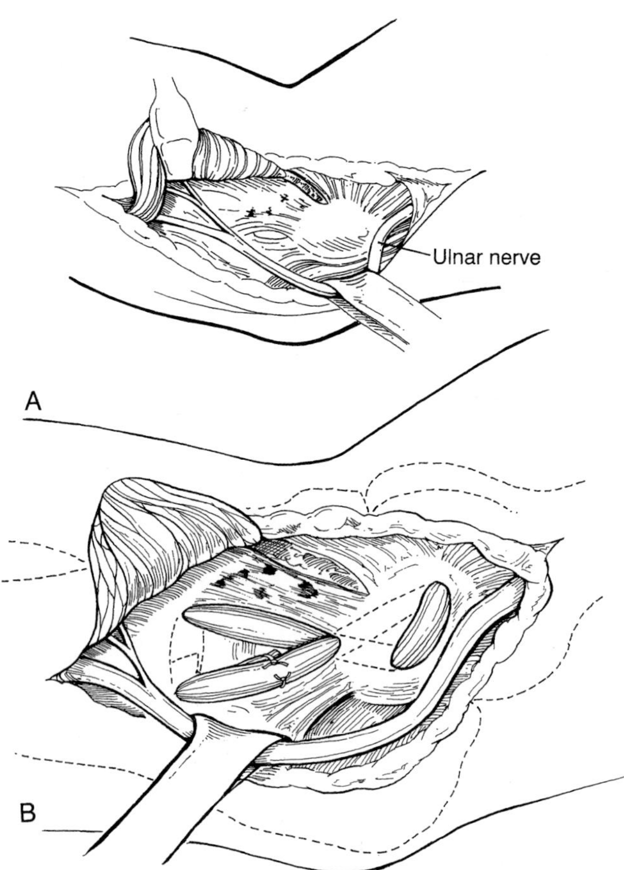

Figure 3–37. Reconstruction of the (medial) ulnar collateral ligament. (From Miller, M.D., Cooper, D.E., and Warner, J.J.P.: Review of Sports Medicine and Arthroscopy. Philadelphia, WB Saunders, 1995, p. 179.)

eral pivot shift test of the elbow (Fig. 3–38). The test is considered positive if the patient experiences apprehension. Reconstruction of the ulnar portion of the lateral collateral ligament is sometimes necessary for recurrent subluxation.

3. Wrist Ligament Instabilities—Include scapholunate instability (dorsal intercalated segment instability), triquetrohamate instability (dorsal or volar intercalated segment instability), and triquetrolunate instability (volar intercalated segment instability) (Fig. 3–39). The Watson test (radial deviation of the hand with volar pressure on the scaphoid) may reproduce pain or a "clunk" in patients with scapholunate instability. Radiographs may demonstrate an increased scapholunate interval as well. The ballotment test (palmar and dorsal displacement of the triquetrum with lunate stabilization using the opposite hand) can produce pain in patients with triquetrolunate instability. Limited arthrodesis is often required for treatment of chronic wrist instabilities.
4. Ligament Injuries in the Hand—Includes collateral ligament injuries (treated with buddy taping) and volar plate injuries (associated with dorsal dislocations), among others. Injury to the ulnar collateral ligament of the thumb is commonly referred to as gamekeeper's, or skier's, thumb. Treatment of the incomplete injury is immobilization. Complete injuries (>15 degrees side-side difference or opening >45 degrees) require operative intervention because of interposition of the adductor aponeurosis between the two torn ends of the ulnar collateral ligament (Fig. 3–40).

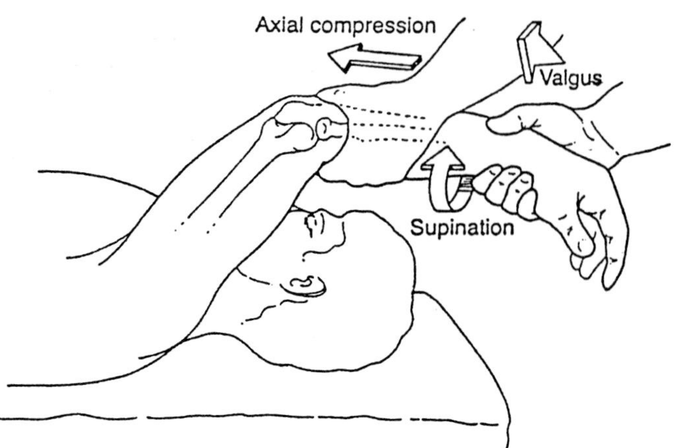

Figure 3–38. Lateral pivot shift test of the elbow for posterolateral rotatory instability. (Redrawn from O'Driscoll, S.W., Bell, D.F., and Morrey, B.F.: Posterolateral instability of the elbow. J. Bone Joint Surg. [Am.] 73:440–446, 1991.)

C. Articular Injuries
1. Medial Epicondyle Injuries—Stress fractures of the medial epicondyle are common in adolescents with repetitive valgus forces in throwing, **Little Leaguer's elbow.** Rest and

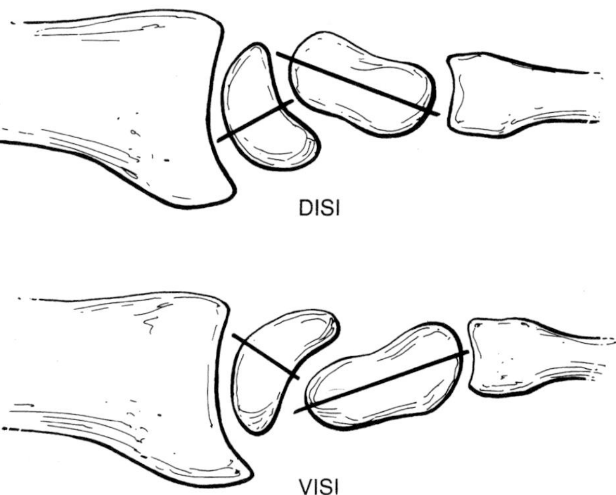

Figure 3–39. Scapholunate instability is associated with a dorsal intercalated instability (DISI) pattern. Triquetrolunate instability may have a volar intercalated instability pattern. Note the increased scapholunate angle (>60 degrees) with the DISI pattern (normal 30 degrees). (From McCue, F.C., and Bruce, J.F.: The wrist. In DeLee, J.C., and Drez, D., Jr., eds.: Orthopaedic Sports Medicine: Principles and Practice. Philadelphia, WB Saunders, 1994, p. 918.)

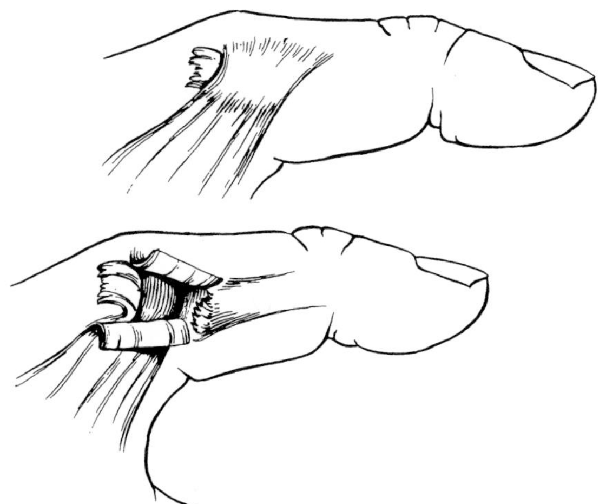

Figure 3–40. Stener's lesion. The adductor aponeurosis separates the two ends of the ulnar collateral ligament, and the aponeurosis must be incised to repair the ligament. (From Green, D.P., and Strickland, J.W.: The hand. In DeLee, J.C., and Drez, D., Jr., eds.: Orthopaedic Sports Medicine: Principles and Practice. Philadelphia, WB Saunders, 1994, p. 976.)

Table 3–3.

Classification of Injuries of the TFCC

Class	Description	Treatment
	Traumatic Lesions (Type 1)	
1A	Horizontal tear adjacent to sigmoid notch[a]	Débridement
1B	Avulsion from ulna ± ulnar styloid fracture	Suture repair
1C	Avulsion from carpus; exposes pisiform	Débridement
1D	Avulsion from sigmoid notch	Débridement
	Degenerative Lesions (Type 2)	
2A	Thinning of TFCC without perforation[b]	
2B	Thinning of disc with chondromalacia	
2C	Perforation of disc with chondromalacia	
2D	Perforation of disc, chondromalacia, partial tear of lunotriquetral ligament	
2E	Perforation of disc, chondromalacia, complete tear of lunotriquetral ligament, ulnocarpal degenerative joint disease	

[a] Most common.

[b] Treatment for degenerative lesions includes débridement of loose degenerated discs, intra-articular resection of the ulnar head, and débridement of lunotriquetral ligament tears with percutaneous pinning of the lunotriquetral joint based on the pathology present.

From Miller M.D., Cooper D.E., Warner J.J.P., et al.: Review of Sports Medicine and Arthroscopy, p. 188. Philadelphia, WB Saunders, 1995.

activity modification can help reduce the incidence of a complete fracture.

2. **Osteochondritis Dissecans**—Related to vascular insufficiency and repetitive microtrauma (compressive forces in pitching), this condition usually affects the **capitellum** but can also involve the radial head. If the fragment is stable, this condition can be treated with activity modification and supportive methods. Arthroscopy may be indicated for separated fragments. Osteochondrosis of the capitellum (Panner's disease) is seen in young children and is associated with a more benign course.
3. Osteoarthritis of the Elbow—This condition, common in football linemen, miners, throwers, and athletes who participate in racket sports, is associated with pain at the endpoint of forced extension or flexion. Arthroscopic débridement, open decompression, distraction arthroplasty, and other procedures may be indicated for advanced cases. The ulnohumeral (Outerbridge-Kashiwagi) arthroplasty may allow decompression with minimal morbidity (Fig. 3–41).
4. Post-traumatic Arthrofibrosis of the Elbow—Presents with loss of motion and dysfunction. Arthroscopic capsular release may be required.
5. Wrist Triangular Fibrocartilage Complex Injuries—Common cause of ulnar wrist pain; tears in this complex can be diagnosed based on arthrography or MRI. Treatment includes débridement or suture repair (Table 3–3).
6. Post-traumatic Problems of the Wrist—Kienböck's disease is avascular necrosis and collapse of the lunate, probably related to overuse and ulnar negative wrist variance. Ulnar lengthening or radial shortening is helpful early, but limited wrist fusions may be

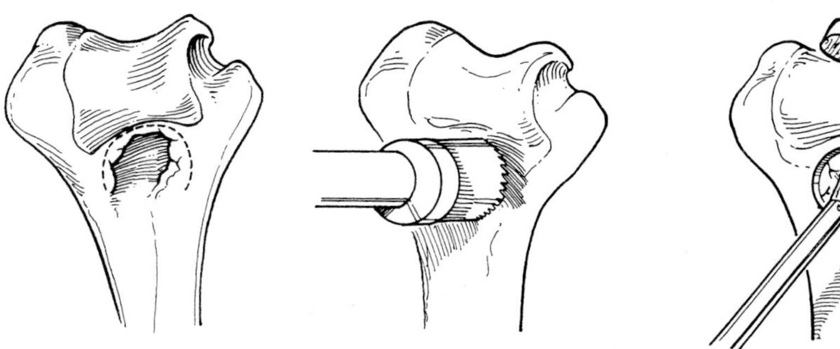

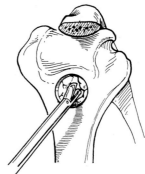

Figure 3–41. Outerbridge-Kashiwagi arthroplasty, performed through a triceps-splitting approach. The coronoid is approached through a Cloward drill hole in the olecranon fossa. The olecranon can also be débrided with this approach. (From Miller, M.D., Cooper, D.E., and Warner, J.J.P.: Review of Sports Medicine and Arthroscopy. Philadelphia, WB Saunders, 1995, p. 180.)

necessary for later stages. Osteochondrosis of the capitate can occur in gymnasts and may respond to débridement or limited fusions. Scaphoid avascular necrosis is relatively common owing to its tenuous blood supply. Bone grafting with internal fixation is usually curative. Unrecognized scapholunate injuries can lead to the development of collapse (scapholunate advanced collapsed [SLAC] wrist), which may require limited, or even total, wrist fusions.

D. Arthroscopy
1. Elbow Arthroscopy—Especially helpful for removing loose bodies, débridement, and synovectomy. Most surgeons prefer supine positioning with a wristholder and traction. Common portals include the anterolateral portal (1 cm distal and 1 cm anterior to the lateral epicondyle), the anteromedial portal (2 cm distal and 2 cm distal to the medial epicondyle), and the posterolateral portal (2 cm proximal to the olecranon, just lateral to the triceps) (Fig. 3–42). The "nick and spread" method is helpful for minimizing neurovascular risks. Recent studies have demonstrated that far proximal portals may reduce these risks.
2. Wrist Arthroscopy—Indications now include triangular fibrocartilage complex débridement, treatment of certain ligamentous injuries, management of ulnar abutment syndrome, and assessing reduction of certain intra-articular fractures. A 2.5- or 3.0-mm arthroscope is commonly used, and the patient is supine with a traction apparatus. Three radiocarpal portals and three midcarpal portals are commonly used. Portals are named in relation to the dorsal compartments of the wrist (Fig. 3–43). The 3–4 radiocarpal portal (located between the extensor pollicis longus and extensor digitorum communis tendons) is usually established first. The 4–5 radiocarpal portal (positioned between the extensor digitorum communis and extensor digiti minimi tendons) is commonly used for instrumentation. The 6R portal (placed just radial to the extensor carpi ulnaris tendon) can be used for visualization or instrumentation. The midcarpal portals include the midcarpal radial portal, the midcarpal ulnar portal, and the scaphotrapezialtrapezoid portal. These portals are used only for disorders involving the midcarpal joints.

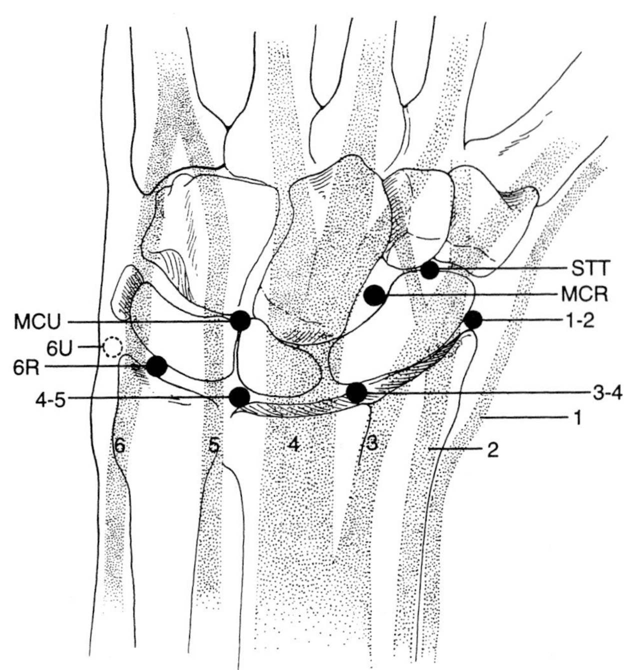

Figure 3–43. Arthroscopic wrist portals. Numbers indicate wrist extensor compartments and associated portals. R = radial; U = ulnar; MCU = midcarpal ulnar; MCR = midcarpal radial; STT = scaphotrapeziotrapezoid. (From Miller, M.D., Osborne J.R., Warner J.J.P., et al.: MRI-Arthroscopy Correlative Atlas, Philadelphia, WB Saunders, 1997, p. 220.)

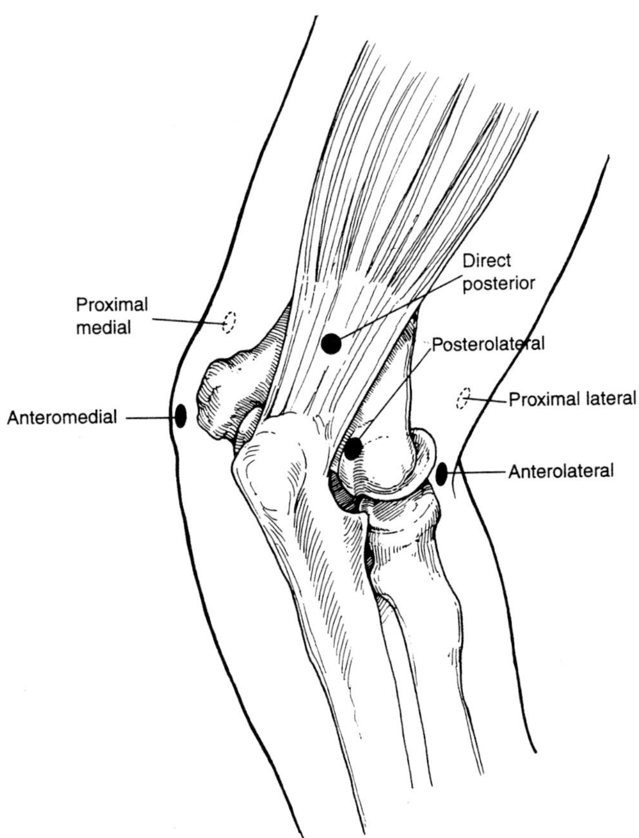

Figure 3–42. Arthroscopic portals for elbow arthroscopy. (From Miller, M.D., Osborne J.R., Warner, J.J.P., et al.: MRI-Arthroscopy Correlative Atlas, Philadelphia, WB Saunders, 1997, p. 197.)

V. Head and Spine Injuries

A. Head Injuries
1. Diffuse Brain Injuries—Includes mild and "classic" cerebral concussion and diffuse axonal injury. Mild concussions occur without loss of consciousness and can be subdivided into three grades as follows (where RTP represents "return to play"):

MILD CONCUSSIONS

Grade	Symptoms	Duration	Recommended RTP
1	Confusion, no amnesia	Minutes	When symptoms resolve
2	Retrograde amnesia	Hours to days	1 Week
3	Amnesia after impact	Days	1 Month

Postconcussion syndrome, characterized by persistent headaches, irritability, confusion, and difficulty concentrating, can occur with grade 2 and 3 mild concussions. "Classic" concussion includes a period of loss of consciousness. If it lasts >5 minutes, head CT should be obtained. Delay in return to play should be 1 week to 1 month after the first episode and for the entire season for a second episode. Diffuse axonal injury occurs with loss of consciousness lasting >6 hours, and athletes who suffer this injury should consider total avoidance of future contact sports.

2. Focal Brain Syndromes—Include contusions, intracranial hematomas, epidural hematomas, and subdural hematomas. CT scanning is helpful for distinguishing these entities (Fig. 3–44). Although epidural hematomas classically are said to be characterized by a period of lucidity followed by loss of consciousness, this sequence may not occur. Surgical treatment of intracranial hematomas may be indicated.
3. Prevention—Head protection, especially with contact sports, equestrian events, hockey, boxing, skating, and skiing, should be encouraged.

B. Cervical Spine Injuries—Catastrophic injury to the cervical spine is unfortunately an all too common event in contact sports (especially football and rugby). Underlying cervical stenosis, or narrowing of the anteroposterior diameter of the spine, can make these injuries worse (Fig. 3–45). Recommendations for return to play for athletes with cervical stenosis with transient symptoms are controversial. Football players who repeatedly use poor tackling techniques can develop a condition known as **spear tackler's spine,** which includes developmental cervical stenosis, loss of lordosis, and other radiographic abnormalities. Return to contact sports should be avoided.

C. Thoracic and Lumbar Spine Injuries—Injuries commonly associated with sports include muscle injury, fractures, disc disease, and spondylolysis/spondylolisthesis. The latter condition is common in football interior lineman and gymnasts. Oblique radiographs, bone scan, and CT are all helpful for establishing the diagnosis. Treatment includes activity modification, bracing, and fusion for high-grade slips.

VI. **Medical Aspects of Sports Medicine**

A. Ergogenic Drugs

1. Anabolic Steroids—Derivatives of testosterone are abused by athletes attempting to increase muscle mass and strength and increase erythropoiesis. Adverse effects include liver dysfunction, hypercholesterolemia, cardiomyopathy, testicular atrophy, gynecomastia, and **irreversible alopecia.** Urine sampling has been the standard for evaluation by the International Olympic Committee.
2. Human Growth Hormone—Made from recombinant DNA; illegal use of this drug is common. Athletes attempting to increase muscle size and weight abuse this drug, which has side effects similar to those of steroids as well as hypertension and gigantism.
3. Other commonly abused drugs include amphetamines, blood doping, diuretics, and laxatives.

B. Cardiac Abnormalities

1. Sudden Cardiac Death—Usually related to an underlying heart condition, especially **hypertrophic cardiomyopathy in young athletes and coronary artery disease in older athletes**. Screening including electrocardiography can identify this problem early.
2. Commotio cordis—Cardiac contusion from a direct blow to the chest (for example, in Little League baseball) has a poor prognosis, even when immediately recognized and treated.

C. Exercise—Done on a regular basis, exercise can decrease heart rate and blood pressure, decrease insulin requirements in diabetics, decrease cardiovascular risk, and increase lean body mass. It has also been shown to reduce cancer risk, osteoporosis, hypercholesterolemia, and hypertension. The aerobic threshold can be determined by measuring oxygen consumption and is useful for evaluating endurance athletes. Sports-specific conditioning involves aerobic and anaerobic conditioning if different proportions are based on the season and the sport. In the off-season, long-distance runs can be helpful to sprinters to increase aerobic recovery capability following sprints. Several exercise categories have been described. Stretching has also been shown to have a beneficial effect.

Exercise	Description	Benefit
Isometric	Muscle tension without change in unit length	Muscle hypertrophy; not endurance
Isotonic	Weight training with a constant resistance through arc of motion	Improved motor
Isokinetic	Weight training with a constant velocity, variable resistance	Increase strength; less time-consuming but more expensive
Plyometric	Rapid shortening	Power generation
Functional	Aerobic fitness	Easily performed

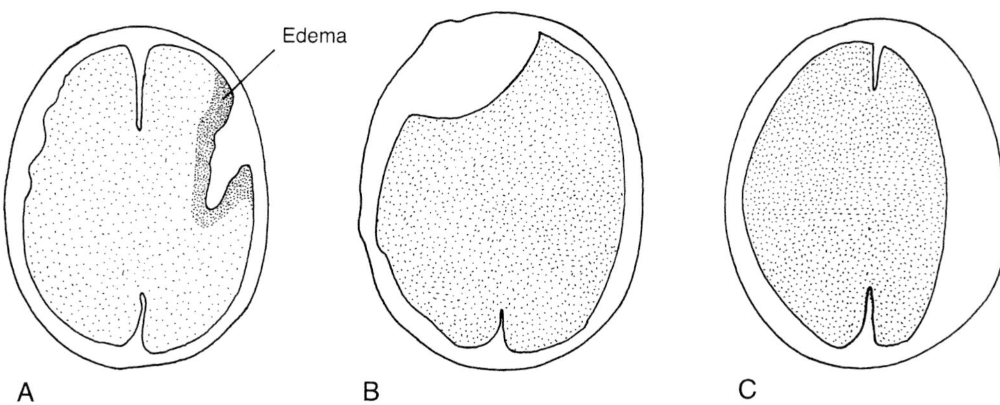

Figure 3–44. CT findings. *A,* Contusion includes a hemorrhagic area and surroundings edema. *B,* Epidural hematomas typically have a biconvex appearance. *C,* Subdural hematomas have a concave or crescentic appearance. (From Miller, M.D., Cooper, D.E., and Warner, J.J.P.: Review of Sports Medicine and Arthroscopy. Philadelphia, WB Saunders, 1995, p. 204.)

D. Female Athlete

1. Physiologic Differences—Women are typically smaller, lighter, and have greater body fat. Lower MVO_2, cardiac output, hemoglobin, and muscular mass/strength are also important considerations. Other differences contribute to the increased incidence of patellofemoral disorders, stress fractures, and knee ACL injuries in females (especially with basketball, soccer, and rugby).
2. Amenorrhea—This problem may be related to a low body fat percentage and/or stress. The incidence approaches 50% in elite runners and is related to stress fractures **(osteopenia) and eating disorders (female athlete triad).** Dietary management and birth control pills are helpful for treating this problem.

E. Muscle—There are two types of muscle, types I and II. Type I muscle is slow-twitch/aerobic and is helpful in endurance sports. Training can increase the number of mitochondria and increased capillary density. Type II muscle is fast-twitch/anaerobis and is helpful for sprinters. It has high contraction speeds, quick relaxation, and low triglycerine stores. Immobilization of muscle results in a shorter position with a decreased ability to generate tension.

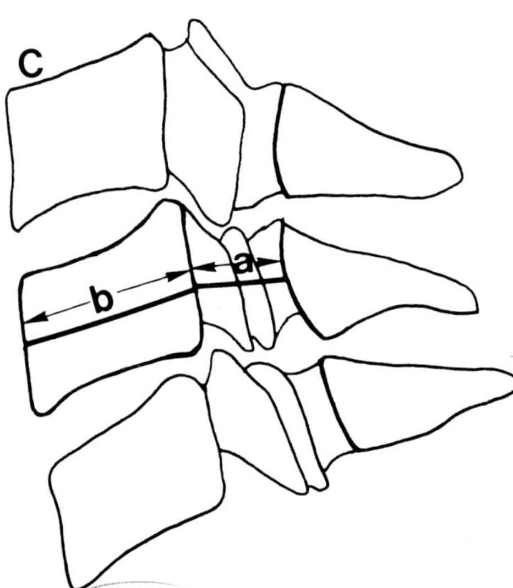

Figure 3–45. Pavlov's ratio (a/b) of <0.8 is consistent with cervical stenosis. (Note that this ratio may not apply to larger individuals.) (From Pavlov, H., and Porter, I.S.: Criteria for cervical instability and stenosis. Op. Tech. Sports Med. 1:170, 1993.)

F. Other Sports Injuries

1. Blunt trauma—Can injure solid organs. These injuries may be subtle and require a high index of suspicion. **The kidney is the most commonly injured organ (especially in boxing), followed by the spleen (injured in football).**
2. Chest Injuries—Can be serious and require immediate on-field action. Decreased breath sounds and hypotension may signify a tension pneumothorax. Treatment entails placing a 14 gauge intravenous needle in the second intercostal space at the midclavicular line and a chest tube. Airway obstructions must also be anticipated and treated. Rib fractures may also occur in contact sports. More commonly, the player may have "had the air knocked out." This is usually related to a problem with the diaphragm.
3. Eye injuries—These injuries are best avoided with proper protection. A hyphema (blood in the eye) is associated with a vitreous or retinal injury in over 50% of cases.

G. Metabolic Issues

1. Dehydration—Fluid and electrolyte loss can lead to decreased cardiovascular function and work capacity. Absorption is increased with solutions with low osmolarity (<10%).
2. Nutritional Supplements—These continue to be a source of controversy. Creatine, one of the more popular supplements, increases the water retention in cells. In-season use can increase the incidence of dehydration and cramps.

Selected Bibiography

Knee

Anatomy and Biomechanics

Arnoczky, S.P.: Anatomy of the anterior cruciate ligament. Clin. Orthop. 172:19–25, 1983.

Arnoczky, S.P., and Warren, R.F.: Microvasculature of the human meniscus. Am. J. Sports Med. 10:90–95, 1982.

Cooper, D.E., Deng, X.H., Burnstein, A.L., et al.: The strength of the central third patellar tendon graft: A biomechanical study. Am. J. Sports Med. 21:818–824, 1993.

Daniel, D.M., Akeson, W.H., and O'Connor, J.J., eds.: Knee Ligaments: Structure, Function, Injury, and Repair. New York, Raven Press, 1990.

Fu, F.H., Harner, C.D., Johnson, D.L., et al.: Biomechanics of knee ligaments: Basic concepts and clinical application. J. Bone Joint Surg. 75:1716–1725, 1993.

Girgis, F.G., Marshall, J.L., and Al Monajem, A.R.S.: The cruciate ligaments of the knee joint: Anatomical, functional and experimental analysis. Clin. Orthop. 106:216–231, 1975.

Noyes, F.R., Butler, D.L., Grood, E.S., et al.: Biomechanical analysis of human ligament grafts used in knee-ligament repairs and reconstructions. J. Bone Joint Surg. [Am.] 66:344–352, 1984.

Seebacher, J.R., Inglis, A.E., Marshall, J.L., et al.: The structure of the posterolateral aspect of the knee. J. Bone Joint Surg. [Am.] 64:536–541, 1982.

Thompson, W.O., Theate, F.L., Fu, F.H., et al.: Tibial meniscal dynamics using three-dimensional reconstruction of magnetic resonance images. Am. J. Sports Med. 19:210–216, 1991.

Warren, L.F., and Marshall, J.L.: The supporting structures and layers of the medial side of the knee. J. Bone Joint Surg. [Am.] 61:56–62, 1979.

Warren, R., Arnoczky, S.P., and Wickiewicz, T.L.: Anatomy of the knee. In Nicholas, J.A., and Hershman, E.B., eds.: The Lower Extremity and Spine in Sports Medicine, St. Louis: CV Mosby, 1986, pp. 657–694.

History and Physical Examination

Fetto, J.F., and Marshall, J.L.: Injury to the anterior cruciate ligament producing the pivot shift sign. J. Bone Joint Surg. [Am.] 61:710–714, 1979.

Fulkerson, J.P., Kalenak, A., Rosenberg, T.D., et al.: Patellofemoral pain. Instr. Course Lect. 41:57–71, 1992.

Galway, R.D., Beaupre, A., and MacIntosh, D.L.: Pivot shift. J. Bone Joint Surg. [Br.] 54:763, 1972.

Hosea, T.M., and Tria, A.J.: Physical examination of the knee: clinical. In Scott, W.N., ed.: Ligament and Extensor Mechanism Injuries of the Knee: Diagnosis and Treatment. St. Louis, CV Mosby, 1991.

Ritchie, J.R., Miller, M.D., and Harner, C.D.: History and physical examination of the knee. In Fu, F.H., Harner, C.D., and Vince, K.G., eds.: Knee Surgery. Baltimore, Williams & Wilkins, 1994.

Slocum, D.B., and Larson, R.L.: Rotatory instability of the knee. J. Bone Joint Surg. [Am.] 50:211, 1968.

Imaging

Blackburne, J.S., and Peel, T.E.: A new method of measuring patellar height. J. Bone Joint Surg. [Br.] 59:241–242, 1977.

Blumensaat, C.: Die lageabweichunger and verrenkungen der kniescheibe. Ergeb. Chir. Orthop. 31:149–223, 1938.

Insall, J., and Salvati, E.: Patella position in the normal knee joint. Radiology 101:101–104, 1971.

Jackson, D.W., Jennings, L.D., Maywood, R.M., et al.: Magnetic resonance imaging of the knee. Am. J. Sports Med. 16:29–38, 1988.

Jackson, R.W.: The painful knee: Arthroscopy or MR Imaging. J. Am. Acad. Orthop. Surg. 4:93–99, 1996.

Merchant, A.C., Mercer, R.L., Jacobsen, R.H., et al.: Roentgenographic analysis of patellofemoral congruence. J. Bone Joint Surg. [Am.] 56:1391–1396, 1974.

Newhouse, K.E., and Rosenberg, T.D.: Basic radiographic examination of the knee. In Fu, F.H., Harner, C.D., and Vince, K.G., eds.: Knee Surgery. Baltimore, Williams & Wilkins, 1994, pp. 313–324.

Rosenberg, T.D., Paulos, L.E., Parker, R.D., et al.: The forty-five degree posteroanterior flexion weight-bearing radiograph of the knee. J. Bone Joint Surg. [Am.] 70:1479–1483, 1988.

Thaete, F.L., and Britton, C.A.: Magnetic resonance imaging. In Fu, F.H., Harner, C.D., and Vince, K.G., eds.: Knee Surgery. Baltimore, Williams & Wilkins, 1994.

Knee Arthroscopy

DeLee, J.C.: Complications of arthroscopy and arthroscopic surgery: Results of a national survey. Arthroscopy 4:214–220, 1988.

DiGiovine, N.M., and Bradley, J.P.: Arthroscopic equipment and setup. In Fu, F.H., Harner, C.D., and Vince, K.G., eds.: Knee Surgery. Baltimore, Williams & Wilkins, 1994.

Gillquist, J.: Arthroscopy of the posterior compartments of the knee. Contemp. Orthop. 10:39–45, 1985.

Johnson, L.L.: Arthroscopic Surgery: Principles and Practice, 3rd ed. St. Louis, CV Mosby, 1986.

O'Connor, R.L.: Arthroscopy in the diagnosis and treatment of acute ligament injuries of the knee. J. Bone Joint Surg. [Am.] 56:333–337, 1974.

Rosenberg, T.D., Paulos, L.E., Parker, R.D., et al.: Arthroscopic surgery of the knee. In Chapman, M.W., ed.: Operative Orthopaedics. Philadelphia, JB Lippincott, 1988, pp. 1585–1604.

Small, N.C.: Complications in arthroscopy: The knee and other joints. Arthroscopy 2:253–258, 1986.

Wantanabe, M., and Takeda, S.: The number 21 arthroscope. J. Jpn. Orthop. Assoc. 34:1041, 1960.

Meniscus

Arnoczky, S.P., Warren, R.F., and Spivak, J.M.: Meniscal repair using an exogenous fibrin clot—An experimental study in dogs. J. Bone Joint Surg. [Am.] 70:1209–1220, 1988.

Baratz, M.E., Fu, F.H., and Mengato, R.: Meniscal tears: The effect of meniscectomy and of repair on intra-articular contact areas and stresses in the human knee. Am. J. Sports Med. 14:270–275, 1986.

Belzer J.P., and Cannon W.D. Meniscus tears: Treatment in the stable and unstable knee. J. Am. Acad. Orthop. Surg. 1:41–47, 1993.

Cannon, W.D., and Vittori, J.M.: The incidence of healing in arthroscopic meniscal repairs in anterior cruciate ligament reconstructed knees versus stable knees. Am. J. Sports Med. 20:176–181, 1992.

DeHaven, K.E., Black, K.P., and Griffiths, H.J.: Open meniscus repair: Technique and two to nine year results. Am. J. Sports Med. 17:788–795, 1989.

Dickhaut, S.C., and DeLee, J.C.: The discoid lateral meniscus syndrome. J. Bone Joint Surg. [Am.] 64:1068–1073, 1982.

Fairbank, T.J.: Knee joint changes after meniscectomy. J. Bone Joint Surg. [Br.] 30:664–670, 1948.

Henning, C.E., Lynch, M.A., Yearout, K.M., et al.: Arthroscopic meniscal repair using an exogenous fibrin clot. Clin. Orthop. 252:64, 1990.

Jordan M.R., Lateral meniscal variants: Evaluation and treatment. J. Am. Acad. Orthop. Surg. 4:191–200, 1996.

Miller, M.D., Ritchie, J.R., Royster, R.M., et al.: Meniscal repair: An experimental study in the goat. Am. J. Sports Med. 23(1):124–128, 1995.

Miller, M.D., Warner, J.J.P., and Harner, C.D.: Mensical repair. In Fu, F.H., Harner, C.D., and Vince, K.G., eds.: Knee Surgery. Baltimore, Williams & Wilkins, 1994.

Neuschwander, D.C., Drez, D., and Finney, T.P.: Lateral meniscal variant with absence of the posterior coronary ligament. J. Bone Joint Surg. [Am.] 74:1186–1190, 1992.

Parisien, J.S.: Arthroscopic treatment of cysts of the menisci: A preliminary report. Clin. Orthop. 257:154–158, 1990.

Warren, R.F.: Meniscectomy and repair in the anterior cruciate ligament–deficient patient. Clin. Orthop. 252:55–63, 1990.

Osteochondral Lesions

Bauer, M., and Jackson, R.W.: Chondral lesions of the femoral condyles: A system of arthroscopic classification. Arthroscopy 4:97–102, 1988.

Buckwalter, J.A., Restoration of injured or degenerated articular cartilage. J. Am. Acad. Orthop. Surg. 2:192–201, 1994.

Buckwalter, J.A., and Mankin, H.J., Articular cartilage (parts I&II). Instructional Course Lectures. J. Bone Joint Surg. 79A:600–632, 1997.

Cahill, B.R.: Osteochondritis dissecans of the knee: Treatment of juvenile and adult forms. J. Am. Acad. Orthop. Surg. 3:237–247, 1995.

Ecker, M.L., and Lotke, P.A.: Spontaneous osteonecrosis of the knee. J. Am. Acad. Orthop. Surg. 2:173–178, 1994.

Guhl, J.: Arthroscopic treatment of osteochondritis dissecans. Clin. Orthop. 167:65–74, 1982.

Mandelbaum, B.R., Browne, J.E., Fu, F.H., et al.: Articular cartilage lesions of the knee: Current concepts. Am. J. Sports Med. 26:853–861, 1998.

Menche, D.S., Vangsness, C.T., Pitman, M, et al.: The treatment of isolated articular cartilage lesions in the young individual. AAOS Instr. Course Lect. 47:505–515, 1998.

Murray, P.B., and Rand, J.A.: Symptomatic valgus knee: The surgical options. J. Am. Acad. Orthop. Surg. 1:1–9, 1993.

Newman, A.P.: Articular cartilage repair: Current concepts. Am. J. Sports Med. 26:309–324, 1998.

O'Driscoll, S.W.: Current concepts review: The healing and regeneration of articular cartilage. J. Bone Joint Surg. 80A:1795–1812, 1998.

Schenck, R.C., and Goodnight, J.M.: Current concepts review: Osteochondritis dissecans. J. Bone Joint Surg. 78A:439–456, 1996.

Synovial Lesions

Curl, W.W.: Popliteal cysts: Historical background and current knowledge. J. Am. Acad. Orthop. Surg. 4:129–133, 1996.

Ewing, J.W.: Plica: Pathologic or not? J. Am. Acad. Orthop. Surg. 1:117–121, 1993.

Flandry, F., and Hughston, J.C.: Current concepts review: Pigmented villonodular synovitis. J. Bone Joint Surg. [Am.] 69:942, 1987.

Knee Ligament Injuries

Albright, J.P., and Brown, A.W.: Management of chronic posterolateral rotatory instability of the knee: Surgical technique for the posterolateral corner sling procedure. AAOS Instr. Course Lect. 47:369–378, 1998.

Carson, E.W., Simonian, P.T., Wickiewicz, T.L., et al: Revision anterior cruciate ligament reconstruction. AAOS Instr. Course Lect. 47:361–368, 1998.

Clancy, W.G., Ray, J.M., and Zoltan, D.J.: Acute tears of the anterior cruciate ligament: Surgical versus conservative treatment. J. Bone Joint Surg. [Am.] 70:1483–1488, 1988.

Cooper, D.E., Warren, R.F., and Warner, J.J.P.: The posterior cruciate ligament and posterolateral structures of the knee: Anatomy, function, and patterns of injury. Instr. Course Lect. 40:249–270, 1991.

Dye, S.F., Wojtys, E.M., Fu, F.H., et al.: Factors contributing to function of the knee joint after injury or reconstruction of the anterior cruciate ligament. J. Bone Joint Surg. 80A:1380–1393, 1998.

Fowler, P.J., and Messieh, S.S.: Isolated posterior cruciate ligament injuries in athletes. Am. J. Sports Med. 15:553–557, 1987.

France, E.P., and Paulos, L.E.: Knee bracing. J. Am. Acad. Orthop. Surg. 2:281–287, 1994.

Frank, C.B.: Ligament healing: Current knowledge and clinical applications. J. Am. Acad. Orthop. Surg. 4:74–83, 1996.

Frank, C.B., and Jackson, D.W.: Current concepts review: The science of reconstruction of the anterior cruciate ligament. J. Bone Joint Surg. 79A:1556–1576, 1997.

Frassica, F.J., Sim, F.H., Staeheli, J.W., et al.: Dislocation of the knee. Clin. Orthop. 263:200–205, 1991.

Good, L., and Johnson, R.J.: The dislocated knee. J. Am. Acad. Orthop. Surg. 3:284–292, 1995.

Harner, C.D., and Hoher, J.: Evaluation and treatment of posterior cruciate ligament injuries: Current concepts. Am. J. Sports Med. 26:471–482, 1998.

Harner, C.D., Irrgang, J.J., Paul, J., et al.: Loss of motion following anterior cruciate ligament reconstruction. Am. J. Sports Med. 20:507–515, 1992.

Howell, S.M., and Taylor, M.A.: Failure of reconstruction of the anterior cruciate ligament due to impingement by the intercondylar roof. J. Bone Joint Surg. [Am.] 75:1044–1055, 1993.

Indelicato, P.A., Isolated medial collateral ligament injuries in the knee. J. Am. Acad. Orthop. Surg. 3:9–14, 1995.

Indelicato, P.A., Hermansdorfer, J., and Huegel, M.: Nonoperative management of complete tears of the medial collateral ligament of the knee in intercollegiate football players. Clin. Orthop. 256:174–177, 1990.

Larson, R.L., and Taillon, M.: Anterior cruciate ligament insufficiency: Principles of treatment. J. Am. Acad. Orthop. Surg. 2:26–35, 1994.

Myers, M.H., and Harvey, J.P.: Traumatic dislocation of the knee joint: A study of eighteen cases. J. Bone Joint Surg. [Am.] 53:16–29, 1971.

Noyes, F.R., Barber-Westin, S.D., Butler, D.L., et al.: The role of allografts in repair and reconstruction of knee joint ligaments and menisci. AAOS Instr. Course Lect. 47:379–396, 1998.

O'Brien, S.J., Warren, R.F., Pavlov, H., et al.: Reconstruction of the chronically insufficient anterior cruciate ligament with the central third of the patellar ligament. J. Bone Joint Surg. [Am.] 73:278–286, 1991.

Paulos, L.E., Rosenberg, T.D., Drawbert, J., et al.: Infrapatellar contracture syndrome: An unrecognized cause of knee stiffness with patellar entrapment and patella infera. Am. J. Sports Med. 15:331–341, 1987.

Shelbourne, K.D., and Nitz, P.: Accelerated rehabilitation after anterior cruciate ligament reconstruction. Am. J. Sports Med. 18:292–299, 1990.

Shelton, W.R., Treacy, S.H., Dukes, A.D., et al.: Use of allografts in knee reconstruction. J. Am. Acad. Orthop. Surg. 6:165–175, 1998.

Sisto, D.J., and Warren, R.F.: Complete knee dislocation: A follow-up study of operative treatment. Clin. Orthop. 198:94–101, 1985.

Sitler, M., Ryan, J., Hopkinson, W., et al.: The efficacy of a prophylactic knee brace to reduce knee injuries in football: A prospective, randomized study at West Point. Am. J. Sports Med. 18:310–315, 1990.

Veltri, D.M., and Warren, R.F.: Isolated and combined posterior cruciate ligament injuries. J. Am. Acad. Orthop. Surg. 1:67–75, 1993.

Anterior Knee Pain

Boden, B.P., Pearsall, A.W., Garrett, W.E., et al.: Patellofemoral instability: Evaluation and management. J. Am. Acad. Orthop. Surg. 5:47–57, 1997.

Cooper, D.E., and DeLee, J.C.: Reflex sympathetic dystrophy of the knee. J. Am. Acad. Orthop. Surg. 2:79–86, 1994.

Cramer, K.E., and Moed, B.R.: Patellar fractures: Contemporary approach to treatment. J. Am. Acad. Orthop. Surg. 5:323–331, 1997.

Fulkerson, J.P.: Anteromedialization of the tibial tuberosity for patellofemoral malalignment. Clin. Orthop. 177:176–181, 1983.

Fulkerson, J.P.: Patellofemoral pain disorders: Evaluation and management. J. Am. Acad. Orthop. Surg. 2:124–132, 1994.

Fulkerson, J.P., and Shea, K.P.: Disorders of patellofemoral alignment: Current concepts review. J. Bone Joint Surg. [Am.] 72:1424–1429, 1990.

James, S.L.: Running injuries to the knee. J. Am. Acad. Orthop. Surg. 3:309–318, 1995.

Kelly, M.A.: Algorithm for anterior knee pain. AAOS Instr. Course Lect. 47:339–343, 1998.

Kilowich, P., Paulos, L., Rosenberg, T., et al.: Lateral release of the patella: Indications and contraindications. Am. J. Sports Med. 18:361, 1990.

Larson, R.L., Cabaud, H.E., Slocum, D.B., et al.: The patellar compression syndrome: Surgical treatment by lateral retinacular release. Clin. Orthop. 134:158–167, 1978.

Matava, M.J.: Patellar tendon ruptures. J. Am. Acad. Orthop. Surg. 4:287–296, 1996.

Merchant, A.: Classification of patellofemoral disorders. Arthroscopy 4:235–240, 1988.

Merchant, A.C., Mercer, R.L., Jacobsen, R.J., et al.: Roentgenographic analysis of patellofemoral congruence. J. Bone Joint Surg. [Am.] 56:1391–1396, 1974.

Childhood and Adolescent Knee Disorders

Andrish, J.T.: Meniscal injuries in children and adolescents: Diagnosis and management. J. Am. Acad. Orthop. Surg. 5:231–237, 1996.

Baxter, M.P., and Wiley, J.J.: Fractures of the tibial spine in children: An evaluation of knee stability. J. Bone Joint Surg. [Br.] 70:228–230, 1988.

Edwards, P.H., and Grana, W.A.: Physical fractures about the knee. J. Am. Acad. Orthop. Surg. 3:63–69, 1995.

Lo, I.K.Y., Bell, D.M., and Fowler, P.J.: Anterior cruciate ligament injuries in the skeletally immature patient. AAOS Instr. Course Lect. 47:351–359, 1998.

McCarroll, J.R., Rettig, A.C., and Shelbourne, K.D.: Anterior cruciate ligament injuries in the young athlete with open physes. Am. J. Sports Med. 16:44–47, 1988.

Meyers, M.H., and McKeever, F.M.: Fractures of the intercondylar eminence of the tibia. J. Bone Joint Surg. [Am.] 41:209–222, 1959.

Micheli, L.J., and Foster, T.E.: Acute knee injuries in the immature athlete. Instr. Course Lect. 42:473–481, 1993.

Ogden, J.A., Tross, R.B., and Murphy, M.J.: Fractures of the tibial tuberosity in adolescents. J. Bone Joint Surg. [Am.] 62:205–215, 1980.

Parker, A.W., Drez, D., and Cooper, J.L.: Anterior cruciate ligament injuries in patients with open physes. Am. J. Sports Med. 22:44–47, 1994.

Riseborough, E.J., Barrett, I.R., and Shapiro, F.: Growth disturbances following distal femoral physeal fracture-separations. J. Bone Joint Surg. [Am.] 65:885–893, 1983.

Stanitski, C.L.: Anterior cruciate ligament injury in the skeletally immature patient: Diagnosis and treatment. J. Am. Acad. Orthop. Surg. 3:146–158, 1995.

Stanitski, C.L.: Patellar instability in the school age athlete. AAOS Instr. Course Lect. 47:345–350, 1998.

Other Lower Extremity Sports Medicine Problems

Nerve Entrapment Syndromes

Baxter, D.E.: Functional nerve disorders in the athlete's foot, ankle, and leg. Instr. Course Lect. 42:185–194, 1993.

Beskin, J.L.: Nerve entrapments of the foot and ankle. J. Am. Acad. Orthop. Surg. 5:261–269, 1997.

Styf, J.: Entrapment of the superficial peroneal nerve: Diagnosis and results of decompression. J. Bone Joint Surg. [Br.] 71:131–135, 1989.

Contusions

Jackson, D.W., and Feagin, J.A.: Quadriceps contusions in young athletes. J. Bone Joint Surg. [Am.] 55:95–105, 1973.

Renstrom, P.A.H.F.: Tendon and muscle injuries in the groin area. Clin. Sports Med. 11:815–831, 1992.

Ryan, J.B., Wheeler, J.H., Hopkinson, W.J., et al.: Quadriceps contusions: West Point update. Am. J. Sports Med. 19:299–304, 1991.

Muscle Injury

Zarins, B., and Ciullo, J.V.: Acute muscle and tendon injuries in athletes. Clin. Sports Med. 2:167, 1983.

Tendon Injuries

Almekinders, L.C.: Tendinitis and other chronic tendinopathies. J. Am. Acad. Orthop. Surg. 6:157–164, 1998.

Bassett, F.H., and Speer, K.P.: Longitudinal rupture of the peroneal tendons. Am. J. Sports Med. 21:354–357, 1993.

Biedert, R.: Dislocation of the tibialis posterior tendon. Am. J. Sports Med. 20:775–776, 1992.

Brage, M.E., and Hansen, S.T.: Traumatic subluxation/dislocation of the peroneal tendons. Foot Ankle 13:423–430, 1992.

Jones, D.C.: Tendon disorders of the foot and ankle. J. Am. Acad. Orthop. Surg. 1:87–94, 1993.

Millar, A.P.: Strains of the posterior calf musculature ("tennis leg"). Am. J. Sports Med. 7:172–174, 1979.

Myerson, M.S., and McGarvey, W.: Disorders of the insertion of the achilles tendon and achilles tendinitis. J. Bone Joint Surg. 80A:1814–1824, 1998.

Ouzounian, T.J., and Myerson, M.S.: Dislocation of the posterior tibial tendon. Foot Ankle 13:215–219, 1992.

Saltzman, C.L., and Tearse, D.S.: Achilles tendon injuries. J. Am. Acad. Orthop. Surg. 6:316–325, 1998.

Sobel, M., Geppert, M.J., Olson, E.J., et al.: The dynamics of peroneus brevis tendon splits: A proposed mechanism, technique of diagnosis, and classification of injury. Foot Ankle 13:413–421, 1992.

Teitz, C.C., Garrett W.E., Miniaci, et al.: Tendon problems in athletic individuals. J. Bone Joint Surg. 79A:138–152, 1997.

Williams, J.G.P.: Achilles tendon lesions in sport. Sports Med. 3:114–135, 1986.

Compartment Syndrome

Beckham, S.G., Grana, W.A., Buckley, P., et al.: A comparison of anterior compartment pressures in competitive runners and cyclists. Am. J. Sports Med. 21:36–40, 1993.

Eisele, S.A., and Sammarco, G.J.: Chronic exertional compartment syndrome. Instr. Course Lect. 42:213–217, 1993.

Pedowitz, R.A., Horgens, A.R., Mubarak, S.J., et al.: Modified criteria for the objective diagnosis of compartment syndrome of the leg. Am. J. Sports Med. 18:35–40, 1990.

Rorabeck, C.H., Bourne, R.B., and Fowler, P.J.: The surgical treatment of exertional compartment syndromes in athletes. J. Bone Joint Surg. [Am.] 65:1245, 1983.

Rorabeck, C.H., Fowler, P.J., and Nitt, L.: The results of fasciotomy in the management of chronic exertional compartment syndrome. Am. J. Sports Med. 16:224–227, 1986.

Stress Fractures

Anderson, E.G.: Fatigue fractures of the foot. Injury 21:274–279, 1990.

Blickenstaff, L.D., and Morris, J.M.: Fatigue fracture of the femoral neck. J. Bone Joint Surg. [Am.] 48:1031, 1966.

Green, N.E., Rogers, R.A., and Lipscomb, A.B.: Nonunions of stress fractures of the tibia. Am. J. Sports Med. 13:171–176, 1985.

Khan, K.M., Fuller, P.J., Brukner, P.D., et al.: Outcome of conservative and surgical management of navicular stress fracture in athletes: Eighty-six cases proven with computerized tomography. Am. J. Sports Med. 20:657–661, 1992.

McBryde, A.M.: Stress fractures in athletes. J. Sports Med. 3:212, 1973.

Rettig, A.C., Shelbourne, K.D., McCarroll, J.R., et al.: The natural history and treatment of delayed union stress fractures of the anterior cortex of the tibia. Am. J. Sports Med. 16:250–255, 1988.

Shin, A.Y., and Gillingham, B.L.: Fatigue fractures of the femoral neck in athletes. J. Am. Acad. Orthop. Surg. 5:293–302, 1997.

Other Hip Disorders

Allen, W.C., and Cope, R.: Coxa saltans: The snapping hip revisited. J. Am. Acad. Orthop. Surg. 3:303–308, 1995.

Clanton, T.O., and Coupe, K.J.: Hamstring strains in athletes: Diagnosis and treatment. J. Am. Acad. Orthop. Surg. 6:237–248, 1998.

Cooper, D.E., Warren, R.F., and Barnes, R.: Traumatic subluxation of the hip resulting in aseptic necrosis and chondrolysis in a professional football player. Am. J. Sports Med. 19:322–324, 1991.

Holmes, J.C., Pruitt, A.L., and Whalen, N.J.: Iliotibial band syndrome in cyclists. Am. J. Sports Med. 21:419–424, 1993.

Martens, M., Libbrecht, P., and Burssens, A.: Surgical treatment of the iliotibial band friction syndrome. Am. J. Sports Med. 17:651–654, 1989.

Other Foot and Ankle Disorders

Baxter, D.E., and Zingas, C.: The foot in running. J. Am. Acad. Orthop. Surg. 3:136–145, 1995.

Churchill, J.A., and Mazur, J.M.: Ankle pain in children: Diagnostic evaluation and clinical decision-making. J. Am. Acad. Orthop. Surg. 3:183–193, 1995.

Colville, M.R.: Surgical treatment of the unstable ankle. J. Am. Acad. Orthop. Surg. 6:368–377, 1998.

Garrick, J.G., and Requa, R.K.: The epidemiology of foot and ankle injuries in sports. Clin. Sports Med. 7:29–36, 1988.

Gill, L.H.: Plantar fasciitis: Diagnosis and conservative management. J. Am. Acad. Orthop. Surg. 5:109–117, 1997.

Hamilton, W.G., Thompson, F.M., and Snow, S.W.: The modified Brostrom procedure for lateral ankle instability. Foot Ankle 14:1–7, 1993.

Hopkinson, W.J., St. Pierre, P., Ryan, J.B., et al.: Syndesmosis sprains of the ankle. Foot Ankle 10:325–330, 1990.

Marotta, J.J., and Micheli, L.J.: Os trigonum impingement in dancers. Am. J. Sports Med. 20:533–536, 1992.

Miller, C.M., Winter, W.G., Bucknell, A.L., et al.: Injuries to the midtarsal joint and lesser tarsal bones. J. Am. Acad. Orthop. Surg. 6:249–258, 1998.

Mizel, M.S., and Yodlowski, M.L.: Disorders of the lesser metatarsophalangeal joints. J. Am. Acad. Orthop. Surg. 3:166–173, 1995.

Renstrom, P.A.F.H.: Persistently painful sprained ankle. J. Am. Acad. Orthop. Surg. 2:270–280, 1994.

Rodeo, S.A., O'Brien, S., Warren, R.F., et al.: Turf toe: An analysis of metatarsal phalangeal joint pain in professional football players. Am. J. Sports Med. 18:280–285, 1990.

Wuest, T.K.: Injuries to the distal lower extremity syndesmosis. J. Am. Acad. Orthop. Surg. 5:172–181, 1997.

Hip and Ankle Arthroscopy

Angermann, P., and Jensen, P.: Osteochondritis dissecans of the talus: Long-term results of surgical treatment. Foot Ankle 10:161–163, 1989.

Basset, F.H., Billy, J.B., and Gates, H.S.: A simple surgical approach to the posteromedial ankle. Am. J. Sports Med. 21:144–146, 1993.

Ferkel, R.D., and Scranton, P.E.: Current concepts review: Arthroscopy of the ankle and foot. J. Bone Joint Surg. [Am.] 75:1233–1243, 1993.

Glick, J.M., Sampson, T.G., Gordon, R.B., et al.: Hip arthroscopy by the lateral approach. Arthroscopy 3:4–12, 1987.

Loomer, R., Fisher, C., Lloyd-Smith, R., et al.: Osteochondral lesions of the talus. Am. J. Sports Med. 21:13–19, 1993.

McCarroll, J.R., Schrader, J.W., Shelbourne, K.D., et al.: Meniscoid lesions of the ankle in soccer players. Am. J. Sports Med. 15:257, 1987.

McCarthy, J.C., Day, B., and Busconi, B.: Hip arthroscopy: Applications and technique. J. Am. Acad. Orthop. Surg. 3:115–122, 1995.

Meislin, R.J., Rose, D.J., Parisien, S., et al.: Arthroscopic treatment of synovial impingement of the ankle. Am. J. Sports Med. 21:186–189, 1993.

Ogilvie-Harris, D.J., Lieverman, I., and Fitsalos, D.: Arthroscopically assisted arthrodesis for osteoarthritic ankles. J. Bone Joint Surg. [Am.] 75:1167–1174, 1993.

Stetson, W.B., and Ferkel, R.D.: Ankle arthroscopy. J. Am. Acad. Orthop. Surg. 4:17–34, 1996.

Stone, J.W.: Osteochondral lestions of the talar dome. J. Am. Acad. Orthop. Surg. 4:63–73, 1996.

Thein, R., and Eichenblat, M.: Arthroscopic treatment of sports-related synovitis of the ankle. Am. J. Sports Med. 20:496–499, 1992.

Shoulder

Anatomy and Biomechanics

Cooper, D.E., Arnoczsky, S.P., O'Brien, S.J., et al.: Anatomy, histology, and vascularity of the glenoid labrum. J. Bone Joint Surg. [Am.] 74:46–52, 1992.

Cooper, D.E., O'Brien, S.J., and Warren, R.F.: Supporting layers of the glenohumeral joint: An anatomic study. Clin. Orthop. 289:144–155, 1993.

Ferrari, D.A.: Capsular ligaments of the shoulder: Anatomical and functional study of the anterior superior capsule. Am. J. Sports Med. 18:20–24, 1990.

Flatow, E.L.: The biomechanics of the acromioclavicular, sternoclavicular, and scapulothoracic joints. Instr. Course Lect. 42:237–245, 1993.

Harryman, D.T. II: Common surgical approaches to the shoulder. Instr. Course Lect. 41:3–11, 1992.

Iannotti, J.P., Gabriel, J.P., Schneck, S.L., et al.: The normal glenohumeral relationships: An anatomical study of one hundred and forty shoulders. J. Bone Joint Surg. [Am.] 74:491–500, 1992.

Kibler, W.B.: The role of the scapula in athletic shoulder function: Current Concepts. Am. J. Sports Med. 26:325–337, 1998.

O'Brien, S.J., Neves, M.C., Rozbruck, S.R., et al.: The anatomy and histology of the inferior glenohumeral ligament complex of the shoulder. Am. J. Sports Med. 18:449, 1990.

O'Connell, P.W., Nuber, G.W., Mileski, R.A., et al.: The contribution of the glenohumeral ligaments to anterior stability of the shoulder joint. Am. J. Sports Med. 18:579–584, 1990.

Warner, J.J.P., Deng, X.H., Warren, R.F., et al.: Static capsuloligamentous restraints to superior-inferior translation of the glenohumeral joint. Am. J. Sports Med. 20:675–685, 1992.

Warner, J.J.P., Deng, X.H., Warren, R.F., et al.: Superior-inferior translation in the intact and vented glenohumeral joint. J. Shoulder Elbow Surg. 2:99–105, 1993.

History and Physical Examination

Altchek, D.W., and Dines, D.M.: Shoulder injuries in the throwing athlete. J. Am. Acad. Orthop. Surg. 3:159–165, 1995.

Gerber, C., and Ganz, R.: Clinical assessment of instability of the shoulder with special reference to anterior and posterior drawer tests. J. Bone Joint Surg. [Br.] 66:551–556, 1984.

Neer, C.S., and Welsh, R.P.: The shoulder in sports. Orthop. Clin. North Am. 8:583–591, 1977.

Imaging of the Shoulder

Beltran, J.: The use of magnetic resonance imaging about the shoulder. J. Shoulder Elbow Surg. 1:287–295, 1992.

Bigliani, L.U., Morrison, D., and April, E.W.: The morphology of the acromion and its relationship to rotator cuff tears. Orthop. Trans. 10:228, 1986.

Garth, W.P., Jr., Slappey, C.E., and Ochs, C.W.: Roentgenographic demonstration of instability of the shoulder: The apical oblique projection—a technical note. J. Bone Joint Surg. [Am.] 66:1450–1453, 1984.

Herzog, R.J.: Magnetic resonance imaging of the shoulder. J. Bone Joint Surg. 79A:934–953, 1997.

Hill, H.A., and Sachs, M.D.: The grooved defect of the humeral head: A frequently unrecognized complication of dislocations of the shoulder joint. Radiology 35:690–700, 1940.

Hobbs, D.W.: Sternoclavicular joint: A new axial radiographic view. Radiology 90:801–802, 1968.

Kozo, O., Yamamuro, T., and Rockwood, C.A.: Use of a thirty-degree caudal tilt radiograph in the shoulder impingement syndrome. J. Shoulder Elbow Surg. 1:246–252, 1992.

Zanca, P.: Shoulder pain: Involvement of the acromioclavicular joint: Analysis of 1000 cases. AJR Am. J. Roentgenol. 112:493–506, 1971.

Arthroscopy of the Shoulder

Altchek, D.W., and Carson, E.W.: Arthroscopic acromioplasty: Indications and technique. AAOS Instr. Course Lect. 47:21–28, 1998.

Bell, R.H.: Arthroscopic distal clavicle resection. AAOS Instr. Course Lect. 47:35–41, 1998.

Caborn, D.M., and Fu, F.H.: Arthroscopic approach and anatomy of the shoulder. Op. Tech. Orthop. 1:126–133, 1991.

Lintner, S.A., and Speer, K.P.: Traumatic anterior glenohumeral instability: The role of arthroscopy. J. Am. Acad. Orthop. Surg. 5:233–239, 1997.

Nisbet, J.K., and Paulos, L.E.: Subacromial bursoscopy. Op. Tech. Orthop. 1:221–228, 1991.

Skyhar, M.J., Altchek, D.W., Warren, R.F., et al.: Shoulder arthroscopy with the patient in the beach chair position. Arthroscopy 4:256–259, 1988.

Wolf, E.M.: Anterior portals in shoulder arthroscopy. Arthroscopy 5:201–208, 1989.

Shoulder Instability

Altchek, D.W., Warren, R.F., Skyhar, M.J., et al.: T-plasty modification of the Bankhart procedure for multidirectional instability of the anterior an inferior types. J. Bone Joint Surg. [Am.] 73:105–112, 1991.

Arciero, R.A., Wheeler, J.H. III, Ryan, J.B., et al.: Arthroscopic Bankart repair for acute, initial anterior shoulder dislocations. Am. J. Sports Med. 22:589–594, 1994.

Cooper, R.A., and Brems, J.J.: The inferior capsular shift procedure for multidirectional instability of the shoulder. J. Bone Joint Surg. [Am.] 74:1516–1521, 1992.

Grana, W.A., Buckley, P.D., and Yates, C.K.: Arthroscopic Bankart suture repair. Am. J. Sports Med. 21:348–353, 1993.

Harryman, D.T. II, Sidles, J.A., Harris, S.L., et al.: Laxity of the normal glenohumeral joint: A quantitative in vivo assessment. J. Shoulder Elbow Surg. 1:66–76, 1992.

Lippit, S., and Matsen, F.A. III: Mechanisms of glenohumeral joint stability. Clin. Orthop. 291:20–28, 1993.

Morgan, C.D., and Bodenstab, A.B.: Arthroscopic Bankart suture repair: Techniques and early results. Arthroscopy 3:111–112, 1982.

Neer, C.S. II, and Foster, C.R.: Inferior capsular shift for involuntary inferior and multidirectional instability of the shoulder: A preliminary report. J. Bone Joint Surg. [Am.] 62:897–908, 1980.

Pollock, R.G., and Bigliani, L.U.: Glenohumeral instability: Evaluation and treatment. J. Am. Acad. Orthop. Surg. 1:24–32, 1993.

Rowe, C.R., Patel, D., and Southmayd, W.W.: The Bankart procedure: A long-term end-result study. J. Bone Joint Surg. [Am.] 55:445–460, 1973.

Schenk, T.J., and Brems, J.J.: Multidirectional instability of the shoulder: Pathophysiology, diagnosis, and management. J. Am. Acad. Orthop. Surg. 6:65–72, 1998.

Turkel, S.J., Panio, M.W., Marshall, J.L., et al.: Stabilizing mechanisms preventing anterior dislocation of the glenohumeral joint. J. Bone Joint Surg. [Am.] 63:1208–1217, 1981.

Zuckerman, J.D., and Matsen, F.A. III: Complications about the glenohumeral joint related to the use of screws and staples. J. Bone Joint Surg. [Am.] 66:175–180, 1984.

Impingement Syndrome/Rotator Cuff

Bigliani, L.U., Cordasco, F.A., McIlveen, S.J., et al.: Operative treatment of failed repairs of the rotator cuff. J. Bone Joint Surg. [Am.] 74:1505–1515, 1992.

Bigliani, L.U., and Levine, W.N.: Current concepts review: Subacromial impingement syndrome. J. Bone Joint Surg. 79A:1854–1868, 1997.

Budoff, J.E., Nirschl, R.P., and Guidi, E.J.: Current concepts review: Debridement of partial-thickness tears of the rotator cuff without acromioplasty. J. Bone Joint Surg. 80A:733–748, 1998.

Caspari, R.B., and Thal, R.: A technique for arthroscopic subacromial decompression. Arthroscopy 8:23–20, 1992.

Cordasco, F.A., and Bigliani, L.U.: The treatment of failed rotator cuff repairs. AAOS Instr. Course Lect. 47:77–86, 1998.

Ellman, H., Kay, S.P., and Worth, M.: Arthroscopic treatment of full-thickness rotator cuff tears: Two to seven year follow-up study. Arthroscopy 9:301–314, 1993.

Flatow, E.L., and Warner, J.J.P.: Instability of the shoulder: Complex problems and failed repairs (part I). J. Bone Joint Surg. 80A:122–140, 1998.

Flatow, E.L., Miniaci, A., Evans, P.J., et al.: Instability of the shoulder: Complex problems and failed repairs (part II). J. Bone Joint Surg. 80A:284–298, 1998.

Gartsman, G.M.: Arthroscopic management of rotator cuff disease. J. Am. Acad. Orthop. Surg. 6:259–266, 1998.

Gerber, C., Terrier, F., and Ganz, R.: The role of the coracoid process in the chronic impingement syndrome. J. Bone Joint Surg. [Br.] 67:703–708, 1985.

Holsbeeck, E.: Subacromial impingement: Open versus arthroscopic decompression. Arthroscopy 8:173–178, 1992.

Ianotti, J.P.: Full-thickness rotator cuff tears: Factors affecting surgical outcome. J. Am. Acad. Orthop. Surg. 2:87–95, 1994.

McConville, O.R., and Iannotti, J.P.: Partial-thickness tears of the rotator cuff: Evaluation and management. J. Am. Acad. Orthop. Surg. 7:32–43, 1999.

Neer, C.S. II: Anterior acromioplasty for the chronic impingement syndrome in the shoulder. J. Bone Joint Surg. [Am.] 54:41–50, 1972.

Rockwood, C.A., Jr., and Lyons, F.R.: Shoulder impingement syndrome: Diagnosis, radiographic evaluation, and treatment with a modified Neer acromioplasty. J. Bone Joint Surg. [Am.] 75:409–424, 1993.

Speer, K.P., Lohnes, J., and Garrett, W.C.: Arthroscopic subacromial decompression: Results in advanced impingement syndrome. Arthroscopy 7:291–296, 1991.

Williams, G.R.: Painful shoulder after surgery for rotator cuff disease. J. Am. Acad. Orthop. Surg. 5:97–108, 1997.

Zeman, C.A., Arcand, M.A., Cantrell, J.S., et al.: The rotator cuff-deficient arthritic shoulder: Diagnosis and surgical management. J. Am. Acad. Orthop. Surg. 6:337–348, 1998.

Biceps Injuries

Andrews, J., Carson, W., and McLeod, W.: Glenoid labrum tears related to the long head of the biceps. Am. J. Sports Med. 13:337–341, 1985.

Froimson, A.I., and Oh, I.: Keyhole tenodesis of biceps origin at the shoulder. Clin. Orthop. 112:245–249, 1974.

Mileski, R.A., and Snyder, S.J.: Superior labral lesions in the shoulder: Pathoanatomy and surgical management. J. Am. Acad. Orthop. Surg. 6:121–131, 1998.

Resch, H., Golser, K., Thoeni, H., et al.: Arthroscopic repair of superior glenoid labral detachment (the SLAP lesion). J. Shoulder Elbow Surg. 2:147–155, 1993.

Snyder, S.J., and Wuh, H.C..K.: Arthroscopic evaluation and treatment of the rotator cuff and superior labrum anterior posterior lesion. Op. Tech. Orthop. 1:207–220, 1991.

Acromioclavicular and Sternoclavicular Injuries

Cahill, B.R.: Osteolysis of the distal part of the clavicle in male athletes. J. Bone Joint Surg. [Am.] 64:1053–1058, 1982.

Gartsman, G.M.: Arthroscopic resection of the acromioclavicular joint. Am. J. Sports Med. 21:71–77, 1993.

Lemos, M.J.: The evaluation and treatment of the injured acromioclavicular joint in athletes: Current concepts. Am. J. Sports Med. 26:137–144, 1998.

Nuber, G.W., and Bowen, M.K.: Acromioclavicular joint injuries and distal clavicle fractures. J. Am. Acad. Orthop. Surg. 5:11–18, 1997.

Richards, R.R.: Acromioclavicular joint injuries. Instr. Course Lect. 42:259–269, 1993.

Rockwood, C.A., Jr., and Young, D.C.: Disorders of the acromioclavicular joint. In Rockwood, C.A., Jr., and Matsen, F.A. III, eds.: The Shoulder, pp. 413–476. Philadelphia, WB Saunders, 1990.

Scavenius, M., and Iverson, B.F.: Nontraumatic clavicular osteolysis in weight lifters. Am. J. Sports Med. 20:463–467, 1992.

Wirth, M.A., and Rockwood, C.A., Jr.: Acute and chronic traumatic injuries of the sternoclavicular joint. J. Am. Acad. Orthop. Surg. 4:268–278, 1996.

Muscle Ruptures

Caughey, M.A., and Welsh, P.: Muscle ruptures affecting the shoulder girdle. In Rockwood, C.A., Jr., and Matsen, F.A. III, eds.: The Shoulder, pp. 863–873. Philadelphia, WB Saunders, 1991.

Gerber, C., and Krushell, R.J.: Isolated rupture of the tendon of the subscapularis muscle. J. Bone Joint Surg. [Br.] 73:389–394, 1991.

Kretzler, H.H., Jr., and Richardson, A.B.: Rupture of the pectoralis major muscle. Am. J. Sports Med. 17:453–458, 1989.

Miller, M.D., Johnson, D.L., Fu, F.H., et al.: Rupture of the pectoralis major muscle in a collegiate football player. Am. J. Sports Med. 21:475–477, 1993.

Wolfe, S.W., Wickiewics, T.L., and Cananaugh, J.T.: Ruptures of the pectoralis major muscle: An anatomic and clinical analysis. Am. J. Sports Med. 20:587–593, 1992.

Calcific Tendinitis and Adhesive Capsulitis

Ark, J.W., Flock, T.J., Flatow, E.L., et al.: Arthroscopic treatment of calcific tendinitis of the shoulder. Arthroscopy 8:183–188, 1992.

Coventry, M.B.: Problem of the painful shoulder. J.A.M.A. 151:177–185, 1953.

Faure, G., and Daculsi, G.: Calcified tendinitis: A review. Ann. Rheum. Dis. 42(suppl):49–53, 1983.

Grey, R.G.: The natural history of "idiopathic" frozen shoulder. J. Bone Joint Surg. [Am.] 60:564, 1978.

Harmon, H.P.: Methods and results in the treatment of 2580 painful shoulders: With special reference to calcific tendinitis and the frozen shoulder. Am. J. Surg. 95:527–544, 1958.

Harryman, D.T. II: Shoulders: Frozen and stiff. Instr. Course Lect. 42:247–257, 1993.

Leffert, R.E.: The frozen shoulder. Instr. Course Lect. 34:199–203, 1985.

Miller, M.D., Wirth, M.A., and Rockwood, C.A., Jr.: Thawing the frozen shoulder: The "patient" patient. Orthopedics (in press).

Murnaghan, J.P.: Adhesive capsulitis of the shoulder: Current concepts and treatment. Orthopaedics 2:153–158, 1988.

Murnaghan, J.P.: Frozen shoulder. In Rockwood, C.A., Jr., and Matsen, F.A. III, eds.: The Shoulder. Philadelphia, WB Saunders, 1990.

Neviaser, J.S.: Adhesive capsulitis and the stiff and painful shoulder. Orthop. Clin. North Am. 2:327–331, 1980.

Neviaser, T.J.: Adhesive capsulitis. In McGinty, J.B., ed.: Operative Arthroscopy, pp. 561–566. New York, Raven Press, 1991.

Neviaser, R.J., and Neviaser, T.J.: The frozen shoulder: Diagnosis and management. Clin. Orthop. 223:59–64, 1987.

Shaffer, B., Tibone, J.E., and Kerlan, R.K.: Frozen shoulder: A long-term follow-up. J. Bone Joint Surg. [Am.] 74:738–746, 1992.

Uthoff, H.K., and Loehr, J.W.: Calcific tendinopathy of the rotator cuff: Pathogenesis, diagnosis, and management. J. Am. Acad. Orthop. Surg. 5:183–191, 1997.

Warner, J.J.P.: Frozen shoulder: Diagnosis and management. J. Am. Acad. Orthop. Surg. 5:130–140, 1997.

Warner, J.J.P., and Greis, P.E.: The treatment of stiffness of the shoulder after repair of the rotator cuff. J. Bone Joint Surg. 79A:1260–1269, 1997.

Nerve Disorders

Black, K.P., and Lombardo, J.A.: Suprascapular nerve injuries with isolated paralysis of the infraspinatus. Am. J. Sports Med. 18:225, 1990.

Burkhead, W.Z., Scheinberg, R.R., and Box, G.: Surgical anatomy of the axillary nerve. J. Shoulder Elbow Surg. 1:31–36, 1992.

Drez, D.: Suprascapular neuropathy in the differential diagnosis of rotator cuff injuries. Am. J. Sports Med. 4:443, 1976.
Fechter, J.D., and Kuschner, S.H.: The thoracic outlet syndrome. Orthopedics 16:1243–1254, 1993.
Kauppila, L.I.: The long thoracic nerve: Possible mechanisms of injury based on autopsy study. J. Shoulder Elbow Surg. 2:244–248, 1993.
Leffert, R.D.: Neurological problems. In Rockwood, C.A., Jr., and Matsen, F.A. III, eds.: The Shoulder, pp. 750–773. Philadelphia, WB Saunders, 1990.
Leffert, R.D.: Thoracic outlet syndrome. J. Am. Acad. Orthop. Surg. 2:317–325, 1994.
Markey, K.L., DiBeneditto, M., and Curl, W.W.: Upper trunk brachial plexopathy: The stinger syndrome. Am. J. Sports Med. 23:650–655, 1993.
Marmor, L., and Bechtal, C.O.: Paralysis of the serratus anterior due to electric shock relieved by transplantation of the pectoralis major muscle. J. Bone Joint Surg. [Am.] 45:156–160, 1983.
Post, M., and Grinblat, E.: Suprascapular nerve entrapment: Diagnosis and results of treatment. J. Shoulder Elbow Surg. 2:190–197, 1993.
Vastamaki, M., and Kauppila, L.I.: Etiologic factors in isolated paralysis of the serratus anterior muscle: A report of 197 cases. J. Shoulder Elbow Surg. 2:244–248, 1993.
Warner, J.J.P., Krushell, R.J., Masquelet, A., et al.: Anatomy and relationships of the suprascapular nerve: Anatomical constraints to mobilization of the supraspinatus and infraspinatus muscles in the management of massive rotator cuff tears. J. Bone Joint Surg. [Am.] 74A:36–45, 1992.

Other Shoulder Disorders

Fees, M., Decker, T., Snyder-Mackler, L, et al.: Upper extremity weight-training modifications for the injured athlete: Current Concepts. Am. J. Sports Med. 26:732–742, 1998.
Goss, T.P.: Scapular fractures and dislocations: Diagnosis and treatment. J. Am. Acad. Orthop. Surg. 3:22–33, 1995.
Green, A.: Current concepts of shoulder arthroplasty. AAOS Instr. Course Lect. 47:127–133, 1998.
Kuhn, J.E., Plancher, K.D., and Hawkins, R.J.: Scapular winging. J. Am. Acad. Orthop. Surg. 3:319–325, 1995.
Kuhn, J.E., Plancher, K.D., and Hawkins, R.J.: Symptomatic scapulothoracic crepitus and bursitis. J. Am. Acad. Orthop. Surg. 6:267–273, 1998.
Matthews, L.S., Wolock, B.S., and Martin, D.F.: Arthroscopic management of degenerative arthritis of the shoulder. In McGinty, J.B., ed.: Operative Arthroscopy, pp. 567–572. New York, Raven Press, 1991.
Miller, M.D., and Warner, J.J.P.: The abduction (weight bearing) radiograph of the shoulder. Poster American Academy of Orthopaedic Surgeons 61st Annual Meeting, New Orleans, 1994.
Schlegel, T.F., and Hawkins, R.J.: Displaced proximal humeral fractures: Evaluation and treatment. J. Am. Acad. Orthop. Surg. 2:54–66, 1994.
Simpson, N.S., and Jupiter, J.B.: Clavicular nonunion and malunion: Evaluation and surgical management. J. Am. Acad. Orthop. Surg. 4:1–8, 1996.

Other Upper Extremity Sports Medicine Problems

Tendon Injuries

Boyd, H.B., and Anderson, L.D.: A method for reinsertion of the distal biceps brachii tendon. J. Bone Joint Surg. [Am.] 43:1041–1043, 1961.
Boyd, H.B., and McLeod, A.C.: Tennis elbow. J. Bone Joint Surg. [Am.] 55:1183, 1973.
Burhkhart, S.S., Wood, M.B., and Linscheid, R.L.: Posttraumatic recurrent subluxation of the extensor carpi ulnaris tendon. J. Hand Surg. 7:1, 1982.
Conrad, R.W.: Tennis elbow. Instr. Course Lect. 35:94–101, 1986.
D'Alessandro, D.F., Shields, C.L., Tibone, J.E., et al.: Repair of distal biceps tendon ruptures in athletes. Am. J. Sports Med. 21:114, 1993.
Froimson, A.I.: Treatment of tennis elbow with forearm support band. J. Bone Joint Surg. [Am.] 53:183, 1971.
Gabel, G.T., and Morrey, B.F.: Tennis elbow. AAOS Instr. Course Lect. 47:165–172, 1998.
Green, D.P., and Strickland, J.W.: The hand. In DeLee, J.C., and Drez, D., Jr., eds.: Orthopaedic Sports Medicine, pp. 945–1017. Philadelphia, WB Saunders, 1993.
Ilfeld, F.W.: Can stroke modification relieve tennis elbow? Clin. Orthop. 276:182–185, 1992.
Jobe, F.W., and Ciccotti, M.G.: Lateral and medial epicondylitis of the elbow. J. Am. Acad. Orthop. Surg. 2:1–8, 1994.
Kiefhaber, T.R., and Stern, P.J.: Upper extremity tendinitis and overuse syndromes in the athlete. Clin. Sports Med. 11:39–55, 1992.
Leddy, J.P.: Soft tissue injuries of the hand in the athlete. AAOS Instr. Course Lect. 47:181–186, 1998.
Leddy, J.P., and Packer, J.W.: Avulsion of the profundus tendon insertion in athletes. J. Hand Surg. 2:66–69, 1977.
Morrey, B.F.: Reoperation of failed surgical treatment of refractory lateral epicondylitis. J. Shoulder Elbow Surg. 1:47–55, 1992.
Moss, J.G., and Steingold, R.F.: The long-term results of mallet finger injury: A retrospective study of one hundred cases. Hand 15:151–154, 1983.
Nirschl, R.P.: Sports and overuse injuries to the elbow. In Morrey, B.F., ed., The Elbow and Its Disorders, 2nd ed., pp. 537–552. Philadelphia, WB Saunders, 1993.
Nirschl, R.P., and Pettrone, F.: Tennis elbow: The surgical treatment of lateral epicondylitis. J. Bone Joint Surg. [Am.] 61:832, 1979.
Regan, W., Wold, L.E., Conrad, R., and Morrey, B.F.: Microscopic histopathology of chronic refractory lateral epicondylitis. Am. J. Sports Med. 20:746–749, 1992.
Rettig, A.C.: Closed tendon injuries of the hand and wrist in the athlete. Clin. Sports Med. 11:77–99, 1992.
Strickland, J.W.: Management of acute flexor tendon injuries. Orthop. Clin. North Am. 14:827–849, 1983.
Tarsney, F.F.: Rupture and avulsion of the triceps. Clin. Orthop. 83:177–183, 1972.
Wood, M.B., and Dobyns, J.H.: Sports-related extraarticular wrist syndromes. Clin. Orthop. 202:93–102, 1986.

Ligamentous Injuries

Alexander, C.E., and Lichtman, D.M.: Ulnar carpal instabilities. Orthop. Clin. North Am. 15:307–320, 1984.
Bednar, J.M., and Osterman, A.L.: Carpal instability: Evaluation and treatment. J. Am. Acad. Orthop. Surg. 1:10–17, 1993.
Bennett, J.B., Green, M.S., and Tullos, H.S.: Surgical management of chronic medial elbow instability. Clin. Orthop. 278:62–68, 1992.
Berger, R.A.: Radial-sided carpal instability. AAOS Instr. Course Lect. 47:219–228, 1998.
Betz, R.R., Browne, E.Z., Perry, G.B., et al.: The complex volar metacarpophalangeal-joint dislocation. J. Bone Joint Surg. [Am.] 64:1374–1375, 1982.
Campbell, C.S.: Gamekeepers thumb. J. Bone Joint Surg. [Br.] 37:148–149, 1955.
Conway, J.E., Jobe, F.W., Glousman, R.E., et al.: Medial instability of the elbow in throwing athletes: Surgical treatment by ulnar collateral ligament repair or reconstruction. J. Bone Joint Surg. [Am.] 74:67, 1992.
Cooney, W.P. III, Linscheid, R.L., and Dobyns, J.H.: Carpal instability: Treatment of ligament injuries of the wrist. Instr. Course Lect. 41:33–44, 1992.
Eaton, R.G., and Malerich, M.M.: Volar plate arthroplasty of the proximal interphalangeal joint: A review of ten years' experience. J. Hand Surg. 5:260–268, 1980.
Green, D.P., and Strickland, J.W.: The hand. In DeLee, J.C., and Drez, D., Jr., eds.: Orthopaedic Sports Medicine, pp. 945–1017. Philadelphia, WB Saunders, 1993.
Habernek, H., and Ortner, F.: The influence of anatomic factors in elbow joint dislocation. Clin. Orthop. 274:226–230, 1992.
Heyman, P.: Injuries to the ulnar collateral ligament of the thumb metacarpophalangeal joint. J. Am. Acad. Orthop. Surg. 5:224–229, 1997.
Hinterman, B., Holzach, P.J., Schultz, M., et al.: Skier's thumb: The significance of bony injuries. Am. J. Sports Med. 21:800–804, 1993.
Isani, A., and Melone, C.P., Jr.: Ligamentous injuries of the hand in athletes. Clin. Sports Med. 5:757–772, 1986.
Jobe, F.W., and Kvitne, R.S.: Elbow instability in the athlete. Instr. Course Lect. 40:17, 1991.
Kaplan, E.B.: Dorsal dislocation of the metacarpophalangeal joint of the index finger. J. Bone Joint Surg. [Am.] 39:1081–1086, 1957.
Kozin, S.H.: Perilunate injuries: Diagnosis and treatment. J. Am. Acad. Orthop. Surg. 6:114–120, 1998.
Light, T.R.: Buttress pinning techniques. Orthop. Rev. 10:49–55, 1981.

Lubahn, J.D., and Cermak, M.B.: Uncommon nerve compression syndromes of the upper extremity. J. Am. Acad. Orthop. Surg. 6:378–386, 1998.

McCue, F.C., and Bruce, J.F.: The wrist. In DeLee, J.C., and Drez, D., Jr., eds.: Orthopaedic Sports Medicine, pp. 913–944. Philadelphia, WB Saunders, 1993.

McElfresh, E.C., Dobyns, J.H., and O'Brien, E.T.: Management of fracture-dislocation of the proximal interphalangeal joints by extension-block splinting. J. Bone Joint Surg. [Am.] 54:1705–1711, 1972.

McLaughlin, H.L.: Complex "locked" dislocation of the metacarpalphalangeal joints. J. Trauma 5:683–688, 1965.

Miller, C.D., and Savoie, F.H. III: Valgus extension injuries of the elbow in the throwing athlete. J. Am. Acad. Orthop. Surg. 2:261–269, 1994.

Morrey, B.F.: Acute and chronic instability of the elbow. J. Am. Acad. Orthop. Surg. 4:117–128, 1996.

Morrey, B.F.: Complex instability of the elbow. J. Bone Joint Surg. 79A:460–469, 1997.

O'Driscoll, S.W., and Morrey, B.F.: Arthroscopy of the elbow: Diagnostic and therapeutic benefits and hazards. J. Bone Joint Surg. [Am.] 74:84–94, 1992.

O'Driscoll, S.W., Morrey, B.F., Korinek, S., et al.: Elbow subluxation and dislocation: A spectrum of instability. Clin. Orthop. 280:17–28, 1992.

Palmer, A.K., and Louis, D.S.: Assessing ulnar instability of the metacarpophalangeal joint of the thumb. J. Hand Surg. 3:542–546, 1978.

Redler, I., and Williams, J.T.: Rupture of a collateral ligament of the proximal interphalangeal joint of the fingers: Analysis of eighteen cases. J. Bone Joint Surg. [Am.] 49:322–326, 1967.

Short, W.H.: Wrist instability. AAOS Instr. Course Lect. 47:203–208, 1998.

Stener, B.: Displacement of the ruptured collateral ligament of the metacarpophalangeal joint of the thumb: A clinical and anatomical study. J. Bone Joint Surg. [Br.] 44:869–879, 1962.

Viegas, S.F.: Ulnar-sided wrist pain and instability. AAOS Instr Course Lect 47:215–218, 1998.

Watson, H.K., and Ballet, F.L.: The SLAC wrist: Scapholunate advanced collapse pattern of degenerative arthritis. J. Hand Surg. 9A:358–365, 1984.

Wilson, F.D., Andrews, J.R., Blackburn, T.A., et al.: Valgus extension overload in the pitching elbow. Am. J. Sports Med. 11:83, 1983.

Articular Injuries

Armstead, R.B., Linscheid, R.L., Dobyns, J.H., et al.: Ulnar lengthening in the treatment of Kienbock's disease. J. Bone Joint Surg. [Am.] 64:170–178, 1982.

Aulicino, P.L., and Siegel, L.: Acute injuries of the distal radioulnar joint. Hand Clin. 7:283–293, 1991.

Bauer, M., Jonsson, K., Josefsson, P.O., and Linden, B.: Osteochondritis dissecans of the elbow: A long-term follow-up study. Clin. Orthop. 284:156–160, 1992.

Bennett, J.B.: Articular injuries in the athlete. In Morrey, B.F., ed.: The Elbow and Its Disorders, 2nd ed., pp. 581–595. Philadelphia, WB Saunders, 1993.

DeHaven, K.E., and Evarts, C.M.: Throwing injuries of the elbow in athletes. Orthop. Clin. North Am. 1:801, 1973.

Dell, P.C.: Traumatic disorders of the distal radioulnar joint. Clin. Sports Med. 11:141–159, 1991.

Gelberman, R.H., Salamon, P.B., Jurist, J.M., et al.: Ulnar variance in Kienbock's disease. J. Bone Joint Surg. [Am.] 57:674–676, 1975.

Morrey, B.F.: Primary arthritis of the elbow treated by ulno-humeral arthroplasty. J. Bone Joint Surg. [Br.] 74:409, 1992.

Murakami, S., and Nakajima, H.: Aseptic necrosis of the capitate bone. Am. J. Sports Med. 12:170–173, 1984.

Nalebuff, E.A., Poehling, G.G., Siegel, D.B., et al.: Wrist and hand: Reconstruction. In Frymoyer, J.W., ed.: Orthopaedic Knowledge Update 4 Home Study Syllabus, pp. 389–402. Rosemont, IL, American Academy of Orthopaedic Surgeons, 1993.

Osterman, A.L.: Arthroscopic débridement of triangular fibrocartilage complex tears. Arthroscopy 6:120–124, 1990.

Palmer, A.K.: Triangular fibrocartilage disorders: Injury patterns and treatment. Arthroscopy 6:125–132, 1990.

Singer, K.M., and Roy, S.P.: Osteochondrosis of the humeral capitellum. Am. J. Sports Med. 12:351–360, 1984.

Watson, H.K., Ryu, J., and DiBella, W.S.: An approach to Kienbock's disease: Triscaphe arthrodesis. J. Hand Surg. 10A:179–187, 1985.

Woodward, A.H., and Bianco, A.J.: Osteochondritis dissecans of the elbow. Clin. Orthop. 110:35, 1975.

Arthroscopy

Adams, B.D.: Endoscopic carpal tunnel release. J. Am. Acad. Orthop. Surg. 2:179–184, 1994.

Andrews, J.R., and Carson, W.G.: Arthroscopy of the elbow. Arthroscopy 1:97, 1985.

Boe, S.: Arthroscopy of the elbow: Diagnosis and extraction of loose bodies. Acta Orthop. Scand. 57:52, 1986.

Carson, W.: Arthroscopy of the elbow. Instr. Course Lect. 37:195, 1988.

Chidgey, L.K.: The distal radioulnar joint: Problems and solutions. J. Am. Acad. Orthop. Surg. 3:95–108, 1995.

Cooney, W.P., Dobyns, J.H., and Linscheid, R.L.: Arthroscopy of the wrist: Anatomy and classification of carpal instability. Arthroscopy 6:133–140, 1990.

Guhl, J.: Arthroscopy and arthroscopic surgery of the elbow. Orthopedics 8:1290, 1985.

Lindenfeld, T.N.: Medial approach in elbow arthroscopy. Am. J. Sports Med. 18:413–417, 1990.

Lynch, G., Meyers, J., Whipple, T., et al.: Neurovascular anatomy and elbow arthroscopy: Inherent risks. Arthroscopy 2:191, 1986.

Osterman, A.L.: Arthroscopic débridement of triangular fibrocartilage complex tears. Arthroscopy 6:120–124, 1990.

Poehling, G.G., Siegel, D.B., Koman, L.A., et al.: Arthroscopy of the wrist and elbow. In DeLee, J.C., and Drez, D., Jr., eds.: Orthopaedic Sports Medicine, pp. 189–214. Philadelphia, WB Saunders, 1993.

Roth, J.H., Poehling, G.G., and Whipple, T.L.: Arthroscopic surgery of the wrist. Instr. Course Lect. 37:183–194, 1988.

Whipple, T.L.: Diagnostic and surgical arthroscopy of the wrist. In Nichols, J.A., and Hershman, E.B., eds.: The Upper Extremity in Sports Medicine, pp. 399–418. St. Louis, CV Mosby, 1990.

Other Upper Extremity Problems

O'Driscoll, S.W.: Elbow arthritis: Treatment options. J. Am. Acad. Orthop. Surg. 2:106–116, 1993.

Rettig, A.C.: Fractures in the hand in athletes. AAOS Instr. Course Lect. 47:187–190, 1998.

Simonian, P.T., and Trumble, T.E.: Scaphoid nonunion. J. Am. Acad. Orthop. Surg. 2:185–191, 1994.

Szabo, R.M., and Steinberg, D.R.: Nerve entrapment syndromes in the wrist. J. Am. Acad. Orthop. Surg. 2:115–123, 1994.

Head and Spine Injuries

Head Injuries

Bruno, L.A.: Focal intracranial hematoma. In Torg, J.S., ed.: Athletic Injuries to the Head, Neck and Face, 2nd ed. St. Louis, Mosby–Year Book, 1991.

Cantu, R.C.: Criteria for return to competition after a closed head injury. In Torg, J.S., ed.: Athletic Injuries to the Head, Neck and Face, 2nd ed., St. Louis, Mosby–Year Book, 1991.

Cantu, R.C.: Guidelines to return to sports after cerebral concussion. Phys. Sports Med. 14:76, 1986.

Gennarelli, T.A.: Head injury mechanisms, and cerebral concussion and diffuse brain injuries. In Torg, J.S., ed.: Athletic Injuries to the Head, Neck and Face, 2nd ed. St. Louis: Mosby–Year Book, 1991.

Jordan, B.D., Tsairis, P., and Warren, R.F.: Sports Neurology. Rockville, MD, Aspen Press, 1989.

Lindsay, K.W., McLatchie, G., Jennett, B.: Serious head injuries in sports. B.M.J. 281:789–791, 1980.

Cervical Spine Injuries

Albright, J.P., Moses, J.M., Feldich, H.G., et al.: Non-fatal cervical spine injuries in interscholastic football. J.A.M.A. 236:1243–1245, 1976.

Bracken, M.D., Shepard, M.J., Collins, W.F., et al.: A randomized, controlled trial of methylprednisolone or naloxone in the treatment of acute spinal cord injury. N. Engl. J. Med. 322:1405, 1990.

Pavlov, H., Torg, J.S., Robie, B., et al.: Cervical spinal stenosis: Determination with vertebral body radio method. Radiology 164:771–775, 1987.

Thompson, R.C.: Current concepts in management of cervical spine fractures and dislocations. Am. J. Sports Med. 3:159, 1975.

Torg, J.S., and Gennarelli, T.A.: Head and cervical spine injuries. In DeLee, J.C., and Drez, D., Jr., eds.: Orthopaedic Sports Medicine: Principles and Practice, pp. 417–462. Philadelphia, WB Saunders, 1994.

Torg, J.S., Pavlov, H., Genuario, S.E., et al.: Neuropraxia of the cervical spinal cord with transient quadriplegia. J. Bone Joint Surg. [Am.] 68:1354–1370, 1986.

Torg, J.S., Sennett, B., Pavlov, H., et al.: Spear tackler's spine: An entity precluding participation in tackle football and collision activities that expose the cervical spine to axial energy inputs. Am. J. Sports Med. 21:640–649, 1993.

Torg, J.S., Sennett, B., Vegso, J.J., et al.: Axial loading injuries to the middle cervical spine segment: An analysis and classification of twenty-five cases. Am. J. Sports Med. 19:6–20, 1991.

Torg, J.S., Vegso, J.J., O'Neill, J., et al.: The epidemiologic, pathologic, biomechanical and cinematographic analysis of football-induced cervical spine trauma. Am. J. Sports Med. 18:50–57, 1990.

White, A.A., Johnson, R.M., and Panjabi, M.M.: Biomechanical analysis of clinical stability in the cervical spine. Clin. Orthop. 109:85–93, 1975.

Thoracic and Lumbar Spine Injuries

Bradford, D.S., and Boachie-Adjei, O.: Treatment of severe spondylolisthesis by anterior and posterior reduction and stabilization: A long-term follow-up study. J. Bone Joint Surg. [Am.] 72:1060, 1990.

Eismont, F.J., and Currier, B.: Surgical management of lumbar intervertebral disc disease. J. Bone Joint Surg. [Am.] 71:1266, 1989.

Eismont, F.J., and Kitchel, S.H.: Thoracolumbar spine. In DeLee, J.C., and Drez, D., Jr., eds.: Orthopaedic Sports Medicine, pp. 1018–1062. Philadelphia, WB Saunders, 1994.

Jackson, D., Wiltse, L., Dingeman, R., et al.: Stress reactions involving the pars interarticularis in young athletes. Am. J. Sports Med. 9:305, 1981.

Keene, J.S., Albert, M.J., Springer, S.L., et al.: Back injuries in college athletes. J. Spinal Disord. 2:190–195, 1989.

Mundt, D.J., Kelsey, J.L., Golden, A.L., et al.: An epidemiological study of sports and weightlifting as possible risk factors for herniated lumbar and cervical discs. Am. J. Sports Med. 21:854–860, 1993.

Medical Aspects

Drugs

Berger, R.G.: Nonsteroidal anti-inflammatory drugs: Making the right choices. J. Am. Acad. Orthop. Surg. 2:255–260, 1994.

Fadale, P.D., and Wiggins, M.E.: Corticosteroid injections: Their use and abuse. J. Am. Acad. Orthop. Surg. 2:133–140, 1994.

Ergogenic Drugs

Aronson, V.: Protein and miscellaneous ergogenic aids. Physician Sports Med. 14:209–212, 1986.

Brien, A.J., and Simon, T.L.: The effects of red blood cell infusion on 10-km race time. J.A.M.A. 257:2761, 1987.

Cowart, V.S.: Human growth hormone: The latest ergogenic aid? Physician Sports Med. 16:175, 1988.

Haupt, H.A.: Anabolic steroids and growth hormone: Current concepts. Am. J. Sports Med. 21:468–474, 1993.

Perlmutter, G., and Lowenthal, D.T.: Use of anabolic steroids by athletes. Am. Fam. Physician 32:208, 1985.

Pope, H.G., Katz, D.L., and Champoux, R.: Anabolic-androgenic steroid use among 1,010 college men. Physician Sports Med. 16:75, 1988.

Robinson, J.B.: Ergogenic drugs in sports. In DeLee, J.C., and Drez, D., Jr., eds.: Orthopaedic Sports Medicine, pp. 294–306. Philadelphia, WB Saunders, 1994.

Cardiovascular

Abraham, P., Chevalier, J-M, Leftheriotis, G., et al.: Lower extremity arterial disease in sports. Am. J. Sports Med. 25:581–584, 1997.

Alpert, S.A., et al.: Athletic heart syndrome. Physician Sports Med. 12:103–107, 1989.

Basilico, F.C.: Cardiovascular disease in athletes: Current concepts. Am. J. Sports Med. 27:108–121, 1999.

Braden, D.S., and Strong, W.B.: Preparticipation screening for sudden cardiac death in high school and college athletes. Physician Sports Med. 16:128–140, 1988.

Finney, T.P., and D'Ambrosia, R.D.: Sudden cardiac death in an athlete. In DeLee, J.C., and Drez, D., Jr., eds.: Orthopaedic Sports Medicine, pp. 404–416. Philadelphia, WB Saunders, 1994.

James, T.N., Froggatt, P., and Marshall, T.K.: Sudden death in young athletes. Ann. Intern. Med. 67:1013–1021, 1967.

Maron, B.J., Epstein, S.E., and Roberts, W.C.: Causes of sudden death in competitive athletes. J. Am. Coll. Cardiol. 7:204–214, 1986.

Maron, B.J., Roberts, W.C., McAllister, H.A., et al.: Sudden death in young athletes. Circulation 62:218–229, 1980.

Van Camp, S.P.: Exercise-related sudden deaths: Risks and causes. Physician Sports Med. 16:97–112, 1988.

Exercise Physiology

Almekinders, L.C., and Oman, J.: Isokinetic muscle testing: It is clinically useful? J. Am. Acad. Orthop. Surg. 2:221–225, 1994.

Cahill, B.R., Misner, J.E., and Boileau, R.A.: The clinical importance of the anaerobic energy system and its assessment in human performance: Current concepts. Am. J. Sports Med. 25:863–872, 1997.

Fleck, S.J., and Schutt, R.C.: Types of strength training. Clin. Sports Med. 4:159–168, 1985.

Katch, F.I., and Drumm, S.S.: Effects of different modes of strength training on body composition and arthropometry. Clin. Sports Med. 5:413–459, 1986.

Kirkendall, D.T., and Garrett, W.E., Jr.: The effects of aging and training on skeletal muscle: Current concepts. Am. J. Sports Med. 26:598–602, 1998.

Lephart, S.M., Pincivero, D.M., Giraldo, J.L., et al.: The role of proprioception in the management and rehabilitation of athletic injuries. Am. J. Sports Med. 25:130–137, 1997.

Paulos, L.E., and Grauer, J.D.: Exercise. In Delee, J.C., and Drez, D., Jr., eds.: Orthopaedic Sports Medicine: Principles and Practice, pp. 228–243. Philadelphia, WB Saunders, 1994.

Pipes, T.V.: Isokinetic vs isotonic strength training an adult men. Med. Sci. Sports 7:262–274, 1975.

Taylor, D.C., Dalton, J.D., Seaber, A.V., et al.: Viscoelastic properties of muscle-tendon units: The biomechanical effects of stretching. Am. J. Sports Med. 18:300–309, 1990.

Yamamoto, S.K., Hartman, C.W., Feagin, J.A., et al.: Functional rehabilitation of the knee: A preliminary study. J. Sports Med. 3:228–291, 1976.

Female Athletes

Barrow, G., and Saha, S.: Menstrual irregularity and stress fractures in collegiate female distance runners. Am. J. Sports Med. 16:209–215, 1988.

Eisenberg, T., and Allen, W.: Injuries in a women's varsity athletic program. Physician Sports Med. 6:112–116, 1978.

Hunter, L., Andrews, J., Clancy, W., et al.: Common orthopaedic problems of the female athlete. Instr. Course Lect. 31:126–152, 1982.

Powers, J.: Characteristic features of injuries in the knee in women. Clin. Orthop. 143:120–124, 1979.

Protzman, R.: Physiologic performance of women compared to men: Observations of cadets at the United States Military Academy. Am. J. Sports Med. 7:191–194, 1979.

Tietz, C.C., Hu, S.S., and Arendt, E.A.: The female athlete: Evaluation and treatment of sportsrelated problems. J. Am. Acad. Orthop. Surg. 5:87–96, 1997.

Voss, L.A., Fadale, P.D., and Hulstyn, M.J.: Exercise-induced loss of bone density in athletes. J. Am. Acad. Orthop. Surg. 6:349–357, 1998.

Whiteside, P.: Men's and women's injuries in comparable sports. Physician Sports Med. 8:130–140, 1980.

Other Lower Extremity Problems

Buckwalter, J.A., and Lane, N.E.: Athletics and osteoarthritis. Am. J. Sports Med. 25:873–881, 1997.

4

Adult Reconstruction

Edward J. McPherson

I. Hip Replacement Surgery

A. Fixation—Total Hip Replacement. The method of long-term fixation of component parts for prosthetic joint replacement is either with cement or biologic interdigitation of bone to the prosthetic interface. The stated reasoning for the trend toward noncemented fixation in total hip replacement (THR) is the reported higher rates of loosening in young active patients. It is thought that the increased cycles and higher stresses applied to the hip joint in young, more active, patients lead to a more rapid failure of cemented components.

1. Cement Fixation—With cement fixation, there is mechanical interlock of methylmethacrylate to the interstices of bone, which is static. If microfractures occur with continued cyclic loading, the cement cannot remodel and will ultimately loosen. In contrast, with noncemented components, there is a biologic fixation to the prosthesis that is dynamic. If microfractures occur with cyclic loading in this system, there is the potential for bone remodeling, thus producing a potentially life-lasting bond. Furthermore, removing cement from the system provides one less interface that can fail.

2. Biologic Fixation—The methods of biologic fixation are either by a porous coated metallic surface that provides bone *ingrowth* fixation or by a grit-blasted metallic surface that provides bone *ongrowth* fixation. With a porous coated surface, pores are created on the metallic surface that allow bone to grow in and secure the prosthesis to host bone. Successful bone ingrowth requires an optimum pore size from 50 to 350 μm (preferably 50–150 microns). *Porosity* of the porous coated surface is important to allow bone to fill into a significant area of the prosthesis, and it should be 40–50%. Increased porosity above this is detrimental, as the porous coated surface would be at risk of shearing off. In addition, *pore depth* is a factor in the strength of the bone-prosthetic interlock. A deeper pore depth into the prosthesis provides greater interface shear strength with loading. Finally, *gaps* between the prosthesis and bone must be kept less than 50 μm.

3. Techniques of Fixation

a. Grit Blasting. With a grit-blasted surface, a metallic surface is roughened with an abrasive spray of particles that pits the metallic surface. The resultant peaks and valleys in the metal surface provide areas of bone to interdigitate and provide stable construct. With this method, the success of the bone ongrowth fixation is related to *surface roughness.* Surface roughness is defined as the average distance from peak to valley on the roughened surface. An increasing surface roughness is directly related to an increase in interface shear strength. The drawback of a grit-blasted surface is that bone fixation occurs only on the surface and therefore requires a more extensive area of coating to secure the prosthesis. Typically, the entire prosthesis needs to be grit-blasted to ensure adequate fixation.

b. Rigid Fixation. Successful bone ingrowth or ongrowth requires initial rigid fixation. Micromotion of the prosthesis must be kept below 150 μm (preferably 50–100 μm), or the prosthesis will be secured only by fibrous tissue (fibrous ingrowth). This will allow continued prosthetic micromotion and pain. If gross motion is allowed, the prosthesis will be encapsulated with fibrous tissue rather than with fibrous ingrowth, and this will cause the prosthesis to settle and remain mechanically unstable. The technique for insertion of noncemented components, therefore, is very important. *Initial rigid fixation* of porous coated implants is usually accomplished by the *press-fit technique*, in which the bone prepared for the acetabular cup or the femoral stem is sized slightly smaller in diameter (usually 1–2 mm undersized). When the component is inserted, the bone expands around the prosthesis, generating hoop stresses that keep the prosthesis in position and minimize micromotion. The other technique is a *"line to line"* fit in which the bone is prepared to the same size as the implant and is secured with additional measures. In the cup, a "line to line" technique requires screws for additional fixation. For the femoral stem, an extensive porous coating along the entire stem is required to obtain an "interference fit." This provides a rough surface over a large area and prevents excessive motion.

c. Cortical Bone Sealing. Another important factor for stable bone ingrowth is to have the implant seated against cortical bone rather than cancellous bone. Although cancellous bone will provide bone ingrowth, it is now known that the mechanical strength of an implant seated onto cortical bone is much stronger. Therefore, in the acetabulum it is important to achieve a good cortical rim fit of the acetabular cup. On the femoral side, it is important that the implant design and surgical preparation allow for cortical contact with the porous coated surface.

d. Surface Coating. Hydroxyapatite (HA) has been used as an adjuvant surface coating on porous coated and grit-blasted surfaces. HA is an osteoconductive agent that allows for more rapid closure of gaps. The HA surface readily receives osteoblasts and, thus, it provides a bidirectional closure of gaps (i.e., bone to prosthesis and prosthesis to bone). HA has been reported to delaminate off the prosthetic interface, and its use may be better suited to porous coated surfaces where the bone-HA is not the sole means of fixation. Successful use of HA as an adjuvant surface coating requires high crystallinity and optimal thickness (approximately 100–150 μm).

The recommended amount of porous coating on a femoral stem is controversial. With proximal porous coating, the porous surface is kept in the metaphyseal and upper metadiaphyseal regions of the femur. With this design concept, proximal bone ingrowth allows proximal bone loading and less stress shielding (Fig. 4–1). Conversely, an extensively coated stem has a porous coating over its entire surface. Most bone ingrowth occurs in the diaphysis, and the weight-bearing forces bypass the proximal femur. As a result, the proximal femur is stress-shielded, leading to loss of bone density. Although stress shielding has been noted in the clinical setting, this observation has not detracted from the long-term success of extensively coated implants. A similar distal loading scenario is seen with cemented femoral stems whereby most load bypasses the proximal femur and exits distally. Dual energy x-ray absorption studies have confirmed proximal bone density loss with extensively coated uncemented femoral stems and with cemented femoral stems.

e. Cement Fixation. Cement fixation for hip replacement surgery requires good technique to provide optimal interdigitation of cement to bone. The technique for cement preparation has undergone several generations of development and is summarized in Table 4–1. With cemented total hip replacement, it is usually the acetabular socket that fails first from loosening. Ranawat, Peters, and

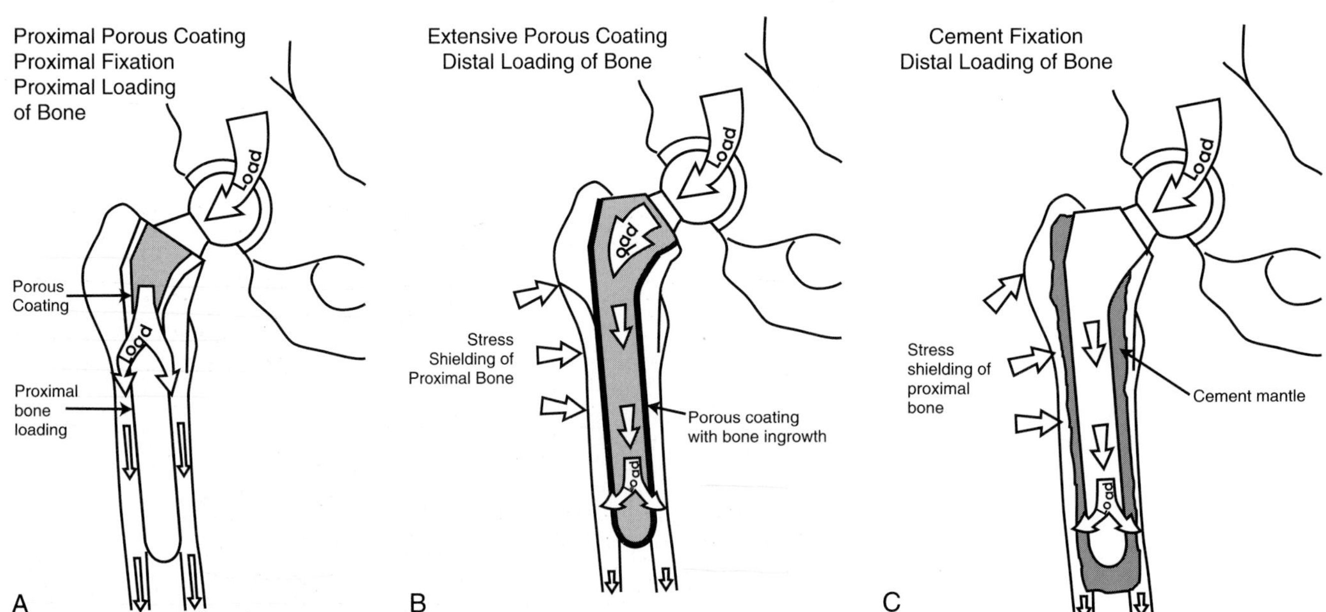

Figure 4–1. Diagram of bone loading in relation to femoral stem fixation. *A*, Proximal porous coating, no cement. *B*, Extensive porous coating, no cement. *C*, Cement.

Table 4–1.

Cement Technique Total Hip Replacement

1st Generation	2nd Generation (began 1975)	3rd Generation (began 1982)
• Finger packing	• Cement gun (began 1971)	• Porosity reduction (vacuum)
• No canal preparation	• Pulsatile lavage	• Pressurization cement
• No cement plug	• Canal preparation (brush and dry)	• Precoat stem
• No cement gun	• Cement restrictor	• Rough surface finish on stem
• No pressurization	• Super alloy stem (forged)	• Stem centralizer
• Cast stem	• Broad and round medial border	
• Narrow medial border on stem	• Collar on stem	
• Sharp edges on stem		

Umlas state that if the subgroups of rheumatoid arthritis (or other similar inflammatory conditions), protrusio deformity, hip dysplasia, and patients with excessive bleeding are excluded, the long-term results of cemented sockets are comparable to those of uncemented sockets.

4. Choice of Fixation
   a. Cemented or Noncemented. The recommended fixation for primary hip arthroplasty remains controversial. The NIH consensus statement for total hip arthroplasty in summary recommends that a cemented femoral component using modern cementing technique, paired with a porous coated hemispherical acetabular component, can give excellent long-term results. This is based on the data showing a higher loosening rate with cemented acetabular sockets compared with those of porous coated noncemented sockets. On the other hand, there are so many different uncemented femoral stem designs and variations of coatings that there is no identified superiority of uncemented femoral stem fixation over cemented femoral stems. The general tendency, however, is to use uncemented femoral stems in younger active patients where cemented stems in this situation have a reported higher loosening rate in long-term follow-up.
   b. Size of Cement Mantle. The size of the cement mantle surrounding the femoral stem is controversial. It is suggested that a minimum of 2 mm of cement thickness be allowed between prosthesis and bone. This would be impractical in narrow canals where a very small stem diameter would be required. A more practical approach is the "two-thirds" rule. With this technique, two-thirds of the canal is displaced by the femoral stem and the other one-third by cement. Cement mantle defects should be avoided. A mantle defect where the prosthesis touches bone creates an area of concentrated stress and is associated with a higher loosening rate (Fig. 4–2).

B. Hip Stability—Primary and Revision Surgery
   1. Dislocation of THR—Evaluation of the dislocated THR is complex and often multifactorial. An understanding of the factors involved in the unstable total hip can provide value to the surgeon in both primary and revision arthroplasty. The dislocation inci-

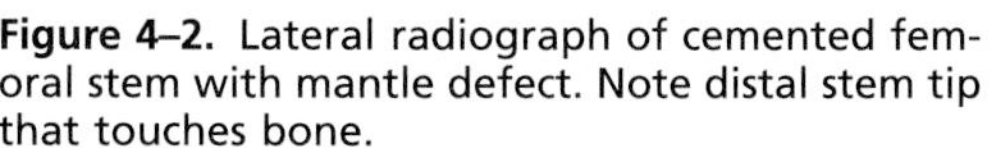

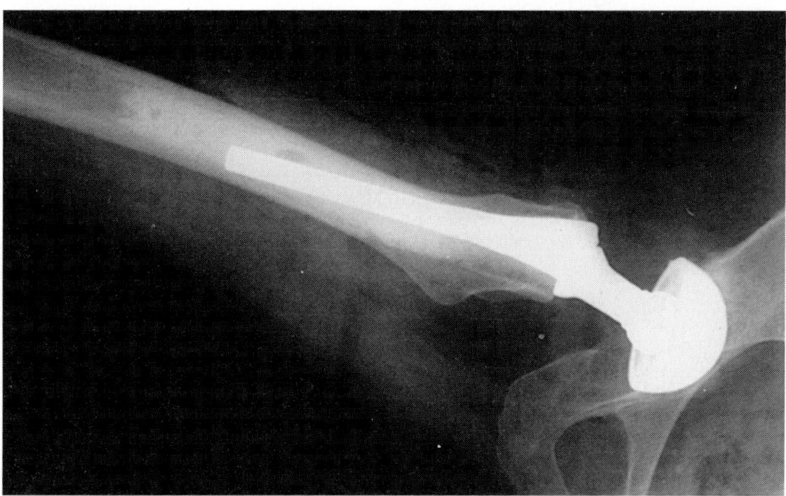

Figure 4–2. Lateral radiograph of cemented femoral stem with mantle defect. Note distal stem tip that touches bone.

dence after primary THR is on average 1–2%, but it has been reported to be as high as 9.5%. Dislocation after revision is higher and is reported as high as 26% in cases of multiple revisions. The highest incidence of dislocation in primary hip arthroplasty is in the subgroup of elderly patients (>80 years old) converted to total hip after failed osteosynthesis for femoral neck fracture. In this subgroup, dislocation incidence in one European study was 82%.

2. Assessment of Hip Stability—The assessment of hip stability involves four major areas: (1) component design, (2) component alignment, (3) soft-tissue tensioning, and (4) soft-tissue function.
   a. Component Design. In the area of component design, the ball cup articulation is most important. The *primary arc range* defines the amount of arc ball and cup articulation moves before impinging and levering out (Fig. 4–3). The major determinant of primary arc range is the *head-neck ratio*. The head-neck ratio is defined as the ratio of the femoral head diameter to the femoral neck diameter. A larger head-neck ratio allows further arc of motion before primary impingement (Fig. 4–4). Another factor affecting component stability is excursion distance. At the point of primary impingement, the head will begin to lever out of the cup. The distance a head must travel to dislocate is defined as excursion. The greater the excursion distance a ball must travel to dislocate when levered out, the more stable the hip. Excursion distance is usually one-half the diameter of the femoral head. Comparing a 32 mm head with a 22 mm head shows that excursion distance is 16 mm compared with 11 mm. In addition, a 32 mm head is more stable because of a more favorable head-neck ratio. Taken to the extreme, the bipolar head is the most inherently stable head because of a very favorable head-neck ratio.

      It is important to know the details of total hip design as it relates to hip stability. The size of the morse taper affects stability by affecting the head-neck ratio. Narrow neck tapers provide more stability via a more favorable head-neck ratio. Conversely, the addition of a collar on a modular femoral head (seen in long neck lengths) increases neck diameter and adversely affects head-neck ratio. Augmented acetabular liners (i.e., hoods) de-

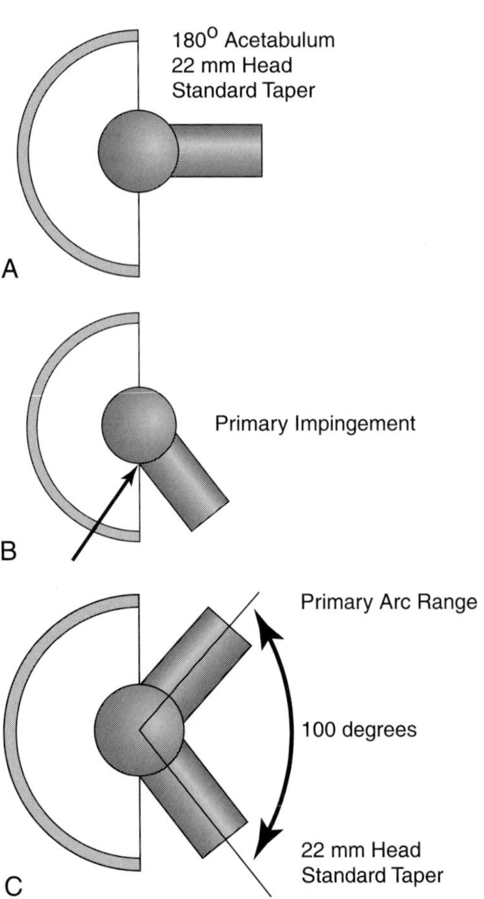

Figure 4–3. Diagram of total hip articulation demonstrating primary arc range. *A*, 22 mm head articulating with 180 degrees polyethylene. *B*, At the end of range, primary impingement occurs. *C*, Primary arc range is the arc of motion allowed between the two ends of primary impingement.

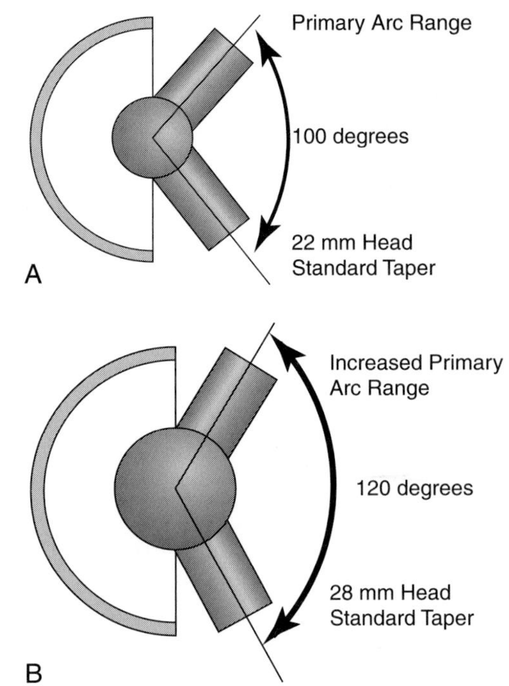

Figure 4–4. Comparison of primary arc range between 22 mm head and 28 mm head. *A*, Primary arc range with 22 mm head. *B*, Primary arc range with 28 mm head. The only change in this illustration is head size. This increases the head to neck ratio, which in turn allows for an increased arc range.

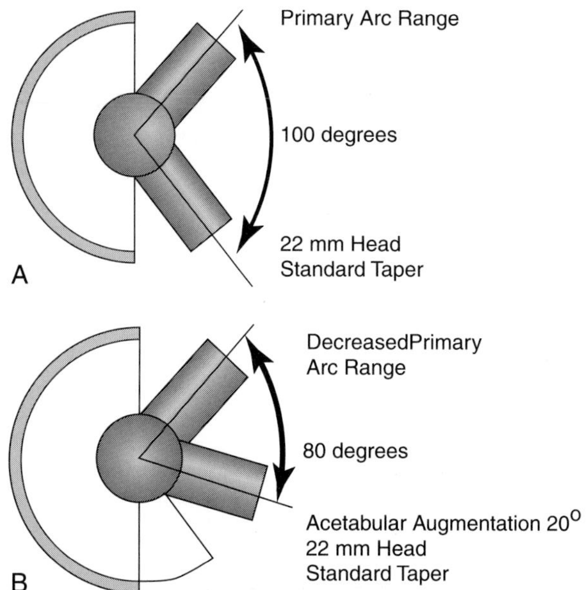

Figure 4–5. Comparison of primary arc range between non-hooded and hooded acetabular liner. *A*, Primary arc range with 22 mm head. *B*, Primary arc range with augmented acetabular liner (i.e., hood). Primary arc range is reduced as a result of the augmented liner.

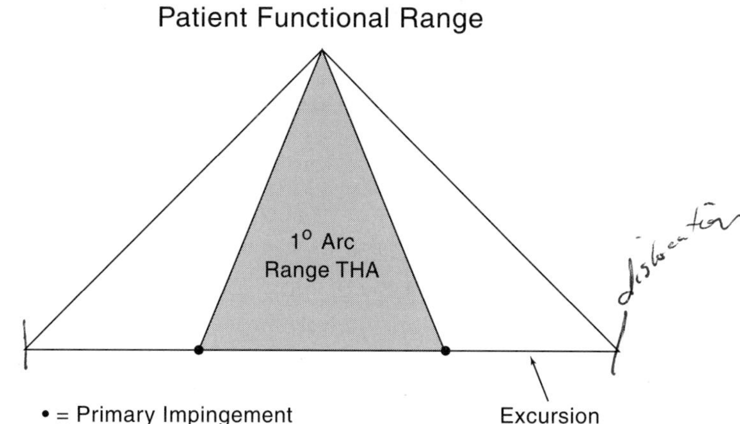

Figure 4–7. Diagram illustrating difference in patient's functional hip range of motion compared with prosthetic range. Because of the smaller heads used in prosthetic replacement, the prosthetic arc range is smaller than native hip range. The prosthetic arc range should be centered within the patient's functional range to minimize dislocation.

crease the primary arc range because the acetabular arc of enclosure is greater than the typical 180-degree arc (Fig. 4–5). The larger the hood, the more likely there will be impingement and excursion. Large hoods should be avoided. A constrained liner that covers almost the entire femoral head provides inherent stability but at a cost. The primary arc range is dramatically reduced (Fig. 4–6). If the patient consistently exceeds this primary arc range, the acetabulum can fail from early mechanical failure. The repetitive impingement imports a levering force on the acetabular component, leading to early loosening.

b. Component Alignment. This is another important area in hip stability. Because the patient's native femoral head is much larger than a prosthetic total hip head, it is more stable and has a larger primary arc range than a prosthetic replacement. Therefore, when inserting acetabular and femoral components, the goal is to center the prosthetic primary arc range in the middle of the patient's functional range (Fig. 4–7). By doing so, if the primary arc range is exceeded, there is still some stability in the excursion distance. Malaligned components do not decrease primary arc range; it is just not centered in the patient's functional range. As a result, on one side of the arc range, the head will suffer excessive excursion and hip dislocation (Fig. 4–8). Because surgeon

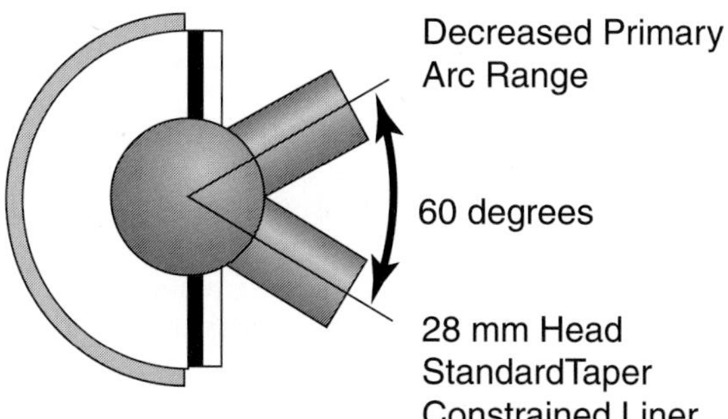

Figure 4–6. Diagram of constrained acetabular liner. A constrained liner covers the femoral head past its equator. This keeps the ball from coming out of socket. This has the adverse effect of severely restricting primary arc range.

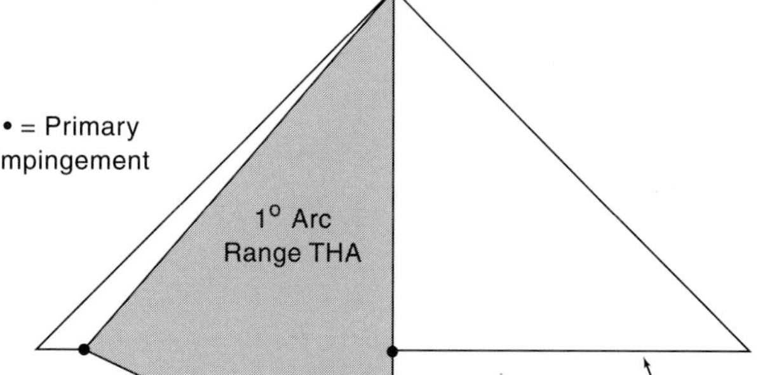

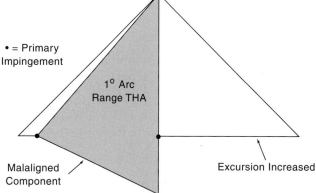

Figure 4–8. Diagram illustrating prosthetic malalignment. In this instance, the prosthetic arc range is positioned to one side of the patient's functional range. On one side of the range, the hip will be very stable. However, on the other side, the patient's arc range will exceed the prosthetic arc range. Primary impingement will occur, followed by head levering, head excursion, and dislocation. If the patient is unwilling to accept limitation of functional range, then recurrent dislocation will result.

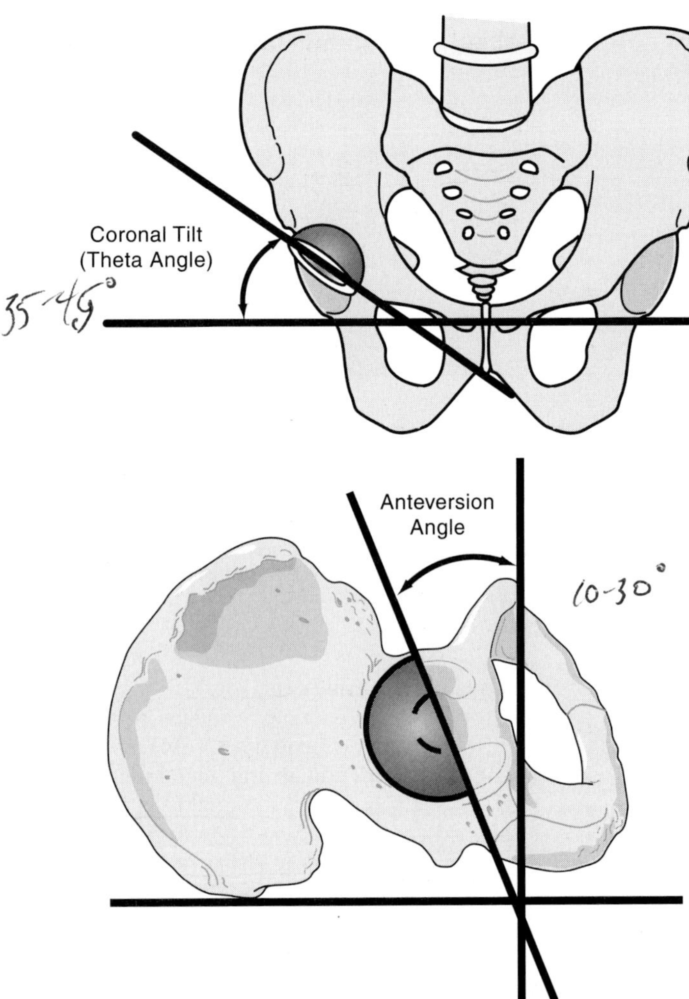

Figure 4–9. Diagram showing acetabular cup position in coronal and sagittal plane. Coronal tilt (also known as theta angle) should be 35–45 degrees. In the sagittal plane, cup anteversion should be 10–25 degrees.

preference and training vary, there is no one correct answer for the proper component position. On the acetabulum, anteversion should be 10–30 degrees, and the theta angle (i.e., coronal tilt) should be 35–45 degrees (Fig. 4–9). Intraoperative trialing is important to ensure that component placement is optimum. The hip must be taken through all extremes of end range to assure stability.

c. Soft-Tissue Tensioning. This factor also plays a critical role in hip stability. Components properly placed may still dislocate if there is inadequate soft-tissue tension to hold the components in place. The major key to hip stability is the abductor complex. This consists primarily of the gluteus medius and minimus. Maintaining the correct tension of this complex will provide optimal stability. *Preoperative templating* should assess *head offset* and *neck length* such that when the prosthetic stem is inserted, appropriate neck length and offset are restored (Fig. 4–10). Restored hip mechanics confers hip stability via optimized abductor tension. Conversely, reduced hip length and offset can lead to instability. A total hip left short in neck length results in a lax abductor complex and may not generate the force required to keep the hip in place. Additionally, a short neck length can cause trochanteric impingement, with abduction and rotation causing the hip to lever out of the socket. Hip stability can also be affected by a decreased offset. With a *narrow offset*, the greater trochanter can again impinge, allowing the hip to lever out of socket. The worst-case scenario would be a total hip with a shortened neck length and a narrow offset. It is very important to template x-rays preoperatively to see if neck length and offset can be adequately restored. If not, a different prosthetic system may be required. In a related issue, greater trochanter deficiency or trochanteric escape (seen after trochanteric osteotomy) often leads to hip instability. With loss of the greater trochanter attachment to

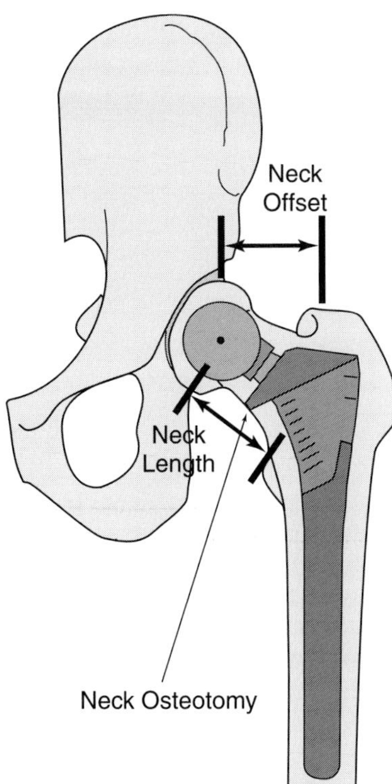

Figure 4–10. Diagram illustrating preoperative templating for proper femoral stem positioning. Prosthetic stem should be positioned such that femoral stem offset (center of head to greater trochanter) matches the native hip. Also, femoral neck length must be restored. Restoring head offset and neck length optimizes abductor tension, providing stability.

the femur, there is loss of abductor power and loss of hip compressive forces. Also, with loss of the greater trochanter, the hip is allowed a greater range of motion, leading to impingement, head excursion, and dislocation.

d. Soft-Tissue Function. This is the last area of concern. What controls the abductor complex and surrounding soft tissues of the hip is the synchronized neurologic firing from the brain delivered through the peripheral nervous system. Any disruption in this system can adversely affect function and hip stability. Soft-tissue function can be broken into two main issues: central and peripheral. *Central issues* involve the brain, brain stem, and spinal cord. Problems in this area can be numerous and include such problems as stroke, cerebellar dysfunction, Parkinson's disease, multiple sclerosis, dementia, cervical stenosis/myelopathy, and psychiatric disorder. The issue common to all of these is the coordinated firing of muscles to keep the hip stable. The problem could be from paralysis, spasticity, or loss of coordinated movements of the surrounding hip musculature. *Peripheral issues* involve the area of the peripheral nerves and muscles that support the hip. Peripheral issues that can affect hip stability include lumbar stenosis, peripheral neuropathy, myopathy, localized soft-tissue trauma, and radiation therapy. The cause of poor soft-tissue function may be multifactorial in the elderly patient. Sometimes, it is difficult preoperatively to ascertain the extent of soft-tissue dysfunction, and it is only after multiple dislocations that one appreciates the significance of these deficits.

3. Management of the Dislocated Total Hip—Treatment of the dislocated total hip depends on the reason for dislocation. Approximately two-thirds of patients with a dislocated total hip can be treated successfully with a closed reduction and a period of hip immobilization. Immobilization can be by means of either a spica cast or brace. A knee immobilizer is effective as well; it keeps the patient from putting the hip in a compromised position. However, immobilization in a brace or cast allows a better chance for soft tissues to heal in a more contracted position. During closed reduction, it is important to take the hip through a full range and assess the positions that make the hip dislocate. If the positions noted are near the extremes of end range, the prognosis for long-term stability is good. On the other hand, if the hip dislocates easily within the patient's functional range, then revision surgery is more likely necessary. As a general rule, if the hip dislocates more than two times, recurrent dislocation is likely, and the hip should be revised to enhance stability.

The surgical options for recurrent dislocation depend on the cause of the dislocation. Although, in many circumstances, the cause of recurrent dislocation is multifactorial, there is usually one main area that stands out. If the total hip components are malaligned, they should be revised, even if they are well fixed. The choice of implants for revision surgery should take into account factors that restore normal hip offset and neck length, and provide an optimal arc range. Optimizing head-neck ratio with a larger head should take priority over polyethylene thickness, if this provides the stability needed for a successful outcome. In some situations, where hip component parts are reasonably aligned, trochanteric osteotomy with distal advancement is a good option (Fig. 4–11). Distal advancement places the abductor complex under tension, providing more hip compressive force. Trochanteric advancement, if performed, is usually accompanied by postoperative immobilization in a spica brace or cast. In the

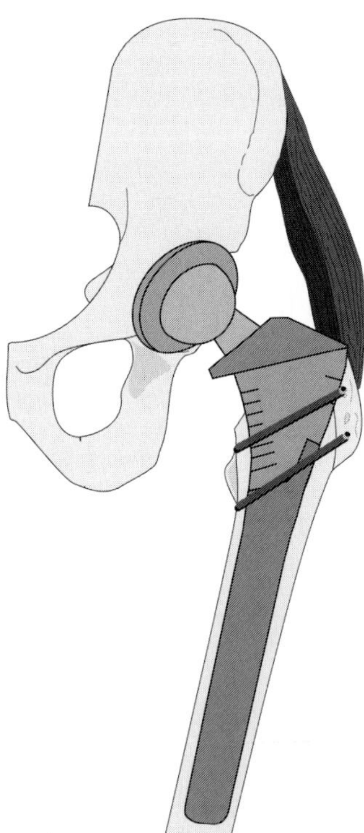

Figure 4–11. Diagram depicting trochanteric advancement. Distal advancement tightens hip abductor complex, restoring compressive force to hip joint.

scenario where a prior trochanteric osteotomy has detached and migrated proximally, reattaching the greater trochanter is not often successful. In the abductor-deficient patient, hip stability may be achieved only by using a larger femoral head and/or a constrained polyethylene liner.

Conversion of a total hip to a hemiarthroplasty with a large femoral head is another solution for hip instability and is more often used when there is soft-tissue deficiency or dysfunction. Conversion to a monopolar or bipolar head cannot be used where the acetabular bone is compromised (i.e., segmental deficiencies). There is a high likelihood of pelvic migration. If the hemiarthroplasty can be seated firmly on the bony acetabular rim and there is acceptable remaining bone stock, then conversion to a hemiarthroplasty is an option. A constrained polyethylene liner is used in a similar fashion where soft-tissue deficiency and dysfunction are the main problem. The advantage of a constrained liner is that it can be used in the reconstructed acetabulum where there is acetabular deficiency. The main problem with a constrained liner is the very limited range of motion it provides. If the patient is not compliant with the limited range, then the acetabular cup may rapidly become mechanically loose from levering forces. Conversion to a constrained liner should not be the first surgical option if other surgical options will take care of the problem. The last surgical option is resection arthroplasty. This option is used when other options have been exhausted. Resection arthroplasty is usually used in the multiply revised patient with significant soft-tissue deficiency along with significant bone loss. Resection arthroplasty is also utilized for the psychiatric patient who purposely dislocates the hip for secondary gratification (e.g., narcotics, hospitalization, etc.).

C. Hip Loosening—Aseptic femoral and acetabular loosening are the most common indications for revision surgery. In cemented hip replacement, the most common reason for revision is failure of the cemented acetabular component. In uncemented total hip replacement, the most common reason for revision is failure of the femoral component (usually from osteolysis). Standard radiographs taken in the same rotational position are required to assess interval changes. Radiographic analysis is based on dividing the acetabular and femoral components into radiographic zones. The acetabulum is divided into three zones as described by DeLee and Charnley. The femoral component is divided into seven zones as described by Gruen, McNeice, and Amstutz (Fig. 4–12). The development of radiolucent lines around these zones (either with cemented or cementless implants) in a progressive fashion suggests loosening. It is important to distinguish progressive radiolucent lines in the femur from the typical age-related expansion of the femoral canal and cortical thinning, which may give the appearance of a progressively widening radiolucency. Age-related radiolucent zones generally do not have the associated sclerotic line seen about loose femoral stems. In addition, radiolucent lines associated with osteolysis tend to be more irregular, with variable areas of cortical thinning and ectasia. With cemented femoral implants, Gruen describes four modes of failure, which are defined and diagrammed in Table 4–2. The acetabular cup is considered loose if there is a radiolucency >2 mm in all three zones, progressive radiolucent lines in zones 1 and 2, or change in component position.

D. Revision Total Hip Replacement—Revision hip surgery is often difficult and complex. The results are less satisfactory than in primary hip replacement. Postoperative complications of infection, dislocation, nerve palsy, cortical perforation, fracture, and deep vein thrombosis are higher than in primary hip replacement. The surgical goals in revision hip replacement are (1) removal of loose components without significant destruction of host bone and tissue, (2) reconstruction of bone defects with bone graft and/or metal augmentation, (3) stable revision implants, and (4) restoration of normal hip center of rotation.

Acetabular reconstruction first requires de-

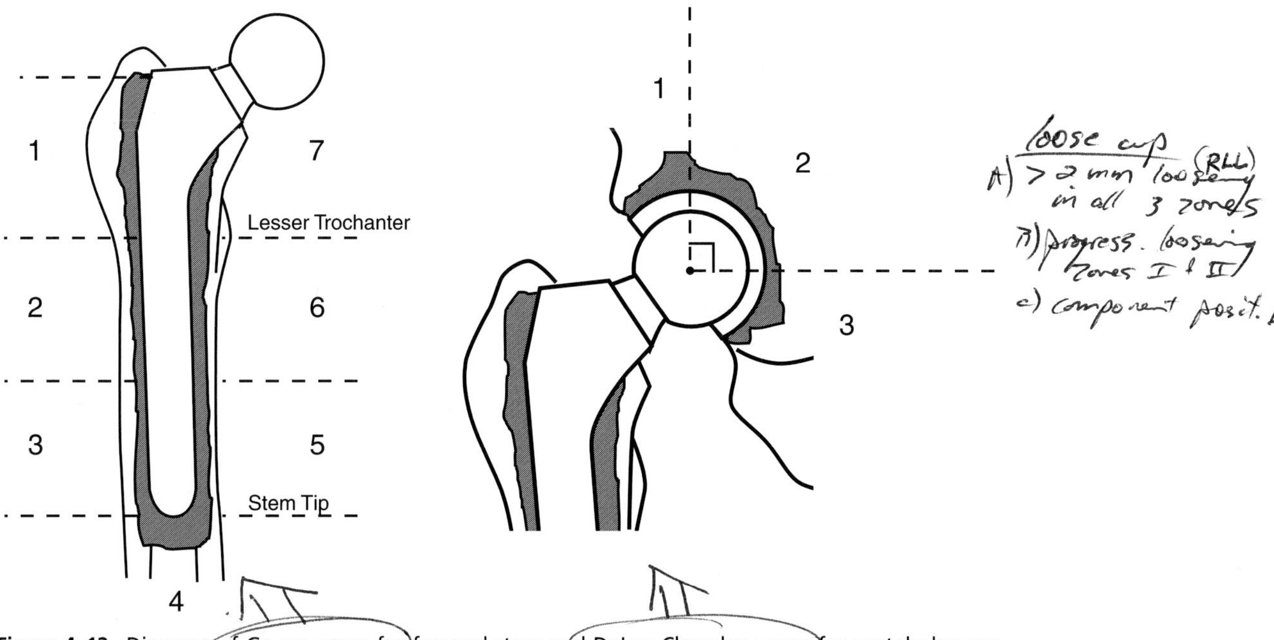

Figure 4–12. Diagram of Gruen zones for femoral stem and DeLee-Charnley zones for acetabular cup.

fining the extent of bone loss. Acetabular defects are classified as follows: (1) *segmental* (type I)—loss of part of the acetabular rim or medial wall; (2) *cavitary* (type II)—volumetric loss in the bony substance of the acetabular cavity; (3) *combined deficiency* (type III)—combination of segmental bone loss and cavitary deficiency; (4) *pelvic discontinuity* (type IV)—complete separation between the superior and inferior acetabulum, usually due to combined deficiencies and fracture; and (5) *arthrodesis* (type V)—obliteration of the acetabulum due to fusion.

1. Revision of Acetabulum—In revision of the acetabulum, a porous coated hemisphere cup secured with superior screws is the preferred choice, provided that the rim is intact. The acetabular rim in the revision situation provides the stability for the acetabular cup when inserted with a press fit technique. Because acetabular bone stock is weakened in revision surgery, superior screws should be placed to augment stability. The correct placement of acetabular screws is important. Figure 4–13 diagrams the safe zones for correct screw placement. Incorrect placement can lead to catastrophic vascular injury or neurologic damage. A porous coated hemisphere cup can still be used with segmental deficiency of the acetabular rim. As a general rule, a hemisphere cup can be utilized

Table 4–2.

Modes of Cemented Femoral Stem Loosening

Mode	Mechanism	Cause	Findings
IA	Pistoning behavior	• Subsidence of stem within cement	• RLL between stem and cement in zones 1 and 2 • Distal cement fracture • Stem displaced distally in cement
IB	Pistoning behavior	• Subsidence of cement mantle and stem within bone	• RLL all 7 zones
II	Medial stem pivot	• Lack of superomedial and inferolateral cement support	• Medial migration proximal stem • Lateral migration distal tip • Cement fracture zones 2 and 6
III	Calcar pivot	• Medial and lateral toggle of distal stem • "Hang up" of stem collar on medial cortex • "Windshield wiper" reaction at distal stem	• Sclerosis and thickening of bone at stem tip • RLL zones 4 and 5
IV	Cantilever bending	• Loss of proximal cement support leaving distal stem still fixed; allows for proximal cantilever bending	• Stem crack or fracture • RLL zones 1 and 2, 6 and 7

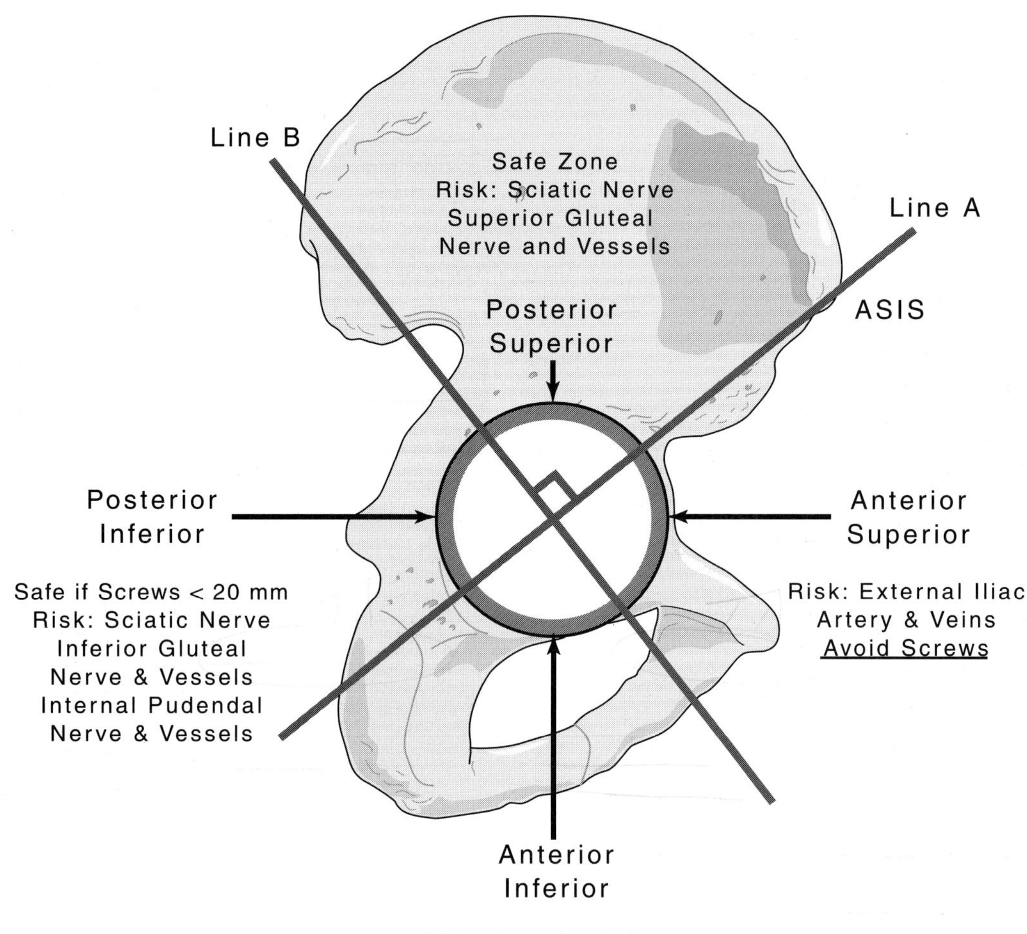

Figure 4–13. Acetabular zones for screw insertion. Line A is formed by drawing line from ASIS to center of acetabular socket. Line B is then drawn perpendicular to A, also passing through center of socket. The posterior-superior quadrant is the preferred zone for screw insertion.

if at least *two-thirds* of the rim is remaining and there is still a good "rim fit." The cup must be secured with screws. Cavitary deficiencies with an intact rim are filled with particulate graft, and the acetabular cup will hold the graft in place.

Acetabular deficiencies that are rim deficient and/or have large cavitary deficiencies will require a structural allograft. A structural allograft (as opposed to particulate graft) is a large solid piece of bone that supports weight-bearing stress. If a cup is placed into a large structural allograft, the failure rate is high. Failure is usually due to graft resorption and subsequent component migration. Failure of cementless components with a large structural allograft is 40–60%. Failure rate with a cemented socket is 40%. A much higher success rate is achieved when the structural allograft is supported by a reconstruction cage (Fig. 4–14). A structural allograft supported by a reconstruction cage is the preferred revision construct if a large structural allograft is to be used. If a reconstruction cage is used, generally an all-polyethylene acetabular component is cemented into the cage.

2. Femoral Bone Defects—Femoral bone defects, like acetabular defects, are primarily either segmental or cavitary. The complete classification of femoral bone deficiencies is as follows: (1) *segmental* (type I)—any loss of bone of the supporting shell of the femur; (2) *cavitary* (type II)—loss of endosteal bone but an intact cortical shell; (3) *combined deficiency* (type III)—combined segmental and cavitary defects; (4) *malalignment* (type IV)—loss of normal femoral geometry due to prior surgery, trauma, or disease; (5) *stenosis* (type V)—occlusion of canal from trauma, fixation devices, or bony hypertrophy; and (6) *femoral discontinuity* (type

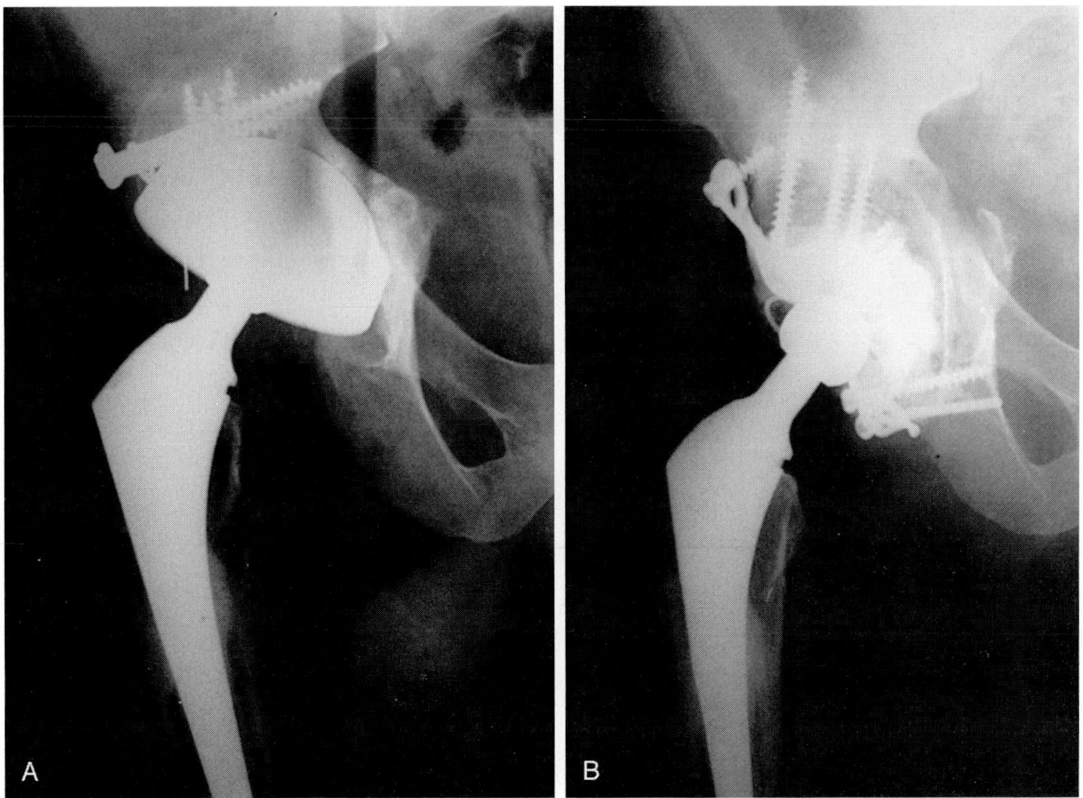

Figure 4–14. X-ray films demonstrating acetabular reconstruction with reconstruction cage and bulk support allograft. *A*, Preoperative radiograph of loose jumbo cup with collapse of superior bone graft. *B*, Postoperative 1 year x-ray film of Birch-Schneider acetabular reconstruction cage for the large segmental acetabular deficiency. A structural allograft is placed superiorly. The cage is secured with screws to the ilium and ischium. A polyethylene acetabular component is then cemented into the cage. This construct enables weight-bearing forces to be partly distributed from the cage to the ilium, allowing allograft to remodel and incorporate to host bone.

VI)—loss of femoral integrity from fracture or nonunion.

With femoral stem revision, the most commonly utilized technique is an uncemented extensively porous coated (or porous coating/grit blast combination) long-stem prosthesis. The revision stem should pass 2–3 cm below the original stem. This is to bypass stress risers that may occur from stem extraction or osteolysis. If there is a femoral cortical violation, the revision stem should pass at least two shaft diameters below the defect. Ectatic, cavitary lesions can be grafted with particulate debris. Segmental deficiencies are usually reconstructed with cortical onlay struts secured with cerclage wires or multifilament cables (Fig. 4–15).

Impaction bone grafting (Ling's technique) can be used in some revision cases where there is a large ectatic canal and narrow, thin cortices (destroyed by osteolysis). This technique uses morselized fresh-frozen allograft packed tightly into the ectatic proximal femur. A smooth tapered stem is cemented into the allograft. This technique requires an intact cortical tube, although small segmental defects can be patched with a wire mesh.

E. Periprosthetic Fracture: Hip—The management of periprosthetic femur fractures depends on the location of the fracture and whether the stem is well-fixed or loose. Femurs with bone ingrowth prosthesis tend to fracture within the first 6 months after implantation. The reason is probable stress risers created by reaming and broaching of the femoral canal. Cemented implants tend to fracture late (5 years on average). Fractures in cemented implants occur most commonly about the stem tip or distal to the prosthesis. In revision cases, fractures tend to occur at the site of cortical defect from previous operations. Fractures also occur when the new stem does not bypass a cortical defect by greater than two cortical diameters.

Fractures that occur where there is a loose prosthesis (cemented or cementless) should be revised using a noncemented ingrowth long-stem prosthesis that bypasses the last cortical defect by two diameters of the femoral shaft.

Treatment of fractures with an intact prosthetic interface depends on the site of fracture and the extent of fracture involvement. A fracture classification (Beals and Tower) with rec-

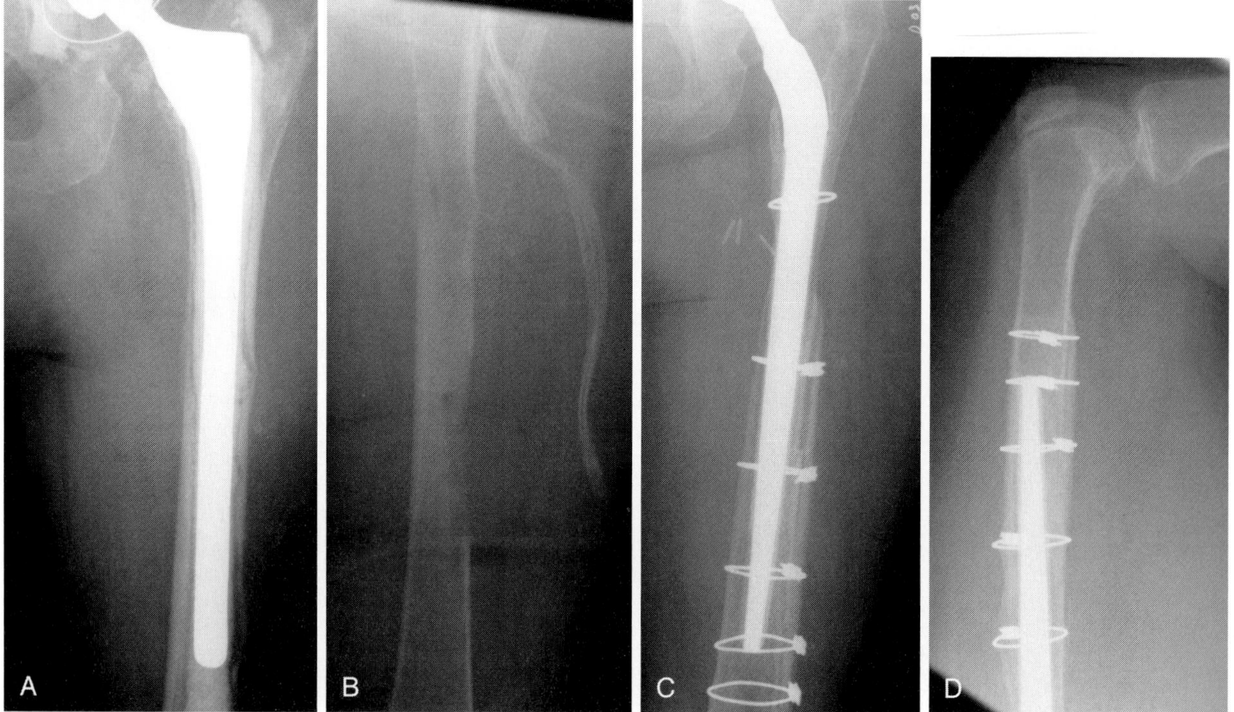

Figure 4–15. X-ray film of long stem revision femoral stem *(A–D)*. Cortical allograft onlay struts are secured with multifilament cables to enforce segmental and cavitary deficiencies.

ommended treatments is reviewed in Table 4–3.

F. Heterotopic Ossification—Heterotopic ossification (HO) after hip replacement surgery most commonly affects males. Predisposing risk factors include hypertrophic osteoarthritis, ankylosing spondylitis, diffuse idiopathic skeletal hyperostosis, post-traumatic arthritis, prior hip fusion, and history of previous development of heterotopic ossification. HO is seen more often with the direct lateral approach to the hip (Harding). If HO is seen in the contralateral hip, the incidence of HO with the ipsilateral hip is high.

Heterotopic ossification limits hip motion when pronounced, but it generally does not cause pain or muscle weakness. Reoperation to remove HO is not recommended unless there

Table 4–3.

Periprosthetic Femur Fracture Classification and Treatment

Stable Prosthetic Interface

Fracture Type	Fracture Location	Recommended Treatment
I	Trochanteric region	Nonoperative
II	Proximal metaphysis/diaphysis not involving stem tip	Nonoperative or cerclage fixation
IIIA	Diaphyseal fracture at stem tip Disruption of prosthetic interface (<25%)	Long-stem ingrowth revision or ORIF: Plate with screws ± cerclage ORIF: Cortical struts with cerclage cables
IIIB	Diaphyseal fracture at stem tip Disruption of prosthetic interface (<25%)	Cemented stem: long-stem ingrowth revision Ingrowth stem: long-stem ingrowth revision or ORIF: Plate with screws ± cerclage ORIF: Cortical struts with cerclage cables
IIIC	Supracondylar fracture at tip of a long-stem prosthesis	Nonoperative if stable or ORIF: Plate with screws ± cerclage ORIF: Custom IM rod extension to prosthesis
IV	Supracondylar fracture distant to stem tip	Nonoperative if stable or ORIF: Plate with screws (must extend proximal to stem tip) ORIF: Supracondylar intramedullary nail
Loose Prosthetic Interface		Long-stem ingrowth revision

is severe restriction of hip range or pain from impingement is severe. Recurrence is likely unless prophylactic measures are taken. Once HO is seen radiographically, there is no treatment to prevent further progression. Instead, treatment for HO is directed toward identifying those patients at high risk for developing HO and treating this subgroup prophylactically.

Prophylactic treatment with low-dose radiation or with certain nonsteroidal anti-inflammatory drugs (NSAIDs) are the two effective treatments for HO. A single dose of 700 cGy (rads) is considered the lowest effective dose for HO. Treatment must be delivered within 72 hours of surgery (preferably within the first 48 hours) to be effective. If noncemented prosthetic components are used, these areas should be shielded from the radiation beam so as not to reduce bone ingrowth potential. Indomethacin is the most commonly used NSAID for heterotopic ossification. Other NSAIDs have also shown effectiveness. The recommended indomethacin dose is 75 mg per day for 6 weeks. The efficacy of indomethacin in preventing recurrent HO after excision is not well documented.

II. Osteolysis and Wear in Prosthetic Joint Replacement—Osteolysis at this time remains the most vexing problem in total joint arthroplasty. In its most basic form, it represents a histiocytic response to wear debris. The process begins with *wear sources* that generate particulate debris, which initiates the osteolytic reaction. The potential wear sources are listed in Figure 4–16. Although any particle can serve as a source of wear debris and cause osteolysis, debris that is known to elicit an enhanced histiocytic response includes ultrahigh molecular-weight polyethylene, polymethylmethacrylate, and cobalt chrome. Because polyethylene is relatively softer than other materials used in joint replacement surgery, it is considered the major source of the osteolytic process by virtue of the

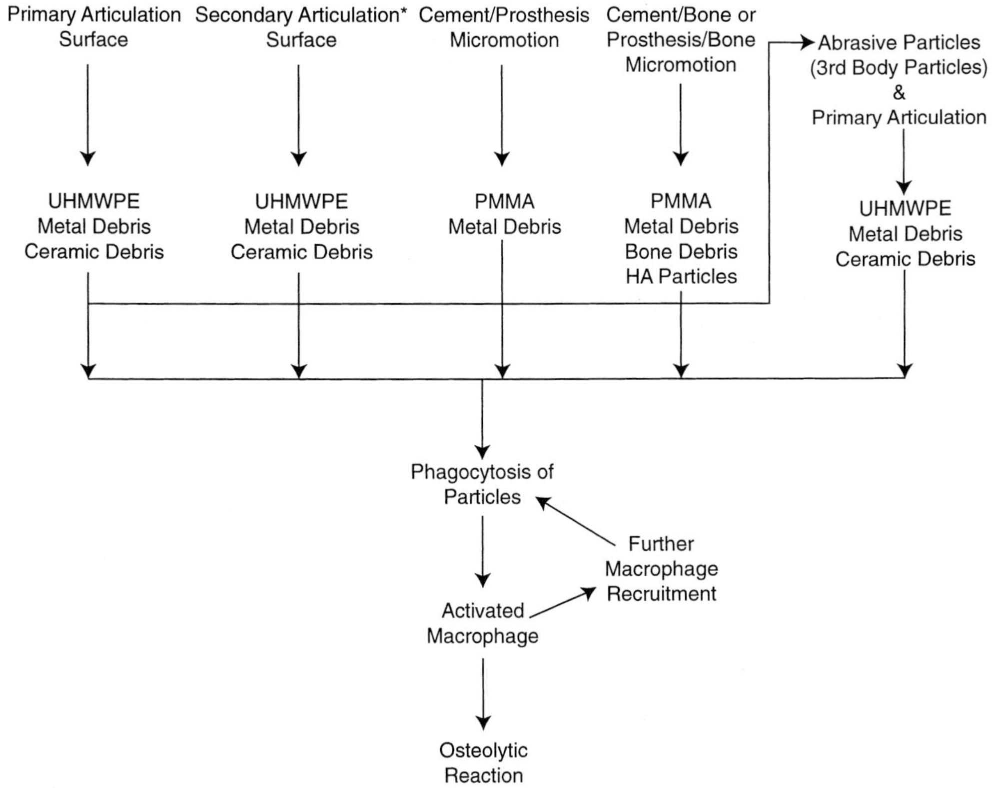

Figure 4–16. Wear in total replacement

volume of polyethylene generated, as compared with other sources. As a result of particle ingestion by the macrophage, the activated macrophage liberates osteolytic factors, including osteoclast-activating factor, oxide radicals, hydrogen peroxide, acid phosphatase, interleukins, and prostaglandins. These factors together assist in the dissolution of bone from around the prosthesis, allowing for prosthetic micromotion that leads to further generation of wear debris. Additional lysis of bone allows for prosthetic macromotion, loosening, and pain.

Once particulate debris is generated and the osteolytic process begins, the inflammatory response generated within the joint produces an increased hydrostatic pressure that allows for dissemination of particulate debris within the *effective joint space*. The effective joint space comprises the potential space where joint fluid can be pumped and thereby allow particle debris to travel (Fig. 4–17). The effective joint space comprises the joint itself along with the surfaces where the prosthesis (or cement) contacts host bone. The size of the particles implicated in osteolysis is very small. The particles are in the micron or submicron range. McKellop suggests that the main culprit in osteolysis is submicron particles of polyethylene.

Wear particles can be generated by *abrasive wear*, in which particles are generated by rough articular surfaces (e.g., scratches, carbide asperites, etc.) either at the primary articulation or other secondary surfaces (backside of polyethylene insert with metal backed shell). *Third-body particles* can generate debris through an abrasive process at articulating surfaces. McKellop also describes the loss of polyethylene at the primary articulation via a process of *adhesive wear*. Polyethylene is produced

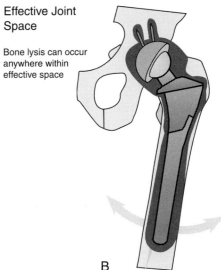

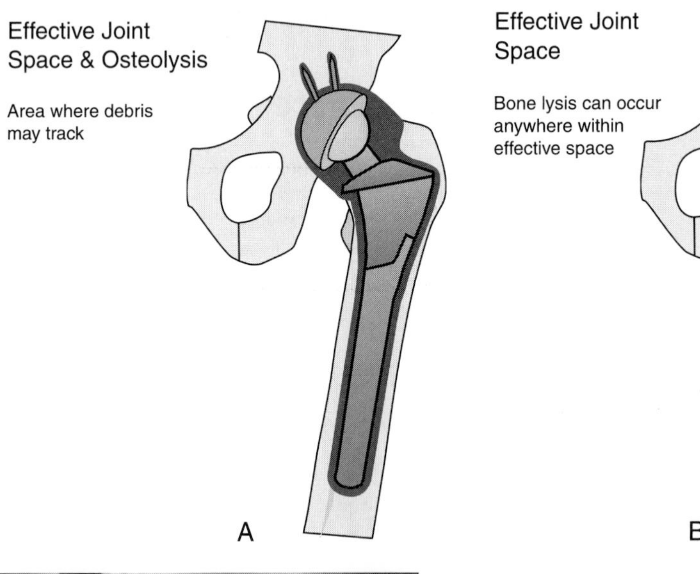

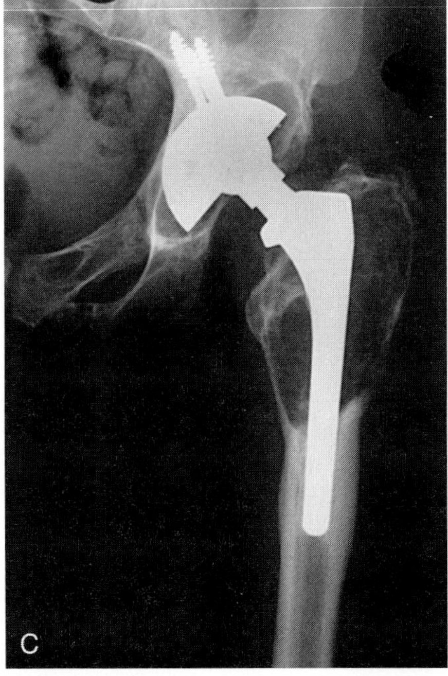

Figure 4–17. Diagram showing effective joint space. *A*, Defines area of effective joint space, which includes any area around prosthetic construct, including screws. *B*, Osteolysis can occur in any region of the effective joint space. Particles are pumped via the path of least resistance. *C*, X-ray film example of massive osteolysis. Note eccentric position of femoral head indicating polyethylene wear.

by the heating of small polyethylene beads into a congealed mass. On its surface, the small submicron beads can be pulled off by the passing of the adjacent articulation surface. The generation of these small particles is significant. The combination of abrasive wear and adhesive wear can generate many billions of particles that are then disseminated throughout the effective joint space. Efforts to minimize osteolysis in total joint replacement are primarily focused on minimizing adhesive wear at the primary articulation and also at minimizing abrasive wear within the total joint construct.

The sterilization process of polyethylene has been implicated as a factor causing high wear rates and rapid polyethylene failure. Polyethylene components sterilized via gamma radiation and stored in an oxygen environment generate oxidized polyethylene that, under repetitive cyclic loading, can delaminate and crack, leading to polyethylene failure. The pathways of gamma-irradiated polyethylene are outlined in Figure 4–18. Gamma-irradiated polyethylene undergoes an intermediate step of free radical formation. At this point, there are four pathways that can be taken: *recombination*, *unsaturation*, *chain scission*, or *cross-linking*. The two important pathways concerning polyethylene wear are chain scission and cross-linking. In the presence of an oxygen environment, oxidized polyethylene is favored. In an environment without oxygen, cross-linking is favored. Cross-linked polyethylene has *improved* resistance to adhesive and abrasive wear and improves wear rates in wear simulator data. The disadvantage of cross-linking polyethylene is that it does diminish the mechanical properties. Therefore, cross-linked polyethylene may fail catastrophically if excessive stresses are applied. Conversely, oxidized polyethylene causes subsurface delamination and cracking, leading to accelerated polyethylene failure. Oxidized polyethylene should be avoided. If polyethylene is gamma-sterilized, modern packaging techniques employ packing in an environment free of oxygen. This is achieved via argon, nitrogen, or vacuum packaging. The other method of sterilization is ethylene oxide gas sterilization, which is not frequently used. The disadvantage of this process is that residues left by the gas sterilization process may have deleterious effects on the surrounding human tissues.

III. Knee Replacement Surgery

A. Surgical Technique—The technical goals of knee replacement surgery are: (1) restoration of *mechanical* alignment, (2) preservation (or

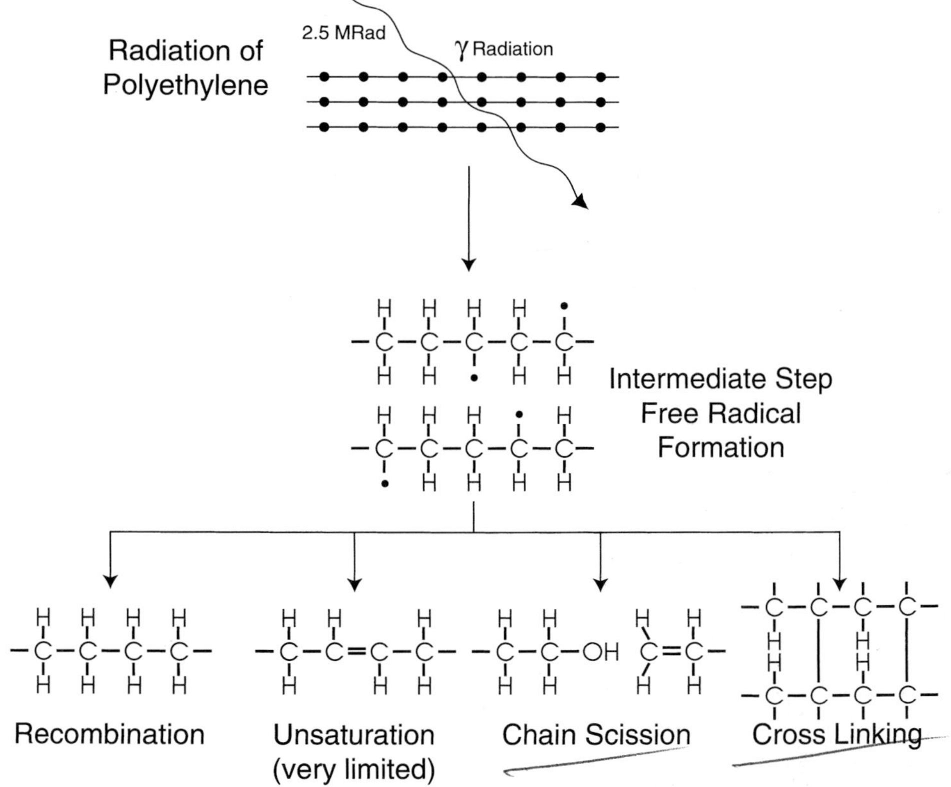

Figure 4–18. Effect of gamma radiation on polyethylene.

Table 4–4.

Recommended Preoperative Radiographs in Knee Replacement Surgery

- Standing full-length anteroposterior radiograph from hip to ankle
- Standing extension lateral on large cassette (14″ × 17″)
- Flexion lateral on large cassette
- Merchant's view

restoration) of the joint line, (3) balanced ligaments, and (4) maintaining or restoring a normal Q angle.

Consistent clinical results are predicated on good preoperative planning, which includes a good clinical examination of the knee along with preoperative radiographs. Preoperative radiographs are used to identify corrections needed in alignment and defects in bone that will require bone grafting or augmentation. Table 4–4 lists the recommended series of preoperative radiographs.

1. Mechanical Alignment—Restoring a neutral mechanical alignment ensures that the forces through the leg pass through the center of the hip, knee, and ankle. Restoring a neutral mechanical alignment in knee replacement surgery allows optimum load share through medial and lateral sides of the components. In a knee replacement where mechanical alignment is not restored, a net varus or valgus moment is created. This places excessive stress on one side of the knee, leading to excessive wear and early failure. Identifying the mechanical axis on preoperative radiographs and with intraoperative instrumentation is essential. Figure 4–19 defines the anatomic and mechanical axes of the femur and tibia. In the femur, the anatomic axis is defined by the medullary canal and most often exits in the intercondylar notch region. The exit of the anatomic axis at the distal end of the femur defines the medullary entry point for the intramedullary rod of the femoral jigs used to prepare the femur. In some cases, the anatomic axis may be located just medial or lateral to the intercondylar notch due to distal femoral bowing deformities. A preoperative standing, full-length radiograph can be used to identify the anatomic axis and femoral entry point. The femoral mechanical axis starts from the center of the femoral head and ends at the point of intersection with the femoral anatomic axis at the intercondylar notch. The angle measured between the femoral anatomic axis and mechanical axis is called the *valgus cut angle*. This can be measured in each case using a standing, anteroposterior full-length radiograph of the leg; in most cases, it measures 5–7 degrees. The goal is to cut the distal femur at an angle perpendicular to the *mechanical axis*. By cutting the distal femur by

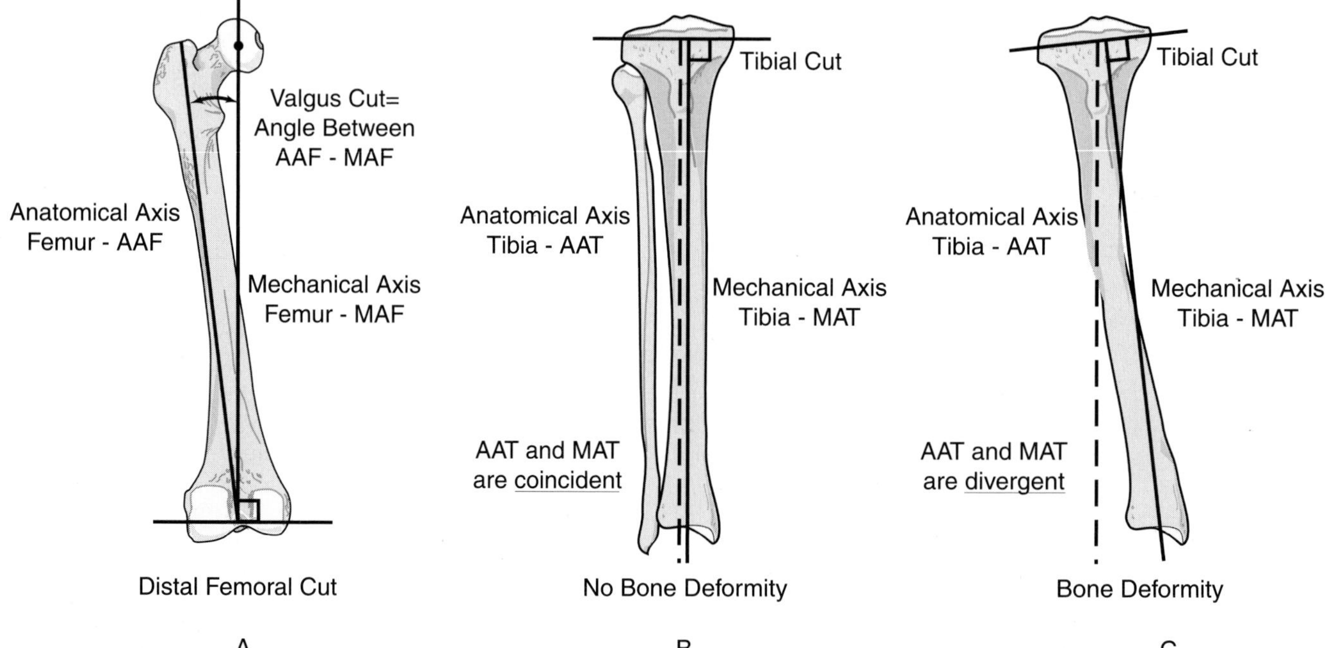

Figure 4–19. Diagram showing mechanical axis and anatomic axis of leg. *A,* In the femur, the anatomic axis follows the femoral shaft, whereas the mechanical axis lies along the line from hip center to knee center (mechanical axis and anatomic axis intersect at knee). *B,* In the tibia, the anatomic axis follows the tibial shaft. Mechanical axis runs from knee center to ankle joint center. When deformities are absent, the tibial anatomic axis and mechanical axis are usually coincident. *C,* When deformities are present, these axes are divergent.

the valgus cut angle, the femoral prosthesis will point toward the center of the femoral head and will be in a mechanically neutral position. Cases in which the valgus cut angle should be measured with a full-length radiograph are patients who are very tall or short, patients who have post-trauma deformities of the femur, and patients who have congenital femoral bow deformities. Patients who are very tall will often have a valgus cut angle less than 5 degrees, whereas patients who are very short may have a valgus cut angle more than 7 degrees.

The anatomic axis of the tibia is a line defining the medullary canal, and in the majority of cases it is coincident with the mechanical axis. The cases in which the tibial anatomic and mechanical axes are disparate are in post-traumatic and congenital bow deformities. The goal in either case is to cut the tibial surface perpendicular to the *mechanical axis* so that the tibial component loads along the mechanical axis. When the tibial anatomic and mechanical axes are coincident, the intramedullary rod will readily assist in determining the correct cut, but in a post-traumatic tibia deformity the medullary rod may not pass. In this instance, an extra medullary guide device placed over the center of the ankle up to the center of the tibia or center of the tibial tubercle will be necessary.

2. Bone Cuts and Alignment—The next technical aspect in knee replacement surgery is to remove sufficient amount of bone so that the prosthesis, when placed, will recreate the original thickness of cartilage and bone. This ensures that the *joint line is recreated*, because knee ligaments play a vital role in knee kinematics. Knee function is optimized when the joint line is preserved. Current total knee instrumentation is capable of providing precise bone cuts, but the surgeon should never be lulled into a sense of complacency. Still, cutting jigs can be pinned improperly or may shift as sawing occurs, causing inaccurate cuts. The surgeon should always double-check cuts and alignment during the trialing process. Furthermore, during the bone cut and trialing process, bone defects should be identified and restored. If not, malalignment may occur. If bone defects are small (≤1 cm), they can be filled with cement. Larger defects may require bone grafts or, more commonly, metallic augmentation, which is provided with many modular knee replacement systems.
3. Maintenance of Q Angle—The next important factor in knee replacement surgery is avoiding techniques that result in an increased Q angle. The most common complications in total knee replacement involve the patellofemoral articulation. An increased Q angle leads to increased lateral subluxation forces, which can adversely affect patellofemoral tracking. The section below will address the technical factors in avoiding abnormal patellofemoral maltracking.
4. Ligament Balancing—Knee ligament balancing is the final important aspect for successful knee replacement. In the degenerative process, ligaments may become scarred and contracted, or they may become stretched from excessive bow deformities. Ligaments must be balanced to provide optimum function and wear for the prosthesis. Balancing must be accomplished in the coronal plane and in the sagittal plane.
   a. Coronal Plane. In the coronal plane, the two deformities are varus and valgus. The basic principle in coronal plane balancing is to *release* on the *concave* side of the deformity and to fill up the convex side until the ligament is taught. Figure 4–20 illustrates the principle for varus and valgus deformities. Table 4–5 lists the structures to be released for varus and valgus deformities. Typically for varus deformities, release of osteophytes and the deep medial collateral ligament (MCL) is all that is required to make the medial and lateral compartments symmetric in size. More significant deformities require the release of the posterior-medial corner along with the attachment of the semimembranosus. For more significant deformities, sequential subperiosteal elevation of the superficial MCL (at the pes anserine region) is required. The ligament cannot be fully released, or it will become incompetent. If over-release occurs, a constrained knee device may be required. The posterior cruciate ligament (PCL) in rare instances may be a deforming factor in significant varus deformities, and one should consider release of the PCL if other releases fail to achieve proper balance. For valgus deformities, release of osteophytes and the lateral capsule off the tibia should be the initial release. If the lateral compartment remains tight, then release of the iliotibial band (either with a Z-type release of the tendon or release off of Gerdy's tubercle) is recommended if the lateral compartment is tight in extension. If the lateral compartment is tight in flexion, then release of the popliteus tendon is recommended. In many situations where the valgus deformity is large (>5 degrees), both the iliotibial band and popliteal tendon need to be released. For severe valgus deformities, balancing may

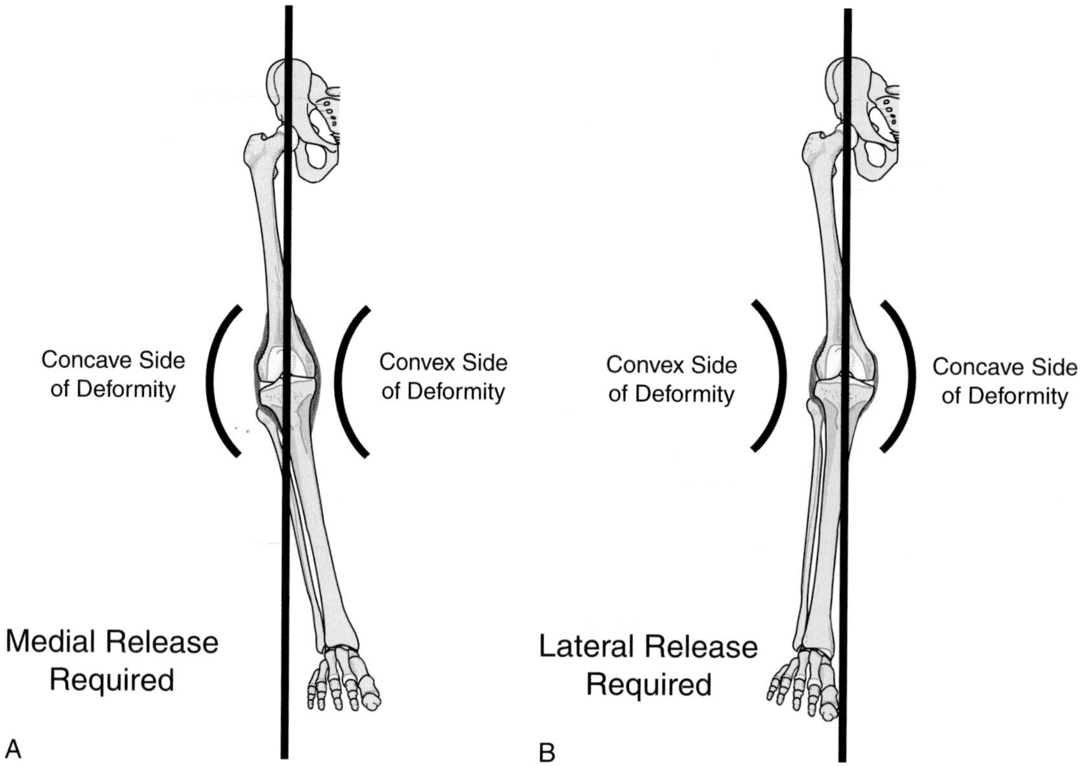

Figure 4–20. Diagram illustrating principle of releases for coronal plane deformities in the knee. *A,* Varus deformity. *B,* Valgus deformity.

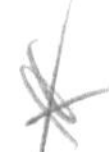

require release of the lateral collateral ligament, and if this is done, then one should strongly consider the use of a constrained-type prosthetic design. Correction of significant valgus deformity places the peroneal nerve on stretch. The deformity *most often* associated with a peroneal nerve palsy is combined valgus deformity with flexion contracture. Correction of both deformities places the nerve on significant stretch. If a postoperative peroneal nerve palsy is noted, initial treatment should be release of all compressive dressings and flexion of the knee.

b. Sagittal Plane. In this plane, balancing becomes more sophisticated. In the sagittal plane, the knee has two radii of curvature, one for the patellofemoral articulation and one for the remaining weight-bearing portion of the knee. The knee, like the hand metacarpal, acts as a modified cam. Stability, in extension and flexion, is provided by different parts of the collateral ligament structures. Balancing in the sagittal plane may require soft-tissue releases but may also require additional bone resection to achieve the correct balance. The goal in sagittal plane balancing is to obtain a gap in extension equal to the gap in flexion. By achieving this goal, the tibial insert, when placed, will be stable throughout the arc of motion. The general rule to follow when balancing the knee in the sagittal plane is as follows: If the gap problem is symmetric (i.e., same problem in flexion and extension): adjust the tibia; if the gap problem is asymmetric (i.e., different problem in flexion and extension): adjust the femur.

The five scenarios for knee balancing are illustrated in Table 4–6.

Table 4–5.

Knee Ligament Balancing Coronal Plane

Varus Deformity Medial Release	Valgus Deformity Lateral Release
• Osteophytes • Deep MCL (meniscotibial ligament) • Posteromedial corner with semimembranosus • Superficial MCL • PCL (rare occasion)	• Osteophytes • Lateral capsule • Iliotibial band • Popliteus • LCL

B. Prosthetic Design—Current total knee prosthetic designs are of three types: unconstrained, constrained nonhinged, and constrained hinged. There are two design types in the unconstrained category, the posterior cruciate retaining and posterior cruciate substituting (often referred to as posterior stabilized) implants.

Table 4–6.

Sagittal Plane Balancing Total Knee Replacement

Scenario	Problem	Solutions
Tight in extension (contracture) Tight in flexion (will not bend fully)	• Symmetric gap • Did not cut enough tibial bone	(1) Cut more proximal tibia
Extension good Flexion loose (large drawer test)	• Asymmetrical gap • Cut too much posterior femur	(1) Increase size of femoral component from anterior to posterior (i.e., go up to next size) (2) Fill up posterior gap with either cement or metal augmentation
Extension tight (contracture) Flexion good	• Asymmetric gap • Did not cut enough distal femur or did not release enough posterior capsule	(1) Release posterior capsule (2) Take off more distal femur bone (1–2 mm at a time)
Extension good Flexion tight (will not bend fully)	• Asymmetric gap • Did not cut enough posterior bone or PCL scarred and too tight (assuming use of a PCL-retaining knee system) • No posterior slope in tibial bone cut (i.e., anterior slope)	(1) Decrease size of femoral component from anterior to posterior (i.e., recut to next smaller size) (2) Recess PCL (3) Check posterior slope of tibia and recut if anterior slope
Extension loose (recurvatum) Flexion good	• Asymmetric gap • Cut too much distal femur or anteroposterior size too big	(1) Distal femoral augmentation (2) Smaller size femur (anteroposterior) that converts to symmetric gap problem (3) Use thicker tibial polyethylene inset and address tight flexion gap

Initial unconstrained total knee resurfacing designs sacrificed both the anterior cruciate ligament (ACL) and PCL ligaments. A drawback of such designs was limited knee flexion (in the range of 95 degrees) and flexion instability. With knee flexion, the femur could dislocate anterior to the tibia.

By preserving the PCL, flexion instability is mitigated as the PCL becomes taut with knee flexion and prevents anterior dislocation of the femur on the tibia (provided adequate knee balancing has been performed). In addition, by preserving the PCL, femoral rollback is produced. Femoral rollback is the posterior shift in the femoral-tibial contact point in the sagittal plane as the knee flexes (Fig. 4–21). The posterior shaft in the femoral-tibial contact point allows the posterior femur to flex further without impinging on the posterior tibia. Femoral rollback is controlled by both the ACL and PCL working in concert, but it can still occur without the ACL to an extent. Total knee prosthetic designs that preserve the PCL do achieve better knee flexion by allowing femoral rollback. The disadvantage of this design is that femoral rollback occurs without the aid of the ACL, and the consequent rollback is a combination of roll and slide. For rollback to occur, the tibial polyethylene needs to be relatively flat, but this has the detrimental effect of

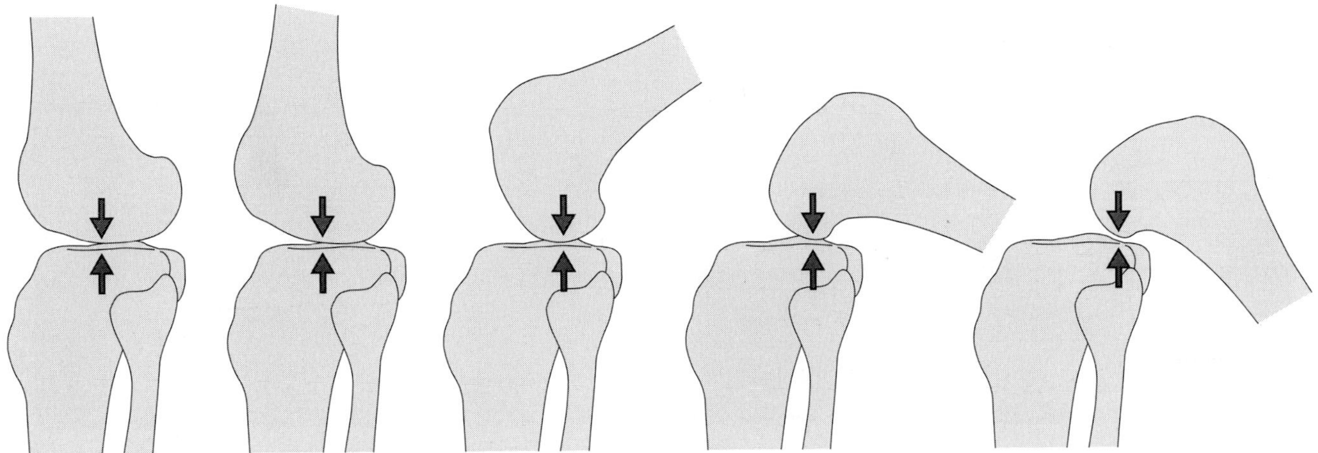

Figure 4–21. Femoral rollback is posterior shift of femoral-tibial contact point as knee flexes. Rollback allows femur to clear tibia to provide further flexion.

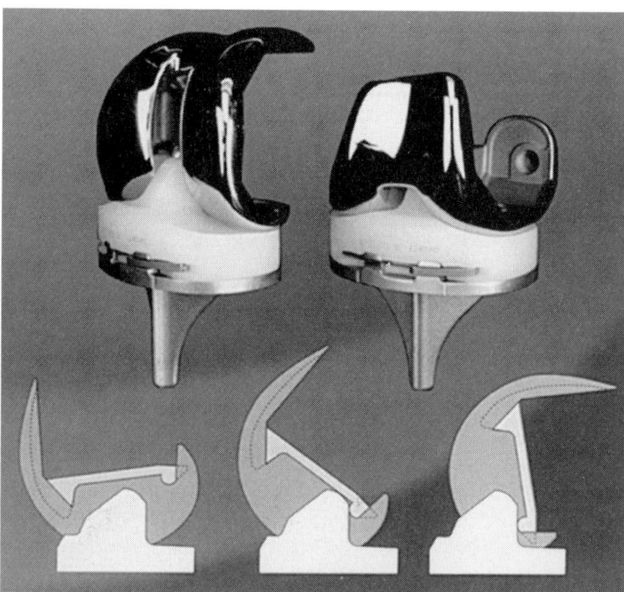

Figure 4–22. Posterior cruciate–substituting (also known as posterior stabilized) knee. Note central polyethylene post and femoral cam device on femur when the knee flexes.

creating high contact stresses. The combination of sliding wear and high contact stresses on the polyethylene can lead to rapid polyethylene wear and failure (see the section on catastrophic wear). To combat this problem, recent PCL-retaining designs contain a more congruent polyethylene insert that allows for less rollback. The more congruent articulation reduces the contact stresses on the polyethylene, but it relegates the PCL to a static stabilizer to prevent anterior dislocation of the femur on the tibia.

Posterior cruciate–substituting implants employ the use of a tibial polyethylene post in the middle of the knee along with a cam situated between the femoral condyles (Fig. 4–22). Depending on the design parameters, the femoral cam will engage against the tibial post at a designated flexion point. At that point, the femur is unable to translate anteriorly, and with further flexion it will mechanically reproduce rollback.

With the knee in the flexed position, the tibial post will prevent the cam from translating anteriorly, thus providing stability. Posterior cruciate–substituting designs do achieve improved knee flexion and allow for mechanical rollback. Because rollback is controlled mechanically, a congruent articulation surface can be used, and this reduces contact stresses on the tibial polyethylene. The disadvantage of the cruciate-substituting design is that knee balancing must be carefully addressed. If the flexion gap is loose, the femur can "jump" over the tibial post and dislocate (Fig. 4–23). If dislocation occurs, reduction requires sedation or general anesthetic, with the reduction maneuver consisting of knee flexion (at 90 degrees), distraction, and posterior force directed on the tibia. Cam jump can occur with hyperflexion even if the knee is well balanced. With a hyperflexed knee, the femur will impinge on the tibia

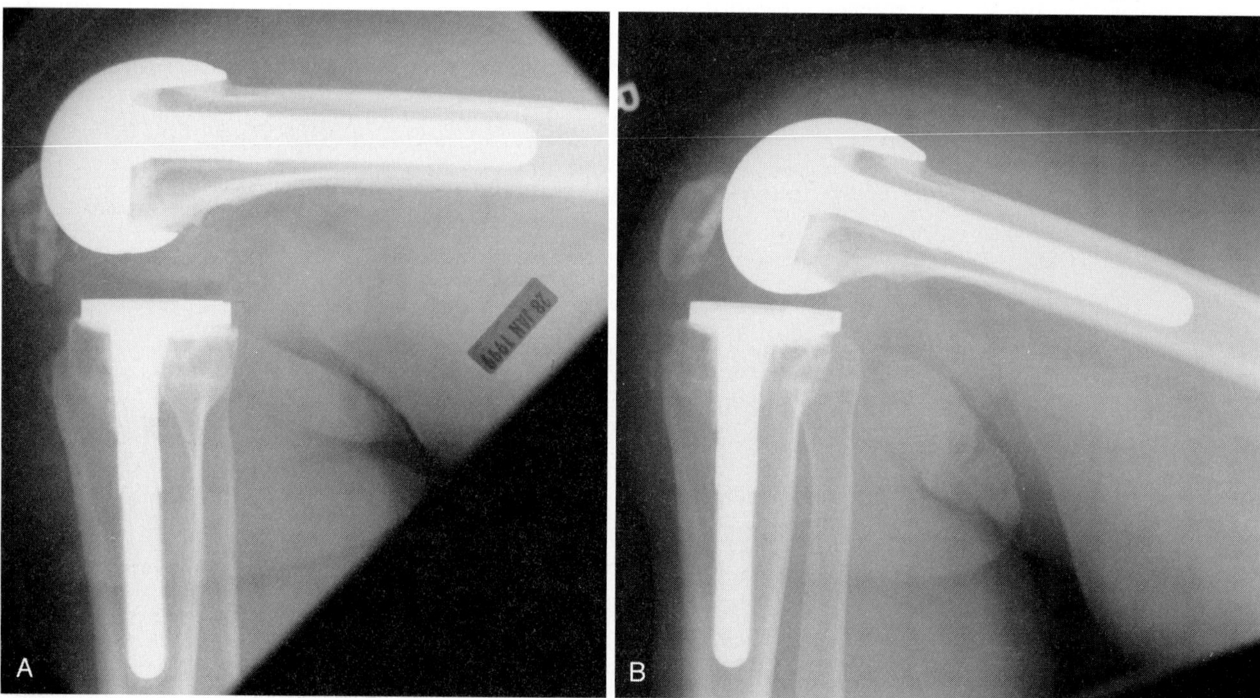

Figure 4–23. Femoral cam jump. *A*, Lateral radiograph of "femoral cam jump." Femur has hyperflexed, allowing cam to rise above tibial post and dislocate anteriorly. Once in this position, it is very difficult to reduce unless an anesthetic is administered. *B*, Postreduction radiograph of same knee.

and lever the femur over the tibial post. Hence, if anticipated knee motion after knee replacement surgery is expected to be beyond 130 degrees, a cruciate-retaining design should be considered. A cruciate-substituting design is favored over a cruciate-retaining design in several situations. First, patients with a previous patellectomy should have a cruciate-substituting prosthesis because the weakened extensor force allows for easier anterior femoral dislocation even if the PCL is retained. Second, patients with *inflammatory arthritis* can have continued inflammatory changes that will cause late PCL ruptures in total knees that retain the PCL. Third, patients with prior trauma with PCL rupture or attenuation should have a posterior stabilized implant. Finally, the last indication for a cruciate-substituting device is over-release of the PCL during knee ligament balancing when using a cruciate-retaining design. If the knee design incorporates a congruent articulation profile, conversion to a cruciate-substituting design may not be necessary. However, if the tibial articular profile is flat, the knee can translate anteriorly and become unstable. In this situation, conversion to a cruciate-substituting device is preferred.

C. Patellofemoral Articulation—The most common complications in total knee replacement involve abnormal patellar tracking. Avoiding patellar problems in knee replacement is essentially an exercise in Q angle management and understanding the technical aspects that alter the knee joint line. The Q angle is the angle formed by the intersection of the extensor mechanism axis above the patella with the axis of the patellar tendon. The significance of the Q angle in knee replacement surgery is that an increased Q angle is associated with increased lateral patellar subluxation forces. An increased Q angle can frequently cause patellofemoral maltracking. The goal in total knee replacement is to maintain a normal Q angle with techniques that *do not compromise* mechanical alignment or ligament stability. Several technical rules in total knee replacement should be followed to prevent abnormal patellar tracking. They are summarized in Table 4–7. First, femoral component internal fixation must be avoided. Internal rotation of the femoral component causes lateral patellar tilt and a net increase in Q angle (Fig. 4–24). The preferred rotational alignment of the femur is slight external rotation to the neutral axis. Normally, the proximal tibia is in slight varus of 3 degrees (Fig. 4–25). In total knee replacement, the tibia is cut at 90 degrees (i.e., perpendicular to the mechanical axis). In order to maintain a symmetric flexion gap, the femoral component must be externally rotated by the same amount to create a symmetric flexion gap. This allows for balanced ligaments in flexion.

Identifying the neutral rotational axis for the femur is not always that easy. Occasionally, landmarks can be damaged during the degenerative process. The three generally accepted landmarks defining a neutral axis are the anteroposterior axis of the femur, the epicondylar axis, and the posterior condylar axis (Fig. 4–26). The anteroposterior axis of the femur is defined as a line running from the center of the trochlear groove to the top of the intercondylar

Table 4–7.

Prevention of Patellofemoral Maltracking

Technical Issues	Guideline	Problems	Preferred Solution
Femoral component rotation	Do not internally rotate femoral component past neutral axis	Internal rotation of femoral component results in net lateral patellar tilt and increased lateral subluxation	Slight external rotation of femoral component
Femoral component position	Do not medialize femoral component	Increases Q angle	Either central or lateralized position
Tibial component rotation	Do not internally rotate tibial component past medial side of tibial tubercle	Internal rotation of tibial component results in net external rotation of tibial tubercle and increases Q angle	Tibial component centered in area between medial border of tibial tubercle and center of tibial tubercle
Mechanical alignment of leg	Do not leave leg with net valgus mechanical alignment of leg (i.e., avoid excess valgus)	Excessive valgus alignment increases Q angle	Femoral and tibial bone cuts that restore a *neutral* mechanical alignment of leg
Patella component position	(1) Avoid lateralization of patellar component on patella	(1) Lateralization of patellar component results in net increase of Q angle	(1) Patellar component placed in center of patella or in medialized position
	(2) Avoid inferior position of patellar component on patella	(2) Inferior positioning can result in relative patella baja	(2) Patellar component placed in center of patella or in superior position
Joint line position	Avoid bone cuts that raise the joint line	Creates or enhances patella baja	Maintain joint line; lower joint line if possible, when baja deformity present

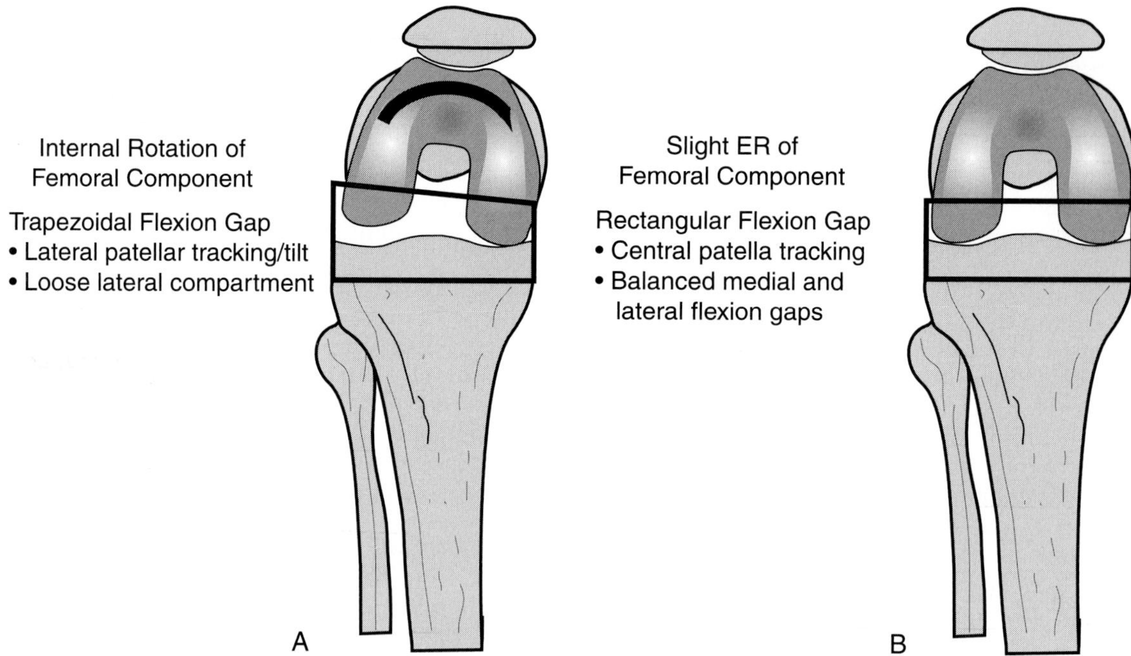

Figure 4–24. Femoral component rotation in coronal plane. *A*, Illustration of femoral component that is placed in internal rotation. Internal rotation of femoral component causes lateral flange of femoral component to push patella medial. Result is increased Q angle. Although the patella is positioned neutral, internal rotation of femoral component gives effect of lateral patellar tilt. In addition, internal rotation of femoral component creates asymmetric flexion gap, making it more difficult to balance the knee. *B*, Femoral component in slight external rotation (ER). This creates symmetric flexion gap, and the trochlear groove matches the patella. Knee is balanced.

notch. The epicondylar axis is considered to be slightly externally rotated to the neutral axis, and the femoral component should parallel the epicondylar axis. The other landmark is the posterior condylar axis, where a line perpendicular to this line defines the neutral axis.

On the tibial side, internal rotation of the tibial component must be avoided. Internal rotation of the tibial component effectively results in relative external rotation of the tibial tubercle. This has the deleterious effect of increasing the Q angle (Fig. 4–27). Anatomic valgus deformities must be corrected back to a normal range (5–8 degrees preferred). The actual goal in total knee replacement is to restore a neutral mechanical alignment. Distal femoral

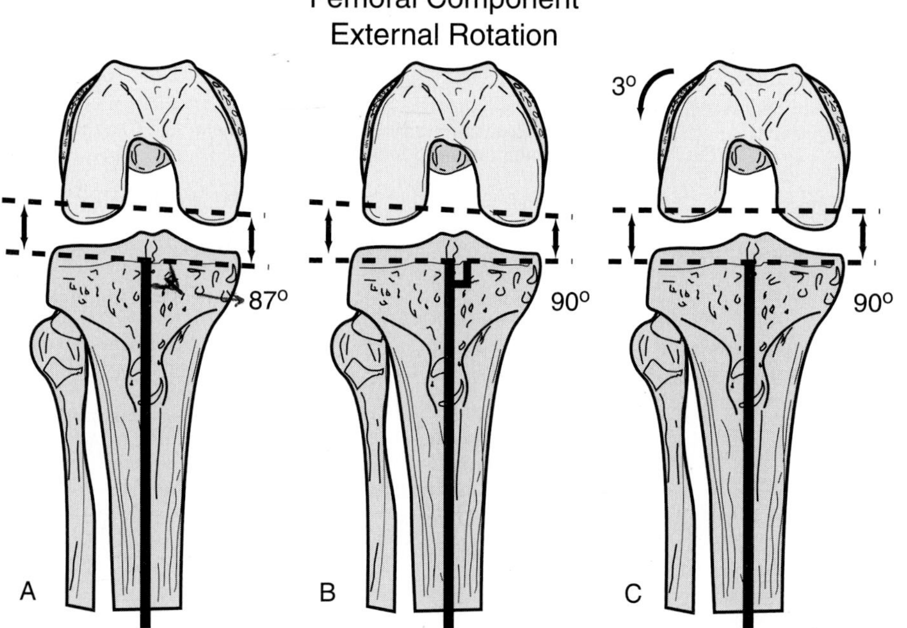

Figure 4–25. Diagrams demonstrating rotational alignment of knee in coronal plane in flexion. *A*, Tibia on average has 3 degrees varus tilt. To match this tilt, medial femoral condyle is slighter bigger in dimension than lateral femoral condyle. *B*, Proximal tibia is cut at 90 degrees, perpendicular to the mechanical axis of the tibia. In flexion, this creates an asymmetric flexion gap of the femur when cut parallel to the posterior femoral condyles. *C*, Anteroposterior (AP) cut of femur made in slight external rotation. AP cut matches tibia cut in flexion, creating symmetric flexion gap. Flexion gap is now balanced.

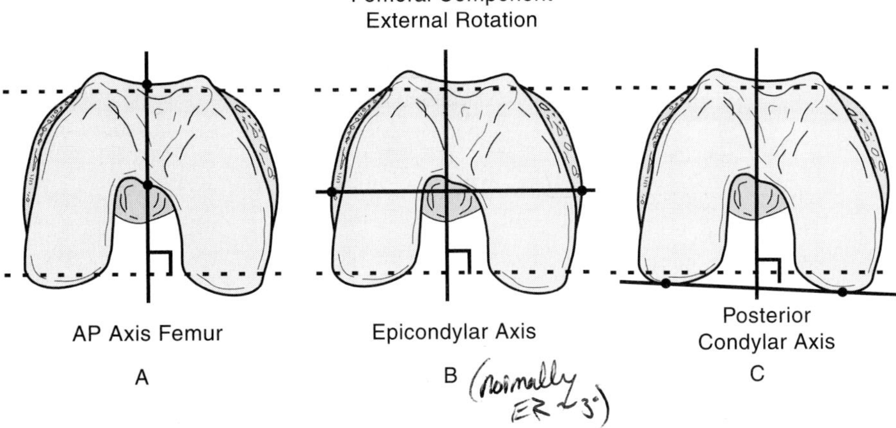

Figure 4–26. Determination of femoral component external rotation. *A*, AP axis: defined by center of trochlear groove and intercondylar notch (dots). AP cut is made perpendicular to this axis. *B*, Epicondylar axis: defined by a line connecting centers of medial and lateral epicondylar (dots). AP cut is made parallel to this axis. *C*, Posterior condylar axis: defined by a line connecting bottom of medial and lateral posterior condyles. AP cut is made in 3 degrees of external rotation to this axis line.

and proximal bone cuts should be made to achieve this goal. If excessive valgus remains, there will be an increased Q angle.

When resurfacing the patella, the desired position of the patellar component is medialized or centralized. A medialized patellar component reduces the Q angle, but it requires the use of a smaller patellar dome (Fig. 4–28). The need for lateral release is less when a small patellar dome is used in a medialized position. Placing a small patellar component in a lateralized position increases the Q angle and lateral subluxation forces. Femoral component position, if it can be adjusted, should be either centered or lateralized. A medialized femoral component places the trochlear groove in a more medial position, which increases the Q angle. Thus, this position should be avoided.

Patella baja (or patella infera) is not an infrequent problem encountered in total knee replacement. Patella baja is a condition manifested by a shortened patellar tendon. With patella baja, knee flexion is limited due to patellar impingement on the tibia as the knee flexes. Patella baja is most frequently seen in patients who have had a proximal tibial osteotomy, tibial tubercle shift or transfer, or prior fracture to the proximal tibia. Patella baja is encountered in various degrees. The solutions are limited. First, when performing a total knee replacement, avoid bone cuts that raise the joint line. Raising the joint line will effectively increase the baja deformity. Conversely, lowering the joint line will decrease the deformity. Lowering the joint line can be achieved by using distal femoral augmentation and cutting off more proximal tibia (Fig. 4–29). Lowering the joint line does not get rid of the deformity entirely, but it does help to provide increased knee flexion. Resurfacing the patella with a small patellar dome placed superiorly can effectively increase patellar tendon length. Inferior bone can be trimmed to prevent impingement. Another useful technique is trimming the anterior tibial polyethylene and patellar polyethylene at the impingement points (Fig. 4–30). This is achieved sharply with a scalpel. It will provide some improved flexion. Only shave polyethylene that does not compromise component stability or patellar tracking. If the baja deformity is severe, one last option is to cut the patella but not resurface. By doing this, there is less patellar impingement, allowing for more knee flexion.

D. Catastrophic Wear: Total Knee Replacement—Catastrophic wear in knee replacement surgery refers to the premature failure of prosthetic implants due to excessive loading, macroscopic failure of polyethylene, and subsequent mechanical loosening (Fig. 4–31). Catastrophic wear does not refer to the long-term effect of microscopic particle debris generation and

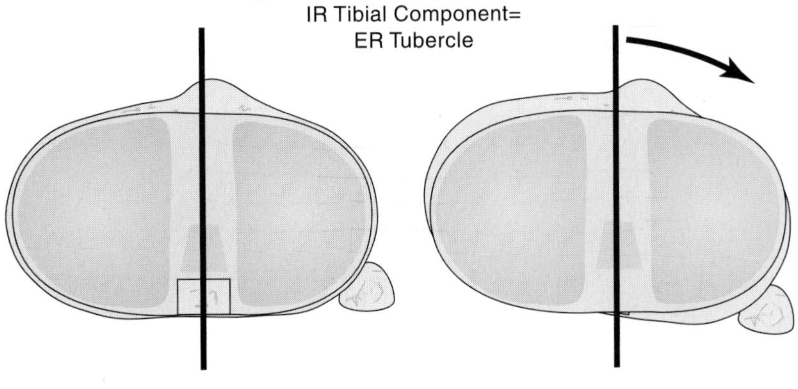

Figure 4–27. Demonstration of tibial component internal rotation. Left diagram shows tibial component centered over medial third of tibial tubercle. This is generally considered the preferred position. Right diagram shows internal rotation of tibial component. This causes a net effect of externally rotating tibial tubercle to lateral side, which increases Q angle.

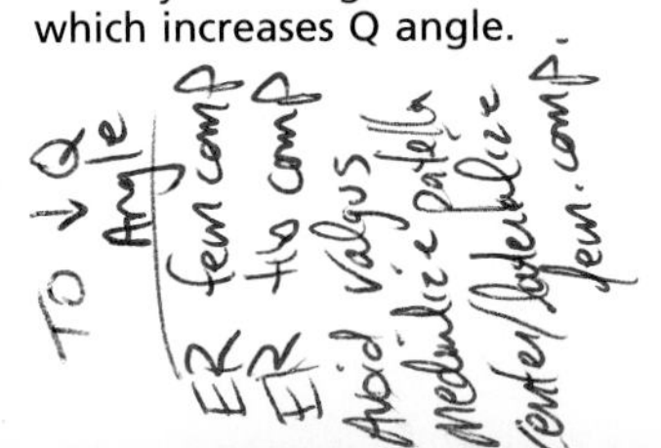

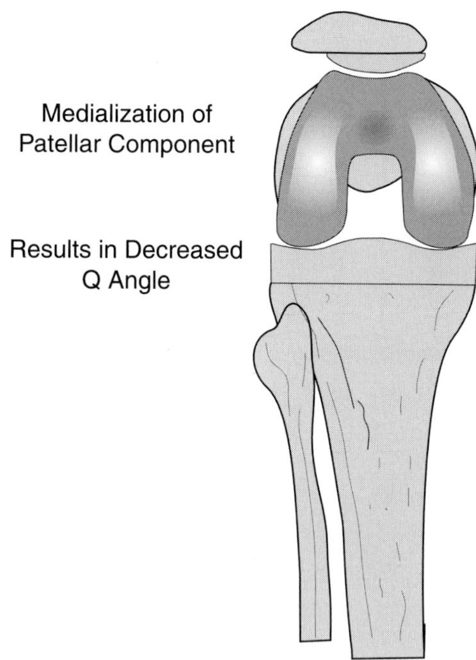

Figure 4–28. Medialization of patellar component. With this technique, a small patella dome is placed on medial side of cut patella (usually centered over trochlear ridge). Because entire patella does not need to be centered in trochlea, the center of the patellar bone is in a lateralized position that reduces Q angle. In addition, lateral retinaculum is more relaxed with patella bone in lateral position.

associated bony osteolysis. It is a problem of large-scale polyethylene failure resulting from a combination of several factors involved in implant design and biomechanics. The problem is seen primarily in total knee replacement, but depending on the situation and conditions, it can also be seen in prosthetic hip and shoulder replacement. The main issues involved in the phenomenon of catastrophic wear are (1) polyethylene thickness, (2) articular geometry, (3) sagittal plane knee kinematics, and (4) polyethylene sterilization.

1. Polyethylene Thickness—Polyethylene thickness is of critical importance in the catastrophic wear process. To keep joint contact stresses below the yield strength of ultrahigh molecular-weight polyethylene (UHMWPE), polyethylene thickness must be at least 8 mm. Thinner sections transmit joint stresses to a localized area only, resulting in microscopic and macroscopic polyethylene failure. It is very important to understand that when placing a tibial polyethylene insert into a metal tray, the polyethylene thickness reported represents the total thickness of the metal tray (usually 2–3 mm) plus the polyethylene. Therefore, in many instances where 8–10 mm polyethylene inserts are used with a metal base tray, the actual polyethylene thickness at the nadir of the convexity on the articular surface may be as thin as 4–7 mm. Consequently, in many cases where thin polyethylene inserts are used, the yield strength of UHMWPE is exceeded. This is seen most often when thin bone-cut resections are used in younger patients to preserve bone stock for future revision. In this scenario, the young active patient will cycle the prosthetic joint at a much higher rate, leading to rapid failure (4–5 years in some instances).
2. Articular Geometry—Another important factor leading to catastrophic failure is articular geometry. A majority of the prosthetic knee implants associated with catastrophic wear have a relatively flat polyethylene articular surface. A flat articular design is disadvantageous in terms of biomechanical loading. With such a design, prosthetic contact areas between the femur and tibia are low, and contact loads are high. Instead, the goal in prosthetic knee design is to *minimize contact loads*; this is achieved by *maximizing surface contact area*. Newer-generation prosthetic knee designs have improved contact areas by increasing articular congruency. This is achieved by increasing congruency in the coronal and sagittal planes. As a result, instead of seeing a flat polyethylene insert, newer components tend to be more "dished" in both the coronal and sagittal planes.
3. Sagittal Plane Knee Kinematics—Sagittal plane kinematics played an important role

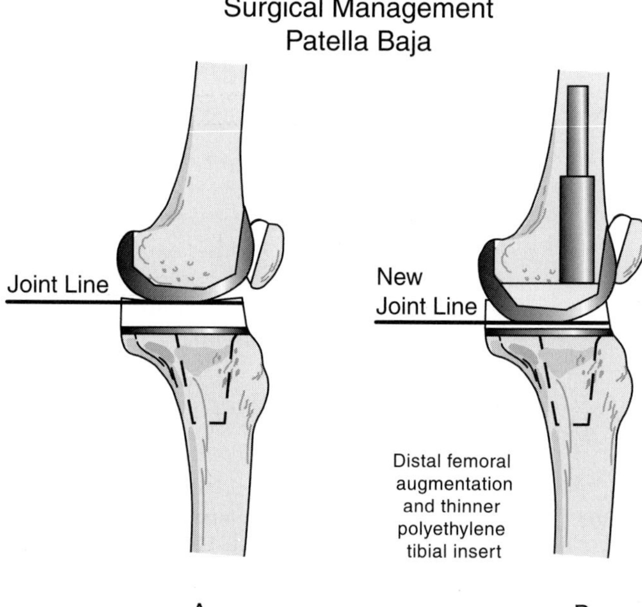

Figure 4–29. Diagram illustrating effect of lowering joint line with distal femoral augmentation to improve baja deformity. *A*, Total knee with baja deformity. *B*, Distal femoral augmentation (augments behind femoral component) has brought joint line inferiorly. Less tibial polyethylene thickness is required. Baja deformity is improved.

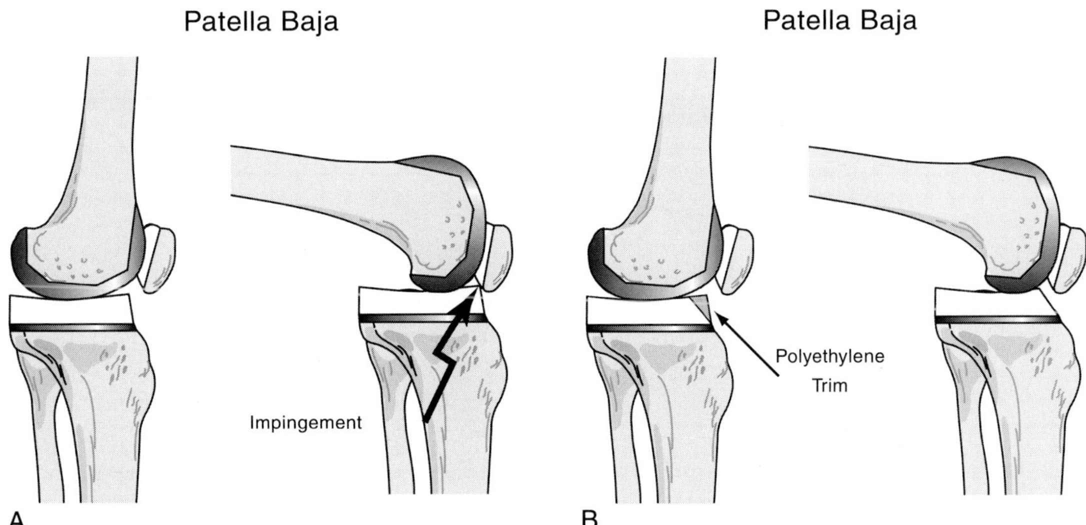

Figure 4–30. Diagram showing technique of trimming polyethylene at impingement points in patella baja. *A,* Total knee with baja deformity. Note impingement of inferior pole of patella component with anterior tibial polyethylene. *B,* Trimming of polyethylene to decrease impingement. Trimming is performed with scalpel and should not compromise articulating surfaces or stability. Trimming provides some improvement (usually up to 10 degrees) in flexion range.

in the design of flat polyethylene inserts. In an effort to improve knee flexion, prosthetic designs utilized the PCL to provide femoral rollback. Femoral rollback is the posterior shift of the femoral tibial contact as the knee flexes (Fig. 4–32). Femoral rollback allows the femur to clear the posterior tibia and bend further. In the native knee, femoral rollback is controlled by both the ACL and PCL. Rollback can still occur without an ACL, but recent fluoroscopic studies observing rollback in PCL-retained total knees show that the posterior rollback is kinetically displeasing. Instead of a smooth gradual roll, there is a combination of forward sliding, backward sliding, and posterior rolling. In addition, to allow the knee to roll back, a flat polyethylene insert is required. The diskinetic sagittal plane movements seen with PCL-retained implants that have flat polyethylene inserts contribute to the catastrophic wear process. Laboratory studies do show that sliding movements (i.e., femoral component translation on the tibia) result in surface and subsurface cracking and significant wear. In contrast, pure rolling movements generated minimal cracking and wear. Therefore, newer prosthetic knee designs incorporate less femoral rollback and provide a more congruent articular polyethylene surface. Knee flexion is achieved with other design techniques, such as a posterior center of rotation, utilizing a posterior slope, or by using a posterior cruciate–substituting knee design.

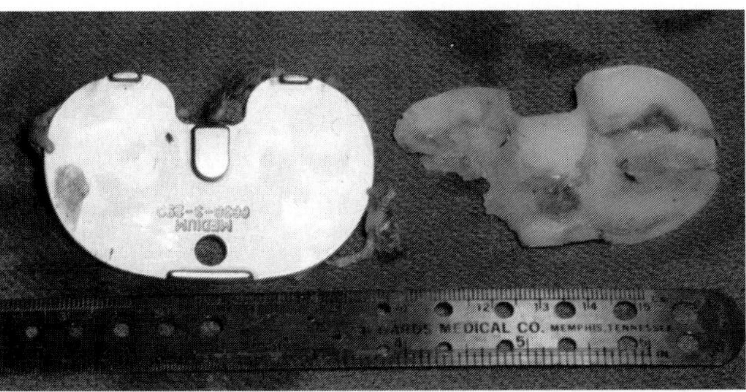

Figure 4–31. Photograph of catastrophic wear of polyethylene in a total knee. Note gross fragmentation of tibial polyethylene.

4. Polyethylene Sterilization—The last major factor in catastrophic wear involves the sterilization of polyethylene. As previously discussed in the section on osteolysis and polyethylene wear, polyethylene components irradiated in an oxygen environment suffer from polyethylene oxidation. Oxidized polyethylene is mechanically weaker, and the threshold for catastrophic wear is lowered. Excessive loading of oxidized polyethylene can result in a rapid polyethylene failure.

The problem of catastrophic wear is multidimensional. The factors involved and the problems encountered are summarized in Table 4–8. The elimination of only one of the problems will not solve the situation; it will only serve to temporarily mitigate or slow the eventual result. Only with an understanding of all factors involved can there be an effective change in component design and manufacturing to prevent this problem from occurring.

E. Rehabilitation—The single most important factor governing the ultimate flexion range

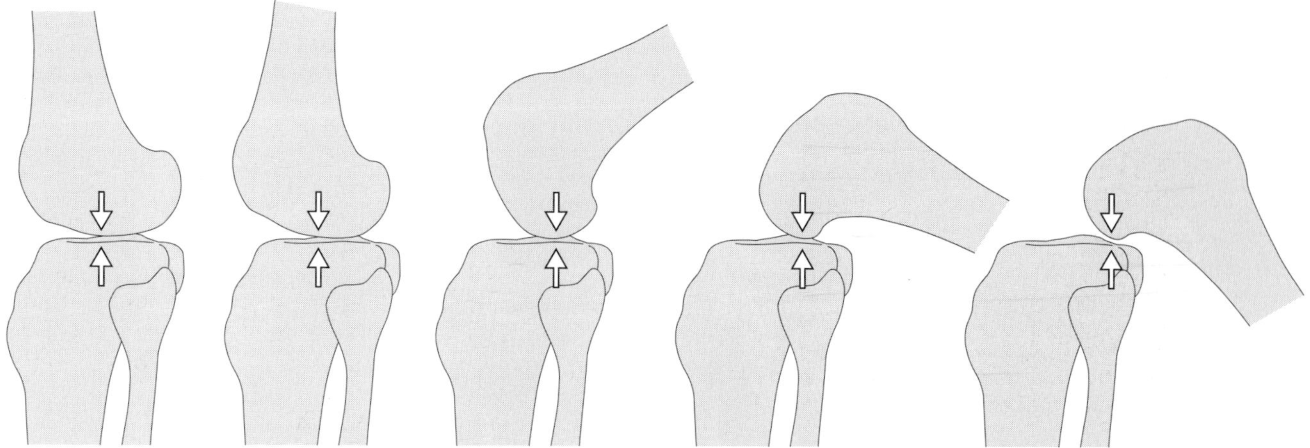

Figure 4–32. Femoral rollback is posterior shift of femoral-tibial contact point as knee flexes. Rollback allows femur to clear tibia to provide further flexion.

after total knee replacement is preoperative flexion range. As a general rule, postoperative flexion range is equal to preoperative flexion range ±10 degrees. Flexion contractures must be corrected at the time of surgery due to the fact that fixed contractures usually do not stretch out. On the other hand, the flexion contractures seen postoperatively that are corrected at the time of surgery (while under anesthesia) are usually due to hamstring tightness and spasm. After an anterior arthrotomy, the quadriceps musculature is not firing vigorously, so there is a relative overpull by the hamstring complex. As knee swelling abates, the quadriceps become more active and will counter hamstring overpull. Almost all postoperative knee flexion contractures due to hamstring overpull will stretch out by 6 months. The few that exist after this time still may stretch out by 1 year. It is important for patients to be diligent with extension and flexion range exercises up to 3 months postoperatively.

Recent studies have also examined flexion closure of total knee wounds as a means of obviating the need for postoperative CPM devices. One study compared knee closure of all wound tissues at 90 degrees, combined with postoperative closed chain (i.e., foot on floor) knee flexion exercises. In the other group, knee closure was in extension and a postoperative CPM device was utilized. Both groups performed equally well, indicating that knee closure in flexion may prove advantageous with postoperative rehabilitation.

F. Patellar Clunk Syndrome—Patellar clunk syndrome is seen with posterior stabilized total knee implants. A fibrous lump of tissue forms on the posterior surface of the quadriceps ten-

Table 4–8.

Catastrophic Wear in Total Knee Replacement

Factors Involved	Problem	Solutions
Polyethylene thickness	Polyethylene <8 mm thickness • Polyethylene ≤8 mm thick will exceed yield strength when loaded	Keep thinnest portion of polyethylene above 8 mm • Thicker tibial cut • All polyethylene tibia (needs to be congruent articulation)
Articular surface design	Flat tibia polyethylene • Low-contact surface area • High-contact stress load	Congruent articular surface design • High contact surface area • Low contact stress load
Kinematics	Femoral rollback with only PCL (no ACL) • Diskinetic motion in sagittal plane • Sliding wear	Minimize rollback with PCL-retained implant • Posterior offset center of rotation for flexion • Posterior slope to improve flexion PCL-substituting implant • Posterior stabilized knee
Polyethylene sterilization	Gamma sterilization in air • Polyethylene oxidation • Diminished mechanical properties of polyethylene • Subsurface cracking and delamination	Gamma sterilization in inert gas or vacuum • Polyethylene cross-linking • Improved wear resistance of polyethylene Alternative bearing surface • Ceramic-to-ceramic • Metal-to-metal (future prospect)

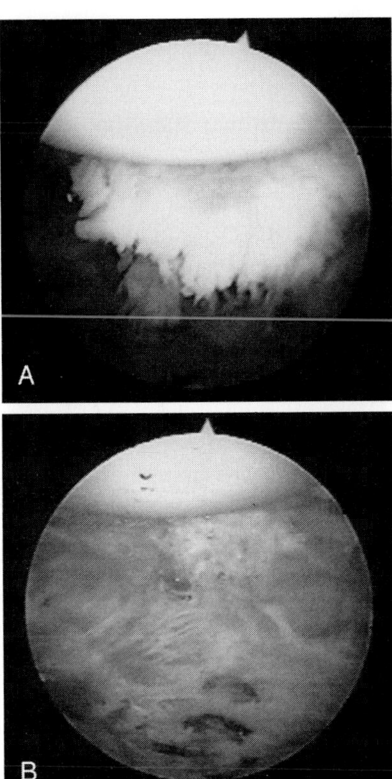

Figure 4–33. Arthroscopic photographs of patient with patellar clunk syndrome. *A*, Cephalad view of patella, showing nodule of fibrous tissue hanging down in front of patella. It is this tissue that gets caught in the central box region of the posterior stabilized femoral component. *B*, Same cephalad view after arthroscopic débridement of fibrous nodule. Patellar clunk resolved postoperatively.

don just above the superior pole of the patella. This nodule of tissue causes symptoms when it gets caught in the box of the posterior stabilized femoral component as the knee comes from flexion into extension. This usually occurs as the knee reaches 30–45 degrees flexion range. As the knee extends further, tension is applied to the entrapped nodule, which subsequently pops out of the box with a palpable and often auditory clunk. The reason for the scar formation is not clear. It may occur from a stimulated healing response from cutting the patella and abrading the adjacent quadriceps tissue. Another proposed reason is the use of a small patellar component that fails to lift the quadriceps tendon away from the anterior edge of the intercondylar notch. Recommended treatment is arthroscopic or open débridement of the nodule (Fig. 4–33).

G. Revision Total Knee Replacement—Aseptic failure of a total knee replacement is caused by several factors. These include component loosening, polyethylene wear (catastrophic wear and osteolysis), ligament instability, and patellofemoral maltracking. Tibial component loosening is more common than femoral component loosening.

The major goals of revision knee surgery are (1) extraction of knee components with minimal bone and soft-tissue destruction, (2) restoration of cavitary and segmental bone defects, (3) restoration of the original joint line as best as possible, (4) balanced knee ligaments, and (5) stable knee components.

The choice of revision knee implants depends on the integrity of the MCL and PCL. If the PCL is attenuated and/or the joint line remains significantly altered, a posterior stabilized implant is recommended. If a PCL-retaining system is used, the option of a posterior stabilized implant should be available at the time of surgery. The integrity of the PCL at the time of revision is often unpredictable. In situations where the MCL is attenuated, additional support for the MCL is required. In this situation, a constrained nonhinged knee is recommended. When there is loss of MCL integrity, a constrained hinged knee with a rotating tibial platform is the best choice (Fig. 4–34).

In many circumstances, the metaphyseal bone in the knee is damaged from mechanical abrasion, osteolysis, or extraction technique.

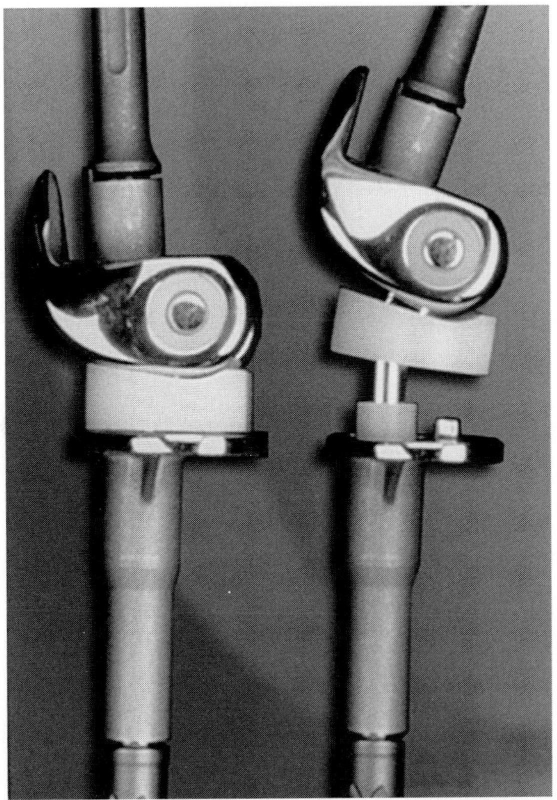

Figure 4–34. Photograph of constrained hinged knee with rotating tibial platform. Tibial polyethylene bearing is mechanically linked to femur via large connecting pin. The tibial polyethylene has a distal extension (called a yoke) that extends into metal tibial tray to allow for some internal and external rotation during the knee gait cycle. This relieves some of rotational forces that would otherwise be placed on the prosthetic bone interface.

When encountered, these areas should be supported with medullary stem extensions, which assist with load share. Cavitary defects can be filled with either particulate bone graft or cement. Generally, contained defects 1 cm or less can be filled with cement. Segmental deficiencies can be reconstructed with metal augments (wedges or blocks) and/or structural bone grafts. Large segmental deficiencies may require bulk support allografts or modular endoprosthetic devices (Fig. 4–35). Almost all revision total knees are cemented at the metaphyseal interfaces. In most cases, stem extensions are noncemented and inserted with a press fit technique.

Reconstruction of the knee after component removal should proceed first with the tibial side. This allows the joint line to be established. A useful guideline in determining the normal joint line is to identify the proximal tip of the fibular head. Generally, the joint line is about 1.5–2 cm above the fibular head. If the contralateral knee is not replaced, a radiograph of the native knee can be used to determine more accurately the distance from fibular head to joint line. Once established, the femur is reconstructed to match the tibia. Balancing is then performed to equalize flexion and extension gaps and to balance medial and lateral gaps. If reconstruction proceeds in this manner, the patellofemoral articulation is usually situated in the appropriate position. Sometimes, patellar baja still occurs and should be addressed accordingly (see the section on patellofemoral tracking).

H. Periprosthetic Fracture: Knee—Supracondylar fractures of the femur occur infrequently (less than 1%). The scenario most likely to cause supracondylar fracture is anterior femoral notching in a patient with weak bone (especially rheumatoid arthritis). Supracondylar fracture can also occur as a result of overexuberant manipulation of a total knee under anesthesia. Nondisplaced fractures are treated with nonoperative management (cast or cast brace). However, if the prosthesis is mechanically loose, then revision to a long-stem prosthesis is required. For fractures that are displaced, there is no one recommended treatment. Open treatment, no matter what method is chosen, is often difficult and demanding. If the total knee implant is mechanically loose or the fracture disrupts the prosthetic interface, revision with a long-stem prosthesis is required. If the implant is solidly fixed, then an attempt should be made to close/reduce the fracture and restore anatomic alignment. If the fracture is stable, then treatment with a cast or cast bone is preferred. If the fracture is unstable, then stabilization with a locked supracondylar nail is pre-

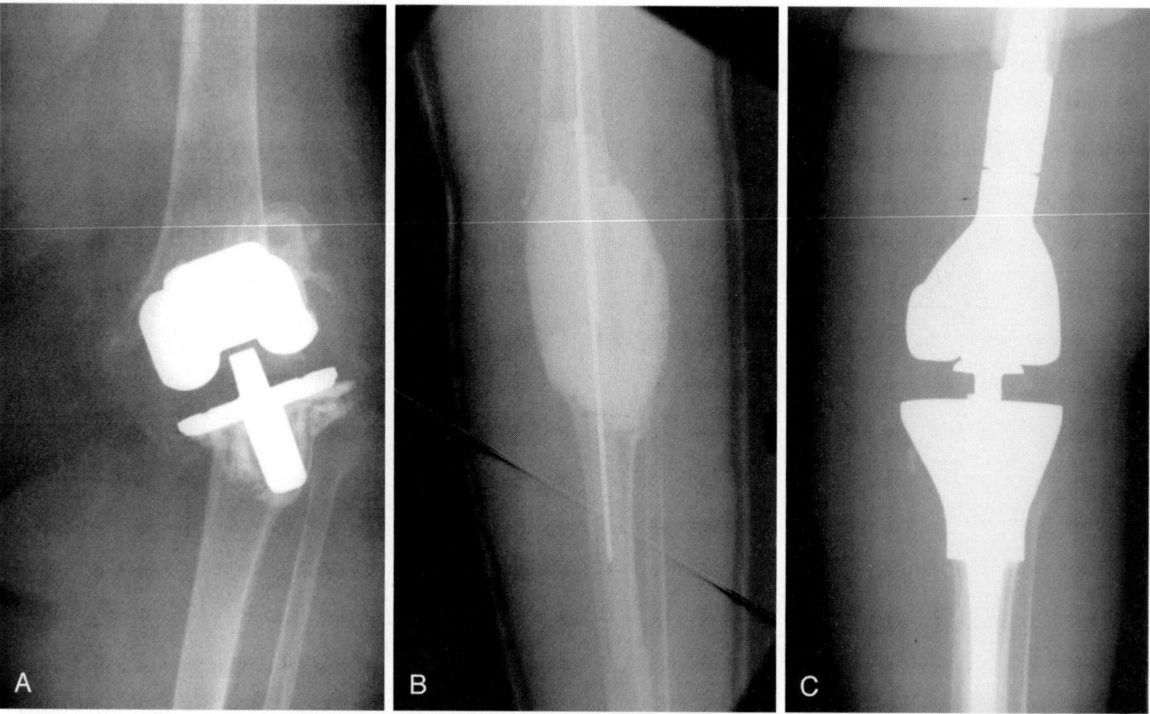

Figure 4–35. X-ray photographs of total knee requiring endoprosthetic components for reconstruction. *A*, Preoperative x-ray film of an infected total knee with significant bone destruction. *B*, X-ray film of knee after resection arthroplasty and placement of a high-dose antibiotic methylmethacrylate spacer. Patellar tendon was necrotic and was resected. *C*, X-ray film of final reconstruction utilizing endoprosthetic components for reconstruction. Knee articulation is a constrained hinged knee with a rotating tibial platform. Extensor mechanism was reconstructed with a medial gastrocnemius rotational flap with an attached achilles tendon (one-half of tendon harvested).

ferred as long as the fracture can be locked proximally and distally. Some total knee designs and sizes may not allow passage of a supracondylar nail because of either a closed intercondylar box or an intercondylar dimension that is too small. In this scenario, open reduction and internal fixation with either a blade plate or supracondylar plate (with bone graft if needed) is the best choice.

Tibia fractures below a total knee are uncommon. Nondisplaced fractures are best treated by immobilization and restricted weight-bearing. Displaced fractures are best handled with a long-stem revision prosthesis.

I. Unicompartmental Knee Replacement—A unicompartmental knee replacement is considered an alternative to osteotomy and total knee replacement when degenerative arthritis involves only one compartment. The preservation of cruciate ligaments and the remaining two knee compartments is purported to result in more normal knee kinematics than in total knee replacement. Females consider unicompartmental knee replacement an attractive option over osteotomy because it does not produce an angular knee deformity like an osteotomy. The requirements for unicompartmental knee replacement include (1) preoperatively correctable varus or valgus deformity back to normal alignment, (2) minimum of 90 degrees of flexion, (3) flexion contracture less than 10 degrees, (4) stress radiographs demonstrating no collapse of opposite knee compartment, and (5) noninflammatory arthritis.

A fixed varus or valgus deformity preoperatively usually indicates a rigid deformity that cannot be balanced adequately with a unicompartmental replacement. A unicompartmental prosthesis placed in a knee with a residual deformity will be overstressed and will likely fail. The tibial component in a unicompartmental knee replacement is usually thin and is subject to rapid wear. Therefore, a unicompartmental replacement should not be used in a high-activity patient or laborer. Heavy weight (over 90 kg) is another contraindication.

IV. Shoulder Replacement Surgery—Although there are similarities to total knee replacement and total hip replacement, total shoulder replacement has its own technical demands that set it apart. First, the range of motion in the shoulder far surpasses the range in either the hip or knee. The success of shoulder replacement surgery is far more dependent on the proper functioning of the soft tissues. Second, the glenoid is far less constrained than the acetabulum, and the forces on the glenoid in shear are significant. This makes the glenoid more prone to mechanical loosening and polyethylene wear.

The two most important factors to take into consideration in shoulder replacement surgery are the condition of the rotator cuff and the amount of glenoid bone stock available for resurfacing. If the rotator cuff is deficient and there is superior migration of the humeral head on preoperative radiographs (Fig. 4–36), glenoid resurfacing is contraindicated. Resurfacing of the glenoid in this circumstance will place excessive stress (in shear) on the superior glenoid and will lead to rapid mechanical loosening and failure. In the situation of a rotator cuff–deficient shoulder with degenerative arthritis, several variations of humeral arthroplasty are recommended. Most common is humeral hemiarthroplasty with a large head that will stay located within the shoulder. A variant of this technique is a bipolar arthroplasty, which has the benefit of providing a stable platform to allow the inner head to rotate with power provided by the deltoid muscle (Fig. 4–37). In either situation, active motion will still be very limited, usually to 60–80 degrees of elevation. A less frequent option is reconstruction of the rotator cuff by superior advancement of the subscapular and teres musculature, with closure of the superior rotator cuff deficiency. This is combined with humeral head resurfacing, using a humeral head of standard size (i.e., same size as the head resected) or slightly smaller. This technique, initially described by Flatow, may provide, in some circumstances, improved active range of motion.

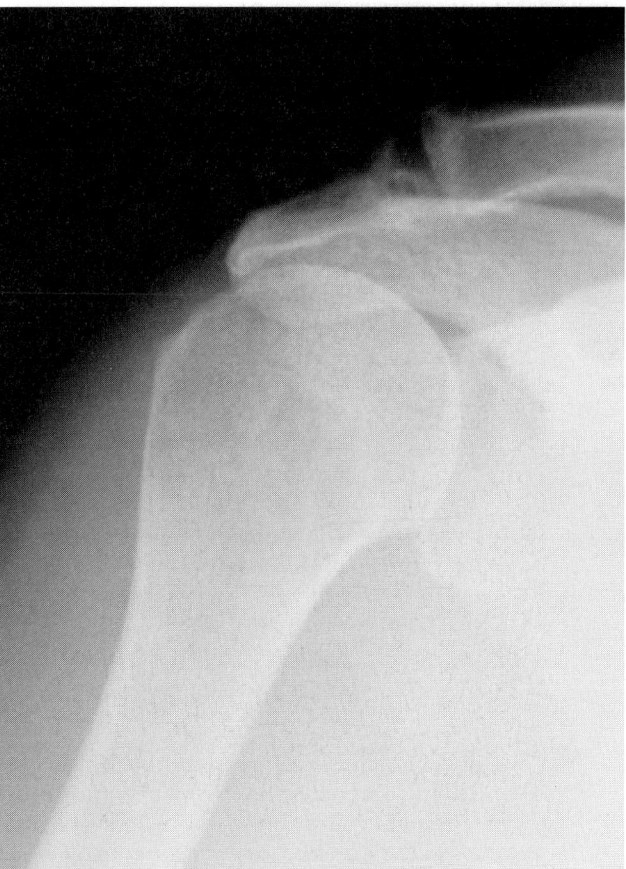

Figure 4–36. X-ray photograph of shoulder with chronic rotator cuff deficiency. With absence of rotator cuff, humeral head articulates with undersurface of acromion. Head does not remain centralized with the glenoid fossa.

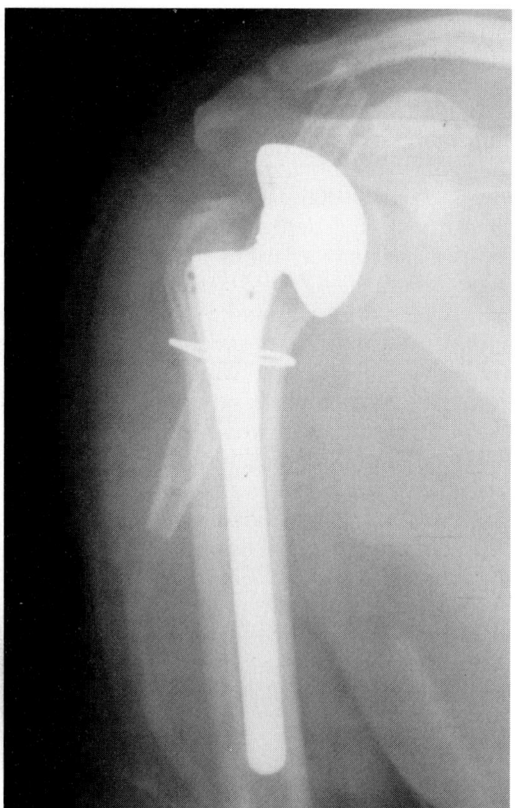

Figure 4–37. Six-month postoperative radiograph of bipolar shoulder hemiarthroplasty for comminuted four-part humeral head fracture. At the time of reconstruction, rotator cuff was attenuated.

The other critical factor when considering shoulder replacement surgery is the integrity of the glenoid. The glenoid fossa is relatively small in size and depth. Mechanical abrasion by the degenerative process may leave little bone and little chance for glenoid resurfacing. A preoperative axillary lateral is an essential part of preoperative evaluation. If the glenoid is eroded down to the coracoid process, glenoid resurfacing is contraindicated. It is also important to assess glenoid version preoperatively. Some suggest using a limited preoperative computed tomography anteversion study to evaluate glenoid version (Fig. 4–38). Patients with osteoarthritis tend to have posterior glenoid erosion and a relative retroversion of the glenoid. This retroversion needs to be corrected intraoperatively back to a neutral version. This is most often accomplished with anterior reaming or, less commonly, with posterior augmentation with bone graft.

It is now generally accepted that an all-polyethylene glenoid component be used if glenoid resurfacing is undertaken. Because the glenoid is relatively small in size and depth, taking away bone during resurfacing arthroplasty is avoided. Preparation for resurfacing usually entails reaming of remaining cartilage and some subchondral bone while glenoid depth is preserved. Keel holes or peg holes are made through the subchondral bone to anchor the prosthesis. As a result, the thickness of the glenoid component used to resurface is small (generally 4–6 mm). If a metal-backed component is used, polyethylene thickness will be significantly reduced and will lead to rapid polyethylene failure.

The choice of humeral stem fixation is similar to that of hip fixation. Successful long-term results can be achieved with cemented stems using modern cement technique (see hip section) or with noncemented porous coated implants. Porous coated noncemented stems have a design rationale similar to that of the hip: proximal porous coating to preserve proximal bone stock versus extensive porous coating that has the potential of stress-shielding in the proximal humerus. When considering the choice of humeral implant and fixation, one should take into consideration that the humeral shaft is not as thick and sturdy as the femur. If revision surgery is required, the humeral shaft is more likely to succumb to the effects of osteolysis and mechanical extraction techniques. Therefore, a proximal porous stem may be favorable in this respect. The positioning of the humeral stem should be in retroversion, generally 20–30 degrees. Its position should allow mating with the glenoid. In a situation in which an amount of glenoid retroversion is accepted, less humeral retroversion is required or else the humeral head will dislocate posteriorly.

V. Prosthetic Joint Infection—Prosthetic joint infection is one of the most devastating complications that can occur in joint replacement surgery. Studies abound as to the correct treatment, but general guidelines are reviewed. Prosthetic joint infection can be divided into three main categories: (1) Early

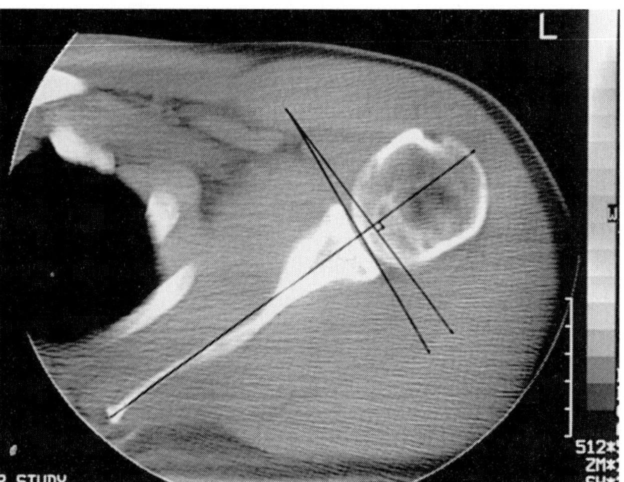

Figure 4–38. Computed tomography anteversion study. A limited scan is performed, obtaining a transverse computed tomographic image of shoulder. A line is then drawn from medial tip of scapula to midpoint of glenoid fossa. A line perpendicular to this defines neutral version. A line drawn from anterior glenoid to posterior glenoid defines the patient's glenoid version. This is then compared with neutral version line. In this example, glenoid has 7 degrees of retroversion.

postoperative infection, (2) hematogenous infection, and (3) late chronic infection. Table 4–9 describes the three categories and recommended treatment options.

A. Early Postoperative Infection—With early postoperative infection, the infection is identified within 4 weeks of the joint replacement surgery. In this setting, the infection is usually confined to within the joint space and has not had sufficient time to burrow under the prosthetic-bone interface and hide. Surgical débridement with component retention is recommended. The prognosis for infection-free recovery is good (usually 90% or greater). Modular parts must be removed to débride the fibrin layer that develops between metal and plastic parts. This fibrin layer can harbor organisms for persistent infection. Postoperative intravenous antibiotics are recommended, usually a minimum of 4–6 weeks' duration. If reinfection occurs, the prosthetic components must be resected.

B. Hematogenous Infection—In hematogenous infection, the prosthetic joint has been in place for a long time. An infection develops at another body site (e.g., necrotic gallbladder, sternal wound infection) that results in a hematogenous seeding of the prosthesis. Usually, the afflicted joint becomes painful and swollen soon after the hematogenous event, but the pain and swelling may be masked by other medical treatments, such as antibiotics and steroids. If the infection persists beyond 4 weeks, it then becomes a late chronic infection. Treatment of an acute hematogenous infection is the same as that of an early postoperative infection. Recurrent infection, if débridement fails, requires surgical extirpation of the prosthetic components.

C. Late Chronic Infection—In a late chronic infection, the infection has been present for more than 4 weeks. The infection has been persistent and has had time to enter the bone-prosthetic interface and hide. Furthermore, in many cases, the bacteria forms a glycocalyx on the implant. Many, but not all, organisms seen with chronic prosthetic infection can develop a glycocalyx. A glycocalyx is a polysaccharide later developed by bacteria that allows other bacteria to adhere to prosthetic implants and seals off some of the bacteria colony from immune system attack. Although some of the glycocalyx can be scrubbed off mechanically, there is no chemical that can be used to safely remove a glycocalyx. Therefore, once an infection is allowed to "take hold" by existing in the prosthetic bone interface and forming a glycocalyx, eradication of the infection requires prosthetic removal along with débridement of infected bone and soft tissue. The bacteria most frequently encountered in chronic prosthetic infection are the coagulase-negative *Staphylococcus* species.

D. Reconstruction of Infected Joint—Once the prosthetic implant has been removed, treatment continues with intravenous antibiotics for 4–6 weeks. Reconstruction of the infected joint thereafter is predicated on a benign clinical examination, a normal serum laboratory analysis (normal WSR and CRP), and aspiration cultures showing no growth. The type of reconstructive process depends on the overall medical/immune condition of the patient and the condition of the local wound. A patient who is ill with multiple medical problems and a compromised immune system will have a higher likelihood for perioperative complications and reinfection. In this situation, leaving the patient with a resection arthroplasty may be the best solution. If the patient's medical/immune condition is good, the choice for the reconstruction depends on the condition of the local wound.

The condition of the local wound is the most important factor in determining the type

Table 4–9.

Prosthetic Joint Infection Classification and Management

Infection Type	Duration	Treatment
Early postoperative infection	≤4 weeks from initial joint replacement	(1) I&D with retention of components • Exchange of modular polyethylene parts • Postoperative IV antibiotics (6 weeks) (2) Resection of components if I&D fails
Hematogenous infection	≤4 weeks from initial hematogenous seeding	(1) I&D with retention of components • Exchange of modular polyethylene parts • Postoperative IV antibiotics (6 weeks) (2) Resection of components if I&D fails
Late chronic infection	>4 weeks from initial joint replacement >4 weeks from initial hematogenous seeding	(1) Two-stage reimplantation with an interval period of IV antibiotics (2) Two-stage arthrodesis with an interval period of IV antibiotics (3) Resection arthroplasty with IV antibiotics postoperatively (4) Amputation

of reconstruction after removal of an infected total joint. With chronic infection, soft tissue and bony tissues are affected by the destructive inflammatory process. This causes bone defects, ligament/tendon loss or attenuation, and muscle loss and/or scarring. If significant soft-tissue destruction has occurred and anticipated function of the joint is going to be poor, then a fusion may be a better reconstructive solution. Amputation is reserved for those patients who are very ill or who have severe soft-tissue destruction where neither a fusion nor reconstructive salvage will help.

Reimplantation arthroplasty is utilized if joint function can be adequately preserved. If soft-tissue deficits are present, a local muscle transfer can be rotated to cover the defect and allow for a tension-free closure. Bone defects can be accommodated with modular revision implants or, in some cases, with modular oncologic implants. Bulk-support allografts are an acceptable alternative for large bone defects. The disadvantage of using an allograft for reconstruction is that the surrounding tissues (damaged by the infection) may have an attenuated blood supply, and the graft may not heal and incorporate. Furthermore, if the allograft is placed in a superficial position (e.g., proximal tibia), the allograft can become easily infected from a minor wound dehiscence or from prolonged drainage. Once the allograft is colonized, eradication of the infection is nearly impossible because the allograft is a dead porous structure in which bacteria can easily hide. In contrast, deficits filled by metallic augmentation have only an outer surface for bacteria to adhere. If colonization does occur, it can be treated successfully with irrigation and débridement.

Antibiotic-loaded cement (polymethylmethacrylate [PMMA]) spacers for prosthetic joint infection have been used to preserve the soft-tissue envelope during the period the prosthetic joint has been resected. The elution of antibiotics from methylmethacrylate depends on porosity of the cement, surface area, and antibiotic concentration. Increased porosity allows for better elution of antibiotics. Some PMMA powders have a larger monomer and, in the solid form, they are more porous. Moreover, the addition of large quantities of antibiotics increases porosity even further. Antibiotic beads have a larger surface area than a block and elute more antibiotics. Higher doses of antibiotics in the cement allow for higher antibiotic elution and longer elution time. Antibiotics that are to be used in PMMA must be heat-stable as the curing process of PMMA generates significantly high temperature to deactivate antibiotics. The common antibiotics used with PMMA for prosthetic joint infection are vancomycin, tobramycin, gentamicin, and cefoxitin.

VI. Osteotomy

A. Hip Osteotomy—In regard to hip dysplasia, rotational pelvic osteotomy is the preferred reconstruction choice if the hip dysplasia primarily involves poor development of the acetabulum. Prerequisites for pelvic rotational osteotomy include the presence of moderate to high-grade dysplasia, good residual joint space thickness, absence of femoral head deformity, and absence of angular femoral head-neck deformity in the coronal plane (i.e., coxa valga). Table 4–10 reviews the choices of pelvic osteotomies. For adults with dysplasia, the preferred pelvic osteotomy is the periacetabular (Ganz et al.) osteotomy. This osteotomy provides a multiplanar correction, and the acetabulum can be medialized. This allows re-creation of a normal hip center of rotation.

The use of femoral intertrochanteric osteotomy should be considered in young patients with arthritic afflictions where hip replacement surgery will result in premature failure due to osteolysis and early loosening. Situations in which femoral osteotomy are useful include certain cases of hip dysplasia, osteonecrosis of the femoral head, femoral head deformities from slip of the capital femoral epiphysis, lateral hip impingement in Perthes' disease, and femoral neck nonunion.

Femoral intertrochanteric varus osteotomy is utilized concomitantly with pelvic rotational osteotomy when there is a prominent coxa valga deformity. Another indication for femoral intertrochanteric osteotomy is management of osteonecrosis of the hip. Defining the extent of the necrotic sector is the dominant variable in predicting outcome for osteotomy. Success is inversely related to the size of the necrotic sector. From numerous studies, it is clear that intertrochanteric osteotomy will fail if more than 50% of the femoral head is involved at the time of surgery. The type of intertrochanteric rotational osteotomy depends on the location of the necrotic lesion within the femoral head. The principle is to rotate the femoral head such that there is viable bone and cartilage articulating with the superior weight-bearing portion of the acetabulum. Therefore, an intact lateral portion of the femoral head is a prerequisite for varus osteotomy. Conversely, an intact medial femoral head is required for valgus osteotomy. A flexion osteotomy is used in those patients with anterior involvement in the sagittal plane. Conversely, an extension osteotomy can be used in those patients with posterior involvement in the sagittal plane. Biplanar corrections are often required (e.g., flexion-valgus intertrochanteric osteotomy).

In certain cases of post-Perthes' adult arthritis, lateral hip impingement occurs causing

Table 4–10.

Review of Pelvic Osteotomies

Procedure	Osteotomy Description	Requirements	Comments
Salter	Innominate (open wedge)	• Congruous acetabular dysplasia • CE angle >12–15 degrees • Anterior and lateral redirection of acetabulum	• Does not always provide good lateral coverage • Used primarily in early youth
Double or triple innominate	Innominate and pubis or innominate and both rami	• CE angle 0–15 degrees • Congruous acetabular dysplasia	• For more advanced dysplasia • Preserves triradiate cartilage • Used primarily in youth
Spherical acetabular osteotomy	Acetabular Subchondral	• Almost any CE angle • Must have closed triradiate cartilage (compromises vascular supply to area) • Congruous acetabular dysplasia	• Medialization of acetabular segment complex and difficult • Capsulotomy contraindicated • Complications of osteonecrosis and intra-articular penetration frequent
Periacetabular osteotomy (Ganz et al.)	Periacetabular	• Almost any CE angle • Congruous acetabular dysplasia	• Capsulotomy is safe (allows look for labral tears) • Medialization of acetabulum is easy • Minimal fixation required; only 2–4 screws • Preferred osteotomy in adult
Chiari's osteotomy	Curved innominate slides iliac shelf over uncovered femoral head and capsule; interposed capsule undergoes metaplasia into cartilage material	• Unstable aspherical joint	• Salvage osteotomy only • Leaves anterior acetabulum uncovered • Abductor lurch common after Chiari's unless trochanteric advancement is performed

pain. In this problem, radiographs show a superior head osteophyte, which impinges against the lateral acetabulum with hip abduction. In this situation, a pure valgus intertrochanteric osteotomy is effective in alleviating the impingement. This is preferable to femoral head cheilectomy or partial femoral head excision.

In the case of slipped capital femoral epiphysis deformities, a valgus-flexion derotational intertrochanteric osteotomy provides a high incidence of success with pain relief and near-normal restoration of biomechanical function. This technique is effective and safe in most deformities and is preferable to the risks incurred with intra-articular femoral neck osteotomies.

The disadvantage of proximal hip osteotomy is the potentially more difficult stem insertion when converting to total hip replacement. This is due to the effects of displacement, rotation, and angulation. Careful preoperative planning is necessary to ensure that the chosen osteotomy will not greatly interface with future hip replacement surgery. Of particular note, flexion osteotomy should not be performed with anterior closing wedges. Such wedges predispose to significant displacement of the distal fragment and compromise future femoral stem insertion. Instead, gaps created by the osteotomy can be easily filled with bone graft and heal with predictable success.

B. Knee Osteotomy—In degenerative arthritis of the knee, varus or valgus deformities are common. This causes an abnormal distribution of weight-bearing stresses through the joint. These deformities concentrate stress either medially or laterally, and the degenerative changes in that compartment are accelerated. The biomechanical goal of a knee osteotomy is to unload the involved joint compartment by correcting the malalignment. Generally, in the knee joint, varus deformity with medial compartment degenerative arthritis is treated with a valgus-producing proximal tibial osteotomy. Valgus deformity with lateral compartment degenerative arthritis is treated with a varus-producing distal femoral supracondylar osteotomy.

Indications for proximal tibial osteotomy are (1) pain and disability resulting from degenerative arthritis that significantly interface with work and recreation, (2) evidence on weight-bearing radiographs of degenerative arthritis confined to one compartment, (3) the ability of the patient to be compliant postoperatively with partial weight-bearing and motivation to carry out a rehabilitation program, and (4) good vascular status without serious arterial insufficiency.

Contraindications to proximal tibial valgus osteotomy are (1) narrowing of lateral compartment cartilage space with stress radiographs, (2) lateral tibial subluxation of more than 1 cm, (3) medial compartment bone loss of more than 2–3 mm, (4) flexion contracture of more than 15 degrees, (5) knee flexion less than 90 degrees, (6) more than 20 degrees of correction needed, and (7) inflammatory arthritis (e.g., rheumatoid arthritis).

In addition, a relative contraindication is a knee that shows a varus thrust. Best results are

Table 4–13.

Staging System for Osteonecrosis of the Hip

Stage	Grade	Criteria
0		X-ray, MRI, and bone scan normal
I		Normal x-ray, abnormal MRI and/or bone scan
II		Abnormal x-ray showing cystic or sclerotic changes in femoral head
III		Subchondral collapse producing *crescent sign*
IV		Flattening of femoral head
V		Joint narrowing with or without acetabular involvement
VI		Advanced degenerative changes
		Quantification of Extent of Involvement
I & II	A	<15% *volume* head involvement on x-ray or MRI
	B	15–30%
	C	>30%
III	A	Subchondral collapse (crescent) beneath <15% of articular surface
	B	Crescent beneath 15–30%
	C	Crescent beneath >30%
IV	A	<15% surface collapse *and* <2 cm depression
	B	15–30% collapse or 2–4 mm depression
	C	>30% collapse or >4 mm depression
V	A	<15% femoral head involvement (same criteria as above)
	B	15–30% of acetabular involvement
	C	>30% involvement

greater trochanter) of the necrotic segment. Curettage of the necrotic segment is taken all the way to subchondral bone. The fibular strut is placed up against subchondral bone, which then heals. This prevents subchondral collapse as the rest of the autogenous bone graft heals. Vascularized fibular strut grafting is generally recommended for earlier stages of ON, but it has been shown to be effective even if some subchondral collapse has occurred. Sometimes, the subchondral bone can even be tapped up to a more congruent position. Vascularized fibular strut grafting is contraindicated when there is "whole head" involvement.

Hip arthroplasty is recommended in advanced stages of ON when degenerative arthritis is present or femoral head collapse is advanced. The choice of hemiarthroplasty versus total hip replacement depends upon activity level, physiologic age, patient compliance, and pre-existing arthritis. Young active patients tend to do less well with hemiarthroplasty due to rapid wear of the acetabular articular cartilage and the development of pain, particularly in the groin. In contrast, an elderly patient whose ON is due to chronic alcohol use and who would be poorly compliant with total hip precautions may be best suited with hemiarthroplasty. Patients with radiographic evidence of acetabular degenerative changes should have a total hip replacement. Hip fusion should be considered in the very young patient who is (or plans to be) in a heavy labor occupation. Additional autogenous bone grafting is required for the necrotic femoral head is necrotic and collapsed. The results of hip fusion for ON are less favorable than cases for degenerative arthritis without ON.

Selected Bibliography

1. Arima, J., Whiteside, L.A., McCarthy, D.S., et al.: Femoral rotational alignment, based on the anterioposterior axis, in total knee arthroplasty in a valgus knee. J. Bone Joint Surg. 77A:1331, 1995.
2. Barrack, R.L., Mulroy, R.D., and Harris W.W.H.: Improved cementing techniques and femoral component loosening in young patients with hip arthroplasty: A 12-year radiographic review. J. Bone Joint Surg. 74B:385, 1992.
3. Beals, R.K., and Tower, S.S.: Periprosthetic fractures of the femur. Clin. Orthop. 327:238, 1996.
4. Bloebaum, R.D., Rubman, M.H., and Hofmann, A.A.: Bone ingrowth into porous-coated tibial components implanted with autograft bone chips: Analysis of ten consecutively retrieved implants, J. Arthroplasty 7:483, 1992.
5. Bobyn, J.D., Pilliar, R.M., Cameron, H.U., et al.: The effect of porous surface configuration on the tensile strength of fixation of implants by bone ingrowth. Clin. Orthop. 149:291, 1980.
6. Bono, J.V., Sanford, L., and Toussaint J.T.: Severe polyethylene wear in total hip arthroplasty: Observations from retrieved AML PLUS hip implants with an ACS polyethylene liner. J. Arthroplasty 9:119, 1994.
7. Brooker, A.F., Bowerman, J.W., Robinson, R.H., et al.: Ectopic ossification following total hip replacement: Incidence and a method of classification. J. Bone Joint Surg. 55A:1629, 1973.
8. Burke, D.W., Gates, E.I., and Harris, W.H.: Centrifugation as a method of improving tensile and fatigue properties of acrylic bone cement. J. Bone Joint Surg. 66A:1265, 1984.
9. Canale, S.T.: Campbell's Operative Orthopaedics, 9th ed. St. Louis, Mosby, 1998.
10. Cappello, W.N.: Femoral component fixation in the 1990s: Hydroxyapatite in total hip arthroplasty: Five-year clinical experience. Orthopedics 17:781, 1994.
11. Cella, J.P., Salvati, E.A., and Sculco, T.P.: Indomethacin for the prevention of heterotopic ossification following total hip arthroplasty: Effectiveness, contraindications and adverse effects. J. Arthroplasty 3:229, 1988.
12. Chandler, H.P., Reineck, F.T., Wixson, R.L., et al.: Total hip replacement in patients younger than thirty years old: A five-year follow-up study. J. Bone Joint Surg. 63A:1426, 1981.
13. Chen, F., Mont, M.A., and Bachner, R.S.: Management of ipsilateral supracondylar femur fractures following total knee arthroplasty. J. Arthroplasty 9:521, 1994.
14. Cofield, R.H., and Briggs, B.T.: Glenohumeral arthrodesis: Operative and long-term functional results. J. Bone Joint Surg. 61A:668, 1979.
15. Collier, J., Mayor, M.B., McNamara, J.L., et al.: Analysis of the failure of 122 polyethylene inserts from uncemented tibial knee components. Clin. Orthop. 273:232, 1991.
16. Cook S.D., Barrack R.L., Thomas K.A., et al.: Quantitative analysis of tissue growth into human porous total hip components. J. Arthroplasty 3:249, 1988.
17. Dall D.M., and Miles, A.W.: Reattachment of the greater trochan-

ter: The use of the trochanter cable-grip system. J. Bone Joint Surg. 65B:55, 1983.

18. D'Antonio, J., McCarthy, J.C., Bargar, W.L., et al.: Classification of femoral abnormalities in total hip arthroplasty. Clin. Orthop. 296:133, 1993.
19. David, A., Eitemuller, J., Muhr, G., et al.: Mechanical and histological evaluation of hydroxyapatite-coated, titanium-coated, and grit-blasted surfaces under weight-bearing conditions. Arch. Orthop. Trauma Surg. 114:112, 1995.
20. Delaunay S, Dussault, R.G., Kaplan, P.A., et al.: Radiographic measurements of dysplastic adult hips. Skeletal Radiol. 26:75, 1997.
21. DeLee, J.G., and Charnley, J.: Radiologic demarcation of cemented sockets in total hip replacement. Clin. Orthop. 121:20, 1976.
22. Ebramzadeh, E., Sarmiento, A., McKellop, H., et al.: The cement mantle in total hip arthroplasty: Analysis of long-term radiographic results. J. Bone Joint Surg. 76A:77, 1994.
23. Emerson, R.H., Head, W.C., and Peters, P.C.: Soft-tissue balance and alignment in medial unicompartmental knee arthroplasty. J. Bone Joint Surg. 74B:807, 1992.
24. Emerson, R.H., Malinin, T.I., Cuellar, A.D., et al.: Cortical allografts in the reconstruction of the femur in revision total hip arthroplasty: A basic science and clinical study. Clin. Orthop. 285:35, 1992.
25. Engh, C.A., and Bobyn, J.D.: The influence of stem size and extent of porous coating on femoral bone resorption after primary cementless hip arthroplasty. Clin. Orthop. 231:7, 1988.
26. Engh, C.A., Bobyn, J.D., and Glassman, A.H.: Porous-coated hip replacement: The factors governing bone ingrowth, stress shielding, and clinical results. J. Bone Joint Surg. 69B:45, 1987.
27. Engh, C.A., Glassman, A.H., Griffin, W.L., et al.: Results of cementless revision for failed cemented total hip arthroplasty. Clin. Orthop. 235:91, 1988.
28. Engh, C.A., Glassman, A.H., and Suthers, K.E.: The case for porous-coated hip implants. Clin. Orthop. 261:63, 1990.
29. Estok, D.M., and Harris, W.H.: Long-term results of cemented femoral revision surgery using second-generation techniques: An average 11.7 year follow-up evaluation. Clin. Orthop. 299:190, 1994.
30. Faris, P.M., Herbst, S.A., Ritter, M.A., et al.: The effect of preoperative knee deformity on the initial results of cruciate-retaining total knee arthroplasty. J. Arthroplasty 7:527, 1992.
31. Feighan, J.E., Goldberg, V.M., Davy, D., et al.: The influence of surface blasting on the incorporation of titanium-alloy implants in a rabbit intramedullary model. J. Bone Joint Surg. 77A:1380, 1995.
32. Foglar, C., and Lindsey, R.W.: C-reactive protein in orthopaedics. Orthopedics 21:687, 1998.
33. Ganz, R., Klaue, K., Vinh, T.S., et al.: A new periacetabular osteotomy for the treatment of hip dysplasias. Clin. Orthop. 232:26, 1988.
34. Greene, N., Holtom, P.D., Warren, C.A., et al.: In vitro elution of tobramycin and vancomycin polymethylmethacrylate beads and spacers from Simplex and Palacos. Am. J. Orthop. 27:201, 1998.
35. Gristina, A.G., and Costerton, J.W.: Bacterial adherence to biomaterials and tissue: The significance of its role in clinical sepsis. J. Bone Joint Surg. 67A:264, 1985.
36. Gruen, T.A., McNeice, G.M., and Amstutz, H.C.: "Modes of failure" of cemented stem-type femoral components: A radiographic analysis of loosening. Clin. Orthop. 141:17, 1979.
37. Hawkins, R.J., and Neer, C.S. II: A functional analysis of shoulder fusions. Clin. Orthop. 223:65, 1987.
38. Healy, W.L., Lo, T.C.M., DeSimone, A.A., et al.: Single-dose irradiation for the prevention of heterotopic ossification after total hip arthroplasty. J. Bone Joint Surg. 77A:590, 1995.
39. Hedley, A.K., Mead, L.P., and Hendren, D.H.: The prevention of heterotopic bone formation following total hip arthroplasty using 600 rad in a single dose. J. Arthroplasty 4:319, 1989.
40. Hofmann, A.A., Bloebaum, R.D., Rubman, M.H., et al.: Microscopic analysis of autograft bone applied at the interface of porous-coated devices in human cancellous bone. Int. Orthop. 16:349, 1992.
41. Holtom, P.D., Warren, C.A., Green, N.W., et al.: Relation of surface area to in vitro elution characteristics of vancomycin-impregnated polymethylmethacrylate spacers. Am. J. Orthop. 27:207, 1998.
42. Hozack, W.J., Rothman, R.H., Booth, R.E., Jr., et al.: The patellar clunk syndrome: A complication of posterior stabilized total knee arthroplasty. Clin. Orthop. 241:203, 1989.
43. Huiskes R: Biomechanical aspects of hydroxylapatite coatings on femoral hip prosthesis. In Manley, M.T., ed.: Hydroxylapatite Coatings in Orthopaedic Surgery. New York, Raven Press, Ltd., 1993.
44. Jones, J.P., Steinberg, M.E., Hungerford, D.S., et al.: Avascular necrosis: Pathogenesis, diagnosis, and treatment. AAOS Instr. Course Lect. 309. San Francisco, 1997.
45. Jonsson, E., Lidgren, L., and Rydholm, U.: Position of shoulder arthrodesis measured with moire photography. Clin. Orthop. 238:117, 1989.
46. Kaplan, S.J., Thomas, W.H., and Poss, R.: Trochanteric advancement for recurrent dislocation after total hip arthroplasty. J. Arthroplasty 2:119, 1987.
47. Kjaersgaard-Andersen, P., and Ritter, M.A.: Short-term treatment with non-steroidal antiinflammatory medications to prevent heterotopic bone formation after total hip arthroplasty: A preliminary report. Clin. Orthop. 279:157, 1992.
48. Kumar, P.J., McPherson, E.J., Dorr, L.D., et al.: Rehabilitation after total knee arthroplasty: A comparison of two rehabilitation techniques. Clin. Orthop. 331:93, 1996.
49. Laskin, R.S., Rieger, M., Schob, C., et al.: The posterior stabilized total knee prosthesis in the knee with severe fixed deformity. J. Knee Surg. 1:199, 1988.
50. Lewonowski, K., Dorr, L.D., McPherson, E.J., et al.: Medialization of the patella in total knee arthroplasty. J. Arthroplasty 12:161, 1997.
51. Livermore, J., Ilstrup, D., and Morrey, B.: Effect of femoral head size on wear of the polyethylene acetabular component. J. Bone Joint Surg. 72A:518, 1990.
52. Lombardi, A.V., Mallory, T.H., Vaughn, B.K., et al.: Dislocation following primary posterior-stabilized total knee arthroplasty. J. Arthroplasty 8:633, 1993.
53. Mantas, J.P., Bloebaum, R.D., Skedros, J.G., et al.: Implications of reference axes used for rotational alignment of the femoral component in primary and revision knee arthroplasty. J. Arthroplasty 7:531, 1992.
54. McPherson, E.J., Patzakis, M.J., Gross, J.E., et al.: Infected total knee arthroplasty: Two-stage reimplantation with a gastrocnemius rotational flap. Clin. Orthop. 341:73, 1997.
55. McPherson, E.J., Tontz, W., Patzakis, M.J., et al.: Outcome of infected total knee utilizing a staging system for prosthetic joint infection. Am. J. Orthop. 28:161, 1999.
56. Nashed, R.S., Becker, D.A., and Gustilo, R.B.: Are cementless acetabular components the cause of excess wear and osteolysis in total hip arthroplasty? Clin. Orthop. 317:19, 1995.
57. National Institutes of Health: Total hip replacement. NIH Consensus Conference, Sept. 2–14; 12:1, 1994.
58. National Institutes of Health: Total hip replacement. NIH Consensus Conference. J.A.M.A. 273:1950, 1995.
59. Nelissen, R.G.H.H., Bauer, T.W., Weidenhielm, R.A., et al.: Revision hip arthroplasty with the use of cement and impaction grafting. J. Bone Joint Surg. 77A:412, 1995.
60. Oh, I., Bourne, R.B., and Harris, W.H.: The femoral cement compactor: An improvement in cementing technique in total hip replacement. J. Bone Joint Surg. 65A:1335, 1983.
61. Otani, T., Whiteside, L.A., and White, S.E.: The effect of axial and torsional loading on strain distribution in the proximal femur as related to cementless total hip arthroplasty. Clin. Orthop. 292:376, 1993.
62. Padgett, D.E., Kull, L., Rosenberg, A., et al.: Revision of the acetabular component without cement after total hip arthroplasty. J. Bone Joint Surg. 75A:663, 1993.
63. Pak, J.H., Paprosky, W.G., Jablonsky, W.S., et al.: Femoral strut allografts in cementless revision total hip arthroplasty. Clin. Orthop. 295:172, 1993.
64. Paprosky, W.G., Perona, P.G., and Lawrence, J.M.: Acetabular defect classification on surgical reconstruction in revision arthroplasty. J. Arthroplasty 9:33, 1994.
65. Peters, C.L., Rivero, D.P., Kull, L.R., et al.: Revision total hip arthroplasty without cement: Subsidence of proximally porous-coated femoral components. J. Bone Joint Surg. 77A:1217, 1995.
66. Poilvache, P.L., Insall, J.N., Scuderi, G.R., et al.: Rotational land-

marks and sizing of the distal femur in total knee arthroplasty. Clin. Orthop. 331:35, 1996.
67. Possai, K.W., Dorr, L.D., and McPherson, E.J.: Metal rings for deficient acetabular bone in total hip replacement. Instr. Course Lect. 45:161, 1996.
68. Ranawat, C.S., Peters, L.E., and Umlas, M.E.: Fixation of the acetabular component. Clin. Orthop. 334:207, 1997.
69. Ritter, M.A., Faris, P.M., and Keating, E.M.: Posterior cruciate ligament balancing during total knee arthroplasty. J. Arthroplasty 3:323, 1988.
70. Rowe, C.R.: Arthrodesis of the shoulder used in treating painful conditions. Clin. Orthop. 173:92, 1983.
71. Santore, R.F., and Murphy, S.B.: Osteotomies about the hip for the prevention and treatment of osteoarthrosis. AAOS Instr. Course Lect. 115. San Francisco, 1997.
72. Schmalzried, T.P., Jasty, M., and Harris, W.H.: Periprosthetic bone loss in total hip arthroplasty: Polyethylene wear debris and the concept of the effective joint space. J. Bone Joint Surg. 74A:849, 1992.
73. Schulte, K.R., Callaghaan, J.J., Kelley, S.S., et al.: The outcome of Charnley total hip arthroplasty with cement after a minimum of twenty year follow-up. J. Bone Joint Surg. 75A:961, 1993.
74. Scott, R.D., Cobb, A.G., McQueary, F.G., et al.: Unicompartmental knee arthoplasty: 8 to 12 year follow-up with survivorship analysis. Clin. Orthop. 271:96, 1991.
75. Scully, S.P., Aaron, R.K., and Urbaniak, J.R.: Survival analysis of hips treated with core decompression or vascularized fibular grafting because of avascular necrosis. J. Bone Joint Surg. 80A:1270, 1998.
76. Serekian P: Process application of hydroxylapatite coatings. In Manley, M.T., ed.: Hydroxylapatite Coatings in Orthopaedic Surgery. New York, Raven Press, Ltd., 1993.
77. Steinberg, M.E., Hayken, G.D., and Steinberg, D.R.: A quantitative system for staging avascular necrosis. J. Bone Joint Surg. 77B:34, 1995.
78. Stern, S.H., Becker, M.W., and Insall, J.N.: Unicondylar knee arthroplasty: An evaluation of selection criteria. Clin. Orthop. 286:143, 1993.
79. Stiehl, J.B., Komistek, R.D., Dennis, D.A., et al.: Fluoroscopic analysis of kinematics after posterior-cruciate-retaining knee arthroplasty. J. Bone Joint Surg. 77B:884, 1995.
80. Tsukayama, D.T., Estrada, R., and Gustilo, R.B.: Infection after total hip arthroplasty. J. Bone Joint Surg. 78A:512, 1996.
81. Vince, K.G., and McPherson, E.J.: The patella in total knee arthroplasty. Orthop. Clin. North Am. 23:675, 1992.
82. Wasielewski, R.C., Cooperstein, L.A., Kruger, M.P., et al.: Acetabular anatomy and the transacetabular fixation of screws in total hip arthroplasty. J. Bone Joint Surg. 72A:501, 1990.
83. Wilson, P.D., Jr., and Gordon, S.L., eds.: NIH Consensus Development Conference: Total hip joint replacement. Bethesda, MD, March 1982. J. Orthop. Res. 1:189, 1983.
84. Wong, M., Eulenberger, J., Schenk, R., et al.: Effect of surface topology on the osteointegration of implant materials in trabecular bone. J. Bio. Mat. Res. 29:1567, 1995.
85. Wroblewski, B.M., Lynch, M., Atkinson, J.R., et al.: External wear of the polyethylene socket in cemented total hip arthroplasty. J. Bone Joint Surg. 69B:61, 1987.
86. Wroblewski, B.M., and Siney, P.D.: Charnley low-friction arthroplasty of the hip: Long-term results. Clin. Orthop. 292:191, 1993.

5

Disorders of the Foot and Ankle

Mark S. Mizel, Mark Sobel, and Amy Jo Ptaszek

This chapter will provide a review of adult foot and ankle deformities. Pediatric and congenital deformities are covered in Chapter 2, Pediatric Orthopaedics.

I. Biomechanics of the Foot and Ankle

A. The Gait Cycle—This brief review of biomechanics assumes a basic knowledge of anatomy of the lower extremity and, specifically, that of the foot and ankle. Should review be necessary, numerous anatomy textbooks are available. The center of mass of the human body displaces in a vertical plane, during the gait cycle. This is necessary, as the distance between the floor and the center of mass must be greater when the center of mass passes over the extended leg during the mid-stance phase of gait than during transmission of body weight from one leg to the other. Horizontal body displacements occur with the rotatory movement of the pelvis as the leg advances. Lateral body displacements occur as the body is shifted slightly over the weight-bearing limb with each step. The total lateral displacement of the body is approximately 5 cm from side to side with each complete gait cycle. This can be increased by walking with the feet more widely separated. **Ground reaction forces for walking reach approximately 1½ times body weight.** The weight-bearing phase of the gait cycle for each leg is divided into multiple parts (Fig. 5–1): heel strike, foot flat, heel off, and toe off. The next cycle of the same foot starts again with heel strike. It should be noted that the contralateral foot goes into toe off very soon after foot flat and enters heel strike soon after the initial foot passes through heel rise. The lower extremity is considered to go through two phases, the stance phase where it is bearing weight and the swing phase where it is being advanced. **The stance phase constitutes approximately 62% and the swing phase 38% of the gait cycle. The stance phase is divided into a double support phase when both feet are on the ground, lasting around 12% of the cycle, followed by a single support phase lasting about 50% of the cycle.** Running includes a period of no weight-bearing on either extremity. Forces generated increase to almost three times body weight.

B. Ankle Axes of Rotation—The ankle axis is directed laterally and posteriorly. Dorsiflexion produces some lateral movement of the foot, and plantar flexion produces some medial movement of the foot (Fig. 5–2). The subtalar joint is a single axis joint that acts as a hinge joint connecting the talus and calcaneus. **The tibia rotates internally during heel strike while the subtalar joint everts, and the calcaneus assumes a slightly valgus position. The tibia rotates externally during push-off while the subtalar joint inverts, and the calcaneus assumes a varus posture.**

C. Energy Absorption—The transverse tarsal articulation (Chopart's joint) consists of the calcaneocuboid joint and the talonavicular

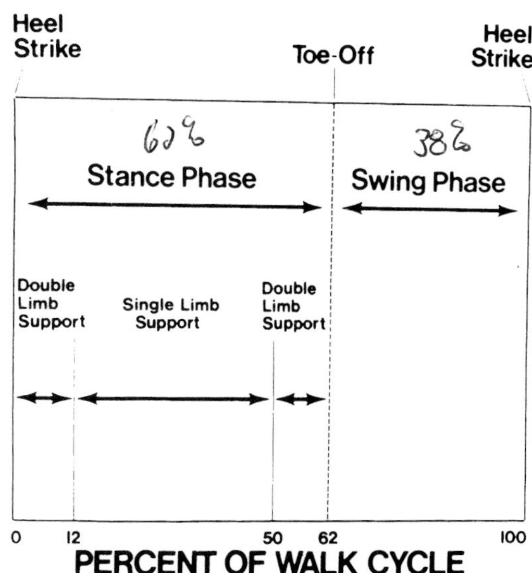

Figure 5–1. Phases of walking cycle. Stance phase constitutes approximately 62% and swing phase 38% of cycle. Stance phase is further divided into two periods of double limb support and one period of single limb support. (From Mann, R.A., and Coughlin, M.J., eds.: Surgery of the Foot and Ankle, 6th ed., vol. 1, p. 15. St. Louis, CV Mosby, 1993.)

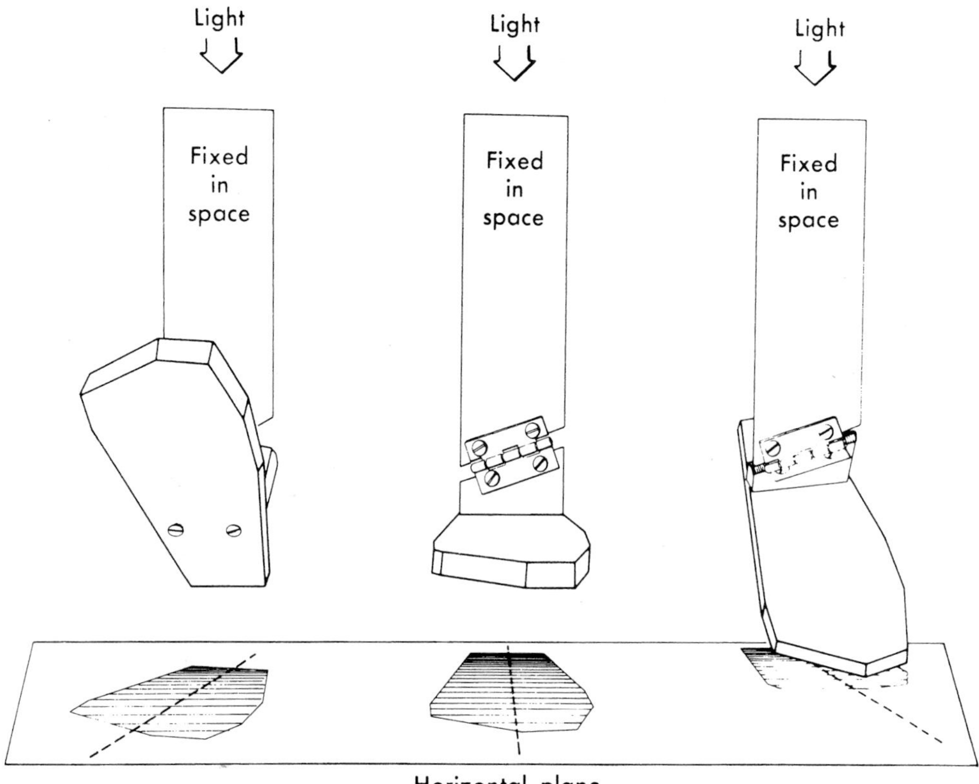

Figure 5–2. Effect of obliquely placed ankle axis on rotation of foot in horizontal plane during plantar flexion and dorsiflexion, with foot free. Displacement is reflected in shadows of foot. (From Mann, R.A., and Coughlin, M.J., eds.: Surgery of the Foot and Ankle, 6th ed., vol. 1, p. 17. St. Louis, CV Mosby, 1993.)

joint. **The transverse tarsal joints are not parallel and thus lock, providing a rigid lever arm for push-off when the subtalar joint inverts. The converse is true with heel strike and foot flat; the subtalar joint everts, and the transverse tarsal joints are parallel and flexible** (Figs. 5–3, 5–4, 5–5). This flexibility is important during the heel strike and the subsequent stance phase of gait, allowing accommodative pronation of the foot, which absorbs some of the energy from heel strike. The anterior compartment of the leg contracts eccentrically (controlled dorsiflexion) at heel strike, lengthening while the gastrocnemius-soleus is quiescent. The gastrocnemius-soleus complex is contracting eccentrically at foot flat, and the anterior tibialis is quiet. The strong gastrocnemius-soleus complex contracts concentrically at heel rise/push-off, and the tibialis anterior (anterior compartment) is quiescent. From heel strike to foot flat there is progressive eversion of the subtalar joint, which unlocks the transverse tarsal joint and causes internal rotation of the tibia. The opposite occurs during heel rise. The plantar aponeurosis originates on the plantar medial aspect of the calcaneus and passes distally, inserting into the base of the flexor mechanism of the toes. It functions as a windlass mechanism, increasing the arch height as the toes dorsiflex during toe off. This is a passive function which aids hindfoot inversion during heel rise. The main invertor of the subtalar joint during heel rise is the posterior tibial tendon, which initiates subtalar inversion.

II. Physical Examination of the Foot and Ankle—A complete examination allows observation of both extremities below the knee and observation of the gait cycle.

A. Neurovascular Examination, Muscle Strength, Tendon Competence—A neurovascular examination is mandatory. Pain in the foot or ankle can be caused by neurologic pathology, such as peripheral neuropathy, peripheral nerve entrapment, or spinal pathology such as a herniated nucleus pulposus. Vascular evaluation should include palpation of the dorsalis pedis and posterior tibial pulses. A formal vascular evaluation to include toe pressures and arterial Doppler examination are necessary if pulses are not palpable or healing potential is questionable.

Active and passive ankle dorsiflexion, plantar flexion, inversion, and eversion should be checked. Bilateral inspection and comparison of motion and strength are helpful. **It is important to check the posterior tibial muscle for inversion strength from an everted position.** The ankle should be

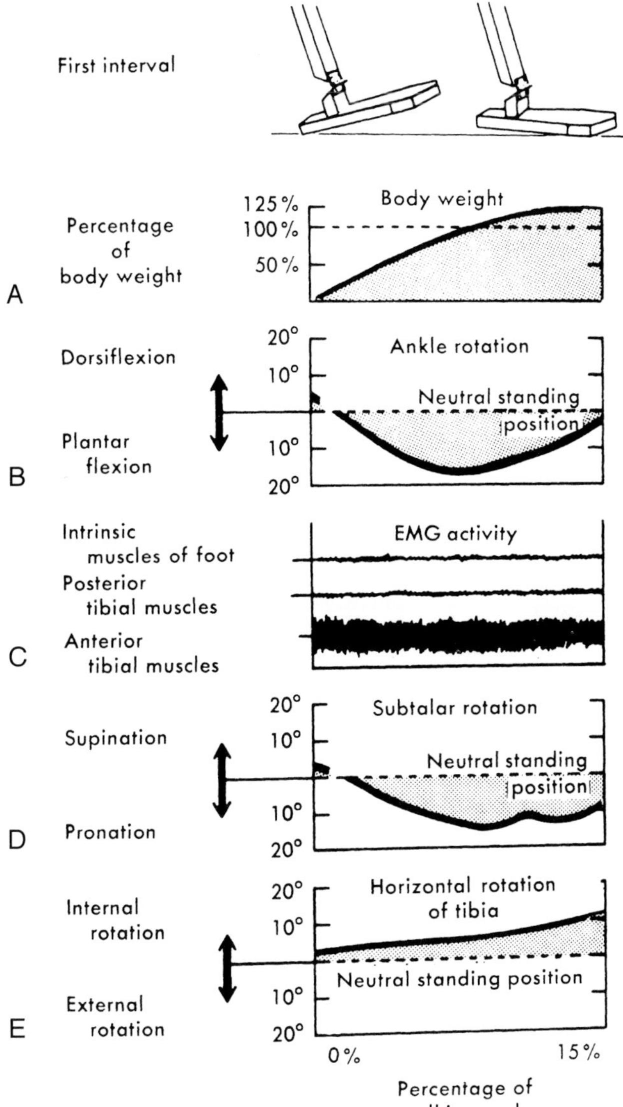

Figure 5–3. Events of first interval of walking, or period that extends from heel strike to foot flat. (From Mann, R.A., and Coughlin, M.J., eds.: Surgery of the Foot and Ankle, 6th ed., vol. 1, p. 29. St. Louis, CV Mosby, 1993.)

plantar-flexed to avoid recruitment of the tibialis anterior. When the ankle is in neutral or inverted, the anterior tibial muscle can function as an inverter along with the posterior tibial muscle. From an everted position, only the posterior tibial tendon functions as an inverter. The ability to initiate heel rise from the stance position is accomplished by the posterior tibial tendon. Hindfoot inversion should occur if the tendon is functional.

B. Joint Motion—Ankle dorsiflexion and plantar flexion (range 20 degrees dorsiflexion to 40 degrees plantar flexion), subtalar inversion and eversion (range 5–20 degrees), and transverse tarsal motion should be checked. Midfoot motion (flexion, abduction) is assessed at the tarsometatarsal joints, specifically the first tarsometatarsal joint.

Test the metatarsophalangeal joints for motion, tenderness, or swelling. Carefully palpate the interdigital spaces. Metatarsophalangeal joints can be tested for stability with the modified drawer sign. Observation of a deviated second or third toe with weight-bearing indicates collateral ligament and/or plantar plate insufficiency.

C. Palpation/Stability—Palpation of the anterolateral and medial ankle ligaments. Test inversion of the ankle in dorsiflexion (to stress the calcaneofibular ligament), and perform an anterior drawer in plantar flexion (to stress the anterior talofibular ligament). Percuss over the tarsal tunnel in an attempt to elicit a Tinel sign suggestive of posterior tibial nerve irritation. Feel the course of all tendon units at rest and as they fire. Palpate the Achilles along its course and insertion for nodularity and thickening.

III. Adult Hallux Valgus

A. **There are multiple intrinsic causes of hallux valgus deformity, including pes planus and metatarsus primus varus. Other causes include rheumatoid arthritis, connective tissue diseases, and disorders such as cerebral palsy. The most common cause is poorly fitted shoewear (i.e. high heels with a narrow toe box).**

B. Pathophysiology—Hallux valgus deformity consists of the great toe in a valgus position (Fig. 5–6). Other anatomic deformities occur concurrently, including the first metatarsal shifting into a varus position. The sesamoid complex shifts laterally relative to the first metatarsal as the first metatarsal drifts into varus. The lateral capsule contracts, and the medial capsule becomes attenuated. The adductor tendon, which inserts into the base of the proximal phalanx and sesamoid complex, tightens. The alignment of the articular surface of the first metatarsal may contribute to the hallux valgus deformity. Unlike the case with an incongruent first metatarsophalangeal joint, the alignment of the articular surface may lead to a similar degree of deformity, but it is secondary to an abnormally laterally sloped distal metatarsal articular angle. The normal angle ranges from 6 to 10 degrees. Increased angle is common in juvenile hallux valgus. In addition, the proximal phalanx may be laterally deviated through the shape of the bone itself, resulting in hallux valgus interphalangeus.

C. Conservative Treatment—Hallux valgus deformities can be well treated with wide-laced (high toe box) shoes. Should concurrent hammer toe or crossover toe deformities exist, extra-depth shoes may be helpful. Stretching the leather over the bunion region can also be beneficial.

D. Surgical Treatment—Surgical management is recommended for painful deformity recal-

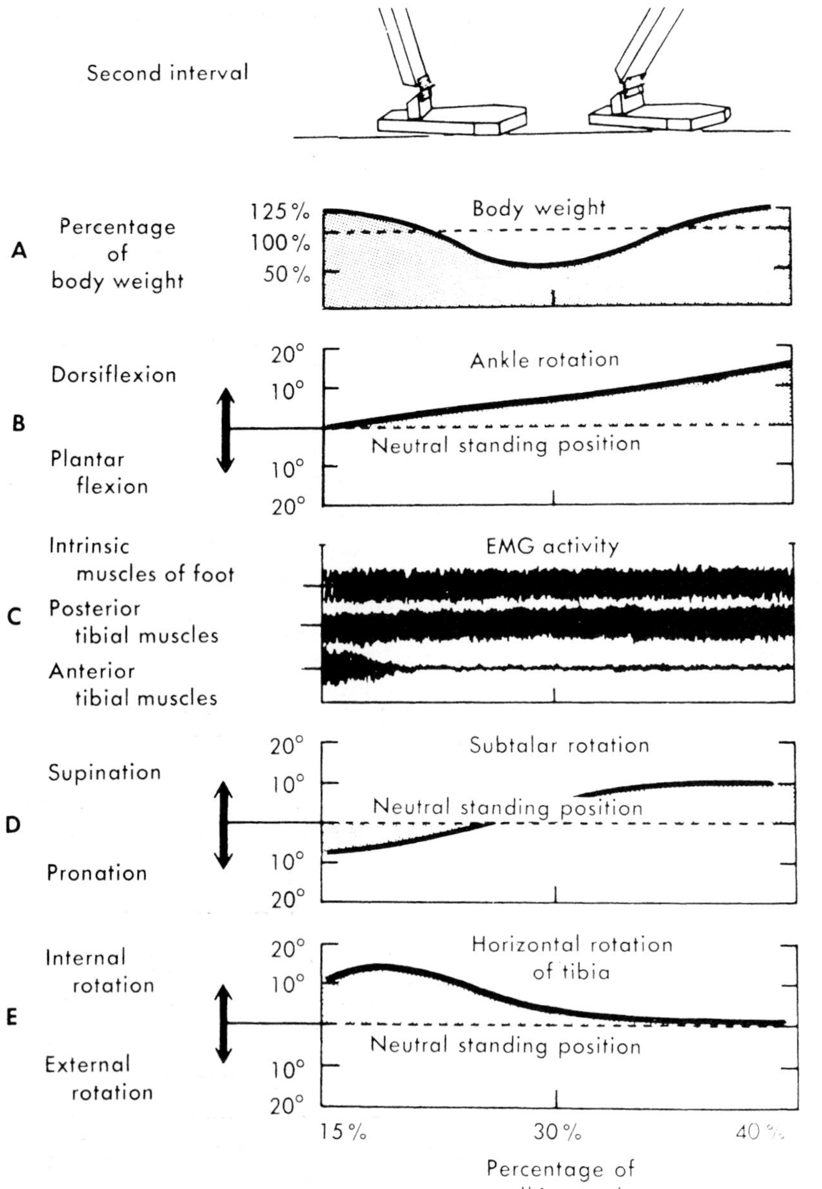

Figure 5–4. Events of second interval of walking, or period of foot flat. (From Mann, R.A., and Coughlin, M.J., eds.: Surgery of the Foot and Ankle, 6th ed., vol. 1, p. 30. St. Louis, CV Mosby, 1993.)

citrant to conservative measure. Treatment algorithms exist as guidelines only, but they may aid in deciding which procedure is appropriate.

Normal metatarsophalangeal joint angle is 9 degrees on average but definitely less than 15 degrees. Intermetatarsal angle is considered abnormal when it is greater than 9 degrees (Fig. 5–7). A variety of procedures for bunion correction have been described (Fig. 5–8).

1. Medial Eminence Resection (Silver's)—This is good for elderly patients with a large medial exostosis. It is important that a minimal hallux valgus angle and a minimal metatarsus primus varus exist (see Fig. 5–8).
2. Distal Soft-Tissue Realignment; Modified McBride's—This is a good operation for mild to moderate deformity with an intermetatarsal angle of less than 15 degrees and hallux valgus less than 35 degrees. It combines a medial exostectomy as well as a release of the lateral capsule and soft tissues and plication of the medial capsule. Modified McBride's means that the fibular sesamoid is *not* excised. The reason for this modification is that **sesamoid excision can be associated with deviation of the hallux, i.e., fibular sesamoid excision can cause a hallux varus deformity; tibial sesamoid excision can cause a hallux valgus deformity; excision of both sesamoids can cause a cock-up deformity and decreased push-off power of the first metatarsophalangeal joint.**

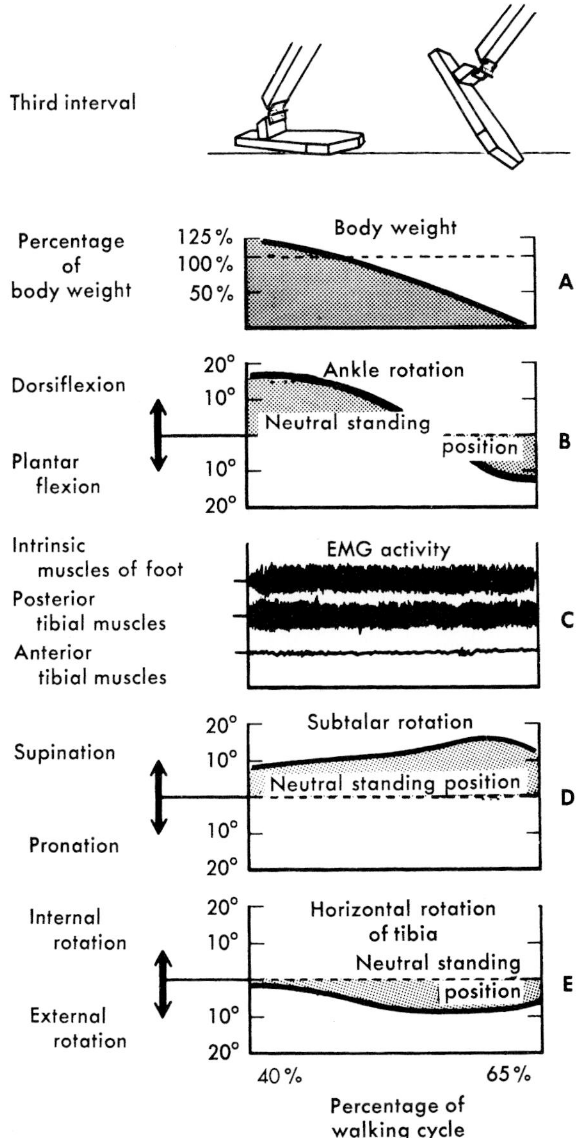

Figure 5–5. Composite of all events of third interval of walking, or period extending from flat to toe off. (From Mann, R.A., and Coughlin, M.J., eds.: Surgery of the Foot and Ankle, 6th ed., vol. 1, p. 31. St. Louis, CV Mosby, 1993.)

3. Distal Metatarsal Osteotomy (Chevron's)—**This procedure is indicated for patients with an intermetatarsal angle of 15 degrees or less and hallux valgus angles less than 35 degrees.** It is performed with a medial exostectomy as well as distal osteotomy and lateral displacement of the metatarsal head. Trimming of the prominent medial metaphysis and a capsulorrhaphy are also performed. An intermetatarsal angle of 16 degrees or greater is a contraindication to the Chevron.
4. Mitchell's Osteotomy—This is indicated for an intermetatarsal angle of less than 20 degrees and hallux valgus angles of less than 40 degrees. It involves a medial incision and resection of the medial eminence as well as an osteotomy cut at a right angle to the long axis of the foot and displacement of the metatarsal. It may be associated with significant shortening of the first metatarsal and subsequent transfer metatarsalgia.
5. Keller's Bunionectomy—This consists of removing the distal metatarsal medial eminence as well as the base of the proximal phalanx. Postoperatively, the joint is stabilized for approximately 6 weeks as fibrous tissue forms. **This procedure is generally indicated for low demand. The common complications include cock-up deformity of the hallux, transfer metatarsalgia, and stress fractures of the lesser metatarsals** that are due to the lack of weight-bearing by the first metatarsophalangeal joint.
6. Proximal Metatarsal Osteotomy—**This can be added to a distal soft-tissue repair to increase the correction that is obtainable.** An osteotomy is often necessary if the intermetatarsal angle is 14 degrees or more. A stiff first metatarsocuneiform joint is another indication. The most popular proximal metatarsal osteotomy performed is a crescentic osteotomy, although a proximal Chevron osteotomy is also effective.
7. First Metatarsal Cuneiform Arthrodesis (Lapidus')—This arthrodesis is indicated if ligamentous laxity is evident with pes planus, if there is increased obliquity of the metacuneiform joint, in certain cases of adolescent hallux valgus, or if there is recurrent deformity.
8. Akin's Procedure—This is a closing wedge osteotomy of the proximal aspect of the proximal phalanx. It is indicated for hallux valgus interphalangeus. It is also indicated for hallux valgus with a congruent joint with insufficient correction after a distal Chevron procedure.
9. First Metatarsophalangeal Arthrodesis—Allows correction of deformity and effective pain relief. Used as both salvage of failed previous procedures and as primary management of hallux valgus in older patients, especially men.

E. Complications of Surgical Procedures
   1. Silver's Bunionectomy—**The disadvantages are high rate of recurrence** and limited applications. It has a low complication rate. If salvage is necessary, an Akin procedure (closing wedge osteotomy of the proximal phalanx) or a modified McBride procedure can be considered. An arthrodesis can act as an effective salvage.
   2. Modified McBride's—**The disadvantage**

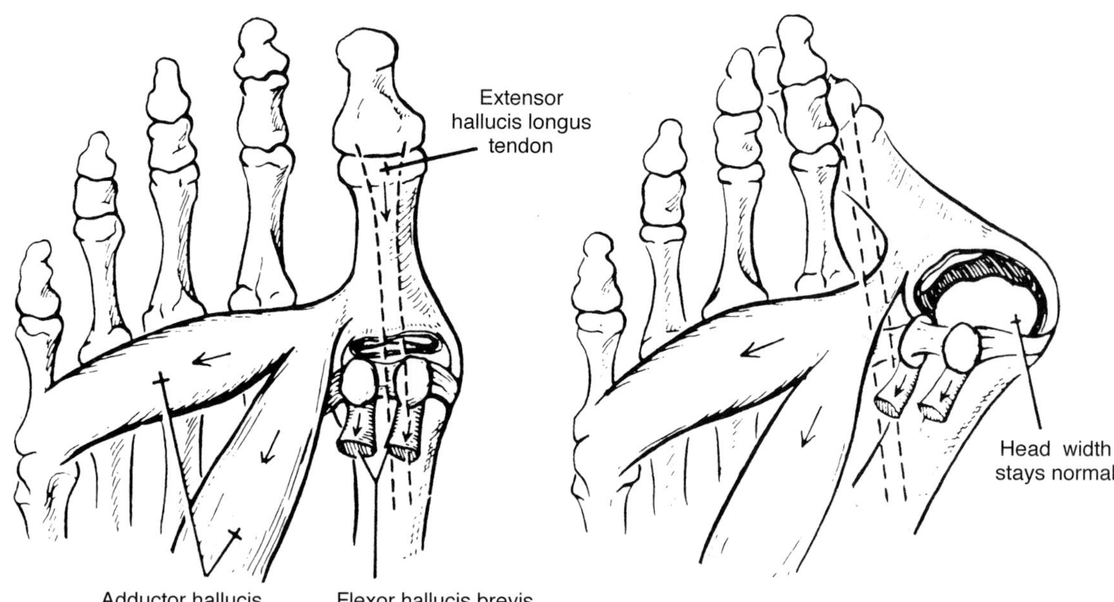

Figure 5–6. Pathophysiology of hallux valgus deformity. Normally, metatarsal head is stabilized within sleeve of ligaments and tendons, which provide stability to joint. As proximal phalanx deviates laterally it places pressure on metatarsal head and deviates medially. It results in attenuation of medial joint capsule and contracture of lateral joint capsule. (From Mann, R.A., and Coughlin, M.J., eds.: Surgery of the Foot and Ankle, 6th ed., vol. 1, p. 184. St. Louis, CV Mosby, 1993.)

is that soft tissue may stretch out, and deformity can recur. Contraindications include the diagnosis of a connective tissue disorder. It should be noted the lateral sesamoid is no longer excised (this is the modification of the original procedure). Salvage can be done with an Akin procedure or a redone McBride with a proximal metatarsal osteotomy. Arthrodesis and Keller's procedure can also be considered. If hallux varus occurs, extensor hallucis longus split transfer can be attempted. If the hallux varus deformity is long-standing, rigid, and/or associated with first metatarsophalangeal degenerative joint disease, an arthrodesis of the first metatarsophalangeal joint (a soft-tissue rebalancing procedure) can be performed.

3. Chevron's Osteotomy—**The disadvantages are limited correction of metatarsus primus varus**, limitation of the amount of correctable deformity, and sometimes age limitations. Pronation of the hallux cannot be corrected. **Avascular necrosis of the metatarsal head can occur after a Chevron osteotomy** and is a devastating complication. Other complications include shortening of the metatarsal, hallux varus, excessive displacement, loss of position of the distal fragment, and nonunion. Salvage of a failed procedure can be performed with an Akin procedure or an arthrodesis.
4. Mitchell's Osteotomy—The disadvantages include a high rate of avascular necrosis, first metatarsal shortening, loss of position of the osteotomy, and the technical difficulty of the procedure. Contraindications include a short first metatarsal or metatarsalgia. Complications include potential shortening and dorsal displacement of the metatarsal head, along with transfer metatarsalgia.
5. Keller's Bunionectomy—The disadvantages include metatarsalgia from lateral weight shifting and weakening of the plantar aponeurosis. Cock-up deformities and recurrence rates are relatively high. Transfer calluses and metatarsal stress fractures can occur.
6. Proximal Metatarsal Osteotomy—The disadvantages include malunion. This includes the possibility of overcorrection, resulting in a hallux varus deformity, as well as dorsiflexion of the first metatarsal, which would impair its ability to bear weight. Nonunion and delayed union in proximal metaphyseal bone are uncommon.
7. First Metacuneiform Arthrodesis—Malposition and nonunion are the most common complications.
8. Hallux Varus—This can be caused by overplication of the medial capsule, overcorrection of the intermetatarsal angle with a metatarsal osteotomy, or over-resection of too much of the medial aspect of the distal first metatarsal. Hallux varus

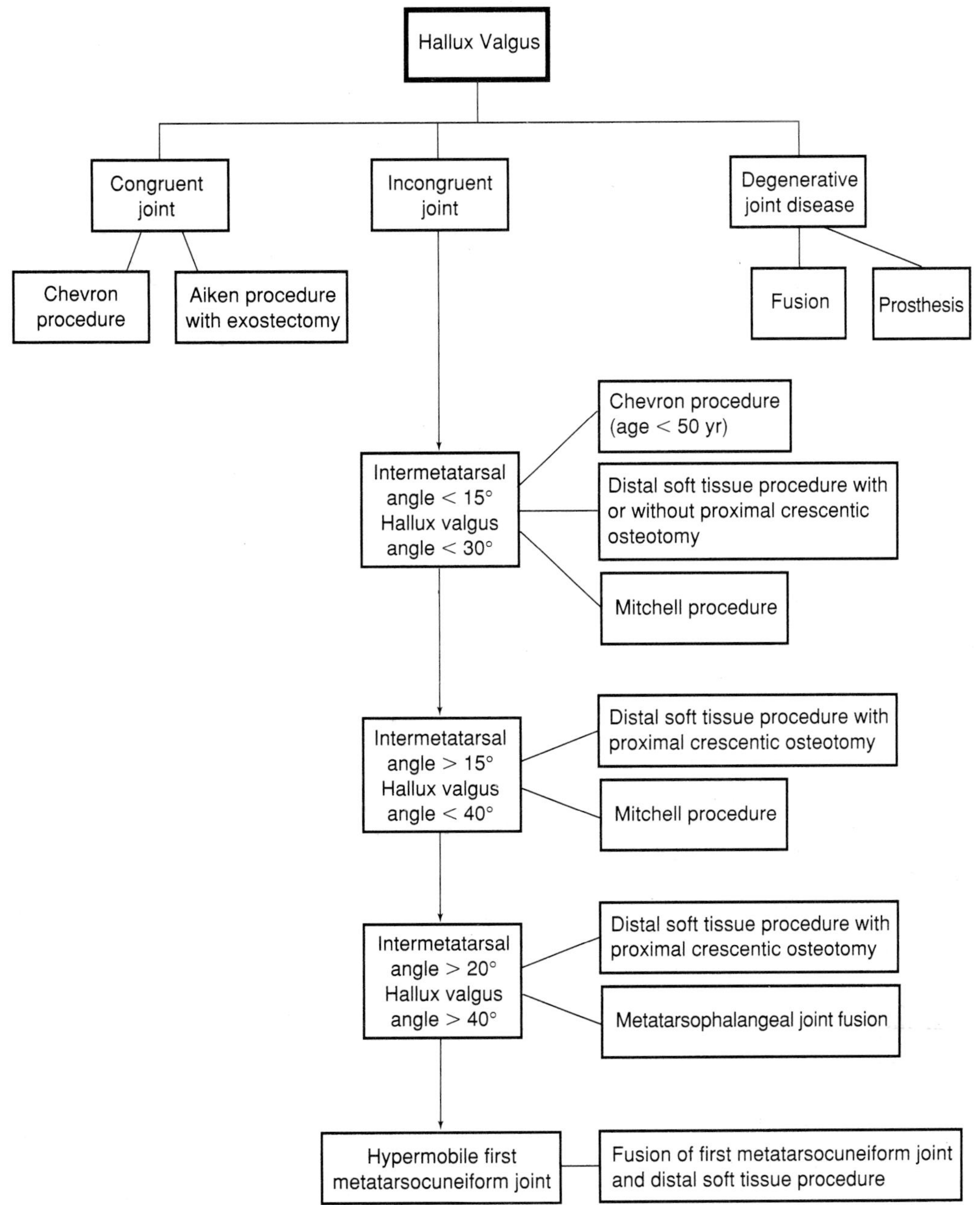

Figure 5–7. (From Mann, R.A., and Coughlin, M.J., eds.: The Video Textbook of Foot and Ankle Surgery, p. 152. St. Louis, Medical Video Productions, 1991.)

can be treated with an extensor tendon transfer (for supple deformity with satisfactory articular surface) or arthrodesis of the first metatarsophalangeal joint.

IV. Lesser Toe Deformities

A. Hammer toe—**A hammer toe is a deformity at the proximal interphalangeal joint (PIP) of a lesser toe (Fig. 5–9). Hammer toe can be fixed or flexible, with a flexible deformity reducible with ankle plantar flexion or dorsal pressure on the plantar surface of the involved lesser metatarsal.**

1. A fixed deformity can be treated with a Duvries arthroplasty, which removes the distal condyles of the proximal phalanx, creating a fibrous joint. This should be held in position with a K-wire or bolster for approximately 2–3 weeks after surgery and then protected for another 3 weeks with taping the PIP joint in extension. Alternatively, arthrodesis of the joint can be accomplished, but this has a high incidence of nonunion.
2. Treatment of a flexible hammer toe must address the contracture of the flexor digitorum longus tendon, which is the presumed cause of this deformity. A standard Duvries arthroplasty of the PIP joint can

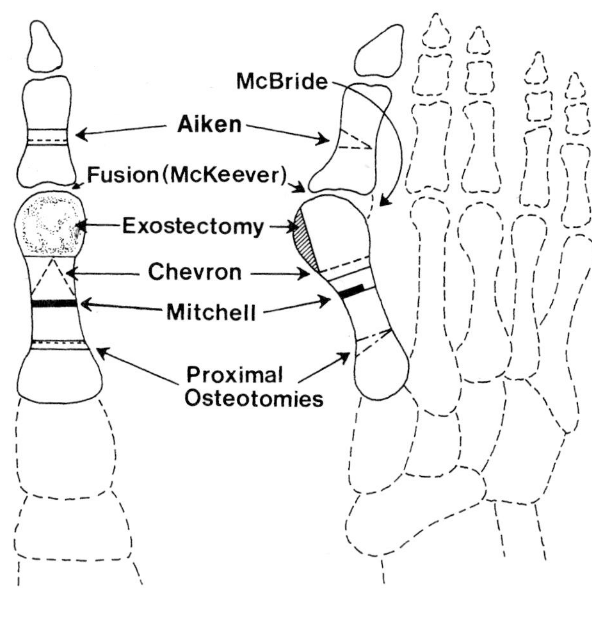

Figure 5–8. Common surgical procedures available for hallux valgus correction.

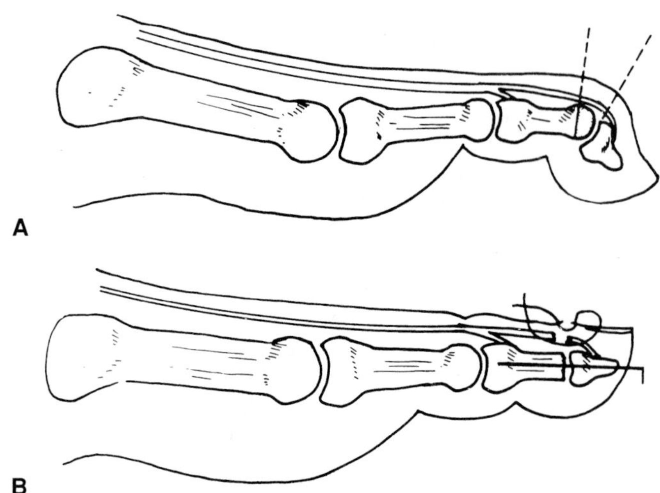

Figure 5–10. *A*, Proposed resection for mallet toe repair. *B*, Alternate means of fixation. Stabilization of toe using vertical mattress suture of 3-0 nylon incorporating two Telfa bolsters. (From Coughlin M.: Orthopedics 10:63–75, 1987.)

be performed along with release of the flexor digitorum longus tendon through the same incision at the level of the PIP joint. Alternatively, a Girdlestone flexor tendon transfer can be performed, releasing the flexor digitorum longus tendon distally, splitting it longitudinally, and transferring the two tails to the dorsal extensor hood, where they are attached.

B. Mallet Toe—**A mallet toe is a flexion deformity of the distal interphalangeal joint (DIP) (Fig 5–10).** This usually presents with either pain or callus formation on the tip of the toe that is striking the ground or on the dorsal DIP joint. If tightness of the flexor digitorum longus tendon is noted, this can be released at the same time after removal of the distal condyles of the middle phalanx. Postoperative care is similar to that for hammer toe.

C. Claw Toe—**A claw toe is a combination of both a hyperdorsiflexion deformity of the metatarsophalangeal joint along with either a hammer toe or mallet toe deformity.** This deformity can be treated at the metatarsophalangeal joint with an arthrotomy and release of the extensor tendon and dorsal capsule as well as release of the medial and lateral collateral ligaments. A Girdlestone flexor tendon transfer can be performed if necessary. Following this, correction of the hammer toe or mallet toe deformity can be accomplished. If the metatarsophalangeal joint is dislocated and deformity is long-standing and/or fixed, a Duvries resection arthroplasty of the metatarsal head may be necessary. This involves excision of the distal 3–4 mm of the metatarsal head.

D. Fifth Toe Deformities—The most common fifth toe deformity is an overlapping fifth toe, which is generally a congenital deformity. The pathologic features involve dorsal and medial contracture of the capsule and extensor tendon as well as of the dorsal skin. Surgical procedures involve the release of the extensor tendon and capsule as well as resolution of the skin contracture. A Duvries procedure consists of a longitudinal dorsal

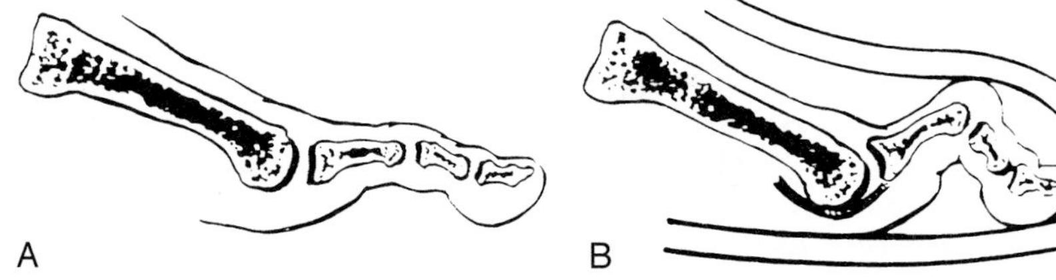

Figure 5–9. *A*, Phalanx extended to normal length. *B*, Bucking of phalanx caused by restriction of end of shoe. Interphalangeal joints and metatarsophalangeal joints become subluxed. Over time, dislocation may occur. (From Mann, R.A., and Coughlin, M.J., eds.: Surgery of the Foot and Ankle, 6th ed., vol. 1, p. 343. St. Louis, CV Mosby, 1993.)

incision, joint and tendon release and, when closure of the skin is performed, it is important to stretch the fibular margin distally and displace the tibial margin proximally. A Wilson V-Y plasty involves making a V-type incision centered over the medial aspect of the fifth toe and extending it into the fourth interspace (Fig. 5–11). After release of the extensor tendon and the dorsal and medial MP joint, the toe is plantar flexed, and the V incision becomes Y-shaped skin flap. This is closed with the toe held in an overcorrected position.

E. Hyperkeratotic Pathology of the Lesser Toes
   1. Hard Corn—A hard corn is a hyperkeratotic skin reaction on the **dorsolateral aspect of the fifth toe, usually at the PIP joint.** This results from the condyle of the proximal phalanx of the fifth toe rubbing against the lateral side of the toe box, with a subsequent skin reaction. Nonsurgical treatment consists of a wider toe box or donut-type skin protectors and trimming the callus with a blade or pumice stone. Should this treatment be unsatisfactory, surgical intervention with removal of the distal condyles of the proximal phalanx is helpful.
   2. Soft Corn—**A soft corn is a hyperkeratotic reaction of the skin between the toes,** which is a result of the pressure of one toe on another with subsequent skin reaction. Nonsurgical treatment consists of a wider toe box in shoewear, as well as lamb's wool, or a foam insert between the toes and trimming the callus. Should this not be satisfactory, removal of the distal condyles of the offending proximal phalanx, as is done in a hammer toe repair, can be performed with or without elliptical excision of the corn and syndactylization. If there is uncertainty as to which bony prominence is the offender, a lead marker can be placed over the soft corn, and an x-ray can be taken.

V. Hyperkeratotic Pathology of the Plantar Foot
   A. Intractable Plantar Keratosis (IPK)—An IPK is a hyperkeratotic skin reaction on the plantar surface of the foot, sometimes referred to as a callus. **It is the result of excess pressure in a small area with a subsequent skin reaction.** It can sometimes be confused with a plantar wart, which is the result of a virus. A plantar wart has pinpoint vessels when trimmed with a blade. An IPK, of necessity, is at a weight-bearing area, whereas a plantar wart is not necessarily so. Several types of IPKs are described.
      1. Discrete IPK
         a. A localized IPK can sometimes be found under a distal plantar metatarsal condyle. This forms a focal or discrete IPK. Nonsurgical options include pads or orthotics to relieve weight-bearing under the region, and surgery, if necessary, can be performed to remove the plantar condyle. A "seed corn"–type IPK (Fig. 5–12) is another form of a focal or discrete IPK caused by invagination of epithelium over which a skin reaction occurs. This IPK becomes narrower and deeper when

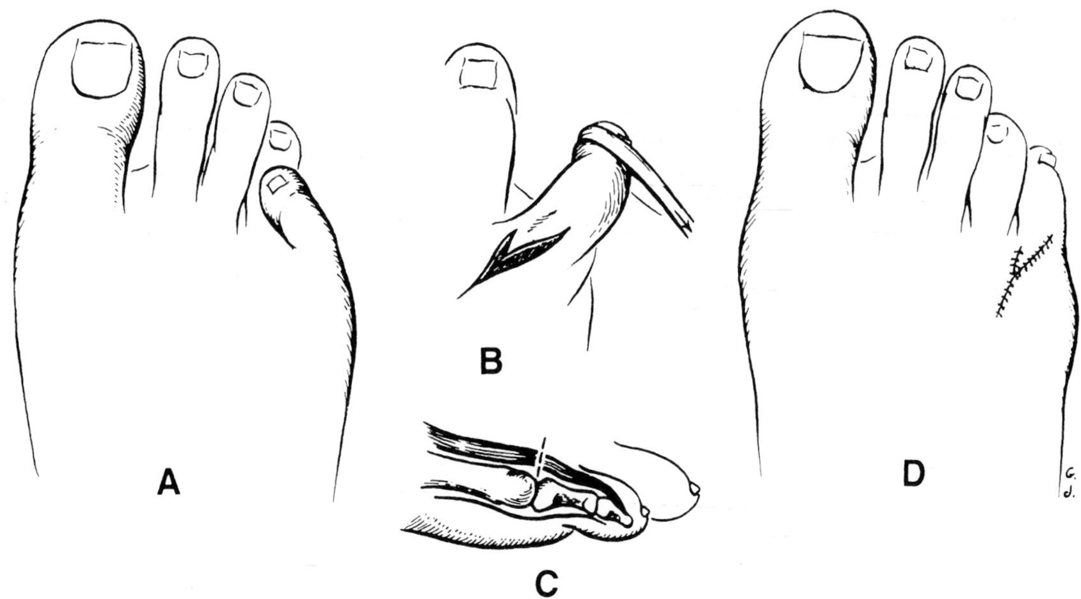

Figure 5–11. Wilson technique for correction of mild-to-moderate overlapping fifth toe. *A*, Preoperative appearance. *B*, Y-Shaped incision over fifth metatarsophalangeal joint. *C*, Sectioning of extensor tendon and dorsal capsule of metatarsophalangeal joint. *D*, Correction of deformity and suturing of skin. (From Mann, R.A., and Coughlin, M.J., eds.: Surgery of the Foot and Ankle, 6th ed., vol. 1, p. 397. St. Louis, CV Mosby, 1993.)

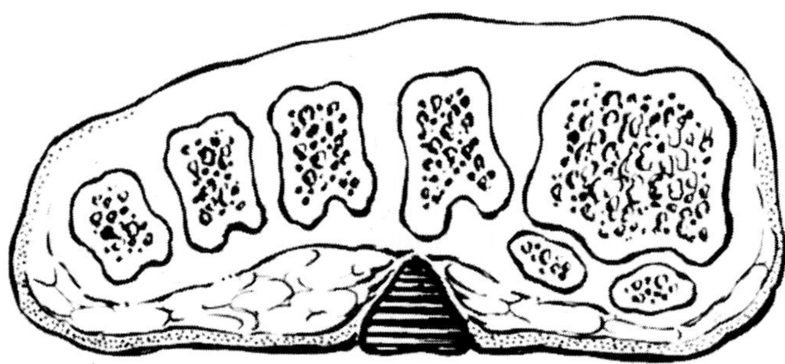

Figure 5–12. Location of a discrete plantar keratosis underneath the prominent fibular condyle. (From Mann, R.A., and Coughlin, M.J., eds.: Surgery of the Foot and Ankle, 6th ed., vol. 1, p. 420. St. Louis, CV Mosby, 1993.)

trimmed down with a blade and is usually cured after one or two trimmings after the "seed corn" is removed.

b. If the focal or discrete lesion is under the first metatarsal head, the lesion may be due to a prominent fibular or tibial sesamoid; if it is refractory to trimming, padding, etc., a sesamoid shaving is the surgical approach.

c. If the focal or discrete lesion is under the interphalangeal joint of the hallux and midline, it may be due to a subhallux sesamoid in the flexor hallucis longus and removed if refractory to padding, trimming, etc.

2. Diffuse IPK—A diffuse IPK is a result of extra weight-bearing in an area of the foot with subsequent skin reaction. This IPK is often treated nonsurgically with metatarsal pads or orthotics. There are numerous causes for this IPK, and the treatment can be specific to the problem. Most common causes: short first metatarsal shaft, long second metatarsal shaft, metatarsal head resection, or a dorsiflexed lesser metatarsal.

B. Bunionette—A bunionette deformity (tailor's bunion) is characterized by a prominence on the lateral distal fifth metatarsal head, which is painful and causes a diffuse callus laterally and occasionally plantarly. Constrictive shoewear and friction between the shoe and the underlying bony structure can lead to the hyperkeratotic reaction. Sometimes the fifth metatarsal can be deviated in a mild plantar position as well as laterally, resulting also in a plantar callus. These are generally of three types.

1. Type 1 consists of an enlarged fifth metatarsal head or lateral condyle. The lateral side of the head can be trimmed, or a distal Chevron-type osteotomy can be performed if conservative measures fail.

2. Type 2 consists of a bunionette deformity with lateral bowing of the fifth metatarsal. Several corrective osteotomies have been described, including the distal Chevron and diaphyseal osteotomies. Proximal osteotomies at the metaphyseal-diaphyseal juncture are generally avoided because of poor healing.

3. Type 3 consists of a bunionette deformity with an abnormally wide 4–5 intermetatarsal angle. A laterally deviated fifth metatarsal (normal 4–5 intermetatarsal angle averages 6 degrees) can be treated with a fifth metatarsal osteotomy. When a plantar callus is present as well as a lateral callus, a diaphyseal osteotomy, oriented so as to shift the metatarsal head both medially and somewhat dorsally, has been found to be associated with symptomatic relief.

VI. Sesamoids and Accessory Bones—Sesamoids under the metatarsal heads are variable from foot to foot and person to person. The most common constant is two sesamoids beneath the first metatarsal heads. One or both can be bipartite. **Of these, 80% of bipartite sesamoids involve the tibial sesamoid. Twenty-five percent of patients have bilateral bipartite tibial sesamoids.** The medial sesamoid is sometimes divided into two, three, or four parts. The lateral sesamoid is rarely divided into more than two. **The sesamoids are encased in the flexor digitorum brevis tendon and help to provide stability to the hallux. One sesamoid rides on either side of the crista of the plantar first metatarsal. The sesamoid ligament interconnects the sesamoids and the intermetatarsal ligament prevents subluxation of the sesamoids from their position in relation to the second metatarsal.** Differentiating between a bipartite sesamoid that is inflamed and a sesamoid fracture can be difficult. Whereas they both remain tender with the great toe in dorsiflexion, the inflamed sesamoid tends to be significantly less tender with palpation with the hallux in plantar flexion. The regular, smooth cortex seen on x-ray film is consistent with a bipartite sesamoid.

A. Accessory Bones—An accessory bone within the posterior tibial tendon is found by x-ray approximately 10% of the time. This bone should be differentiated from an accessory navicular. An os peroneum in the peroneus longus is found in approximately 5% of feet by x-ray. Osteochondritis dissecans can occur in the os peroneum and can be quite painful (Fig. 5–13). Rupture of the peroneus longus tendon can occur and be noted by proximal migration of the os peroneum on x-ray film. An os trigonum can be found posterior to the talus and can cause posterior impingement, which presents with posterior ankle pain with extremes of ankle plantar flexion.

VII. Neurologic Disorders

A. Interdigital Neuritis (IDN)—IDN (Morton's

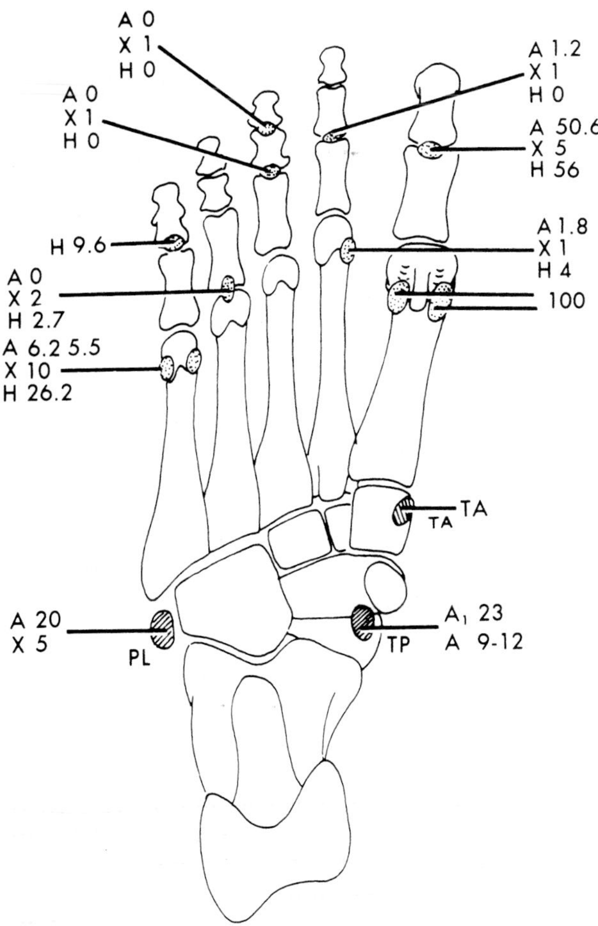

Figure 5–13. Sesamoids of the foot. Frequency of occurrence based on anatomic evaluation (A), histoembryologic investigation (H), and radiographic investigation (X). (From Mann, R.A., and Coughlin, M.J., eds.: Surgery of the Foot and Ankle, 6th ed., vol. 1, p. 500. St. Louis, CV Mosby, 1993.)

neuroma) usually occurs in the second or third interdigital space (Fig. 5–14). It is rare in the first and fourth interdigital space and is bilateral 15% of the time. It is believed to be the probable result of continuous trauma/traction in the region. Positive physical findings include tenderness in the involved interdigital space, differential sensory loss, and pain with compression of the metatarsal heads. Differential diagnoses include plantar fasciitis, tarsal tunnel syndrome, metatarsal stress fracture, and synovitis of the metatarsophalangeal joint.

1. Nonsurgical treatment includes metatarsal pads, soft-soled wide-laced shoes, and local corticosteroid injection.
2. Surgical treatment consists of excision of the nerve with resection of the intermetatarsal ligament and is 80% successful. Most surgeons prefer a dorsal approach for neuritis that has not previously been operated on.

B. Recurrent Neuroma—A neuroma can recur from 1 to 4 years after the initial surgery. Clinical symptoms are similar to those of the initial preoperative pain, and nonsurgical treatment remains similar. Surgical excision of a recurrent neuroma involves a longer dorsal incision than an initial neuroma. Careful dissection proximally should be undertaken to enhance exposure and ensure removal of adequate nerve tissue. Many surgeons prefer a plantar incision and approach for recurrent neuroma. However, plantar incisions have been associated with painful scars, oftentimes worse than the initial problem.

C. Tarsal Tunnel Syndrome—Tarsal tunnel syndrome involves compression of the posterior tibial nerve from intrinsic and/or extrinsic causes. Mass effect within the tunnel is the usual cause. **The tarsal tunnel syndrome can be caused by a ganglion of one of the tendon sheaths, a lipoma within the tarsal canal, an exostosis or bony fracture fragment, or enlarged venous complex or neurologic pathology such as a neurilemoma of the posterior tibial nerve.** Tarsal tunnel syndrome should be confirmed with a positive electromyogram and nerve conduction velocity in addition to magnetic res-

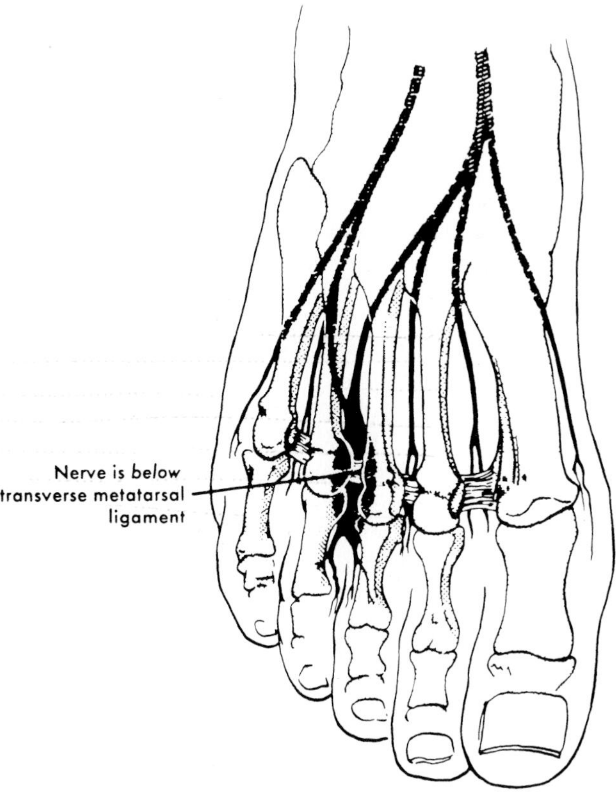

Figure 5–14. Third branch of medial plantar nerve. Note that it courses in a plantar direction under the transverse metatarsal ligament. (From Mann, R.A., and Coughlin, M.J., eds.: Surgery of the Foot and Ankle, 6th ed., vol. 1, p. 546. St. Louis, CV Mosby, 1993.)

onance imaging (MRI) to evaluate mass effect prior to surgical release.

D. Incisional Neuromas—A neuroma over the dorsum of the foot can be quite disabling as there is little soft-tissue protection over this area. Shoewear can cause a continuous pressure and pain in the region. The general anatomy of nerves on the dorsum of the foot has tremendous variability, and the surgeon must exercise great care because of this variation. The patient usually complains of localized pain, sometimes radicular in nature. The patient is often comfortable when ambulating without shoes. Physical examination reveals a scar as well as a localized area of tenderness.

Nonsurgical treatment consists of pads to protect the area of the tender neuroma. Resection of the nerve will leave an area of anesthesia and possibly dysesthesia, but this can often be an improvement over the initial condition by placing the new nerve ending in an area not continuously irritated by shoewear or ankle motion.

E. Central Nervous System Disorders

1. Stroke

a. Orthoses management is indicated in either stroke or a traumatic brain injury where weak plantar flexors of the ankle allow dorsiflexion during the stance phase of gait. A stiff ankle foot orthosis (AFO) with the ankle in neutral can be quite helpful. Weak ankle dorsiflexion can also be helped with an AFO. Impaired proprioception in the ankle or knee can also often be helped with an AFO.

b. Surgical correction should not take place until the neurologic status has stabilized. **In a patient injured by a cerebral vascular accident, variable recovery usually occurs over 6 months. With traumatic brain injury, improvement can continue for 18 months or more. An incomplete spinal cord injury can continue to improve for 12 months.** Cerebral palsy does not progress. However, function problems and deformities may change because of growth of the affected limb, with changing soft-tissue contractures or bony deformities. Flexion deformities of the toes are not uncommon and can often be treated with flexor tendon release or Girdlestone-Taylor flexor tendon transfer. When contractures exist, release of the contracted tissues or decompression by resection of bone might be necessary. With an isolated equinus contracture, Achilles tendon lengthening can be enough to restore a plantargrade foot.

1. A relatively common deformity of gait following a stroke or traumatic brain injury is an equinovarus deformity during swing and stance. There are five muscles that can produce this deformity. These include the anterior tibialis, flexor hallux longus and posterior tibialis, flexor digitorum longus, and the gastrocnemius-soleus complex. The posterior tibialis is rarely over-reactive in the stance phase.

2. Split Anterior Tibial Tendon Transfer—This can help enhance ankle dorsiflexion as well as balance the foot out of inversion to a more neutral position.

F. Charcot-Marie-Tooth disease (Hereditary Motor Sensory Neuropathy)—This disease is a hereditary neurologic disorder characterized by weakness of the peroneal muscles and progressive weakness of the intrinsic muscles of the foot, dorsiflexors of the foot and toes, and plantar flexors. In general, the peroneus longus overpowers the peroneus brevis, the posterior tibialis tendon is stronger than the tibialis anterior tendon, and intrinsic imbalance occurs. The end presentation of this syndrome is usually clawing of the toes, forefoot varus with a plantar flexed first ray, midfoot and hindfoot cavus, and ankle equinus. Lateral ankle instability is a common associated finding if hindfoot varus is present. Intrinsic weakness of the muscles of the hand is an associated finding.

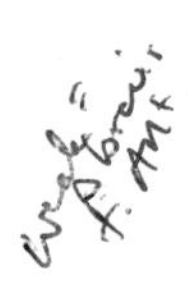

1. The disease is inherited as a sex-linked recessive, autosomal-dominant or autosomal-recessive mechanism. Males are affected more than females, and the age of onset of symptoms varies with the genetic cause, with autosomal-recessive presenting early, usually at less than 10 years of age. The sex-linked recessive inheritance usually presents in the second decade, and autosomal-dominant inheritance presents in the third decade. The earlier the onset of symptoms, the more severe the clinical presentation.

2. Treatment consists initially of orthoses management supporting the foot in a plantar-grade position. A plastic AFO may be sufficient. An important diagnostic point consists of evaluating whether the patient's symptomatology involves primarily the hindfoot, forefoot, or both. With forefoot disorder, plantar flexion of the first metatarsal is the primary problem. The pathologic condition is usually quite obvious, if present. The Coleman

block test is helpful in differentiating fixed from flexible hindfoot varus deformities. Procedures including Achilles tendon lengthening, split anterior tibial tendon transfer, plantar fascia release, and claw toe procedures as previously described can often be helpful. A Jones procedure (hallux interphalangeal arthrodesis and transfer of the extensor hallucis longus tendon into the distal first metatarsal) can be helpful in elevating the first ray. First metatarsal dorsiflexing osteotomy is sometimes also necessary. A Dwyer calcaneal osteotomy can be performed for fixed hindfoot varus deformity. If the varus deformity is flexible, a tenodesis of the peroneus brevis to the longus can be performed.

G. Peripheral Nerve Injuries
   1. A minor peripheral nerve injury is a neuropraxia, involving a local conduction block with continuity of the axon. Prognosis for recovery is good.
   2. Axonotmesis is more serious and involves loss of axonal continuity with an intact endoneural tube. There is good potential for reinnervation.
   3. Neurotmesis is complete severance of the nerve. Spontaneous regeneration does not occur.
   4. The most common peripheral nerve injured in the lower extremity is the common peroneal nerve. If spontaneous function does not recur 3–6 months after a compression injury, surgical exploration should be considered. Penetrating injuries can be explored approximately 1 month after injury, which allows for demarcation of the injury. Nonsurgical treatment consists of an AFO.
      a. Motor injury to the common peroneal usually results in paralysis of the muscles of the anterior and lateral compartments (ankle and toe dorsiflexors and ankle evertors). Plantar flexion of the first ray by the peroneus longus is also lost.
      b. Sensory loss usually involves the dorsum of the foot and is not considered clinically important.
      c. The most common transfer for this motor deficiency is a transfer of the posterior tibialis through the interosseous membrane to the dorsum of the foot.

H. Postpolio Syndrome—Postpolio syndrome is characterized by progressive weakness and fatigue in motor groups affected by polio. It often presents approximately 30 years after the initial onset of infectious poliomyelitis. This is considered probably the result of excessive muscle action during walking and chronic overuse of weakened muscles. Other theories include activation of latent poliovirus in the anterior horn cells or progression of polio to a variation of amyotrophic lateral sclerosis. Treatment often consists of changes in lifestyle, reducing demands on symptomatic muscles. The use of equipment such as wheelchairs, crutches, walkers, or canes can be of assistance. In addition to this, AFOs with locked ankle dorsiflexion or plantar flexion stops can be helpful. Occasionally, hindfoot arthrodesis may be necessary for stability.

VIII. Arthritic Disease
   A. Crystal Disease
      1. Gout—Gout is a systemic disease of altered purine metabolism with subsequent sodium urate crystal precipitation into synovial fluids. This results in an inflammatory response or deposition of these crystals into tophi or both. These tophi can cause periarticular destruction, which is often found as a manifestation of the chronic disease. The disease is more frequently seen in men than in women, and approximately 50–75% of the initial attacks occur in the great toe metatarsophalangeal joint. Diagnosis is often made by the identification of sodium urate crystals, but it can be inferred on the basis of clinical examination, serum uric acid, or the response to treatment with colchicine. Allopurinol can be used to prevent further attacks. Approximately 10% of the patients with untreated gout develop chronic tophaceous deposits in the soft tissues, followed by destruction of the joints. One of the distinguishing features of gouty arthritis is the destructive bony lesions remote from the articular surface. Treatment of an acute attack is symptomatic, with elevation and rest. Colchicine or nonsteroidal anti-inflammatory drugs (NSAIDs) are also helpful. Symptomatic tophi can be excised with curettage. Medical treatment can sometimes result in dissolution of tophi.
      2. Pseudogout—Chondrocalcinosis, also known as pseudogout, results from the deposition of calcium pyrophosphate. It can become symptomatic when crystals are shed into a joint where they can lead to phagocytosis and enzyme release by leukocytes. The resulting painful inflammatory response can cause significant pain. The talonavicular and subtalar joints are more often implicated in the foot, and the end result often resembles advanced degenerative arthritis. Treatment consists of NSAIDs. When joint destruction is significant, surgical treatments used in degenerative arthritis can be indicated.

B. Seronegative Diseases—The three seronegative spondyloarthropathies—psoriatic arthritis, Reiter's disease syndrome, and ankylosing spondylitis—have clinical and radiologic manifestations that are different from rheumatoid arthritis. Radiologic differences are (1) intra-articular ankylosis, (2) calcification within the adventitia, and (3) the lack of osteopenia. Clinically, all of these can present with painful heel syndrome or Achilles tendinitis, whereas rheumatoid arthritis does not.
   1. Psoriatic arthritis can antedate by years the skin lesions of psoriasis in approximately 20% of patients. There is often symmetric involvement of hands and feet, and cuticle changes are not uncommon (splitting nails). Involvement of the distal interphlanageal joints and dorsal tuft resorption can also be seen. Destruction of the proximal phalanges can produce a "cup and saucer" appearance of a destroyed joint. There is a 25% correlation of HLA-B27 in patients with psoriasis and peripheral arthritis.
   2. Reiter's Syndrome—This syndrome consists of conjunctivitis, urethritis, and symmetric arthritis (possibly a painful heel). It is much more common in males and correlates often (95%) with a positive HLA-B27. Lower extremities are usually involved, and "sausage toes" are common. Radiographic changes can range from nothing to soft-tissue swelling. Occasionally, demineralization can be noted at the PIP joints. Heel pain can be a presenting symptom.
   3. Ankylosing spondylitis has its main effect on the axial skeleton. Manifestations within the foot and ankle are relatively minor compared with these and often involve attachments of tendons and ligaments to the calcaneus. Manifestations similar, but less intense, can be seen in the metatarsophalangeal joints. There is a 90% correlation with HLA-B27.

C. Lyme Disease—Lyme disease is caused by the **spirochete** *Borrelia burgdorferi.* It is transmitted by **an arthropod-borne tick *Ixodes dammini* that can infect deer and other animals**. Endemic areas include the northeastern part of the United States, Minnesota, Oregon, and California. The infection presents in stages, including a target-shaped skin rash, fever, and systemic disease, although these do not always occur. Late manifestations in the musculoskeletal system masquerade as tendinitis, internal derangement of the joint, or overuse syndrome. Symptoms are not helped by steroid injections, physical therapy, or arthroscopy. **Positive blood study results for titres to Lyme disease are the method of diagnosis, and a high level of suspicion in endemic areas is appropriate.** Treatment with antibiotics results in resolutions of symptoms or improvement.

D. Degenerative Joint Disease—This usually occurs in the middle-aged and elderly populations, but it can also occur following trauma or osteochondritis dissecans. Obesity and high levels of physical activity are also found to correlate with this disease. The actual cause of the degenerative changes is uncertain, but biochemical changes within the articular cartilage have been noted. Nonsurgical treatment is aimed at reducing stress or motion. NSAIDs can be helpful as well as weight loss, activity modification, and properly fitted shoes. Orthotics can be helpful in removing stresses from rigid or painful areas. An AFO can sometimes be helpful. Surgical treatments are limited to patients with a great deal of pain, and techniques usually involve arthrodesis, excisional arthroplasty or, occasionally, osteotomy. Implants within the foot and ankle have had disappointing results.

E. Rheumatoid Arthritis—This is a systemic disease affecting synovial tissues; it is often symmetric in pattern but can be extra-articular. There is thought to be a predilection among those with HLA-DR4. Females are affected three times more often than males.
   1. Diagnosis is based on clinical, laboratory, and roentgenographic findings. Approximately 17% of rheumatoid arthritis begins in the feet. The forefoot is involved more commonly than the hindfoot. This may be asymmetric, but progression to symmetric involvement often occurs.
      a. Pathophysiology—The basic pathologic change is chronic synovitis that invades and destroys the bone, capsular tissue, cartilage, and ligamentous structures, causing a loss of stability of the joint as well as destroying the smooth articular surface. Mechanical stresses applied to the weakened supporting structures result in deformity. The magnitude of the deformity usually depends on the length of time the disease has been present.
      b. Forefoot Changes—Approximately 90% of patients with rheumatoid arthritis have forefoot involvement, and approximately 15% of them first present with forefoot pain. As the metatarsophalangeal joints lose their competence, the toes sublux dorsally and dislocate dorsally at the metatarsophalangeal joints, pulling the plantar fat pad distally with them so it becomes an anterior rather than a plantar struc-

ture. The hallux often deforms into a severe valgus deformity, helping to dorsally displace the lesser toes. Many rheumatoid forefoot deformities have interphalangeal joint hyperextension. Hallux varus is a less common deformity of the great toe.

c. Midfoot Changes—The midfoot is not usually severely involved. Chronic synovitis can occur with eventual loss of the joint space.

d. Hindfoot Changes—Hindfoot deformity is probably the result of destruction of the ligaments and soft tissues supporting the hindfoot. The subtalar joint collapses into valgus, and the talonavicular joint subluxes into abduction, creating a forefoot abduction deformity. Posterior tibial tendon destruction can also result in a flat foot deformity.

e. Surgical Treatment—In rheumatoid arthritis, soft-tissue repairs tend to do poorly, and arthrodeses and bony resection are usually necessary. The timing of surgery is extremely variable among patients.

1. Hallux valgus deformities in patients with rheumatoid arthritis can be treated with arthrodesis, a Keller-type procedure (excisional arthroplasty), or Silastic implant (fraught with problems). All of these, except for arthrodesis, have a high recurrence rate, and are not recommended.
2. Forefoot Reconstruction—The aim of forefoot reconstruction is to provide a stable medial post via arthrodesis of the first metatarsophalangeal joint. The other goal in forefoot reconstruction is to reduce the plantar fat pad to its proper plantar position. This is usually done with a Hoffman-type procedure, which involves removal of the metatarsal heads, allowing the plantar fat pad to relocate. Extensor tenotomy or removal of the proximal aspect of the proximal phalanges helps to decompress the area.
3. The hindfoot responds well to arthrodesis, either with an isolated subtalar arthrodesis or a triple arthrodesis, depending on the involvement of the talonavicular and calcaneocuboid joint.

F. Treatment for Specific Arthritic Joints

1. Interphalangeal Joint—Arthritis of the interphalangeal joint can be treated with a stiffened shoe to prevent motion, or arthrodesis, of the joint.
2. First MP Joint (Hallux Rigidus)—Degenerative arthritis of the first metatarsophalangeal joint usually produces a dorsal and/or lateral osteophyte. Dorsiflexion of the great toe, as in heel rise, produces pain from both the arthritis and the bone-on-bone bumping of the osteophytes. Limitation of motion of the MP joint is usually significant. A number of treatments are available for this.

   a. **Cheilectomy removes the dorsal and lateral osteophytes** off the distal metatarsal and proximal phalanx, allowing greatly increased motion. The degenerative arthritis continues to exist, but the bone-on-bone bumping of the proximal phalanx against the osteophytes is resolved, and this appears to satisfy most patients. Aim for 70 degrees of dorsiflexion intraoperatively, and get approximately half of that at 2 months.

   b. A Silastic implant can be helpful in resolving the degenerative arthritis pain, but this involves all the pitfalls of a Silastic implant (transfer metatarsalgia, breakage, silicone synovitis, variable stability, cock-up toe, and stress fracture).

   c. Arthrodesis of the first metatarsophalangeal joint can resolve the pain of degenerative arthritis but at the cost of the loss of motion, the loss of pivoting sports, and the loss of ability to wear high heels if desired.

   d. A closing wedge osteotomy of the proximal phalanx can be performed to bring the toe into greater dorsiflexion.
3. First Metatarsal Cuneiform Joint—This can be treated with a steel shank stiffener to decrease the motion of the joint and NSAIDs. If these are unsuccessful, arthrodesis of the joint can be accomplished. Rigid internal fixation is helpful in achieving fusion.
4. Talonavicular Joint—Nonsurgical treatment for arthritis in this joint consists of a University of California Biomechanics Laboratory–type insert or polypropylene AFO. If unsatisfactory, an isolated talonavicular arthrodesis is helpful in the rheumatoid patient or in a patient with a sedentary lifestyle. For a more active patient, a double (talonavicular and calcaneocuboid) or triple arthrodesis will be necessary.

IX. Arthrodeses of the Foot and Ankle—There are many techniques of arthrodeses of the foot and ankle as well as many methods of internal fixation.

A. Ankle Arthrodesis (Fig. 5–15)—Ankle arthrodesis is indicated for arthritis that produces pain or deformity. Ankle arthrodesis should be in a neutral position regarding

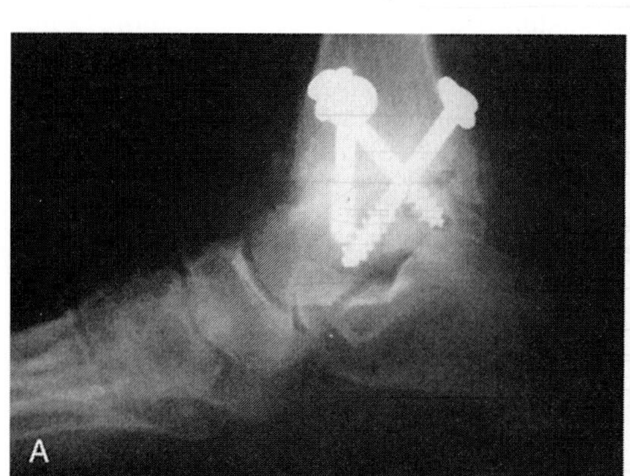

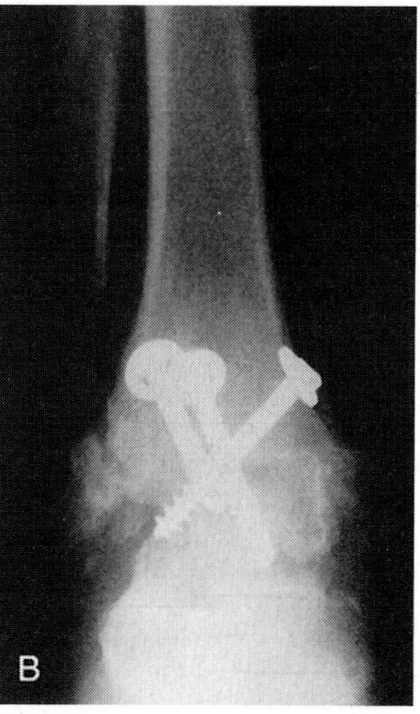

Figure 5–15. Ankle arthrodesis technique with screw fixation. *A*, Lateral view. *B*, Anteroposterior view. (Myerson, M., ed.: Arthrodesis procedures. Foot and Ankle Clinics. Philadelphia, WB Saunders, 1996.)

dorsiflexion and plantar flexion. Approximately 10 degrees of equinus is appropriate for a patient with osteomyelitis, polio, or other neurologic disease in which the patient otherwise cannot stabilize the knee. Varus/valgus alignment should be approximately 5 degrees of valgus, and rotation should be similar to that of the contralateral limb, usually approximately 7 degrees of external rotation. A stiff ankle cushioned heel may be a helpful hindfoot cushion. For failed total ankle arthrodesis, the patient may require a tibiocalcaneal arthrodesis positioned in 5–10 degrees of dorsiflexion.

B. Subtalar Arthrodesis—For isolated subtalar arthritis, subtalar arthrodesis is an appropriate procedure. Subtalar arthrodesis should be placed in approximately 5 degrees of valgus. Up to 10 degrees is well tolerated, but a greater amount can result in lateral impingement against the fibula. Varus alignment is very poorly tolerated because it locks Chopart's joint.

C. Talonavicular Arthrodesis—Arthrodesis of the talonavicular joint results in loss of motion of the calcaneocuboid joint as well as significant loss of motion in the subtalar joint. Talonavicular arthrodesis is usually satisfactory in sedentary-type patients, including those with rheumatoid arthritis. For a patient with a higher level of activities, a calcaneocuboid arthrodesis should be performed concurrently to add stability to the construct. The position of arthrodesis should be with the calcaneus in 5 degrees of valgus and the forefoot in a neutral position so that the long axis of the talus is aligned with the long axis of the first metatarsal.

D. Double Arthrodesis—Double arthrodesis consists of arthrodesis of the calcaneocuboid joint as well as the talonavicular joint (Chopart's joint). The effect of this arthrodesis is the same as that of a triple arthrodesis, as it also restricts subtalar motion. Position of the heel is very important when a double arthrodesis is performed because there will be little or no motion following it. The subtalar joint should be placed in 5 degrees of valgus, and Chopart's joint should be manipulated to provide a plantar-grade foot (neutral) with respect to varus/valgus and abduction/adduction of the forefoot.

E. Triple Arthrodesis (Fig. 5–16)—Triple arthrodesis is arthrodesis of the calcaneocuboid joint, talonavicular joint, and subtalar joint. It prevents inversion, eversion, abduction, and adduction. The talonavicular joint is the one most likely to suffer a nonunion.

F. Tarsometatarsal Arthrodesis—This is sometimes indicated for degenerative changes or following injury to the plantar metatarsal cuneiform ligaments. If no deformity exists, an in situ arthrodesis is appropriate. If there is deformity or subluxation, reduction of all planes should be carried out before arthrodesis.

G. Metatarsophalangeal Joint Arthrodesis—This procedure is indicated for repair of hallux valgus in a patient with rheumatoid arthritis or other significant soft-tissue disease or neuromuscular disorder. It is also satisfactory for severe hallux valgus deformity and hallux rigidus or as a salvage procedure for a failed bunion surgery. The great toe should be in approximately 10–20 degrees of valgus and approximately 10–15 degrees of dorsiflexion relative to the plantar aspect of the foot and neutral rotation. Various means of internal fixation are used, including interfragmentary screws, dorsal plates, or a combination of both. Steinman's pin fixation is also used. Complications include nonunion and malunion.

H. Interphalangeal Joint Arthrodesis of the

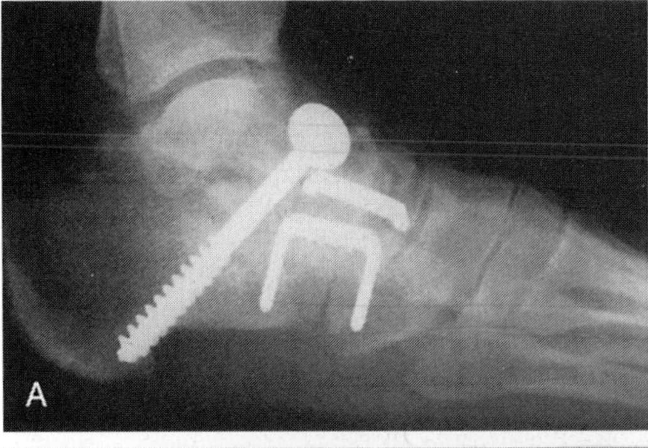

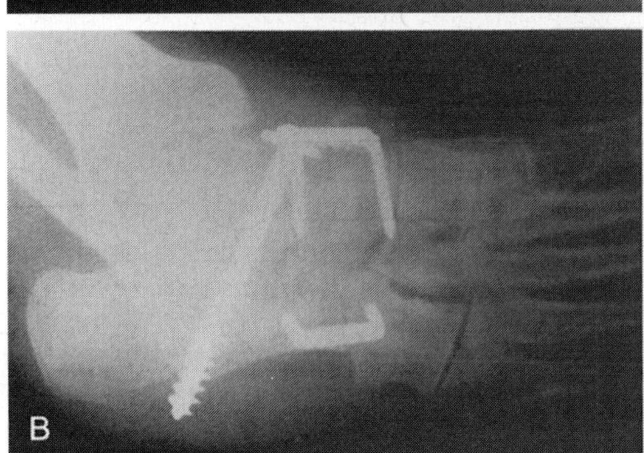

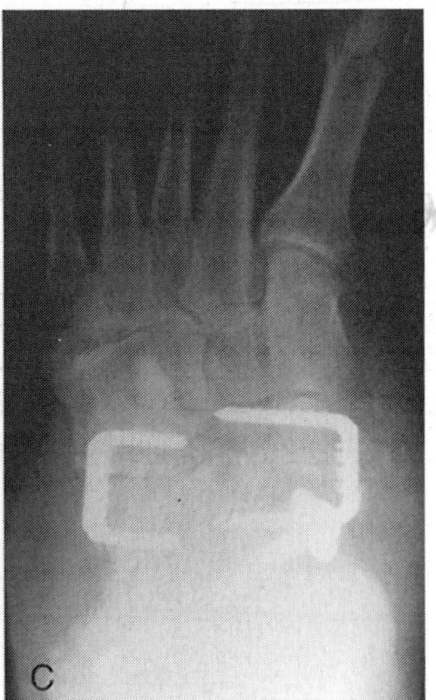

Figure 5–16. Triple arthrodesis technique. *A*, Anteroposterior view. *B*, Oblique view. *C*, Lateral view. (Myerson, M., ed.: Arthrodesis procedures. Foot and Ankle Clinics. Philadelphia, WB Saunders, 1996.)

Hallux—Indications for arthrodesis of the interphalangeal joint of the hallux include arthritis, flexion deformity, or loss of competence of the extensor hallucis longus tendon. The joint should be arthrodesed in approximately 5 degrees of plantar flexion with neutral varus or valgus orientation.

X. Postural Disorders in Adults
   A. Congenital Flat Foot
      1. Congenital flat foot is divided into two categories, flexible and fixed. Flexible flat feet are pronated with weight-bearing but with non–weight-bearing reconstitute an arch. These are almost always nonpathologic; however, they can be caused by a tight heel cord. Tendoachilles tightness is most adequately assessed with the subtalar joint in neutral or inversion.
      2. Rigid flat feet are pronated regardless of weight-bearing status. They are likely pathologic but not necessarily symptomatic. Causes include tarsal coalition, congenital vertical talus, and arthrogryposis.
   B. Acquired Flat Foot—**Acquired flat foot in the adult has multiple potential causes. Posterior tibial tendon dysfunction, rheumatoid arthritis, and Charcot's neuroarthropathy with subsequent collapse and primary degenerative joint disease of the tarsometatarsal joints are the most common causes. Severe trauma including calcaneus fractures, Lisfranc's fracture dislocations or acquired neuromuscular imbalance from polio, and peripheral nerve injury or trauma to the muscles of the leg can also cause this deformity. Lateral column lengthening and medial displacement calcaneal osteotomy may be beneficial for refractory cases.**
   C. Pes Cavus—Pes cavus is usually caused by neuromuscular disorder, although it can also be caused by congenital or traumatic entities. The patient with pes cavus should have a thorough neurologic evaluation, including computed tomography (CT) or MRI of the spine. The disease can affect the hindfoot, the forefoot, or both. The Coleman block test can evaluate whether a hindfoot varus deformity is fixed or flexible, which guides surgical treatment.
      1. Neuromuscular diseases causing pes cavus can include diseases such as muscular dystrophy, peripheral and lumbosacral spinal nerve problems including Charcot-Marie-Tooth disease, spinal dysraphism, polyneuritis, and spinal tumor. Anterior horn cell disease such as poliomyelitis can cause muscular imbalance as well as central nervous system diseases such as Friedreich's ataxia and cerebellar disease.
      2. Congenital causes include residual clubfoot, arthrogryposis, and idiopathic causes.
      3. Traumatic causes include the residuals of compartment syndrome, crush injuries to the lower extremity, severe burns, and malunions of fractures of the foot.

XI. Tendon Disorders

A. Achilles Tendon—The most common Achilles tendon disorder is a rupture. Antecedent tendinitis/tendinosis occurs in up to 15% of ruptures. Up to 75% of all ruptures during sports-related activities happen in patients between 30 and 40 years old. Most ruptures occur in the watershed area about 4 cm proximal to the calcaneal insertion. Reported rerupture rates without surgery approach 14% (range 4–50%), whereas rerupture with surgical repair averages about 1.5% (range 0–7%). Strength is diminished by about 20% relative to the normal contralateral extremity without repair and roughly 10% with surgical repair. Surgical repair may allow for early range of motion. Closed management usually consists of casting in slight plantar flexion with gradual dorsiflexion. Symptomatic, chronic ruptures often require augmentation. The flexor digitorum longus tendon and flexor hallucis longus tendon have been used.

B. Peroneal Tendon—The peroneal tendons can have traumatic dislocation or, less commonly, traumatic rupture. Attenuation of the superior peroneal retinaculum can allow subluxation of the tendons around the posterior fibula region. **Chronic subluxation can lead to longitudinal splitting of the peroneus brevis over the sharp posterior ridge of the fibula.** This tendon should be repaired if a laceration occurs. Any associated lateral ankle instability can also be addressed with a modified Brostrom, near-anatomic ligamentous repair (Fig. 5–17).

C. Flexor Hallucis Longus—The flexor hallucis longus tendon should be repaired if lacerated.

D. Stenosing Tenosynovitis—Stenosing tenosynovitis can result from swelling within the tendon, and the flexor hallucis longus is the most commonly involved tendon in the foot. This may present with triggering of the hallux. This usually occurs at the tarsal retinaculum posterior to the medial malleolus as well as where the tendon passes through the sesamoids, inserting into the distal phalanx of the hallux. Treatment consists of immobilization to reduce the inflammation followed by physical therapy for stretching of the hallux. The use of NSAIDs or possibly steroid injection can be helpful. If this fails, surgical treatment for decompression of the area can be carried out.

E. Extensor Tendons—**Lacerations of the extensor tendons (extensor hallucis longus and extensor digitorum longus) should be surgically repaired.** Extensor tendinitis can be diagnosed by producing pain with active dorsiflexion and passive plantar flexion of the toes.

F. Posterior Tibial Tendon—Incompetence of the posterior tibial tendon can produce both **a hindfoot valgus and forefoot abduction deformity**. This gives rise to the **"too many toes sign"** that is visualized on the affected side when the patient is viewed from behind. Patients often complain about pain in the midfoot region early on and sometimes describe instability in gait.

Physical examination is remarkable for weakness in inversion from an everted position. In addition, the patient has difficulty or is unable to stand on tiptoes on only the affected side. If capable, heel inversion

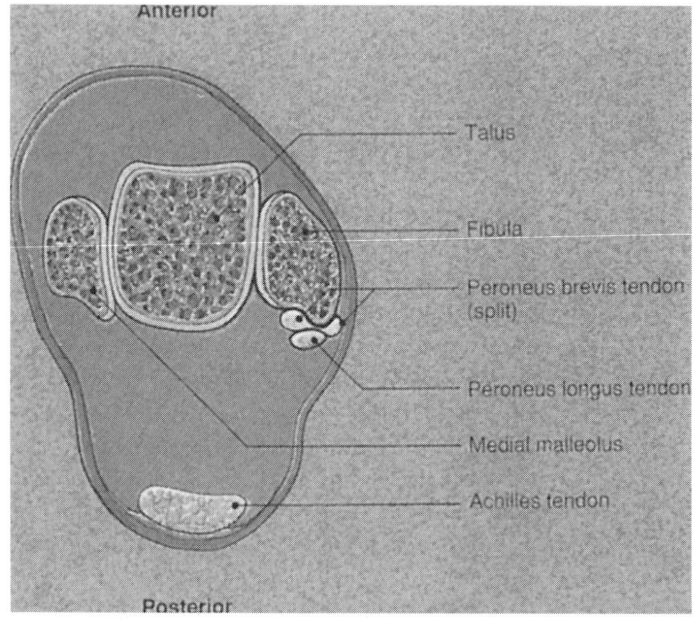

Figure 5–17. Cross-section of the peroneal tendons at the level of the fibular groove showing the mechanism of injury. The peroneus brevis is compressed by the longus, which lies posterior, into the sharp edge of the fibula. Such compression results in splitting of the peroneus brevis tendon. The superior peroneal retinaculum is not shown. (From Yodlowski, M., and Mizel, M.: Reconstruction of peroneus brevis pathology. Op. Tech. Orthop. 4(3):147, 1994.)

will not occur. **Hindfoot valgus and midfoot collapse are common findings as the disease progresses. Anterolateral ankle and/or sinus tarsi pain may ensue with chronicity secondary to impingement and arthrosis.**

Nonsurgical treatment consists of a University of California Biomechanics Laboratory insert, medial wedge, or an AFO that locks the hindfoot and midfoot. Surgical treatment varies with the stage of the dysfunction and remains controversial. Hindfoot arthrodesis is effective management of rigid deformity with arthrosis. Reconstruction of the posterior tibial tendon with the flexor digitorum longus tendon through a hole in the navicular or medial cuneiform with lateral column lengthening and/or medial calcaneal slide is another surgical option for supple deformity.

XII. Heel Pain

A. Plantar Heel Pain—Plantar heel pain has multiple causes.

1. Neurologic causes include tarsal tunnel syndrome, herniated nucleus pulposus, and spinal stenosis. Entrapment or irritation of the medial or lateral branches of the posterior tibial nerves can cause heel pain. Additionally, the nerve to the abductor digiti quinti can be irritated as it passes through the abductor hallucis. This is commonly seen in the athletic population. A peripheral neuropathy is an uncommon cause.
2. Bony disorders include stress fractures of the calcaneus from overuse. Calcification at the origin of the flexor digitorum brevis (reactive heel spur) is rarely a cause of pain, but a fracture at the base of a "heel spur" can be a cause of pain.
3. Soft-tissue problems such as plantar fasciitis or inflammation of the plantar heel pad can cause pain. Treatment includes stretching, heel cushions, NSAIDs, casting, and night splints. Rigid-soled shoes, steel sole stiffener, and rocker-bottom shoes can be helpful as well.

B. Posterior Heel Pain

1. Posterior heel pain can be caused by retrocalcaneal bursitis, Hagland's disease, or insertional Achilles tendinitis. It presents with pain and tenderness in the superior-posterior portion of the calcaneus at the area of the insertion of the Achilles tendon or more proximally on the tendon.
2. Posterior heel pain can be treated nonsurgically with NSAIDs, a heel lift, or cast immobilization. Surgical procedures are not commonly necessary. Excision of the retrocalcaneal bursa and superior bony prominence or Achilles tendon débridement may be necessary in some cases.

XIII. Infections of the Foot and Ankle

A. Bacterial Infections

1. Soft-Tissue Infections—Superficial lesions such as blisters or scratches are most commonly caused by *Staphylococcus aureus* and beta-hemolytic streptococci. Puncture wounds of the foot can cause osteomyelitis, osteochondritis, and septic arthritis. If a puncture wound causes an infection, evaluation and treatment should be aggressive, with consideration of a bone scan and possibly CT if clinically considered necessary. If there is abscess formation or a septic joint, surgical débridement (through a dorsal approach if possible) should be performed. If there is osteomyelitis of a sesamoid, it should be removed. Parenteral antibiotics are usually necessary. ***Pseudomonas* is the most common organism if the puncture wound is through a sneaker. *S. aureus* is otherwise the most common organism. Cat and dog bites can result in an infection from *Pasteurella multocida*.** Antibiotics should be administered if a cat or dog bite occurs. *P. multocida* is usually covered by penicillin but cephalosporins will cover *P. multocida* as well as *S. aureus*.
2. Joint Infections—These are usually caused by *S. aureus*, although in the young adult *Neisseria gonorrhoeae* is not common. Treatment of joint infections usually involves parenteral antibiotics and repeated aspirations. If the infection does not improve after several days, surgical intervention should be considered.
3. Bone Infections
   a. Diagnosis is similar to elsewhere in the skeleton. Diagnostic studies, including bone scan, CT scan, or MRI, can be helpful.
   b. Treatment usually involves surgical débridement and treatment with parenteral antibiotics.
4. Diabetic Foot Infections—Infected feet in the diabetic population account for 15% of the admissions of diabetic patients. More than 5% of diabetic patients eventually require amputation below the knee. The peripheral neuropathy they often develop prevents them from taking appropriate protective care of their limb, and the large- and small-vessel diseases make healing more difficult. *S. aureus* is the most common bacteria, but polymicrobial infections are not uncommon. Wound culture from the surface may be inaccurate, and if possible an aspiration or deep culture should be obtained. Parenteral

antibiotics should be used unless the infection is relatively mild. Hyperbaric oxygen treatment has not been proved to be of additional benefit.

Evaluation should give consideration to vascular status/depth of ischemia, quantification of neuropathy via monofilament testing, nutritional status, and medical management/control of diabetes. Should profusion be poor, possible revascularization or amputation might be appropriate. Débridement and drainage should be carried out as would be done in a nondiabetic foot. Brachial/ankle systolic pressure ratio of 0.45 or higher, toe pressures greater than 30 mm Hg, serum albumin greater than 3.5 mg/dL, and total lymphocyte count greater than 1500 are good prognostic indicators for healing.

B. Mycobacterial Infections
   1. Tuberculosis—Tuberculosis in the foot is very rare.
   2. Atypical Mycobacteria—Atypical mycobacteria is quite rare in the foot. *Mycobacterium avium-intracellulare* is seen in patients with AIDS. ***Mycobacterium marinum*** **is found in patients exposed to infections with marine life.**

C. Fungal Infections
   1. Tinea pedis is a common fungal infection of the skin and cuticles in the foot. It can present with scaling, itching, and blisters and is often found on the sole and in the interdigital spaces. Local skin infection can be treated with topical agents, and nail infection can be treated with oral griseofulvin. Treatment with griseofulvin can take 8 months to a year, and significant potential complications can occur with this medication. Given these complications, this treatment is often inappropriate due to the low-level symptoms usually present. Several relatively new treatments are available (terbinafine, itraconazole) that appear to have significantly less toxicity, but long-term results are not yet available.
   2. Mycetoma—This fungus can cause Madura foot, a chronic foot infection. This condition is rare in developed countries.

XIV. The Diabetic Foot

A. Pathophysiology—**The primary cause of the diabetic foot is peripheral neuropathy.** This allows excess pressure to cause soft-tissue disorder while remaining undetected. The often coexisting circulatory impairment delays or prevents healing. **Diabetics tend to develop arteriosclerotic disease at an earlier age, which is more diffuse, affecting both upper and lower extremities.** The aorta and iliac and femoral arteries are often involved, and vascular evaluation for large-vessel disease should be carried out in diabetics with nonhealing ulcers or infection. Incidence in males and females is the same. Effects of neurologic disorders include lesser toe deformities, ischemic clawing, and dry, flaking skin.

B. Clinical Problems and Treatment—A nonhealing plantar ulcer is a serious problem. It usually results from excess pressure due to bony prominence. Treatment consists of relieving the pressure with orthotic devices or pads, braces, or a total contact cast. If nonsurgical treatment is unsuccessful, removal of prominent condyles or resection of the offending bony structure can be considered. If osteomyelitis exists, excision of the infected bone or partial amputation should be performed as needed. If an ulcer is present under the heel and this cannot be resolved, a partial calcanectomy can sometimes be helpful. A Syme amputation might be necessary, which requires less energy consumption during ambulation than amputation below the knee.
   1. Infections fall into the general categories of cellulitis, abscess, and osteomyelitis. Cellulitis should be treated with parenteral antibiotics. An abscess needs irrigation and débridement as well as packing and appropriate wound care. Osteomyelitis in the foot, if it exists, requires excision of the infected bone. Partial amputation of a digit, ray, or part of the foot may be necessary for exposed bone or tendon. **In the case of suspected infection in a diabetic foot, it is important to evaluate the foot for possible Charcot's changes.**
   2. **The differential diagnosis between infection and a neuropathic joint may be difficult to make.** Charcot's joints (ankle, subtalar joint, midtarsal joint, and tarsometatarsal joints) are warm and erythematous, mimicking infection. Treatment includes total contact casting or a wooden shoe, depending on the deformity present. During the initial stages, these Charcot joints are quite swollen, and weight-bearing should be avoided. **A biopsy is not indicated,** and assistance in differential diagnosis between a Charcot joint and an infectious process can be aided by laboratory evaluation (complete blood cell count, erythrocyte sedimentation rate) as well as an indium scan or MRI, which can reveal bony changes consistent with osteomyelitis. If the soft-tissue envelope is intact, the likelihood of deep infection is diminished. The goal of treatment is to obtain a durable, plantigrade foot that will probably necessitate prolonged casting or bracing.

3. Table 5–1 shows classifications for diabetic foot lesions.

XV. Amputations of the Foot and Ankle

A. Surgical Techniques

1. Tourniquet—There is no contraindication to a tourniquet in diabetic patients.
2. Wound Closure—In partial foot amputations, removal of slightly more bone than originally intended might be necessary to achieve wound closure. In the case of infection, delayed primary closure can be considered.
3. The level of amputation should be at a level to preserve as much viable bony architecture as is reasonable under the circumstances. Vascular evaluation of the larger vessels of the extremity is appropriate as improvement of enlarged blood vessels may allow for a higher level of amputation.

B. Amputation Levels

1. With amputation of the great toe it is better to save the proximal aspect of the proximal phalanx if possible. This helps to preserve some function of the plantar fascia.
2. Preservation of part of the lesser toes gives the advantage of the remaining residual toe, which can serve to prevent adjacent toes from drifting towards each other.
3. Ray amputation can be successful in the case of infection, gangrene, or trauma. **Complications of this occur with increased weight-bearing on the remaining metatarsals.**
4. Transmetatarsal amputation is well tolerated, allowing ambulation in off-the-shelf shoes with a forefoot filler. The most common complication is ulceration of the stump.
5. Chopart's amputation, an amputation through the calcaneocuboid and talonavicular joint, must be accompanied by a release of the Achilles tendon to prevent a plantar flexion contracture. Ambulation requires an AFO.

XVI. Toenail Pathology

A. Systemic Nail Pathology

1. Psoriasis—Changes in the cuticles of a patient with psoriasis often look similar to those with fungal infection. Toenail changes include stippling and pitting.
2. Dermatitis—Dermatitis, if chronic, can result in maladies in the nail plate. Transverse ridging and scaling can occur along with discoloration. Causes include allergic reactions to solvents, dyes, nail polish, detergents, and other chemicals. **Pigmentation under the cuticle can be caused by malignant melanoma.** Another cause of darkening under the cuticle

Table 5–1.

Depth/Ischemic Classification for Diabetic Foot Lesions

Grade	Definition	Treatment
Depth Classification		
0	The "at risk" foot. Previous ulcer or neuropathy with deformity that may cause new ulceration	Patient education, regular examination, appropriate shoewear and insoles
1	Superficial ulceration, not infected	External pressure relief: total contact cast, walking brace, special shoewear, etc.
2	Deep ulceration exposing tendon or joint (with or without superficial infection)	Surgical débridement—wound care—pressure relief if closes and converts to grade 1 (PRN antibiotics)
3	Extensive ulceration with exposed bone, and/or deep infection (i.e., osteomyelitis or abscess)	Surgical débridement—ray or partial foot amputations—IV antibiotics—pressure relief if wound converts to grade 1
Ischemia Classification		
A	Not ischemic	Adequate vascularity for healing
B	Ischemic without gangrene	Vascular evaluation (Doppler, $TcPO_2$, arteriogram, etc.)—vascular reconstruction PRN
C	Partial (forefoot) gangrene	Vascular evaluation—vascular reconstruction—partial foot amputation
D	Complete foot gangrene	Vascular evaluation—major extremity amputation with possible proximal vascular reconstruction

PRN = per res necessita.
From Brodsky, J. W.: The diabetic foot. In Mann, R.A., and Coughlin, M.J., eds.: Surgery of the Foot and Ankle. St. Louis, Mosby–Yearbook, 1992.

is Addison's disease. Ingrown toenail (onychocryptosis) occurs when the border of the cuticle pierces the adjacent skin at the border of the cuticle. This soft-tissue irritation leads to localized edema and often cellulitis or small abscess formation. Treatment is antibiotics for any cellulitis or abscess along with removal of the offending piece of cuticle, which is acting as a foreign body. If the problem continues to recur, **a Winograd procedure for permanent ablation of the border of the cuticle can be considered.**

XVII. Ankle Sprains

A. Lateral Ankle Sprains—Lateral ankle sprains account for 90% of all ankle sprains. **The anterior talofibular ligament alone is involved in approximately two-thirds of ankle sprains and in another 25% together with the calcaneofibular ligament.**

1. Evaluation of the **anterior talofibular ligament is done with palpation in the sinus tarsi region as well as inversion of the ankle in plantar flexion. Evaluation of the calcaneofibular ligament is performed with inversion of the ankle in dorsiflexion.** The anterior drawer sign is done with the ankle in mild plantar flexion with the tibia stabilized and the hindfoot drawn forward. Anterior subluxation of the talus under the tibia is consistent with an incompetent anterior talofibular ligament.
2. **Differential diagnosis of lateral ankle sprains includes osteochondral fractures of the talus, fracture at the base of the fifth metatarsal, fracture of the lateral process of the talus, peroneal tendinitis/tear, and fracture of the anterior process of the calcaneus.** Fractures of the lateral malleolus and syndesmosis injuries can also produce significant lateral ankle pain.
3. Treatment of **Acute** Ankle Sprains
   a. Nonoperative treatment is the treatment of choice for the majority of ankle sprains. It is indicated for all mild or moderate injuries and most severe ankle sprains. Rest, immobilization, cold, and elevation are the basics of treatment. Immobilization can take the form of an Ace bandage or UNA boot, taping of the ankle to prevent inversion, an ankle brace to prevent inversion, or a cast.
   b. Surgical treatment is controversial. It is recommended at this time only for high-profile athletes with severe injuries.
4. In patients with **chronic** lateral ankle sprains or instability, careful evaluation should be made to detect any occult bony tenderness or cartilaginous or neurologic disorder. Inversion stress views, both in dorsiflexion and plantar flexion, can be helpful. Bone scans can reveal unsuspected fractures. Arthroscopy can be considered, where many times débridement of soft tissue from the anterolateral ankle can relieve symptoms consistent with impingement. Reconstruction using the peroneus brevis tendon and the plantaris tendons and tightening of the ligaments (Brostrom's procedure) have all been successfully used. The anatomic Brostrom ligament repair appears to be the most mechanically stable and is now favored in primary reconstructive efforts.

XVIII. Arthroscopy of the Foot and Ankle

A. Indications and Contraindications—Indications include unexplained pain, instability, stiffness, popping, osteochondral injury, or bony impingement. Some fractures may be fixed arthroscopically. Contraindications include active infection and vascular insufficiency. Ankle arthroscopy has been shown to be useful with synovitis, anterolateral soft-tissue impingement, and treatment of osteochondral fractures. Arthroscopic ankle arthrodesis and treatment of osteochondral fractures have been performed.

Complications include injuries to a branch of the superficial peroneal nerve with the anterolateral portal and to the saphenous nerve with the anteromedial portal.

B. Arthroscopic Portals—Anteromedial and anterolateral portals are commonly used. An anterocentral portal is sometimes used, and it is placed between the tendons of the extensor digitorum communis to decrease the potential injury to neurovascular structures. Posterolateral portals are sometimes indicated. Posteromedial portals are not used because of the potential for injury to the posterior tibial nerve, and trans-Achilles tendon portals are not used because of postoperative tendinitis.

XIX. Soft-Tissue Trauma and Compartment Syndromes

A. Acute Compartment Syndrome—With numerous separate compartments made up of inelastic fascial structures, the foot is susceptible to compartment syndromes, as is the leg. This can occur after an injury, with subsequent edema and increase in intracompartmental pressure; crush injuries and fractures are frequent causes. Diagnosis often reveals a palpable dorsalis pedis and posterior tibial pulse. Pain caused by a compartment syndrome does not decrease with immobilization, and the pain can be exacerbated with passive dorsiflexion of the toes (stretching the intrinsic muscles of the foot). During evaluation of the patient, the foot should be kept elevated at the level of the heart. Pressure measuring devices should be used to measure the intracompartmental pressure. Fasciotomy should be performed if pressure is more than 30 mm Hg. Fasciotomy is often performed through two dorsal incisions and one medial incision. The deep calcaneal compartment of the quadratus plantae often has the most elevated pressure.

B. Chronic Compartment Syndrome—If an acute compartment syndrome is left untreated, intrinsic muscles suffer ischemia and necrosis. This produces lesser toe deformities with hyperdorsiflexion at the metatarsophalangeal joint and hyperplantarflexion deformities at the PIP and DIP joints, as the extrinsic muscles overcome the remaining power of the intrinsics. Sensory deficit is a result of local injury to nerves and often also exists.

XX. Fractures and Dislocations of the Ankle—Ankle fractures were classified by Lauge-Hansen. He divided them into supination-adduction, supination-external rotation, pronation-abduction, and pronation-external rotation. The Weber classification done by the AO group is based on the level of the fibula fracture in relation to the plafond. Type A is at or level with the plafond. Type B is a spiral fracture beginning at the level of the plafond and extending proximally. Type C is a fracture above the syndesmosis. Weber's B or C injuries require evaluation of the syndesmosis as fixation can be necessary. If a Weber B fracture has more than 1.5 mm of syndesmotic widening, it should be treated with open reduction internal fixation.

XXI. Fractures and Dislocations of the Foot

A. Calcaneus Fractures—Calcaneus fractures are evaluated radiologically using Bohler's angle, which ranges 25–40 degrees, as well as the angle of Gissane, which normally ranges from 120–145 degrees. The subtalar joint can be evaluated with Broden's view, and the entire calcaneus is evaluated for possible surgical intervention using a CT scan in two planes. A Harris axial view demonstrates posterior facet depression and displacement as well as varus malalignment of the heel. A CT scan in both axial and coronal planes is helpful for preoperative planning.

1. Extra-articular Fractures—Usually do well when treated nonsurgically.
2. Anterior Process of the Calcaneus Fracture—Usually do well when treated nonsurgically with cast immobilization. If pain persists, excision of the fragment is usually successful. Hindfoot arthrodesis is considered a last step to relieve pain.
3. Tuberosity Fractures (Beak and Avulsion Fractures)—Displaced beak fractures (without Achilles tendon involvement) can often be reduced, closed, and immobilized. If there is a possibility of skin necrosis and an unsatisfactory closed reduction, open reduction should be considered. Displaced avulsion fractures (with involvement of the Achilles tendon) usually require reduction with open reduction and internal fixation.
4. Fractures of the Sustentaculum Tali—Usually do not need surgical intervention. The hallux should be frequently passively dorsiflexed to maintain motion of the flexor hallucis longus tendon, which passes just inferior to the sustentaculum.
5. Fractures of the Body Involving the Posterior Facet—Often treated with open reduction and internal fixation. A lateral approach is popular at this time, but some authors prefer a medial approach, and others prefer a combined approach.

B. Talus Fractures

1. The potential complications for talus fractures include avascular necrosis as well as degenerative changes of the ankle and subtalar joints. Displaced talar neck fractures require open reduction and internal fixation. Nonunion and malunion are other complications.
2. Osteochondral fractures, if acute, are treated with either immobilization or excision and drilling, depending on the severity of the fracture. For long-standing lesions, excision of the fragment and drilling to bleeding bone is recommended. This can often be done arthroscopically.
3. Fractures of the lateral process of the talus can be treated with immobilization, open reduction and internal fixation, or excision, depending on the severity of the fracture and the size and displacement of the fragment as well as the chronicity of the problem.

C. Metatarsal Fractures—Displaced and/or angulated fractures have some propensity for malunion that may lead to metatarsalgia secondary to shortening and plantar prominence. These should be fixed with either closed pinning and/or open reduction and internal fixation. True **Jones' fractures** occur at the proximal diaphysis of the fifth metatarsal. **These are treated with cast immobilization and non–weight-bearing. This fracture is in an area of poor vascularity.** If a nonunion occurs, this may require late treatment with internal fixation and bone grafting. High-performance athletes are sometimes treated directly with internal fixation.

D. Subtalar Dislocations—Subtalar dislocations involve a dislocation of the subtalar joint as well as of the talonavicular joint. Open subtalar joint dislocations should be taken to the operating room and irrigated and débrided before reduction. These dislocations are classified as medial, lateral, anterior, and posterior, according to which position the dislocated calcaneus has taken. The latter two are extremely rare.

1. Medial Dislocation—A medial dislocation involves an injury of the lateral ankle ligaments, with the calcaneus dislocated medially. **The talonavicular joint is dislocated so the talar head is dislocated laterally. Closed reduction may be impossible if the talar neck gets entrapped by the extensor retinaculum or peroneal tendons or there is impaction of the talus onto the lateral aspect of the navicular.**
2. Lateral Dislocation—**With the calcaneus dislocated laterally, the talar head and neck dislocate medially. Failure of closed reduction can be caused by the talar neck and head entangled in the posterior tibial tendon or flexor digitorum longus tendon or by a small fracture involving the head of the talus.**

E. Lisfranc's Joint Injury—There is no ligament between the base of the first and second metatarsal. **The second metatarsal is attached obliquely to the first cuneiform by an interosseous ligament termed Lisfranc's ligament.** The base of the second metatarsal keys into the middle cuneiform, providing stability in the midfoot analogous to the Roman arch effect. Diagnosis of these injuries can be subtle. Lisfranc's midfoot strains may occur without evidence of fracture and should be immobilized. Stress views and/or CT evaluation may aid the evaluation. These fracture dislocations should be reduced and treated with screw fixation, with hardware to be removed after ligamentous healing occurs. Chronic pain or dysfunction from missed or undertreated cases may lead to early degenerative arthrosis, which is a significant cause of morbidity.

Selected Bibliography

Mann, R.A.: Biomechanics of the foot. In Atlas of Orthotics: Biomechanical Principles and Application, pp. 257–266. St. Louis, CV Mosby, 1975.

Anatomy

Sarrafian, S.K.: Functional anatomy of the foot and ankle. In Sarrafian, S.K., ed.: Anatomy of the Foot and Ankle, 2nd ed. Philadelphia, JB Lippincott, 1993.

Biomechanics

Buck, P., Morrey, B.F., and Chao, E.Y.S.: The optimum position of arthrodesis of the ankle: A gait study of the knee and ankle. J. Bone Joint Surg. [Am.] 69:1052–1062, 1987.

Inman, V.T.: The Joints of the Ankle. Baltimore, Williams & Wilkins, 1976.

Johnson, J.E.: Axis of rotation of the ankle. In Stiehl, J.B., ed.: Inman's Joints of the Ankle. Baltimore, Williams & Wilkins, 1991.

Mann, R.A.: Biomechanics of the foot and ankle. In Surgery of the Foot and Ankle, vol. 1, pp. 3–43. St. Louis, Mosby 1993.

Gait

Sarrafian, S.K.: Functional anatomy of the foot and ankle. In Sarrafian, S.K., ed.: Anatomy of the Foot and Ankle, pp. 574–577. Philadelphia, JB Lippincott, 1993.

Nerves

Mann, R.A.: The tarsal tunnel syndrome. Orthop. Clin. North Am. 5:109, 1974.

Mann, R.A., and Reynold, J.: Interdigital neuroma: A critical analysis. Foot Ankle 3:238, 1983.

Diabetes

Wagner, F.W.: The dysvascular foot: A system for diagnosis and treatment. Foot Ankle 2:84–122, 1982.

Walker, S.R.: The contact casting and chronic diabetic neuropathic foot ulcerations: Healing rates by wound location. Arch. Phys. Med. Rehabil. 68:217–221, 1987.

Waters, R.L., Perry, J., Antonelli, E.E., et al.: Energy cost of walking of amputee: The influence of level of amputation. J. Bone Joint Surg. [Am.] 58:42–46, 1976.

Arthritis—Forefoot

Mann, R.A., and Coughlin, M.J.: The rheumatoid forefoot: A review of the literature and method of treatment. Orthop. Rev. 8:105, 1979.

Mann, R.A., and Oates, J.C.: Arthrodesis of the first metatarsophalangeal joint. Foot Ankle 1:159, 1980.

Mann, R.A., and Thompson, F.M.: Arthrodesis of the first metatarsophalangeal joint for hallux valgus in rheumatoid arthritis. J. Bone Joint Surg. [Am.] 66:687, 1984.

Mann, R.A., and Clanton, T.O.: Hallux rigidus: Treatment by cheilectomy. J. Bone Joint Surg. [Am.] 70A:400–406, 1988.

Shereff, M., and Jahss, M.: Complications of Silastic implant arthroplasty in the hallux. Foot Ankle 1:95, 1980.

Arthritis—Hindfoot/Ankle

Buck, P., Morrey, B.F., and Chao, E.Y.S.: The optimum position of arthrodesis of the ankle. J. Bone Joint Surg. [Am.] 69:1052–1062, 1987.

Elbaor, J.E., Thomas, W.H., Weinfeld, M.S., et al.: Talonavicular arthrodesis for rheumatoid arthritis of the hindfoot. Orthop. Clin. North Am. 7:821–826, 1976.

Fogel, G.R., Katoh, Y., Rand, J.A., et al.: Talonavicular arthrodesis for isolated arthrosis: 9.5 year results and gait analysis. Foot Ankle 3:105–113, 1982.

Iwata, H., Yasuhara, N., Kawashima, K., et al.: Arthrodesis of the ankle joint with rheumatoid arthritis: Experience with the transfibular approach. Clin. Orthop. 153:189–193, 1980.

Mann, R.A.: Surgical implications of biomechanics of the foot and ankle. Clin. Orthop. 146:1–118, 1980.

Mazur, J.M., Schwartz, E., and Simon, S.R.: Ankle arthrodesis: Long-term follow-up with gait analysis. J. Bone Joint Surg. [Am.] 61:964–975, 1979.

Bunions

Bordelon, R.L.: Evaluation and operative procedures for hallux valgus deformity. Orthopedics 10:37–44, 1987.

Coughlin, M.J.: Arthrodesis of the first metatarsophalangeal joint. Orthop. Rev. 19:177–186, 1990.

Coughlin, M.J., and Mann, R.A.: Arthrodesis of the first metatarsophalangeal joint as salvage for the failed Keller procedure. J. Bone Joint Surg. [Am.] 69:68–75, 1987.

Coughlin, M.J., and Mann, R.A.: The pathophysiology of the juvenile bunion. Instr. Course Lect. 36:123–136, 1987.

Mann, R.A.: Complications in surgery of the foot. Orthop. Clin. North Am. 7:851, 1976.

Mann, R.A.: Hallux valgus. Instr. Course Lect. 35:339–353, 1986.

Mann, R.A.: Treatment of the bunion deformity. Orthopedics 10:49–56, 1987.

Mann, R.A., and Coughlin, M.J.: Hallux valgus—etiology, anatomy, treatment, and surgical considerations. Clin. Orthop. 157:31–41, 1981.

Mann, R.A., and Coughlin, M.J.: Hallux valgus and complications of hallux valgus. In Mann, R.A., ed.: Surgery of the Foot, 5th ed., pp. 66–130. St. Louis, CV Mosby, 1986.

Mann, R.A., and Oates, J.C.: Arthrodesis of the first metatarsophalangeal joint. Foot Ankle 1:159–166, 1980.

Mitchell, C.L., Fleming, J.L., Allen, R., et al.: Osteotomy-bunionectomy for hallux valgus. J. Bone Joint Surg. [Am.] 40:41, 1958.

Silver, D.: The operative treatment of hallux valgus. J. Bone Joint Surg. 5:225–232, 1923.

Lesser Toes

Coughlin, M.J.: Crossover second toe deformity. Foot Ankle 8:29–39, 1987.

Coughlin, M.J.: Second metatarsophalangeal joint instability in the athlete. Foot Ankle 14:309–319, 1993.

Coughlin, M.J.: Subluxation and dislocation of the second metatarsalphalangeal joint. Orthop. Clin. North Am. 20:535–551, 1989.

Coughlin, M.J., and Mann, R.A.: Lesser toe deformities. Instr. Course Lect. 36:137–159, 1987.

Coughlin, M.J., and Mann, R.A.: Lesser toe deformities. In Mann, R.A., and Coughlin, M.J., eds.: Surgery of the Foot and Ankle, 6th ed. St. Louis, CV Mosby, 1993.

Mizel, M.S.: Correction of hammertoe and mallet toe deformities: Operative techniques. Orthopedics 2:188–194, 1992.

Sangeorzan, B.J., Benirschke, S.K., Mosca, V., et al.: Displaced intra-articular fractures of the tarsal navicular. J. Bone Joint Surg. [Am.] 71:1504–1510, 1989.

Intractable Plantar Keratosis

Bordelon, L.R.: Orthotics, shoes and braces. Orthop. Clin. North Am. 20:751–757, 1989.

Brodsky, J.W., Kourosh, S., Stills, M., et al. Objective evaluation of insert material for diabetic and athletic footwear. Foot Ankle 9:111–116, 1988.

Holmes, G.B., and Timmerman, L.: A quantitative assessment of the effect of metatarsal pads on plantar pressures. Foot Ankle 11:141–145, 1990.

Mann, R.A., and Coughlin, M.J.: Keratotic disorders of the plantar skin. In Mann, R.A., and Coughlin, M.J., eds.: Surgery of the Foot and Ankle, CV Mosby, 1993.

Mann, R.A., and Duvries, H.L.: Intractable plantar keratosis. Orthop. Clin. North Am. 4:67–73, 1973.

Mann, R.A., and Wapner, K.L.: Tibial sesamoid shaving for treatment of intractable plantar keratosis. Foot Ankle 13:196–198, 1992.

Achilles Tendon

Cetti, R.: Rupture of the Achilles tendon: Operative vs. non-operative options. Foot Ankle 2(3): 1997.

Tendon Injury

Hamilton, W.G.: Stenosing tenosynovitis of the flexor hallucis longus tendon and posterior impingement upon the os trigonum in ballet dancers. Foot Ankle 3:74–80, 1982.

Inglis, A.E., Scott, W.N., Sculo, T.P., et al.: Ruptures of the tendon Achilles: An objective assessment of surgical and non-surgical treatment. J. Bone Joint Surg. [Am.] 52:990–993, 1976.

6

Hand and Microsurgery

Steven M. Topper

I. **Anatomy and Pathophysiology** (see also Chapter 11, Anatomy)

A. **Limb Embryology**—The limb bud appears during the fourth week of gestation. At 33 days the hand is a paddle without individual digits. Digital separation begins at 47 days (7 weeks) and is complete by 54 days (8 weeks). At 7 weeks the condensation that will give rise to each of the bones of the hand is evident. (See Chapter 11, Anatomy, for ossification order of carpal and digital bones.)*

B. **Dorsal Compartments of the Wrist**

Comp	Tendons	Associated Pathologic Conditions
1	EPB/APL	De Quervain's tenosynovitis
2	ECRL/ECRB	Intersection syndrome
3	EPL	Drummer's wrist and traumatic rupture with distal radius fracture
4	EIP/EDC	Extensor tenosynovitis
5	EDM	Vaughn-Jackson syndrome (ischemic rupture in rheumatics)
6	ECU	Snapping ECU (unstable ECU subsheath)

C. **Joint Flexion and Extension**

Joint	Flexion	Extension
MCP	IO, lumbricals	EDC (sagittal bands)
PIP	FDS, FDP	Lumbricals (lateral bands) EDC (central slip)
DIP	FDP	EDC (terminal tendon) ORL (Landsmeer's ligament)

D. **Relationships**

1. The extensor indicis proprius (EIP), extensor digiti minimi (EDM), and extensor pollicis longus (EPL) are all ulnar to the extensor digitorum communis (EDC) and extensor pollicis brevis (EPB), respectively. The extensor carpi radialis brevis (ECRB) (central wrist extensor) is also ulnar to the extensor carpi radialis longus (ECRL) at the level of the wrist.

2. Digital cutaneous ligaments: **C**leland's ligament: dorsal (**C**eiling). **G**rayson's ligament: volar (**G**round), stabilizes the neurovascular bundle with finger flexion and extension.

3. There are four dorsal **interosseous (IO)** abductors (DAB) with insertions on the index finger, long finger (both ways; radial and ulnar), and ring finger. There are three palmar adductors that adduct the index finger, ring finger, and small finger. These muscles also flex the metacarpophalangeal (MCP) and contribute to proximal interphalangeal (PIP) extension through the lateral bands.

4. The **lumbrical muscles** originate on a tendon flexor digitorum profundus (FDP) and insert on a tendon (*radial lateral band of the extensor expansion*). It is the only muscle in the body with this distinction. It therefore is able to relax its own antagonist (FDP), which is also a singularly held distinction. The radial two lumbricals are innervated by the median nerve and the ulnar two by the ulnar nerve.

5. The thenar and hypothenar abductors are superficial; the opponens muscles are deep. The flexor pollicis brevis has dual innervation: The median nerve innervates the superficial head and the ulnar nerve innervates the deep head. This branch of the ulnar nerve is its terminal branch. The remainder of the thenar muscles are innervated by the median nerve alone. The hypothenar muscles are innervated by the ulnar nerve. *The abductor pollicis brevis is primarily responsible for palmar abduction of the thumb.*

6. The superficial arch is distal, and the ulnar artery is its predominant supply. The deep arch is proximal and is primarily fed by the deep branch of the radial artery. The classic complete (codominant) arch is present in only a third of patients—hence the importance of the Allen test. *The deep branch of the radial artery becomes the deep arch as it passes between the two heads of the first dorsal interosseous muscle.* The princeps pollicis artery is the continuation of the deep branch of the radial artery after it gives off the branch to the deep arch. This

*I would like to acknowledge the following surgeons for their previous contributions to the development of this chapter: Mark D. Miller, M.D., and James F. Bruce, M.D.

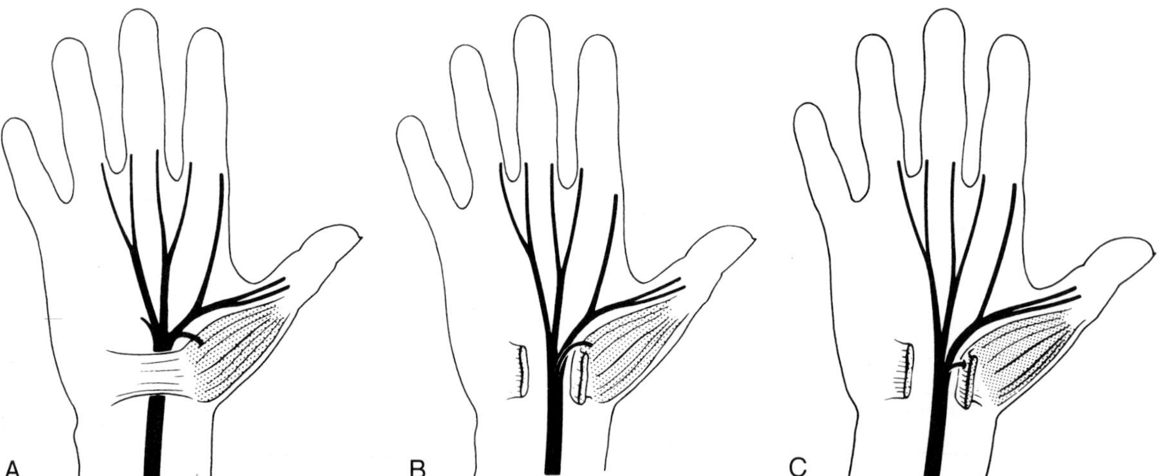

Figure 6–1. Variations in median nerve anatomy in the carpal tunnel. *A,* Extraligamentous and recurrent, the most common. *B,* Subligamentous branching of a recurrent median nerve. *C,* Transligamentous course of the recurrent branch of the median nerve. (From Lanz, U.: Anatomical variations of the median nerve in the carpal tunnel. J. Hand Surg. 2A:44–53, 1977.)

then bifurcates into the thumb digital arteries after giving off the branch to the radial side of the index finger (radialis indicis). There are three common digital arteries in the second through the fourth web spaces that bifurcate into the proper digital arteries. The digital artery to the ulnar side of the small finger is the first branch off the superficial arch.* Arteries are volar to the nerve in the palm and dorsal in the digit.

7. There are nine flexor tendons and one nerve (median n.) in the carpal tunnel. The flexor pollicis longus is the most radial structure. The palmar cutaneous branch of the median nerve usually lies between the palmaris longus and the flexor carpi radialis at the level of the wrist flexion crease. The usual pattern of the recurrent motor branch of the median nerve is extraligamentous branching and recurrent innervation (50%). Other relatively common patterns include subligamentous branching with recurrent innervation (30%) and transligamentous branching and innervation (20%). Other variations are extremely rare (Fig. 6–1).
8. Flexor Pulley System—Cruciate pulleys: No. 3 at the level of the joints; they primarily facilitate sheath collapse and expansion during digital motion. Annular pulleys: No. 5 located between the joints. *A2 and A4 are critical to preserve* so as to prevent bowstringing of the tendons with digital flexion (these are the ones that derive their origin from bone proximal and middle phalanx, respectively).
9. The Oblique Retinacular Ligament (of Landsmeer) (Fig. 6–2) originates from the periosteum of the proximal phalanx and the A2 and C1 pulleys. It inserts into the terminal tendon. *It functions to link PIP and distal interphalangeal joint (DIP) extension.* As the PIP joint extends, the volarly

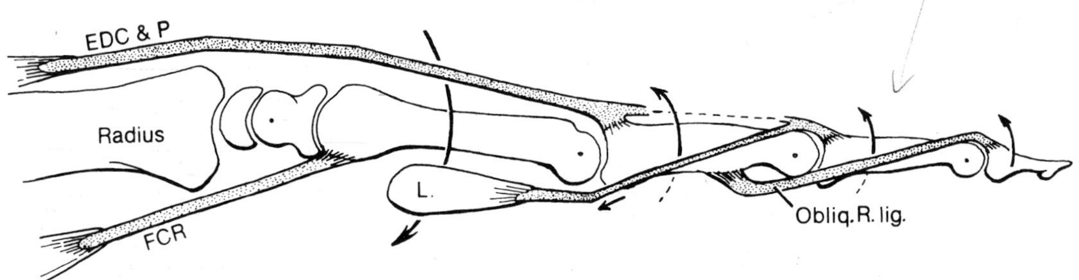

Figure 6–2. As the wrist is flexed by the flexor carpi radialis (FCR) and the flexor carpi ulnaris, tone is increased in the extensor digitorum communis and proprius systems (EDC and P), thus passively bringing the metacarpophalangeal joint into extension. Extension of this joint increases the tone in the intrinsic system, represented here by the lumbrical (L), by tenodesis action, thereby extending the proximal interphalangeal joint. The oblique retinacular ligament (Obliq.R.lig.) will tenodese the distal joint into extension by a similar mechanism. (From Green, D.P., Hotchkiss, R.M., and Pederson, W.C.: Green's Operative Hand Surgery, 4th ed. New York, Churchill-Livingstone, 1999. Adapted from Littler, J.W., Burton, R.I., and Eaton, R.G.: The dynamics of digital extension. AAOS Sound Slide Program 467, 468, 1976.)

positioned ligament at this joint tightens. As it tightens, it pulls on the terminal tendon as it is positioned dorsally at the level of the DIP joint.

10. Small Finger Variations—Flexor digitorum superficialis (FDS) is absent in a third of the population; that is why comparison with the opposite side is important when evaluating for an FDS laceration in a small finger. EDC may be absent in half, and extension is achieved via the EDM.

E. **Pathophysiology**

1. Intrinsic Minus or Claw Hand—This condition is secondary to ulnar/median nerve palsy or Volkmann's ischemic contracture. Musculotendinous weakness or tightness leads to an imbalance of forces, yielding MCP hyperextension and IP joint flexion (Fig. 6–3). This characteristic posture results in deformity with loss of ability to perform prehensile grasp and diminished grip and pinch strength. Operative treatment is directed at preventing MCP joint hyperextension either by a passive tenodesis or an active tendon transfer.

2. Intrinsic Plus Hand—This is caused by intrinsic tightness. This is generally a result of trauma or distal joint malalignment, as occurs in rheumatoid arthritis (RA). The Bunnell test differentiates intrinsic from extrinsic tightness. A positive test result for intrinsic tightness is demonstrated when there is less IP flexion with MCP joints (MPJs) hyperextended (which puts the volarly oriented intrinsics on stretch) compared with when MPJs are flexed (which puts the dorsally oriented extrinsics on stretch) (Fig. 6–4). The intrinsic plus position is characterized by MPJ flexion and interphalangeal joint (IPJ) extension. Depending on the degree of tightness, passive stretching exercises are indicated. Otherwise, operative treatment is directed at loosening the intrinsics, either by a distal release when the deformity is severe involving both the MPJs and IPJs or when the intrinsic muscles are fibrotic and dysfunctional, or by a proximal muscle slide when the intrinsics are spastic or have remaining useful function.

3. Lumbrical Plus Finger—This disorder is characterized by paradoxic extension of the IPJs while attempting to flex the finger. It is caused by retracted FDP tendon and lumbrical origin by laceration of the FDP tendon, distal digital amputation, reconstruction of the FDP with a loose tendon graft, or adhesion of the lumbrical to the FDP tendon distal to the MPJ. The lumbrical muscle belly essentially becomes a continuation of the FDP tendon (Fig. 6–5). When the FDP contracts to flex the finger,

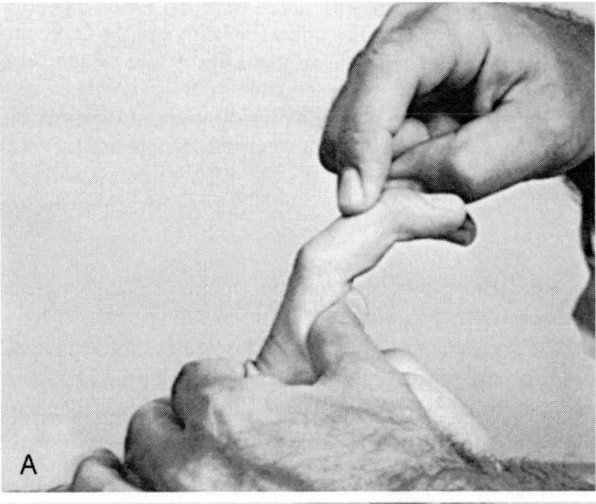

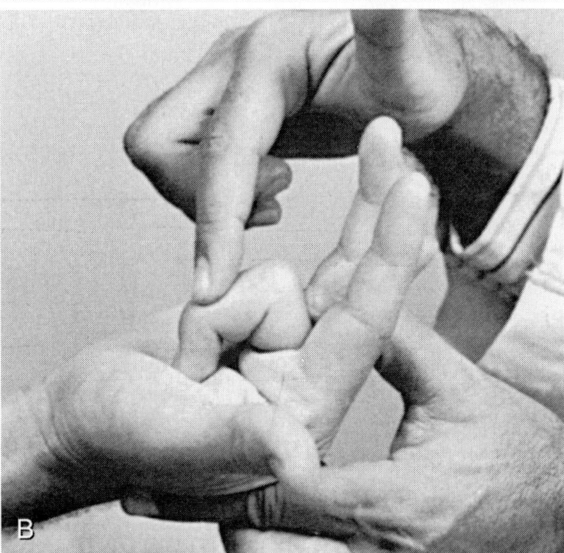

Figure 6–4. Intrinsic contracture with positive Bunnel tightness test. *A,* MCP hyperextension: restricted PIP flexion. *B,* MCP flexion: normal PIP flexion. (From Green, D.P., Hotchkiss, R.M., and Pederson, W.C.: Green's Operative Hand Surgery, 4th ed. New York, Churchill-Livingstone, 1998.)

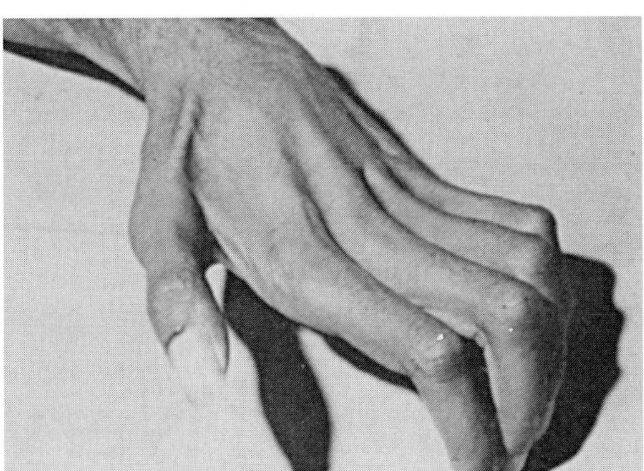

Figure 6–3. A combined median-ulnar palsy with intrinsic motor atrophy and atrophy of the volar pulps of the digits. There is a flat transverse palmar arch and clawing of the fingers. An adduction contracture has developed in the thumb. (From Green, D.P., Hotchkiss, R.M., and Pederson, W.C.: Green's Operative Hand Surgery, 4th ed. New York, Churchill-Livingstone, 1998.)

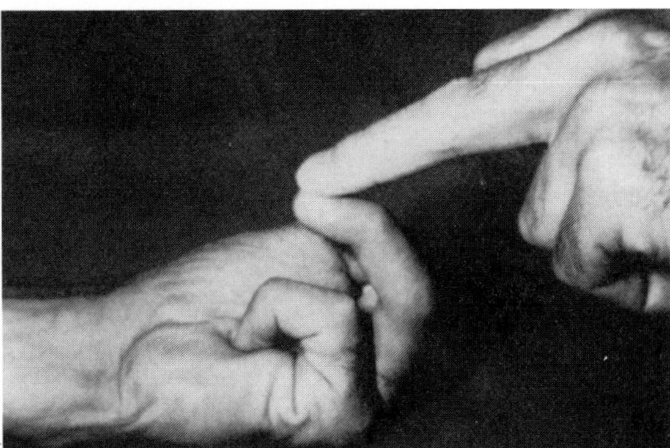

Figure 6–5. Lumbrical plus finger. With attempted flexion the ring finger paradoxically extends against the resistance of the examiner's finger. (From Lister, G.: The Hand: Diagnosis and Indications, 3rd ed. Edinburgh, Churchill-Livingstone, 1993.)

it pulls on the lumbrical, which inserts on the radial lateral band of the extensor expansion. Therefore, the IP joints extend. This problem is treated by lysis of the lumbrical tendon in the finger or by repair of the FDP to its insertion under correct tension.

4. Swan neck deformity is characterized by hyperextension of the PIP joint and flexion of the DIP joint (Fig. 6–6). It is caused by an imbalance of forces at the PIP joint and a lax volar plate. Improper balance results from MPJ volar sublux (as occurs in rheumatoid patients), mallet finger, laceration or transfer of FDS, and intrinsic contracture. As the PIP joint hyperextends, transverse retinacular ligaments tether the conjoined lateral bands, restricting their excursion and effect on the distal IPJ. Double ring splints can be used to prevent hyperextension of the PIP joint. Operative treatment options include FDS tenodesis or spiral oblique retinacular ligament reconstruction or proximal Fowler (central slip) tenotomy.
5. Boutonnière deformity is characterized by the opposite posture of the finger, with PIP flexion and DIP hyperextension (Fig. 6–7). It is caused by central slip rupture or attenuation (secondary to capsular distension like in RA), laceration, or traumatic disruption. Volar subluxation of the lateral bands due to incompetence or disruption of the triangular ligament leads to increasing deformity as the lateral bands become a flexor of the PIP, with the majority of their forces being transmitted to the DIP joint, resulting in hyperextension of the DIP. The Elson test is helpful in diagnosing an acute boutonnière before deformity is evident. The PIP joint is bent 90 degrees over the edge of a table. With resisted middle phalanx extension, the DIP joint goes into rigid extension because all the forces are distributed to the terminal tendon through the intact lateral bands. The lateral bands are no longer tethered dorsally by the triangular ligament but rather are subluxated volarly by flexing the proximal interphalangeal joint (PIPJ) over the edge of a table (positive test result described; a negative test result is demonstrated when the distal interphalangeal joint [DIPJ] remains floppy with this maneuver). If recognized early before contractures and in the acute healing phase, an extension splint that allows active DIP flexion exercises is effective. Chronic cases are treated with a distal Fowler (terminal tendon) tenotomy or a secondary tendon reconstruction (Tendon graft, Littler, Matev) only after passive joint motion is restored.
6. The quadrigia effect involves an active flexion lag in fingers adjacent to a digit with an injured, adheased, or improperly repaired FDP tendon. It is due to the tethering of the normal FDP tendons by the injured or repaired FDP because they all share a common muscle belly. As the injured digit reaches its maximum flexion, the FDP tendons in adjacent digits can have no further proximal excursion as all forces of the common muscle belly are being expended on the injured and tethered digit. It is treated by correcting the problem in the injured digit.

II. **Compressive Neuropathies**

A. Introduction

1. **Phases of Compressive Neuropathy**
   a. Early—Intermittent symptoms; responds favorably to nonoperative approach, splints, avoiding aggravating activities and corticosteroid injections.
   b. Intermediate—Constant symptoms; responds favorably to decompression of the involved nerve at the sight or sights of entrapment.
   c. Late—Characterized by long-standing constant symptoms and motor deficit. Endoneurial fibrosis rather than ischemia is the predominant process. Decompression can halt the progression of the disease; however, improvement in symptoms is inconsistent.
2. Double Crush Phenomenon—Normal axon function is dependent on factors synthesized in the nerve cell body. Blockage of axonal transport at one point makes the entire axon more susceptible to compression elsewhere. Outcome of surgical decompression may be disappointing unless all points of compression are addressed. It is logical to start with less complex distal releases first.
3. Etiology of Compressive Neuropathy
   a. Systemic/Inflammatory (diabetes, alco-

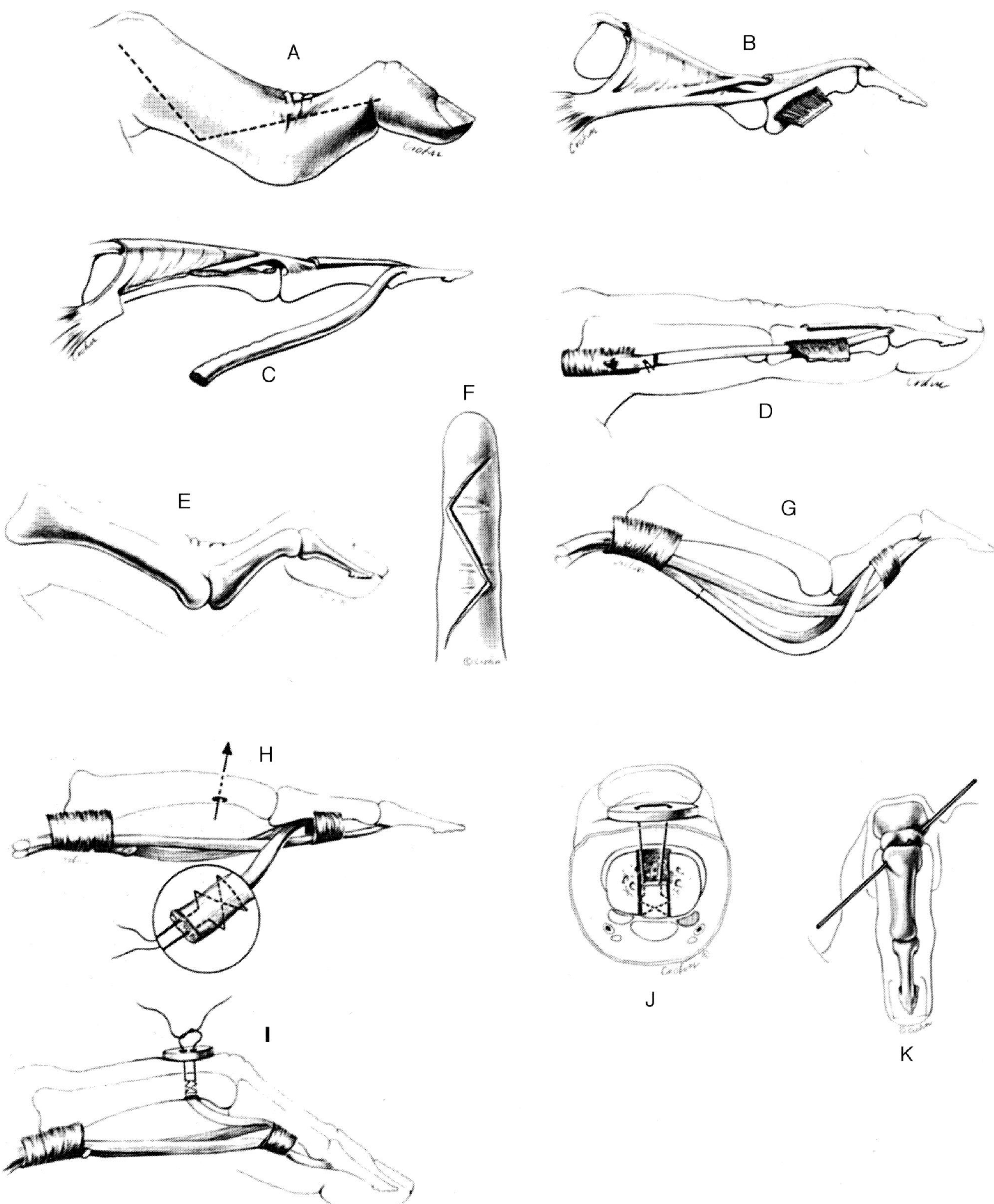

Figure 6–6. *A–D,* Littler oblique retinacular ligament reconstruction. *E–K,* Littler superficialis tenodesis. (From Green, D.P., Hotchkiss, R.M., and Pederson, W.C.: Green's Operative Hand Surgery, 4th ed. New York, Churchill Livingstone, 1998. Parts *A–D* adapted from Littler, J.W.: The finger extensor mechanism. Surg. Clin. North Am. 47:415–432, 1967; Parts *E–K* adapted from Burton, R.I.: The hand. In Goldstein, L.A., and Dickerson, R.C., eds.: Atlas of Orthopaedic Surgery, 2nd ed. St. Louis, Mosby, 1981, pp. 137–170.)

symptoms. Provocative tests for specific sites of compression are: resisted elbow flexion with forearm supination (bicipital aponeurosis), resisted forearm pronation with elbow extended (two heads of PT), isolated long finger PIP joint flexion (FDS origin). An elbow film is a mandatory preoperative examination. EMG and NCV are helpful. This condition usually responds to a nonoperative approach of rest splinting and NSAIDs (3–6 months). Failing this, a global decompression of all potential sites of compression yields a variable treatment outcome.

3. Anterior Interosseous Nerve (AIN) Compressive Neuropathy—This syndrome involves **motor loss without sensory involvement** (AIN innervated muscles: radial two FDP, flexor pollicus longus (FPL), pronator quadratus (PQ) plus or minus anterior forearm pain (see Fig. 6–8). The FDP and FPL are tested by asking the patient to make the "A OK" sign *(precision tip to tip pinch)*. PQ involvement is tested by resisted pronation with the elbow maximally flexed. Bilateral AIN palsy may indicate Parsonage-Turner syndrome (viral brachial neuritis), especially if motor loss was preceded by intense pain in the shoulder region. EMG/NCV is helpful in confirming the diagnosis. It is important to rule out a tendon disruption if only one finger is weak (Mannerfelt-Norman syndrome: FPL rupture). Sources of compression include: fibrous bands within the pronator teres, FDS arcade, edge of the lacertus fibrosus, enlarged bicipital bursa, Gantzer's muscle (accessory head of the FPL). Nonoperative treatment involves: tincture of time and elbow splinting in 90 degrees of flexion (8–12 weeks). Surgical decompression is recommended failing a trial of nonoperative management; results are generally satisfactory if done within 3–6 months from the onset of symptoms.

C. **Ulnar Nerve**

1. Cubital tunnel syndrome is due to compression of the ulnar nerve from the arcade of Struthers (which must be excised when the nerve is transposed anteriorly) through the cubital tunnel retinaculum to the point where the nerve proceeds through the two heads of the flexor carpi ulnaris (FCU). It presents with paresthesias over small finger and ulnar half of the ring finger and ulnar dorsal hand. Weakness of the intrinsics with a positive Froment's sign (FPL compensating for paralyzed thumb adductor) or Jeanne's sign (compensatory hyperextension of thumb MP joint) and/or weakness of the ulnar two FDP (Pollock's test) can also be seen. Examination findings include a positive Tinel sign over the cubital tunnel and positive elbow flexion test result (60 seconds). Sources of compression include: fascial bands, tumors, ganglions, the anconeus epitrochlearis, cubitus valgus, bony spurs, and a medial epicondyle nonunion. EMG/NCV is helpful in establishing the diagnosis. Nonoperative treatment includes NSAIDs, activity modifications, night-time extension splint (effective in 50% of cases). A number of surgical procedures are used for this disorder, including: release of the cubital tunnel retinaculum, medial epicondylectomy, or anterior transposition (subcutaneous, submuscular, intramuscular). Generally, any technique yields 80–90% good results when symptoms are intermittent and denervation has not occurred. Better results with fewer recurrences are seen with anterior submuscular transposition in cases with moderate (continuous symptoms) and severe (evidence of denervation) compression. **Poor prognosis correlates most closely with intrinsic atrophy.**

2. Ulnar Tunnel Syndrome—This is due to ulnar nerve compression in Guyon's canal. The roof of the tunnel is the volar carpal ligament. The floor is the transverse carpal ligament and the pisohamate ligament. The ulnar wall is the hook of hamate, and the radial wall is the pisiform and ADM muscle belly. Symptoms may be pure motor, sensory, or mixed based on location of compression within the tunnel. Pain is more infrequent when compared with CTS. Causative factors include: ganglia from the triquetrohamate joint (85% nontraumatic cases), nonunited hook of the hamate fracture, ulnar artery thrombosis, anomalous muscle, and palmaris brevis hypertrophy. The ulnar tunnel is divided into three zones (Fig. 6–9).

Zone 1: proximal to bifurcation of the nerve and associated with mixed motor sensory symptoms.

Zone 2: surrounds deep motor branch and has motor symptoms only. Ganglia and hook-of-hamate pathology are the most likely etiology in zones 1 and 2.

Zone 3: surrounds superficial sensory branch and has sensory symptoms only. *Thrombosis of the ulnar artery is the most likely etiology in zone 3.*

Treatment: identifying the etiology is the key to treatment. CT for hook-of-hamate fracture, MRI for ganglion cyst, Doppler ultrasound for ulnar artery thrombosis. Nonoperative treatment if warranted includes: avoiding aggravating activities, splints, and NSAIDs. Operative treatment

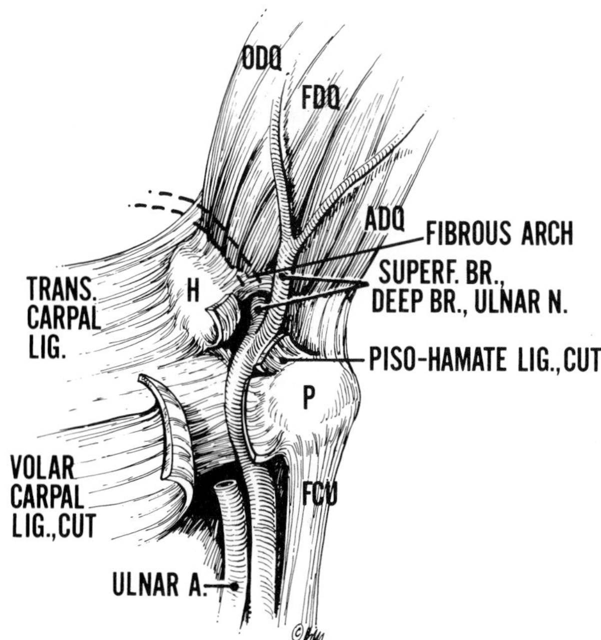

Figure 6–9. The ulnar nerve courses through Guyon's canal between the volar carpal ligament and the transverse carpal ligament. (P, pisiform; H, hamate.) (From Green, D.P., Hotchkiss, R.M., and Pederson, W.C.: Green's Operative Hand Surgery, 4th ed. New York, Churchill Livingstone, 1998.)

involves treating the underlying cause and decompressing the area of entrapment.

D. **Radial Nerve**

1. Arm—Although rare, the radial nerve can be compressed by a fibrous arch from the lateral head of the triceps (also remember the Holstein-Lewis fracture pattern at the junction of the middle and distal third of radius). Clinical findings include weakness of posterior interosseous nerve (PIN) and proximally innervated muscles (Henry's mobile wad). Also, radial sensory symptoms may be present. EMG and NCV are very helpful. Observation for up to 3 months is warranted; if no recovery, surgical decompression is indicated.
2. Posterior Interosseous Nerve Compression Syndrome—Symptoms include pain at the lateral elbow and weakness with radial drift with wrist extension (ECRL innervated higher than the PIN takeoff). This nerve carries no sensory fibers for cutaneous innervation; however, it does carry sensory fibers from the dorsal wrist capsule. The PIN innervates the ECRB, supinator, extensor indicis proprius, ECU, EDC, EDM, APL, EPB, and EPL. EMG is usually diagnostic. Anatomic sites of compression include: thickened fascia at radiocapitellar joint, radial artery recurrent leash of Henry, edge of ECRB, arcade of Frohse, and distal edge of the supinator (Fig. 6–10). Unusual causes include: chronic radial head dislocation, fractured radial head or neck, rheumatoid synovitis of the radiocapitellar joint, or mass (lipoma, ganglion) at the elbow. It is treated by avoiding aggravating activities and with NSAIDs. If this fails to provide recovery in 3 months, surgical decompression is warranted. 85% good to excellent results can be expected from surgical decompression.
3. Radial Tunnel Syndrome *is a pain-only problem without motor or sensory dysfunction.* It involves the same nerve as PIN syndrome, same sights of entrapment, but a different presentation and a different response to treatment. Provocative tests include: long finger extension test (positive result if pressure over P1 of the long finger reproduces pain at the edge of the ECRB) and the resisted supination test. **EMG/NCV is not helpful in this condition**. The chief differential is lateral epicondylitis (coexists in 5% of patients). In radial tunnel syndrome the maximum tenderness is distal to the radial head in a line from the lateral epicondyle through the radial head to a point 2–3 cm more distal over the radial tunnel. A long

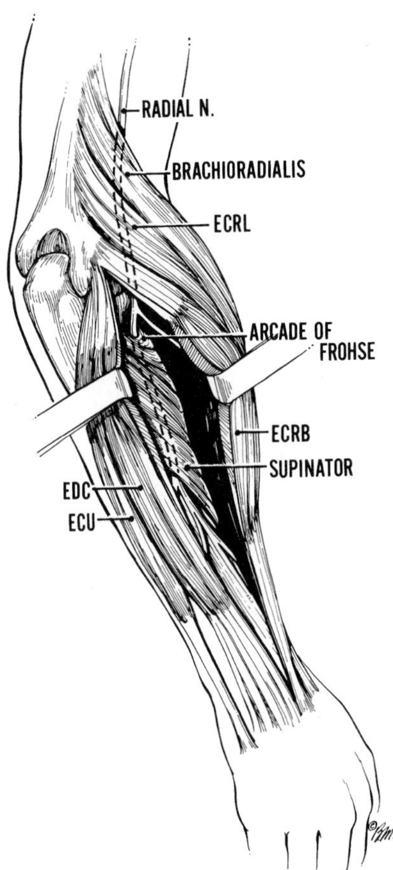

Figure 6–10. Extension of the posterior Thompson approach to the radial tunnel. (From Green, D.P., Hotchkiss, R.M., and Pederson, W.C.: Green's Operative Hand Surgery, 4th ed. New York, Churchill Livingstone, 1998.)

nonoperative approach is warranted (1 year), including: activity modification, temporary splinting, NSAIDs, and other modalities of therapy. Operative release is often disappointing, with only 51% good-to-excellent results reported and maximal recovery after surgery not until 9–18 months after surgery.

4. Wartenberg's Syndrome (cheiralgia paresthetica) is a compressive neuropathy of the sensory branch of the radial nerve. It is compressed between the brachioradialis (BR) and extensor carpi radialis longus (ECRL) with forearm pronation (by a scissor-like action between the tendons). Symptoms include pain, numbness, and paresthesias over radiodorsal hand. The provocative tests include forceful forearm pronation (60 seconds) and a positive Tinel's sign over the nerve. This condition is treated by rest, NSAIDs, avoiding aggravating activities, and wrist splints. Surgical decompression is warranted failing a 6-month trial nonoperative treatment.

E. **Other Compressive Neuropathies**

1. Suprascapular Nerve Entrapment Syndrome (SENS) presents with acute onset of deep, diffuse, posterolateral shoulder pain. It occurs after trauma or aggressive athletic activity. The most consistent finding is pain with palpation over suprascapular notch. EMG/NCV is very helpful in establishing the diagnosis. Spinati muscle atrophy is also common, usually because of a delay in diagnosis. The current trend is toward early surgical decompression through the posterior approach.

2. Thoracic Outlet Syndrome—There are two types: vascular and neurogenic. The vascular variety involves subclavian artery disease or aneurysm and is easily diagnosed by examination and imaging (angiogram). The neurogenic variety is infrequent and diagnosed by clinical examination alone (EMG/NCV rarely helpful). A cervical spine film should be taken to rule out a cervical rib. Chest radiograph is taken to rule out a Pancoast tumor. The provocative tests (Wright's hyperabduction maneuver, Adson's test, at attention test, elevation test) are rarely helpful because results are often abnormal in normal subjects. Sights of compression include a cervical rib, anterior scalene muscle, congenital fibrous bands, or the sternocleidomastoid muscle. A therapy approach is tried first, focusing on shoulder girdle strengthening and proper posture and relaxation techniques. The favored surgical procedure if necessary is a transaxillary first rib resection with 90% good-to-excellent results reported. Complication rates from the procedure are significant.

III. **Tendon Injuries**

A. **Extensor Tendons**—Description and treatment based on zones (Table 6–1). In general, partial lacerations (<50%) should be treated with early motion. Repair of partial lacerations actually impairs tendon healing and precipitates unnecessary adhesions. Traditionally, extensor tendon repairs have been managed with postoperative immobilization. The current trend is toward early mobilization (at 3 postoperative days) in a dynamic splint, particularly with multiple tendon lacerations beneath the extensor retinaculum or when there are associated injuries. This new trend is applicable to injuries in zones V–VIII. Its usefulness in zones II–IV is less clear, where traditional postoperative immobilization is usually satisfactory.

1. Zone I (Mallet Finger) represents a disruption of the terminal tendon. Treatment involves extension splinting for 6 weeks (80% good-to-excellent results reported). Greater complication rates are seen with a dorsal splint, and hyperextension should be avoided. Mallet fingers associated with a fracture are generally treated in an extension splint unless the distal phalanx is volarly subluxated, in which case reduction of the distal fragment should be done. The chronic mallet finger can be treated as a fresh injury up to 4 weeks out. When the time from injury is beyond that and the joint is supple, congruent, and without arthritis, repair, imbrication, or reconstruction of the terminal tendon (joint then held extended 6–8 weeks) is indicated. If the joint is otherwise, the best option is a DIP fusion. Loss of terminal tendon insertion causes proximal migration of the extensor apparatus with transfer of forces to the PIPJ. If volar plate is lax or attenuates over time, a swan neck deformity can develop in conjunction with the mallet finger. The favored technique for correction of this

Table 6–1.

Tendon Zones of Injury Extensor

Zone	Finger	Thumb
I	DIP joint	IP joint
II	Middle phalanx	Proximal phalanx
III	PIP joint	MP joint
IV	Proximal phalanx	Metacarpal
V	MP joint	CMC joint radial styloid
VI	Metacarpal	
VII	Dorsal wrist retinaculum	
VIII	Distal forearm	
IX	Mid and proximal forearm	

problem is a spiral oblique retinacular ligament reconstruction. Other options include a sublimis tenodesis or a Fowler central slip tenotomy.

2. Zone II (Finger: Middle Phalanx and Thumb: Proximal Phalanx)—The mechanism of injury usually involves laceration or crush. Insignificant (<50%) disruptions of the tendon are treated with skin and wound care and mobilization at 7–10 days from injury. Significant (>50%) disruptions are treated with suture repair and static splinting in extension for 4–6 weeks. Dynamic splinting can be considered in cooperative patients.
3. Zone III (Boutonnière Finger PIPJ, Thumb MPJ)—The three components of the acute boutonnière deformity include (1) disruption of the central slip, (2) attenuation of the triangular ligament, and (3) volar migration of the lateral bands. Diagnostic tests include the Elson test or evidence of a 15- to 20-degree (or greater) loss of active extension of the PIPJ with the wrist and MPJs fully flexed. Treatment of the acute boutonnière involves splinting the PIPJ in full extension for 6 weeks with active DIP joint flexion exercises. Holding the PIP joint in full extension reduces the separation of the ends of the central slip. Active flexion of the DIP joint draws the lateral bands distally and dorsally, further coapting the disrupted tendon ends. Indications for operative intervention include a displaced avulsion fracture or an open wound requiring irrigation and débridement (I&D) anyway. When there is loss of tendon substance, this is managed by free tendon graft or a flap of the extensor mechanism turned distally like an Achilles tendon repair. Treatment of a chronic boutonnière deformity is best done after the joint has full passive mobility. If this cannot be accomplished with therapy and splints, it may need to be done in a two-stage surgical procedure with the first stage being a joint release. Options include a soft-tissue release (distal Fowler tenotomy: release of the extensor mechanism at the junction of the middle and proximal thirds of the middle phalanx, which leaves the oblique retinacular ligament [ORL] intact; the lateral bands slide proximally, increasing extensor tone at the PIPJ and the intact ORL, which provides extensor tone at DIPJ), or a secondary tendon reconstruction such as excision of scar tissue and direct repair of central slip or VY advancement, free tendon graft, lateral band transfer procedure: Littler (ulnar lateral band through radial lateral band to P2) or Matev (ulnar lateral band transferred to distal stump radial lateral band, proximal stump radial lateral band brought through central slip and anchored at the dorsal base of P2) (Fig. 6–11).
4. Zone IV (Proximal Phalanx of Finger and Thumb MC)—These are managed similar to zone II injuries.
5. Zone III and IV (Thumb)—The EPB and EPL are easily distinguishable at this level. Significant disruptions (>50%) are repaired with a core suture. Postoperatively it is splinted with the wrist and MPJ in extension for 3–4 weeks, then mobilization is started.
6. Zone V (MP Joint)—Beware of the human bite wounds at this level. Lacerations involving >50% of the tendon substance should be repaired. Early mobilization in a dynamic extension outrigger splint is encouraged.
7. Traumatic Dislocation of the Extensor Tendon (Sagittal Band Rupture)—This is seen after laceration or forceful resisted flexion or extension injuries. *The long finger is the most commonly involved digit.* If

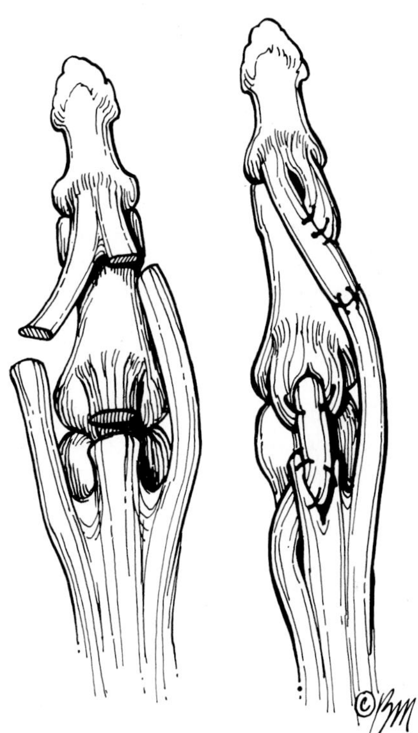

Figure 6–11. Matev reconstruction of the central slip. The radial lateral band is incised over the middle phalanx, then freed and brought through the central tendon at the PIP joint, inserting it into the base of the middle phalanx. The ulnar lateral tendon is then advanced into the distal portion of the radial lateral tendon and remnant of central tendon at the DIP joint. (From Green, D.P.: Operative Hand Surgery, 3rd ed. New York, Churchill Livingstone, 1993. Adapted from Swanson, A.B.: Flexible Implant Resection Arthroplasty in the Hand and Extremities. St. Louis, Mosby, 1973.)

diagnosed early (within a week) it may be treated with extension splint for 6 weeks. If diagnosis is delayed, direct repair is indicated. If the sagittal band cannot be mobilized for direct repair, an extrinsic extensor centralization procedure is done.

8. Zone VI (Metacarpal)—Significant lacerations (>50%) are repaired with core suture, and dynamic splint mobilization is started early. There is an excellent prognosis for tendon repairs at this level.
9. Zone VII (Wrist)—Lacerations at this level are associated with damage to the extensor retinaculum. Repair of significant lacerations with a core suture technique is advised. It is no longer recommended to excise portions of the extensor retinaculum over the repair sites; instead, early dynamic splint mobilization is advised.
10. Zone VIII (Distal Forearm)—These disruptions are at the level of the musculotendinous junction. The tendons obviously hold suture well, but sutures in muscle risk ischemia and failure. Remember that tendons originate from a fibrous septa that runs several centimeters within the muscle belly. This is the tissue that will hold a stitch. Postoperatively, static immobilization of the wrist in extension (40–45 degrees) and the MPJs in flexion (15–20 degrees) for 2 weeks; dynamic splint mobilization of the MPJs is then started at 2 weeks while maintaining the wrist in extension for an additional 2 weeks.
11. Zone IX (Proximal Forearm)—These disruptions are often secondary to penetrating trauma and are associated with neurovascular injury, which adversely affects the prognosis. Repair is done with figure-of-eight Vicryl or tendon grafts placed through the epimysium. After repair, the elbow and wrist are immobilized for 4 weeks in flexion and extension, respectively.

B. **Flexor Tendons**—Description and treatment based on zones (Fig. 6–12). Tendon healing is divided into three phases: (1) Inflammatory (0–5 days): characterized by cellular proliferation that functions to debris. (2) Fibroblastic (5–28 days): fibroblastic proliferation and synthesis of randomly organized collagen. There is also neoangiogenesis and fibronectin production, which acts as a chemotactic factor for the fibroblasts. (3) Remodeling (>28 days): realignment of collagen fibers and cross-linking along lines of stress. **Tendon repairs are the weakest between postoperative days 6 and 12.** Tendon structure compared with ligament: *Tendons have more collagen and are less viscoelastic*. They have more organized collagen strands and deform less under an applied load. Both fail in a nonlinear fashion.

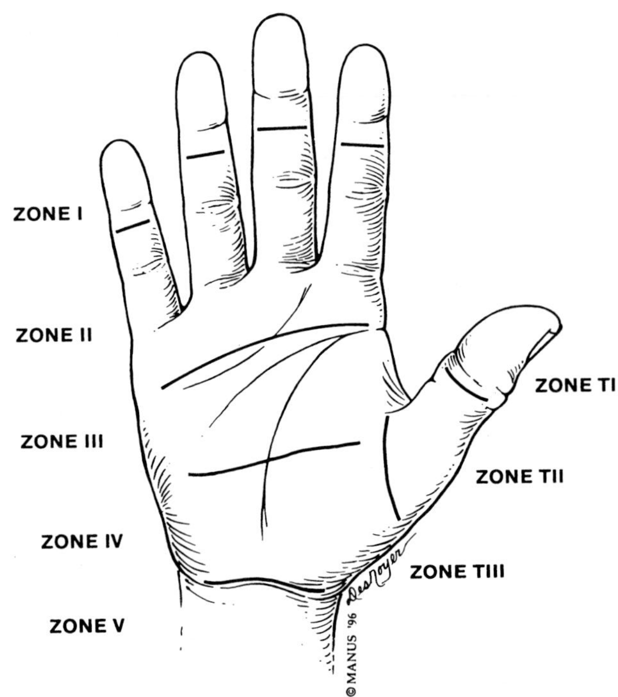

Figure 6–12. Zones of tendon injury. (From Green, D.H., Hotchkiss, R.M., and Pederson, W.C.: Green's Operative Hand Surgery, 4th ed. New York, Churchill Livingstone, 1998.)

1. Zone I (Distal to FDS Insertion)—Only FDP injured, direct repair is advocated. Profundus advancement of 1 cm or greater carries a risk of flexion contracture or inducing a quadrigia effect. Early patient-assisted passive range of motion (PROM) (Duran program) contributes to elongation of the repair and a 35% complication rate and should be avoided. Kleinert's protocol (dynamic splint assisted PROM) is preferred at this level. This can also be a result of an avulsion injury (rugger jersey finger) (Table 6–2).
2. Zone II (Within the Finger Flexor Retinaculum)—Also known as "no man's land" because for years repair of both tendons was thought to be fruitless. At this level both tendons (FDS/FDP) are injured. Repair of both tendons is now advocated, followed by an early mobilization program (Kleinert, Duran). The tendon laceration may be at a different level than the skin laceration depending on the position of the finger when laceration occurred.
3. Zone III (The Palm)—Concomitant neurovascular injury is likely, which dramatically diminishes the expected result. Good results from direct repair is usual because of absence of the retinacular structures.
4. Zone IV (The Carpal Tunnel)—Close

Table 6–2.

Leddy Classification of Profundus Avulsions

Type	Tendon Retraction Level	Repair	Interval/Treatment
I	Palm	(Disvascular)	7–10 days
II (most common)	PIPJ (held by vinculum longus)		3 mo
III	A4 pulley (held by bony avulsion fragment)	ORIF fragment	
IIIa	Type III but profundus also avulses off fracture fragment	Treatment based on level of tendon retraction	

quarters and synovial sheaths make postoperative adhesions likely. *The transverse carpal ligament should be repaired in a lengthened fashion,* which prevents bowstringing and allows for immobilization of the wrist in flexion.

5. Zone V (Wrist and Forearm)—Repairs in this zone have a favorable prognosis. The results are diminished when there is concomitant neurovascular injury.
6. Thumb—End-to-end repair of the FPL is advocated. It is recommended to work outside of zone III (beneath the thenar muscles) so as to avoid injury to the recurrent motor branch of the median nerve. The oblique pulley is the most important but, if necessary, either the A1 or the oblique pulley may be incised to facilitate repair. One of them should be preserved or bowstringing of the tendon will result.
7. Suture Technique—Core grasping suture: **Number of grasping loops not as significant as the number of suture strands that cross the repair site.** Circumferential epitendinous suture not only improves tendon gliding but also improves the strength of the repair and allows for less *gap formation, which is the initial event in repair failure.*
8. Sheath repair remains controversial. It supposedly takes advantage of the synovial pathway for tendon nutrition. However, clinical results with sheath repair are about the same as without. Most hand surgeons close the sheath if possible but will not go to great lengths to do so.
9. Postoperative controlled mobilization has been the major advance that has improved results of repair in zone II. It limits restrictive adhesions and improves tendon-healing biology. The two typically used protocols are the (1) Kleinert (active extension, dynamic splint assisted passive flexion). The Mayo synergistic splint is now favored because it incorporates active wrist motion improving overall tendon excursion. (2) Duran (active extension, patient-assisted passive flexion). Both programs essentially employ controlled motion for 6 weeks.
10. Flexor Tendon Reconstruction—Primary tendon graft is rarely used secondary to improved results with primary repair. A one-stage reconstruction is only advocated if the flexor sheath is pristine and the digit has full passive motion. Otherwise a two-stage procedure is advocated. A temporary silicone tendon implant is used to create a favorable bed for tendon graft. Active implants are available but provide little clinical benefit over the standard passive rod. Stage one is followed by a 3- to 4-month interval to allow for achieving tissue stability before the biologic tendon graft is placed. Total active motion of 260 degrees is usually achievable. Available grafts include the palmaris longus, which is most often used (absent in 15% of upper extremities [UEs]). The plantaris is an alternative if a longer graft is needed (absent in 19%). Otherwise a long toe extensor can be used.
11. Grafting Through an Intact Superficialis—If the patient can demonstrate a need, it may be considered (e.g., concert pianist, hand surgeon). Occasionally this is indicated in the small finger, where 34% of people have an incompetent FDS. In general it is avoided, but DIPJ fusion may be necessary if the joint is unstable.
12. Tenolysis may be indicated when there is a discrepancy between active and passive motion after therapy and the soft tissues have stabilized. Ideally it should be deferred until all adjacent joints have full passive motion. It is important to preserve critical pulleys (A2 and A4) during tenolysis. Postoperative therapy is extensive.
13. Pulley Reconstruction—Ideally one pulley should be placed proximal and distal to each joint requiring pulley reconstruction. Considerable force is placed on the reconstructed pulley: 3 N force on the fingertip generates 107 N force on the pulley. Available techniques include: triple loop (favored), fibrous rim method, belt loop method, FDS tail method.

IV. **Hand Infections**—Can involve any tissue type and a wide variety of pathogens. Early recognition and appropriate treatment followed by vigorous therapy are the keys to successful treatment.

A. Paronychia/Eponychia are the most common infections in the hand. These are infections of the nail fold and are most commonly caused by *Staphylococcus aureus*. It is treated by I&D including partial or total nail plate removal, oral antibiotics, and dressing changes. It is important to preserve the eponychial fold by placing material between the skin and the nail bed after débridement.

B. Felon—An infection of the finger tip pulp. It is similarly treated with I&D through midlateral incisions (the "fish-mouth" incision carries a risk of tip necrosis). It is important to break up the septa to adequately decompress the fingertip; otherwise, local compartment syndrome can occur. This is usually treated with IV antibiotics. Incisions are usually placed on the ulnar side except on the thumb and small finger, where they are placed on the radial side.

C. Human Bite—This is a potential serious infection that should be treated with I&D, especially if joints or tendon sheaths are violated. It most commonly involves the third or fourth MCP joints (fist to mouth). The most common organisms isolated are alpha-hemolytic strep and *S. aureus*. The incidence of *Eikenella corrodens* varies from 7% to 29%. Antibiotics of choice include ampicillin—sulbactam or Augmentin.

D. Dog and Cat Bites—Also potentially serious injuries often requiring I&D. The frequency of various isolates is as follows: alpha-hemolytic strep (46%), *Pasteurella multocida* (26%), *S. aureus* (13%), anaerobes (41%). Devastating infections causing digital necrosis can arise from the DF-2 organism. The drugs of choice include ampicillin—sulbactam or Augmentin. DF-2 infections are usually managed with penicillin.

E. Suppurative Flexor Tenosynovitis—An infection of the flexor tendon sheath. The cardinal clinical signs were described by Kanavel: flexed posture, fusiform swelling, pain with passive extension, and flexor sheath tenderness. If recognized early the patient can be admitted and treated with IV antibiotics. If the signs improve within the first 24 hours, surgery may be avoided. Otherwise, the treatment of choice is I&D and IV antibiotics. Many different incisions have been described; however, the principle is thorough irrigation of the involved tendon sheath. Continuous drip irrigation with an indwelling catheter carries a risk for compartment syndrome. The classic "horseshoe abscess" is based on proximal connection of thumb and small finger flexor sheaths in Parona's space (potential space between pronator quadratus and FDP tendons). Spread of infection into deep spaces is as follows: index and thumb to thenar space; long, ring, and small to midpalmar space; small can also spread into the ulnar bursa.

F. Herpetic Whitlow—Occurs with increased frequency in medical/dental personnel. It is a viral infection caused by herpes simplex virus. It presents clinically with pain followed by erythema, which then develops into a small vesicular rash, which may coalesce to form a bullae. The process is self-limited, usually resolving in 3–4 weeks. I&D is not recommended because rates of secondary bacterial infection are high.

G. Deep Potential Space Infections—**Collar button abscess** occurs in the web space between digits. It is treated by I&D with volar and dorsal incisions, which avoid incising the skin in the web, and IV antibiotics. **Midpalmar space infections** are rare. Clinically there is a loss of midline contour of the hand and palmar pain elicited with flexion of the long, ring, and small fingers. It is similarly treated with I&D and IV antibiotics. The **thenar space infection** presents with pain and swelling over the thenar eminence exacerbated by flexion of thumb and index finger. I&D and IV antibiotics are also required. The **hypothenar space infection** is also rare but it is treated the same way.

H. Necrotizing Fasciitis—Results from streptococci infection (gram-negative cocci known as Meleney's disease) or as a result of clostridia (gram-positive rod). Group A beta-hemolytic streptococci is the most common organism. Suspicion of this condition should be raised in host compromised patients (diabetes, CA). It requires emergency radical débridement and broad-spectrum antibiotic coverage started empirically to include: penicillin, clindamycin, metronidazole, and an aminoglycoside. Hemodynamic monitoring is a must. Amputation may be necessary because the average mortality rate is 32.2%. Hyperbaric oxygen is helpful when anaerobic organisms are present.

I. Fungal Infection—Serious infections are seen most frequently in host compromised patients. These infections are divided into three categories: cutaneous, subcutaneous, and deep. **Cutaneous**: Chronic infection of the nail fold most commonly caused by *Candida albicans*. It is treated with topical antifungals. Onychomycosis is a destructive, deforming infection of the nail plate most commonly caused by *Trichophyton rubrum*. This is also treated with topical antifungal agents; systemic therapy with griseofulvin or ketoconazole may be necessary. **Subcutaneous**: Most commonly caused by *Sporothrix schenckii*. It follows penetrating injury while handling plants or soil (rose thorn). It starts with a papule at the site of inoculation, with subsequent lesions developing along lymphatic channels. The treatment is potassium iodine supersaturated solution irrigation. **Deep:** Involves three forms: tenosynovial infection, septic arthritis, osteomyelitis. Treatment is based on fungal cultures and involves surgical débridement and an IV antifungal such as amphotericin B. True pathogens include: histoplasmosis, blastomycosis, coccidioidomycosis. Opportunistic infections include: aspergillosis, candidiasis, mucormycosis, cryptococcosis.

J. Atypical Mycobacterial Infections—These organisms are widely distributed in the environment but are infrequent human pathogens. The most common infecting organisms include: *M. marinum*, *M. kansasii*, *M. terrae*, *M. avium-intracellulare.* Musculoskeletal manifestations involve the wrist and hand in 50% of cases. *M. marinum:* proliferates in fresh and salt water enclosures. *M. avium-intracellulare:* found in soil, water, poultry (most frequently isolated organism in terminal AIDS patients). *M. kansasii* and *M. terrae:* found in soil. The diagnosis is based on biopsy for histopathology. Cultures and sensitivities are a must, and they require special medium at exact temperatures (**32°C**). A CXR is mandatory to rule out hematogenous spread. Treatment generally requires surgical débridement and oral antibiotics. Rifampin, ethambutol, or tetracycline is the drug of choice.

K. Hand Infection and HIV—Virulence of organism enhanced by immunocompromised state. The following organisms are frequent isolates: Viral (**herpes simplex**, cytomegalovirus), fungal (candidiasis, *Cryptococcus*, histoplasmosis, aspergillosis), protozoal, mycobacteria. Herpes simplex is the overall most common hand infection in AIDS patients.

V. **Vascular Occlusion/Disease**

A. Evaluation techniques include the **three-phase bone scan**—Phase I (pictures taken within 2 minutes: extremity arteriogram); Phase II (pictures at 5–10 minutes: soft-tissue images demonstrating cellulitis or synovial inflammation); Phase III (pictures taken at 2–3 hours: these are the bone images; reflex sympathetic dystrophy is demonstrated by a diffusely positive phase III image that does not correlate with positive phase I and II studies; osteomyelitis is also seen in this phase); Phase IV (delayed 24-hour films are useful to differentiate osteomyelitis from adjacent cellulitis if there is a question). **Segmental limb pressures** are done with a blood pressure cuff 1.2 × the diameter of the extremity and a 10-Mhz Doppler probe. A difference of 20 mm Hg between arms is abnormal. A difference of 1 mm Hg between fingers is abnormal. The sensitivity of the test is increased if also done after exercise. A **duplex scan** visualizes arterial intimal lesions, true and false aneurysms, and AV fistulas. **Photoplethysmography** demonstrates arterial insufficiency when there is a loss of the dicrotic notch or a decreased rate of rise in the systolic peak. **Cold stimulation testing** demonstrates autonomic vascular dysfunction because patients with arterial disease require more than 20 minutes to return to preexposure temperatures when submersed for 20 seconds in ice water, whereas normals experience return in 10 minutes. The **arteriogram** remains the *gold standard* for elucidating the nature and extent of thrombotic and embolic disease. It is invasive with antecedent risks; therefore, it is generally considered a preoperative test. **Ultrasound duplex imaging** is emerging as a noninvasive test with near equal sensitivity and specificity in experienced hands.

B. Compartment Syndrome—Caused by increased pressure in a closed fascial space leading to tissue ischemia, death, and fibrosis. Findings include the 5 Ps: pain, pallor, pulselessness, paresthesias, and paralysis. *Pain accentuated with passive stretch is the most sensitive indicator.* Compartment pressures are diagnostic when pressures are 30 mm Hg, indicating that immediate fasciotomy is required (use a lower threshold in hypotensive patients—20 mm Hg). Muscle viability is determined by the 4 Cs: color, consistency, contractility, capacity to bleed.

C. Volkmann's Ischemic Contracture—A posttraumatic wrist, hand, and forearm contracture resulting from death and fibrosis of forearm musculature. *The most severely involved muscles are the FDP and FPL.* Three varieties and their treatment have been described (Table 6–3).

D. **Occlusive Vascular Disease**—Can be caused by arterial trauma, emboli, atherosclerosis, or

Table 6–3.

Stages of Volkmann's Ischemic Contracture

Type	Affected Muscles	Treatment
Mild	Wrist flexors	Dynamic splinting, tendon lengthening
Moderate	Wrist and digital flexors	Excision necrotic muscle, neurolysis (median, ulnar), BR to FPL and ECRL to FDP tendon transfers, distal slide of viable flexors (usually FDS)
Severe	Flexors and extensors	Excision necrotic muscle, neurolysis, tendon transfers; may need functioning free muscle transfer if insufficient motors are available for transfer

a variety of systemic diseases. It presents with claudication, paresthesias, and cold intolerance. It tends to be unilateral, whereas vasospastic disease tends to be bilateral.

1. Post-traumatic—Most common in upper extremity is the hypothenar hammer syndrome, which is thrombosis of the ulnar artery as it emerges from Guyon's canal. Thrombus irritates the peri-adventitial sympathetic fibers, inducing vasospasm distally, which further embarrasses circulation; embolization can also occur and will *most likely affect the ring finger* because of the angle of take-off of the common digital arteries of the third and fourth webs. Options for treatment include resection of the thrombosed segment, effecting a local sympathectomy, or resection and reconstruction (with vein graft). Some advocate intraoperative digital brachial index (DBI) measurements to determine whether reconstruction is necessary. (DBI ≤0.7 would be an indication for reconstruction). It has been suggested in the literature that re-establishing circulation may diminish cold intolerance.
2. Embolic Disease—Upper-extremity emboli compose 20% of all arterial emboli; of these 70% are of cardiac origin. Occasionally emboli are derived from the subclavian system as a result of thoracic outlet syndrome. Once recognized, the patient is heparinized and embolectomy is performed if possible. Heparin is continued for 7–10 days followed by 3 months of warfarin. If the vessels affected are too small for embolectomy, streptokinase and urokinase have been shown to be beneficial, especially if done within 36 hours of occlusion. Tissue-plasminogen activator is currently the favored thrombolytic agent because of its specificity for the clot and long-lasting effect. If the emboli are from a proximal aneurysm, this is treated with resection of the aneurysm and reconstruction of the vessel. Sympathectomy will only relieve vasospasm and not prevent further embolization.
3. **Arteritis and Other Systemic Diseases**
   a. **Thromboangiitis Obliterans** (Buerger's Disease)—A vasculitis seen in smokers that initially involves distal vessels and progresses proximally. The treatment is simple for the doctor and hard for the patient: STOP SMOKING. Ischemic lesions are treated with wound care and amputation if necessary.
   b. **Giant Cell Arteritis**—Mainly involves arteries of the head and aortic branches in older women. In the upper extremity, involvement of the subclavian and axillary artery is seen. When associated with myalgias and arthralgias, it constitutes the syndrome known as *polymyalgia rheumatica*. Temporal artery biopsy is diagnostic. Treatment is with high-dose steroids and arterial reconstruction if ischemia persists.
   c. **Takayasu's Arteritis**—Also involves the subclavian and axillary artery but is more prevalent in young women. Intimal proliferation is responsible for the arterial stenosis. This condition has variable response to steroids.
   d. **Polyarteritis Nodosa**—A necrotizing arteritis associated with aneurysmal dilatations of small vessels. These lesions have a predilection for bifurcations and tend to occur at the level of the bifurcation of the common digital arteries in the upper extremity.
   e. **Connective Tissue Disorders** (Lupus, Scleroderma, RA)—Can cause segmental arterial occlusion from deposition of antigen-antibody complexes in the vascular endothelium. This usually occurs at the level of the digital arteries and presents with ischemia with superimposed vasospastic disease. Treatment involves getting the underlying disease process under control and treating the vasospasm as described later.
   f. **Atherosclerosis**—Usually involves the subclavian and axillary arteries and is more common on the left side (3:1). Proximal subclavian occlusions can induce a subclavian steal syndrome wherein blood is shunted away from the brain stem by a reversal of flow in the vertebral artery to meet the upper extremity demands. In proximal subclavian occlusions (proximal to vertebral artery), CNS symptoms are more common; with distal subclavian occlusions, arm claudication is more common. Digital ischemia is more frequently caused by emboli than by distal plaques. This is treated with extra-anatomic bypass of the subclavian artery.

E. **Vasospastic Disease**—Symptoms include periodic digital ischemia brought on by cold temperatures or other sympathetic stimuli to include emotional stress or pain. Initially fingers blanch (white), followed closely by cyanosis (blue) as deoxygenated blood pools during persistent vasospasm. The final ruborous (red) appearance is associated with vasodilation and is coincident with burning pain and dysesthesias.

1. **Raynaud's**
   a. **Phenomenon**: Episodic digital ischemia with typical color changes and dysesthesias.
   b. **Syndrome**: When Raynaud's phenomenon occurs as a result of a disease (Table 6–4). These patients are generally older than those with Raynaud's disease, trophic changes are usually present, pulses

Table 6–4.

Causes of Secondary Vasospastic Disorder

1. Connective tissue disease: scleroderma (incidence of Raynaud's 80–90%), SLE (incidence 18–26%), dermatomyositis (incidence 30%), RA (incidence 11%)
2. Occlusive arterial disease
3. Neurovascular compression: thoracic outlet syndrome
4. Hematologic abnormalities: cryoproteinemia, polycythemia, paraproteinemia
5. Occupational trauma: percussion and vibratory tool workers
6. Drugs and toxins: sympathomimetics, ergot compounds, beta-adrenergic blockers
7. CNS disease: syringomyelia, poliomyelitis, tumors/infarcts
8. Miscellaneous: RSD, malignant disease

are often absent, the problem is usually asymmetric, and an angiogram often demonstrates a lesion.

c. **Disease**: Primary vasospastic disorder that is usually seen in young women. In order to make the diagnosis, symptoms and characteristics must satisfy Allen and Brown's criteria: (1) intermittent attacks of discoloration of the acral parts, (2) bilateral involvement, (3) absence of clinical arterial occlusion, (4) gangrene or atrophic changes are rare, (5) symptoms present for 2 years, (6) absence of previous disease to which vascular reactivity can be attributed, (7) a predominance in women.

Treatment is focused on the underlying disease (if known) and a common-sense approach such as: avoid cold exposure and stop smoking. Medical intervention includes: intra-arterial reserpine (*does not help ulcer healing*), calcium channel blockers, or drugs aimed at improving blood elements (aspirin [A.S.A.], dipyridamole [Persantine], pentoxifylline [Trental]). Thermal biofeedback is helpful in 67–92% of patients. Microvascular reconstruction can be helpful if a damaged or occluded area can be identified and the underlying disease can be controlled. Digital sympathectomy can be considered after proving it will be of benefit with pulse volume recordings before and after local sympathetic block.

F. Reflex Sympathetic Dystrophy—Neurologic dysfunction following trauma, prolonged immobilization, surgery, or disease characterized by intense/exaggerated pain, vasomotor disturbance, delayed functional recovery, hyperhidrosis, swelling, osteopenia, and trophic skin changes. It is caused by sustained efferent sympathetic nerve activity perpetuated in a reflex arc. If it is associated with a definable nerve injury it is known as causalgia. The stages have been described by Lankford and Evans (Table 6–5).

Diagnosis—Four cardinal signs include: disproportionate amount of pain, swelling, stiffness, discoloration. Relief with sympathetic blockade is diagnostic. Thermography, radiographs, and a three-phase bone scan are also helpful. *Early diagnosis is critical to successful treatment.* Treatment includes physical therapy (pain-free AROM, fluidotherapy, transcutaneous electrical nerve simulation). Sympathectomy, either chemical (four blocks of the stellate ganglion) or surgical (if persistent symptoms after four blocks or symptoms >6 months' duration), can be curative. Prevention is the key (avoiding nerve injury, tight dressings, or prolonged immobilization).

G. Frostbite—Rapid rewarming (40–44°C water baths) is done with analgesia, tetanus prophylaxis, antibiotics, and wound care. Delay amputation until complete demarcation and mummification has occurred. Active and passive ROM and functional splinting are done from the start. Surgical sympathectomy may be required for late persistent vasospastic disease. Anticoagulation, dextran, and intra-arterial reserpine are not useful.

VI. **Replantation/Microsurgery**

A. Traumatic Amputation

1. Favorable indications for replantation
   a. Almost any part in a child
   b. Multiple digits
   c. Individual digit distal to the FDS insertion
   d. Thumb
   e. Wrist or proximal
2. Unfavorable indications for replantation
   a. Individual finger proximal to FDS insertion
   b. Crushed or mangled parts
   c. Amputations at multiple levels
   d. Arteriosclerotic vessels
   e. Other serious injury or disease
   f. Mentally unstable patients
   g. Signs of severe vessel trauma (red line

Table 6–5.

Stages

Stage	Onset (Months)	Findings
Acute	0–3	Pain, swelling, warmth, redness, decreased ROM, normal radiographs, positive three-phase bone scan, hyperhidrosis
Subacute	3–12	Worse pain, cyanosis, dry skin, worse stiffness, atrophy of skin, osteopenia on radiograph
Chronic	>12	Diminished pain, fibrosis, glossy skin that is dry and cool, joint contractures, extreme osteopenia

sign: branch tears along vessel; ribbon sign: elastic recoil from traction media and intima usually separated)

3. Care of the Amputated Part—Replantation is not recommended if warm ischemia time is >6 hours for level proximal to the carpus or >12 hours for a digit. Cool ischemia times of <12 hours proximal to carpus or <24 hours for a digit; retain the option for replantation. The amputated part should be wrapped in moist gauze (lactated Ringer's solution); this is placed in a sealed plastic bag, which is then placed on regular ice (not dry ice).
4. Operative Sequence of Replantation—(1) bone, (2) extensor tendons, (3) flexor tendons, (4) arteries, (5) nerves, (6) veins, (7) skin. *For multiple amputations, the structure-by-structure technique is faster and has a higher viability rate.* The priority for digit replantation is thumb, long, ring, small, index.
5. Postoperative Care Includes—Warm room (80°F), adequate hydration, aspirin, dipyridamole, low-molecular-weight dextran 30–40 mL/hr, and heparin if necessary. There is a higher incidence of postoperative hemorrhage when two anticoagulants are used with aspirin rather than one (53% rate rather than 2% rate). Nicotine, caffeine, and chocolate are not allowed.
6. Monitoring—Close observation of color, capillary refill, and Doppler pulse remains the most reliable method. Skin surface temperature is a noninvasive, reproducible, and safe method to aid close observation. A drop in temperature >2°C in 1 hour or temperature below 30°C indicates decreased digital perfusion.
7. Arterial Insufficiency—If arterial insufficiency develops: release constricting bandages, place the extremity in a dependent position, consider heparinization, consider stellate ganglion blockade, explore early if these maneuvers don't work. Thrombosis secondary to vasospasm is the most frequent cause for early replant failure. If this happens, revision of the anastomosis will likely be required.
8. Inadequate Venous Outflow—Causes part engorgement, diminished inflow, and eventually part loss. It is treated with extremity elevation. If this fails to resolve the problem, leeches are tried (they produce the anticoagulant hirudin, which yields 8–12 hours of sustained bleeding; *Aeromonas hydrophila* infection is a risk). If leeches are not available or tolerated by the patient or nursing staff, heparin-soaked pledgets can be used. A last resort is a surgical arteriovenous anastomosis.
9. Complications—No. 1, infection; No. 2, cold intolerance (which can last up to 2 years post replantation). *Smoking causes a more pronounced effect on vasoconstriction in the replanted digit compared with the normal digit.*
10. Forearm and Arm Replantations—Muscle necrosis leads to *myoglobinuria, which can precipitate renal failure and threaten the patient's life;* infection is also prevalent because of the difficulty in obtaining a sufficient débridement. Arterial inflow is established early (usually before skeletal stabilization), using shunts if necessary, to minimize ischemia time. Fasciotomies are always performed. Fastidious débridement and second-look surgery in 72 hours are necessary. Blood loss during the procedure must be closely monitored.

B. Ring Avulsion Injuries—Classified based on the extent of the injury (Urbaniak)
   1. Class 1: Circulation adequate, standard bone and soft-tissue treatment.
   2. Class 2: Circulation inadequate, vessel repair preserves viability (others have divided 2 into 2A: no additional bone tendon nerve injury, and 2B: these additional injuries are present).
   3. Class 3: Complete degloving or complete amputation.

   Advances in technique with interposition grafts have improved results with replantation of these injuries. In general, class 2B and 3 injuries are better treated with amputation. The most common complication after successful replantation is cold intolerance (30–70% incidence).

C. Finger Tip Amputations—The goal is to provide a sensate, durable tip with adequate bony support for the nail. It is generally agreed that when the surface area lost is 1 cm^2 and there is no bone exposed, healing by secondary intention yields a satisfactory result. For many this is the treatment of choice whenever there is no bone exposed. Others argue that wound contraction will draw the nail down over the tip, causing a hook-nail deformity. It is universally agreed that any type of closure that draws the nail bed curving over the tip will lead to a hook nail deformity, so *tight tip closures should be avoided.* If for some reason healing by secondary intention is judged not to be a satisfactory option, full-thickness skin graft from the hypothenar eminence is a good choice. If bone is exposed it may be rongeured back so long as the bone loss does not compromise the support of the nail bed. If rongeuring the bone is judged to be a bad choice, a coverage procedure is indicated because exposed bone will impede healing by secondary intention. Straight or dorsally angulated amputations are best covered with a volar VY advancement flap or a double lateral VY advancement flap of Kutler (Fig. 6–13). The volar arterialized advancement flap of Moberg is a reasonable choice in the thumb, but it leads to excessive joint stiffness in a finger. A volarly angled amputation is covered with a cross finger flap, a thenar crease flap, or a thenar H flap. The thenar crease and thenar H flaps can lead to joint contractures in adults because the PIP joint is held in flexion for 2 weeks before the pedicle is divided. These flaps are generally best reserved for young people. Other more complex flaps such as the second dorsal metacarpal artery island flap (comes with a nerve and is sometimes used for thumb tip coverage) or the homodigital island flap (must prove that both digital arteries are intact before harvesting this flap) are available if the aforementioned choices are judged to be insufficient or less desirable.

D. Microsurgery

1. Wound Classification—It is important to obtain early consultation (first 48 hours) from the reconstructive surgeon who may be assisting with wound management. It is generally accepted that limb salvage is not indicated when a sensate limb is not achievable, when adequate débridement is not achievable, and when a limb with sufficient mobility and stability is not achievable. The single most important procedure is early aggressive wound débridement (ideally within 6 hours of injury). Several classification systems are available that aide in wound assessment and therefore treatment decisions. The mangled extremity severity score (MESS) provides a guide to determining the expected outcome from a limb salvage attempt by weighing the energy of injury, limb ischemia, hemodynamic status, and the patient's age (Table 6–6). A MESS score >7 is a relative contraindication to limb salvage, whereas a score <4 indicates a limb with a good prognosis if salvaged. The current literature suggests that this system is not as useful for upper extremity trauma. The Gustilo classification of open fractures (see Chapter 10) remains a useful tool because it emphasizes the condition of the soft-tissue envelope. Wounds that have a compromised soft-tissue envelope are more likely to develop infection (Gustilo types I–IIIA 12% infection rate, Gustilo types IIIB and IIIC 56% infection rate) and are also more likely to go on to nonunion.
2. Timing of Wound Coverage—Early coverage of traumatic wounds has the following advantages: lower flap failure rate, effects of fibrosis minimized, easier flap planning and vessel anastomoses, less vascular spasm and the veins are easier to work with, lower infection rates, diminished time of hospitalization, less tissue desiccation, fewer number of overall surgeries to final result. Godina noted in a large series of complex lower extremity trauma cases an advantage to early soft-tissue coverage. Wounds that were covered in less than 6 days had the fewest complications (0.7%). Those covered between 6 days and 3 months had the highest failure rate (17.5%). Those that were covered after 3 months when the wound had stabilized had an intermediate result (9% failure rate). Lister has noted similar findings in complex upper extremity trauma.
3. The Reconstructive Ladder—The goal is to restore the limb to useful function while diminishing morbidity using the simplest methods that are judged to be appropriate for the wound in question. Primary closure is considered first. If this is not an option, successively more complex methods are considered: delayed primary closure, skin grafting, rotation flap, and finally free flap coverage.
   a. Primary Wound Closure—Undue tension causes local tissue ischemia and wound dehiscence or compartment syndrome. Wounds that are clean, with minimal bacterial contamination, and that are less than 6 hours old are usually safe to close primarily.
   b. Secondary Wound Closure—Closure by wound granulation and epithelialization. This requires regular dressing changes and is associated with contraction over time. The Papino graft (filling the defect with cancellous bone graft) is intended to stimulate this process when bone is exposed. This method poses some danger of late infection when devascularized tissues are present within the wound (such as bone stripped of its periosteum). Granulation can occur over exposed implants, but it takes a very long time.
   c. Skin Grafts—Require a well vascularized bed in order for them to take. Split-thickness grafts are 0.012–0.025 inches thick. The thinner the graft, the more wound contraction will occur. Donor sites re-epithelialize because dermal papillae are left behind. Once it is re-epithelialized it can be used for skin graft again if needed. Meshing a split-thickness graft increases the surface area that can be covered and allows for egress of hematoma. Failure of skin grafting is caused by shear, hematoma, and infection. Full-thickness grafts have a higher failure rate than split-thickness grafts, but they yield a better cosmetic result

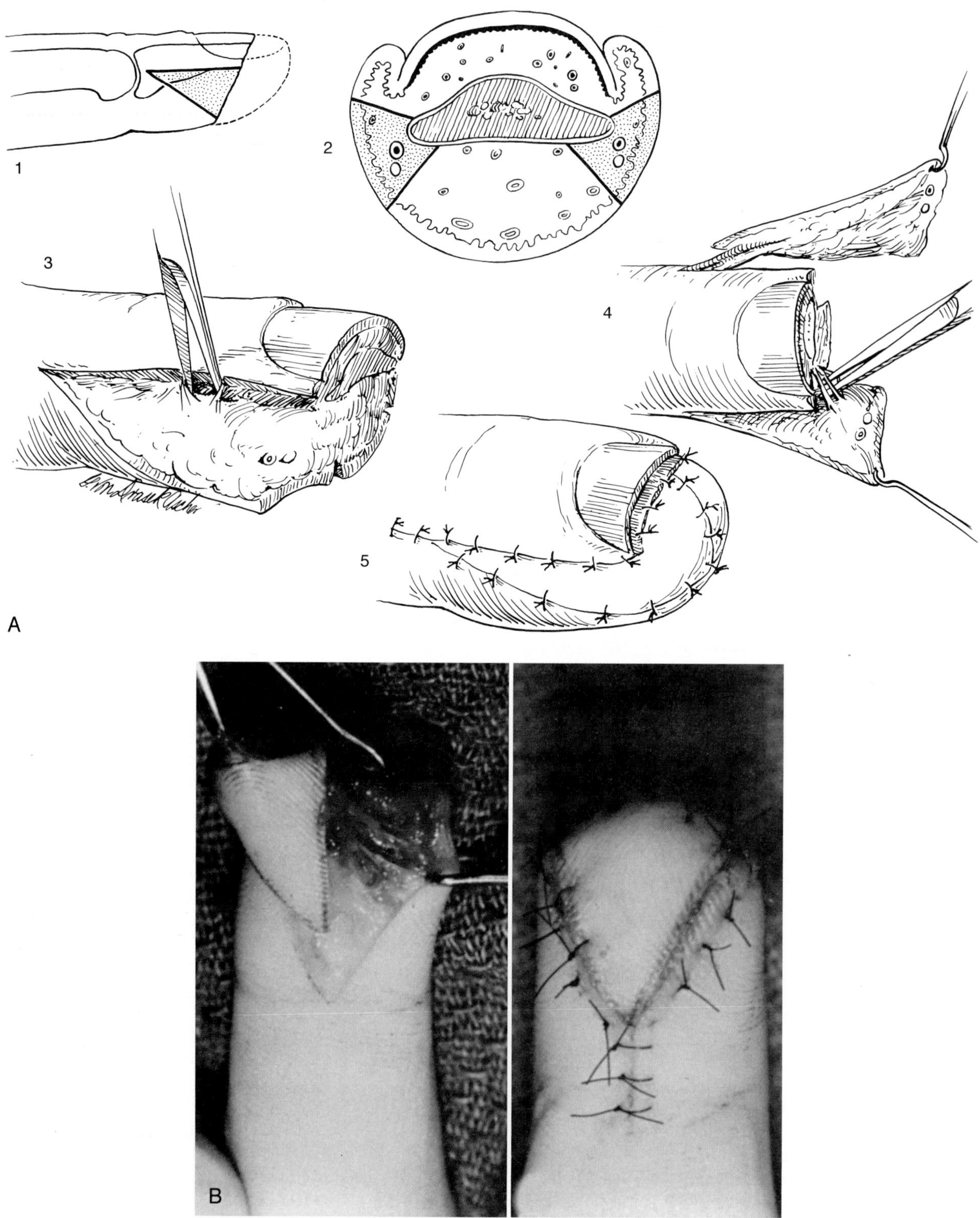

Figure 6–13. *A,* Kutler double lateral V-Y advancements. (1) The advancement flaps are designed over the neurovascular pedicles and carried right down to the bone (2). The fibrous septa are defined and (3) divided, permitting free mobilization (4) on the neurovascular pedicles alone. The flaps then advance readily to the midline (5). *B,* The volar V-Y advancement flap. (From Green, D.H., Hotchkiss, R.M., and Pederson, W.C.: Green's Operative Hand Surgery, 4th ed. New York, Churchill Livingstone, 1998.)

Table 6–6.

Mangled Extremity Severity Score

Criteria	Score
Energy of Injury	
Low	1
Medium	2
High	3
Massive	4
Ischemia*	
No ischemia	0
Decreased pulses	1
Thready pulses	2
No pulses	3
Shock	
Normal	0
Transient	1
Prolonged	2
Age	
<30 yrs	0
30–50 yrs	1
>50 yrs	2

*Ischemia score doubles when warm ischemia time >6 hrs.

and are generally more durable than split-thickness grafts. *Full-thickness grafts do not contract* and for that reason are preferable to cover hand defects, except for the dorsum of the hand, where a nonmeshed split-thickness graft yields the best results. Full-thickness grafts regain better sensibility because of more retained sensory receptors.

d. Flap Reconstruction—A flap is a unit of tissue that is supported by blood vessels and is moved from a donor site to a recipient site to cover a defect of tissue. This unit can be composed of one or several tissue types to include: Skin, fascia, muscle, tendon, nerve, and bone. A flap composed of more than one tissue type is called a composite flap. Flap reconstruction has some biologic advantages, such as lower secondary infection rates and higher bone union rates. This relates to a flap's ability to improve a portion of the soft-tissue envelope by virtue of the fact that it is vascularized. Flaps are indicated when the wound has exposed tissue such as bone (stripped of its periosteum), tendons (stripped of paratenon), cartilage, or orthopaedic implants that cannot revascularize a skin graft. They are also indicated when a skin graft may impair later reconstruction or be subject to excessive exposure and repeated ulceration. Flaps can be classified by their vascular supply, tissue type, and donor site location and method of transfer.

1) Classification according to blood supply
   a) Axial pattern flaps have a single arteriovenous pedicle (types include: peninsular [pedicle and overlying skin] rotation flap, island [pedicle only] rotation flap, free flap).
   b) Random pattern flaps are supported by the microcirculation with no single arteriovenous system (e.g., Z-plasty).
   c) Venous flaps involve flow though the venous system only where the distal vein in the flap is hooked up to a donor artery and the proximal vein in the flap is hooked up to a recipient vein.
2) Classification according to tissue type
   a) Cutaneous flaps include skin and subcutaneous tissue (e.g., thenar H flap).
   b) Fascia and fasciocutaneous flaps include fascia with or without the overlying skin (e.g., radial forearm flap).
   c) Muscle and musculocutaneous flaps involve perforators supplied via the pedicle that allow harvesting with overlying skin if needed (e.g., latissimus dorsi). If the motor nerve is not preserved, a muscle flap will atrophy to about 50% of its original size.
   d) Bone and osteocutaneous flaps (e.g., fibula with or without overlying skin).
   e) Composite flaps are composed of several tissue types, allowing for single-stage reconstructions (e.g., free toe transfer).
   f) Innervated flaps involve a tissue unit with its nerve supply. These can involve a motor nerve (e.g., gracilis flap: motor branch of obturator nerve) or a sensory nerve (e.g., lateral arm flap: posterior cutaneous nerve of the arm).
3) Classification according to mobilization
   a) Local—Transposition flaps are geometric in their design and can be random pattern (rhomboid flap) or axial pattern (first dorsal metacarpal artery island flap) regarding their blood supply. A Z-plasty is a form of a transposition flap. The lengths of the limbs of a Z-plasty should always be the same. The angles can vary. As the angle increases, so does the lengthening that occurs along the line of the

central limb. The commonly used 60-degree angle theoretically yields a 75% lengthening along the line of the central limb. If sufficient skin is not available for one large Z-plasty, they can be done in series. *The longitudinal gain is aggregate, whereas the transverse loss is not.* Rotation flaps are not geometric and are all random pattern regarding their blood supply. (*It is important not to make a random pattern flap longer than the width of the base so as not to exceed the capacity of the microcirculation.*) Advancement flaps advance in a straight line to fill the defect; they can also be either random pattern (VY advancement flap) or axial pattern (Moberg's advancement flap).

b) Distant—Flaps can be transferred either in stages or in a single stage as a free tissue transfer. Flaps transferred in stages are raised from their anatomic location and placed in the defect without dividing the base (groin flap). Neovascularization occurs from the wound bed into the graft. After this (usually at 14–21 days), the pedicle of the flap is divided and inset into the defect. Free flaps are all axial pattern. They are raised on the pedicle, which is then divided and reanastamosed to donor vessels in the same operation. *It is important to remember that the anastomoses should be done out of the zone of injury.*

4. Causes of Flap Failure—The main cause is inadequate arterial blood flow. Often vasospasm is the culprit leading to thrombosis at the anastomosis. Other factors that compromise inflow include hypotension, compression, hematoma, edema, infection, hypothermia, and vasoconstrictive agents such as nicotine. Outflow problems can also lead to the demise of a flap. In this situation the flap will become engorged with blood as evidenced by a purple discoloration and brisk capillary refill. Eventually, altered hemodynamic pressure differentials can compromise inflow, leading to flap failure.
5. Thumb Reconstruction—*The wrap-around procedure: best duplicates thumb appearance and size.* The great toe transfer: provides mobility and growth potential, and it is very stable. The second toe transfer: provides mobility and growth potential, but it is the least stable. The great and second toe transfers have the same vascular pedicle: first dorsal metatarsal artery, a branch of the dorsalis pedis, runs superficially in 78% of cases. In 22% of cases it arises deeply from the descending branch of the dorsalis pedis artery to ascend in the first metatarsal space, coursing beneath or through the first dorsal interosseous muscle. Indications include traumatic loss and congenital deficiency. If pollicization of a damaged digit that is not useful in its orthotopic location is an option, this is preferable over toe-to-hand transfer. The wrap-around procedure is preferred when loss is distal to a mobile MCP joint in an adult. The great toe transfer is otherwise preferred because of its stability. The second toe transfer is useful when length is needed, requiring the MCP joint and a portion of the second metatarsal. Harvesting the great toe MCP joint should be avoided. Osteoplastic reconstruction is considered in patients who are not good candidates for microarterial anastomosis if no option for pollicization exists.
6. Microsurgical Bone Reconstruction—Donor sites include any expendable bone with an identifiable vascular pedicle (most commonly used are the fibula and the anterior iliac crest). The free fibula is based on the peroneal artery pedicle and is useful for diaphyseal reconstruction. The free iliac crest is based on the deep circumflex iliac vessels and is useful for metaphyseal reconstruction. Indications include extensive post-traumatic defects (>6–8 cm, best results), post-tumor intercalary resection, osteomyelitis (worst results), congenital pseudoarthrosis of the tibia or ulna, resistant nonunions, failed prior conventional bone graft, postirradiation fractures, allograft nonunion, avascular necrosis. Success rates average 88% overall. The best results are in nonseptic cases. Adjuvant radiation and chemotherapy adversely effect results. Average time to union is 6 months.
7. Microsurgical Joint Transfer—Remains controversial. Donor sites include the MTP or PIPJ of the second toe. Indications include a destroyed PIPJ or MCP joint in a child with associated epiphyseal plate injury or in young active persons who are not candidates for conventional arthroplasty. A limited but useful ROM with good lateral stability can usually be achieved (adult 32 degrees, child 37 degrees). The chief complication is the limited ROM.
8. Microsurgical Functioning Free Muscle Transfer—The most frequently used donor is the gracilis muscle (nerve; anterior division of obturator; vessel; branch of medial femoral circumflex artery). Alternatives associated with success include the latissimus dorsi, pectoralis major, rectus femoris, semitendinosis, and medial gastrocnemius. The chief indication is restoration of active

digital flexion in a severe Volkmann ischemic contracture. Prerequisites include full passive motion of the digits and wrist and a stable wrist joint. Results are markedly better if the intrinsics are intact. Overall, 83% of patients have return of some degree of useful function. Other indications include brachial plexus palsy reconstruction.

9. Defects Over the Tibia—A gastrocnemius flap is used for wounds over the proximal third (medial head for medial and midline defects, lateral head for lateral defects). A soleus flap is used for wounds in the middle one third of the leg if the soleus is in good condition. Free flaps are generally used for wounds over the distal third of the leg if a fasciocutaneous pedicle flap such as the sural artery island flap is not available. Free flaps are also used for extensive defects, particularly when the gastrocnemius and soleus are damaged. Getting the anastomoses out of the zone of injury can be challenging in extensive lower extremity trauma.

VII. Wrist Pain/Instability

A. Introduction—Wrist Evaluation

1. Functional ROM

Motion	Degrees
Dorsiflexion	40
Volarflexion	40
Radioulnar deviation arc	40

2. Examination involves bilateral functional assessment, including: ROM, digital flexion/extension lags, sensibility, grip strength, and provocative maneuvers.

Provocative Maneuvers

Eponym	Tests For Instability At:
Watson test	Scapholunate (SL) interval
Regan test	Lunotriquetral (LT) interval
Klienman test	Dynamic assessment LT instability
Lichtman test	Dynamic assessment of midcarpal instability
TFCC grind	Assessment for TFCC pathology
ECU snap	Assessment for unstable ECU
Piano key sign	DRUJ instability

3. Plain radiographs

Interval	Normal Angle, Gap, or Relationship
SL angle	30–60 degrees (average 47 degrees)
Capitolunate angle	0–15 degrees
Radiolunate angle	−25 to +10 degrees
SL gap	<3 mm

4. Arthroscopy—Has been shown to be more sensitive and specific than arthrography and as least as sensitive and specific as arthrotomy. Other valuable diagnostic tests include: fluoroscopic motion studies (dynamic instability), bone scan (infection, RSD), MRI (avascular necrosis [AVN], ligament disruptions, tumors), CT scan (fractures, structural abnormalities), and diagnostic injections. Arthrography has fallen out of favor because of its lack of specificity.

5. Kinematics—The proximal carpal row (scaphoid, lunate, and triquetrum) flexes in radial deviation and extends in ulnar deviation. There are two main theories as to why this happens. Radial side theory (Linschied): With radial deviation there is a rotational moment on the scaphoid via forces applied by the radius and the trapezium, which favors flexion. In ulnar deviation the radioscaphocapitate and scaphotrapezial ligaments tighten, lifting the scaphoid into extension. Ulnar side theory (Weber): With radial deviation the triquetrum moves to the dorsoradial facet of the helicoid hamate joint. This flexes the lunate and the scaphoid via forces transmitted through the interosseous ligaments. In ulnar deviation the triquetrum translates to the volar ulnar facet of the hamate, subsequently extending the rest of the proximal carpal row. There is probably truth to both of these theories, with both mechanisms contributing to motion of the proximal carpal row, the radial theory being predominant in radial deviation and the ulnar theory being predominant in ulnar deviation (author's opinion).

B. Wrist Instability—Classification; this helps to localize the instability based on established patterns recognizable on plain radiographs. The advent of arthroscopy of the wrist and MRI have identified lesser degrees of instability amenable to treatment, usually with less invasive methods than open surgery.

1. CID (Carpal Instability Dissociative)—Disruption of an intercarpal ligament within a carpal row.

a. Dorsal Intercalated Segment Instability (DISI)—Disruption of the scapholunate ligament or unstable fracture of the scaphoid. Usually there is associated disruption of the volar radiocarpal ligaments. Other causes associated with DISI include Kienbock's disease and distal radius malunions. Pertinent radiographic findings include a scapholunate (SL) gap >3 mm on PA view with clenched fist (Terry Thomas' sign). There can be a break in Gilula's arc at the scapholunate interval, although this is not always abnormal. There also may be a cortical ring sign. An SL angle >60 degrees on neutral rotation lateral and an abnormal radiolunate angle are also seen. An unstable scaphoid fracture is associated with malalignment in flexion and scaphoid foreshortening—the so-called humpback deformity. It is seen radiographically by displacement >1 mm, SL angle >60 degrees, capitolunate (CL) angle >15 degrees. Current treatment recommendations for a scapholunate instability with DISI are repair of the scapholunate ligament (linkage procedure) if possible (effective up to 17 months from injury in one study). If the ligament is not repairable, a stabilization procedure such as a scaphotrapezialtrapezoidal (triscaphe) (STT) fusion (scapholunocapitate or scaphocapitate are also favored fusions) is advised. Reconstruction of the ligament with a tendon weave is currently not advised because of high incidence of late failure. A number of bone retinaculum reconstructions are currently under investigation. Early reports suggest that they are effective for dynamic instability. A Blatt dorsal capsulodesis is often added to a ligament repair and remains a viable alternative for a chronic instability when ligament repair is not feasible. Unstable scaphoid fractures are best treated by open reduction, internal fixation (ORIF).

b. Volar Intercalated Segment Instability (VISI)—Involves disruption of the lunotriquetral interosseous ligament. A static instability pattern will not be evident unless the dorsal radiocarpal ligament is also disrupted (Viegas S) as well as the ulnocapitate ligament (Trumble T). Pertinent radiographic findings include a break in Gilula's arc on the PA view and a radiolunate or capitolunate angle >15 degrees. Arthroscopy is helpful in establishing this diagnosis. Options for treatment include multiple pin fixation (dynamic instability) or fusion of the lunotriquetral (LT) interval (static instability). In patients with additional ulnar positive variation and ulnocarpal impaction, both the LT instability and the ulnocarpal impaction are well managed with an ulnar-shortening osteotomy. Ligament reconstructions have fallen out of favor because of late recurrent instability.

c. Axial Carpal Instability—Secondary to violent trauma causing intercarpal disruption of the proximal and distal rows as well as the intermetacarpal bases in a longitudinal fashion. These injuries have been classified by Garcia-Elias into axial-radial, axial-ulnar, and combined. They are treated with reduction and pinning as well as prolonged casting.

2. CIND (Carpal Instability Nondissociative)—Ligamentous disruption leading to instability between rows (radiocarpal or midcarpal). These patients present with complaints of subluxations that may or may not be painful but give them a feeling of giving way and an unreliable clunking wrist. Generally, these patients are ligamentously lax but it also occurs after trauma. Cineradiographic examination will show a sudden shift of the proximal carpal row (DISI or VISI) with active radial or ulnar deviation. Nonoperative management with 6–8 weeks of immobilization is tried first; if this fails the most reliable option for treatment is a fusion across the unstable joint. Again the ligament reconstruction approach does not yield lasting results in most series.

3. CIC (Carpal Instability Combined)—Ligamentous disruption both within and between rows.
   a. Classic example is the perilunate dislocation. The arc of this injury can course through bone (i.e., trans-scaphoid or transradial styloid perilunar injury), which is known as the greater arc. When the disruption courses though ligaments around the lunate, this is known as the lesser arc. It can involve a combination of both the greater and lesser arcs. Radiographs will demonstrate breaks in Gilula's arcs as well as signs of instability in the involved intervals as previously described. Mayfield described four stages of perilunar instability proceeding from radial to ulnar around the lunate involving the following joints: (1) SL, (2) SL and CL, (3) SL and CL and LT, (4) lunate dislocates from the radiocarpal joint, usually in a volar direction. This injury is treated by open reduction pin fixation and a prolonged period of casting (8–12 weeks). The efficacy of direct repair of the disrupted volar ligaments has not been definitively shown to be beneficial. **Poor outcome correlates most closely with a persistently elevated scapholunate gap.**
   b. Scaphocapitate Syndrome—This is an uncommon variant of the perilunate dissociation wherein the arc of injury proceeds through the neck of the capitate and the proximal fragment rotates 90–180 degrees. This obviously could lead to a midcarpal arthritis problem if not recognized and dealt with. If recognized early, treat with open reduction and

fixation of the capitate fragment. If recognized late, options include excision of the fragment with or without interposition grafts, silicone replacement versus ORIF if the cartilage is still good, or a midcarpal fusion may be necessary.

C. Limited Arthrodesis—Most reliable way to correct instability if the patient is willing to sacrifice motion. Fusion across a joint or interval is associated with the following percentage loss of motion: radiocarpal, 55–60%; midcarpal, 20–35%; between two bones in the same row, 10–20%.

D. Other Common Causes of Wrist Pain

1. Scaphoid Fracture

a. The major blood supply is from the radial artery, branches of which enter at the dorsal ridge and supply the proximal 80% of the bone. There is another group of vessels, which are branches of the superficial palmar branch of the radial artery, that enter the bone in the distal tubercle and supply the distal 30%. Because of the end-artery arrangement of the vascular supply, fractures of the proximal fifth of the scaphoid are associated with an AVN rate of 100%; those of the proximal one third are associated with an AVN rate of 33%.

b. Incidence of Fracture Location Within the Bone—Waist, 65%; proximal third, 25%; distal third, 10%

c. Treatment—A bone scan has a specificity of 98% and a sensitivity of 100% and is therefore the best test to diagnose an occult scaphoid fracture. It should be positive within 24 hours of injury. The vast majority of stable scaphoid fractures are well treated by casting. It is important to start immobilization early because nonunion rates are significantly increased when immobilization is delayed beyond 4 weeks from fracture. The type of cast is controversial, and literature support can be found for nearly anything; therefore, this remains surgeon's preference. However Gellman and coworkers (*Journal of Bone and Joint Surgery* 71A:347, 1989) demonstrated that time to union and rates of delayed union and nonunion are diminished with a long arm thumb spica cast. There is evidence that pulsed electromagnetic fields are helpful with delayed unions. Unstable scaphoid fractures have a higher incidence of nonunion and malunion (which can be problematic) and are best treated by early ORIF. Criteria for instability include: displacement greater than 1 mm, capitolunate angle greater than 15 degrees, or a scapholunate angle greater than 60 degrees. Vertical oblique fractures and comminuted fractures are inherently unstable and should be watched closely if nonoperative treatment is selected.

2. Scaphoid Nonunion—Can lead to advanced collapse and progressive arthritis. Two types of bone grafts are generally used to treat this problem: the inlay (Russe) graft, which has a union rate of 92% and is used in nonunions not associated with adjacent carpal collapse and excessive flexion deformity (humpback scaphoid); and the interposition (Fisk) graft, which is an opening wedge graft designed to restore scaphoid length and angulation. This will usually correct the adjacent carpal instability. Union rates are reported as between 72% and 95%. The most reliable sign of a vascular proximal pole is punctate bleeding at the time of surgery. If bleeding is obvious, the union rate is 92%; if bleeding is questionable, the union rate is 71%; if there is no bleeding, the union rate is 0%. After successful surgery, the progression of arthritis is slower but still occurs in 40–50% of patients. It is therefore desirable to attempt to obtain union.

3. Scapholunate Advanced Collapse (SLAC Wrist)—Progressive arthritis due to scapholunate interval disruption with flexion deformity of the scaphoid and DISI of the proximal carpal row. As a consequence of the instability, concentric joint surfaces are malaligned, leading to force concentration and arthritis. Watson has classified SLAC into three stages (Fig. 6–14): stage I: arthritis between the scaphoid and radial styloid; stage II: arthritis between the scaphoid and the entire scaphoid facet of the radius (in Scaphoid Nonunion Advanced Collapse [SNAC], the proximal pole of the scaphoid and corresponding surface of the radius are spared from arthritis because they are not loaded); stage III: stages I and II plus arthritis between the capitate and lunate. Options for treatment are based on stage: stage I: radial styloidectomy and scaphoid stabilization (e.g., STT fusion); stage II: scaphoid excision and four-corner fusion, proximal row carpectomy, wrist fusion; stage III: scaphoid excision and four-corner fusion, wrist fusion. *Results of treatment:* wrist fusion: best pain relief and good grip strength, no motion; proximal row carpectomy: best motion, worst grip strength and pain relief; scaphoid excision four-corner fusion: a good compromise between the other two.

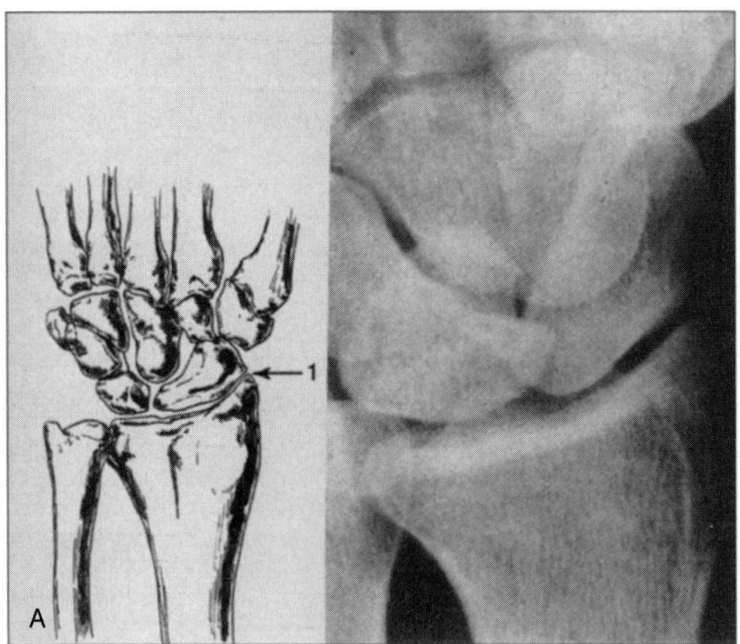

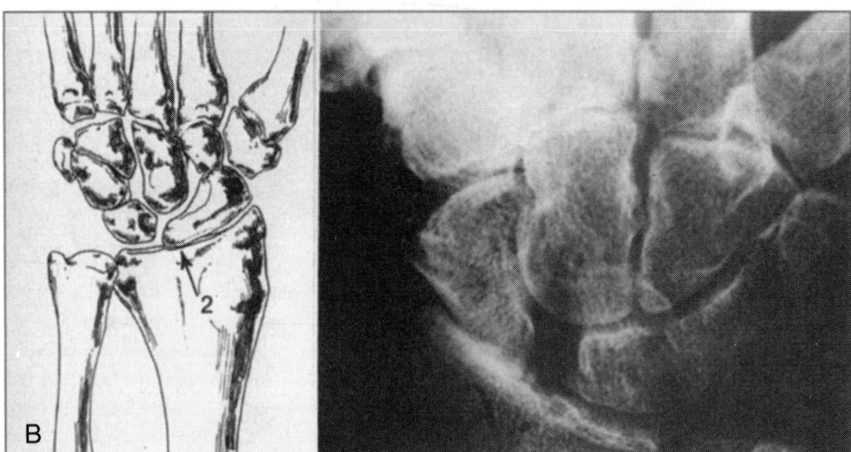

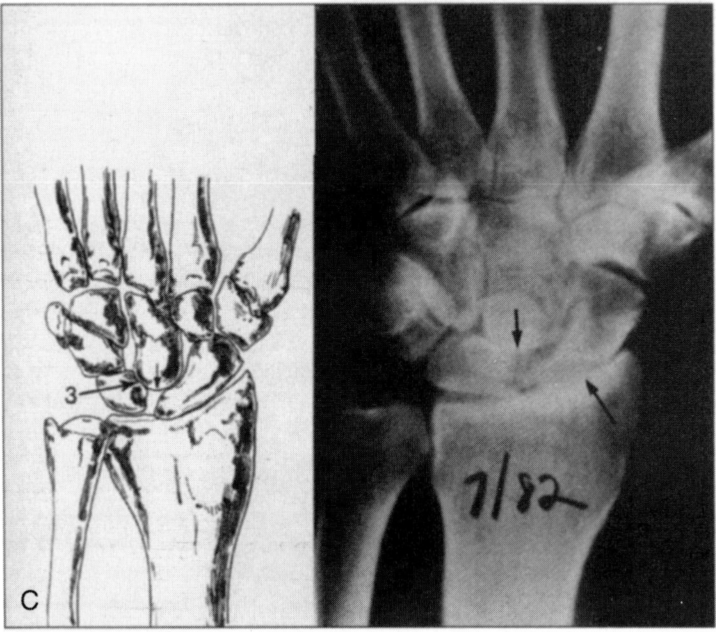

Figure 6–14. Scapholunate advanced collapse. *A,* Early degenerative changes noted at the tip of the radial styloid and distal-radial aspect of the scaphoid (arrow) (stage I.) *B,* Degenerative process has progressed to articular surface between distal radius and scaphoid (arrow); radiograph on the right shows scapholunate dissociation, joint cartilage loss, and osteophyte formations (stage II.) *C,* Progression of degeneration from the radioscaphoid (arrow pointing up on the right) to the capitolunate articulation (arrow pointing down on the right) with preservation of the radiolunate joint (stage III.) (From Watson, H.K., and Ballet, F.L.: The SLAC wrist: Scapholunate advanced collapse pattern of degenerative arthritis. J. Hand Surg. [Am.] 9:358–365, 1984.)

4. Hamate Hook Fracture—Presents with history of blunt trauma to the palm, usually sports-associated with a club (golf club, tennis racket); they also often have paresthesias involving the ring and small fingers. A CT scan is the best test to confirm the diagnosis. It is treated with excision of fracture fragment. ORIF can be done but has little benefit. When evaluating be aware of the bipartite hamate (os hamuli proprius); smooth cortical surfaces are the clue.
5. Scaphoid Trapezium Trapezoid (STT) Arthritis—Second most common degenerative condition in the wrist. It is well treated with an STT fusion after a trial of nonoperative management to include splints, NSAIDs, and steroid injections.
6. AVN of the Scaphoid (Preiser's Disease)—A rare condition. The diagnosis is based on radiographic evidence of sclerosis and fragmentation of the proximal pole of the scaphoid without evidence of fracture. The average age of onset is 40years. It is treated with immobilization, which is effective in 20% of cases. Operative treatment includes drilling, revascularization, allograft replacement, a salvage procedure such as proximal row carpectomy, or scaphoid excision and four-corner fusion.
7. AVN of the Capitate—Also rare with only sporadic case reports. It is treated with immobilization. If this fails, excision of the necrotic portion and tendon interposition arthroplasty has had good early results.
8. Kienbock's Disease (Avascular Necrosis of the Lunate)—The etiology remains controversial but involves both biomechanical and anatomic factors that create a lunate at risk that is susceptible to repetitive microtrauma. The principle biomechanical factor is negative ulnar variation. Anatomic factors include the shape of the lunate bone and the type of vascular supply. Lunates with a proximal ulnar apex (type I) tend to coexist with ulnar negative variation, whereas lunates that are square (type II) or rectangular (type III) are seen in ulna-neutral or ulna-positive variation, receptively. Patterns of blood supply of the lunate and their incidence: Y (60%), I (30%), X (10%). The radiographic stages are described in Table 6–7.

Table 6–7.

Radiographic Stages of Kienbock's Disease

Stage	Characteristics
1	No visible changes in the lunate, changes seen on MRI
2	Sclerosis of the lunate
3A	Sclerosis and fragmentation of the lunate
3B	Stage 3A with fixed rotation of the scaphoid
4	Degenerative arthritis of the adjacent intercarpal joints

Treatment: Initial treatment of stage 1 is immobilization and anti-inflammatories; 50% of patients treated in this manner have continued daily symptoms. Failing a trial of nonoperative management or initial presentation of a more advanced stage, the condition is generally treated operatively. Revascularization procedures have encouraging early results; however, long-term follow-up is lacking and the results do not appear to be better than less technical alternatives. The recommended treatment for stage 1–3A is a joint leveling procedure. Radial shortenings and ulnar lengthenings have similar results, but the nonunion rate for ulnar lengthenings is higher. Patients who are initially ulnar-neutral can be treated with a wedge osteotomy of the radius or an intercarpal fusion (STT, SC). Stage 3B requires dealing with the intercarpal collapse pattern (DISI). This is usually done with a limited intercarpal fusion (STT). Stage 4 is treated with wrist fusion, limited intercarpal fusion, or proximal row carpectomy in an attempt to obliterate or remove the arthritic portions of the joint. Effects of various procedures on radiolunate loads (percentage decrease): STT fusion (3%), scaphocapitate fusion (12%), capitohamate fusion (0%), ulnar lengthening or radial shortening of 4 mm (45%), capitate shortening and capitohamate arthrodesis (66%, but radioscaphoid load increases by 26%).
9. TFCC Anatomy—Dorsal radioulnar ligament, volar radioulnar ligament, articular disk, meniscus homologue, ulnar collateral ligament, ECU subsheath, origins of the ulnolunate and lunotriquetral ligaments. The periphery is well vascularized, whereas the radial central portion is relatively avascular (Fig. 6–15).
10. Classification of TFCC abnormalities—Treatment of class 1 lesions (Table 6–8): All traumatic lesions of the TFCC are initially managed with immobilization and anti-inflammatory medication if seen acutely and are not associated with instability patterns, subluxations, or displaced fractures on radiograph. Failing this, persistent symptoms usually require operative treatment. Arthroscopic repair or resection of the torn portion is possible for type 1A and 1B lesions. Types 1C and 1D are usually managed with an arthroscopically assisted limited open repair.

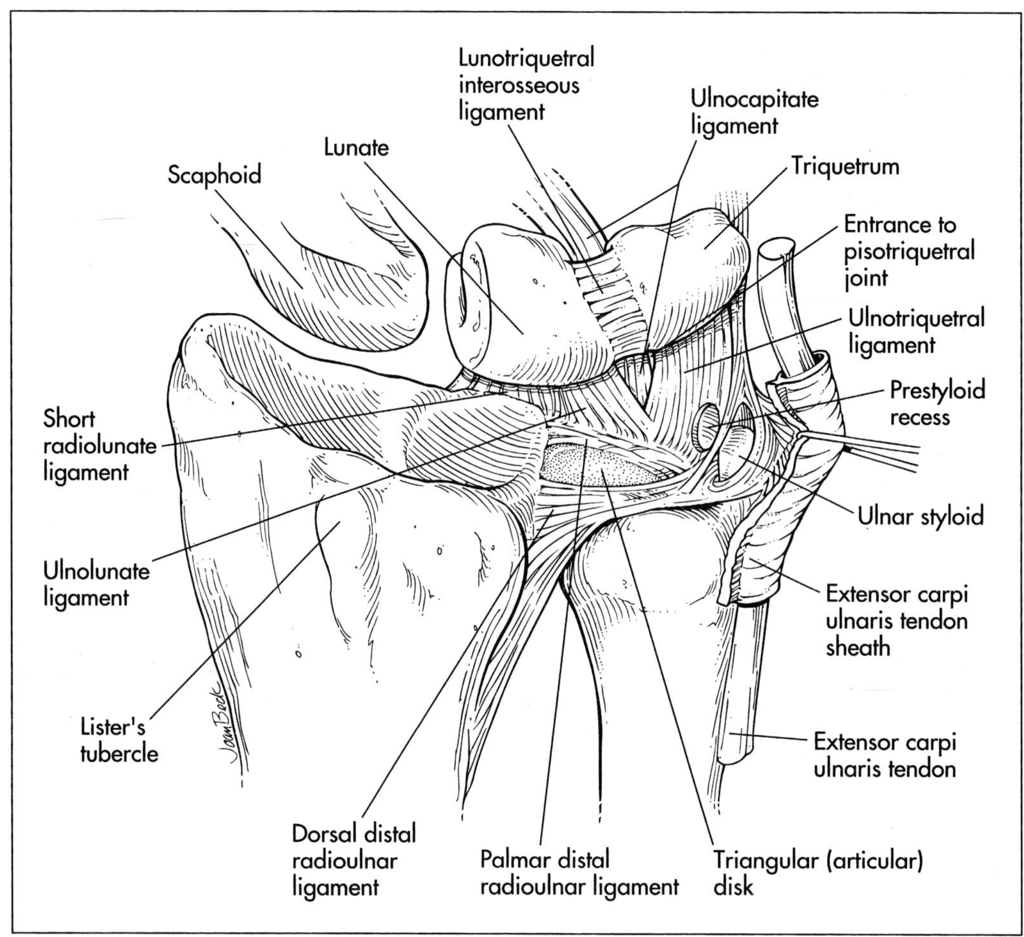

Figure 6–15. Anatomy of the TFCC. (From Cooney, W.P., Linscheid, R.L., and Dobyns, J.H.: The Wrist: Diagnosis and Operative Treatment. St. Louis, Mosby, 1998.)

Treatment of class 2 lesions (Table 6–9): These abnormalities represent a pathologic progression of disease associated with ulnar-positive variation and impaction between the ulnar head and proximal pole of the lunate. Nonoperative treatment is tried first with immobilization, NSAIDs, and avoidance of aggravating activities (steroid injections are also worthwhile). Surgical treatment involves decompression of the ulnocarpal articulation. This has been traditionally done with a diaphyseal ulnar shortening. This approach has the additional advantage of tightening the ulnocarpal ligaments and is recommended when concomitant LT instability is present. Other options not requiring osteotomy include the wafer (class 2A–C) or arthroscopic wafer (class 2C) resections of the ulnar head (2–4 mm). Class 2E lesions are managed with limited ulnar head resections as described by Bowers or Watson or a Suave-Kapandji procedure (arthrodesis of DRUJ and cre-

Table 6–8.

Class 1: Traumatic TFCC Injuries

Class	Characteristics	Treatment
1A	Central perforation or tear	Resection of unstable flap back to a stable rim
1B	Ulnar avulsion with or without ulnar styloid fracture	Repair of the rim to its origin at the ulnar styloid
1C	Distal avulsion (origins of UL and UT ligaments)	Advancement of the distal volar rim to the triquetrum (bone anchor)
1D	Radial avulsion (involving the dorsal and/or volar radioulnar ligaments)	Direct repair to the radius to preserve the TFCC contribution to DRUJ stability

Table 6–9.

Class 2: Degenerative TFCC Tears (Ulnocarpal Impaction Syndrome)

Class	Characteristics
2A	TFCC wear (thinning)
2B	2A + lunate and/or ulnar chondromalacia
2C	TFCC perforation + lunate and/or ulnar chondromalacia
2D	2C + LT ligament disruption
2E	2D + ulnocarpal and DRUJ arthritis

ation of a proximal pseudoarthrosis at the level of the ulnar neck). Darrach's resection of the distal ulna is considered a salvage procedure because of problems with impingement and instability of the residual ulnar stump.

11. Ulnar Styloid Impaction Syndrome—Seen in patients with excessively long ulnar styloids. Impaction occurs between the styloid tip and the triquetrum. Excessive ulnar styloid length is determined by subtracting the ulnar variance from the ulnar styloid length and dividing this by the width of the ulnar head (ulnar styloid process index >0.22 is elevated). This pathologic entity is treated with avoidance of aggravating activities, NSAIDs, and cortisone injections. Failing this, excellent results have been reported with partial ulnar styloidectomy.
12. Tendinitis
    a. DeQuervain's Tenosynovitis—A stenosing tenosynovial inflammation of the first dorsal compartment of the wrist. It is most common in women 30–50 years old. The provocative examination maneuver is the Finkelstein test (wrist ulnar deviation with the thumb held in patient's clenched fist). It is initially managed with splints, activity modification, NSAIDs, and steroid injections. Surgical treatment involves release of the first dorsal compartment on its dorsal side. Surgical pitfalls include injury to the sensory branch of the radial nerve or failure to recognize and decompress the EPB lying in a separate compartment.
    b. Flexor Carpi Radialis Tendinitis—Occurs where the flexor carpi radialis tendon passes under the ridge on the trapezium. It is usually well managed with a brief period of immobilization and NSAIDs or a steroid injection. Surgical decompression is rarely necessary.
    c. Intersection Syndrome—An inflammation of a potential space between the thumb outriggers (APL, EPB) and the radial wrist extensors. An inflamed bursa in this region has been found in some patients. It tends to occur after repetitive wrist dorsiflexion activities in the work place. Examination often reveals crepitus over the area with resisted wrist dorsiflexion and thumb extension. It is treated with a wrist splint and a steroid injection. Recalcitrant cases are managed by surgical débridement of the area. Some have suggested that this condition is really a tenosynovitis of the second dorsal compartment and that release of this compartment is an important part of the procedure.
    d. Snapping Extensor Carpi Ulnaris (ECU)—The sixth dorsal compartment is unique because it has a subsheath that is critical to the stability of the ECU. When these fibers, which also contribute to the TFCC, are attenuated, the ECU can subluxate in an ulnar and volar direction. This snapping of the ECU can lead to tendinitis. Treatment involves the usual trial of nonoperative means to include a splint that restricts forearm pronation and supination. Failing this, reconstruction of the ECU subsheath is indicated.
13. Ganglions–Ganglion Cysts—Account for 60–70% of soft-tissue tumors of the hand. These synovial cysts appear predominantly on the dorsum of the wrist (70%). In this location the origin is almost always from the scapholunate ligament. They also are seen on the volar wrist (20%), deriving their origin from the radiocarpal or STT joints. They are also seen on the volar aspect of a digit at the metacarpal phalangeal flexion crease (volar retinacular ganglion cyst). The cyst fluid is a gelatinous (apple jelly)-like material with a high concentration of hyaluronic acid. Recurrence rates after aspiration are between 15% and 20%. When they are properly excised with a swath of joint capsule surrounding the stalk of the cyst, *recurrence rates are less than 10%.*

VIII. Arthritis

A. Radiographic Differentiation Osteoarthritis/RA

OA	RA
Osteophytes	No osteophytes
Sclerosis	Osteopenia
Asymmetric	Symmetric
Subchondral cysts	Juxta-articular erosions

B. Osteoarthritis (OA)—Common locations in upper extremities include the trapeziometacarpal joint of the thumb, DIP joint (Heberden's nodes), carpus (STT, pisotriquetral joint), and less commonly the PIP joint (Bouchard's nodes). Primary OA tends to occur in females >40 years old, and there is a questionable genetic predisposition.

1. Mucous Cyst—A ganglion type cyst emanating from an arthritic DIPJ. Nail deformity is common. Rupture is dangerous because there is a direct communication with the joint that could lead to septic arthritis. Spontaneous resolution occurs in 20–60% of patients. Surgical treatment is indicated in an impending rupture; skin coverage can be an issue, and local rotational flap may be needed.
2. DIP Joint OA—Patients complain of pain, deformity, and appearance. Treatment is fusion of the joint. Most reliable technique regarding fusion rates is 90-90 interosseous wires.
3. PIP Joint OA—Same complaints as DIP joint OA. Treatment is fusion, especially for the index finger, to preserve pinch strength. Silicone replacement arthroplasty can be considered for the other digits. Recommended position for small joint arthrodesis is described in Table 6–10.
4. Thumb Basilar Arthritis (CMCJ)
   a. Anatomy—This joint is a biconcave saddle joint. Important ligaments include the anterior oblique (holds the Bennett's fracture fragment), intermetacarpal ligament, posterior oblique ligament, dorsoradial capsule (this is the ligament that disrupts in a dorsal CMCJ dislocation from trauma). Joint reactive force is 13 × applied pinch force.
   b. Classification (Eaton et al., 1984)
      I Pre-arthritis (slight joint space widening)
      II Slight narrowing CMCJ
      III Marked narrowing CMCJ (STT not involved)
      IV Pantrapezial arthritis
   c. Physical Findings—Include swelling, painful CMC grind test, and crepitus. Metacarpal adduction and web space contractures develop late.
   d. Treatment—Nonoperative measures include NSAIDs, splints, and steroid injections. Failing a trial of nonoperative treatment, operative options include arthrodesis (stages II, III) of the CMCJ, which may be a good choice for the heavy laborer. The advantages include good pain relief, stability, and length preservation. Disadvantages include decreased ROM, nonunion rate of 12%, and the STT joint not treated. Resection interposition arthroplasty (stages II, III, IV) has emerged as the favored approach in most patients. Reconstruction of the anterior oblique ligament function has prevented excessive shortening of the thumb ray, which was a problem with the simple anchovy procedure. Though shortening of the ray with pinch has been documented, this does not correlate with deterioration of the clinical result. If the MCP joint hyperextends beyond 30 degrees, this must be addressed as well with capsulodesis, EPB tendon transfer, or sesamoid fusion; otherwise a swan neck deformity will develop over time. Silicone replacement arthroplasty is still done because symptom relief is good and length and stability are maintained. The disadvantages to this approach include particulate synovitis with endosteal absorption, subluxation/dislocation of the implant, implant fracture, and cold flow deformation of the implant.
5. Erosive OA—Is seen in middle-aged women (F/M ratio = 10:1). The arthritis is confined to the IP joints. Radiographs demonstrate cartilage destruction, osteophytes, and subchondral erosions ("gull wing deformity"). The disease is self-limited, and patients are relatively asymptomatic; after 10 years of intermittently acute disease, bony ankylosis can occur late in 10–15% of patients. Occasionally fusions can be used to correct deformity.
6. Pulmonary Hypertrophic Osteoarthropathy—Periosteal new bone formation in association with clubbing of the fingers. Patients complain of diffuse pain with morning joint stiffness. Up to 12% of patients with bronchogenic carcinoma have it.

C. Inflammatory Arthritis
1. Arthritis Mutilans—Seen in patients with RA or psoriatic arthritis. Digits develop gross instability with bone loss (pencil-in-cup deformity, wind chime fingers). It is treated by restoring length and stability with interposition bone graft and fusion.
2. Rheumatoid Arthritis (RA)
   a. Rheumatoid Nodules—Seen in 20–25% of patients with RA. *They constitute the*

Table 6–10.

Position for Small Joint Arthrodesis

DIP	10–20 degrees of flexion
PIP	30–45 degrees of flexion, cascading from index to small finger in 5-degree increments
Thumb MCP	15 degrees of flexion 10 degrees of pronation
Thumb CMC	30–40 degrees of palmar abduction 30–35 degrees of radial abduction 15 degrees of pronation

Stage	Characteristic	Treatment
I	Synovitis	Medical
II	Persistent synovitis	Synovectomy
III	Fixed deformities	Reconstruction

most common extra-articular manifestation of the disease and are associated with aggressive disease. They are usually found over the olecranon, ulnar border of forearm, and over IP joints dorsally. Symptoms include esthetic compromise, pain, and ulcerations. Treatment involves corticosteroids or surgical excision. Both are associated with a high recurrence rate and incidence of breakdown or ulceration.

b. Caput Ulnae Syndrome—Synovitis in the DRUJ leads to capsular and ligamentous stretching and bone and cartilage damage. As the ECU subsheath stretches the ECU will subluxate into a volar and ulnar position. This leads to supination of the carpus away from the ulnar head, further stretching dorsal restraints. This developing instability allows the ulna to subluxate in a dorsal direction. When this occurs, it adds to increased pressures in the overlying extensor compartments, which are already elevated by synovitis. This increased pressure causes ischemic necrosis and rupture of the extensor tendons ("Vaughn-Jackson syndrome"). Alternatively, the tendon can also rupture via attrition over sharp bone. If this problem is recognized before the ulna subluxates, synovectomy can dramatically slow the disease process. Darrach resection of ulnar head remains the gold standard for treating this problem. The distal ulnar stump is stabilized with volar capsule. The ECU is relocated dorsally with a retinacular flap. The Suave-Kapandji ulnar pseudoarthrosis has the advantage of preserving the TFCC and ulnar buttress and is therefore a good option in younger patients before the carpus has slid in an ulnar direction. Silicone ulnar head replacement is out.

c. Sudden Loss of Ability to Extend the Digits—Differential diagnosis includes tendon rupture (loss of passive tenodesis), subluxation of extensors into ulnar valleys (inspection), subluxation of MCP joints (radiographs), PIN compressive neuropathy at the elbow secondary to synovitis (can still extend the wrist actively and tenodesis effect intact). Can have multiple causes, which makes the diagnosis challenging.

d. Tendon Rupture—EDM is the most common, followed by EDC to ring and small finger, followed by the EPL. MP joints are passively correctable but can't be actively maintained, no tenodesis effect, and the tendon defect is usually palpable. It is treated with dorsal tenosynovectomy, Darrach's procedure and primary repair (rarely possible), tendon transfer (Table 6–11), or intercalated tendon graft.

e. Attritional Rupture of the Flexor Pollicis Longus (Mannerfelt-Norman syndrome)—*Most common flexor tendon rupture in RA.* It requires exploration because a spike of bone in the carpal tunnel can go on to rupture the index flexors. It is treated with interposition graft or an FDS tendon transfer.

f. Radiocarpal Destruction—Synovitis causes capsular distension and previously mentioned changes in the DRUJ lead to supination, radial rotation, and ulnar and volar translocation of the carpus. Scapholunate disruption can lead to rotatory subluxation of the scaphoid and carpal collapse. When this is seen before significant destruction has occurred, synovectomy is the treatment of choice. Transfer of the ECRL to ECU can redistribute forces to diminish radial rotation and volar subluxation (Clayton's procedure). Fifty to 60% of patients so treated have arrest of the destruction at the wrist. A radiolunate fusion is a good intermediate choice, particularly after a previous Darrach resection of the ulna. It centralizes the lunate and diminishes further ulnar and volar subluxation. Wrist arthrodesis remains the gold standard for advanced disease. Bilateral fusions are not contraindicated. Total wrist arthroplasty is an option in low-demand patients with adequate bone stock, minimal deformity, and intact

Table 6–11.

Commonly Used Extensor Tendon Transfers

Ruptured Tendon	Transfer
EPL	EIP to EPL
EDM	Just leave it and deal with tenosynovitis and caput ulnae
EDM and EDC5	EIP to EDC5
EDM, EDC5, EDC4	EDC4 side to side to EDC3, EIP to EDM
Multiple	Motor choices are EIP, FDS (ring), wrist extensor or flexor

Table 6–12.

Treatment of Rheumatoid Swan Neck Deformity

Type	Description	Treatment
Type I	PIP supple in all MP positions	Proximal Fowler's tenotomy, sublimis tenodesis, SORL reconstruction
Type II	PIP flexion limited with MP hyperextension	Intrinsic release and/or reconstruction MP joint
Type III	PIP flexion limited in all MP positions	Closed manipulation with or without pinning
Type IV	Rigid deformity with ankylosis on radiograph	Arthrodesis

extensors. Silicone replacement arthroplasty had a reoperation rate of 41% at postoperative 5.8 years in one study. The biaxial prosthesis (metal and plastic) had a 24% failure rate at 6.5 years in one study.

g. Etiology of MPJ Ulnar Drift
   1) Joint synovitis leads to stretching of the radial hood sagittal fibers, which are weaker than their ulnar counterparts.
   2) The extrinsic extensors drift into the ulnar valleys.
   3) The lax collateral ligaments from joint synovitis permit ulnar deviation.
   4) Synovitis damage in the joint further destabilizes it.
   5) The ulnar intrinsics contract and become an ulnar and volar deforming force.
   6) Radial rotation of the wrist alters the vector of pull on the extrinsic extensors toward the ulnar direction.
   7) Flexor sheath synovitis distends the flexor retinaculum, allowing the flexors to shift in an ulnar direction.
   8) Descent of the ring and small finger metacarpals, from altered pull of the ECU, contributes to the ulnovolar deforming forces, transmitting it through the juncturae tendons and the intervolar plate ligaments.

h. Treatment of MP Joint Disease—Early: synovectomy, extensor tendon centralization, ulnar intrinsic release with or without crossed intrinsic transfer. Late: arthroplasty. Long-term results from MP arthroplasty: overall patient satisfaction 70%, total arc of motion 40 degrees, implant breakage rate variable (10–20%), recurrent ulnar drift (6–10 degrees), infection and particulate synovitis are rare.

i. PIP Swan Neck Deformities—Caused by multiple factors that lead to an imbalance of forces and can include: terminal tendon rupture and DIP mallet, synovitis attenuation volar plate, FDS rupture, intrinsic tightness from MPJ disease (Table 6–12).

j. PIP Boutonnière Deformity—Synovitis leads to attenuation of central slip, volar subluxation of lateral bands, tightness of transverse retinacular ligament, and volar plate contracture (Table 6–13).

k. Rheumatoid Thumb Deformity

   Treatment thumb deformity—Type 1: stage 1 (MP and IP passively correctable): synovectomy and extensor hood reconstruction. Stage 2 (MP fixed IP passively correctable): MP joint fusion or arthroplasty. Stage 3 (fixed MP and IP): IP fusion MP arthroplasty or IP and MP fusion if CMC is normal.

   Type 2: determine stage of involvement at CMC and MP and treat based on recommendations for types 1 and 3.

   Type 3: stage 1 (CMC pain minimal deformity): splinting/medical management or CMC arthroplasty. Stage 2 (passively correctable CMC and MP): CMC arthroplasty, MP fusion or tenodesis. Stage 3 (CMC dislocation fixed MP and adducted thumb): CMC hemiarthroplasty, MP fusion, first web release. Hemiarthroplasty is the preferred CMC arthroplasty.

   Type 4: stage 1 (passively correctable deformities): synovectomy, UCL reconstruction, adductor fascia release. Stage 2

Table 6–13.

Treatment of Rheumatoid Boutonnière Deformity

Stage	Description	Treatment
Stage I	Synovitis and mild deformity	Synovectomy, splints and lateral band, or distal Fowler's tenotomy
Stage II	Moderate deformity (30–40 degrees flexion), but passive extension is possible	Synovectomy, combined with central slip reconstruction, lateral band reconstruction, or distal Fowler's tenotomy
Stage III	Fixed flexion contracture	Arthoplasty or fusion

Type	Description	Disease Location
Type 1	Boutonnière	MPJ (dorsal capsule)
Type 2	Type 1 with CMC joint subluxation	MPJ and CMC
Type 3	Swan neck	CMC (adducted MC)
Type 4	Gamekeeper	MPJ (UCL)
Type 5	Swan neck with disease at the MPJ, CMC OK	MPJ (volar plate)

(fixed deformity): MP arthroplasty (with UCL reconstruction) or fusion.

Type 5: MP stabilized in flexion by volar capsulodesis or fusion.

3. Gout—90% occur in men, primary is idiopathic, secondary is associated with diseases with high metabolic turnover such as psoriasis, hemolytic anemia, leukemia, hyperparathyroidism, drugs. *Monosodium urate crystals* are seen.

   Eighty percent of patients with elevated uric acid levels never have a gout attack. *The diagnosis can only be made by joint aspiration and inspection for crystals.* Radiographic findings include soft-tissue densities (tophi), intra-articular erosions at the joint margins, extra-articular erosions (punched-out appearance with overhanging lip). Treat acute attacks with IM injection ACTH (40 U) or indomethacin. Cyclosporin A, used in transplant surgery, impairs renal urate clearance and can precipitate a gout attack.
4. CPPD (Pseudogout)—*Calcium pyrophosphate dehydrate crystals.* Associated diseases include hemochromatosis, hyperparathyroidism, gout, RA, hypophosphatemia, systemic lupus erythematosus, ochronosis, Wilson's disease (copper deposition), hemophilia. Chondrocalcinosis is present in 7% of patients. Long-term dialysis can cause a pyrophosphate-like arthropathy. Can cause pseudorheumatoid acute wrist inflammation mimicking sepsis. Radiographs show calcification of fibrocartilage structures such as the TFCC. It is treated with ACTH injection, splints for comfort. Recurrent cases managed with colchicine 0.6 mg PO BID. Surgery is rarely necessary.
5. SLE (Systemic Lupus Erythematosus)—90% of these patients have arthritis in a rheumatoid-like pattern. Other characteristics include marked joint laxity, deformity, Raynaud's phenomenon, facial butterfly rash, positive ANA, high titer of anti-DNA antibodies. Treatment is primarily medical (corticosteroids). Splinting is usually not successful, and soft-tissue reconstructions tend to stretch out. Fusions are the most reliable procedures in these patients; however, success has been reported with MCP arthroplasties.
6. Scleroderma (Systemic Sclerosis)—Hand manifestations include Raynaud's phenomenon in 90% of these patients, PIP flexion contractures, skin ulcers, septic arthritis, and calcific deposits. CREST (Calcinosis, Raynaud's, Esophageal problems, Sclerodactyly, Telangiectasia) is a form of the disease. Surgical involvement usually deals with refractory Raynaud's with periadventitial digital sympathectomy. Arthrodesis is helpful for PIP flexion deformities with dorsal skin ulcers over fixed flexed joints. Symptomatic calcific deposits (calcinosis circumscripta) can be treated by débridement. Refractory finger tip ulcers are best treated with conservative tip amputation.
7. Psoriatic Arthritis (Seronegative Spondyloarthropathy)—Skin manifestations precede joint involvement by several years. RA and ANA tests are usually negative, human leukocyte antigen studies are often positive. Clinical manifestations include onychodystrophy, distal phalanx acrolysis, PIP fusions, MCP erosions, and wrist fusions. The arthritis can be isolated to DIP joint and is differentiated from degenerative joint disease (DJD) by centripetal erosions, which actually cause joint space widening advancing to pencil-in-cup deformity, in which there is a whittling of the middle phalanx and widening of the base of the distal phalanx. Treatment is primarily medical, with methotrexate usually yielding excellent relief. Surgery is indicated when destroyed, unstable, or stiff joints cause significant functional problems. They may benefit from either resection arthroplasty or fusion.
8. Juvenile Rheumatoid Arthritis—There are three clinical types: (1) systemic or Still's disease, (2) polyarticular, and (3) pauciarticular. Laboratory studies are not diagnostic. Hand involvement is most common in the polyarticular variant. Unlike the adult variety, deformities are wrist ulnar deviation and flexion with MCP stiffness in an extended position. Nonoperative treatment is favored so as to avoid damaging open growth plates. Splinting can aid autofusions in progress to fuse in a functional position. Tenosynovectomy can provide pain relief but usually doesn't improve motion. Corrective osteotomies are usually deferred until skeletal maturity.

IX. **Dupuytren's Disease**—Luck has divided this into three stages: (1) proliferative stage: large myofibroblasts, minimal extracellular matrix, with a lot of cellular gap junctions, very vascular; (2) involutional stage: dense myofibroblast network, ratio of type III to type I collagen increased; (3) residual stage: myofibroblasts disappear and a smaller population of fibrocytes become the predominant cell line. The offending cell is the myofibroblast, characterized by cytoplasmic monofilament bundles composed of cytoskeletal proteins. The cell of origin remains obscure. Other cells that contribute to contraction include the "mobile fibroblasts." Involved fascial components include the peritendinous bands, spiral bands, natatory ligaments, Grayson's ligaments, Cleland's ligaments, and lateral digital sheath (Fig. 6–16). Named cords include the central cord, spiral cord, lateral cord, retrovascular cord, abductor digiti minimi cord, and first web space intercommissural cord (Fig. 6–17). The *spiral cord* is composed of the peritendinous aponeurosis, spiral band, lateral digital sheath, and Grayson's ligament. *The only part of the web coalescence not involved in the spiral cord is the natatory ligament.* The spiral cord always puts the neurovascular bundle at risk. As IP contracture increases, the neurovascular bundle is pushed volarly, proximally, and toward the midline. The incidence is higher in Northern Europeans and persons of Celtic origin. Disease onset is rare before the age of 40. The male/female ratio has been reported to be from 2:1 to 10:1. There is a high incidence of Dupuytren's in the HIV-positive population (increased activity oxygen free radicals). It is inherited as an autosomal dominant trait with variable penetrance (accounting for the fact that only 10% of patients have a positive family history). Dupuytren's diathesis is associated with aggressive early onset of the disease involving hands, feet, (Lederhosen's disease) and the penis (Peyronie's disease). Disease associations include alcoholism, diabetes, epilepsy, and chronic pulmonary disease. Occupational hand trauma does not bring on the disease, but it can possibly exacerbate it by microtrauma to early nodules. Nonoperative treatment such as tabletop extension exercises, vitamin E, and splints are proven to be ineffective. Corticosteroid injections in nodules not associated with a cord can slow down the progression of the disease (Ketchum). Indications for surgery include MP flexion contracture of ≥30 degrees and/or PIP flexion contractures greater than 30 degrees. The current trend is to move away from early surgery for PIP flexion contractures. Regional palmar fasciotomy of involved rays through various skin incisions is the currently favored surgical intervention. Segmental aponeurectomies have been shown to be as effective as regional fasciotomies in two studies. Total palmar fasciotomy is no longer favored because it does not completely prevent

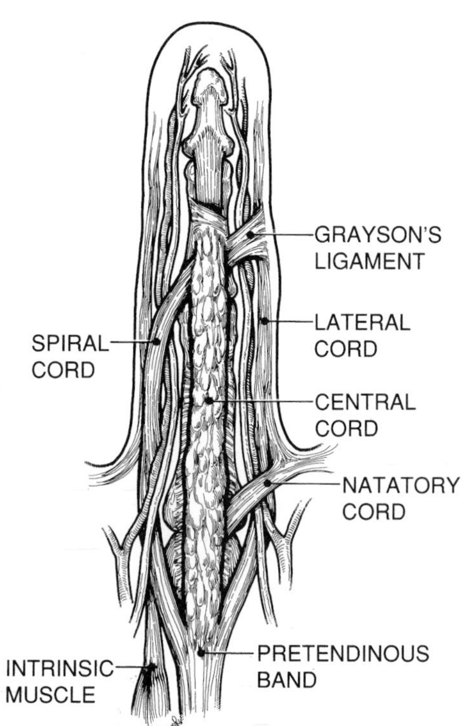

Figure 6–17. The change in the normal fascia bands to diseased cords. (From Green, D.H., Hotchkiss, R.M., and Pederson, W.C.: Green's Operative Hand Surgery, 4th ed. New York, Churchill Livingstone, 1998. Courtesy of Dr. R.M. McFarlane.)

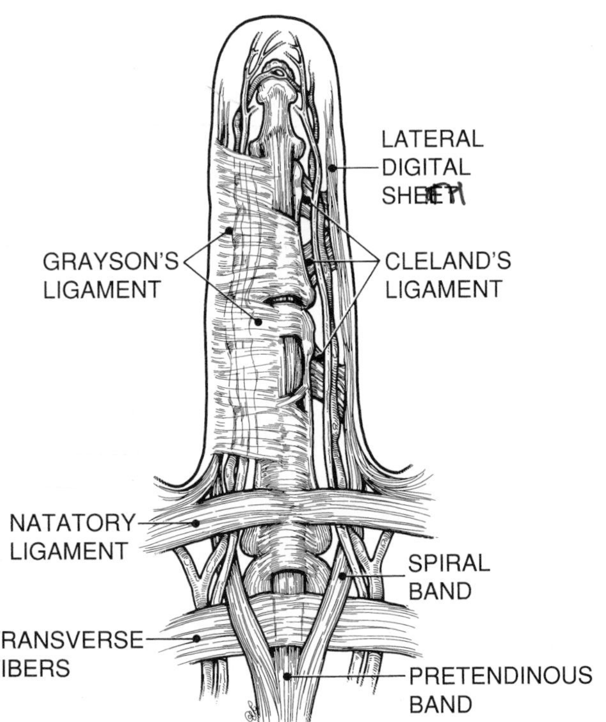

Figure 6–16. Parts of the normal digital fascia that become diseased. Grayson's ligament, shown on the left, is an almost continuous sheet of thin fascia in the same plane as the natatory ligament. Cleland's ligaments, shown on the right, do not become diseased. The lateral digital sheet receives fibers from the natatory ligament as well as the spiral band. The spiral bands pass on either side of the MP joint, deep to the neurovascular bundles, to reach the side of the finger. (From McFarlane, R.M.: Patterns of the diseased fascia in the fingers in Dupuytren's contracture. Plast. Reconstr. Surg. 54:31–44, 1974.)

recurrence and it has a high complication rate. The open palm technique of McCash may be the procedure of choice in older patients that are at high risk for stiffness. Leaving the wounds open prevents edema, hematoma, and pain and allows for early motion. It takes a long time for the wounds to heal (6–8 weeks). Dermofasciectomy is generally reserved for those patients who have a strong diathesis or a recurrence. Skin grafting of residual defects remains controversial. If possible it is best to wait until the disease reaches the involutional stage because recurrence rates are lower. *The best predictor of central neurovascular bundle displacement is the presence of a PIP joint flexion contracture (77% positive predictive value)*; second is the presence of an interdigital soft-tissue mass (71% positive predictive value). Meticulous hemostasis is essential because hematoma is the most common complication of Dupuytren's surgery. Active motion is generally started 5–7 days postoperatively. A night-time extension splint is worn for 6 months. Continuous passive motion (CPM) has not been shown to be helpful. Long-term recurrence rates are around 50%. Flare reactions are more common in women. Concomitant CTR increases incidence of postoperative flare reaction.

X. **Nerve Injury/Paralysis/Tendon Transfers**—Classification (Seddon, 1943): type 1 (neuropraxia): nerve contusion involving conduction block without wallerian degeneration. There is a variable order of recovery and the prognosis is excellent. Type 2 (axonotmesis): conduction block with wallerian degeneration. Axons and myelin sheaths degenerate but endoneural tubes remain intact. Sequential order of neurologic return at a rate dependent on the magnitude of injury is usual. Type 3 (neurotmesis): conduction block with all layers of the nerve disrupted and wallerian degeneration. No recovery without operative repair can be expected. There is an orderly sequence of return at a rate of 1 mm/day in adults and 3–5 mm/day in children after successful repair. Classification (Sunderlands, 1951): first degree: same as neuropraxia. Second degree: same as axonotmesis. Third degree: *most variable degree of ultimate recovery*, axonal injury associated with endoneurial scarring. Fourth degree: nerve is in continuity, but at the level of injury there is complete scarring across the nerve, preventing regeneration. Tinel's sign is present at the level of injury, but it does not move distally with time. Fifth degree: same as neurotmesis. After transection of a peripheral nerve, the distal segment undergoes wallerian degeneration (axoplasm and myelin are degraded and removed by phagocytosis). Existing Schwann's cells that produce myelin proliferate and line up on the basement membrane. This distal tube receives sprouting axons. The nerve cell body swells and enlarges, and the rate of structural protein production increases. There are multiple sprouts from each proximal axon, which connect into the distal stump and migrate at a rate of 1 mm/day. **Age is the single most important factor influencing the success of nerve recovery, with a noticeable change after the age of 30.** The level of injury is the second most important factor. Distal repairs have a better prognosis than proximal ones. The nature of the injury, with sharp lacerations doing better than crush avulsion injuries, is also noteworthy. Delayed repairs yield a loss of 1% of neural function for each week beyond the third week from injury (time limit: 18 months for repair). Specificity of regenerating axons depends on deletion of erroneously migrating motor axons after initial random regeneration along both motor and sensory pathways. Nerve growth factors are thought to effect the rate of nerve regeneration but not specificity. EMG tests the innervation of muscle. Signs of denervation are fibrillations, and these can be seen as early as 2–4 weeks post injury. Technique of nerve repair: epineural: epineurium repaired in a tension free fashion. Fasicular: repairs the perineural sheaths. This has not been demonstrated to improve functional results clinically or experimentally. Group fascicular (three indications): median nerve in the distal third of the forearm, ulnar nerve in the distal third of the forearm, and the sciatic nerve in the thigh. If the gap is >2.5 cm, nerve grafting is usually necessary. Fibrin glue provides for better histologic result, but functional results are statistically the same as with suture anastomosis. Schwann's cells in the nerve graft survive and are eventually replaced by Schwann's cells migrating from either end of the graft.

1. Brachial Plexus Palsy—It is still a good idea to draw out the plexus when you see a patient or open a test book and break the evaluation down into its component parts. It is better to do this before the question is asked because this limits confusion and anxiety.

   Any one patient can have any and all degrees of injury at any level along the plexus. Because of the straight-line course, the lower elements of the plexus C8 and T1 roots tend to suffer the most severe injury. It is important to assess the energy

Leffert Classification

I	Open
II	Closed
IIA	Supraclavicular Preganglionic: nonrepairable, psuedomeningocele, denervation dorsal neck, Horner's syndrome, no neuroma Postganglionic: roots remain intact, + neuromas, psuedomeningoceles do not develop
IIB	Infraclavicular
III	Radiation therapy
IV	Obstetric
IVA	Erb's (upper root)—waiter tip hand
IVB	Klumpke's (lower root)
IVC	Mixed

of the injury via the history because high-energy injuries are associated with more severe damage, such as rupture of plexal segments and root avulsions. The goal is to determine the extent of nerve injury and from this decide whether early surgical intervention is indicated or a period of further observation for recovery is warranted. Important signs of injury severity include: Horner's sign on the affected side, which usually shows up 3–4 days after injury and correlates with C8 and or T1 root avulsions. Severe pain in an anesthetic limb correlates with root avulsion because it represents deafferentation and the presence or absence of rhomboid; serratus anterior function can also help delimit level of the injury. A standard and complete motor sensory evaluation is documented to assist with preoperative planning and recovery assessment. Radiographs of the cervical spine, chest clavicle, and scapula are done. Inspiration and expiration chest radiograph can demonstrate a paralyzed diaphragm, indicating a severe upper root injury. Fracture of the transverse processes indicates a high-energy injury with likely root avulsion. Scapulothoracic dissociation is often associated with root avulsion and major vascular injury. CT and MRI are both useful, and they have largely supplanted traditional myelography. MRI demonstrates: T2—highlights the fat content of the cervical spinal cord and nerve roots (empty sleeves); T1—highlights the water content that is present in a pseudomeningocele. Findings consistent with significant injury include pseudomeningocele, empty root sleeves, and cord shift away from midline. Sensory and motor evoked potentials are more useful than standard EMG and NCV. They should be done 3–6 weeks postinjury to allow wallerian degeneration to occur. Stimulation is done over Erb's point, and recordings are taken over the cortex with scalp electrodes. Positive readings provide evidence of roots that are in continuity with the spinal cord. Negative readings cannot differentiate among avulsion, rupture, or axonotmesis. Modern series indicate that there is a reverse relationship between time from injury to operation and outcome. Even in cases with total clinical brachial-plexopathy, less than 24% of patients have avulsion of all five roots. Therefore, there should almost always be something to repair or graft; if not, nerve transfers can be done. Immediate surgical exploration is indicated in penetrating trauma and iatrogenic injuries. One study showed that many patients with gunshot wounds to the plexus improved with time. Therefore, it is reasonable to wait these out for 3 months in the absence of a major vascular injury. Early surgical intervention (3 weeks–3 months postinjury) is indicated in patients with total or near-total plexus involvement or patients with less than this but a high-energy injury. It is clear that recovery in this situation is improved by neurologic repair or reconstruction. The delayed surgical approach (3–6 months postinjury) is reserved for patients with low-energy injuries and/or patients with partial upper level palsy. It is preferable to wait this out for a while and observe for recovery. If recovery plateaus early on, surgery would be warranted. *The best clinical sign of improvement and effective nerve regeneration is an advancing Tinel sign.* If surgery is going to be done at all, it should be done within the first 6 months after injury, if possible. An isolated C8–T1 injury in an adult is best treated with early tendon transfers. The problem is that the distance between the injury site and the hand intrinsic muscles makes reinnervation over that distance virtually impossible. The surgical priorities of repair are as follows: (1) elbow flexion (musculocutaneous n.), (2) shoulder stabilization (suprascapular n.), (3) brachiothoracic pinch (pectoral nerve), (4) sensation in C6–C7 distribution (lateral cord), (5) wrist extension and finger flexion (lateral and posterior cords). Direct repair is infrequently possible without excessive traction; therefore, nerve grafts are often used. Donor sites include the sural, medial brachial, and medial antebrachial cutaneous nerves. Vascularized nerve graft includes the ulnar nerve when there is proven avulsion of C8 and T1. The nerve is mobilized on its branches from the superior ulnar collateral artery. Nerve regeneration appears to be quicker, but ultimate recovery is not significantly affected. Nerve transfer is indicated when there are an insufficient number of proximal axon resources (i.e., multiple root avulsions). In this circumstance it is necessary to turn to extraplexal sources to get axons. Commonly used sources include the spinal accessory nerve (1700 axons), intercostal nerve (1300 axons), motor branches of cervical plexus (3400–4000 axons), contralateral lateral pectoral nerve (400–600 axons). In general, repair and reconstruction does improve the prognosis. Infraclavicular injuries have a better prognosis than supraclavicular, the fewer the avulsed roots the better. Results of nerve transfer thus far have been mixed.

2. Obstetrical Brachial Plexopathy—Associated with a high birth weight (>4000 g), difficult presentation (shoulder dystocia),

cephalopelvic disproportion, and forceps delivery. The muscle grading system used to evaluate these patients is as follows: M0—no contraction; M1—contraction without movement; M2—contraction with slight movement; M3—complete movement. Complete recovery ispossible if the biceps and deltoid are graded M1 by 2 months. Results though still good are incomplete if biceps and deltoid don't contract until 3.5 months. If biceps is not graded M3 by 5 months, results will be highly unsatisfactory. Early surgery is indicated if, at 1 month, the arm is completely flail and Horner's sign is present. If at 1 month the hand shows signs of recovery but the shoulder does not, there is still a chance for spontaneous recovery. If at 3 months biceps function is evident, surgery is not recommended. In cases in which there is no biceps function, an EMG is obtained. Total absence of electrical evidence of reinnervation indicates corresponding root avulsion. In indicated cases, the results of surgical reconstruction are far better than the expectant approach. Reinnervation of the hand intrinsics is possible in infants, unlike adults. The results of nerve grafting are better in infants than they are in adults. Palliative treatment of the sequelae of birth palsies is difficult, and the results are rarely satisfactory.

3. Tendon Transfers—Indicated to replace a paralyzed muscle, replace ruptured or avulsed tendon or muscle, and restore balance to a paralyzed hand (i.e., cerebral palsy). Tendon transfers are generally deferred until tissue equilibrium is achieved, passive mobility is restored, and donors with adequate power and excursion are available. Important definitions and relationships to understand include: force that is proportional to the cross-sectional area of the muscle, amplitude (see Table 6–14) that is proportional to length of the muscle, work capacity that is equal to force times the length (F × L), and power that is work per unit of time. Other important principles include selecting a motor that is expendable in its orthotopic location. Synergistic transfers are easier to rehabilitate. The motor will decrease one grade in strength after transfer. A straight line of pull is best. Transfers should have only one function per motor unit. Try to restore sensibility before transfer, if possible. The selection of a transfer is based on a careful assessment of the patient. The key questions are (1) what is missing, (2) what is available for transfer, and (3) how are these best combined. This plus a familiarity with classic transfers will usually lead to an acceptable solution or, in the case of a test, the right answer (Table 6–15).

4. Cerebral Palsy—The typical deformities include wrist and finger flexion, thumb in palm deformity, forearm pronation, and elbow flexion. Initial management involves physical therapy and night-time extension splints. Botulinum toxin is temporarily effective when severe spasticity is present. The best results are in children with spastic contractures, an IQ of 50–70 or higher, and the ability to place the hand on the knee or head within 5 seconds. Children with motion disorders do not do well with surgery. The better the sensibility, the better patients will do with surgery. In poor surgical candidates, surgery is done for hygiene alone and involves (1) shoulder derotational osteotomy or lengthening of subscapular and/or pectoralis; (2) elbow: when contracture is >60 degrees, biceps/brachialis lengthening capsulotomy; musculocutaneous nerve neurectomy can help for mild contracture <30 degrees; flexor pronator slide is not a good procedure for function because it corrects too many problems, not allowing for independent adjustment; (3) wrist: arthrodesis (SIMPLIFY THE MACHINE); and (4) fingers: superficialis to profundus transfer and FPL lengthening. Surgery for the good candidate is aimed at improving function. Wrist extension is classically achieved with the Green transfer (FCU to ECRB around the ulnar border of the forearm). This should only be done in patients who have active digital extension with the wrist positioned in neutral preoperatively; otherwise, overcorrection may impair digital release. Other available motors include the brachioradialis. Overcorrection with this transfer is not a frequent problem and it exhibits a multiplier effect with elbow motion. The ECU is another option. This transfer can also diminish hyperulnar deviation, especially when combined with a fractional lengthening of the FCU. It can also be transferred to the EDC if digital extensors are weak. Inadequate release is corrected with a flexor lengthening. Z-lengthening is probably the most controlled method, with 1 degree of extension achieved for each 0.5 mm of lengthening. Tendon transfers to the extensors are indicated only when there are no significant

Table 6–14.

Amplitude (the 3-5-7 Rule)

Wrist flexors or extensors	33 mm
EDC, FPL, EPL	50 mm
FDS/FDP	70 mm

Table 6–15.

Classic Tendon Transfers

Palsy	Loss	Transfer
Radial	Wrist extension	Pronator teres to ECRB
	Finger extension	FCU to EDC II–V
		FCR to EDC II–V
		FDS III to EPL and EIP, FDS IV to EDC III–V
	Thumb extension	Palmaris longus to EPL
Low ulnar	Hand intrinsics (interosseous and ulnar lumbricals)	FDS to radial lateral band
		ECRL to lateral band
		EDQ EIP to lateral band
		FCR + graft to lateral band
		Metacarpal phalangeal capsulodesis
	Thumb adduction	ECRL + graft to adductor pollicis
		Brachioradialis + graft to adductor pollicis
	Index abduction	EIP to first dorsal interosseous
		Abductor pollicis longus to first dorsal interosseous
		ECRL to first dorsal interosseous
High ulnar	Low problems + FDP	Suture to functioning FDP index and long index and long finger
	Ring and small	
Low median	Opposition	FDS ring to abductor pollicis brevis (FCU pulley)
		EIP to thumb proximal phalanx (routed around the ulna for line of pull)
		Abductor digiti quinti to abductor pollicis brevis
		Palmaris longus to abductor pollicis brevis
High median	Thumb IP flexion	Brachioradialis to flexor pollicis longus
	Index and long finger flexion	Suture to functioning FDP ring and small or ECRL to FDP index and long if additional power needed
	Plus opposition transfer	
Low median and ulnar	Thumb adduction	ECRB + graft to abductor tubercle of thumb
	Thumb abduction	EIP to abductor pollicis brevis
	Index abduction	Abductor pollicis longus to first dorsal interosseous
	Clawed fingers	Brachioradialis + four-tailed free graft to the A2 pulley
	Volar sensibility	Neurovascular island flap from back of hand
High median and ulnar	Thumb adduction	ECRB + graft to abductor tubercle of thumb
	Thumb IP flexion	Brachioradialis to FPL
	Thumb abduction	EIP to abductor pollicis brevis
	Index abduction	Abductor pollicis longus to first dorsal interosseous
	Finger flexion	ECRL to FDP
	Clawed fingers	Tenodesis of all MP joints with free tendon graft from dorsal carpal ligament routed deep to transverse metacarpal ligament to extensor apparatus
	Wrist flexion	ECU to FCU
	Volar sensibility	Neurovascular island flap from back of hand

joint contractures and when there is a muscle available for transfer that is only active in the release phase. The other alternative is to transfer the FDS through the interosseous membrane. Favored muscles include FCU, ECU, and ECRB. Thumb in palm deformity is treated surgically with release or lengthening of the adductor pollicis, first dorsal interosseous, flexor pollicis brevis, and flexor pollicis longus. Web space deepening plasty and augmentation of thumb extension and abduction with transfer of brachioradialis, palmaris longus, or flexor digitorum sublimis is also done. When the metacarpal phalangeal joint is unstable in hyperextension, this is managed with a volar capsulodesis or an arthrodesis. For spastic thumb in palm deformity with interphalangeal hyperextension, the EPL is redirected along the axis of the first dorsal compartment.

XI. **Congenital Hand Disorders**

A. Failure of Part Formation

1. Transverse absence relates to all congenital amputations, including: true transverse absence, constriction ring syndrome, and symbrachydactyly (unilateral, nongenetic, and no foot involvement). Surgical management of transverse absence includes any or all of the following: free phalangeal transfer, ulnar postreconstruction, and free toe to hand transfer. Free phalangeal transfer is a good choice when (1) there is suitable soft-tissue envelope (symbrachydactyly), (2) there is adequate proximal bony support, and (3) the child is <15 months old because survival of the growth plate diminishes with age. Intact periosteum and collateral ligament repair improve survival and function. Ulnar postconstruction is a good choice when there is not an adequate soft-tissue envelope. This procedure involves distrac-

tion manoplasty followed by interposition corticocancellous graft or on-top plasty with an adjacent metacarpal. The goal is to provide for opposable posts for rudimentary pinch. Toe to hand transfer should be carefully considered in all cases. Although survival is possible, the vestigial nature of the structures used to motor the transferred toe make functional results usually poor. The exception to this is in amputation due to constriction ring syndrome that mimics trauma, wherein functional results are much better because there are suitable proximal parts to connect to the transferred toe.

2. Longitudinal Absence
   a. Radial Club Hand—Both extremities affected in 50–72% of cases. Associated anomalies include: Holt-Oram syndrome, TAR (thrombocytopenia-absent radii), Fanconi's anemia, and VATER syndrome. Classification: stage I, deficient distal radial epiphysis; stage II, complete but short = hypoplasia; stage III, present proximally = partial aplasia; stage IV, completely absent = total aplasia. The humerus is often short in these children. The ulna is curved and thick and only 60% of normal length. Carpal bone fusion and absence is also seen. Treatment begins with early passive motion therapy. If elbow motion can be achieved so that centralization will benefit the patient, this can be done. Centralization involves any or all of the following and is done at 6–12 months of age: resection of varying amounts of carpus, shortening of the ECU, and, when necessary, angular osteotomy of the ulna. It is important to preserve the distal ulnar physis. In children with particularly resistant stiffness, a two-stage centralization utilizing a distraction external fixator in the first stage is indicated.
   b. Ulnar Club Hand—Less common than radial club hand. It is not associated with cardiac or hematologic problems. The wrist is stable, and the elbow is the problem. Ulnar digits are often absent and, if present, are syndactylized. Classification: stage I, hypoplasia of the ulna; stage II, partial aplasia of the ulna; stage III, total aplasia of the ulna; stage IV, radiohumeral synostosis. Ulnar club hand is treated with syndactyly release and digital rotation osteotomies done early (12–18 months of age). In type IV, an osteotomy of the radius may be necessary to obtain elbow motion. This is generally reserved for those children who have bilateral deformity and those with severe elbow flexion contractures and/or fixed hyperpronation deformity ("hand on flank"). Type II may be associated with a radial head dislocation, which may require radial head resection and creation of a one-bone forearm. A fibrocartilaginous band connecting the carpus to the ulna is present in types II and IV. There is considerable controversy over the benefit of resecting this abnormal structure.
   c. Cleft Hand—The true cleft hand is often bilateral and familial and it involves the feet and has associated absent metacarpals, differentiating it from symbrachydactyly. The severity of this anomaly varies widely from a cleft between middle and ring fingers to oligodactylous (absent) radial digits and syndactylous ulnar digits. Cleft closure and thumb web construction are the top priorities. Syndactyly, when present, should be released early because it is between digits of different lengths andgrowth potential. Thumb reconstruction may require anything from web space deepening, to tendon transfers, to rotational osteotomies, to toe to hand transfer. Web deepening should not precede cleft closure because it may compromise flaps for the cleft closure. Transverse bones should be removed because they widen the cleft with growth.

B. Failure of Part Differentiation
   1. Radioulnar Synostosis—Bilateral in 60% of cases. Examination reveals fixed pronation deformity exceeding 50 degrees in 50% of cases. The radius is heavy and bowed, whereas the ulna is straight and narrow. When this disorder is unilateral and minor, it is best not to intervene. If pronation deformity is significant, a rotational osteotomy is done through the synostosis at age 5, setting the forearm at 10–20 degrees of pronation. If it is bilateral, the dominant side is set at 30–45 degrees of pronation, and the nondominant side is set at 20–35 degrees of supination.
   2. Symphalangism (Congenital Digital Stiffness)—Hereditary symphalangism is autosomal dominant and associated with correctable hearing loss. It is more common in the ulnar digits. Nonhereditary symphalangism is seen with syndactyly, Apert's syndrome, and Poland's syndrome. Indications for surgery in infancy do not exist. Appearance and function can sometimes be improved by angular osteotomies in adolescence.
   3. Camptodactyly (Congenital Digital Flexion Deformity)—Usually occurs at the PIP joint in the small finger. There are two

types. Type I is seen in infancy and affects the sexes equally. Type II is seen in adolescent girls. This is rarely a functional problem, though the deformity gets worse during the adolescent growth spurt. It is due to abnormal lumbrical insertion or an abnormal FDS origin and/or insertion. If full PIP extension can be achieved actively with the MCP held in flexion and there are no profound secondary radiographic changes, the digit can be explored and the abnormal tendon can be transferred to the radial lateral band. If associated with arthrogryposis, the anatomic abnormalities are more complex. Skin grafts, tendon lengthening, and capsulotomy can yield limited improvement. **Kirner's deformity** is a specific deformity involving an apex dorsal and ulnar curvature of the distal phalanx. Epiphyseal arrest or osteochondrosis has been implicated as an etiologic factor. Operative treatment while the epiphysis is open is generally avoided; however, there is one report of successful results with hemiepiphysiodesis. If a functional problem exists after skeletal maturity, corrective osteotomies can improve the angular deviation.

4. Clinodactyly (Congenital Curvature of the Digit in the Radioulnar Plane)—There are three types: type I, minor angulation—normal length (very common); type II, minor angulation, short phalanx—present in 25% of children with Down's syndrome and 3% of others; type III, marked angulation—delta phalanx. The delta phalanx has a C-shaped epiphysis and longitudinally bracketed diaphysis. When the involved digit is too long, especially when the delta phalanx is an extra bone, early excision is done. When the delta phalanx replaces a normal digit of a consequently short finger, opening wedge osteotomy is done.
5. Flexed Thumb—The two main causes are congenital trigger thumb and congenital clasped thumb.
   a. Congenital Trigger Thumb—Involves flexion at the IP joint only. If it does not resolve spontaneously, it will respond to A1 pulley release. This is usually deferred until the child is 6–12 months old.
   b. Congenital Clasped Thumb—Exhibits deficient active thumb extension and slight limitation of passive extension. The types are differentiated based on passive mobility. Supple clasped thumbs are a result of a weak or absent EPL and EPB. The rigid variety is associated with hypoplastic extensors, MCP joint contractures, ulnar collateral ligament deficiency, thenar muscle hypoplasia, and inadequate first web space skin. This condition is initially treated with splinting for 3–6 months. If the child does not experience active extension or if significant flexion contractures exist, surgery is indicated. The supple variety is treated with a tendon transfer to the EPL. Complex cases may require any or all of the following: capsular release MPJ/CMC, muscular release of ADP/flexor pollicis brevis/first DIO, FPL Z-lengthening, extensor tendon transfer, opposition transfer, first web space deepening plasty.
6. Arthrogryposis (Congenital Curved Joints)—Due to a defect in the motor unit as a whole at some point between the anterior horn cell and the muscle itself. It may be either neurogenic (90%) or myopathic (10%). The resultant immobility in fetal life produces the characteristic joint contractures, which tend to be symmetric. Classification: type I, single localized deformity (e.g., forearm pronation, complex clasped thumb); type II, full expression (absence of shoulder musculature, thin tubular limbs, elbows extended, wrists flexed and ulnarly deviated, fingers fixed in intrinsic plus, thumb adducted, no flexion creases); type III, same as type II plus polydactyly and involvement of systems other than neuromuscular. In type I cases, correction of isolated deformity is usually achieved surgically. Type II cases are treated with therapy, splints, and serial casts to diminish contractures. Tendon transfers to replace essential motors are deferred until passive joint mobility is restored. The main goals in these children are one elbow that extends, one elbow that flexes, and wrist extension. Occasional arthrodesis of PIP joints is required to improve digital posture.
7. Syndactyly—**The most common congenital hand anomaly.** Syndactyly is classified based on the absence (simple) or presence (complex) of bony connections and whether the joining extends to the tip of the finger (complete) or stops somewhere short of that (incomplete). Acrosyndactyly refers to fusion between the more distal portions of the digit with proximal fenestrations as is seen in constriction ring syndrome. When syndactyly presents alone, it is autosomal dominant with reduced penetrance and variable expression yielding a positive family history in 10–40% of cases. Syndactyly ray involvement is remembered with the mnemonic "5,15,50,30" and is as follows: thumb-index (5%), index-middle (15%), middle-ring (50%), ring-small (30%). Generally, syndactylized digits are released at around 1 year of age. The exceptions to

this rule are in acrosyndactyly, in which distal releases should be accomplished in the neonatal period, and in syndactyly between rays of unequal length, which should not be delayed beyond 6 months. Both sides of the same digit are never separated on the same day so as to protect the circulation. The new web is constructed with a local skin flap. Full-thickness skin grafts are always required to obtain sufficient coverage. **Poland's syndrome** is a rare nongenetic disorder characterized by four things: (1) unilateral short fingers, (2) *simple complete syndactyly*, (3) hand hypoplasia, and (4) ipsilateral absence of the sternocostal head of the pectoralis major. **Apert's syndrome** includes the following anomalies: acrocephaly, hypertelorism, bilateral complex syndactyly with symphalangism. In this condition the index, middle, and ring fingers often share a common nail. Simple syndactyly between small and ring fingers is present. There is usually a deficient thumb web with a shortened and radially deviated thumb and a delta proximal phalanx. The general approach is to release the border digits before age 1, with construction of two digits out of the central three 6 months later.

C. Duplication

1. Preaxial Polydactyly (Thumb Duplication)—Usually unilateral and sporadic and not associated with syndromes except in type VII. Type VII associations include: Holt-Oram syndrome, Fanconi's anemia, Blackfan-Diamond anemia, hypoplastic anemia, imperforate anus, cleft palate, and tibia defects. Wassel has classified this condition based on the complete or incomplete duplication of each phalanx (Table 6–16).

   The goal of surgical correction is to construct a thumb that is at least 80% of the size of the contralateral normal thumb. A type 1 combination is known as the Bilhaut-Celoquet procedure. It involves removing the central composite tissue segments from each thumb and combining the two into one. Though this seems the logical thing to do, there are significant problems with this approach. These problems include: stiffness residua (from tendon scarring and nonlevel joints), size or angular deformity (from physeal arrest), and nail deformity (from germinal matrix scarring). Generally, this procedure is avoided unless there is no other way to obtain a thumb of sufficient size. The type II combination involves preserving the skeleton and nail of one of the thumbs and augmenting this with soft tissues from the other thumb. This allows for obtaining good size match and tendon and ligament balance. This, if possible, is generally the favored approach. In Wassel types IV and VI, the ulnar thumb is retained so that integrity of the all-important ulnar collateral ligament is maintained. It is important to trim the metacarpal head on the side of skeletal excision to avoid an unsightly prominence. Division of anomalous tendon insertions, radial collateral ligament reconstruction, and reattachment of the intrinsics are also done. The type III combination (segmental digital transfer or "on-top plasty") is sometimes done for types V, VI, and VII when there is a clearly superior proximal segment on one digit and a clearly superior distal segment on the other digit. This involves a transfer of the superior distal segment to the superior proximal segment on a neurovascular pedicle with retained tendons.

2. Postaxial Polydactyly (Small Finger Duplication)—There are two types: type A, well-formed digit, and type B, a rudimentary skin tag. This disorder is 10 times more common in African Americans compared with whites. Associated anomalies are rare in African Americans because the condition is inherited as an autosomal dominant trait. In Caucasians, however, a thorough genetic and physical work-up is needed. Virtually every body system and 17 chromosome abnormalities have been associated with postaxial polydactyly in whites. Vestigal digits are either tied off in the nursery or amputated before 1 year of age. The type A digit is managed with a type 2 combination with preservation of the radial digit and appropriate augmentation of soft-tissue structures from the ulnar digit.

3. Central Polydactyly—Most commonly associated with syndactyly. Early surgery is indicated to prevent angular deformity with growth. Impaired motion may result

Table 6–16.

Preaxial Polydactyly Thumb Classification

Type	Description	Frequency
I	Bifid distal phalanx	2%
II	Duplicated distal phalanx	15%
III	Bifid proximal phalanx	6%
IV	**Duplicated proximal phalanx**	**43% (most common)**
V	Bifid metacarpal	10%
VI	Duplicated metacarpal	4%
VII	Triphalangia	20%

from interposed digit or symphalangism of adjacent digits. Tendons, nerves, and vessels may be shared to the point that only one finger from three skeletons may be obtainable. Angular deviation may require ligament reconstruction, osteotomy, or both.

D. Overgrowth—Macrodactyly is a nonhereditary congenital digital enlargement. Ninety percent are unilateral, 70% involve more than one digit. The adult analog is lipofibromatous hamartoma of the median nerve. Affected digits correspond with anatomic neural innervation, with median nerve being the most common. Angular deviation, joint stiffness, and involved nerve compression syndromes also occur. Classification: static—present at birth and growth is linear with other digits; progressive—not always evident at birth, but growth compared with normal digits is exponential. The severely affected single digit is best amputated. When the thumb or multiple digits are involved, the following procedures may offer improvement: epiphyseal ablation, angular and/or shortening osteotomies, longitudinal narrowing osteotomies, nerve stripping and defatting. All are associated with the following risks: increased stiffness and impaired neurovascular status.

E. Undergrowth—Thumb hypoplasia has been classified by Blauth (Table 6–17).

Type I requires no treatment. Types IIIB–V are best treated with pollicization. Types II and IIIA are treated with reconstruction, addressing the following issues: stabilization of the MCP joint ulnar collateral ligament, web deepening plasty, opponens transfer if opposition is insufficient (Huber's transfer has the following advantages: amplitude and direction of pull are equal to replaced motors, tension is automatically set, thenar eminence will have a more normal appearance), extrinsic flexor and extensor exploration with correction of any anomalies to include tendon graft, if needed.

F. Constriction Ring Syndrome—Occurs sporadically with no evidence of hereditary predisposition. It manifests in four ways: (1) simple constriction rings, (2) rings with distal deformity with or without lymphedema, (3) acrosyndactyly, and (4) amputations. Early (neonatal period) surgery is indicated when edema may jeopardize circulation. Release is accomplished with multiple circumferential Z-plasties. Acrosyndactyly is managed by early release, preferably in the neonatal period.

G. Congenital Dislocation of the Radial Head—Clues suggestive of congenital dislocation rather than post-traumatic include: bilateral involvement, other congenital anomalies, familial occurrence, irreducible by closed means. Some helpful radiographic clues include: hypoplastic capitellum, short ulna with long radius, and a convex radial head. Sixty percent of the time this occurs with malformation syndromes or connective tissue disorders. In 40% of cases, the defect is isolated. The inheritance pattern can be dominant or recessive. The only accepted surgical indications are pain, limited motion, or cosmetic dissatisfaction. In these instances, radial head excision is indicated once the child reaches skeletal maturity.

H. Madelung's Deformity—Results from a disruption of the volar ulnar epiphysis of the distal radius. As the child grows, the distal radius exhibits excessive radial inclination and radiopalmar tilt. Symptoms arise form ulnocarpal impaction, restricted forearm rotation, and median nerve irritation and usually do not present until the child is an adolescent. Corrective osteotomies of the radius with or without distal ulna recession are the preferred operative approach. Severe deformities may benefit from a distraction external fixator so as not to compromise circulation or nerve function with a single-stage correction.

XII. **Hand Tumors** (See also Chapter 8, Orthopaedic Pathology)

A. Benign Tumors

1. Localized Nodular Tenosynovitis (Xanthoma, Localized PVNS, Giant Cell Tumor of Tendon Sheath)—Age range 10–75. This is a firm, lobulated, nontender mass usually located on the volar surface of the fingers. Joint involvement occurs in 20% of cases, with bone erosions 10% of the time. Marginal excision is the treatment of choice. The recurrence rate is 10%. Pathology: gross; solid, tan, lobulated mass; micro: collagen stroma, giant cells, polyhedral histiocytes, hemosiderin.
2. Neurolemmoma—Most common solitary peripheral nerve tumor. It has a Schwann cell origin. The age range is 20–70. These tumors are not associated with sensory/motor deficit. They are eccentric in the

Table 6–17.

Blauth's Classification of Thumb Hypoplasia

Type I:	Minor hypoplasia, all structures present, just a small thumb
Type II:	Adduction contracture, MCP joint ulnar collateral ligament instability, thenar hypoplasia, normal skeleton with respect to articulations
Type IIIA:	Extensive intrinsic and extrinsic musculotendinous deficiencies, intact CMC joint
Type IIIB:	Extensive intrinsic and extrinsic musculotendinous deficiencies, basal metacarpal aplasia, CMC joint not intact
Type IV:	Total or subtotal aplasia of the metacarpal, rudimentary phalanges, thumb attached to hand by skin bridge (pouce flottant)
Type V:	Complete absence of the thumb

nerve and encapsulated. They can therefore be shelled out of the nerve without disrupting axons as opposed to neurofibroma. The treatment is marginal excision.

3. Glomus Tumor—A tumor of perivascular temperature regulating bodies; 75% occur in the hand; 50% of these are subungual, and 50% occur with erosions in the distal phalanx. Nail ridging is a common finding. The symptom complex involves the following triad: pain, cold intolerance, and exquisite tenderness to touch. MRI is helpful in making the diagnosis. Treatment is marginal excision.
4. Epidermal Inclusion Cyst—A common, painless, slow-growing mass emanating from a penetrating injury that drives keratinizing epithelium into subcutaneous tissues. It is treated with marginal excision and has a low recurrence rate.
5. Ganglion—**Most common hand mass**. Presentation may occur in a variety of areas such as the dorsum of the wrist, volar wrist, DIP joint (mucous cyst), digital flexor retinaculum. These lesions are firm, well-circumscribed, often fixed to deep tissue but not to the overlying skin, and they transilluminate. Surgical excision requires adequate exposure to delineate the joint of origin so that the stalk and a portion of the adjacent capsule can be excised. *Volar wrist cysts have a higher recurrence rate than dorsal cysts after surgical excision.* Nonoperative management such as aspiration has a higher recurrence rate than surgery but most often is tried prior to surgery because the risk is extremely low. Arthroscopic ganglionectomy is being studied as to its efficacy in several centers.
6. Calcinosis—May be secondary to degeneration. Symptoms include pain and erythema. Treatment includes rest, heat, and anti-inflammatory medication or injection. Surgical excision of large deposits is indicated in refractory cases. Calcinosis circumscripta can be seen in SLE, RA, and scleroderma, and it may be associated with Raynaud's phenomenon.
7. Dejerine-Sottas Disease—Localized swelling of a peripheral nerve due to hypertrophic interstitial neuropathy. Usually seen in the median nerve, and it may require carpal tunnel release. The lesion cannot be shelled out of the nerve without sacrificing axons.
8. Turret Exostosis—Traumatic subperiosteal hemorrhage that leads to extraperiosteal new bone formation. These lesions can be symptomatic if they form under the nail or under the extensor expansion on a digit. They are treated with excision after the bone matures so as to minimize recurrence.
9. Carpometacarpal Boss—This represents a degenerative osteophyte located at the index and long finger CMC joint. Symptomatic lesions are best treated with excision and CMC fusion.
10. Enchondroma—The age range is 10–60. It is a benign cartilage tumor causing a radiolucent lobulated mass in the diaphyseal and/or metaphyseal portions of the bone. It is usually seen in the metacarpal, proximal, and middle phalanges and is rare in the distal phalanx. It causes symmetric fusiform expansion of the bone with endosteal scalloping and calcifications within the mass. It is most often incidentally noted in association with a pathologic fracture or other hand trauma. If noted with a pathologic fracture through the tumor, the fracture is managed in a standard fashion. Once the fracture is healed, the treatment is curettage and bone grafting of the lesion if it is symptomatic or associated with more than one pathologic fracture.
11. Osteoid Osteoma—The age range is 10–30. Location is more common in the phalanx but it also occurs in the carpus. Classically, the pain is worse with alcohol and better with aspirin, except in fingertips, where aspirin does not seem to help. The diagnosis is often difficult but plain films, bone scans, tomograms, and MRI are all helpful in localizing the nidus. Treatment involves excision of the nidus.
12. Giant Cell Tumor of Bone—These lesions are not entirely benign and can occasionally be very aggressive. The age range is in the third decade of life. Symptoms can include pain, but it also noted incidentally when investigating other hand trauma. It is typically located in tubular bones (epiphyseal region); the third most common location is the distal radius. It is multicentric 18% of the time; cortical thinning and breakthrough can be seen on radiograph. Curettage alone has a high recurrence rate of 20–80%. Intercalary resection or amputation may be needed, especially when cortical breakthrough is visible. If there is no breakthrough, curettage and packing with polymethacrylate can be successful. If intercalary resection is done, the distal radius can be effectively reconstructed with a free fibula graft (either vascularized or nonvascularized).
13. Pigmented Subungual Lesions—Should go through usual blood break-down color

changes and grow distally with the nail. If not, biopsy is indicated because there is a risk of subungual melanoma.

14. Melanoma—Lesions <1 mm thick are treated with local resection with a 1-cm margin. Lesions that are thicker should undergo sentinel node biopsy even if nodes are negative clinically. If the biopsy is positive, radical node dissection is done. If the nodes are positive clinically, node dissection is done.

B. Malignancies—Rare in the hand. The most common primary malignancy is squamous cell carcinoma. The most common bony malignancy is chondrosarcoma. The most common metastasis to the hand is lung CA, and the most common location is distal phalanx. The most common primary sarcoma is epithelioid sarcoma.

XIII. **Nails**

A. Structure—The ventral germinal matrix produces the largest amount of nail keratin. The sterile matrix lies under the nail. The lunula is the junction of the sterile and germinal matrix. The hyponychium lies between distal nail and tip skin and is a barrier to microorganisms. The eponychium is the distal margin of the nail fold, whereas the perionychium is the lateral margin.

B. Nail Bed Injury—The best results are from early accurate repair. Though there are conflicting reports in the literature; a subungual hematoma involving >50% of the surface area of the nail is often associated with a significant nail bed injury. Removal of nail and repair of the nail bed with a 6-0 absorbable stitch is indicated in this circumstance. Distal phalanx fractures with step-off of the dorsal cortex are associated with nail deformity. They should be reduced. The nail plate or synthetic substitute should be replaced after nail bed repair to preserve the eponychial fold and to diminish postoperative pain. If the nail bed is avulsed, the avulsed segment can be replaced, if available, as a free nail bed graft. Other options include: a reversed dermal graft, nail matrix graft from the toe, or a split-thickness matrix graft from injured finger or a toe. As a secondary reconstructive effort, a vascularized wraparound flap can be considered in selected patients.

C. Split Nail Deformity—Reconstruction requires excision of scarred nail bed and dorsal roof. Small defects can be closed primarily. Larger defects require full- or split-thickness toenail bed graft or a reverse dermal graft.

D. Hook Nail Deformity—Caused by loss of bony support or aggressive tip closure that brings the nail bed over the tip of the finger. The nail plate will follow the bed over the edge like a lemming over the cliff. It is treated by replacing the sterile matrix to the dorsum of the finger and tip closure with a local flap. The antenna procedure is a method in which the sterile matrix is suspended on K wires and volar soft-tissue loss is replaced with a cross-finger flap. In recalcitrant cases, a vascularized composite flap from the toe can be considered.

XIV. **Elbow**

A. Anatomy—The articular geometry of the ulnohumeral joint provides significant stability to the elbow, particularly when the joint is in extension. Primary ligament stability comes from the anterior band of the medial collateral ligament. The ulnar lateral collateral ligament provides stability to the radiocapitellar joint. When this ligament is incompetent, posterolateral rotatory instability can develop. The functional range of motion of the elbow is 30–130 degrees with 50 degrees of pronation and 50 degrees of supination.

B. Distal Biceps Tendon Rupture—Rare condition but is generally seen in young, active males. When identified, the tendon should be repaired because there is a significant loss of power forearm supination and elbow flexion. Traditionally, the two-incision approach has been used (Boyd and Anderson); however, a single anterior approach utilizing suture anchors is gaining in popularity. Early reports are inconclusive but would suggest that there may be a diminished incidence of radioulnar synostosis with a single incision.

C. Epicondylitis

1. Lateral (Tennis Elbow)—A common inflammation of the origin of the ECRB tendon. Typically, an insufficient healing response occurs, leaving the origin vulnerable to secondary injury. In that light it can be a difficult problem to treat, requiring patience. Tenderness over the lateral epicondyle and pain reproduced with resisted wrist extension that is worse when the elbow is also in extension are the clinical clues. Nonoperative measures include: rest, NSAIDs, a counterforce brace (strap), and corticosteroid injections. It is usually a good idea to engage in a prolonged course of nonoperative treatment (9–12 months) because the vast majority of patients will get better. Recalcitrant cases are managed with release of the ECRB origin from the lateral epicondyle and débridement of "granulation tissue." It is important to remember that in 5% of these cases, there will be a coexistent radial tunnel syndrome that should also be released to be complete.
2. Medial (Golfer's Elbow)—This disorder is less common. It is also best treated with a long trial of nonoperative treatment. Refractory cases often respond to débride-

ment of the medial epicondyle and reattachment of the flexor-pronator group. It is important to rule out cubital tunnel syndrome preoperatively so that an opportunity to transpose the ulnar nerve is not missed.

D. Rheumatoid Elbow—Principally, these patients are managed medically and with cortisone injections. When these measures lose their efficacy or joint destruction yields mechanical problems, surgical measures can be considered.
   1. Synovectomy—Radial head excision done through a lateral approach is effective in properly selected patients. Patients with stability and remaining articular cartilage and uncontrollable painful synovitis will do the best after synovectomy. Arthoscopic synovectomy with a limited exposure for radial head excision has also been done with similar success.
   2. Interposition Arthroplasty—Yields results that are less predictable than with total elbow arthroplasty. It remains a reasonable choice for young, active patients, with 75–80% good results having been reported. It involves resection and contouring the articular surfaces, which are then covered with fascia. Many use a distraction external fixator to allow for early motion in a controlled fashion to diminish instability and encourage a useful arc of motion.
   3. Total Elbow Arthroplasty—Has emerged as a reliable procedure for advanced stages of RA of the elbow. The principal indications are pain, loss of motion, and instability. The semi-constrained design is associated with the best results and implant survival rates. It is also used in properly selected post-traumatic arthritis cases, with good results.

E. Stiff Elbow—Principally managed with physical therapy to include the use of a dynamic splint. Contractures that are primarily intrinsic (secondary to intra-articular arthritis) are best managed with either total elbow arthroplasty or distraction interposition arthroplasty, depending on the patient's activity level and age. Intrinsic contractures that involve only the olecranon and the olecranon fossa can be well treated with osteophyte excision and clearing the olecranon fossa with a Cloward drill. Contractures that are primarily extrinsic (secondary to capsular contractures) are well managed with extrinsic capsular release. A technique called the "column procedure" has been described, which allows for a safe anterior and posterior capsular release through a single lateral approach, with reliable good results reported.

Selected Readings

Anatomy and Pathophysiology

Smith, R.J.: Intrinsic muscles of the fingers: Function, dysfunction and surgical reconstruction. AAOS Instructional Course Lectures, Vol. 24. St. Louis, C.V. Mosby, 1975, pp. 200–220.

Compressive Neuropathy

Agee, J.M., McCarroll, H.R., Tortosa, R., et al.: Endoscopic release of the carpal tunnel: A randomized prospective multicenter study. J. Hand Surg. [Am.] 17:987–995, 1992.
Buch-Jaeger, N., and Foucher, G.: Correlation of clinical signs with nerve conduction tests in the diagnosis of carpal tunnel syndrome. J. Hand Surg. [Br.] 19:720–724, 1994.
Dellon, A.L.: Review of results for ulnar nerve entrapment at the elbow. J. Hand Surg. [Am.] 14:688–670, 1989.
Gelberman, R.H., Pfeffer, G.B., Galbraith, R.T., et al.: Results of treatment of severe carpal tunnel syndrome without internal neurolysis of the median nerve. J. Bone Joint Surg. [Am.] 69:896–903, 1987.
Gundberg, A.B.: Carpal tunnel decompression in spite of normal electromyography. J. Hand Surg. 8:348–349, 1983.
Hartz, C.R., Linschied, R.L., Gramse, R.R., et al.: The pronator teres syndrome: Compressive neuropathy of the median nerve. J. Bone Joint Surg. [Am.] 63:885–890, 1981.
Learmonth, J.R.: A technique for transplanting the ulnar nerve. Surg. Gynecol. Obstet. 75:92–93, 1942.
Leffert, R.D.: Anterior submuscular transposition of the ulnar nerve. J. Hand Surg. 7:147–155, 1982.
Ritts, G.D.: Radial tunnel syndrome: A 10 yr surgical experience. Clin. Orthop. 219:201–205, 1987.
Spinner, M.: The anterior interosseous nerve syndrome. J. Bone Joint Surg. [Am.] 52:84–94, 1970.
Wood, V.E.: Thoracic outlet syndrome. Orthop. Clin. North Am. 19:131–146, 1988.

Tendon Injuries

Bishop, A.T., Topper, S.M., and Bettinger, P.C.: Flexor mechanism reconstruction and rehabilitation. In Peimer, C.A., ed.: Surgery of the Hand and Upper Extremity. New York, McGraw Hill, 1996, pp. 1133–1162.
Gelberman, R.H., Vande Berg, J.S., Lundborg, G.N., et al.: Flexor tendon healing and restoration of the gliding surface. J. Bone Joint Surg. [Am.] 65:70–80, 1983.
LaSalle, W.E., and Strickland, J.W.: An evaluation of the two stage flexor tendon reconstruction technique. J. Hand Surg. 8:263–267, 1983.
Leddy, J.P., and Packer, J.W.: Avulsion of the profundus tendon insertion in athletes. J. Hand Surg. 2:66–69, 1977.
Lister, G.D., Kleinert, H.E., Kutz, J.E., et al.: Primary flexor tendon repair followed by immediate controlled mobilization. J. Hand Surg. 2:441–451, 1977.
Manske, P.R.: Nutrient pathways of flexor tendons in primates. J. Hand Surg. 7:436–444, 1982.
Manske, P.R., Gelberman, R.H., Vande Berg, J.S., et al.: Intrinsic flexor tendon repair. J. Bone Joint Surg. [Am.] 66:385–396, 1984.
Parkes, A.: The lumbrical plus finger. J. Bone Joint Surg. [Br.] 53:236–239, 1971.
Stern, P.J., and Kastrup, J.J.: Complications and prognosis of treatment of mallet finger. J. Hand Surg. [Am.] 13A:329–334, 1988.
Strickland, J.W., and Glogovac, S.V.: Digital function following flexor tendon repair in zone II: A comparison of immobilization and controlled passive motion techniques. J. Hand Surg. 5:537–543, 1980.
Verdan, C.: Syndrome of quadrigia. Surg. Clin. North Am. 40:425–426, 1966.
Wehbe, M.A., and Schneider, L.H.: Mallet fractures. J. Bone Joint Surg. [Am.] 66:658–669, 1984.

Hand Infections

Chuinard, R.G., and D'Ambrosia, R.D.: Human bite infections of the hand. J. Bone Joint Surg. [Am.] 59:416–418, 1977.
Glickel, S.Z.: Hand infections in patients with acquired immunodeficiency syndrome. J. Hand Surg. [Am.] 13:770–775, 1988.

Gunther, S.F., Elliott, R.C., Brand, R.L., et al.: Experience with atypical mycobacterial infection in the deep structures of the hand. J. Hand Surg. 2:90–96, 1977.

Hitchcock, T.F., and Amadio, P.C.: Fungal infections. Hand Clin. 5:599–611, 1989.

Louis, D.S., and Silva, J. Jr.: Herpetic whitlow: Herpetic infections of the digits. J. Hand Surg. 4:90–94, 1979.

Neviaser, R.J.: Closed tendon sheath irrigation for pyogenic flexor tenosynovitis. J. Hand Surg. 3:462–466, 1978.

Schecter, W., Meyer, A., Schecter, G., et al.: Necrotizing fasciitis of the upper extremity. J. Hand Surg. 7:15–19, 1982.

Vascular Occlusion/Disease

Flatt, A.E.: Digital artery sympathectomy. J. Hand Surg. 5:550–556, 1980.

Jones, N.F.: Accute and chronic ischemia of the hand: Pathophysiology, treatment, and prognosis. J. Hand Surg. [Am.] 16:1074–1083, 1991.

Koman, L.A., and Urbaniak, J.R.: Ulnar artery insufficiency—a guide to treatment. J. Hand Surg. 6:16–24, 1981.

Tsuge, K.: Treatment of established Volkmann's contracture. J. Bone Joint Surg. [Am.] 57:925–929, 1975.

Replantation

Nissenbaum, M.: Class IIA ring avulsion injuries: An absolute indication for microvascular repair. J. Hand Surg. [Am.] 9:810–815, 1984.

Russell, R.C., O'Brien, B., Morrison, W.A., et al.: The late functional results of upper limb revascularization and replantation. J. Hand Surg. [Am.] 9:623–633, 1984.

Schlenker, J.D., Kleinert, H.E., and Tsai, T.: Methods and results of replantation following traumatic amputation of the thumb in sixty-four patients. J. Hand Surg. 5:63–70, 1980.

Tamai, S.: Twenty years' experience of limb replantation—review of 293 upper extremity replants. J. Hand Surg. 7:549–555, 1982.

Urbaniak, J.R., Evans, J.P., and Bright, D.S.: Microvascular management of ring avulsion injuries. J. Hand Surg. 6:25–30, 1981.

Urbaniak, J.R., Roth, J.H., Nunley, J.A., et al.: The results of replantation after amputation of a single finger. J. Bone Joint Surg. [Am.] 67:611–619, 1985.

Microsurgery

Godina, M.: Early microsurgical reconstruction of complex trauma of the extremities. Plast. Reconstr. Surg. 78:285–292, 1986.

Hans, C.S., Wood, M.B., Bishop, A.T., et al.: Vascularized bone transfer. J. Bone Joint Surg. [Am.] 74:1441–1449, 1992.

Lister, G., et al.: Emergency free flaps to the upper extremity. J. Hand Surg. [Am.] 13:22–28, 1988.

Lister, G.D., Kallisman, M., and Tsai, T.: Reconstruction of the hand with free microvascular toe to hand transfer: Experience with 54 toe transfers. Plast. Reconstr. Surg. 71:372–384, 1983.

Manktelow, R.T., Zuker, R.M., and McKee, N.H.: Functioning free muscle transplantation. J. Hand Surg. [Am.] 9:32–39, 1984.

Matev, I.B.: Thumb reconstruction through metacarpal bone lengthening. J. Hand Surg. 5:482–487, 1980.

Morrison, W.A., O'Brien B, and MacLeod, A.M.: Thumb reconstruction with a free neurovascular wrap-around flap from the big toe. J. Hand Surg. 5:575–583, 1980.

Scheker, L.R., Kleinert, H.E., and Hanel, D.P.: Lateral arm composite tissue transfer to ipsilateral hand defects. J. Hand Surg. [Am.] 12:665–672, 1987.

Stern, P.J., and Lister, G.D.: Pollicization after traumatic amputation of the thumb. Clin. Orthop. 155:85–94, 1981.

Wood, M.B., and Irons, G.B.: Upper extremity free skin flaps transfer: Results and utility compared with conventional distant pedicle skin flaps. Ann. Plast. Surg. 11:523–526, 1983.

Wrist Pain/Instability

Chun, S., and Palmer, A.K.: The ulnar impaction syndrome: Follow-up of ulnar shortening osteotomy. J. Hand Surg. [Am.] 18:46–53, 1993.

Cooney, W.P.: Evaluation of chronic wrist pain by arthrography, arthroscopy and arthrotomy. J. Hand Surg. 18:815–822, 1993.

Fernandez, D.L.: A technique for anterior wedge-shaped grafts for scaphoid nonunions with carpal instability. J. Hand Surg. [Am.] 9:733–737, 1984.

Gelberman, R.H., et al.: The vascularity of the lunate bone and Kienbock's disease. J. Hand Surg. 5:272–278, 1980.

Gelberman, R.H., Wolock, B.S., and Siegel, D.B.: Current concepts review: Fractures and non-unions of the carpal scaphoid. J. Bone Joint Surg. [Am.] 71:1560–1565, 1989.

Green, D.P.: The effect of avascular necrosis on Russe bone grafting for scaphoid nonunion. J. Hand Surg. [Am.] 10:597, 1985.

Green, D.P., and O'Brien, E.T.: Classification and management of carpal dislocations. Clin. Orthop. 149:55–72, 1980.

Herbert, T.J., and Fischer, W.E.: Management of the fractured scaphoid using a new bone screw. J. Bone Joint Surg. [Br.] 66:114–123, 1984.

Horii, E., Garcia-Elias, M., Bishop, A.T., et al.: Effect of force transmission across the carpus in procedures used to treat Kienbock's disease. J. Hand Surg. [Am.] 15:393–400, 1990.

Joseph, R.B., Linschied, R.L., Dobyns, J.H., et al.: Chronic sprains of the carpometacarpal joints. J. Hand Surg. 6:172–180, 1981.

Lavernia, C.J., Cohen, M.S., and Taleisnik, J.: Treatment of scapholunate dissociation by ligamentous repair and capsulodesis. J. Hand Surg. [Am.] 17:354–359, 1992.

Linschied, R.L., Dobyns, J.H., Beabout, J.W., et al.: Traumatic instability of the wrist: Diagnosis, classification and pathomechanics. J. Bone Joint Surg. [Am.] 54:1612–1632, 1972.

Mayfield, J.K., Johnson, R.P., and Kilcoyne, R.K.: Carpal dislocations: Pathomechanics and progressive perilunar instability. J. Hand Surg. 5:226–241, 1980.

Palmer, A.K.: Triangular fibrocartilage complex lesions: A classification. J. Hand Surg. [Am.] 14:594–606, 1989.

Regan, D.S., Linschied, R.L., and Dobyns, J.H.: Lunotriquetral sprains. J. Hand Surg. [Am.] 9:502–514, 1984.

Ruby, L.K., Stinson, J., and Belsky, M.R.: The natural history of scaphoid nonunion. J. Bone Joint Surg. [Am.] 67:428–432, 1985.

Taleisnik, J.: Post-traumatic carpal instability. Clin. Orthop. 149:73–82, 1980.

Topper, S.M., Wood, M.B., and Cooney, W.P.: Athletic injuries of the wrist. In Cooney, W.P., Linschied, R.L., and Dobyns, J.H. (eds.): The Wrist: Diagnosis and Operative Treatment. St. Louis, Mosby-Year Book, 1998, pp. 1030–1074.

Topper, S.M., Wood, M.B., and Ruby, L.K.: Ulnar styloid impaction syndrome. J. Hand Surg. [Am.] 22:699–704, 1997.

Trousdale, R.T., Amadio, P.C., Cooney, W.P., et al.: Radio-ulnar dissociation. J. Bone Joint Surg. [Am.] 74:1486–1497, 1992.

Trumble, T., Glisson, R.R., Seaber, A.V., et al.: A biomechanical comparison of methods for treating Kienbock's disease. J. Hand Surg. [Am.] 11:88–93, 1986.

Viegas, S.F., Patterson, R.M., Peterson, P.D., et al.: Ulnar sided perilunate instability: An anatomic and biomechanical study. J. Hand Surg. [Am.] 15:268–278, 1990.

Watson, H.K., and Ballet, F.L.: The SLAC wrist: Scapholunate advanced collapse pattern of degenerative arthritis. J. Hand Surg. [Am.] 9:358–365, 1984.

Watson, H.K., and Hempton, R.F.: Limited wrist arthrodesis: 1. The triscaphoid joint. J. Hand Surg. 5:320–327, 1980.

Weiss, A.P., Weiland, A.J., Moore, J.R., et al.: Radial shortening for Kienbock disease. J. Bone Joint Surg. [Am.] 73:384–391, 1991.

Arthritis

Bamberger, H.B., Stern, P.J., Kiefhaber, T.R., et al.: Trapeziometacarpal joint arthrodesis: A functional evaluation. J. Hand Surg. [Am.] 17:605–611, 1992.

Brown, F.E., and Brown, M.L.: Long-term results after tenosynovectomy to treat the rheumatoid hand. J. Hand Surg. [Am.] 13:704–708, 1988.

Burton, R.I., and Pellegrini, V.D., Jr.: Surgical management of basal joint arthritis of the thumb. Part II: Ligament reconstruction with tendon interposition arthroplasty. J. Hand Surg. [Am.] 11:324–332, 1986.

Carroll, R.E., and Hill, N.A.: Arthrodesis of the carpometacarpal joint of the thumb. J. Bone Joint Surg. [Br.] 55:292–294, 1973.

Cobb, T.K., and Bechenbaugh, R.D.: Biaxial total-wrist arthroplasty. J. Hand Surg. [Am.] 21:1011, 1996.

Eaton, R.G., Lane, L.B., Litter, J.W., et al.: Ligament reconstruction for the painful thumb carpometacarpal joint: A long-term assessment. J. Hand Surg. [Am.] 9:692–699, 1984.

Imbriglia, J.E., Broudy, A.S., Hagberg, W.C., et al.: Proximal row carpectomy: Clinical evaluation. J. Hand Surg. [Am.] 15:426–430, 1990.

Kirschenbaum, D., Schneider, L.H., Adams, D.C., et al.: Arthroplasty of the metacarpophalangeal joints with use of silicone rubber implants in patients who have rheumatoid arthritis. J. Bone Joint Surg. [Am.] 75:3–12, 1993.

Mannerfelt, L., and Norman, O.: Attritional ruptures of the flexor tendons in RA caused by bony spurs in the carpal tunnel. J. Bone Joint Surg. [Br.] 51:270, 1969.

Millender, L.H., and Nalebuff, E.A.: Arthrodesis of the rheumatoid wrist. J. Bone Joint Surg. [Am.] 55:1026–1034, 1973.

Nalebuff, E.A., and Garrett, J.: Opera-glass hand in rheumatoid arthritis. J. Hand Surg. 1:210–220, 1976.

Dupuytren's Disease

Hill, N.A.: Current concepts review: Dupuytren's contracture. J. Bone Joint Surg. [Am.] 67:1439–1443, 1985.

McFarlane, R.M.: The current status of Dupuytren's disease. J. Hand Surg. 8:703–709, 1983.

Schneider, L.H., Hankin, F.M., and Eisenberg, T.: Surgery of Dupuytren's disease: A review of the open palm method. J. Hand Surg. [Am.] 11:23–27, 1986.

Seyfer, A., and Hueston, J.: Dupuytren's contracture. Hand Clin. 7:617–776, 1991.

Strickland, J.W., and Bassett, R.L.: The isolated digital cord in Dupuytren's contracture: Anatomy and clinical significance. J. Hand Surg. [Am.] 10:118–124, 1985.

Nerve Injury, Tendon Transfers, Paralysis

Aziz, W., Singer, R.M., and Wolff, T.W.: Transfer of the trapezius for flail shoulder after brachial plexus injury. J. Bone Joint Surg. [Br.] 72:701–704, 1990.

Brand, P.: Biomechanics of tendon transfers. Hand Clin. 4:137–154, 1988.

Dellon, A.L., Curtis, R.M., and Edgerton, M.T.: Reeducation of sensation in the hand after nerve inury and repair. Plast. Reconstr. Surg. 53:297–305, 1974.

Eversmann, W.W.: Tendon transfers for combined nerve injuries. Hand Clin. 4:187–199, 1988.

Freehafer, A.A.: Tendon transfers in patients with cervical spinal cord injury. J. Hand Surg. [Am.] 16:804–809, 1991.

Gaul, J.S., Jr.: Intrinsic motor recovery: A long term study of ulnar nerve injury. J. Hand Surg. 7:502–508, 1982.

Gilbert, A., and Razaboni, R.: Indications and results of brachial plexus surgery in obstetrical palsy. Orthop. Clin. North Am. 19:91, 1988.

Hentz, V.R., Brown, M., and Keoshian, L.A.: Upper limb reconstruction in quadriplegia: Functional assessment and proposed treatment modifications. J. Hand Surg. 8:119–131, 1983.

House, J.H., and Shannon, M.A.: Restoration of strong grasp and lateral pinch in tetraplegia: A comparison of two methods of thumb control in each patient. J. Hand Surg. [Am.] 10:22–29, 1985.

Inglis, A.E., and Cooper, W.: Release of the flexor-pronator origin for flexion deformities of the hand and wrist in spastic paralysis. J. Bone Joint Surg. [Am.] 48:847–857, 1966.

Keenan, M.E., Korchek, J.I., Botte, M.J., et al.: Results of transfer of the flexor digitorum superficialis tendons to the flexor digitorum profundus in adults with acquired spasticity of the hand. J. Bone Joint Surg. [Am.] 69:1127–1132, 1987.

Kline, D.G.: Civilian gunshot wounds to the brachial plexus. J. Neurosurg. 70:166–174, 1989.

Leffert, R.D.: Clinical diagnosis, testing, and electromyographic study in brachial plexus traction injuries. Orthop. Clin. North Am. 237:24–31, 1988.

Millesi, H., Meissl, G., and Berger, A.: Further experience with interfascicular grafting of the median ulnar and radial nerves. J. Bone Joint Surg. [Am.] 58:209–218, 1976.

Riordan, D.C.: Tendon transfers in hand surgery. J. Hand Surg. 8:748–753, 1983.

Seddon, H.: Three types of nerve injury. Brain 66:237–288, 1943.

Sedel, L.: The results of surgical repair of brachial plexus injuries. J. Bone Joint Surg. [Br.] 64:54–66, 1982.

Skoff, H., and Woodbury, D.F.: Current concepts review: Management of the upper extremity in cerebral palsy. J. Bone Joint Surg. [Am.] 67:500–503, 1985.

Smith, R.J.: Tendon Transfers of the Hand and Forearm. Boston, Little, Brown, 1987.

Stern, P.J., and Caudle, R.J.: Tendon transfers for elbow flexion. Hand Clin. 4:297–307, 1988.

Stewart, J.D.: Electrodiagnostic techniques. Hand Clin. 2:677, 1986.

Sunderland, S.: A classification of peripheral nerve injuries producing loss of function. Brain 74:491–516, 1951.

Szabo, R.M., and Gelberman, R.H.: Operative treatment of cerebral palsy. Hand Clin. 1:525–543, 1985.

Terzis, J., Faibisoff, B., and Williams, H.B.: The nerve gap: Suture under tension vs. graft. Plast. Reconstr. Surg. 56:166–170, 1975.

Congenital Hand Disorders

Buck-Gramcko, D.: Congenital malformations [Editorial]. J. Hand Surg. [Am.] 15:150–152, 1990.

Buck-Gramcko, D.: Pollicization of the index finger. J. Bone Joint Surg. [Am.] 53:1605–1617, 1971.

Buck-Gramcko, D.: Radialization as a new treatment for radial club hand. J. Hand Surg. [Am.] 10:964–968, 1985.

Cleary, J.E., and Omer, G.E.: Congenital proximal radioulnar synostosis. J. Bone Joint Surg. [Am.] 67:539–545, 1985.

Eaton, C.J., and Lister, G.D.: Syndactyly. Hand Clin. 6:555–575, 1990.

Eaton, C.J., and Lister, G.D.: Toe transfer for congenital hand defects. Microsurgery 12:186–195, 1991.

Gilbert, A.: Toe transfers for congenital hand defects. J. Hand Surg. 7:118–124, 1982.

Klienman, W.B.: Management of thumb hypoplasia. Hand Clin. 6:617–641, 1990.

Lamb, D.W.: Radial club hand. J. Bone Joint Surg. [Am.] 59:1–13, 1977.

Light, T.R., and Manske, P.R.: Congenital malformations and deformities of the hand. AAOS Instr. Course Lect. 38:31–71, 1989.

Manske, P.R.: Thumb reconstruction. Hand Clin. 8:1–196, 1992.

Marks, T.W., and Bayne, L.G.: Polydactyly of the thumb: Abnormal anatomy and treatment. J. Hand Surg. 3:107–116, 1978.

Miller, J.K., Wenner, S.M., and Kruger, L.M.: Ulnar deficiency. J. Hand Surg. [Am.] 11:822–829, 1986.

Siegert, J.J., Cooney, W.P., and Dobyns, J.H.: Management of simple camptodactyly. J. Hand Surg. [Br.] 15:181–189, 1990.

Swanson, A.B.: A classification for congenital limb malformation. J. Hand Surg. 8:693–702, 1983.

Tada, K., and Yonenobu, K.: Duplication of the thumb: A retrospective review of 237 cases. J. Bone Joint Surg. [Am.] 65:584–598, 1983.

Tsuge, K.: Treatment of macrodactyly. J. Hand Surg. [Am.] 10:968–969, 1985.

Upton, J., and Tan, C.: Correction of constriction rings. J. Hand Surg. [Am.] 16:947–953, 1991.

Weckesser, E.C.: Congenital clasped thumb. J. Bone Joint Surg. [Am.] 37:1417–1428, 1968.

Hand Tumors

Amadio, P.C., and Lombardi, R.M.: Metastatic tumors of the hand. J. Hand Surg. [Am.] 12:311, 1987.

Angelides, A.B., and Wallace, P.F.: The dorsal ganglion of the wrist: Its pathogenesis, gross and microscopic anatomy, and surgical treatment. J. Hand Surg. 1:228–235, 1976.

Carroll, R.E., and Berman, A.T.: Glomus tumors of the hand. J. Bone Joint Surg. [Am.] 54:691–703, 1972.

Creighton, J., Peimer, C., Mindell, E., et al.: Primary malignant tumors of the upper extremity: Retrospective analysis of one hundred twenty six cases. J. Hand Surg. [Am.] 10:808–814, 1985.

Doyle, L.K., Ruby, L.K., Nalebuff, E.A., et al.: Osteoid Osteoma of the hand. J. Hand Surg. [Am.] 10:408–410, 1985.

Fleegler, E.J., and Zeinowicz, R.J.: Tumors of the perionychium. Hand Clin. 1:128, 1990.

Frassica, F.J., Amadio, P.C., Wold, L.E., et al.: Primary malignant bone tumors of the hand. J. Hand Surg. [Am.] 14:1022, 1989.

Kuur, E., Hansen, S.L., and Lindequist, S.: Treatment of solitary enchondromas in fingers. J. Hand Surg. [Br.] 14:109–112, 1989.

Moore, J.R., Weiland, A.J., and Curtis, R.M.: Localized nodular tenosynovitis: Experience with 115 cases. J. Hand Surg. [Am.] 9:412–417, 1984.

Rock, M., Pritchard, D., and Unni, K.: Metastases from histologically benign giant cell tumor of bone. J. Bone Joint Surg. [Am.] 64:269–274, 1984.

Steinberg, B., Gelberman, R.H., Mankin, H., et al.: Epithelioid sarcoma in the upper extremity. J. Bone Joint Surg. [Am.] 74:28–35, 1992.

Strickland, J.W., and Steichen, J.B.: Nerve tumors of the hand and forearm. J. Hand Surg. 2:285–291, 1977.

Nails

Ashbell, T.S., Kleinert, H.K., Putcha, S., et al.: The deformed fingernail, a frequent result of failure to repair nail bed injuries. J. Trauma 7:177–190, 1967.
Louis, D.S., Palmer, A.K., and Burney, R.E.: Open treatment of digital tip injuries. J.A.M.A. 244:697–698, 1980.
Schenck, R., and Cheema, T.A.: Hypothenar skin grafts for fingertip reconstruction. J. Hand Surg. [Am.] 9:750–753, 1984.
Shephard, G.H.: Treatment of nail bed avulsions with split thickness nail bed grafts. J. Hand Surg. 8:49–54, 1983.
Shibata, M., Seki, T., Yoshizu, T., et al.: Microsurgical toenail transfer to the hand. J. Plast. Reconstr. Surg. 88:102–109, 1991.
Zook, E.G., Guy,, R.J., and Russell, R.C.: A study of nail bed injuries: Causes, treatment, and prognosis. J. Hand Surg. [Am.] 9:247–252, 1984.
Zook, E.G., Van Beek, A.L., Russell, R.C., et al.: Anatomy and physiology of the perionychium: A review of the literature and anatomic study. J. Hand Surg. 5:528–536, 1980.

Elbow

Boyd, H.B., and Anderson, M.D.: A method for reinsertion of the distal biceps brachii tendon. J. Bone Joint Surg. [Am.] 43:1041, 1961.
Ferlic, D.C., Patchett, C.E., and Clayton, M.L.: Elbow synovectomy in rheumatoid arthritis: Long term results. Clin. Orthop. 220:119–125, 1987.
Mansat, P., and Morrey, B.F.: The column procedure: A limited lateral approach for extrinsic contracture of the elbow. J. Bone Joint Surg. [Am.] 80:1603–1615, 1998.
Morrey, B.F., Askew, L.J., An, K.N., et al.: A biomechanical study of normal elbow motion. J. Bone Joint Surg. [Am.] 63:872, 1981.
Nirschl, R.P., and Pettrone, F.A.: Tennis elbow. J. Bone Joint Surg. [Am.] 61:832–839, 1979.
O'Driscoll, S.W., Bell, D.F., and Morrey, B.F.: Posterolateral rotatory instability of the elbow. J. Bone Joint Surg. [Am.] 73:440, 1991.

7

Spine

William C. Lauerman and Michael E. Goldsmith

I. Introduction

A. Anatomy—See Chapter 12, Anatomy.

B. History and Physical Examination (Table 7–1)—A complete history is critical to fully assess complaints, including evaluation of localized pain (trauma, tumor, infection), mechanical pain (instability, discogenic disease), radicular pain (herniated nucleus pulposus [HNP] versus stenosis), night pain (tumor), and associated symptoms such as fevers and weight loss (infection, tumor). The physical examination must be complete to evaluate both the spine and the neurologic function of the extremities. Localized hip and shoulder pathologic conditions may simulate spine disease and must also be evaluated. The examination must include the following:

Examination	Features
Inspection	Overall alignment in sagittal and coronal planes, balanced posture
Gait	Wide-based (myelopathy), forward-leaning (stenosis), antalgic
Palpation	Localized posterior swelling (trauma), acute gibbus deformity, tenderness
Range of motion	Flexion/extension, lateral bend, full vs. limited
Neurologic assessment	Motor, sensory, reflexes, long tract signs (Tables 7–2, 7–4)
Special tests	Straight-leg raise, Spurling's test, Waddell's signs of inorganic pathology

C. Objective Tests—Plain radiographs after 6 weeks and occasionally dynamic flexion/extension views (instability). Computed tomography (CT) scans with fine cuts ± myelographic dye (bony anatomy) and magnetic resonance imaging (MRI) scans (soft tissue, tumor, infection) are excellent for further imaging. Bone scan, helpful in evaluating metastatic disease, may be negative with multiple myeloma. Laboratory evaluation: C-reactive protein and erythrocyte sedimentation rate for infection, metabolic screen, serum/urine protein electrophoresis for myeloma, complete blood count (often normal white blood cell count with infection, anemia with myeloma).

D. Back Pain—Ubiquitous complaint, second only to upper respiratory infection as cause of office visits, with 60–80% lifetime prevalence. Standard work-up, beginning with taking history (most important) and progressing to physical examination (see Table 7–1). Radiographic and laboratory studies rarely help in diagnosis. Some important considerations in the evaluation of back pain are presented below.

1. Age—Children may be affected by congenital or, more commonly, developmental disorders, infection, or primary tumors. Young adults are more likely to suffer from disc disease, spondylolisthesis, or acute fractures. In older adults, spinal stenosis, metastatic disease, and osteopenic compression fractures are more common.
2. Radicular Signs and Symptoms—Often associated with disc herniation or spinal stenosis. Intraspinal pathologic conditions or other entities associated with cord or root impingement may be responsible. Herpes zoster is a rare cause of lumbar radiculopathy with pain preceding the skin eruption.
3. Systemic Symptoms—Careful history-taking can lead to the diagnosis of metabolic disease, ankylosing spondylitis, tumor, or infection (confirmed with laboratory studies). Associated signs and symptoms may be essential to the diagnosis (e.g., ophthalmologic symptoms with spondyloarthropathies; other joint involvement with rheumatoid arthritis [RA] or osteoarthritis). Metastatic tumor should be suspected in patients with a history of cancer, pain at rest, or unexplained weight loss, and in those older than age 50.
4. Referred Pain—"Back pain" can often be viscerogenic, vascular, or related to other skeletal areas (especially with hip arthritis). Careful history-taking and physical examination are essential. Common areas of referred back pain include peptic ulcer disease, cholecystitis, nephrolithiasis, pancreatitis, pelvic inflammatory disease, and dissecting aortic aneurysm.
5. Psychogenic—Psychological disturbances play an important role in some patients with chronic low back disorders. Evidence of secondary gain (especially compensation or litigation) and inappropriate (Waddell's) signs, symptoms, and maneuvers (Burn's test) can help identify these patients. Nevertheless,

Table 7–1.

Differential Diagnosis of Disorders in the L-Spine

Evaluation	Back Strain	HNP	Spinal Stenosis	Spondylo-listhesis/ Instability	Tumor	Spondylo-arthropathy	Metabolic	Infection
Predominant pain (leg versus back)	Back	Leg	Leg	Back	Back	Back	Back	Back
Constitutional symptoms				+	+		+	
Tension sign		+						
Neurologic examination		+	+ After stress					
Plain x-ray studies			+	+	±	+	+	±
Lateral motion x-ray studies				+				
CT scan		+	+		+			+
Myelogram		+	+					
Bone scan					+	+	+	+
ESR					+	+		+
Ca/P/alk phos					+			

From Weinstein, J.N., and Wiesel, S.W.: The Lumbar Spine. Philadelphia, WB Saunders, 1990, p. 360.

one must be wary of real pathologic conditions, even in such patients.

6. History of Back Pain—Perhaps the most important risk factor for future pain, especially with frequent disabling episodes and short intervals between episodes. Compensation work situations, smoking, and age over 30 years are also associated with development of persistent disabling lower back pain. The incidence of disabling pain actually declines after age 60.

II. Cervical Spine

A. Cervical Spondylosis—Chronic disc degeneration and associated facet arthropathy. Resultant syndromes include discogenic neck pain (mechanical pain), radiculopathy (root compromise), myelopathy (cord compression), and combinations. Cervical spondylosis typically begins at age 40–50, is seen in men > women, and most commonly occurs at the C5–C6 > C6–C7 levels. Risk factors include frequent lifting, cigarette smoking, and a history of excessive driving.

1. Pathoanatomy—Involves the disc and four other articulations (Fig. 7–1): two facet joints and two false uncovertebral joints (of Luschka). The cervical cord becomes compromised when the diameter of the canal (normally about 17 mm) is reduced to less than 13 mm. With neck extension, the cord is pinched between the degenerative disc and spondylotic bar anteriorly and the hypertrophic facets and infolded ligamentum flavum posteriorly. With neck flexion, the canal dimension increases slightly to relieve pressure on the cord. Progressive collapse of the cervical discs results in loss of normal lordosis of the cervical spine and chronic anterior cord compression across the kyphotic spine/anterior chondro-osseous spurs. Spondylotic changes in the foramina primarily from chondro-osseous spurs of the joints of Luschka may restrict motion and may lead to nerve root compression. Soft-disc herniation is usually posterolateral, between the posterior edge of the uncinate process and the lateral edge of the posterior longitudinal ligament, resulting in acute radiculopathy. Anterior herniation may cause dysphagia (rare). Myelopathy may be seen with large central herniation or spondylotic bars with a congenitally narrow canal. Ossification of the posterior longitudinal ligament, resulting in cervical stenosis and myelopathy, is common in Asians but may also be seen in non-Asians.

2. Signs and Symptoms—Degenerative discogenic neck pain may present with the insidious onset of neck pain without neurologic signs or symptoms, exacerbated by excess vertebral motion. Occipital headache is common. Radiculopathy can involve one or multiple roots, and symptoms include neck, shoulder, and arm pain, paresthesias, and numbness. Findings may overlap because of intraneural intersegmental connections of sensory nerve roots. Mechanical stress, such

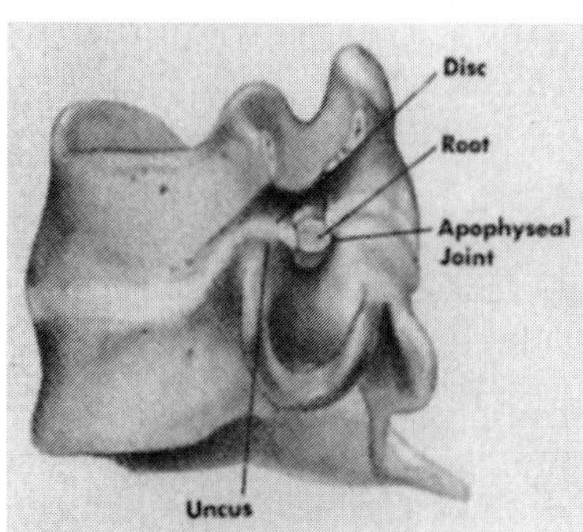

Figure 7–1. Cervical root impingement. (From Rothman, R.H., and Simeon, F.A.: The Spine, 2nd ed. Philadelphia, WB Saunders, 1982, p. 452.)

Table 7–2.

Findings in Nerve Root Compression

Level	Root	Muscles Affected	Sensory Loss	Reflex
C3–C4	C4	Scapular	Lateral neck, shoulder	None
C4–C5	C5	Deltoid, biceps	Lateral arm	Biceps
C5–C6[a]	C6	Wrist extensors, biceps, triceps (supination)	Radial forearm	Brachioradialis
C6–C7	C7	Triceps, wrist flexors (pronation)	Middle finger	Triceps
C7–C8	C8	Finger flexors, interossei	Ulnar hand	None
C8–T1	T1	Interossei	Ulnar forearm	None

[a]Most common.

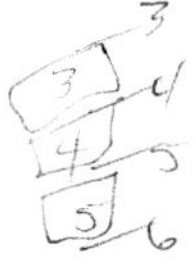

as excessive vertebral motion, in particular rotation and lateral bend with a vertical compressive force (Spurling's test), may exacerbate these symptoms. The lower nerve root at a given level is usually affected (Table 7–2). Myelopathy may be characterized by weakness (upper > lower extremity), decreased manual dexterity, ataxic broad-based shuffling gait, sensory changes, spasticity and, rarely, urinary retention. The most worrisome complaint is lower-extremity weakness (corticospinal tracts). Patients may complain of urinary urgency or frequency. "Myelopathy hand" and the "finger escape sign" (small finger spontaneously abducts because of weak intrinsics) suggest cervical myelopathy. Upper motor neuron findings such as hyperreflexia, Hoffmann's sign, inverted radial reflex (ipsilateral finger flexion with elicitation of the brachioradialis reflex), clonus, or Babinski's sign may be present. Additionally, the upper extremities may have radicular (lower motor neuron) signs along with the myelopathic signs. Funicular pain, characterized by central burning and stinging (± Lhermitte's phenomenon (radiating lightning-like sensations down the back with neck flexion) may also be present with myelopathy.

3. Diagnosis—Largely based on history and physical examination. Plain radiographs, including oblique views, should be studied for changes in Luschka and facet joints, osteophytes (bars), and disc space narrowing. However, radiographic changes of the degenerated cervical spine may not correlate with symptoms: 70% of patients by the age of 70 will have degenerative changes on x-ray film. CT-myelography or MRI demonstrates neural compressive pathology well, although false-positive MRI scans are common: 25% of asymptomatic patients over age 40 will have findings of either HNP or foraminal stenosis on cervical MRI. Therefore correlation with history and physical examination is critical. MRI is also useful for detecting intrinsic changes in the spinal cord (myelomalacia—area of bright signal in the cord on T2) as well as disc degeneration. Discography is controversial and is rarely used for cervical spine disorders. Electrodiagnostic studies have a high false-negative rate but may be helpful in select cases for differentiating peripheral nerve compression from more central compression and diseases such as amyotrophic lateral sclerosis.
4. Treatment—Nonsteroidal anti-inflammatory drugs (NSAIDs), moist heat, exercises, use of a cervical collar, cervical traction, and pain clinic modalities are helpful in most cases of discogenic neck pain and radiculopathy. Indications for surgery include myelopathy with motor/gait impairment or radiculopathy with persistent disabling pain and weakness. Surgery for discogenic neck pain is less rewarding. Anterior Smith-Robinson diskectomy and block fusion is preferred over the Cloward dowel for involvement of one or two interspaces. The Cloward technique is associated with a higher rate of kyphosis secondary to settling. Posterior foraminotomy is useful for single-level radiculopathy with a lateral soft-disc herniation. For multilevel spondylosis and myelopathy, more extensive decompression is necessary. The anterior approach involves excision of osteophytes and multiple vertebrectomies with a strut graft fusion plus or minus instrumentation. Anterior plating may increase fusion rate in multilevel diskectomies with fusion and will protect a strut graft in multilevel corpectomies. Posterior approaches include canal-expansive laminoplasty (commonly used for ossification of the posterior longitudinal ligament), which can help decrease the incidence of instability associated with multilevel laminectomy. Overall alignment should be lordotic for this approach to be successful. Multilevel laminectomy may fail owing to failure to adequately relieve anterior compression or secondary to progressive kyphosis, which may require anterior decompression and fusion with a strut graft for salvage. Complications of the anterior approach include neurologic injury (<1%), pseudarthrosis of 12% for single-level fusions, 30% for multilevel fusions (treated with posterior wiring or plating and

arthrodesis if symptomatic), upper airway obstruction after multilevel corpectomy, or injury to other neck structures, including the recurrent laryngeal nerve, which is increased if the right-side approach is used. Complications of laminectomy include subluxation if facets are sacrificed, leading to a swan neck deformity, muscle ischemia, and direct spinal cord injury with quadriparesis. Radicular symptoms may be alleviated after decompression, but gait changes may not.

B. Cervical Stenosis—May be congenital or acquired (traumatic, degenerative). Absolute (anteroposterior canal diameter <10 mm) or relative (10–13 mm diameter) stenosis predisposes the patient to the development of radiculopathy, myelopathy, or both from relatively minor soft- or hard-disc pathology or trauma. Pavlov's (Torg's) ratio (canal/vertebral body width) should be 1.0. A ratio <0.80 or a sagittal diameter of <13 mm is considered a significant risk factor for later neurologic involvement. Minor trauma such as hyperextension may lead to a central cord syndrome, even without overt skeletal injury. In relative stenosis, radicular symptoms usually predominate. CT scan and MRI (including flexion and extension studies) are helpful. Evaluation may include somatosensory evoked potentials, which help identify cord compromise in absolute stenosis. Surgery may serve a prophylactic function but is usually reserved for patients who develop myelopathy or radiculopathy. Surgical approaches are similar to those described above.

C. Rheumatoid Spondylitis—Cervical spine involvement is common in RA (up to 90%) and is more common with long-standing disease and multiple joint involvement. Neck pain, decreased range of motion, crepitation, and occipital headaches are the most common complaints. Neurologic impairment in patients with RA usually occurs gradually (weakness, decreased sensation, hyperreflexia) and is often overlooked or attributed to other joint disease. Surgery may not be successful in reversing significant neurologic deterioration, especially if a tight spinal canal is present. Therefore it is essential to look for subtle signs of early neurologic involvement and to assess the space available for the cord (SAC). Indications for surgical stabilization include instability, pain, neurologic deficit due to neural compression, impending neurologic deficit (based on objective studies), or some combination. Patients with RA should have flexion/extension films before elective surgery.

1. Atlantoaxial Subluxation—Most common, 50–80% of cases. Usually a result of pannus formation at the synovial joints between the dens and the ring of C1, resulting in destruction of the transverse ligament, the dens, or both. Anterior subluxation of C1 on C2 is most common, but posterior and lateral subluxation can also occur. Findings on examination may include limitation of motion, upper motor neuron signs, and detection of a "clunk" with neck flexion (Sharp's and Purser's sign [not recommended]). Plain radiographs to include patient-controlled flexion and extension views are evaluated to determine the anterior atlantodens interval as well as the SAC, which is the posterior atlantodens interval. Instability is present with a 3.5 mm atlantodens interval difference on flexion and extension views, although radiographic instability in RA is common and is not an indication for surgery. A 7 mm difference may imply disruption of the alar ligaments. A difference of >9–10 mm or SAC of <14 mm is associated with an increased risk of neurologic injury and usually requires surgical treatment. Progressive neurologic impairment and progressive instability are also indications for surgical stabilization, usually a posterior C1–C2 fusion and wiring with halo vest stabilization. Transarticular screw fixation (Magerl's) across C1–C2 has been described and may eliminate the need for halo immobilization. Atlantoaxial subluxation that is not reducible may require removal of the posterior arch of C1 for cord decompression followed by occiput–C2 fusion. Neurologic impairment with RA has been classified by Ranawat.

Grade	Characteristics
I	Subjective paresthesias
II	Subjective weakness; upper motor neuron findings
III	Objective weakness; upper motor neuron findings (A = ambulatory; B = nonambulatory)

Surgery is less successful in patients with severe (Ranawat IIIB) neurologic deficits. Complications include pseudarthrosis (20%) and recurring myelopathy. The pseudarthrosis rate may be lessened by extending the fusion to the occiput. An atlantodens interval of >7–10 mm or a posterior space of <13 mm is a relative contraindication to surgery in other areas, and the spine should be stabilized first.

2. Cranial Settling (Basilar Invagination)—Least common. Cranial migration of the dens from erosion and bone loss between the occiput and C1–C2. Measurement techniques are shown in Figure 7–2. Landmarks may be difficult to identify, with Ranawat's line probably the most easily reproducible. Progressive cranial migration (>5 mm) or neurologic compromise may require operative intervention (occiput–C2 fusion).

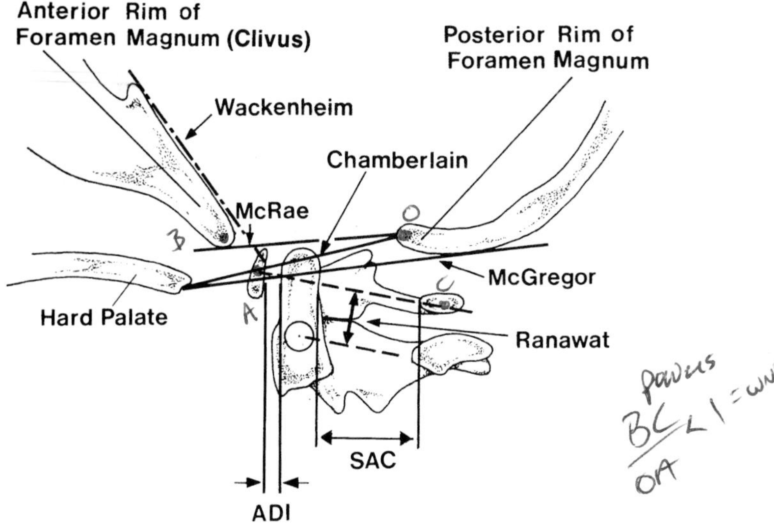

Figure 7–2. Common measurements in C1–C2 disorders.

Somatosensory evoked potentials may be helpful in evaluation. When brain stem compromise is significant with functional impairment, transoral or anterior retropharyngeal odontoid resection may be required.

3. Lower Cervical Spine—Occurs in 20% of cases. Because the joints of Luschka and facet joints are affected by RA, subluxation may occur at multiple levels. Lower cervical spine involvement is more common in males, with steroid use, with seropositive RA, in patients with rheumatoid nodules, and in those with severe RA. Subaxial subluxation of >4 mm or >20% of the body is indicative of cord compression. The cervical height index (cervical body height/width) of <2.00 approaches 100% sensitivity and specificity in predicting neurologic compromise. Posterior fusion and wiring is sometimes required for subluxation >4 mm with intractable pain and neurologic compromise.

D. Cervical Spine and Cord Injuries

1. Introduction—Spinal cord injuries occur most commonly in young males involved in motor vehicle accidents, falls, and diving accidents. Gunshot wounds are an increasing cause. Findings may be subtle; the significant morbidity and mortality rates associated with missed injuries have led to current emphasis on cervical spine protection after polytrauma. Missed cervical spine injuries are most common in the presence of decreased level of consciousness, alcohol/drug intoxication, head injury, and in patients with multiple injuries. Facial injuries, hypotension, and localized tenderness or spasm should be sought. Careful neurologic examination to document the lowest remaining functional level and to assess for the possibility of sacral sparing, or sparing of posterior column function indicating an incomplete spinal cord injury, is essential. Neurologic level by American Spine Association standards is defined as the most caudal level with normal motor and sensory function bilaterally. Initial treatment with large doses of methylprednisolone (30 mg/kg initially and 5.4 mg/kg each hour for the next 23 hours) has been shown to improve neurologic recovery if initiated within the first 8 hours after injury. Spinal shock usually involves a 24- to 72-hour period of paralysis, hypotonia, and areflexia. At its conclusion, the progressive onset of spasticity, hyperreflexia, and clonus develops over days to weeks. The return of the bulbocavernosus reflex (anal sphincter contraction in response to squeezing the glans penis or tugging on the Foley catheter) signifies the end of spinal shock, and for complete injuries further neurologic improvement is minimal. Prognosis with incomplete spinal cord injury is unaffected by the bulbocavernosus reflex. Injuries below the thoracolumbar level (conus or cauda equina) may permanently interrupt the bulbocavernosus reflex. Neurogenic shock (secondary to loss of sympathetic tone) can be differentiated from hypovolemic shock based on the presence of relative bradycardia in neurogenic shock, in contrast to the presence of tachycardia and hypotension with hypovolemic shock. Swan-Ganz monitoring is helpful in this setting as neurogenic and hypovolemic shock often occur concurrently. Hypovolemic shock is treated with fluid resuscitation, whereas selective vasopressors are effective in neurogenic shock.

2. Prognosis—The Frankel classification is useful when considering functional recovery from spinal cord injury.

Frankel Grade	Function
A	Complete paralysis
B	Sensory function only below injury level
C	Incomplete motor function (grade 1–2/5) below injury level
D	Fair to good motor function (grade 3–4/5) below injury level
E	Normal function (grade 5/5)

3. Radiographic Evaluation—Includes complete cervical spine series (C1–T1; multiple-level injuries are common [10–20%]), obliques (facet subluxation, dislocations, fractures); tomograms (dens fractures and facet joint injuries) may be helpful. On the lateral, 85% of C-spine fractures are detected. CT scanning is useful for evaluating C1 fractures and

assessing bone in the canal but may miss an axial plane fracture (type II odontoid). Myelography may be used in patients with an otherwise unexplained neurologic deficit. MRI has advantages for demonstrating posterior ligamentous disruption, disc herniation, canal compromise, and the status of the spinal cord.

4. Cord Injuries—May be complete (no function below a given level) or incomplete (with some sparing of distal function). Most cord injury is due to contusion or compression, not transection. With complete injuries, an improvement of one nerve root level can be expected in 80% of the patients, and approximately 20% recover two functioning root levels. Several categories of incomplete lesions exist. These syndromes are classified based on the area of the spinal cord that has been the most severely damaged. Central cord syndrome is the most common and is usually seen in patients with pre-existing cervical spondylosis who sustain a hyperextension injury. The cord is compressed by osteophytes anteriorly and by the infolded ligamentum flavum posteriorly. The cord is injured in the central gray matter, which results in proportionately greater loss of motor function to the upper extremities than to the lower extremities, with variable sensory sparing. The second most common cord injury is anterior cord syndrome, in which the damage is primarily in the anterior two-thirds of the cord, sparing the posterior columns (proprioception and vibratory sensation). These patients demonstrate greater motor loss in the legs than in the arms. CT scan may demonstrate bony fragments compressing the anterior cord. The anterior cord syndrome has the worst prognosis. The rare Brown-Séquard syndrome damages half of the cord, causing ipsilateral motor loss, position/proprioception loss, contralateral pain, and temperature loss (usually two levels below the insult). This injury, usually the result of penetrating trauma, carries the best prognosis. Posterior cord syndrome spares only a few tracts anteriorly (with only crude touch sensation remaining). It is very rare; in fact, some authors do not believe that it exists. Single-root lesions can occur at the level of the fracture, most commonly C5 or C6, leading to deltoid or biceps weakness; and they are usually unilateral. A summary of the syndromes is presented in Table 7–3.

5. Specific Cervical Spine Injuries—The reader is referred to Chapter 10, Adult Trauma, for classification and treatment of cervical spine injuries.

6. Treatment—Discussed in Chapter 10, Adult Trauma. It basically includes immobilization (collar for undisplaced, stable fractures; skeletal traction, halo vest, or surgery for unstable fractures) and immediate application of skeletal traction to realign the spine in the presence of a displaced fracture with or without neurologic injury. Skeletal traction requires the placement of Gardner-Wells tongs (pins parallel to the external auditory meatus) and the addition of 5–10 pounds initially, with 5–7 pounds per cervical level with sequential radiographs between the additions of weight. If necessary, anterior decompression for incomplete injuries with persistent cord compression (can lead to improvement of one to three levels, even with complete injuries) and stabilization may be indicated. Late decompression for up to 1 year may be effective in improving root return. Laminectomies are contraindicated except in the rare case of posterior compression from a fractured lamina. Gunshot wounds are treated nonoperatively except with esophageal or colonic perforation.

7. Complications—Numerous; include neurologic injury, nonunion, and malunion. Autonomic dysreflexia can follow cervical and upper thoracic spinal cord injuries. It is commonly related to bladder overdistention or fecal impaction and manifests with pounding headache (from severe hypertension), anxiety, profuse head and neck sweating, nasal obstruction, and blurred vision. Urinary catheterization or rectal disimpaction and supportive treatment usually relieve symp-

Table 7–3.

Spinal Cord Injury Syndromes

Syndrome	Pathology	Characteristics	Prognosis
Central	Age >50, extension injuries	Affects upper > lower extremities, motor and sensory loss	Fair
Anterior	Flexion-compression (vertebral A)	Incomplete motor and some sensory loss	Poor
Brown-Séquard	Penetrating trauma	Loss of ipsilateral motor function, contralateral pain and temperature sensation	Best
Root	Foramina compression/herniated nucleus pulposus	Based on level—weakness	Good
Complete	Burst/canal compression	No function below injury level	Poor

toms. If not, nifedipine (10 mg) is given sublingually immediately, followed by phenoxybenzamine (Dibenzyline) (10 mg) administered daily for prophylaxis. Instability in the cervical spine can occur late and is associated with >3.5 mm of subluxation and >11 degrees of difference in angulation between adjacent motion segments.

E. Sports-Related Cervical Spine Injuries

1. Burner's Syndrome—Common injury associated with stretching the upper brachial plexus by bending the neck away from the depressed shoulder or neck extension toward the painful shoulder in the setting of foraminal stenosis (root irritation). Athlete will complain of burning dysesthesia with weakness in the involved extremity. Fracture or acute HNP should be ruled out. The athlete with a neck injury should be transported for cervical pain, tenderness, or neurologic symptoms.
2. Transient Quadriplegia—Most commonly seen after axial load injury (spearing), but may also be seen after forced hyperextension or hyperflexion. Presents with bilateral burning paresthesia and weakness or paralysis. High association with cervical stenosis (Torg ratio <0.8) as well as instability, HNP, and congenital fusions. No definitive association with future permanent neurologic injury. Patients with concurrent pathologic conditions, including instability, HNP, degenerative changes, or symptoms that lasted more than 36 hours, should be prohibited from contact sports.

F. Other Cervical Spine Problems—Ankylosing spondylitis and neuromyopathic conditions can cause severe flexion deformities of the cervical spine. Patients with ankylosing spondylitis must be carefully evaluated for silent fractures because of the problem of pseudarthrosis and progressive kyphotic deformity. Severe chin-on-chest deformity in ankylosing spondylitis, with the inability to look straight ahead, occasionally represents a major functional limitation and is often associated with severe hip flexion contractures as well as a flexion deformity of the lumbar spine. Treatment usually begins by addressing the hip and lumbar disorder first but may ultimately require cervicothoracic laminectomy, osteotomy, and fusion for correction of the neck deformity. This procedure is performed under local anesthesia with brief general anesthesia, and immobilization postoperatively is carried out in a halo cast. Traction, surgical release of contracted sternocleidomastoid muscles, and posterior fusion are sometimes required for severe neuromyopathic conditions.

III. Thoracic/Lumbar Spine

A. HNP

1. Introduction—Disc degeneration with aging includes loss of water content, annular tears, and myxomatous changes, resulting in herniation of nuclear material. Changes in proteoglycan metabolism, secondary immunologic factors, and structural factors also play a role. Discs can protrude (bulging nucleus, intact annulus), extrude (through the annulus but confined by the posterior longitudinal ligament), or be sequestrated (disc material free in canal) (Fig. 7–3). HNP is usually a disease of young and middle-age adults; the disc nucleus desiccates and is less likely to herniate in older patients.
2. Thoracic Disc Disease—Relatively uncommon (<1% of all HNPs), it usually involves the mid to lower thoracic levels, with T11–T12 being the most common and 75% occurring between T8–T12. Thoracic HNP is divided between central and lateral herniations and is usually secondary to torsional motions. It usually presents with the onset of back or chest pain that may progress to radicular symptoms (band-like chest or abdominal discomfort, numbness, paresthesias, leg pain) and/or myelopathy (sensory changes, paraparesis, bowel/bladder/sexual dysfunction). Physical findings may be difficult to elicit but may include localized tenderness, sensory pinprick level, upper motor neuron signs with leg hyperreflexia, weakness, and abnormal rectal examination. Radiographs may show disc narrowing and calcification or osteophytic lipping. Underlying Scheuermann's disease may predispose patients to develop HNP. Myelo-CT or MRI should demonstrate thoracic HNP. MRI is useful for ruling out cord disorder, but there is a high false-positive rate, requiring close clinical correlation. Immobilization, analgesics, and nerve blocks are sometimes helpful for radiculopathy. Surgery, usually through an anterior transthoracic approach or costotransversectomy (including anterior diskectomy and hemicorpectomy as needed), is recommended in the presence of myelopathy or persistent unremitting pain with documented pathologic conditions. Thorascopic diskectomy can also be employed. Posterior approach to a thoracic HNP is contraindicated because of the high rate of neurologic injury.
3. Lumbar Disc Disease—Major cause of increased morbidity and causes major financial impact in the United States. Most often involves the L4–L5 disc (the "backache disc"), followed closely by L5–S1. Most herniations are posterolateral (where the posterior longitudinal ligament is the weakest) and may present with back pain and nerve root pain/sciatica involving the lower nerve root at that level. Central prolapse is usually associated with back pain only; however, acute insults may precipitate a cauda equina compression syndrome (Fig. 7–4). This syndrome is a surgical emergency that most commonly pre-

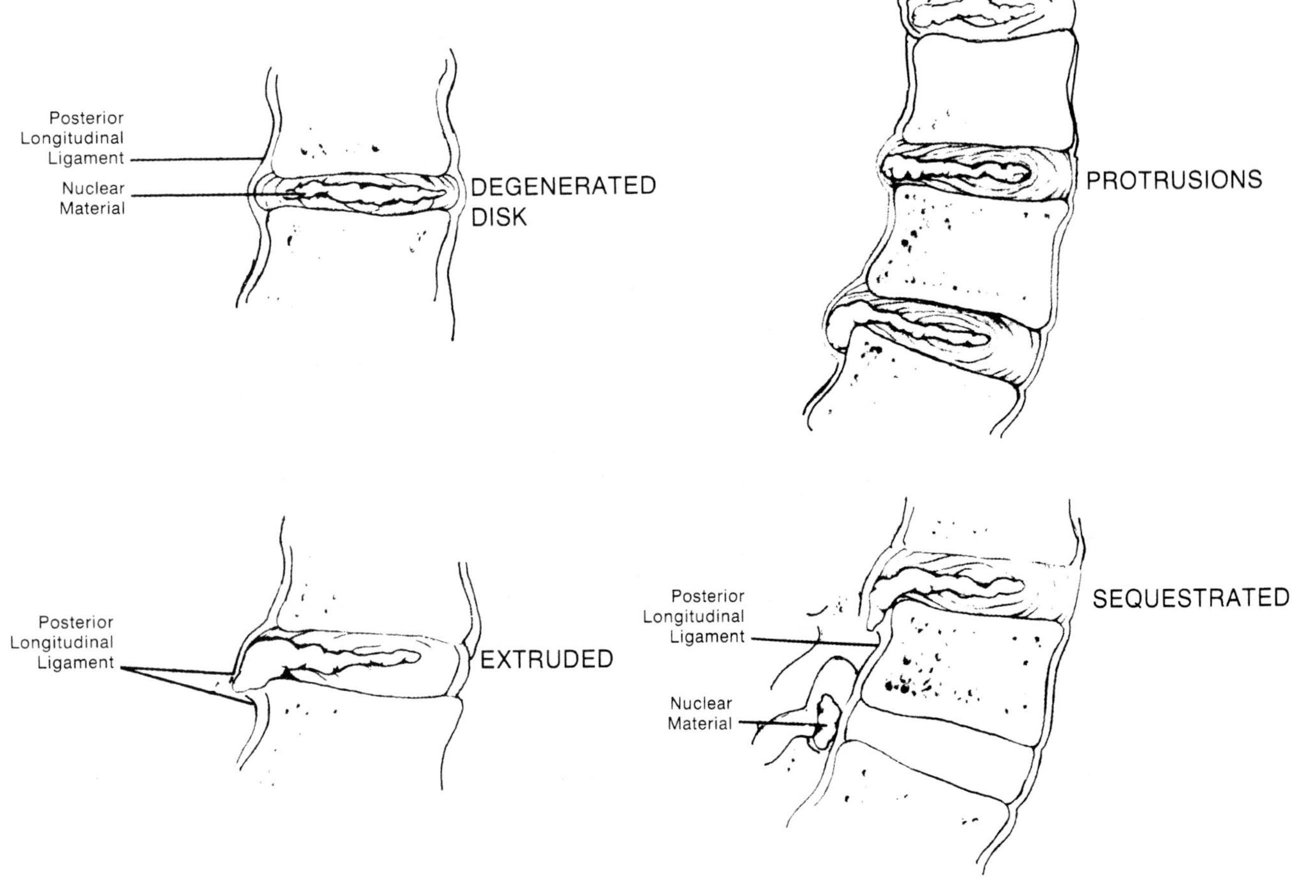

Figure 7–3. Nomenclature for disc pathology. (From Wiltse, L.L.: Lumbosacral spine reconstruction. In Orthopaedic Knowledge Update I. Chicago, American Academy of Orthopaedic Surgeons, 1984, p. 247.)

sents with bilateral buttock and lower-extremity pain as well as bowel or bladder dysfunction (usually urinary retention), saddle anesthesia, and varying degrees of loss of lower-extremity motor or sensory function. Digital rectal examination and evaluation of perianal sensation are important for the immediate diagnosis. Immediate myelography (or MRI) and surgery (if the test results are positive) are indicated to arrest progression of neurologic loss.

a. History and Physical Examination—An acute injury or precipitating event should be sought, and the location of symptoms (especially pain radiating to the extremity), character of pain, postural changes (neurogenic claudication), effect of increased intrathecal pressure, and a complete review of symptoms (including psychiatric history) should be elicited. Occupational risks, such as jobs requiring prolonged sitting and repetitive lifting, are also important factors. Intradiscal pressure is lowest when lying supine and highest when sitting and flexed forward with weights in hands. Referred pain in mesodermal tissues of the same embryologic origin, often to the buttocks or posterior thighs, must be differentiated from true radicular pain due to nerve root impingement, with symptoms that typically reach distal to the knee. Psychosocial evaluation, pain drawings, and psychological testing are helpful in some cases. The finding of an "inverted V" triad of hysteria, hypochondriasis, and depression on the Minnesota Multiphasic Personality Inventory has been identified as a significant adverse risk factor in lumbar disc surgery. Physical examination should include observation (change in posture, gait), palpation of the posterior spine (spasm, localized tenderness), measurement of range of motion (decreased flexion), hip examination, vascular evaluation (distal pulses), abdominal and rectal examination, and neurologic evaluation. Tension signs such as straight-leg raising or the bowstring sign (L4–L5 or L5–S1) and the femoral nerve stretch test (L2–L3 or L3–L4) are important findings that suggest HNP and are essential when considering a patient for diskectomy. A positive contralateral straight-leg raising test

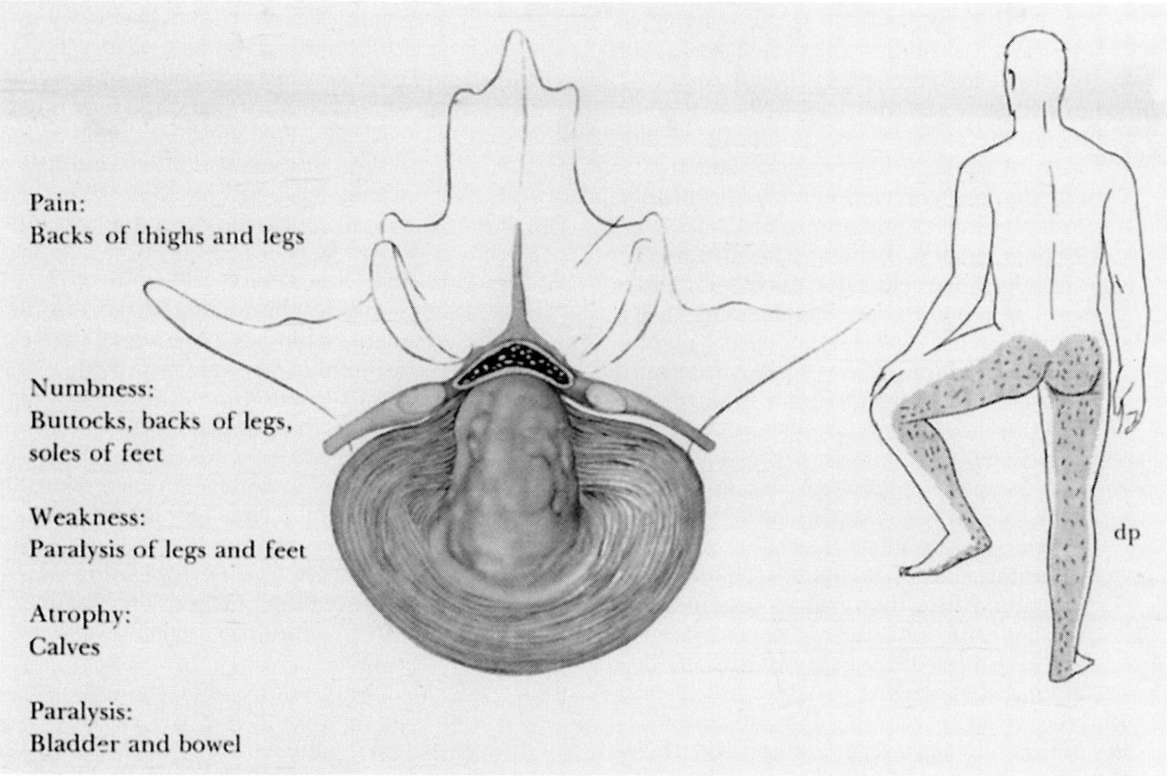

Figure 7–4. Cauda equina syndrome. (From DePalma, A.F., and Rothman, R.H.: The Intervertebral Disc. Philadelphia, WB Saunders, 1970, p. 194.)

is most specific for HNP. Specific findings by level are presented in Table 7–4. A large central disc herniation at one level may impinge on more than one nerve root. Inappropriate signs and symptoms (Waddell's) are also important to note. Inappropriate symptoms include pain at the tip of the "tailbone," pain plus numbness, or giving way of the whole leg. Nonorganic physical signs include tenderness with light touch in nonanatomic areas, simulation (light axial loading), distraction testing, pain with pelvic rotation, negative sitting (and positive supine) straight-leg raising test results, regional nonanatomic disturbances (such as a stocking-glove distribution), and overreaction.

b. Diagnostic Tests—Plain radiographs are indicated before proceeding with special tests to rule out other disorders, such as isthmic defects. However, most plain radiographic findings are nonspecific, and plain radiography can usually be deferred for 6 weeks. Myelography, CT, or MRI is effective when used as a confirming study. CT is noninvasive and helpful for demonstrating bony stenosis and identifying lateral pathologic conditions. Combined with myelography (invasive), imaging of neural compression may be improved. MRI is superior for identifying cord disorders, neural tumors, and far lateral discs. It is noninvasive, involves no ionizing radiation, and gives a "myelogram" effect on the T2 images. Multiplanar views allow imaging of central, foraminal, and extraforaminal stenosis. In addition, MRI demonstrates the state of hydration

Table 7–4.

Findings in Lumbar Disc Disease

Level	Nerve Root	Sensory Loss	Motor Loss	Reflex Loss
L1–L3	L2, L3	Anterior thigh	Hip flexors	None
L3–L4	L4	Medial calf	Quadriceps, tibialis anterior	Knee jerk
L4–L5	L5	Lateral calf, dorsal foot	EDL, EHL	None
L5–S1	S1	Posterior calf, plantar foot	Gastrocnemius/soleus	Ankle jerk
S2–S4	S2, S3, S4	Perianal	Bowel/bladder	Cremasteric

of the discs and visualizes the marrow of the vertebral bodies, thus representing an excellent modality to screen for tumor or infection. False-positive MRI scans are common (35% of those <40 years old; 93% of those >60 years old) and therefore require correlation with the history and physical examination. Electromyelographic studies (which demonstrate fibrillations 3 weeks after nerve root pressure) are not usually helpful and rarely provide more information than a good physical examination. Thermography does not have proven efficacy in the evaluation of disc disease.

c. Treatment—Short-term bed rest (2 days) with support underneath the knees and neck, NSAIDs or aspirin, moist heat, and progressive ambulation are successful in returning most patients to their normal function. More than half of patients who present with low back pain recover in 1 week, and 90% recover within 1–3 months. One-half of patients with sciatica recover in 1 month. This treatment is followed by back rehabilitation and fitness programs. Aerobic conditioning and education are the most important factors in avoiding missed work days due to disc disease and in returning patients to work. Instruction should include avoiding rotation and flexion due to increased disc pressure associated with these activities. If patients fail to improve within 6 weeks of conservative care, further evaluation is indicated. Those patients with predominantly low back pain should undergo a bone scan and medical work-up to rule out spinal tumors or infection. If these study results are normal, back rehabilitation is continued. In patients who have predominantly leg pain (sciatica) who fail conservative therapy, a trial of lumbar epidural steroids may be helpful, although it has not been proved effective in controlled studies. Additional studies (CT [± myelogram] or MRI) are undertaken in patients who after 6–12 weeks continue to be symptomatic with pain, neurologic deficit, or positive nerve tension signs. These studies are, as a rule, preoperative tests and should be done to confirm clinical suspicions. Patients with positive study results, neurologic findings, tension signs, and predominantly sciatic symptoms without mitigating psychosocial factors are the best candidates for surgical diskectomy. Standard partial laminotomy and diskectomy are most commonly performed. Operative positioning requires the abdomen to be free to decrease pressure on the inferior vena cava and consequently on the epidural veins. With proper indications, 95% of patients have initially good or excellent results, although as many as 15–20% of patients have significant backache on long-term follow-up. Microdiskectomy decreases visualization of herniated or extruded disc fragments and lateral root stenosis, and some authors report a higher complication rate, including infection. Percutaneous diskectomy currently has limited indications in the treatment of lumbar disc disease, with no long-term follow-up studies proving its efficacy. It is contraindicated in the presence of a sequestered fragment or spinal stenosis. Intradiscal enzyme therapy has fallen out of favor because of its questionable efficacy and serious complications (anaphylaxis and transverse myelitis). Indications for its use for disc herniations are similar to those for surgery (leg pain, tension signs, neurologic deficits, positive study results).

d. Complications—Fortunately rare but can be devastating.

4. Vascular Injury—May occur during attempts at disc removal if curettes are allowed to penetrate the anterior longitudinal ligament. Intraoperative pulsatile bleeding due to deep penetration is treated with rapid wound closure, intravenous (IV) fluids and blood, repositioning the patient, and a transabdominal approach to find and stop the source of bleeding. Mortality may exceed 50%. Late sequelae of vascular injuries may include delayed hemorrhage, false aneurysm, or arteriovenous fistula formation.
5. Nerve Root Injury—More common with anomalous nerve roots. Dural tears should be repaired primarily when they occur in order to avoid the development of a pseudomeningocele or spinal fluid fistula. Adequate exposure, as well as hemostasis, lighting, magnification, and careful surgical technique, is important for diminishing the incidence of the "battered root syndrome."
6. Failed Back Syndrome—Often the result of poor patient selection, but other causes include recurrent herniation (usually acute recurrence of signs/symptoms following a 6- to 12-month pain-free interval), herniation at another level, discitis (3–6 weeks postoperatively, with rapid onset of severe back pain), unrecognized lateral stenosis (may be most common), and vertebral instability. Epidural fibrosis occurs at about 3 months postoperatively, and there may be associated leg pain. Epidural fibrosis is related to hemorrhage and surgical trauma and responds poorly to re-exploration. Scar can best be differentiated from recurrent HNP with a gadolinium-enhanced MRI.

7. Dural Tear—More common during revision surgery and should be repaired immediately if it is recognized. Fibrin adhesive sealant may be a useful adjunct for effecting dural closure. Bed rest and subarachnoid drain placement is advocated if cerebrospinal fluid leak is suspected postoperatively.
8. Infection—(Approximately 1% in open diskectomy.) Similar to infection elsewhere. Increased risk in diabetics. Incision and drainage and removal of loose graft may be required.
9. Cauda Equina Syndrome—Secondary to extruded disc, surgical trauma, hematoma. Suspect with postoperative urinary retention. Digital rectal examination is used to diagnose initially. Further imaging may be necessary.

B. Discogenic Back Pain—Hard or "dark" disc disease. Patients complain of back pain greater than leg pain. Patients may have a paucity of physical findings, no radiculopathy, and negative tension signs. X-ray films may show disc-space narrowing, but this is nondiagnostic. MRI reveals decreased signal intensity in the disc space on T2 (dark disc). Discography is a useful preoperative study to correlate MRI findings with a clinically significant pain progenitor. The study should be performed at multiple levels to include all abnormal levels on MRI and one or more normal levels. The procedure should elicit pain similar, after injection, to that usually described by the patient and should lack pain at the normal level. Treatment consists of conservative therapy with NSAIDs, therapy, and conditioning. If extended nonoperative treatment has failed, and if the patient has a positive MRI and discogram, interbody fusion can be performed either from an anterior or retroperitoneal approach or through a posterior midline (posterior lumbar interbody fusion) or posterior transforaminal approach. Fusion is performed with either nonstructural (chip posterior lumbar interbody fusion) or structural constructs (femoral ring allografts or interbody fusion cages).

C. Lumbar Segmental Instability—Present when normal loads produce abnormal spinal motion. The most common symptom is mechanical back pain, although "dynamic" stenosis can occur, leading to leg symptoms. The most consistent clinical sign is the "instability catch" (sudden, painful snapping with extension from flexed position). Degenerative lumbar disc disease is indicated by disc space narrowing. A combination of annulus damage and disc space narrowing may cause reduction in the disc's ability to resist rotatory forces. Continuing degeneration or facet subluxation may then lead to instability. Radiographically, traction spurs (horizontal and below disc margin [versus syndesmophyte]), angular changes >10 degrees (20 degrees at L5–S1) on flexion films, and translatory motion >3–4 mm (6 mm at L5–S1) with flexion-extension views are all characteristic of lumbar instability but are difficult to quantify and may not correlate with clinical symptoms. Iatrogenic instability can occur after removal of a total of one or more facet joints during surgery. Surgical treatment options do not have clearly defined indications but include posterolateral fusion, posterior lumbar interbody fusion (posterior lumbar interbody fusion—graft is "keyed" into the intervertebral space), and anterior interbody fusion. Posterior lumbar interbody fusion is associated with a high incidence of pseudarthrosis and neurologic injury. Internal fixation, utilizing pedicle screw fixation in rod or plate constructs, is gaining popularity as an adjunct in lumbar spine fusion surgery, but the efficacy of these implants, particularly when the added cost and potential complications are considered, remains unproven.

D. Spinal Stenosis
1. Introduction—Spinal stenosis is narrowing of the spinal canal or neural foramina, producing nerve root compression, root ischemia, and a variable syndrome of back and leg pain. Central stenosis produces compression of the thecal sac, whereas lateral stenosis involves compression of individual nerve roots either in the subarticular (lateral) recess (by the medial overgrowth of the superior articular facet at a given facet joint) or in the intervertebral foramen. Stenosis usually does not become symptomatic until patients reach late middle age; it affects men twice as often as women.
2. Central Stenosis
   a. Introduction—Can be congenital (idiopathic or developmental in achondroplastic dwarfs) or acquired. Acquired stenosis, the most common type, is usually degenerative owing to enlargement of osteoarthritic facets with medial encroachment, but it can be secondary to degenerative spondylolisthesis, post-traumatic, postsurgical, or due to various disease processes (e.g., Paget's, fluorosis). Pre-existing "trefoil" canal shapes, a congenitally narrow canal, or medially placed facets may limit the ability to tolerate minor acquired encroachment (Fig. 7–5). Central stenosis represents compression of the thecal sac, with absolute stenosis defined as a cross-sectional area of <100 mm^2 or <10 mm of anteroposterior diameter as seen on CT cross-section. Soft tissue (ligamentum flavum and disc) may contribute as much as 40% to thecal sac compression. Central stenosis is more common in men because their spinal canal is smaller at the L3–L5 levels than is that of women and afflicts an older population than does lateral recess stenosis.
   b. Symptoms—Include insidious pain and paresthesias with ambulation and exten-

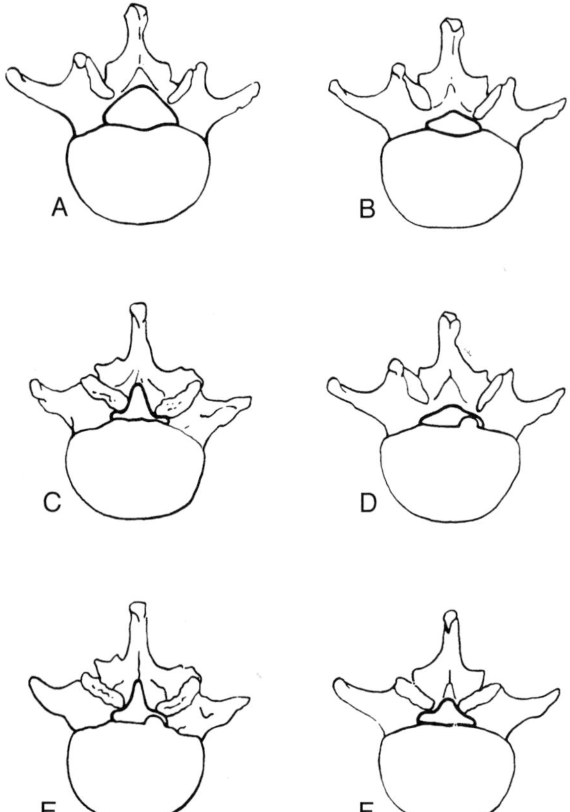

Figure 7–5. Spinal stenosis. *A,* Normal. *B,* Congenital stenosis. *C,* Degenerative stenosis. *D,* Congenital stenosis with disc herniation. *E,* Degenerative stenosis with disc herniation. *F,* Congenital and degenerative stenosis. (From Arnoldi, C.C., et al.: Lumbar spinal stenosis and nerve root entrapment syndromes. Clin. Orthop. 115:4, 1976.)

sion, relieved by lying supine or with flexion of the spine. Patients commonly complain of lower-extremity pain, numbness, or "giving way." A history of radiating leg pain in a true dermatomal distribution, although typical in patients with HNP, is relatively uncommon in those with spinal stenosis. Neurogenic claudication, which occurs in about 50% of patients with stenosis, usually can be differentiated from vascular claudication by history.

Activity	Vascular Claudication	Neurogenic Claudication
Walking	Distal-proximal pain, calf pain	Proximal-distal thigh pain
Uphill walking	Symptoms develop sooner	Symptoms develop later
Rest	Relief with sitting or bending	
Bicycling	Symptoms develop	Symptoms do not develop
Lying flat	Relief	May exacerbate symptoms

Physical examination is also important. Patients with stenosis may have pain with extension, typically have normal pulses, and may have neurologic findings. Abnormal neurologic findings, however, or positive tension signs are seen in fewer than one-half of patients. Neurologic findings not otherwise obvious are sometimes demonstrated with a "stress test" (walking until symptoms occur).

c. Imaging—Further work-up may include plain radiographs on which disc degeneration, interspace narrowing, medially placed facets, and flattening of the lordotic curve are commonly seen; subluxation and degenerative changes of the facet joints may be seen. Plain CT, postmyelo-CT, and MRI are standard imaging modalities. Careful inspection of these studies is necessary to assess lateral nerve root entrapment by medial hypertrophy of the superior facet, the tip of the superior facet, osteophyte formation off the posterior vertebral body (uncinate spur), or a combination of these problems. Central stenosis is a diminution in the area of the thecal sac and is produced by thickening of the ligamentum flavum and/or posterior protrusion of the disc, in combination with enlarged facet joints. Simply looking for the "bony" measurements results in underestimating the degree of stenosis; soft-tissue contribution to thecal sac narrowing must be considered. Bone scan or MRI may help to rule out malignancy. Electromyelographic studies or somatosensory evoked potentials may be used, but sensitivity is variable and depends on the examiner.

d. Treatment—Rest, isometric abdominal exercises, pelvic tilt, Williams' flexion exercises, NSAIDs, and weight reduction are important in management of patients with stenosis. Lumbar epidural steroids may be helpful for short-term relief but have not shown efficacy in controlled studies. Surgery is indicated in patients with positive study results and persistent, unacceptably impaired quality of life. Adequate decompression of the identified disorder should include laminectomy and partial medial facetectomy, which can usually be done without destabilizing the spine, thus avoiding fusion. Fusion is indicated in patients with surgical instability (removal of one facet or more), pars defects (including postsurgical) with disc disease, symptomatic radiographic instability, degenerative or isthmic spondylolisthesis, and degenerative scoliosis.

3. Lateral Stenosis—Impingement of nerve roots lateral to the thecal sac as they pass through the lateral recess and into the neural

foramen. Often associated with facet joint arthropathy (superior articular process enlargement) and disc disease (Fig. 7–6). The three-joint complex (disc and both facets) must be considered when evaluating lateral stenosis. Nerve root compression can occur at more than one level and must be completely decompressed to relieve symptoms. Compression can be subarticular (lateral recess stenosis), which consists of compression between the medial aspect of a hypertrophic superior articular facet and the posterior aspect of the vertebral body and disc. Hypertrophy of the ligamentum flavum and/or ventral facet joint capsule and vertebral body osteophyte/disc exacerbates the stenosis. Foraminal stenosis can be produced by intraforaminal disc protrusion, impingement of the tip of the superior facet, uncinate spurring, or a combination. Subarticular stenosis, which is more common, affects the traversing (lower) nerve root, whereas foraminal stenosis affects the exiting (upper) root at a motion segment. Lateral stenosis is most frequently seen in combination with central stenosis but can appear as an isolated entity usually involving middle-aged or even young adults with symptoms of radicular pain unrelieved by rest and without tension signs. Lower lumbar areas are most commonly involved because the foramina size decreases as the nerve root size increases. Pain may be the result of intraneural edema and demyelination. Substance P may be released as a response to spinal nerve root irritation. After failure of nonoperative treatment, decompression of the hypertrophied lamina and ligamentum flavum and partial facetectomy are usually successful. Fusion may be necessary if instability is present or created.

4. Extraforaminal Lateral Root Compression ("Far Out Syndrome" [Wiltse's])—Involves L5 root impingement between the sacral ala and the L5 transverse process. It is usually seen in degenerative scoliosis, isthmic spondylolisthesis, or extraforaminal herniated discs. It must be specifically sought on special radiographs (25 degree caudocephalic [Ferguson's] view) or CT.

E. Spondylolysis and Spondylolisthesis
   1. Spondylolysis—Defect in the pars interarticularis. It is the most common cause of low back pain in children and adolescents. The defect in the pars is thought to be a fatigue fracture from repetitive hyperextension stresses (most common in gymnasts, football linemen), to which there may be a hereditary predisposition. Plain lateral radiographs demonstrate 80% of lesions, with another 15% visible on oblique radiographs, which show a defect in the "neck of the Scottie dog" as described by Lachapelle (Fig. 7–7). CT, bone scan and, more recently, single positron emission computed tomography scanning may be helpful in identifying subtle defects; increased uptake is more compatible with acute lesions that have the potential to heal. Bracing or casting (a single thigh pantaloon spica) has been advocated for acute lesions, but treatment is usually aimed at symptomatic relief rather than fracture healing and includes activity restriction, flexion exercises, and bracing. Nonunion is common and may have normal scans.
   2. Spondylolisthesis—Forward slippage of one vertebra on another. Can be classified into six types (Newman, Wiltse, McNab) (Table 7–5; Figs. 7–8, 7–9). Severity of slip in spondylolisthesis is based on the amount or degree (as compared with S1 width): I, 0–25%; II, 25–50%; III, 50–75%; IV, >75%; V, >100% (spondyloptosis). Other measurements, including the sacral inclination (normally >30 degrees) and the slip angle (normally >0 degrees), are also useful for quantifying lumbopelvic deformity, which af-

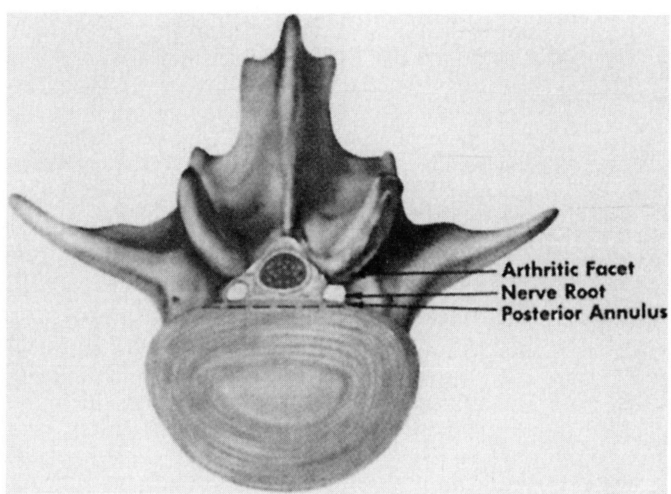

Figure 7–6. Lateral stenosis. Note nerve root entrapment laterally on the right by arthritic facet and bulging posterior annulus. (From Rothman, R.H., and Simeon, F.A.: The Spine, 2nd ed. Philadelphia, WB Saunders, 1982, p. 194.)

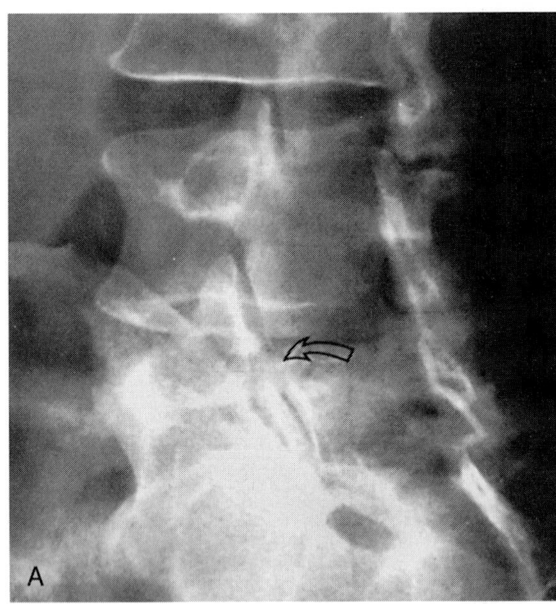

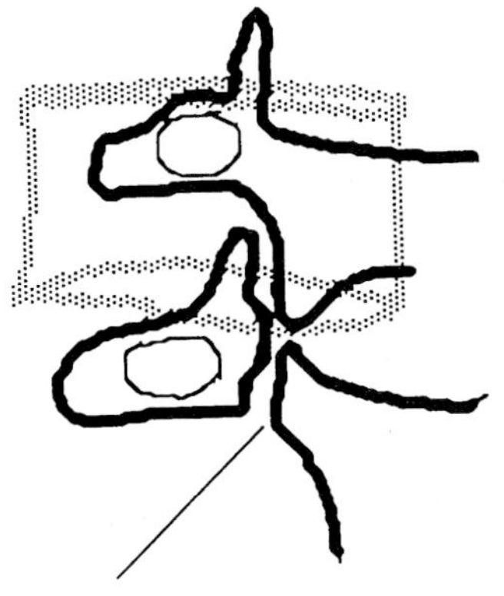

Figure 7–7. Spondylolysis. Note disruption of "collar on Scottie dog." (From Helms, C.A.: Fundamentals of Skeletal Radiology. Philadelphia, WB Saunders, 1989, p. 101.)

fects cosmesis as well as prognosis (Fig. 7–10).

3. Childhood Spondylolisthesis—Usually at L5–S1, is typically type II, and usually presents with back pain (instability), hamstring tightness, deformity, or alteration in gait ("pelvic waddle"). Although the onset of symptoms may occur at any time in life, screening studies identify the occurrence of the slippage as being most common at 4–6 years. Spondylolisthesis is most common in whites, boys, and youngsters involved in hyperextension activities, and it is remarkably common in Eskimos (>50%). It is thought to result from shear stress at the pars interarticularis associated with repetitive hyperextension. Severe slips are rare and are associated with radicular findings (L5), cauda equina dysfunction, kyphosis of the lumbosacral junction, and "heart-shaped" buttocks. Spina bifida occulta, thoracic hyperkyphosis, and Scheuermann's disease are associated with spondylolisthesis.
   a. Low-Grade Disease (<50% Slip)—Spondylolysis or mild spondylolisthesis may require bone scan or CT for diagnosis and usually responds to nonoperative treatment consisting of activity modification and exercise. Adolescents with a grade I slip may return to normal activities, including contact sports, once they are asymptomatic. Those with asymptomatic grade II spondylolisthesis are restricted from activities such as gymnastics or football. Progression is uncommon, but risk factors include young age at presentation, female gender, a slip angle of >10 degrees (see Fig. 7–10), a high-grade slip, and a dome-shaped or significantly inclined sacrum (>30 degrees beyond vertical). Furthermore, patients with type I or congenital spondylolisthesis are at higher risk for slip progression and the development of cauda equina dysfunction because the neural arch is intact. Patients with a greater than 25% slip, or with L4–5 or L3–4 spondylolisthesis, have a higher risk of low back pain than the general population. Surgery for patients with a low-grade slip generally consists of L5–S1 posterolateral fusion in situ and is usually reserved for those with intractable pain

Table 7–5.

Types of Spondylolisthesis

Class	Type	Age	Pathology/Other
I	Congenital	Child	Congenital dysplasia of S1 superior facet
II	Isthmic[a]	5–50	Predisposition leading to elongation/fracture of pars (L5–S1)
III	Degenerative	Older	Facet arthrosis leading to subluxation (L4–L5)
IV	Traumatic	Young	Acute fracture/other than pars
V	Pathologic	Any	Incompetence of bony elements
VI	Postsurgical	Adult	Excessive resection of neural arches/facets

[a]Most common.

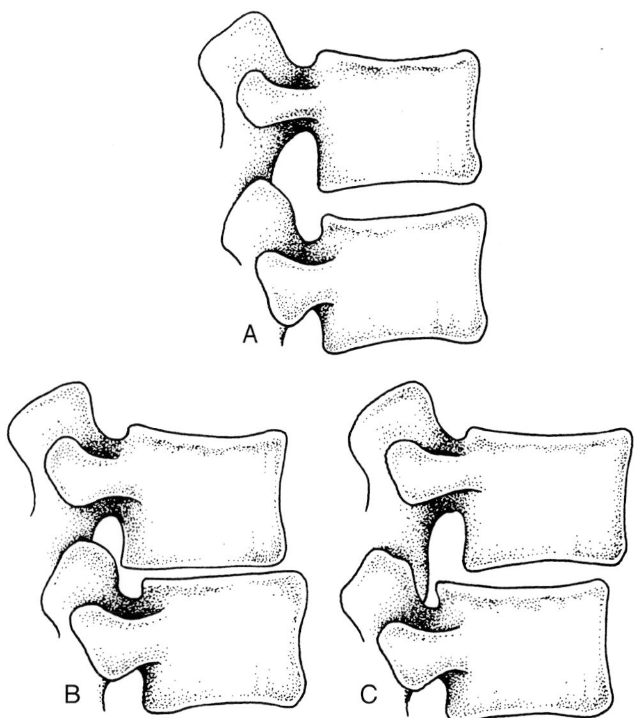

Figure 7–8. Degenerative spondylolisthesis. *A,* Normal. *B,* Retrolisthesis—disc narrowing is greater than posterior joint degeneration. *C,* Anterolisthesis—posterior joints are more degenerated than the disc. (From Weinstein, J.N., and Wiesel, S.W.: The Lumbar Spine. Philadelphia, WB Saunders, 1990, p. 84.)

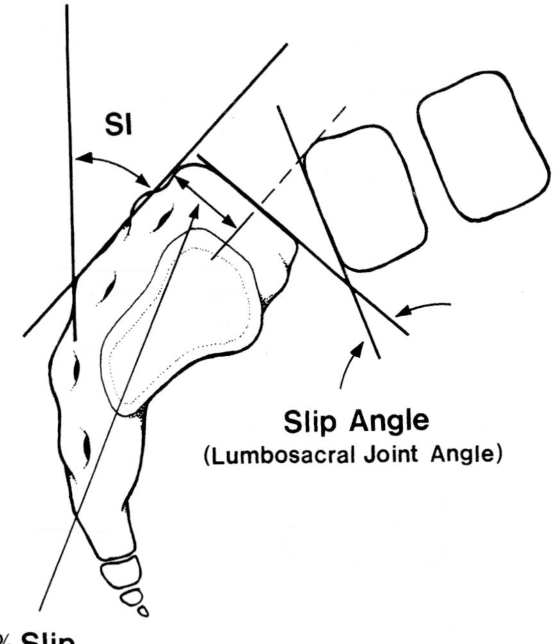

Figure 7–10. Measurements used for evaluation of spondylolisthesis. (Modified from Wiltse, L.L., and Winter, R.B.: Terminology and measurement of spondylolisthesis. J. Bone Joint Surg. [Am.] 65:768–772, 1983.)

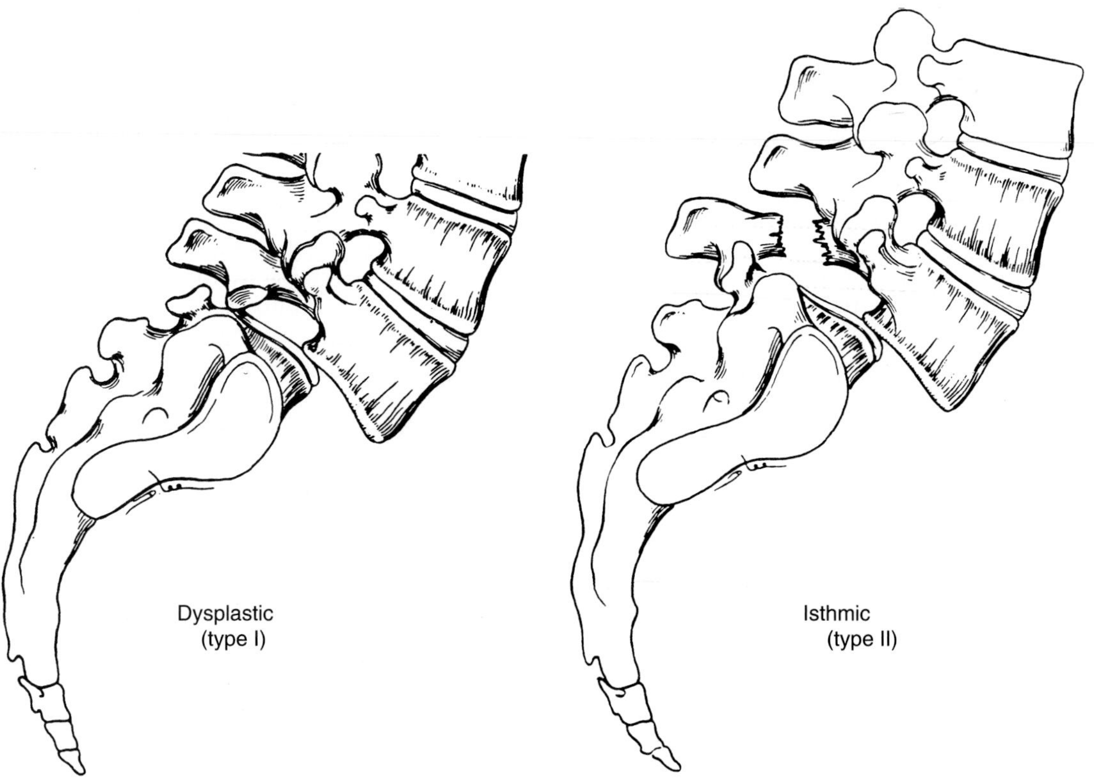

Figure 7–9. Spondylolisthesis. (From Rothman, R.H., and Simeon, F.A.: The Spine, 2nd ed. Philadelphia, WB Saunders, 1982, p. 264.)

who have failed nonoperative treatment or those demonstrating progressive slippage. Wiltse has popularized a paraspinal splitting approach to the lumbar transverse process and sacral alae that is frequently utilized in this setting. L5 radiculopathy is uncommon in children with low-grade slips and rarely if ever requires decompression. Repair of the pars defect utilizing a lag screw (Buck's) or tension band wiring (Bradford's) with bone grafting has been reported. It may be indicated in young patients with slippage less than 25% and a pars defect at L4 or above.

b. Grades III and IV Spondylolisthesis and Spondyloptosis (Grade V)—Commonly cause neurologic abnormalities. L5–S1 isthmic spondylolisthesis causes an L5 radiculopathy (contrast with S1 radiculopathy in L5–S1 HNP). Prophylactic fusion is recommended in children with slippage of more than 50%. It often requires bilateral posterolateral fusion in situ, usually at L4–S1 (L5 is too far anterior to effect L5–S1 fusion) without instrumentation. Nerve root exploration is controversial but is usually limited to children with clear-cut radicular pain or significant weakness. Reduction of spondylolisthesis has been associated with a 20–30% incidence of L5 root injuries and should be utilized cautiously. A cosmetically unacceptable deformity and L5–S1 kyphosis so severe that the posterior fusion mass from L4 to the sacrum would be under tension without reversal of the kyphosis are the most commonly cited indications. Close neurologic monitoring should be done during the procedure and for several days afterward to identify postoperative neuropathy. Posterior decompression, fibular interbody fusion, and posterolateral fusion without reduction has been reported with excellent long-term results (Bohlman's). "Spondylolisthetic crisis" is seen in patients with severe slips, increasing pain, and hamstring tightness. The Gill procedure, consisting of removal of the loose elements without fusion, is contraindicated in children and is rarely performed in adults.

4. Degenerative Spondylolisthesis—More commonly involves African Americans, diabetics, and women over age 40; it is most common at the L4–L5 level (see Fig. 7–8). It is reported to be more common in patients with transitional L5 vertebrae and with sagitally oriented facet joints. Degenerative spondylolisthesis frequently causes L5 radiculopathy owing to root compression in the lateral recess between the hypertrophic and subluxated inferior facet of L4 and the posterosuperior body of L5. The operative treatment of degenerative spondylolisthesis involves decompression of the nerve roots and stabilization by posterolateral fusion.The addition of hardware is controversial and may be indicated for concurrent scoliotic deformity, severe slips, and failed fusions.

5. Adult Isthmic Spondylolisthesis—Although the significance of isthmic spondylolisthesis in an adult is controversial, it remains a common indication for surgery. Nonoperative treatment includes rest, corset, NSAIDs, and flexion exercises. It is essential to assess for other common sources of back pain before assuming that spondylolisthesis is the cause; MRI scanning is a useful tool in this setting. Isthmic L5–S1 spondylolisthesis frequently causes radicular symptoms in the adult, resulting from compression of the exiting L5 root in the L5–S1 foramen; compression may involve hypertrophic fibrous repair tissue at the pars defect, uncinate spur formation off the posterior L5 body, and bulging of the L5–S1 disc. Operative treatment is favored in the presence of radicular symptoms and usually involves thorough foraminal decompression and fusion, with or without pedicular screw fixation. Compromised results in workers' compensation patients have been reported.

F. Thoracolumbar Injuries

1. Introduction—The thoracolumbar spine is the most common site for vertebral column injuries. Although the classification and treatment of these injuries is included in Chapter 10, Trauma, some points need to be emphasized here. The upper thoracic spine (T1–T10) is stabilized by the ribs and the facet orientation, as well as the sternum, and is less susceptible to trauma. At the thoracolumbar junction, however, there is a fulcrum of increased motion, and this area is more commonly affected by spinal trauma. Two anatomic points also bear noting: (1) the middle T-spine is a vascular "watershed" area, and vascular insult can lead to cord ischemia; and (2) the spinal cord ends and the cauda equina begins at the level of L1–L2, so lesions below the L1 level carry a better prognosis because nerve roots, not cord, are affected.

2. Stable Versus Unstable Injuries—The three-column system (Denis') has been proposed for evaluating spinal injuries and determining which are stable or unstable. The anterior column is composed of the anterior longitudinal ligament and the anterior two-thirds of the annulus and vertebral body. The middle column consists of the posterior third of the body and annulus and the posterior longitudinal ligament. The posterior column comprises the pedicles, facets, spinous processes, and posterior ligaments, including the inter-

spinous and supraspinous ligaments, ligamentum flavum, and facet capsules. Disruption of the middle column (seen as widening of the interpedicular distances on anteroposterior radiographs or a change in height of the posterior cortex of the body on lateral views) suggests an unstable injury that may require operative fixation. In addition, disruption of the posterior ligamentous complex in the face of anterior fracture or dislocation is a strong indication of instability and of the potential need for surgical stabilization. Exceptions may include the upper thoracic spine, which is inherently more stable, and bony Chance's fractures. Compression fractures of three sequential vertebrae lead to an increase in risk of post-traumatic kyphosis.

3. Treatment—May be either operative or nonoperative (bracing or casting) for stable fractures, with a well-aligned spine with less than 20–30 degrees of kyphosis and no neurologic compromise. Operative intervention includes decompression for progressive neurologic deficit (emergency) or for incomplete neurologic deficit. May be accomplished anteriorly via vertebrectomy and stabilization or posteriorly via a transpedicular route. Posterior instrumentation with restoration of height and sagittal alignment may decompress the canal by repositioning the "posterolateral complex." Historically, posterior instrumentation and fusion have extended three levels above and two levels below the injury to stabilize the fracture. A recent alternative is the "rod-long, fuse-short" technique, allowing fusion across only two motion segments but requiring implant removal. Constructs are created either in compression (fracture/dislocations, Chance's fractures, or shear fractures) or in distraction (burst fractures) to reduce and stabilize the injury. Newer, more rigid segmental systems with multiple hooks, wires, and screws or rod-sleeve constructs have supplanted the standard Harrington system and allow maintenance of the normal sagittal contour of the spine. Pedicle screw systems are available that purport to limit instrumentation levels to one above and one below the injury. High rates of screw breakage have been reported, and the concepts regarding fusion levels and constructs are in evolution. The goals of surgery include stabilization of the fracture and preservation or improvement of neural function in all patients, as well as more rapid entry into rehabilitation and a shorter hospital stay for patients with complete injuries. Rehabilitation following spinal cord injury is discussed more fully in Chapter 9, Rehabilitation.
4. Complications—The most common long-term complication of a thoracolumbar fracture, treated with or without surgery, is pain. Unfortunately, the relationship between chronic pain and "stability," deformity, pseudarthrosis, and many other factors is unclear. Various types of post-traumatic deformity are noted, including scoliosis caudal to a complete injury (an age-related phenomenon with 100% occurrence in those <10 years old) and progressive kyphosis (common with unrecognized posterior ligamentous injury). Symptomatic flat back of the lumbar spine results in a forward flexed posture and easy fatigue (occurs with uncontoured distraction instrumentation). Other complications include late progressive neurologic loss and pain due to the development of post-traumatic syringomyelia. Late development of a neuropathic spine with gross bony destruction and bony spicules in the soft tissue has also been described.

G. Other Thoracolumbar Disorders

1. Destructive Spondyloarthropathy—Seen in hemodialysis patients with chronic renal failure. Typically involves three adjacent vertebrae with two intervening discs. Changes include subluxation, degeneration, and narrowing of the disc height. Although the process may resemble infection, it probably represents crystal or amyloid deposition.
2. Facet Syndrome—Inflammation or degeneration of the lumbar facet joints. May cause pain that is characteristically in the low back, with radiation down one or both buttocks and posterior thighs that is worse with extension. Selective injections of local anesthetic can be helpful in the diagnosis of this condition, but anesthetic/steroid injections into the facet joint as a treatment modality are less effective (<20% with excellent pain relief). The significance of the facet syndrome is debated, and no widely accepted treatment regimen exists. There is no proof that surgery (facet rhizotomy or fusion) is beneficial.
3. Diffuse Idiopathic Skeletal Hyperostosis (DISH)—Also known by the eponym Forestier's disease, this entity is defined by the presence of nonmarginal syndesmophytes (differentiated from ankylosing spondylitis, which has marginal syndesmophytes [Fig. 7–11]) at three successive levels. DISH can occur anywhere in the spine but is most common in the T-spine and is more often seen on the right side. DISH is associated with chronic lower back pain and is more common in patients with diabetes and gout. The prevalence of DISH has been found to be as high as 28% in autopsy specimens. Although there appears to be no relationship between DISH and spinal pain, DISH is associated with extraspinal ossification at several joints, including an increased risk of heterotopic ossification following total hip surgery.

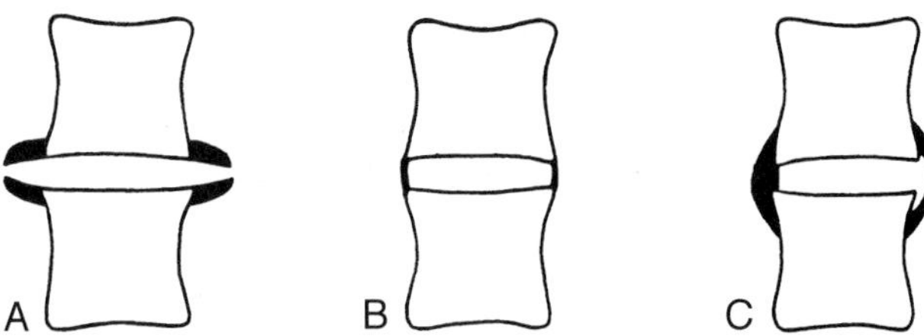

Figure 7–11. Differential diagnoses of *(A)* osteophytes (degenerative joint disease), *(B)* marginal syndesmophytes (ankylosing spondylitis), and *(C)* nonmarginal syndesmophytes (DISH). (From Rothman, R.H., and Simeon, F.A.: The Spine, 2nd ed. Philadelphia, WB Saunders, 1982, p. 924.)

4. Ankylosing Spondylitis—HLA-B27–positive patients are usually young men who present with insidious onset of back and hip pain during the third or fourth decade of life. Sacroiliac joint obliteration and marginal syndesmophytes allow radiographic differentiation from DISH. Ankylosing spondylitis may result in fixed cervical, thoracic, or lumbar hyperkyphosis. It occasionally causes marked functional limitation, primarily due to the inability of affected patients to face forward. Extension osteotomy and fusion of the lumbar spine with compression instrumentation can successfully balance the head over the sacrum. Assessment for hip flexion contractures or cervicothoracic kyphosis is mandatory. The cervical spine may be corrected by a C7–T1 osteotomy and fusion under local anesthesia. Complications of osteotomies include nonunion, loss of correction, and neurologic and aortic injury.
5. Adult Scoliosis—Usually defined as scoliosis in patients over age 20, it is more symptomatic than its childhood counterpart (discussed in Chapter 2, Pediatric Orthopaedics). Cause is usually idiopathic but can also be neuromuscular, degenerative (secondary to degenerative disc disease or osteoporosis), post-traumatic, or postsurgical. Curves are usually thoracic (secondary to unrecognized adolescent scoliosis) or lumbar/thoracolumbar (degenerative). Although the association between pain and scoliosis is controversial, back pain is the most common presenting complaint and appears to be related to curve severity and location (lumbar curves more painful). Pain usually begins in the convexity of the curve and later moves to the concavity, reflecting a more refractory condition. Radicular pain and stenosis can occur and may require surgical decompression. Other complaints include cosmetic deformity, cardiopulmonary problems (thoracic curves >60–65 degrees may alter pulmonary function tests; curves >90 degrees may affect mortality), and neurologic symptoms (secondary to stenosis). There is no demonstrated association between curve progression and pregnancy. Progression is unlikely in curves <30 degrees. Right thoracic curves ≥50 degrees are at highest risk for progression (usually 1 degree/year), followed by right lumbar curves. Myelography with CT or MRI is useful for the evaluation of nerve root compression in stenosis. MRI, facet injections, and/or discography may be utilized to evaluate symptoms in the lumbar spine. Nonoperative treatment includes NSAIDs, weight reduction, therapy, muscle strengthening, facet joint injections, and orthotics (used with activity). The uncertain correlation between adult scoliosis and back pain makes conservative management, including a thorough evaluation for other common causes of back pain, essential. Surgery is usually reserved for symptomatic curves >50–60 degrees in young adults and up to 90 degrees and beyond in older patients, for progressive curves, for patients with cardiopulmonary compromise (worsening pulmonary function tests in severe curves), and for patients with refractory spinal stenosis. Operative risk is high (up to 25% complication rate in older patients), and complications include pseudarthrosis (15% with posterior fusion only, highest risk in lumbar spine), urinary tract infection, instrumentation problems, infection (up to 5%), and neurologic deficits. Additionally, long convalescence is usually required. Combined anterior release and fusion and posterior fusion and instrumentation may be beneficial for large (>70 degrees), more rigid curves (as determined on side-bending films) or curves in the lumbar spine. Preservation of normal sagittal alignment with fusion is critical. Fusion to the sacrum is associated with more complications (pseudarthrosis, instrumentation failure, loss of normal lordosis, and pain) and should be avoided when possible. Achieving a successful result, including fusion to the sacrum, is enhanced by combined anterior and posterior fusion. The ideal implant for instrumentation in these cases has not been found; commonly used instrumentation for sacral fixation includes Galveston's fixation and sacral pedicle or alar screw constructs. Clinical and experimental evidence exists demonstrating the benefit of structural interbody grafting (femoral ring allograft or mesh cage), at L5–S1 and L4–5, to decrease the stress on the sacropelvic fixation.
6. Postlaminectomy Deformity—Progressive deformity (usually kyphosis) due to a prior wide laminectomy. Laminectomy in children is followed by a high risk (90%) of deformity. Fusion plus internal fixation may be considered prophylactic for young patients who re-

quire extensive decompression. Fusion utilizing pedicular screw fixation is best for reconstruction in the adult lumbar spine.

H. Kyphosis

1. Introduction—Kyphosis in adults may be idiopathic (old Scheuermann's), post-traumatic, secondary to trauma or ankylosing spondylitis, or a result of metabolic bone disease. Progressive kyphosis secondary to multiple osteoporotic compression fractures (occur secondary to loss of vertical trabeculae in vertebral body) is usually treated with exercises, bracing, and medical management of the underlying bone disease. Surgical attempts at correction and stabilization are marked by high complication rate. An underlying malignancy as a cause of the osteopenia should be considered; evaluation with MRI is sensitive for determining the presence of tumor.
2. Nontraumatic Adult Kyphosis—Severe idiopathic or congenital kyphosis may be a source of back pain in the adult, particularly when present in the thoracolumbar or lumbar spine. When the symptoms fail to respond to nonoperative management (see Adult Scoliosis, above), posterior instrumentation and fusion of the entire kyphotic segment, utilizing a compression implant, may be indicated. Anterior fusion in conjunction is performed for curves not correcting to 55 degrees or less on hyperextension lateral radiographs.
3. Post-traumatic Kyphosis—May be seen following fractures of the thoracolumbar spine treated nonoperatively, particularly when the posterior ligamentous complex has been disrupted; fractures treated by laminectomy without fusion; and fractures for which fusion has been performed unsuccessfully. Progressive kyphosis may produce pain at the fracture site, with radiating leg pain and/or neurologic dysfunction if there is associated neural compression. Operative options include posterior fusion with compression instrumentation for milder deformities; combined anterior and posterior osteotomies, instrumentation, and fusion for more severe deformities; and anterior spinal cord or cauda equina decompression combined with posterior instrumentation and fusion for cases involving neurologic dysfunction.

IV. Sacrum and Coccyx

A. Sacroiliac Joint Pain—Elicited with the patient lying on the affected side without support (Gaenslen's test); direct compression; or flexion, abduction, and external rotation (flexion, abduction, and external rotation, i.e., Faber or Patrick's test). Local injections may have a diagnostic and therapeutic role. Orthotic management (trochanteric cinch) can be helpful. Fusion is not indicated unless an infection is present.

B. Idiopathic Coccygodynia—Painful coccyx may be associated with psychological conditions. Four types have been identified (Postacchini and Massobrio).

Type	Coccyx Morphology	Coccygodynia
I	Slight forward curve, apex dorsal	Rare
II	Marked curve, apex ventral	Common
III	Sharp angulation between coccyx segments	Common
IV	Ventral subluxation of segments (sacrococcygeal or coccycoccygeal)	Common

Treatment of coccygodynia should be conservative, with a donut pillow and NSAIDs. Local steroid injection is occasionally utilized for resistant cases. Complete or partial coccygectomy may relieve symptoms of type III or IV disorder but is a last resort and is associated with a high complication and failure rate.

C. Sacral Insufficiency Fracture—Occurs in older patients with osteopenia, often without a history of trauma. Complaints include low back and groin pain. Diagnosed with technetium bone scan (H-shaped uptake pattern is diagnostic) or CT scan. Treatment is nonoperative with rest, analgesics, and ambulatory aids until symptoms resolve.

V. Spine Tumors and Infections

A. Introduction—The spine is a frequent site of metastasis, and certain tumors with a predilection for the spine have unique manifestations in vertebrae. Tumors of the vertebral body include histiocytosis X, giant cell tumor, chordoma, osteosarcoma, hemangioma, metastatic disease, and marrow cell tumors. Tumors of the posterior elements include aneurysmal bone cysts, osteoblastoma, and osteoid osteoma. Radiographic changes include absent pedicle, cortical erosion or expansion, and vertebral collapse. Bone scans can be helpful in cases of protracted back pain or night pain. MRI is also useful: malignant tumors have decreased T1 and increased T2 intensity, the sensitivity of which is increased with use of gadolinium. Malignant tumors occur more commonly in lower (lumbar > thoracic > cervical) spinal levels and in the vertebral body. Complete surgical excision is difficult and usually consists of tumor debulking and stabilization. Adjuvant therapy is essential. For more details on these tumors, refer to Chapter 8, Orthopaedic Pathology.

B. Metastasis—Most common tumors of the spine, with spread to the vertebral body first and later to the pedicles. "Red flags" for possible spinal metastasis include a history of cancer, recent unexplained weight loss, night pain, and age >50 years. Most tumors are osteolytic and are not demonstrated on plain films until >30% destruction of the vertebral body has occurred. Breast, lung, and prostate metastases are most common, the latter being blastic. CT-guided needle biopsy is often possible, and surgery for diagnosis can be avoided. Poor prognosis is associated with neurologic dysfunction, proximal lesions, long duration of symptoms, and rapid growth of the metastasis. Radiation therapy and chemotherapy are the mainstays of treatment unless the tumor is destabilizing and progressive or causes spinal cord or cauda equina dysfunction. Radiosensitivity varies among primary tumor types: prostate and lymphoid tumors are quite radiosensitive; breast cancer is 70% sensitive, 30% are resistant; gastrointestinal and renal cell tumors are quite radioresistant. Surgical indications include progressive neurologic dysfunction unresponsive to radiation therapy, persistent pain despite radiation therapy, need for a diagnostic biopsy, and pathologic fracture/dislocation. In cases of neurologic deficit and/or spinal instability, anterior decompression and stabilization (preserving intact posterior structures) have a role and may result in recovery of neurologic function. Posterior stabilization or a circumferential approach is indicated in cases with multiple levels of destruction, involvement of both anterior and posterior columns, or translational instability. Life expectancy should play an important role as to whether surgical treatment is performed. Methyl methacrylate may be useful as an anterior strut but should only be utilized as an adjunct because of the high complication rate. Iliac crest graft is favored if life expectancy is >6 months. Anterior internal fixation may be indicated to maximize immediate stability and rehabilitation.

C. Primary Tumors
   1. Osteoid Osteoma and Osteoblastoma—Common in the spine. May present with painful scoliosis in a child. Pain is typically relieved by aspirin. Bone scan can help localize the level, and thin-cut CT scans can direct surgical excision. Scoliosis (the lesion is typically at the apex of the convexity) resolves with early resection (within 18 months) in a child <11 years of age. If no scoliosis exists, NSAIDs are the mainstay of treatment. If they do not alleviate the pain, resection may be required. Osteoblastomas typically occur in the posterior elements in older patients, with neurologic involvement in more than half. This presentation typically requires resection and posterior fusion.
   2. Aneurysmal Bone Cyst—May represent degeneration of other, more aggressive tumors. These cysts typically occur during the second decade of life. They occur in the posterior elements but may also involve the anterior elements. Treatment is excision and/or radiation therapy.
   3. Hemangioma—Typically seen in asymptomatic patients. Symptomatic patients over age 40 may present after small spinal fractures. Classically has "jailhouse striations" on plain films and "spikes of bone" demonstrated on CT. Vertebrae are typically normally sized and not expanded (as in Paget's disease). Treatment is observation or radiation therapy in cases of persistent pain after pathologic fracture. Anterior resection and fusion are reserved for refractory cases or pathologic collapse and neural compression, but massive bleeding may be encountered.
   4. Eosinophilic Granuloma—Usually seen in children younger than 10 years old. Seen more often in the thoracic spine; may present with progressive back pain. Classically causes vertebral flattening (vertebra plana—Calve's disease), which is seen on lateral radiographs. Biopsy may be required for diagnosis unless the radiographic picture is classic or histiocytosis has already been diagnosed. Chemotherapy is useful for the systemic form. Bracing may be indicated in children to prevent progressive kyphosis. Low-dose radiation therapy may be indicated in the presence of neurologic deficits; otherwise, symptoms are usually self-limited. At least 50% reconstitution of vertebral height may be expected.
   5. Giant Cell Tumor—Most commonly seen in the fourth and fifth decades of life. Destroys the vertebral body in an expansile fashion. Surgical excision and bone grafting comprise the usual recommended treatment. High recurrence rate is reported. Radiation therapy should be avoided because of the possibility of malignant degeneration of the tumor.
   6. Plasmacytoma/Multiple Myeloma—Also common in the spine, causing osteopenic, lytic lesions. Pain, pathologic fractures, and diffuse osteoporosis are common. Increased calcium and decreased hematocrit levels are common, as well as abnormal protein studies. Treatment is radiation therapy (3000–4000 cGy ± chemotherapy). Surgery is reserved for instability and patients with refractory neurologic symptoms.
   7. Chordoma—Classically a slow-growing lytic lesion in the midline of the anterior sacrum or the base of the skull. May occur in other vertebrae (cervical most common). These tumors may present with intra-abdominal complaints and a presacral mass. Radiation therapy and surgery are favored. Surgical excision can include up to half of the sacral roots (i.e., all roots on one side) and still maintain bowel and bladder function. Recurrence rate is high, but aggressive attempts at surgical exci-

sion are indicated. Although a "cure" is rare, patients typically survive 10–15 years after diagnosis.

8. Osteochondroma—Arises in the posterior elements. It is seen commonly in the cervical spine. Treatment is excision, which may be necessary to rule out sarcomatous changes.
9. Neurofibroma—Can present with enlarged intervertebral foramina seen on oblique radiographs.
10. Malignant Primary Skeletal Lesions—Osteosarcoma, Ewing's sarcoma, and chondrosarcoma are uncommon in the spine. When they do occur they are associated with a poor prognosis. Chemotherapy and irradiation are the mainstays of treatment, but aggressive surgical excision may have a role. Lesions may actually be metastases, which are treated palliatively.
11. Lymphoma—Can present with "ivory" vertebrae. Usually associated with a systemic disease, lymphoma is treated after histologic diagnosis by irradiation and/or chemotherapy.

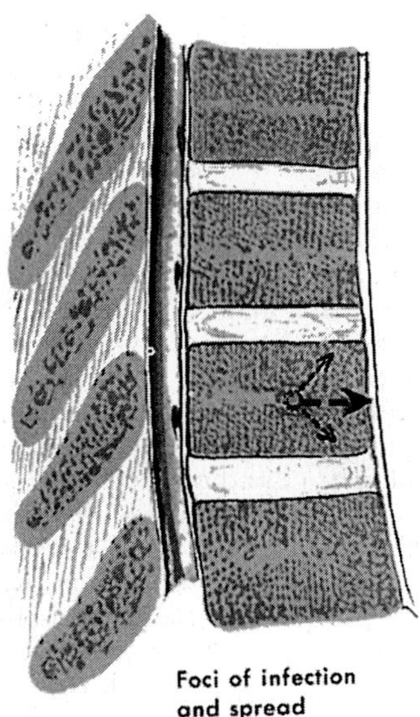

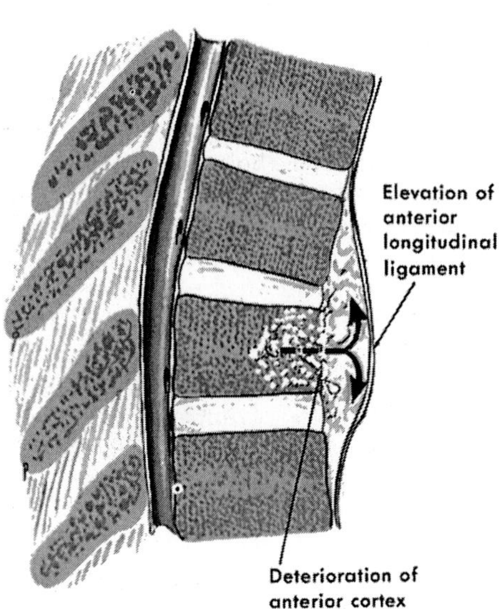

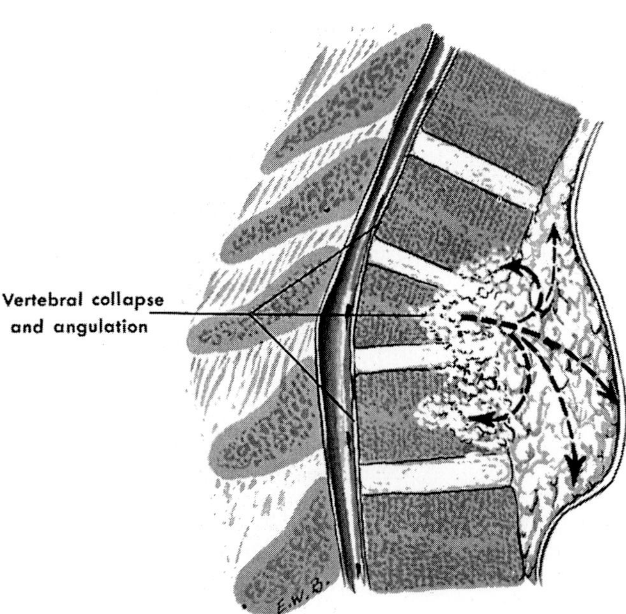

Figure 7–12. Pathogenesis of spinal tuberculosis. (From Tachdjian, M.O.: Pediatric Orthopaedics, 2nd ed. Philadelphia, WB Saunders, 1990, p. 1450.)

D. Spinal Infections

1. Disc Space Infection—Blood-borne infection can invade primarily the disc space in children. *Staphylococcus aureus* is the most common offender, but gram-negative organisms are common in older patients. Children (mean age 7, although all age groups are affected) commonly present with inability to walk, stand, or sit; back pain/tenderness; and restricted spine range of motion. Laboratory studies may be normal except for an elevated erythrocyte sedimentation rate and white blood cell count. Radiographic findings include disc space narrowing and endplate erosion, but these findings do not occur until 10 days to 2 weeks, and their absence is unreliable. MRI scan is the diagnostic test of choice, although bone scan is also useful in the diagnosis. Treatment includes bed rest (traction, however, is contraindicated), immobilization, and antibiotics.
2. Pyogenic Vertebral Osteomyelitis—Seen with increasing frequency but still associated with a significant (6–12 week) delay in diagnosis. Older debilitated patients and IV drug addicts are at increased risk. A history of pneumonia, urinary tract infection, skin infection, or immunologic compromise (transplant patients) is common. The organism is usually hematogenous in origin. A history of unremitting spinal pain at any level is characteristic, and tenderness, spasm, and loss of motion are seen. Forty percent of neurologic deficits are seen in older patients, in patients with infections at more cephalad levels of the spine, and in patients with debilitating systemic illnesses, such as diabetes or RA, and in patients with delayed diagnoses. Plain radiographic findings include osteopenia, paraspinous soft-tissue swelling (loss of psoas shadow), erosion of the vertebral endplates, and disc destruction. Disc destruction, seen on plain radiographs or MRI, is atypical of neoplasms. Bone scanning is sensitive for a destructive process. MRI is both sensitive for detecting infection and specific in differentiating infection from tumor. Gadolinium enhances sensitivity. Tissue diagnosis via blood cultures or aspirate of the infection is mandatory; when made, 6–12 weeks of IV antibiotics is the treatment of choice. Bracing may be used adjunctively. Open biopsy is indicated when a tissue diagnosis has not been made, and an anterior approach or costotransversectomy is utilized. Anterior débridement and strut grafting are reserved for refractory cases, typically associated with abscess formation, or cases involving neurologic deterioration, extensive bony destruction, or marked deformity.
3. Spinal Tuberculosis (Pott's Disease)—The most common extrapulmonary location of tuberculosis is in the spine. Originating in the metaphysis of the vertebral body and spreading under the anterior longitudinal ligament, spinal tuberculosis can cause destruction of several contiguous levels or can result in skip lesions (15%) or abscess formation (50%) (Fig. 7–12). On early plain x-ray, vertebral body destruction anteriorly, with preservation of the disc, distinguishes tuberculosis from pyogenic infection. About two-thirds of patients have abnormal chest radiographs, and 20% have a negative PPD test or are anergic. Severe kyphosis, sinus formation, and (Pott's) paraplegia are late sequelae. Spinal cord injury may occur secondary to direct pressure from the abscess, bony sequestra (good prognosis) or, rarely, meningomyelitis (poor prognosis). Radical anterior débridement of the infection followed by autogenous strut grafting (Hong Kong procedure) is the accepted surgical treatment in most centers. Advantages include less progressive kyphosis, earlier healing, and decrease in sinus formation. Adjuvant chemotherapy beginning 10 days before surgery is recommended. In cases without severe kyphosis or neurologic deficit, adjuvant chemotherapy and bracing remain a viable treatment option, particularly in centers not equipped for major anterior spinal surgery.

Selected Bibliography

Reviews

General Information

Boden, S.D.: The use of radiographic imaging studies in the evaluation of patients who have degenerative disorders of the lumbar spine. J. Bone Joint Surg. [Am.] 78:114–125, 1996.

Boden, S.D., and Wiesel, S.W.: Lumbar spine imaging: Role in clinical decision making. J. Am. Acad. Orthop. Surg. 4:238–248, 1996.

Cervical Spondylosis, Stenosis

Bohlman, H.H.: Cervical spondylosis and myelopathy. AAOS Instr. Course Lect. 44:81–98, 1995.

Law, M.D., Bernhardt, M., and White, A.A.: Evaluation and management of cervical spondylotic myelopathy. AAOS Instr. Course Lect. 44:99–110, 1995.

Levine, M.J., Albert, T.J., and Smith, M.D.: Cervical radiculopathy: Diagnosis and nonoperative management. J. Am. Acad. Orthop. Surg. 4:305–316, 1996.

Rheumatoid Spondylitis

Monsey, R.D.: Rheumatoid arthritis of the cervical spine. J. Am. Acad. Orthop. Surg. 5:240–248, 1997.

Cervical Spine Injury

Botte, M.J., Byrne, T.P., Abrams, R.A., et al.: Halo skeletal fixation: Techniques of application and prevention of complications. J. Am. Acad. Orthop. Surg. 4:44–53, 1996.

Slucky, A.V., and Eismont, F.J.: Treatment of acute injury of the cervical spine. AAOS Instr. Course Lect. 44:67–80, 1995.

Disc Disease

Eismont, F.J., and Currier, B.: Current concepts review: Surgical management of lumbar intervertebral-disc disease. J. Bone Joint Surg. [Am.] 71:1266, 1989.

Lumbar Stenosis

Spivak, J.M.: Degenerative lumbar spinal stenosis. J. Bone Joint Surg. [Am.] 80:1053–1067, 1998.

Spondylolisthesis

Hensinger, R.N.: Current concepts review: Spondylolysis and spondylolisthesis in children and adolescents. J. Bone Joint Surg. [Am.] 71:1098, 1989.

Larsen, J.M., and Capen, D.A.: Pseudarthrosis of the lumbar spine. J. Am. Acad. Orthop. Surg. 5:153–162, 1997.

Lauerman, W.C., and Cain, J.E.: Isthmic spondylolisthesis in the adult. J. Am. Acad. Orthop. Surg. 4:201–208, 1996.

Thoracolumbar Injury

Bohlman, H.H.: Current concepts review: Treatment of fractures and dislocations of the thoracic and lumbar spine. J. Bone Joint Surg. [Am.] 67:165, 1985.

Slucky, A.V., and Potter, H.G.: Use of magnetic resonance imaging in spinal trauma: Indications, techniques, and utility. J. Am. Acad. Orthop. Surg. 6(3):134–145, 1998.

Deformity

Bradford, D.S.: Adult scoliosis: Current concepts of treatment. Clin. Orthop. 229:70, 1988.

Tribus, C.B.: Scheuermann's kyphosis in adolescents and adults: Diagnosis and management. J. Am. Acad. Orthop. Surg. 6:36–43, 1998.

Other

Kambin, P., McCullen, G., Parke, W., et al.: Minimally invasive arthroscopic spinal surgery. AAOS Instr. Course Lect. 46:143–161, 1997.

Regan, J.J., Yuan, H., and McCullen, G.: Minimally invasive approaches to the spine. AAOS Instr. Course Lect. 46:127–141, 1997.

Recent Articles

General Information

Sidhu, K.S., and Herkowitz, H.H.: Spinal instrumentation in the management of degenerative disorders of the lumbar spine. Clin Orthop 335:39–53, 1997.

Back Pain

Jensen, M.E.: MRI of the lumbar spine in people without back pain. N. Engl. J. Med. 331:69, 1994.

Cervical Spondylosis, Stenosis

Bernhardt, M., Hynes, R.A., Blume, H.W., et al.: Cervical spondylotic myelopathy. J. Bone Joint Surg. [Am.] 75:119, 1993.

Bohlman, H.H., Emery, S.E., Goodfellow, D.B., et al.: Robinson anterior cervical diskectomy and arthrodesis for cervical radiculopathy. J. Bone Joint Surg. [Am.] 75:1298–1307, 1993.

Emery, S.E., Bohlman, H.H., Bolesta, M.J., et al.: Anterior cervical decompression and arthrodesis for the treatment of cervical spondylotic myelopathy: Two to seven year follow-up. J. Bone Joint Surg. [Am.] 80:941–951, 1998.

Ghanayem, A.J., Leventhal, M., and Bohlman, H.H.: Osteoarthrosis of the atlanto-axial joints: Long-term follow-up after treatment with arthrodesis. J. Bone Joint Surg. [Am.] 78:1300–1308, 1996.

Iwasaki, M., and Ebara, S.: Expansive laminoplasty for cervical radiculomyelopathy due to soft disc herniation. Spine 21:32–38, 1996.

Johnson, M.J., and Lucas, G.L.: Value of cervical spine radiographs as a screening tool. Clin Orthop. 340:102–108, 1997.

McAfee, P.C., Hohlman, H.H., Ducker, T.B., et al.: One-stage anterior cervical decompression and posterior stabilization: A study of one hundred patients with minimum two years of follow-up. J. Bone Joint Surg. [Am.] 77:1791, 1995.

Zdeblick, T.A., Hughes, S.S., Riew, K.D., et al.: Failed anterior cervical discectomy and arthrodesis: Anaylsis and treatment of thirty-five patients. J. Bone Joint Surg. [Am.] 79:523–532, 1997.

Rheumatoid Spondylitis

Boden, S.D., Dodge, L.D., Bohlman, H.H., et al.: Rheumatoid arthritis of the cervical spine: A long-term analysis with predictors of paralysis and recovery. J. Bone Joint Surg. [Am.] 75:1282, 1993.

Cervical Spine Injury

Anderson, P.A., and Bohlman, H.H.: Anterior decompression and arthrodesis of the cervical spine: Long-term motor improvement. Part II—Improvement in complete traumatic quadriplegia. J. Bone Joint Surg. [Am.] 74:683–692, 1992.

Bohlman, H.H., and Anderson, P.A.: Anterior decompression and arthrodesis of the cervical spine: Long term motor improvement. Part I—Improvement in incomplete traumatic quadriparesis. J. Bone Joint Surg. [Am.] 74:671–682, 1992.

McAfee, P.C., Bohlman H.H., Ducker, T.B., et al.: One-stage anterior cervical decompression and posterior stabilization. J. Bone Joint Surg. [Am.] 77:1791, 1995.

Torg, J.S., Naranja, R.J., Pavlov, H., et al.: The relationship of developmental narrowing of the cervical spinal canal to reversible and irreversible injury of the cervical spinal cord in football players: An epidemiological study. J. Bone Joint Surg. [Am.] 78:1308–1314, 1996.

Disc Disease

Atlas, S.J., Deyo, R.A., Keller, R.B., et al.: The Maine lumbar spine study: Part II. Spine 21:1777–1786, 1996.

Ethier, D.E., Cain, J.E., Yaszemski, M.J., et al.: The influence of annulotomy selection on disc competence: A biomechanical, radiographic, and histologic analysis. Spine 19:2071–2076, 1994.

Komori, H., and Shinomiya, K.: The natural history of HNP with radiculopathy. Spine 21:225–229, 1996.

Lumbar Stenosis

Grob, D., Humke, T., and Dvorak, J.: Degenerative lumbar spinal stenosis: Decompression with and without arthrodesis. J. Bone Joint Surg. [Am.] 77:1036–1041, 1995.

Katz, J.N., and Lipson, S.J.: Seven to ten year outcome of decompressive surgery for degenerative lumbar spinal stenosis. Spine 21:92–98, 1996.

Stewart, G., and Sachs, B.L.: Patient outcomes after reoperation on the lumbar spine. J. Bone Joint Surg. [Am.] 78:706–711, 1996.

Spondylolisthesis

Boden, S.D., Schimandle, J.H., Hutton, W.C.: The use of an osteoinductive growth factor for lumbar spinal fusion: Study of dose, carrier, and species. Spine 20:2633–2644, 1995.

Boden, S.D., Schimandle, J.H., Hutton, W.C., et al.: The use of an osteoinductive growth factor for lumbar spinal fusion: Biology of spinal fusion. Spine 20:2626–2632, 1995.

Carpenter, C.T., and Dietz, J.W.: Repair of a pseudarthrosis of the lumbar spine: A functional outcome study. J. Bone Joint Surg. [Am.] 78:712–720, 1996.

Carragee, E.J.: Single-level posterolateral arthrodesis, with or without posterior decompression, for the treatment of isthmic spondylolisthesis in adults: A prospective, randomized study. J. Bone Joint Surg. [Am.] 79:1175–1180, 1997.

Fischgrund, J.S., Mackay, M., Herkowitz, H.N., et al.: Degenerative lumbar spondylolisthesis with spinal stenosis: A prospective, randomized study comparing decompressive laminectomy and arthrodesis with and without spinal instrumentation. Spine 22:2807–2812, 1997.

Goel, V.K., and Gilbertson, L.G.: Basic science of spinal instrumentation. Clin. Orthop. 335:10–31, 1997.

Guanciale, A.F., Dinsay, J.M., and Watkins, R.G.: Lumbar lordosis in spinal fusion. Spine 21:964–969, 1996.

Herkowitz, H.N., and Kurz, L.T.: Degenerative lumbar spondylolisthesis with spinal stenosis: A prospective study comparing decompression with decompression and intertransverse process arthrodesis. J. Bone Joint Surg. [Am.] 73:802–808, 1991.

Kanayama, M., Cunningham, B.W., Weis, J.C., et al.: Maturation of the posterolateral spinal fusion and its effect on load-sharing of spinal instrumentation. An in vivo sheep model. J. Bone Joint Surg. [Am.] 79:1710–1720, 1997.

Thomsen, K., and Christensen, F.B.: The effect of pedicle screw instrumentation on functional outcome and fusion rates in posterolateral lumbar spinal fusion: A prospective, randomized clinical study. Spine 22:2813–2822, 1997.

Zdeblick, T.: A prospective randomized study of lumbar fusion. Spine 18:983–991, 1993.

Thoracolumbar Injury

Delamarter, R.B., Sherman, J., and Carr, J.B.: Pathophysiology of spinal cord injury: Recovery after immediate and delayed decompression. J. Bone Joint Surg. [Am.] 77:1042, 1995.

Kaneda, K., and Taneichi, H.: Anterior decompression and stabilization with the Kaneda device for thoracolumbar burst fractures associated with neurological deficits. J. Bone Joint Surg. [Am.] 79:69–83, 1997.

Deformity

Dickson, J.H., and Mirkovic, S.: Results of operative treatment of idiopathic scoliosis in adults. J. Bone Joint Surg. [Am.] 77:513–523, 1995.

Infections, Tumors

Bauer, H.C.: Posterior decompression and stabilization for spinal metastases: Analysis of sixty-seven consecutive patients. J. Bone Joint Surg. [Am.] 79:514–522, 1997.

Carragee, E.J.: Pyogenic vertebral osteomyelitis. J. Bone Joint Surg. [Am.] 79:874–880, 1997.

Complications

Klein, J.D., and Hey, L.A.: Perioperative nutrition and postoperative complications in patients undergoing spinal surgery. Spine 21:2676–2682, 1996.

McDonnell, M.F., and Glassman, S.D.: Perioperative complications of anterior procedures on the spine. J. Bone Joint Surg. [Am.] 78:839–847, 1996.

Classic Articles

General Information

Boden, S.D., Davis, D.O., Dina, T.S., et al.: Abnormal magnetic resonance scans of the lumbar spine in asymptomatic subjects. J. Bone Joint Surg. [Am.] 72:403, 1990.

Boden, S.D., McCown, P.R., Davis, D.O., et al.: Abnormal MRI scans of cervical spine in asymptomatic subjects: A prospective investigation. J. Bone Joint Surg. [Am.] 72:1178–1184, 1990.

Dommisse, G.F.: The blood supply of the spinal cord. J. Bone Joint Surg. [Br.] 56:225, 1974.

Garfin, S.R., Bottle, M.J., Walters, R.L., et al.: Complications in the use of the halo fixation device. J. Bone Joint Surg. [Am.] 68:320, 1986.

Macnab, I.: The blood supply of the lumbar spine and its application to the technique of intertransverse lumbar fusion. J. Bone Joint Surg. [Br.] 53:628, 1971.

White, A.A. III, Johnson, R.M., Panjabi, M.M., et al.: Biomechanical analysis of clinical stability in the cervical spine. Clin. Orthop. 109:85–96, 1975.

Wiesel, S.W., Tsourmas, N., Feffer, H.L., et al.: A study of computer-assisted tomography: The incidence of positive CAT scans in an asymptomatic group of patients. Spine 9:549, 1984.

Back Pain

Deyo, R.H., Diehl, A.K., and Rosenthal M.: How many days of bed rest for acute low back pain? A randomized clinical trial. N. Engl. J. Med. 315:1064–1070, 1986.

Deyo, R.A., and Tsui-Wu, Y.J.: Descriptive epidemiology of low back pain and its related medical care in the United States. Spine 12:264–268, 1987.

Frymoyer, J.W.: Back pain and sciatica. N. Engl. J. Med. 318:291–300, 1988.

Frymoyer, J.W., Pope, M.H., Clements, J.H., et al.: Risk factors in low back pain: An epidemiological survey. J. Bone Joint Surg. [Am.] 65:213–218, 1983.

Nachemson, A.: Work for all: For those with low back pain as well. Clin. Orthop. 179:77–85, 1983.

Cervical Spondylosis, Stenosis

Fielding, J.W., Hensinger, R.N., and Hawkins, R.J.: Os odontoideum. J. Bone Joint Surg. [Am.] 62:376, 1980.

Gore, D.R., and Sepic, S.B.: Anterior cervical fusion for degenerated or protruded discs: A review of one hundred forty-six patients. Spine 9:667–671, 1984.

Gore, D.R., Sepic, S.B., Gardner, G.M., et al.: Neck pain: A long-term follow-up of 205 patients. Spine 12:1–5, 1987.

Herkowitz, H.N., Kurz, L.T., and Overholt, D.P.: Surgical management of cervical soft disk herniation: A comparison between anterior and posterior approach. Spine 15:1026–1030, 1990.

Hirabayashi, K., and Satomi, K.: Operative procedure and results of expansive open-door laminoplasty. Spine 13:870–876, 1988.

Robinson, R.A., and Smith, G.W.: Anterior lateral cervical disc removal in interbody fusion for cervical disc disease. Bull. Johns Hopkins Hosp. 96:223–224, 1955.

Smith, G.W., and Robinson, R.A.: The treatment of certain cervical spine disorders by anterior removal of the intervertebral disk and interbody fusion. J. Bone Joint Surg. [Am.] 40:607–623, 1958.

Zdeblick, T.A., and Bohlman, H.H.: Cervical kyphosis and myelopathy: Treatment by anterior corpectomy and strut-grating. J. Bone Joint Surg. [Am.] 71:170, 1989.

Rheumatoid Spondylitis

Brooks, A.L., and Jenkins, E.B.: Atlanto-axial arthrodesis by the wedge compression method. J. Bone Joint Surg. [Am.] 60:279, 1978.

Clark, C.R., Goetz, D.D., and Menezes, A.H.: Arthrodesis of the cervical spine in rheumatoid arthritis. J. Bone Joint Surg. [Am.] 71:381–392, 1989.

Kraus, D.R., Peppleman, W.C., Agrwal, A.K., et al.: Incidence of subaxial subluxation in patients with generalized rheumatoid arthritis who have had previous occipital cervical fusions. Spine 16S:486–489, 1991.

Pellicci, P.M., Ranawat, C.S., Tsairis, P., et al.: A prospective study of the progression of rheumatoid arthritis of the cervical spine. J. Bone Joint Surg. [Am.] 63:342, 1981.

Rana, N.A.: Natural history of atlanto-axial subluxation in rheumatoid arthritis. Spine 14:1054–1056, 1989.

Ranawat, C.S., O'Leary, P., Pellicci, P., et al.: Cervical spine fusion in rheumatoid arthritis. J. Bone Joint Surg. [Am.] 61:1003, 1979.

Slatis, P., Santavirta, S., Sandelin, J., et al.: Cranial subluxation of the odontoid process in rheumatoid arthritis. J. Bone Joint Surg. [Am.] 71:189, 1989.

Zoma, A., Sturrock, R.D., Fisher, W.D., et al.: Surgical stabilization of the rheumatoid cervical spine: A review of indications and results. J. Bone Joint Surg. [Br.] 69:8–12, 1987.

Cervical Spine Injury

Allen, B.L., Jr., Ferguson, R.L., Lehmann, T.R., et al.: A mechanistic classification of closed, indirect fractures and dislocation of the lower cervical spine. Spine 7:1–27, 1982.

Anderson, L.D., and D'Alozono, R.T.: Fractures of the odontoid process of the axis. J. Bone Joint Surg. [Am.] 56:1663, 1974.

Bohlman, H.H.: Acute fractures and dislocations of the cervical spine: An analysis of 300 hospitalized patients and review of the literature. J. Bone Joint Surg. [Am.] 61:1119–1142, 1979.

Bohlman, H.H., and Eismont, F.J.: Surgical techniques of anterior decompression and fusion for spinal cord injuries. Clin. Orthop. 154:57, 1981.

Clark, C.R., and White, A.A. III: Fractures of the dens: A multicenter study. J. Bone Joint Surg. [Am.] 67:1340–1348, 1985.

Fielding, J.W., and Hawkins, R.J.: Atlanto-axial rotatory fixation: Fixed rotatory subluxation of the atlanto-axial joint. J. Bone Joint Surg. [Am.] 59:37, 1977.

Gallie, W.E.: Fractures and dislocations of the cervical spine. Am. J. Surg. 46:495, 1939.

Johnson, R.M., Hart, D.L., Simmons, E.F., et al.: Cervical orthoses: A study comparing their effectiveness in restricting cervical motion in normal subjects. J. Bone Joint Surg. [Am.] 59:332, 1977.

Kang, J.E., Figgie, M.P., and Bohlman, H.H.: Sagittal measurements of the cervical spine in subaxial fractures and dislocations: An analysis of two hundred eighty-eight patients with and without neurologic deficits. J. Bone Joint Surg. [Am.] 76:1617–1628, 1994.

Levine, A.M., and Edwards, C.C.: The management of traumatic spondylolisthesis of the axis. J. Bone Joint Surg. [Am.] 67:217–226, 1985.

Stauffer, E.S.: Wiring techniques of the posterior cervical spine for the treatment of trauma. Orthopaedics 11:1543, 1988.

Torg, S., Pavlov, H., Genuario, S.E., et al.: Neurapraxia on the cervical spinal cord with transient quadriplegia. J. Bone Joint Surg. [Am.] 68:1354–1370, 1986.

Disc Disease

Albrand, O.W., and Corkill, G.: Thoracic disc herniation: Treatment and prognosis. Spine 4:41–46, 1979.

Bell, G.R., and Rothman, R.H.: The conservative treatment of sciatica. Spine 9:54–56, 1984.

Bohlman, H.H., and Zdeblick, T.A.: Anterior excision of herniated thoracic discs. J. Bone Joint Surg. [Am.] 70:1038, 1988.

Crawshaw, C., Frazer, A.M., Merriam, W.F., et al.: A comparison of surgery and chemonucleolysis in the treatment of sciatica: A prospective randomized trial. Spine 9:195–198, 1984.

Hanley, E.N., and Shapiro, D.E.: The development of low back pain after excision of a lumbar disk. J. Bone Joint Surg. [Am.] 71:719–721, 1989.

Kostuik, J.P., Harrington, I., Alexander, D., et al.: Cauda equina syndrome and lumbar disc herniation. J. Bone Joint Surg. [Am.] 68:386, 1986.

Nachemson, A.L., and Rydevik, B.: Chemonucleolysis for sciatica: A critical review. Acta Orthop. Scand. 59:56, 1988.

Waddell, G., Kummell, E.G., Lotto, W.M., et al.: Failed lumbar disk surgery and repeat surgery following industrial injuries. J. Bone Joint Surg. [Am.] 61:201–207, 1979.

Weber, H.: Lumbar disc herniation: A controlled, prospective study with ten years of observation. Spine 8:131, 1983.

Lumbar Stenosis

Kirkaldy-Willis, W.H.: The relationship of structural pathology to the nerve root. Spine 9:49–52, 1984.

Kirkaldy-Willis, W.H., Wedge, J.H., Yong-Hing, K., et al.: Pathology and pathogenesis of lumbar spondylosis and stenosis. Spine 4:319, 1978.

Spengler, D.M.: Current concepts review: Degenerative stenosis of the lumbar spine. J. Bone Joint Surg. [Am.] 69:305, 1987.

Spondylolisthesis

Boxall, D., Bradford, D.S., Winter, R.B., et al.: Management of severe spondylolisthesis in children and adolescents. J. Bone Joint Surg. [Am.] 61:479, 1979.

Bradford, D.S.: Closed reduction of spondylolisthesis and experience in 22 patients. Spine 13:580, 1988.

Bradford, D.S., and Boachie-Adjei, O.: Treatment of severe spondylolisthesis by anterior and posterior reduction and stabilization: A long-term follow-up study. J. Bone Joint Surg. [Am.] 72:1060, 1990.

Farfan, H.: The pathological anatomy of degenerative spondylolisthesis: A cadaver study. Spine 5:412–418, 1980.

Frederickson, B.W., Baker, D., McHolick, W.J., et al.: The natural history of spondylolysis and spondylolisthesis. J. Bone Joint Surg. [Am.] 66:699–707, 1984.

Gill, G.G., Manning, J.G., and White, H.L.: Surgical treatment of spondylolisthesis without spine fusion. J. Bone Joint Surg. [Am.] 37:493, 1955.

Harris, I.E., and Weinstein, S.D.: Long-term follow-up of patients with grade III and IV spondylolisthesis: Treatment with and without posterior fusion. J. Bone Joint Surg. [Am.] 69:960–969, 1987.

Ogilvie, J.W., and Sherman, J.: Spondylolysis in Scheuermann's disease. Spine 12:251–253, 1987.

Osterman, K., Lindholm, T.S., and Laurent, L.E.: Late results of removal of the loose posterior element (Gill's operation) in the treatment of lytic lumbar spondylolisthesis. Clin. Orthop. 117:121, 1976.

Peek, R.D., Wiltse, L.L., Reynolds, J.B., et al.: In situ arthrodesis without decompression for grade III or IV isthmic spondylolisthesis in adults who have severe sciatica. J. Bone Joint Surg. [Am.] 71:62, 1989.

Saraste, H: The etiology of spondyloysis: A retrospective radiographic study. Acta Orthop. Scand. 56:253, 1985.

Wiltse, L.L., and Winter, R.B.: Terminology and measurement of spondylolisthesis. J. Bone Joint Surg. [Am.] 65:768–772, 1983.

Wiltse, L.L., Guyer, R.D., Spencer, C.W., et al.: Alar transverse process impingement of the L5 spinal nerve: The far-out syndrome. Spine 9:31, 1984.

Thoracolumbar Injury

An, H.S., Vaccaro, A., Cotler, J.M., et al.: Low lumbar burst fractures: Comparison among body cast, Harrington rod, Luque rod, and Steffee plate. Spine 16:S440–S444, 1991.

Bohlman, H.H., and Eismont, F.J.: Surgical techniques of anterior decompression and fusion for spinal cord injuries. Clin. Orthop. 154:57, 1981.

Bracken, M.B., Shepard, M.J., Collins, W.F., et al.: A randomized, controlled trial of methylprednisolone or naloxone in the treatment of acute spinal cord injury. N. Engl. J. Med. 322:1405, 1990.

Cain, J.E., DeJung, J.T., Divenberg, A.S., et al.: Pathomechanical analysis of thoracolumbar burst fracture reduction: A calf spine model. Spine 18:1640–1647, 1993.

Cammissa, F.P., Jr., Eismont, F.J., and Green, B.A.: Dural laceration occurring with burst fractures and associated laminar fractures. J. Bone Joint Surg. [Am.] 71:1044–1052, 1989.

Denis, F.: The three-column spine and its significance in the classification of acute thoracolumbar spinal injuries. Spine 8:817–831, 1983.

Ferguson, R.L., and Allen, B.L., Jr.: A mechanistic classification of thoracolumbar spine fractures. Clin. Orthop. 189:77, 1984.

Holdsworth, F.W.: Fractures, dislocations, and fracture-dislocations of the spine. J. Bone Joint Surg. [Am.] 52:1534, 1970.

Kaneda, K., Abumi, K., and Fujiya, M.: Burst fractures with neurologic deficits of the thoracolumbar-lumbar spine: Results of anterior decompression and stabilization with anterior instrumentation. Spine 9:788, 1984.

McAfee, P.C., Bohlman, H.H., and Yuan, H.A.: Anterior decompression of traumatic thoracolumbar fractures with incomplete neurologic deficit using a retroperitoneal approach. J. Bone Joint Surg. [Am.] 67:89–104, 1985.

Mumfred, J., Weinstein, J.N., Spratt, K.F., et al.: Thoracolumbar burst fractures: The clinical efficacy and outcome of nonoperative management. Spine 18:955–970, 1993.

Transfeldt, E.E., White, D., Bradford, D.S., et al.: Delayed anterior decompression in patients with spinal cord and cauda equina injuries of the thoracolumbar spine. Spine 15:953, 1990.

Deformity

Allen, B.L., Jr., and Ferguson, R.L.: The Galveston technique of pelvic fixation with L-rod instrumentation of the spine. Spine 9:388, 1984.

Bradford, D.S., Ganjavian, S., and Antonious, D.: Anterior strut-grafting for the treatment of kyphosis: Review of experience with forty-eight patients. J. Bone Joint Surg. [Am.] 64:680, 1982.

Bradford, D.S., Moe, J.H., Montalvo, F.J., et al.: Scheuermann's kyphosis and roundback deformity: Results of Milwaukee brace treatment. J. Bone Joint Surg. [Am.] 56:740, 1974.

Jackson, R.P., Simmons, E.H., and Stripinis, D.: Incidence and severity of back pain in adult idiopathic scoliosis. Spine 8:749, 1983.

Lauerman, W.C., Bradford, D.S., Ogilvie, J.W., et al.: Results of lumbar pseudarthrosis repair. J. Spinal Disord. 5:128–136, 1992.

Lauerman, W.C., Bradford, D.S., Transfeld, E.E., et al.: Management of pseudarthrosis after arthrodesis of the spine for idiopathic scoliosis. J. Bone Joint Surg. [Am.] 73:222–236, 1991.

Luque, E.R.: Segmental spinal instrumentation of the lumbar spine. Clin. Orthop. 203:126–134, 1986.

Murray, P.M., Weinstein, S.L., and Spratt, K.F.: The natural history and long term follow-up of Scheuermann's kyphosis. J. Bone Joint Surg. [Am.] 75:236–248, 1993.

Nachemson, A.: Adult scoliosis and back pain. Spine 4:513–517, 1979.

Sponseller, P.D., Cohen, M.S., Nachemson, A.L., et al.: Results of surgical treatment of adults with idiopathic scoliosis. J. Bone Joint Surg. [Am.] 69:667–675, 1987.

Swank, S., Lonstein, J.E., Moe, J.H., et al.: Surgical treatment of adult scoliosis: A review of two hundred and twenty-two cases. J. Bone Joint Surg. [Am.] 63:268, 1981.

Weinstein, S.L., and Ponseti, I.V.: Curve progression in idiopathic scoliosis. J. Bone Joint Surg. [Am.] 65:447–455, 1983.

Winter, R.B., Lonstein, J.E., and Denis, F.: Pain patterns in adult scoliosis. Orthop. Clin. North Am. 19:339, 1988.

Sacrum

Denis, F., Davis, S., and Comfort, T.: Sacral fractures: An important problem retrospective analysis of 236 cases. Clin. Orthop. 227:67–81, 1988.

Newhouse, K.E., El-Khoury, G.Y., and Buckwalter, J.A.: Occult sacral fractures in osteopenic patients. J. Bone Joint Surg. [Am.] 75:1472–1477, 1992.

Postacchini, F., and Massobrio, M.: Idiopathic coccygodynia: Analysis of fifty-one operative cases and a radiographic study of the normal coccyx. J. Bone Joint Surg. [Am.] 65:1116–1124, 1983.

Infections, Tumors

Allen, A.R., and Stevenson, A.W.: A ten-year follow-up of combined drug therapy and early fusion in bone tuberculosis. J. Bone Joint Surg. [Am.] 49:1001, 1967.

Batson, O.B.: The function of the vertebral veins and their role in the spread of metastases. Ann. Surg. 112:138–149, 1940.

Bohlman, H.H., Sachs, B.L., Carter, J.R., et al.: Primary neoplasms of the cervical spine: Diagnosis and treatment of twenty three patients. J. Bone Joint Surg. [Am.] 68:483, 1986.

Constans, J.P., Devitiis, E.D., Donzelli, R., et al.: Spinal metastases with neurological manifestations: Review of 600 cases. J. Neurosurg. 59:111, 1983.

Eismont, F.J., Bohlman, H.H., Soni, P.L., et al.: Pyogenic and fungal vertebral osteomyelitis with paralysis. J. Bone Joint Surg. [Am.] 65:19–29, 1983.

Emery, S.E., Chan, D.P.K., and Woodward, H.R.: Treatment of hematogenous pyogenic vertebral osteomyelitis with anterior débridement and primary bone grafting. Spine 14:284, 1989.

Hodgson, A.R., Stock, F.E., Fang, H.S.Y., et al.: Anterior spinal fusion: The operative approach and pathological findings in 412 patients with Pott's disease of the spine. Br. J. Surg. 48:172, 1960.

Kostulk, J.P., Errica, T.J., Gleason, T.F., et al.: Spinal stabilization of vertebral column tumors. Spine 13:250, 1988.

McAfee, P.C., and Bohlman, H.H.: One-stage anterior cervical decompression and posterior stabilization with circumferential arthrodesis: A study of twenty-four patients who had a traumatic or neoplastic lesion. J. Bone Joint Surg. [Am.] 71:78, 1989.

Paus, B.: Tumor, tuberculosis and osteomyelitis on the spine: Differential diagnostic aspects. Acta Orthop. Scand. 44:372, 1973.

Siegal, T., Tiqva, P., and Siegal, T.: Vertebral body resection for epidural compression by malignant tumors: Results of forty-seven consecutive operative procedures. J. Bone Joint Surg. [Am.] 67:375–382, 1985.

Weinstein, J.N., and MacLain, R.F.: Primary tumors of the spine. Spine 12:843–851, 1987.

Complications

Deyo, R.A., Cherkin, D.C., Loeser, J.D., et al.: Morbidity and mortality in association with operation on the lumbar spine. J. Bone Joint Surg. [Am.] 74:536, 1992.

Eismont, F.J., Wiesel, S.W., and Rothman, R.H.: The treatment of dural tears associated with spinal surgery. J. Bone Joint Surg. [Am.] 63:1132, 1981.

Farey, I.D., McAfee, P.C., Davis, R.F., et al.: Pseudarthrosis of the cervical spine after anterior arthrodesis: Treatment by posterior nerve-root decompression, stabilization and arthrodesis. J. Bone Joint Surg. [Am.] 72:1171, 1990.

Flynn, J.C., and Price, C.T.: Sexual complications of anterior fusion of the lumbar spine. Spine 9:489, 1984.

Graham, J.J.: Complications of cervical spine surgery: A five-year report on a survey of the membership of the Cervical Spine Research Society by the morbidity and mortality committee. Spine 14:1046–1050, 1989.

Kurz, L.T., Garfin, S.F., and Both, R.E.: Harvesting autologous iliac bone grafts: A review of complications and techniques. Spine 14:1324–1331, 1989.

Simpson, J.M., Silveri, C.P., Balderston, M.D., et al.: The results of operation on the lumbar spine in patients who have diabetes mellitus. J. Bone Joint Surg. [Am.] 75:1823–1829, 1993.

Other

Detwiler, K.N., Loftus, C.M., Godersky, J.C., et al.: Management of cervical spine injuries in patients with ankylosing spondylitis. J. Neurosurg. 72:210, 1990.

Graham, B., and Can Peteghem, P.K.: Fractures of the spine in ankylosing spondylitis: Diagnosis, treatment, and complications. Spine 14:803–807, 1989.

Simmons, E.H.: Kyphotic deformity of the spine in ankylosing spondylitis. Clin. Orthop. 128:65–77, 1977.

8

Orthopaedic Pathology

Frank J. Frassica, Deborah Anne Frassica,
and Edward F. McCarthy, Jr.

I. Introduction

A. Nomenclature—Primary bone lesions can be broadly classified into three types: malignant bone tumors (sarcomas), benign bone tumors, and lesions that simulate bone tumors (reactive and miscellaneous conditions). Common lesions that occur in bone but are not of mesenchymal origin include metastatic bone disease, myeloma, and lymphoma. A common classification system for bone tumors is shown in Table 8–1. Sarcomas are malignant neoplasms of connective tissue (mesenchymal) origin. Sarcomas generally exhibit rapid growth in a centripetal fashion and invade adjacent normal tissues. Each year in the United Stases there are about 2000 new bone sarcomas. High-grade malignant bone tumors tend to destroy the overlying cortex and spread into the soft tissues. Low-grade tumors are generally contained within the cortex or a surrounding periosteal rim. Sarcomas metastasize primarily via the hematogenous route, with the lungs being the most common site. Benign bone tumors may be small and have a limited growth potential or may be large and destructive. Tumor simulators and reactive conditions are processes that occur in bone but are not true neoplasms (e.g., osteomyelitis, aneurysmal bone cyst, bone island).

Table 8–1.

Classification of Primary Tumors of Bone[a]

Histology Type	Benign	Malignant
Hematopoietic		Myeloma Lymphoma
Chondrogenic	Osteochondroma Chondroma	Primary chondrosarcoma Secondary chondrosarcoma
	Chondroblastoma	Dedifferentiated chondrosarcoma
	Chondromyxoid fibroma	Mesenchymal chondrosarcoma Clear cell chondrosarcoma
Osteogenic	Osteoid osteoma Benign osteoblastoma	Osteosarcoma Parosteal osteosarcoma Periosteal osteosarcoma
Unknown origin	Giant cell tumor	Ewing's tumor
	(Fibrous) histiocytoma	Malignant giant cell tumor Adamantinoma
Fibrogenic	Fibroma Desmoplastic fibroma	Fibrosarcoma Malignant fibrous histiocytoma
Notochordal		Chordoma
Vascular	Hemangioma	Hemangioendothelioma Hemangiopericytoma
Lipogenic	Lipoma	
Neurogenic	Neurilemoma	

[a]Classification is based on that advocated by Lichtenstein, L.: Classification of primary tumors of bone. Cancer 4:335–341, 1951.

B. Staging—Staging systems may be useful for developing evaluation strategies, planning treatment, and predicting prognosis. For musculoskeletal lesions the staging system of the Musculoskeletal Tumor Society (also called the Enneking system) is the most popular and useful. There are two systems: one for malignant lesions and one for benign lesions. For malignant lesions, the system is based on knowing the histologic grade of the lesion (low or high), the anatomic features (intracompartmental or extracompartmental), and the absence (M_0) or presence (M_1) of metastases.

1. Grade—Most malignant lesions are high-grade (G_2) (potential for distant metastases is $\geq$25%). Low-grade malignant (G_1) lesions are less common, with less than 25% chance of distant metastases. Grading of tumors requires a morphologic range, and most grading systems are based on four grades: grade 1, well differentiated; grade 2, less well differentiated; grades 3 and 4, poorly differentiated. Grading can be difficult and is based on nuclear anaplasia (degree of loss of structural differentiation), pleomorphism (variations in size and shape), and nuclear hyperchromasia (increased nuclear staining). Commonly graded lesions are shown in Table 8–2.
2. Tumor Site—The plain radiographs and special studies, such as computed tomography (CT) and magnetic resonance imaging (MRI) scans, are inspected to determine whether the tumor is situated within the bone compartment (intracompartmental, or T_1) or has left the confines of the bone (extracompartmental, or T_2).
3. Metastases—For most lesions a chest radiograph and CT scan of the chest are per-

Table 8–2.

Typical Low-Grade and High-Grade Bone and Soft-Tissue Tumors

Low-Grade	High-Grade
Bone	
Parosteal osteosarcoma	Intramedullary (classic) osteosarcoma
Primary chondrosarcoma	Postradiation sarcoma
Secondary chondrosarcoma	Paget's sarcoma
Hemangioendothelioma	Fibrosarcoma
Chordoma	Malignant fibrous histiocytoma
Adamantinoma	
Soft Tissue	
Myxoid liposarcoma	Malignant fibrous histiocytoma
Lipoma-like liposarcoma	Pleomorphic liposarcoma
Angiomatoid malignant fibrous histiocytoma	Synovial sarcoma
	Rhabdomyosarcoma
	Alveolar cell sarcoma

formed to search for pulmonary lesions. A technetium bone scan is used to exclude the presence of other bone lesions.

4. The staging system can be synthesized into six distinct stages (Table 8–3).

C. Evaluation

1. Clinical Presentation—Most patients with bone tumors present with musculoskeletal pain. The pain is similar whether the bone destruction is secondary to a primary mesenchymal tumor (e.g., osteosarcoma, chondrosarcoma) or due to metastatic bone disease, myeloma, or lymphoma. The pain is typically deep-seated and dull and may resemble a toothache. Initially, the pain may be intermittent and related to activity, a work injury, or a sporting injury. The pain usually progresses in intensity and becomes constant. Many patients experience pain at night. As the pain progresses, it is not relieved by nonsteroidal anti-inflammatory drugs (NSAIDs) or gentle narcotics. Most patients with a high-grade sarcoma will present with a 1–3 month history of pain. In contrast, with low-grade tumors such as chondrosarcoma, adamantinoma, and chordoma, there may be a long history of mild to moderate pain.
2. Physical Examination—Patients with suspected bone tumors should be examined carefully. The affected site is inspected for soft-tissue masses, overlying skin changes, adenopathy, and general musculoskeletal condition. When metastatic disease is suspected, the thyroid gland, abdomen, prostate, and breasts should be examined as appropriate.
3. Radiography—Plain radiographs in two planes are the first radiographic examinations to be performed. When the clinician suspects malignancy, and the radiographs are normal, selected studies may follow. Technetium bone scans are an excellent modality to search for occult malignancies. In patients with myeloma for whom scan results may be negative, a skeletal survey is more sensitive. MRI is an excellent modality for screening the spine for occult metastases, myeloma, or lymphoma. A chest radiograph should be obtained in all age groups when the clinician suspects a malignant lesion. The radiographs must be inspected carefully in order to formulate a working diagnosis. The working diagnosis then guides the clinician during further evaluation and treatment. Formulation of the differential diagnosis is based on several clinical and radiographic parameters.
   a. Age of the Patient—Knowledge of common diseases in defined age groups is the first step. Certain diseases are uncommon in particular age groups (Table 8–4).
   b. Number of Bone Lesions—Is the process monostotic or polyostotic? If there are multiple destructive lesions in the middle to older patients (ages 40–80), the most likely diagnosis is metastatic bone disease, multiple myeloma, or lymphoma. In the

Table 8–3.

Staging System of the Musculoskeletal Tumor Society (Enneking System)

Stage	GTM	Description
I-A	$G_1T_1M_0$	Low grade Intracompartmental No metastases
I-B	$G_1T_2M_0$	Low grade Extracompartmental No metastases
II-A	$G_2T_1M_0$	High grade Intracompartmental No metastases
II-B	$G_2T_2M_0$	High grade Extracompartmental No metastases
III-A	$G_{1/2}T_1M_1$	Any grade Intracompartmental With metastases
III-B	$G_{1/2}T_2M_1$	Any grade Extracompartmental With metastases

Grade system (G): low grade (G_1) and high grade (G_2). High-grade lesions are intermediate in grade between low-grade, well-differentiated tumors and high-grade, undifferentiated tumors.

Tumor size (T): Determined using specialized procedures, including radiography, tomography, nuclear studies, CT, and MRI. Compartments are used to describe the tumor site. Usually compartments are easily defined based on fascial borders in the extremities. Of note, the skin and subcutaneous tissues are classified as a compartment, and the periosseous potential space between cortical bone and muscle is often considered as a compartment as well. T_0 lesions are confined within the capsule and within its compartment of origin. T_1 tumors have extracapsular extension into the reactive zone around it, but both the tumor and the reactive zone are confined within the compartment of origin. T_2 lesions extend beyond the anatomic compartment of origin by direct extension or otherwise (e.g., trauma, surgical seeding). Tumors that involve major neurovascular bundles are almost always classified as T_2 lesions.

Metastases (M): Regional and distal metastases both have an ominous prognosis; therefore the distinction is simply between no metastases (M_0) or the presence of metastases (M_1).

Table 8–4.

Age Distribution of Various Bone Lesions

Age	Malignant	Benign
Birth to 5 Years	Leukemia Metastatic neuroblastoma Metastatic rhabdomyosarcoma	Osteomyelitis Osteofibrous dysplasia
10–25 Years	Osteosarcoma Ewing's tumor Leukemia	Eosinophilic granuloma Osteomyelitis Enchondroma Fibrous dysplasia
40–80 Years	Metastatic bone disease Myeloma Lymphoma Paget's sarcoma Postradiation sarcoma	Hyperparathyroidism Paget's disease Mastocytosis

young patient (ages 15–40), multiple lytic and oval lesions are most likely a vascular tumor (hemangioendothelioma). In children below age 5, multiple destructive lesions may represent metastatic neuroblastoma or Wilms' tumor. Histiocytosis X may also lead to multiple lesions in the young patient. Fibrous dysplasia and Paget's disease may present with multiple lesions in all age groups.

c. Anatomic Location Within Bone—Certain lesions have a predilection for occurring within a certain bone or a particular location. Adamantinoma is a malignant tumor that most commonly occurs in the tibia in young patients. Chondroblastoma most commonly occurs within the epiphysis of long bones. Giant cell tumor typically begins in the metaphysis and extends through the epiphysis to lie just below the cartilage. Ewing's tumor, in many cases, involves the diaphysis. Osteogenic sarcoma most commonly occurs in the metaphysis of the distal femur and proximal tibia but occurs within the diaphysis in about 7% of patients with long-bone lesions.

d. Effect of the Lesion on Bone—High-grade malignant lesions generally spread rapidly through the medullary cavity. Cortical bone destruction occurs early, and the process spreads into the adjacent soft tissues. Low-grade malignant lesions tend to spread slowly, but they can also destroy the cortical bone and produce a soft-tissue mass.

e. Response of the Bone to the Lesion—With high-grade lesions, there is often little ability of the host bone to contain the process; the result is rapid destruction of cortical bone and the presence of a soft-tissue mass. In contrast with low-grade lesions, the host bone can often contain the lesion with a thickened cortex or rim of periosteal bone. With benign or low-grade lesions, there is often a thick periosteal response about the lesion.

f. Matrix Characteristics—If the lesion produces a matrix, it is helpful to determine whether the matrix is cartilage calcification or mineralization of osteoid. Cartilage calcification often appears stippled or may show arcs or rings; osteoid mineralization is often cloud-like.

4. Laboratory Studies—They are often nonspecific. There are a set of routine studies that should be obtained for all patients when there is not an obvious diagnosis (Table 8–5). The studies can be grouped into those for younger patients (up to age 40) and those for older patients (40–80 years).

5. Biopsy—It is generally performed after complete evaluation of the patient. It is of great benefit to both pathologist and surgeon to have a narrow working diagnosis, as it allows accurate interpretation of the frozen section analysis and allows definitive treatment of some lesions based on the frozen section. There are several surgical principles which the clinician must follow.

a. The orientation and location of the biopsy tract is critically important. If the lesion proves to be malignant, the entire biopsy tract must be removed with the underlying lesion. Transverse incisions should be avoided (Fig. 8–1).

b. The surgeon must maintain meticulous hemostasis to prevent hematoma formation and subcutaneous hemorrhage. When possible, biopsies are done through muscles so the muscle layer can be closed tightly. Tourniquets are utilized to obtain tissue in a bloodless field and then are released so bleeding points can be controlled. Avitene, Gelfoam, and Thrombostat sprays are used as necessary. If hemostasis cannot be achieved, a small drain should be brought out of the corner of the wound to prevent hematoma formation. A compression dressing is routinely used on the extremities.

Table 8–5.

Laboratory Evaluations for Young and Middle-Aged Patients

Age 5–40 Years
- Complete blood count with differential
- Peripheral blood smear
- Erythrocyte sedimentation rate

Age 40–80 Years
- Complete blood count with differential
- Erythrocyte sedimentation rate
- Chemistry group: calcium and phosphate
- Serum or urine protein electrophoresis
- Urinalysis

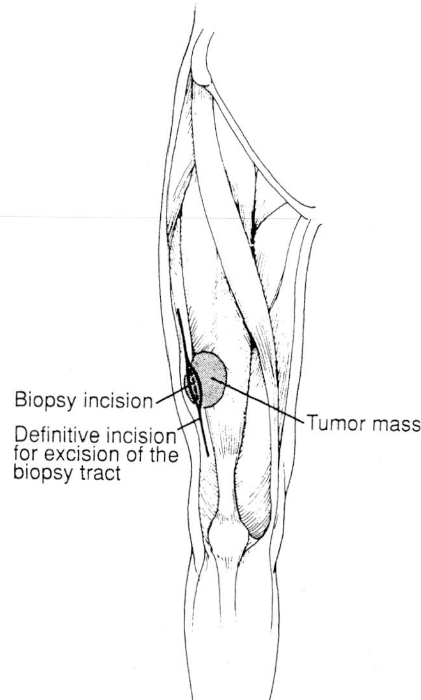

Figure 8–1. Lesion in the lateral aspect of the quadriceps mechanism. A short longitudinal incision is made over the lesion. Prior to incising the skin a second incision line should be drawn to demonstrate how the biopsy tract can be removed at the time of the definitive surgery. (From Sim, F.H., Frassica, F.J., and Frassica, D.A.: Soft tissue tumors: diagnosis, evaluation and management. AAOS 2:209, 1994. Copyright 1994 American Academy of Orthopaedic Surgeons. Reprinted with permission.)

c. A frozen section analysis is done on all biopsy samples to ensure that adequate diagnostic tissue is obtained. Prior to biopsy, the surgeon should review the radiographs with the pathologist to plan the biopsy site. When possible, the soft-tissue component should be sampled rather than the bony component.
d. It is an important tenet to remember that all biopsy samples should be submitted for bacteriologic analysis if the frozen section does not reveal a neoplasm. Antibiotics should not be delivered until the cultures are obtained.
e. Needle biopsy is an excellent method for achieving a tissue diagnosis and providing minimal tissue disruption. However, open biopsy remains the most reliable technique for avoiding incorrect diagnoses. When the nature of the lesion is obvious based on the radiographic features, and adequate tissue can be obtained with needle biopsy, the needle biopsy technique can be safely utilized. The pathologist must be experienced and comfortable with the small sample of tissue.

6. Surgical Procedures—The goal of treatment of malignant bone tumors is to remove the lesion with minimal risk of local recurrence. Limb salvage is performed when two essential criteria are met: (1) local control of the lesion must be at least equal to that of amputation surgery; and (2) the limb that has been saved must be functional. A wide surgical margin (a cuff of normal tissue around the tumor) is the surgical goal. Surgical procedures are graded according to the system of the Musculoskeletal Tumor Society (Fig. 8–2).
   a. Intralesional—The plane of dissection goes directly through the tumor. When dealing with malignant mesenchymal tumors, an intralesional margin results in 100% local recurrence.
   b. Marginal—A marginal line of resection goes through the reactive zone of the tumor; the reactive zone contains inflammatory cells, edema, fibrous tissue, and satellites of tumor cells. When resecting malignant mesenchymal tumors, a plane of dissection through the reactive zone will probably result in a local recurrence rate of 25–50%.
   c. Wide—A wide surgical resection is accomplished when the entire tumor is removed with a cuff of normal tissue. The local recurrence rate drops below 10% when such a surgical margin is achieved.
   d. Radical—A radical margin is achieved when the entire tumor and its compartment (all surrounding muscles, ligaments, and connective tissues) are removed.
7. Adjuvant Therapy
   a. Chemotherapy—Multiagent chemotherapy has a significant impact on both the

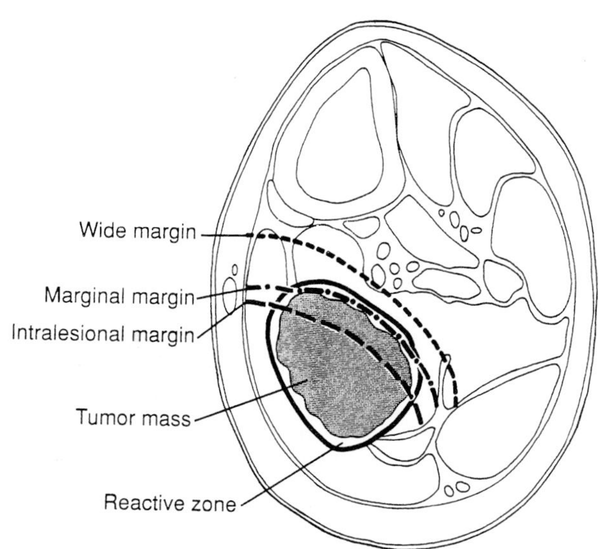

Figure 8–2. Types of surgical margin. An intralesional line of resection enters the substance of the tumor. A marginal line of resection travels through the reactive zone of the tumor. A wide surgical margin removes the tumor with a cuff of normal tissue. (From Sim, F.H., Frassica, F.J., and Frassica, D.A.: Soft tissue tumors: diagnosis, evaluation and management. AAOS 2:209, 1994. Copyright 1994 American Academy of Orthopaedic Surgeons. Reprinted with permission.)

efficacy of limb salvage and disease-free survival for osteogenic sarcoma and Ewing's tumor. Most protocols utilize preoperative regimens (called neoadjuvant chemotherapy) for 8–12 weeks. Patients are then restaged and, if appropriate, limb salvage is performed. Patients then undergo maintenance chemotherapy for 6–12 months. Patients who present with localized disease have up to a 60–70% long-term disease-free survival with the combination of multiagent chemotherapy and surgery (osteosarcoma and Ewing's tumor).

b. Radiation Therapy—External beam irradiation is utilized for local control of Ewing's tumor, lymphoma, myeloma, and metastatic bone disease. It is also utilized as an adjunct for the treatment of soft-tissue sarcomas, in which it is used in combination with surgery. The role of surgery in the treatment of Ewing's tumor is evolving. In some centers, chemotherapy and surgery are the major forms of treatment, whereas in others traditional chemotherapy and external beam irradiation are preferred.

(1) Postirradiation sarcoma is a devastating complication in which a spindle sarcoma occurs within the field of irradiation for a previous malignancy (e.g., Ewing's tumor, breast cancer, Hodgkin's disease). The histology is usually that of an osteosarcoma, fibrosarcoma, or malignant fibrous histiocytoma. Postirradiation sarcomas are probably more frequent in patients who undergo intensive chemotherapy (especially with alkylating agents) and irradiation.

(2) Late stress fractures also may occur in weight-bearing bones to which high-dose irradiation has been applied. The subtrochanteric region and the diaphysis of the femur are common sites.

II. Soft-Tissue Tumors

A. Introduction—Soft-tissue tumors are common. Patients may present with small lumps or large masses. Soft-tissue tumors can be broadly classified as benign, malignant (sarcomas), or reactive tumor-like conditions (Table 8–6). Lesions are classified according to the direction of differentiation of the lesion—whether the tumor is tending to produce collagen (fibrous lesion), fat, or cartilage.

1. Benign Soft-Tissue Tumors—They may occur in all age groups. The lesions vary in their biologic behavior, from tumors that are asymptomatic and self-limited (Enneking stage 1—inactive) to growing and symptomatic (Enneking stage 2—active). Occasionally, benign lesions grow rapidly and invade adjacent tissues (Enneking stage 3—aggressive).

2. Malignant Soft-Tissue Tumors (Sarcomas)—Sarcomas are rare tumors of mesenchymal origin. In the United States each year there are approximately 7000 new cases of soft-tissue sarcomas. Patients often present with an enlarging painless or painful soft-tissue mass. Most sarcomas are large (>5 cm), deep, and firm in character. In some instances they are small and may be present for a long time prior to recognition. Lesions that may be initially small include synovial sarcoma, epithelioid sarcoma, and clear cell sarcoma. Initial radiographic evaluation begins with plain radiographs in two planes. MRI scans are the best imaging modality to define the anatomy and to help characterize the lesion. When a mass is judged to be indeterminate, an open incisional or needle biopsy is performed. Radiation therapy is an important adjunct to surgery in the treatment of soft-tissue sarcomas. The ionizing irradiation can be delivered preoperatively, perioperatively with brachytherapy afterloading tubes, or postoperatively. Treatment regimens are often designed to use combinations of the three types of preoperative, postoperative, and external beam irradiation.

B. Tumors of Fibrous Tissue—Fibrous tumors are common, and there is a wide range, from small self-limited benign conditions to aggressive, invasive benign tumors. The malignant fibrous tumors are fibrosarcoma and malignant fibrous histiocytoma.

1. Calcifying Aponeurotic Fibroma—This entity presents as a slowly growing, painless mass in the hands and feet in children and young adults, ages 3–30 (Enzinger). Radiographs may reveal a faint mass with stippling. Histologic examination shows a fibrous tumor with centrally located areas of calcification and cartilage formation. Local excision often results in recurrence (in up to 50% of cases); however, the condition appears to resolve with maturity.

2. Fibromatosis

a. Palmar (Dupuytren's) and Plantar (Ledderhosen) Fibromatosis—These disorders consist of firm nodules of fibroblasts and collagen that develop in the palmar and plantar fascia. The nodules and fascia hypertrophy, producing contractures.

b. Extra-abdominal Desmoid Tumor—It is the most locally invasive of all benign soft-tissue tumors. It commonly occurs in adolescents and young adults. On palpation, the tumor has a distinctive "rock-hard" character. Multiple lesions may be present in the same extremity. Histologically, the tumor consists of well-differentiated fibroblasts and abundant collagen. The lesion infiltrates adjacent tissues. Surgical

group of tumors, having in common the presence of lipoblasts (signet ring–type cells) in the tissue. Liposarcomas virtually never occur in the subcutaneous tissues. Liposarcomas are classified into the following several types:

Well-differentiated liposarcoma
- Lipoma-like
- Sclerosing
- Inflammatory
- Dedifferentiated

Myxoid liposarcoma
- Round cell liposarcoma
- Pleomorphic liposarcoma

Liposarcomas range in biologic behavior from that of very low-grade tumors (well differentiated) to very high-grade tumors (poorly differentiated). Well-differentiated liposarcomas can be difficult to distinguish from benign lipomas. The name "well-differentiated lipoma-like liposarcoma," attests to this difficulty (grade 1 liposarcoma). Grade 1 liposarcomas virtually never metastasize. Other authors believe these lesions are benign and classify them as an "atypical lipoma." High-grade liposarcomas behave similarly to other high-grade sarcomas, with a propensity for local recurrence and metastasis. Low-grade lesions are treated with wide local resection. Radiotherapy is utilized as an adjunct depending on the adequacy of the surgical margin. High-grade liposarcomas are treated with both wide excision and radiotherapy for large lesions (>5 cm).

D. Tumors of Neural Tissue—The two benign neural tumors are neurilemoma and neurofibroma. Their malignant counterpart is neurofibrosarcoma.
   1. Neurilemoma (Benign Schwannoma)—This lesion is a benign nerve-sheath tumor. It occurs in the young to middle-aged adult (20–50 years) and is usually asymptomatic except for the presence of the mass. The tumor grows slowly and may wax and wane in size (cystic change). MRI studies demonstrate an eccentric mass arising from a peripheral nerve. Histologically, the lesion is composed of Antoni's A and B areas.
      a. Antoni's A—Compact spindle cells, usually having twisted nuclei, indistinct cytoplasm, and occasionally clear intranuclear vacuoles. When the lesion is highly differentiated, there may be nuclear palisading, whorling of cells, and Verocay's bodies.
      b. Antoni's B—Less orderly and cellular, the cells are arranged haphazardly in the loosely textured matrix (with microcystic change, inflammatory cells, and delicate collagen fibers); large irregularly spaced vessels.
      c. When the lesion is predominantly cellular (Antoni's A), the tumor may be confused with a sarcoma. Treatment consists in removing the eccentric mass while leaving the nerve intact.
   2. Neurofibroma—It may be solitary or multiple (neurofibromatosis). Most are superficial, grow slowly, and are painless. When they involve a major nerve, they may expand it in a fusiform fashion. Histologically, there are interlacing bundles of elongated cells with wavy, dark-staining nuclei. The cells are associated with wire-like strands of collagen (Enzinger). Small to moderate amounts of mucoid material separate the cells and collagen. Treatment consists of excision with a marginal margin. Neurofibromatosis (von Recklinghausen's disease) is an autosomal dominant trait, with both a peripheral and central form of the disease. In addition to neurofibromas, patients have café au lait spots and variable skeletal abnormalities (nonossifying fibromas, scoliosis, and long-bone bowing). Malignant change occurs in 5–30% of patients.
   3. Neurofibrosarcoma—This is a rare tumor that arises de novo or in the setting of neurofibromatosis. Neurofibrosarcomas are high-grade sarcomas and are treated in a fashion similar to other high-grade sarcomas.

E. Tumors of Muscle Tissue—They are uncommon tumors ranging from benign leiomyoma and rhabdomyoma to the malignant entities of leiomyosarcoma and rhabdomyosarcoma. The benign entities seldom occur on the extremities.
   1. Leiomyosarcoma—It may present as a small nodule or a large extremity mass. The lesions may or may not be associated with blood vessels. They may be either low- or high-grade and are treated as other low- and high-grade sarcomas.
   2. Rhabdomyosarcoma—This highly malignant tumor is most common in young patients (<20 years of age). The tumor is the most common sarcoma in young patients and may grow rapidly. Histologically, the lesion is composed of spindle cells in parallel bundles, multinucleated giant cells, and racquet-shaped cells. The histologic hallmark is the appearance of cross striations within the tumor cells (rhabdomyoblasts). Rhabdomyoblasts may be difficult to find. Rhabdomyosarcomas are sensitive to multiagent chemotherapy. Wide surgical resection is performed after induction chemotherapy. External beam irradiation plays a prominent rôle in this tumor.

F. Vascular Tumors—Hemangiomas and glomus tumors are the two principal benign entities, and hemangiopericytoma and angiosarcoma are the less common malignant entities.
   1. Hemangioma—This soft-tissue tumor is commonly seen in children and adults. The lesion may occur in a cutaneous, subcutaneous, or intramuscular location. Patients with

large tumors complain of symptoms of vascular engorgement (aching, heaviness, swelling). MRI scans demonstrate a heterogeneous lesion with numerous small blood vessels and fatty infiltration. Plain radiographs may reveal small phleboliths. Nonoperative treatment is chosen if local measures adequately control discomfort: NSAIDs, vascular stockings, and activity modification. Wide surgical resection is utilized for resistant cases, but the local recurrence rate is high.

2. Hemangiopericytoma—This rare tumor of the pericytes of blood vessels appears in benign and malignant forms. Within the malignant group there is a morphologic range from intermediate- to high-grade malignancy. Patients present with a slowly enlarging painless mass. Treatment is based on the grade of the lesion.
3. Angiosarcoma—In this rare tumor the tumor cells resemble the endothelium of blood vessels. Treatment depends on the grade and location of the lesion.

G. Synovial Disorders—These entities include benign conditions, such as ganglia, and synovial proliferative disorders, such as pigmented villonodular synovitis and synovial chondromatosis.

1. Ganglia—It presents as an outpouching of the synovial lining of an adjacent joint. The most common locations include the wrist, foot, and knee. The cyst is filled with gelatinous, mucoid material. Histologically, the cyst wall is made up of paucicellular connective tissue without a true epithelial lining.
2. Pigmented Villonodular Synovitis—This reactive condition (not a true neoplasm) is characterized by an exuberant proliferation of synovial villi and nodules. The process may occur locally within a joint or diffusely. The knee is most commonly affected, followed by the hip and shoulder. Patients present with pain and swelling in the affected joint. Arthrocentesis demonstrates a bloody effusion. Cystic erosions may occur on both sides of the joint. Histologically, there are highly vascular villi lined with plump, hyperplastic synovial cells, hemosiderin-stained multinucleated giant cells, and chronic inflammatory cells. Treatment is aimed at complete synovectomy. Local recurrence is common.
3. Giant Cell Tumor of Tendon Sheath—This benign nodular tumor occurs along the tendon sheaths of the hands and feet. Histologically, the lesion is moderately cellular (sheets of rounded or polygonal cells). There are hypocellular collagenized zones (Enzinger). Multinucleated giant cells are common, as are xanthoma cells. Treatment consists in resection with a marginal margin.
4. Synovial Chondromatosis—This lesion may occur within a joint, ranging in appearance from metaplasia of the synovial tissue to firm nodules of cartilage. The lesion typically affects young adults who present with pain, stiffness, and swelling. Radiographs may demonstrate fine stippled calcification. Treatment consists in removing the loose bodies and synovectomy.
5. Synovial Sarcoma—This highly malignant tumor occurs in close proximity to joints but rarely arises from an intra-articular location. The tumor may be present for years or present as a rapidly enlarging mass. Synovial sarcoma is the most common sarcoma in the foot. Radiographs may show mineralization within the lesion (in up to 25% of cases). Histologically, the tumor is biphasic, with an epithelial component and a spindle cell component. The epithelial component may show epithelial cells that form glands or nests, or they may line cyst-like spaces. Regional lymph nodes may be involved. All synovial sarcomas are high-grade lesions. Wide surgical resection with adjuvant radiotherapy is the most common method of treatment.

H. Other Rare Sarcomas

1. Epithelioid Sarcoma—This rare nodular tumor commonly occurs in the upper extremity of young adults. It may also occur about the buttock/thigh, knee, or foot. Epithelioid sarcoma is the most common sarcoma in the hand. The lesion may ulcerate and mimic a granuloma or rheumatoid nodule. Lymph node metastases may occur. Histologically, the cells range from ovoid to polygonal, with deeply eosinophilic cytoplasm (Enzinger). Cellular pleomorphism is minimal. The lesions are often misdiagnosed as benign processes. Wide surgical resection is necessary to prevent local recurrence.
2. Clear Cell Sarcoma—This tumor presents as a slowly growing mass associated with tendons or aponeuroses. The lesion most commonly occurs about the foot and ankle but may also involve the knee, thigh, or hand. Microscopically, it is characterized by compact nests or fascicles of rounded or fusiform cells with clear cytoplasm (Enzinger). Multinucleated giant cells are common. Wide surgical resection with adjuvant irradiation is the treatment of choice.
3. Alveolar Cell Sarcoma—It presents as a slowly growing, painless mass in young adults (age 15–35 years). It most commonly occurs in the anterior thigh. Microscopically, it appears as dense fibrous trabeculae dividing the tumor into an organoid or nest-like arrangement (Enzinger). Cells are large and rounded and contain one or more vesicular nuclei with small nucleoli. Vascular invasion is prominent. Treatment is wide surgical resection with adjuvant irradiation in selected cases.

I. Post-Traumatic Conditions

1. Hematoma—Hematoma may occur after

trauma to the extremity. The lesion organizes and resolves with time.

2. Myositis Ossificans (Heterotopic Ossification)—It occurs after single or repetitive episodes of trauma. Occasionally, patients cannot recall the traumatic episode. The most common locations are over the diaphyseal segment of long bones (in the midaspect of the muscle bellies). As maturation progresses, radiographs show peripheral mineralization with a central lucent area. In most cases the lesion is not attached to the underlying bone, but in some cases it may become fixed to the periosteal surface. Histologically, there is a zonal pattern with mature, trabecular bone at the periphery and immature tissue in the center. When the diagnosis is apparent, nonoperative treatment is all that is necessary.

III. Bone Tumors

A. Introduction—All bone lesions can be subdivided into three groups: benign bone neoplasms, malignant bone neoplasms, and non-neoplastic lesions (also called tumor-like conditions, tumor simulators, and reactive conditions). Lesions can be further subclassified into processes that begin in the bone (intramedullary lesions) and processes that clearly begin outside the intramedullary cavity (surface lesions).

B. Bone-Producing Lesions—There are only three lesions in which the tumor cells produce osteoid: osteoid osteoma, osteoblastoma, and osteosarcoma.

1. Osteoid Osteoma (Fig. 8–3)—This self-limited benign bone lesion produces pain in young patients (ages 5–30 years, although all age groups may be affected). Patients present with pain that increases with time. Most patients have pain at night, which may be strikingly relieved by salicylates. The pain may be referred to an adjacent joint, and when the lesion is intracapsular, it may simulate arthritis. The tumor may produce painful scoliosis, growth disturbances, and flexion contractures. Common locations include the proximal femur, tibial diaphysis, and spine (Fig. 8–4). The radiographs usually show intensely reactive bone and a radiolucent nidus. It may be possible to detect the lesion with special studies only, such as tomograms, CTs, or MRI scans, because of the intense sclerosis. The nidus is by definition always <1.5 cm, although the area of reactive bone sclerosis may be quite long. Technetium bone scan results are always positive and show intense focal uptake. Microscopically, there is a distinct demarcation between the nidus and the reactive bone. The nidus consists of an interlacing network of osteoid trabeculae with variable mineralization. The trabecular organization is haphazard, and the greatest degree of mineralization is in the center of the lesion. Treatment consists in complete removal of the nidus (en bloc excision) or curettage of the nidus with hand and power instruments. Patients may also be treated nonoperatively with aspirin or NSAIDs. About 50% of patients treated with NSAIDs will have their lesions burn out with no further medical or surgical treatment necessary. A new treatment that is gaining popularity is percutaneous radiofrequency ablation of the osteoid osteoma. Under CT guidance, a radio frequency probe is placed into the lesion, and the nidus is heated up to 80°C. About 90% of selected patients can be successfully treated with radio frequency ablation.

2. Osteoblastoma (Fig. 8–5)—This rare bone-producing tumor can attain a large size and is not self-limited as is osteoid osteoma. Patients present with pain, and when the lesion involves the spine, neurologic symptoms may be present. Common locations include the spine, proximal humerus, and hip (see Fig. 8–5). Radiographically, there is bone destruction with or without the characteristic reactive bone formation in osteoid osteoma. The bone destruction occasionally has a moth-eaten or permeative character simulating a malignancy. Histologically, the lesions show regularly-shaped nuclei containing little chromatin but abundant cytoplasm (Dahlin). The tissue is loosely arranged with numerous blood vessels. The lesion does not permeate the normal trabecula bones but, rather, merges with them. Treatment consists in excision with at least a marginal line of resection.

3. Osteosarcoma—Spindle cell neoplasms that produce osteoid are arbitrarily classified as osteosarcomas. There are many types of osteosarcoma (Table 8–7 and Fig. 8–6). The lesions that must be recognized (in order to have a reasonable grasp on the entity osteosarcoma) include high-grade intramedullary osteosarcoma (ordinary or classic osteosarcoma), parosteal osteosarcoma, periosteal osteosarcoma,

Table 8–7.

Classification of Osteosarcoma

High-grade central osteosarcoma
Low-grade central osteosarcoma
Telangiectatic osteosarcoma
Surface osteosarcomas
  Parosteal osteosarcoma
  Periosteal osteosarcoma
  High-grade surface osteosarcoma
Osteosarcoma of the jaw
Multicentric osteosarcoma
Secondary osteosarcomas
  Osteosarcoma in Paget's disease
  Postradiation osteosarcoma
  Dedifferentiated chondrosarcoma
Osteosarcoma derived from benign precursors

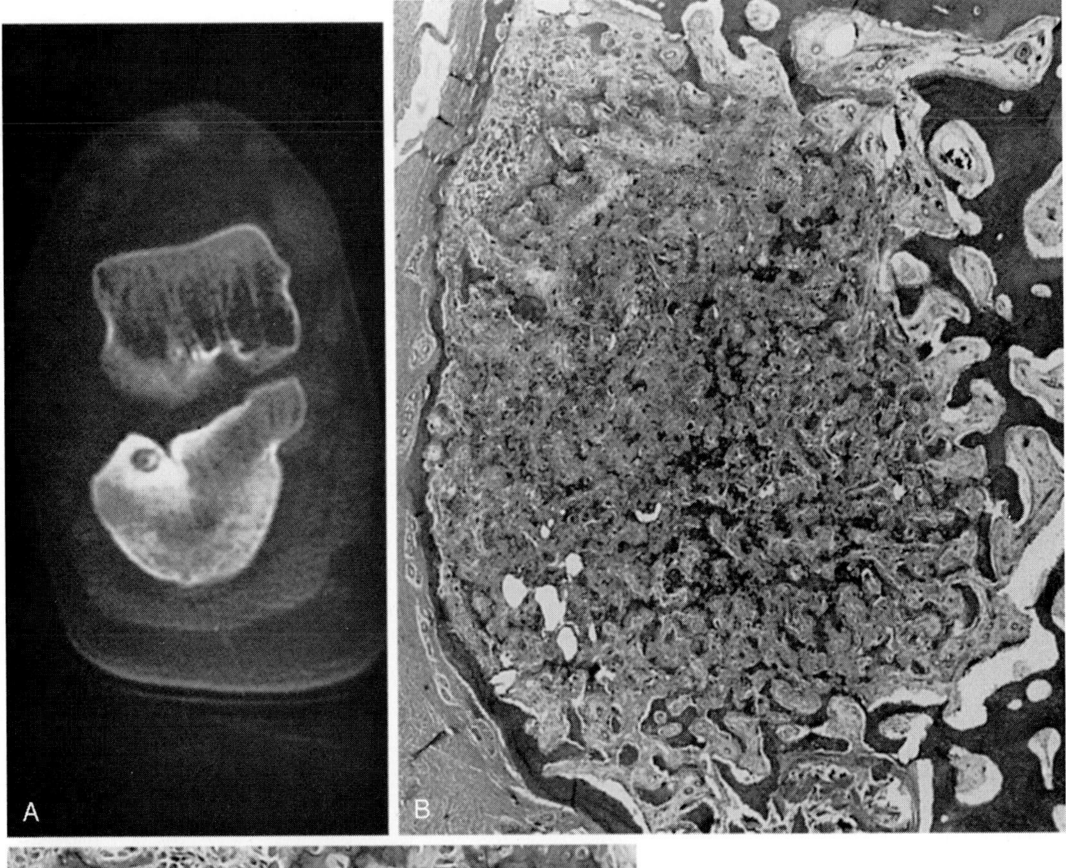

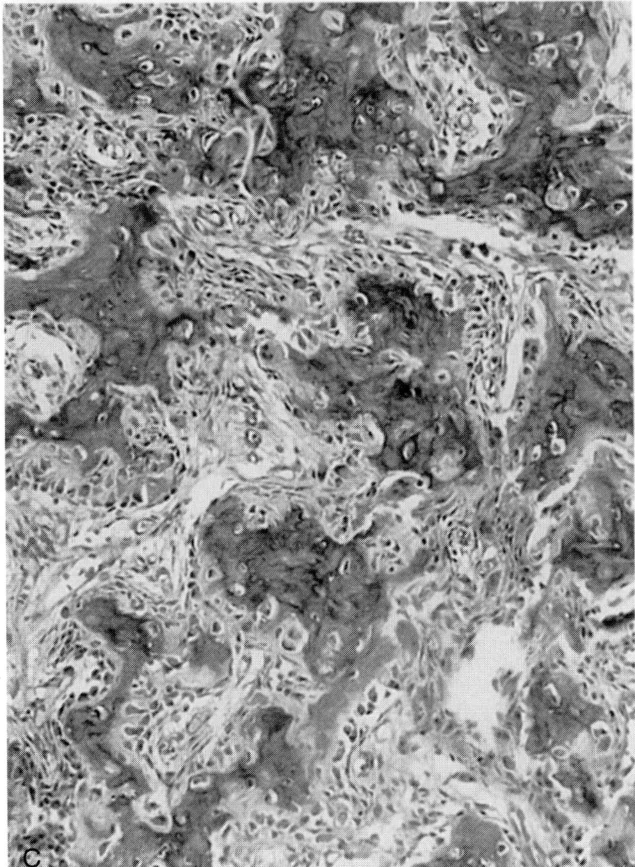

Figure 8–3. Osteoid osteoma of the calcaneus. *A,* Radiograph shows a well-circumscribed lytic lesion with dense surrounding bone and a central nidus. *B,* Low-power photomicrograph (×25) shows the nidus. *C,* Higher-power photomicrograph (×160) shows mineralizing new bone with a loose fibrovascular stroma.

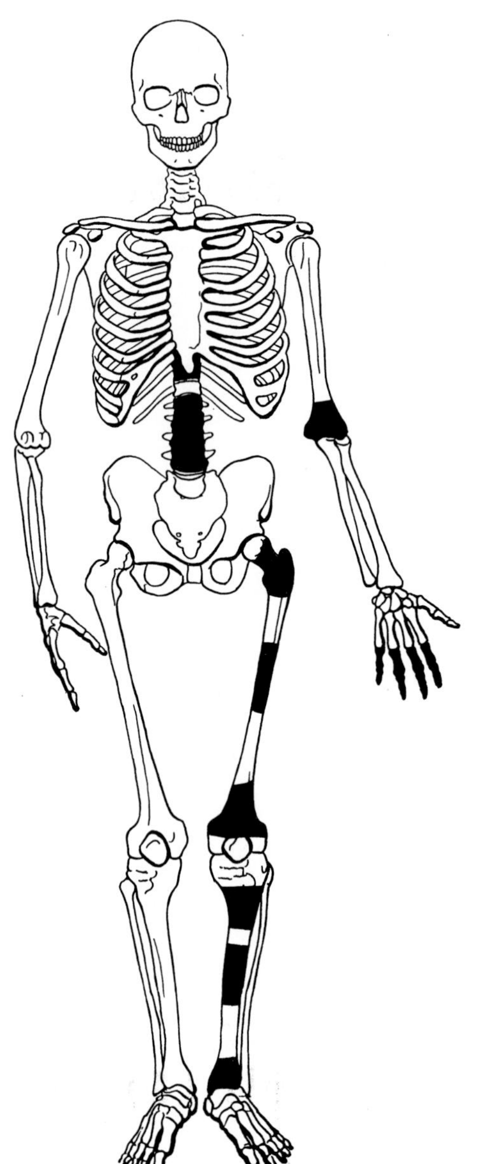

Figure 8–4. Skeletal distribution of the most common sites of osteoid osteoma. (From McCarthy, E.F., and Frassica, F.J.: Pathology of Bone and Joint Disorders. Philadelphia, WB Saunders, 1998.)

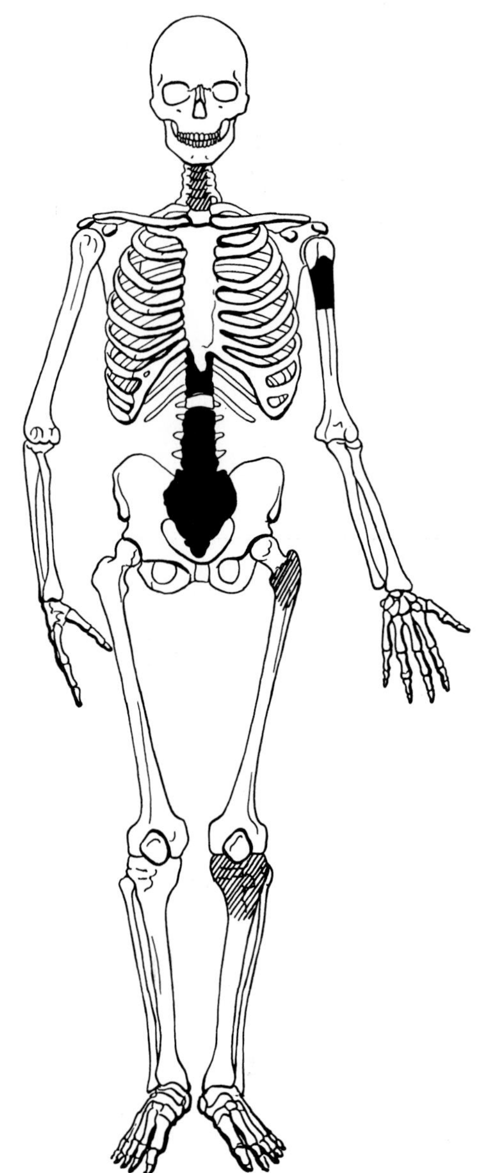

Figure 8–5. Skeletal distribution of the most common sites of osteoblastoma. (From McCarthy, E.F., and Frassica, F.J.: Pathology of Bone and Joint Disorders. Philadelphia, WB Saunders, 1998.)

telangiectatic osteosarcoma, osteosarcoma occurring with Paget's disease, and osteosarcoma following irradiation (see Fig. 8–6).

a. High-Grade Intramedullary Osteosarcoma (Fig. 8–7)—Also called ordinary or classic osteosarcoma, it is the most common type of osteosarcoma and most commonly occurs about the knee in children and young adults (Fig. 8–8). Other common sites include the proximal humerus, proximal femur, and pelvis. Patients present primarily with pain. More than 90% of intramedullary osteosarcomas are high-grade and penetrate the cortex early to form a soft-tissue mass (stage IIB lesion). About 10–20% of patients have pulmonary metastases at presentation. Plain radiographs demonstrate a lesion in which there is bone destruction and bone formation. Occasionally, the lesion is purely sclerotic or lytic. MRI or CT scans are useful for defining the anatomy of the lesion in regard to intramedullary extension, involvement of neurovascular structures, and muscle invasion. Histologically, two criteria are utilized: (1) the tumor cells produce osteoid, and (2) the stroma cells are frankly malignant. The lesions may be highly heterogeneous in appearance, with some lesions being predominantly chondroblastic, osteoblastic, or fibroblastic. Other lesions may contain large numbers of giant cells or predominantly small cells rather than spindle cells. Telangiectatic osteosarcoma is a type in which the lesional tissue can be described as a bag of blood with few cellular elements. The cellular elements present are highly malignant in appearance. The radiographic features of telangiectatic osteosarcoma are those of a destructive, lytic, expansile lesion. Telangiectatic osteosarcomas occur in the same locations

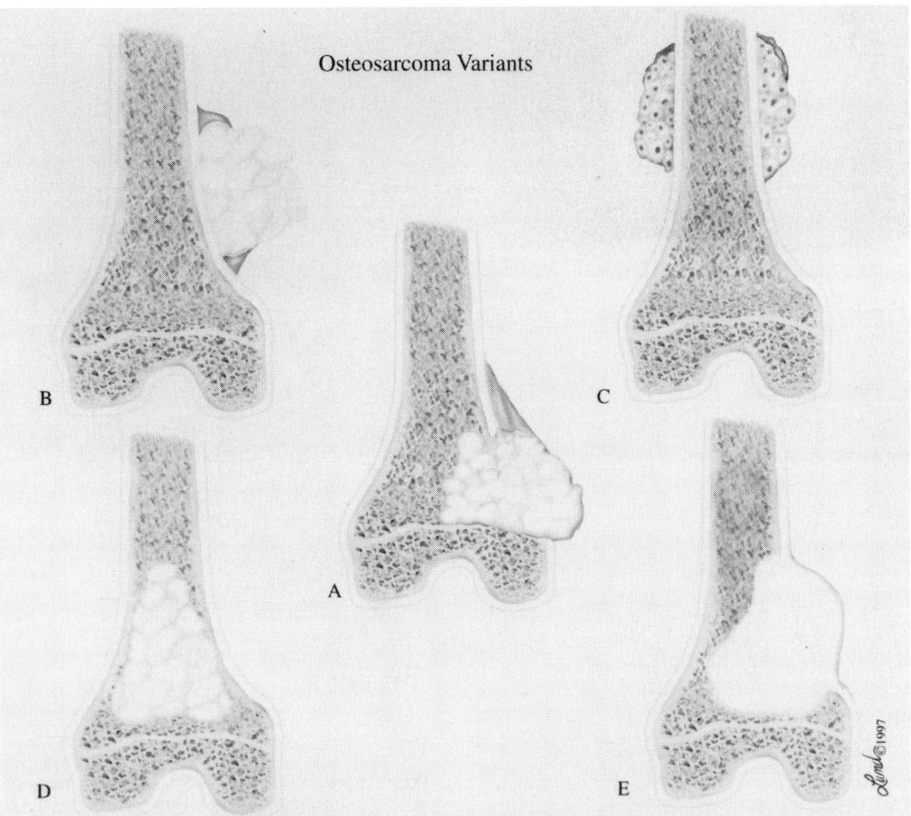

Figure 8–6. Artist's depiction of the different types of osteosarcoma of bone. The two left-hand figures depict the low-grade variants of osteosarcoma: parosteal osteosarcoma and well-differentiated intramedullary osteosarcoma. Parosteal osteosarcoma arises from the surface of the bone with a broad cortical attachment. The tumor grows in a lobulated fashion. In contrast, well-differentiated intramedullary osteosarcoma stays within the medullary cavity and usually does not break through the cortex. Both of these lesions are heavily mineralized. In contrast, the center figure shows a destructive process that has destroyed the distal metaphysis and extended into the soft tissues. The cortical bone destruction and extension into the soft tissues is typical of a high-grade intramedullary osteosarcoma. The figure in the top right, which shows a lesion arising from the cortex with a lobular pattern suggestive of cartilage, is a periosteal osteosarcoma. In this surface tumor there is osteoid production by the cells, but there is a predominance of cartilage. The figure in the bottom right shows a very destructive lytic lesion with no bone production. The overlying cortex has been destroyed with extension into the soft tissues. This pattern of bone destruction occurs in telangiectatic osteosarcoma. (From McCarthy, E.F., and Frassica, F.J.: Pathology of Bone and Joint Disorders. Philadelphia, WB Saunders, 1998.)

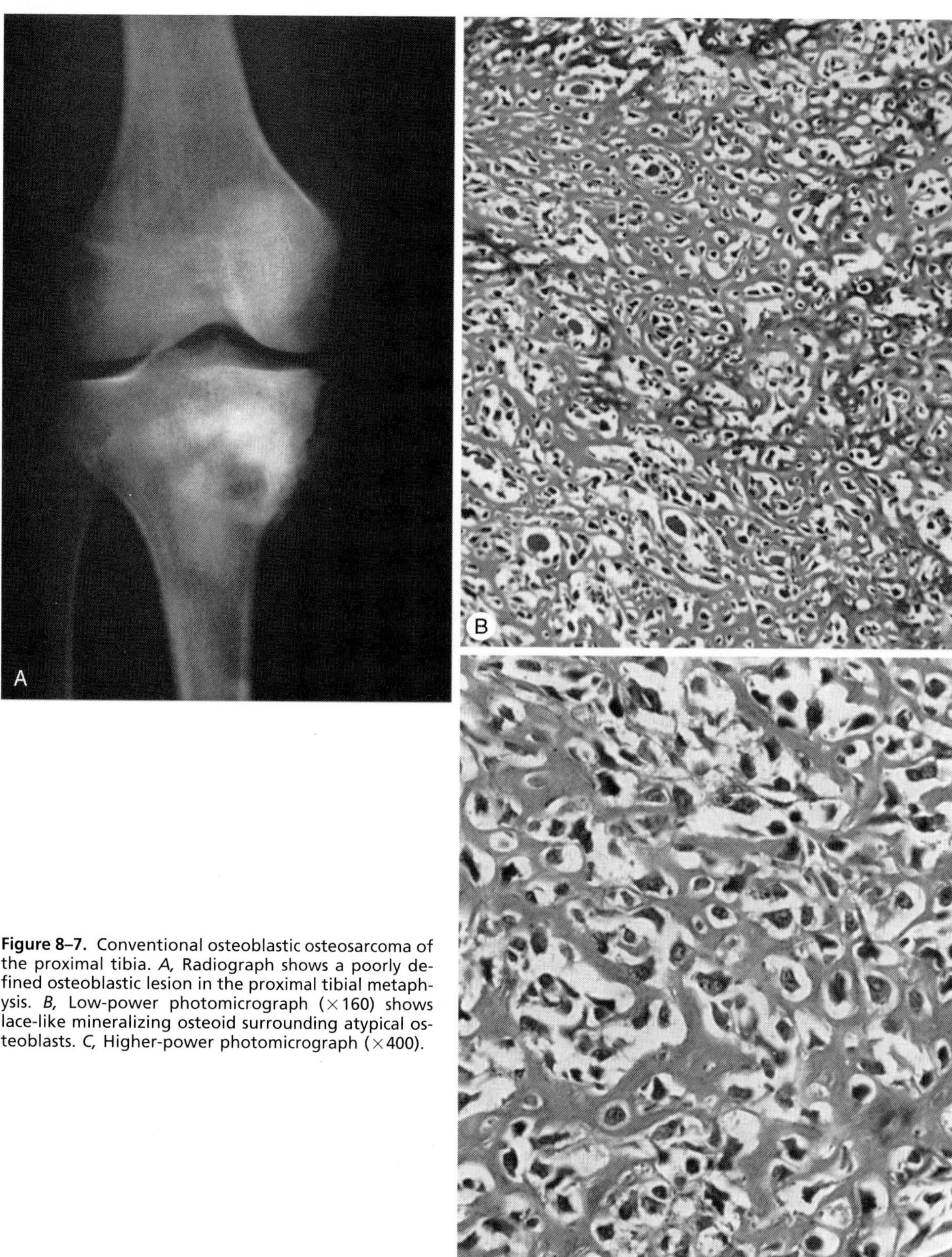

Figure 8–7. Conventional osteoblastic osteosarcoma of the proximal tibia. *A,* Radiograph shows a poorly defined osteoblastic lesion in the proximal tibial metaphysis. *B,* Low-power photomicrograph (×160) shows lace-like mineralizing osteoid surrounding atypical osteoblasts. *C,* Higher-power photomicrograph (×400).

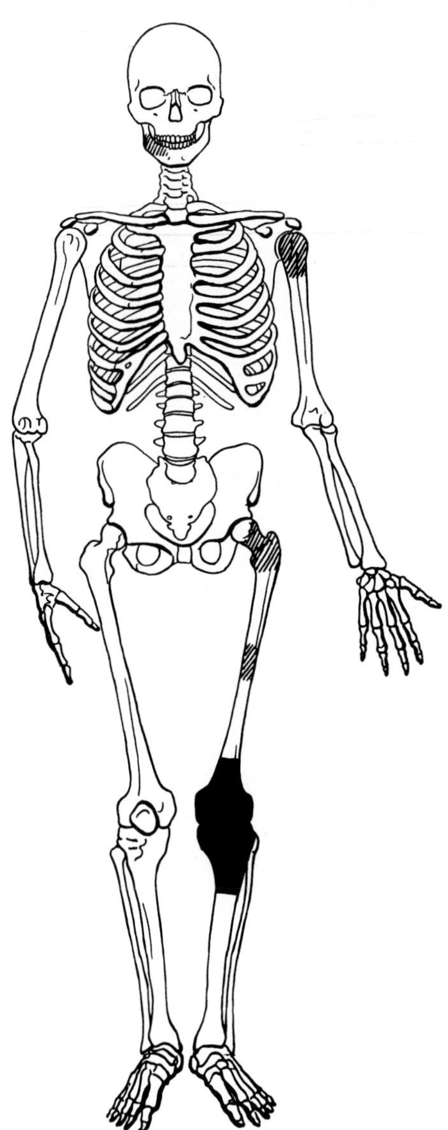

Figure 8–8. Conventional osteosarcoma locations. (From McCarthy, E.F., and Frassica, F.J.: Pathology of Bone and Joint Disorders. Philadelphia, WB Saunders, 1998.)

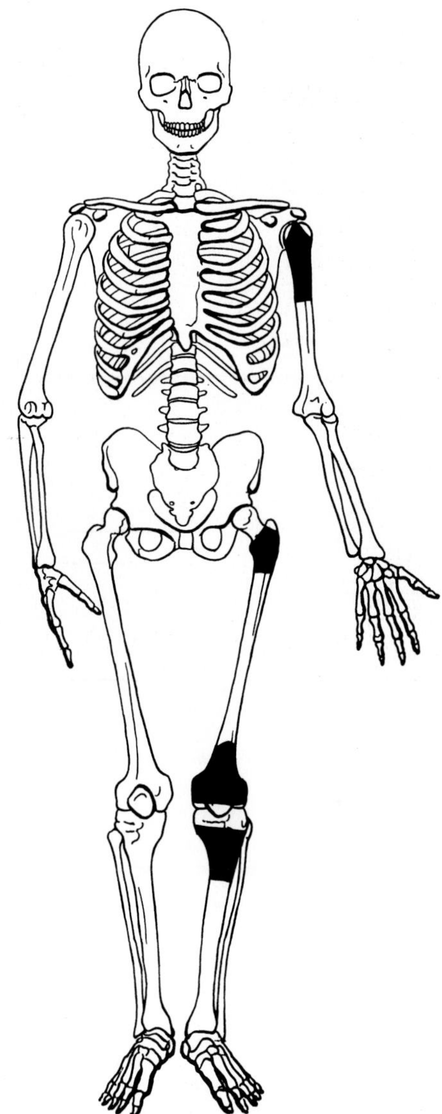

Figure 8–9. Telangiectatic osteosarcoma locations. (From McCarthy, E.F., and Frassica, F.J.: Pathology of Bone and Joint Disorders. Philadelphia, WB Saunders, 1998.)

as aneurysmal bone cysts, and their radiographic appearances can be confused (Fig. 8–9). Historically, osteosarcoma was treated by amputation; long-term studies show a survival of only 10–20%, with the pulmonary system being the most common site of failure. Multiagent chemotherapy has dramatically improved long-term survival and the potential for limb salvage. It effectively destroys the malignant cells,

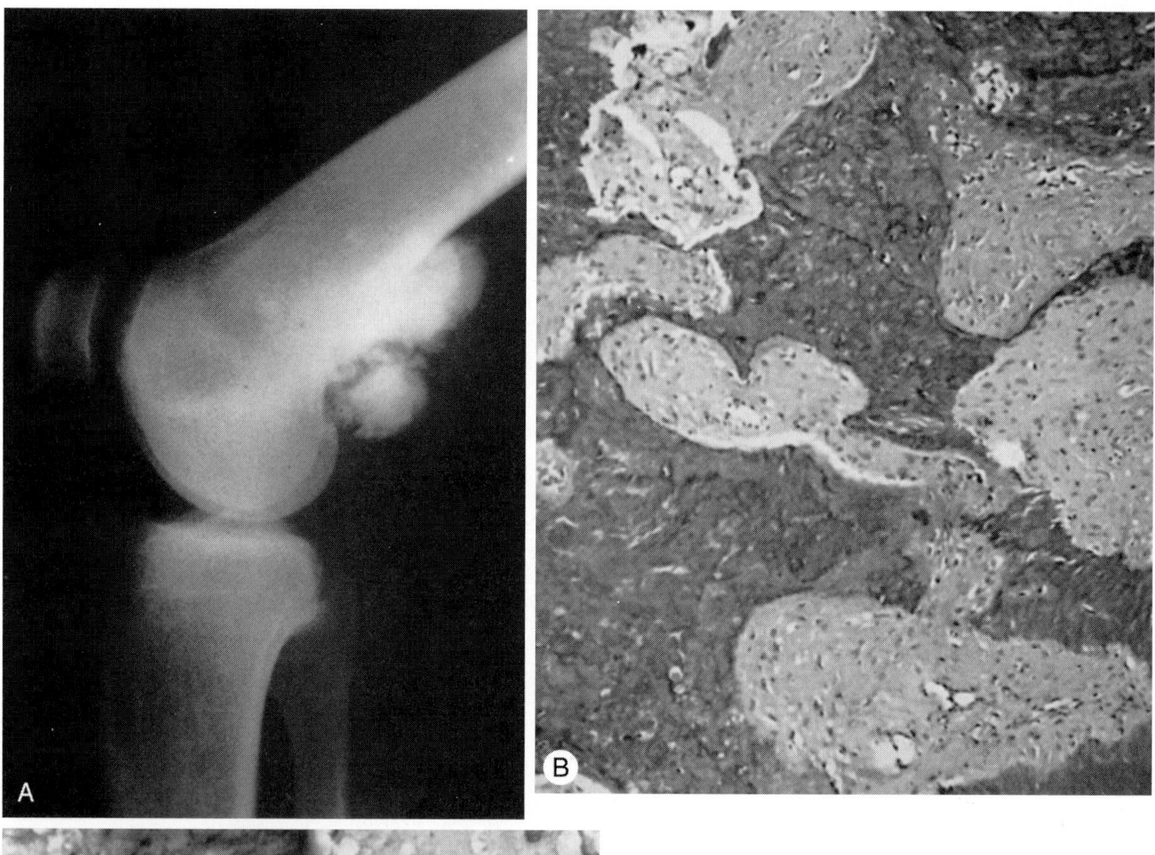

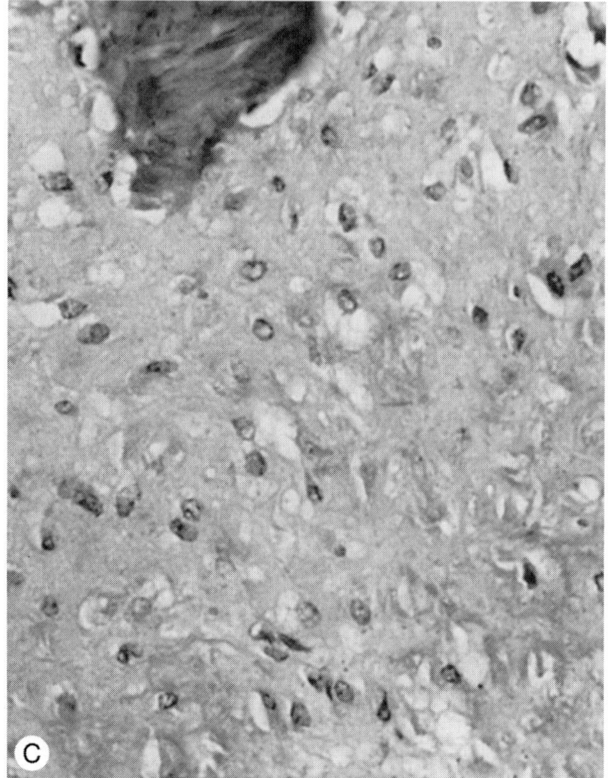

Figure 8–10. Parosteal osteosarcoma of the distal femur. *A,* Radiograph shows an exophytic bony mass in the posterior distal femur. *B,* Low-power photomicrograph (×160) shows plates of new bone in a fibrous matrix. *C,* Higher-power photomicrograph (×400) shows a fibrous stroma with atypical cells.

and in many patients there is total necrosis of the tumor. The chemotherapy kills both the micrometastases that are present in 80–90% of the patients at presentation and sterilizes the reactive zone around the tumor. Preoperative chemotherapy is delivered for 8–12 weeks, followed by resection of the tumor. Staging studies are performed at the end of chemotherapy to ensure that the lesion is resectable. Maintenance chemotherapy is then given for 6–12 months. Long-term survival is approximately 60–70% with these regimens.

b. Parosteal Osteosarcoma (Fig. 8–10)—This low-grade osteosarcoma occurs on the surface of the metaphysis of long bones. Patients often complain of a painless mass. The most common sites are the posterior aspect of the distal femur, proximal tibia, and proximal humerus (Fig. 8–11); the lesion is more common in females than in males. The radiographic appearance is characteristic in that it demonstrates a heavily ossified, often lobulated mass arising from the cortex. Histologically, the most prominent feature is regularly-arranged osseous trabeculae (Dahlin). Between the nearly normal trabeculae are slightly atypical spindle cells. At the periphery of the tumor are spindle cells, which typically invade skeletal muscle. Interestingly, cartilage is frequently present and may be arranged as a cap over the lesion. Treatment of parosteal osteosarcoma is wide surgical resection, which is usually curative. In approximately one-sixth of the lesions that appear radiographically to be parosteal osteosarcoma, there is a high-grade component. In this setting the lesion is called a dedifferentiated parosteal osteosarcoma. For typical low-grade parosteal osteosarcomas, chemotherapy or irradiation is not needed; however, the prognosis is much worse for dedifferentiated parosteal osteosarcomas, and multiagent chemotherapy is an important component of therapy. When local control has been achieved in parosteal osteosarcoma, the prognosis is excellent, with >95% long-term survival. Invasion into the medullary cavity does not adversely affect long-term survival. Dedifferentiation is a poor prognostic factor.

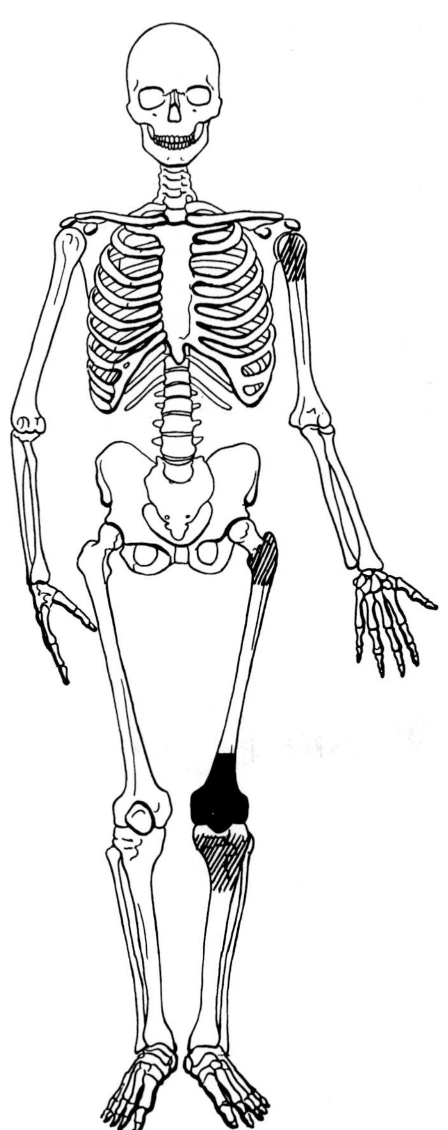

Figure 8–11. Skeletal distribution of the most common sites of parosteal osteosarcoma. (From McCarthy, E.F., and Frassica, F.J.: Pathology of Bone and Joint Disorders. Philadelphia, WB Saunders, 1998.)

c. Periosteal Osteosarcoma (Fig. 8–12)—This rare surface form of osteosarcoma occurs most commonly in the diaphysis of long bones (typically the femur or tibia) (Fig. 8–13). The radiographic appearance is fairly constant; a sunburst-type lesion rests on a saucerized cortical depression. Histologically, the lesion is predominantly chondroblastic, and the grade of the lesion is intermediate (grade 2 or 3). Highly anaplastic regions are not found. The prognosis for periosteal osteosarcoma is intermediate between parosteal osteosarcoma (very low-grade) and high-grade intramedullary osteosarcoma. Preoperative chemotherapy, wide surgical resection, and maintenance chemotherapy comprise the preferred treatment. The risk of pulmonary metastases is between 20 and 35%.

C. Chondrogenic Lesions—The principal benign cartilage lesions are chondromas, osteochondroma, chondromyxoid fibroma, and chondroblastoma (Fig. 8–14). The common malignant cartilage tumors are intramedullary chondrosarcoma and dedifferentiated chondrosarcoma. Clear cell chondrosarcoma and mesenchymal chondrosarcoma are rare forms.

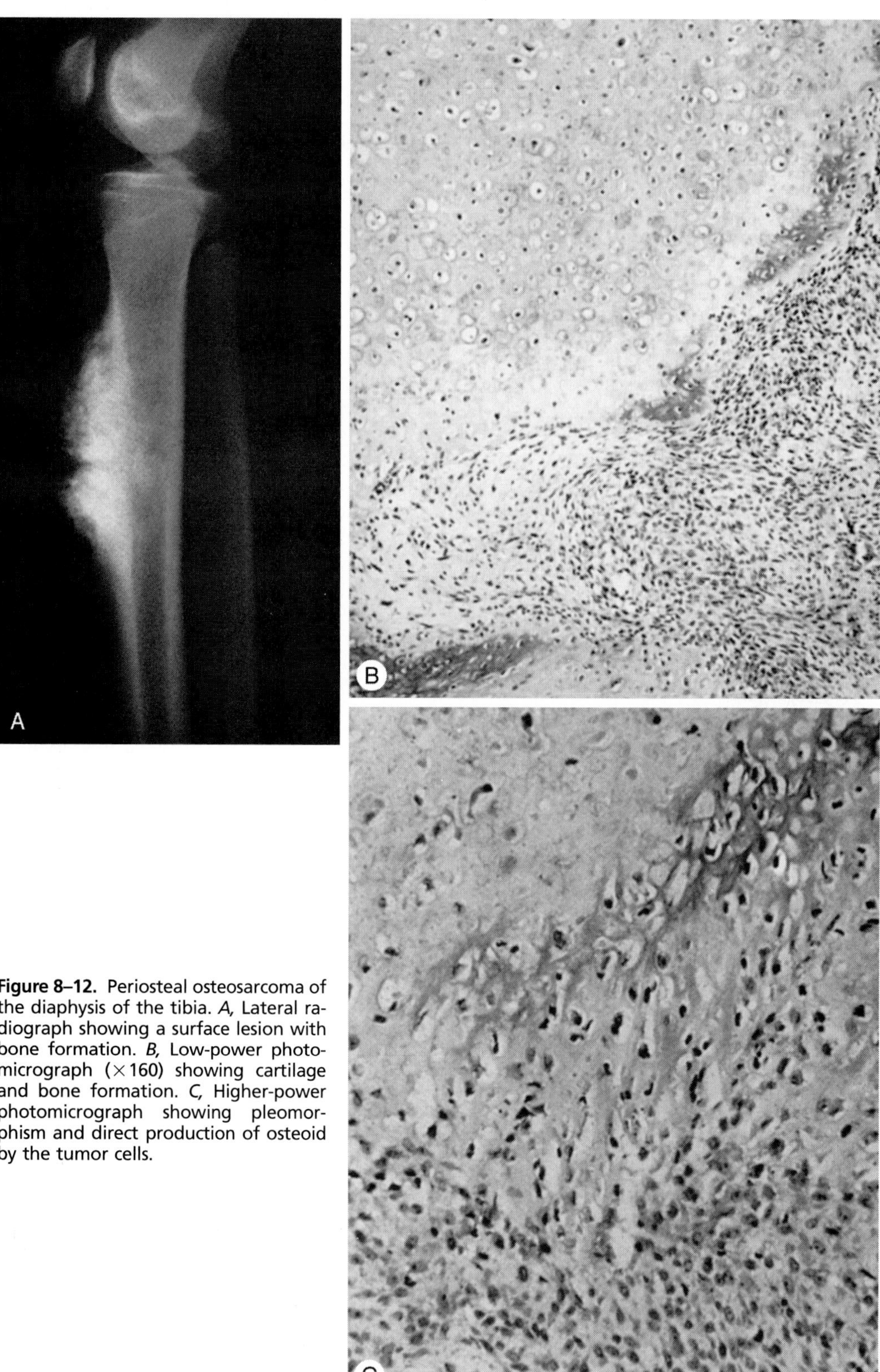

Figure 8–12. Periosteal osteosarcoma of the diaphysis of the tibia. *A,* Lateral radiograph showing a surface lesion with bone formation. *B,* Low-power photomicrograph (×160) showing cartilage and bone formation. *C,* Higher-power photomicrograph showing pleomorphism and direct production of osteoid by the tumor cells.

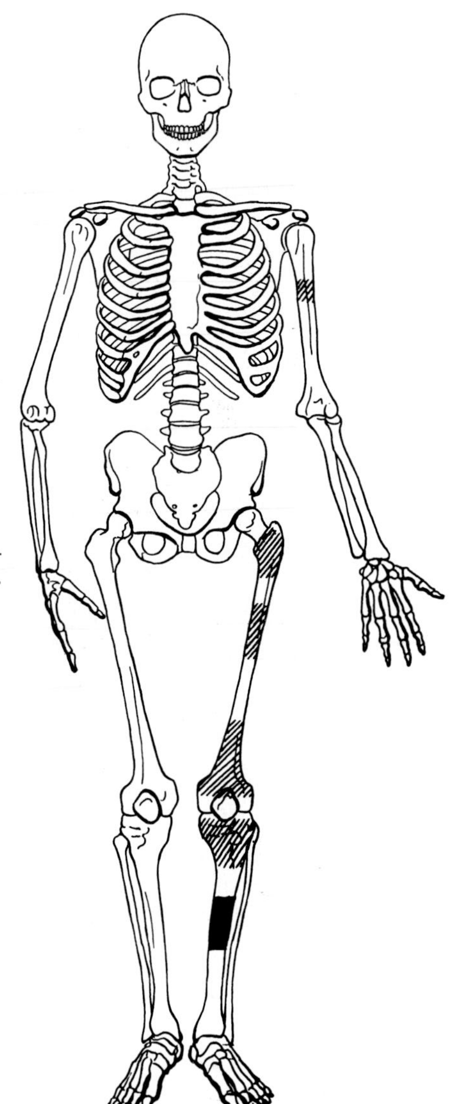

Figure 8–13. Skeletal distribution of the most common sites of periosteal osteosarcoma. (From McCarthy, E.F., and Frassica, F.J.: Pathology of Bone and Joint Disorders. Philadelphia, WB Saunders, 1998.)

1. Chondromas (Fig. 8–15)—These benign cartilage tumors may occur in the medullary cavity or on the surface of the bone (periosteal chondroma). Enchondromas are benign cartilage lesions that are most commonly localized in the metaphysis of long bones, especially the proximal femur and humerus and the distal femur (Fig. 8–16). They are common in the hand, where they usually occur in the diaphysis (Dahlin). Pathologic fractures in the hand are common. Involvement of the epiphysis is rare. Most enchondromas are asymptomatic. Radiographically, in long bones there may be a prominent stippled or mottled calcified appearance. Occasionally, active lesions are purely lytic without evidence of mineralization. Most enchondromas require no treatment other than observation. Histologically, they are composed of small cells that lie in lacunar spaces. The lesion is usually hypocellular, and the cells have a bland appearance (no pleomorphism, anaplasia, or hyperchromasia). In contrast, lesions in the hand may be hypercellular and display worrisome histologic features. When lesions are not causing pain, serial radiographs are obtained to ensure that the lesions are inactive (not growing). Radiographs are obtained at 3 months and 1 year after presentation. In contrast, periosteal chondromas occur on the surface of long bones (Fig. 8–17). They most commonly occur on the surface of the distal femur, proximal humerus, and proximal femur (Fig. 8–18). Usually, there is a well-demarcated cortical defect and a slight overhang of the cortical edges. About one-third of periosteal chondromas have a mineralized cartilaginous matrix on the radiograph, whereas two-thirds have no apparent radiographic mineralization. When surgical treatment is necessary, enchondromas are treated by curettage and bone grafting. Periosteal

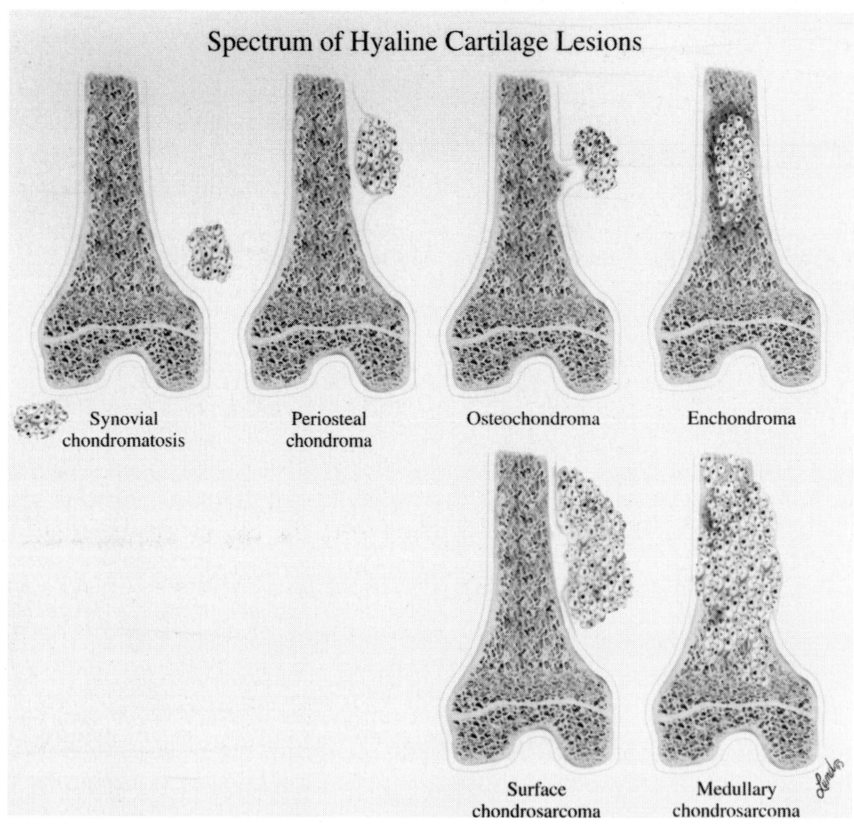

Figure 8–14. Artist's depiction of the common types of cartilage tumors. The top left figure shows the lobular pattern of cartilage in synovial chondromatosis. The second figure from the left demonstrates a surface tumor of bone composed of mature cartilage that sits in a saucer-shaped depression on the bone's surface. These lesions are called periosteal chondromas. The next lesion (third from the left) shows a surface tumor in which the cortices are continuous between the surface lesion and the host cortex. On top of the bone sits a thin rim of cartilage (1–3 mm). This lesion is called an osteochondroma and is one of the most common benign cartilage tumors. The fourth lesion from the left represents an enchondroma. Notice that this benign cartilage tumor sits in the medullary cavity in a quiescent manner. There are no cortical changes such as erosions, cortical thickening, or cortical bone destruction. In contrast, the lesion on the bottom right shows destruction of the cortex and extension into the soft tissues. This is a medullary chondrosarcoma with active growth. In this instance, the cartilage is growing and destroying the bone rather than being quiescent. (From McCarthy, E.F., and Frassica, F.J.: Pathology of Bone and Joint Disorders. Philadelphia, WB Saunders, 1998.)

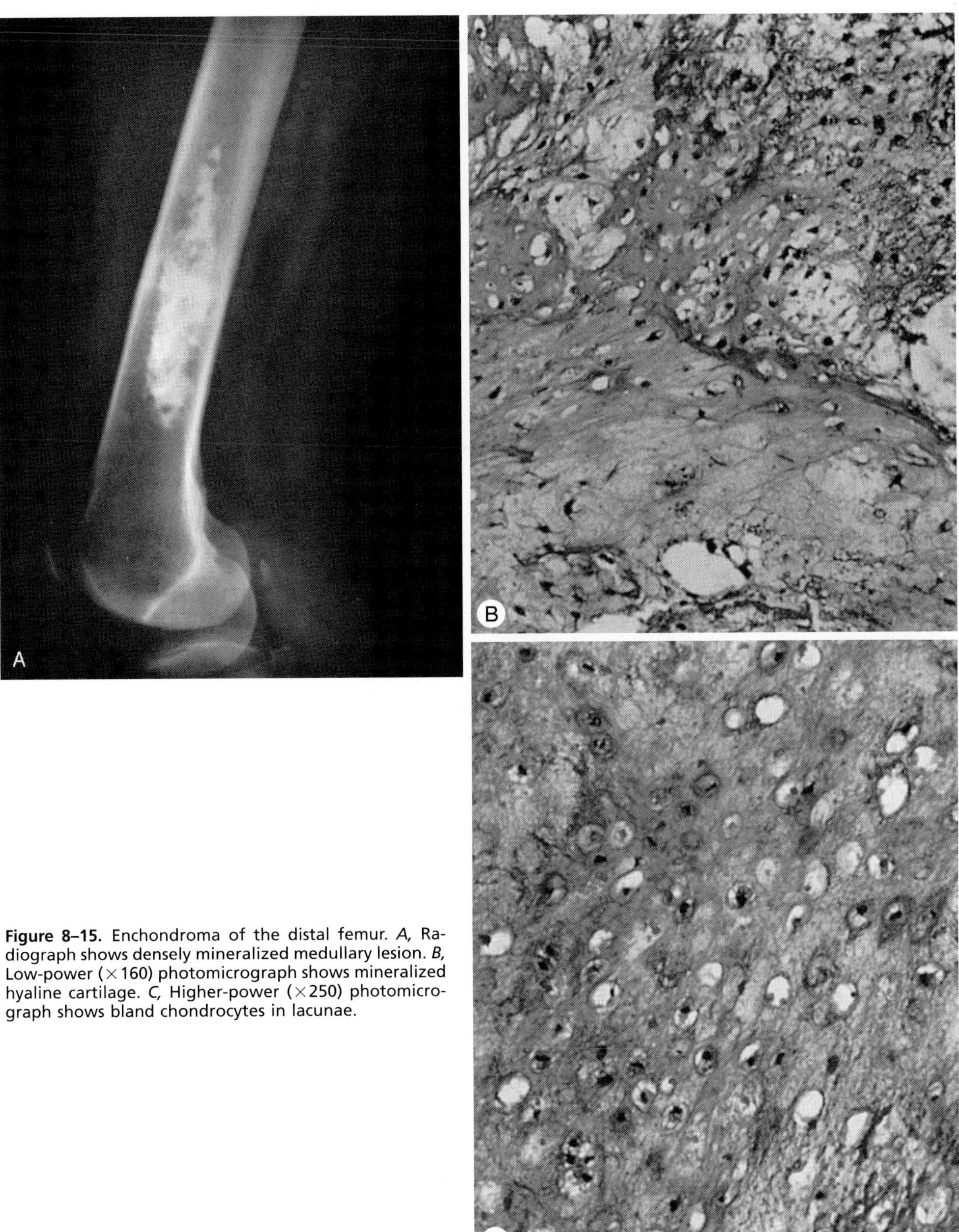

Figure 8–15. Enchondroma of the distal femur. *A,* Radiograph shows densely mineralized medullary lesion. *B,* Low-power (×160) photomicrograph shows mineralized hyaline cartilage. *C,* Higher-power (×250) photomicrograph shows bland chondrocytes in lacunae.

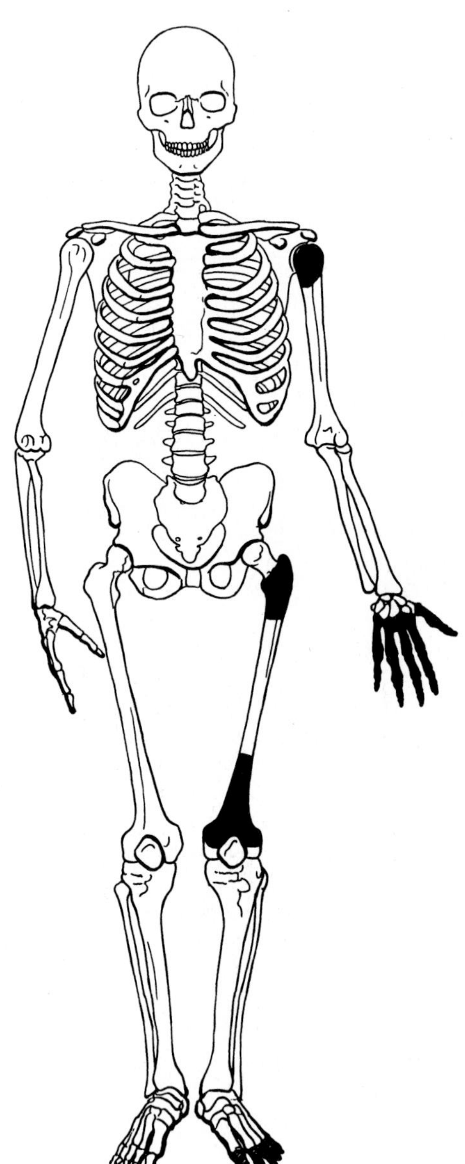

Figure 8–16. Skeletal distribution of the most common sites of enchondromas. Note the common location in the phalanges of the hand, the proximal humerus, and distal femur. (From McCarthy, E.F., and Frassica, F.J.: Pathology of Bone and Joint Disorders. Philadelphia, WB Saunders, 1998.)

chondromas are usually excised with a marginal margin. Enchondromas may be multiple in the same extremity. When there are many lesions, when the involved bones are dysplastic, and when the lesions tend to unilaterality, the diagnosis of multiple enchondromatosis, or Ollier's disease, is made. If soft-tissue angiomas are also present, the patient has Maffucci's syndrome. Chondrosarcomas virtually never occur in the setting of a previous enchondroma; however, patients with multiple enchondromatosis are at increased risk (Ollier's disease, 30%; Maffucci's syndrome, 100%). Patients with multiple enchondromatosis also have an increased risk of visceral malignancies, such as astrocytomas, and gastrointestinal malignancies.

2. Osteochondroma (Fig. 8–19)—These benign surface lesions probably arise secondary to aberrant cartilage on the surface of bone (Dahlin). Patients usually present with a painless mass or incidentally when a radiograph is obtained for another reason. They most commonly occur about the knee, proximal femur, and proximal humerus (Fig. 8–20). The characteristic appearance is a surface lesion in which the cortex of the lesion and the underlying cortex are continuous; the medullary cavity of the host bone also flows into (is continuous with) the osteochondroma. The osteochondroma may have a narrow stalk (pedunculated) or a broad base (sessile). These lesions typically occur at the site of tendon insertions, and the affected bone is abnormally wide (Dahlin). Histologically, the underlying cortex is covered by a thin cap of cartilage. Grossly, the cartilage cap is usually only 2–3 mm thick. In a growing child the cap may exceed 1–2 cm. Histologically, the chondrocytes are arranged in linear clusters

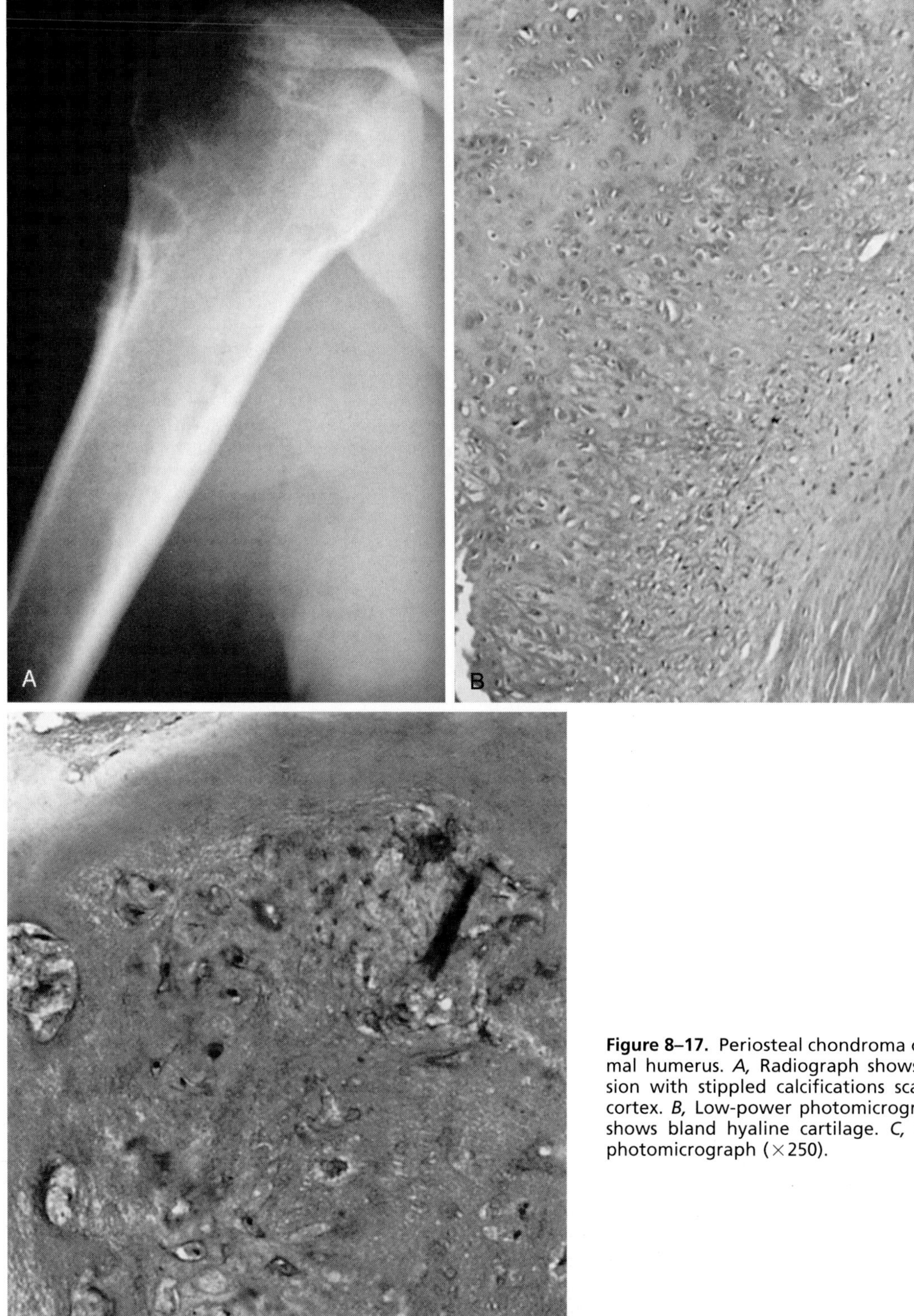

Figure 8–17. Periosteal chondroma of the proximal humerus. *A,* Radiograph shows surface lesion with stippled calcifications scalloping the cortex. *B,* Low-power photomicrograph (×100) shows bland hyaline cartilage. *C,* High-power photomicrograph (×250).

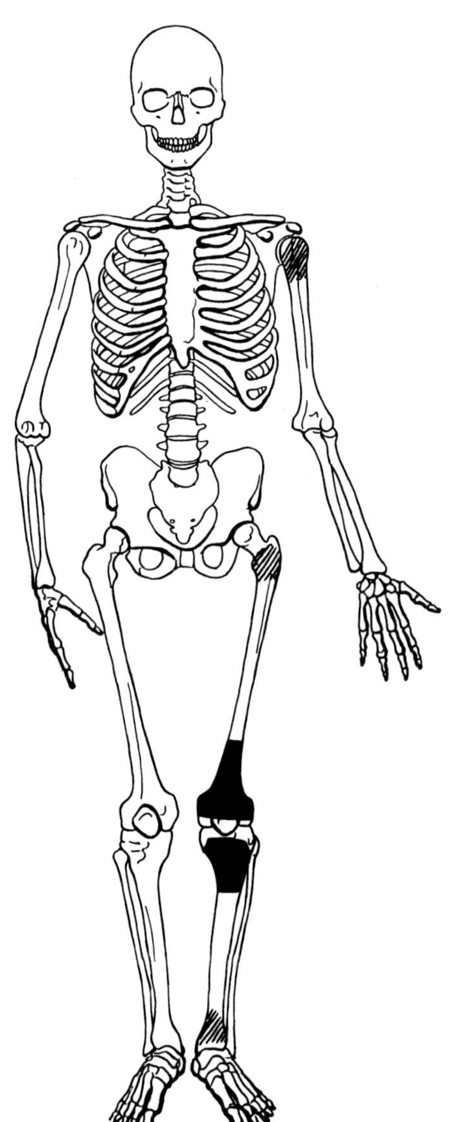

Figure 8–20. Skeletal distribution of the most common sites of osteochondromas. (From McCarthy, E.F., and Frassica, F.J.: Pathology of Bone and Joint Disorders. Philadelphia, WB Saunders, 1998.)

droblasts. There are scattered multinucleated giant cells throughout the lesion and zones of chondroid substance. Mitotic figures may be found. Chondroblastomas are treated by curettage (intralesional margin) and bone grafting. About 2% of benign chondroblastomas metastasize to the lungs.

4. Chondromyxoid Fibroma (Fig. 8–23)—These rare benign cartilage tumors contain variable amounts of chondroid, fibromatoid, and myxoid elements. The lesion is more common in males and tends to involve long bones (especially the tibia). The pelvis and distal femur are other common locations (Fig. 8–24). Patients present with pain of variable duration (months to years). Radiographically, there is a lytic, destructive lesion that is eccentric and sharply demarcated from the adjacent normal bone. Usually, no matrix mineralization is seen radiographically. The tumor grows in lobules, and there is often a condensation of cells at the periphery of the lobules. The chondroid element may vary from small to heavy concentrations. Treatment is resection with a marginal line of resection.
5. Intramedullary Chondrosarcoma (Fig. 8–25)—These common malignant neoplasms of cartilage cells occur in adults and the older age groups. The most common locations include the shoulder and pelvic girdles, knee, and spine. Patients may present with pain or a mass. Plain radiographs are usually diagnostic, with bone destruction, thickening of the cortex, and mineralization consistent with cartilage within the lesion (Fig. 8–26). About 85% of patients will have prominent cortical changes. A soft-tissue mass is often present in patients who have had symptoms for a long time. It may be extremely difficult to differentiate malignant cartilage based on histologic features alone. The clinical, radio-

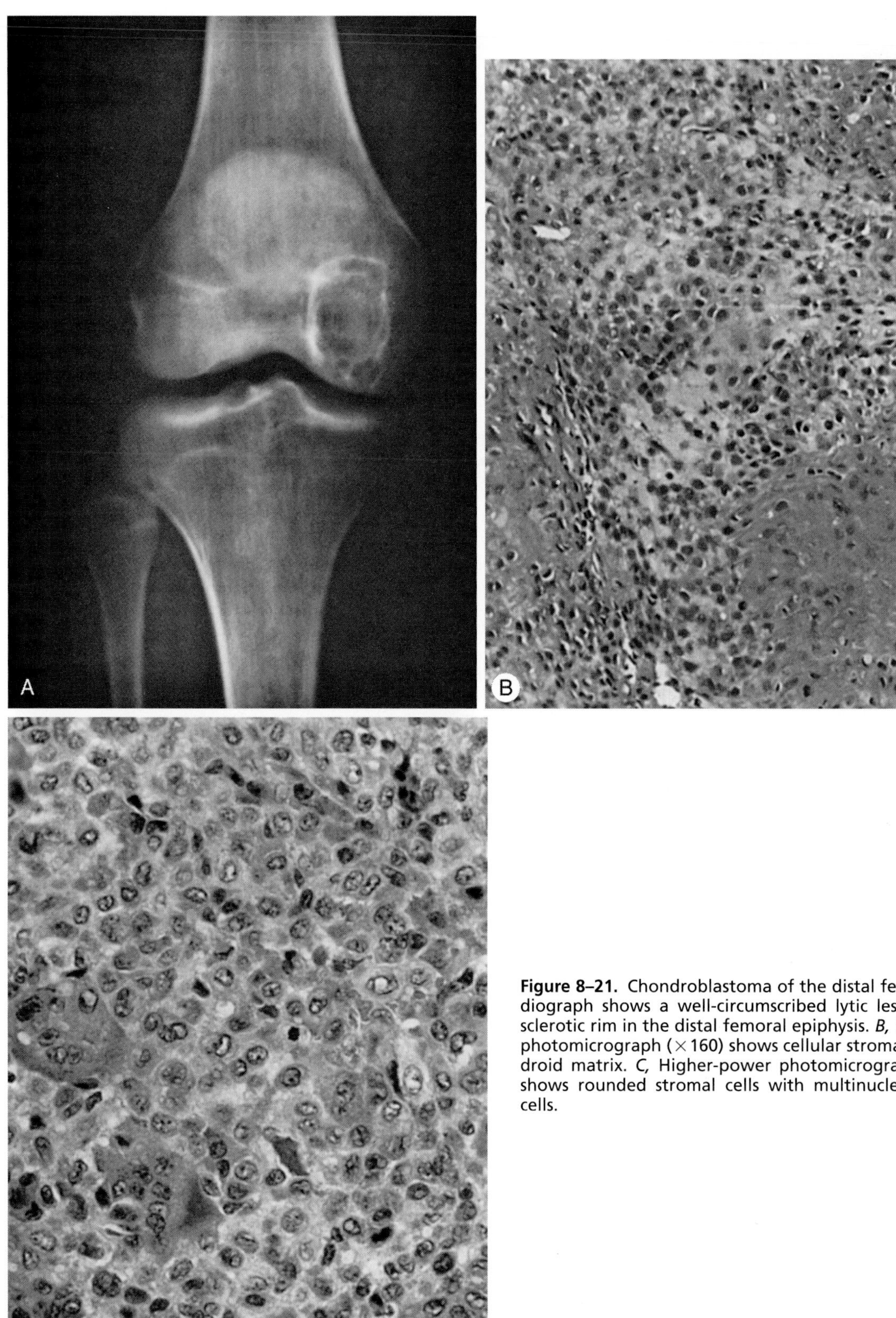

Figure 8–21. Chondroblastoma of the distal femur. *A,* Radiograph shows a well-circumscribed lytic lesion with a sclerotic rim in the distal femoral epiphysis. *B,* Low-power photomicrograph (×160) shows cellular stroma in a chondroid matrix. *C,* Higher-power photomicrograph (×400) shows rounded stromal cells with multinucleated giant cells.

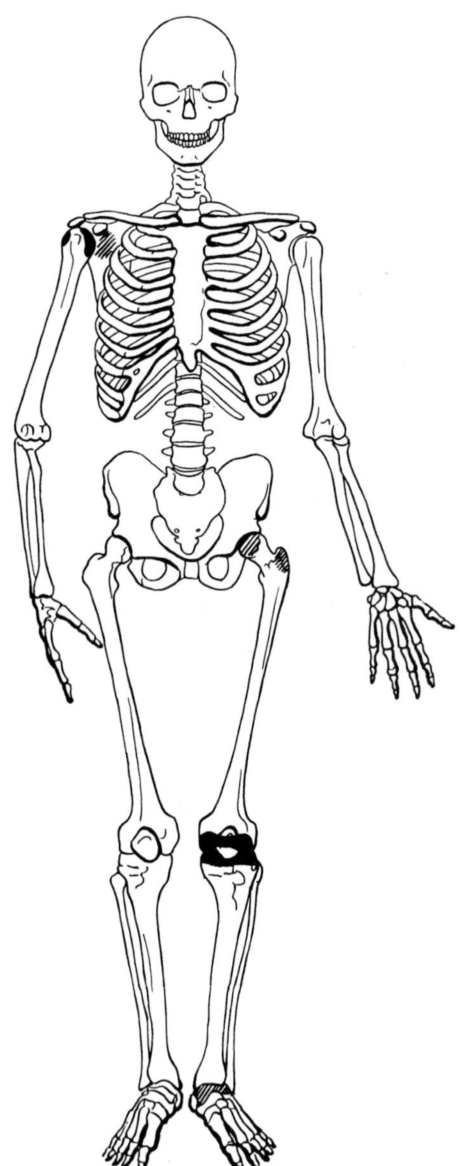

Figure 8–22. Skeletal distribution of the most common sites of chondroblastomas. Chondroblastomas begin exclusively in either the epiphysis or apophysis. They commonly occur in the distal femur, proximal tibia, femoral head, greater trochanteric apophysis, and the proximal humeral epiphysis. When they occur in the proximal humeral epiphysis, the eponym "Codman's tumor" is used. (From McCarthy, E.F., and Frassica, F.J.: Pathology of Bone and Joint Disorders. Philadelphia, WB Saunders, 1998.)

graphic, and histologic features of a particular lesion must be combined to avoid incorrect diagnoses. The criteria for the diagnosis of malignancy are difficult: (1) many cells with plump nuclei, (2) more than an occasional cell with two such nuclei, and (3) especially giant cartilage cells with large single or multiple nuclei with clumps of chromatin (Dahlin). Chondromas of the hand, lesions in patients with Ollier's disease and Maffucci's syndrome, and periosteal chondromas may have atypical histopathologic features; however, their behavior is that of a benign cartilage lesion and, hence, they are not malignant lesions. In these lesions there may be hypercellularity and worrisome nuclear features; however, the biologic behavior is innocent. More than 90% of chondrosarcomas are grade 1 or grade 2 lesions. Grade 4 lesions do not occur; when this degree of malignancy is observed, the lesion is most likely a chondroblastic osteosarcoma. Treatment consists of wide surgical resection. For typical low-grade (grades 1 and 2) chondrosarcoma there is no role for chemotherapy or irradiation.

6. Dedifferentiated Chondrosarcoma (Fig. 8–27)—These lesions are the most malignant cartilage tumors. They have a bimorphic histologic and radiographic appearance. Histologically, there is a low-grade cartilage component that is intimately associated with a high-grade spindle cell sarcoma (osteosarcoma, fibrosarcoma, malignant fibrous histiocytoma). The most common locations include the distal and proximal femur and the proximal humerus (Fig. 8–28). Radiographically, in more than 80% of the lesions there is a typical chondrosarcoma with a superimposed highly destructive area. Patients present with a picture similar to that of low-grade chon-

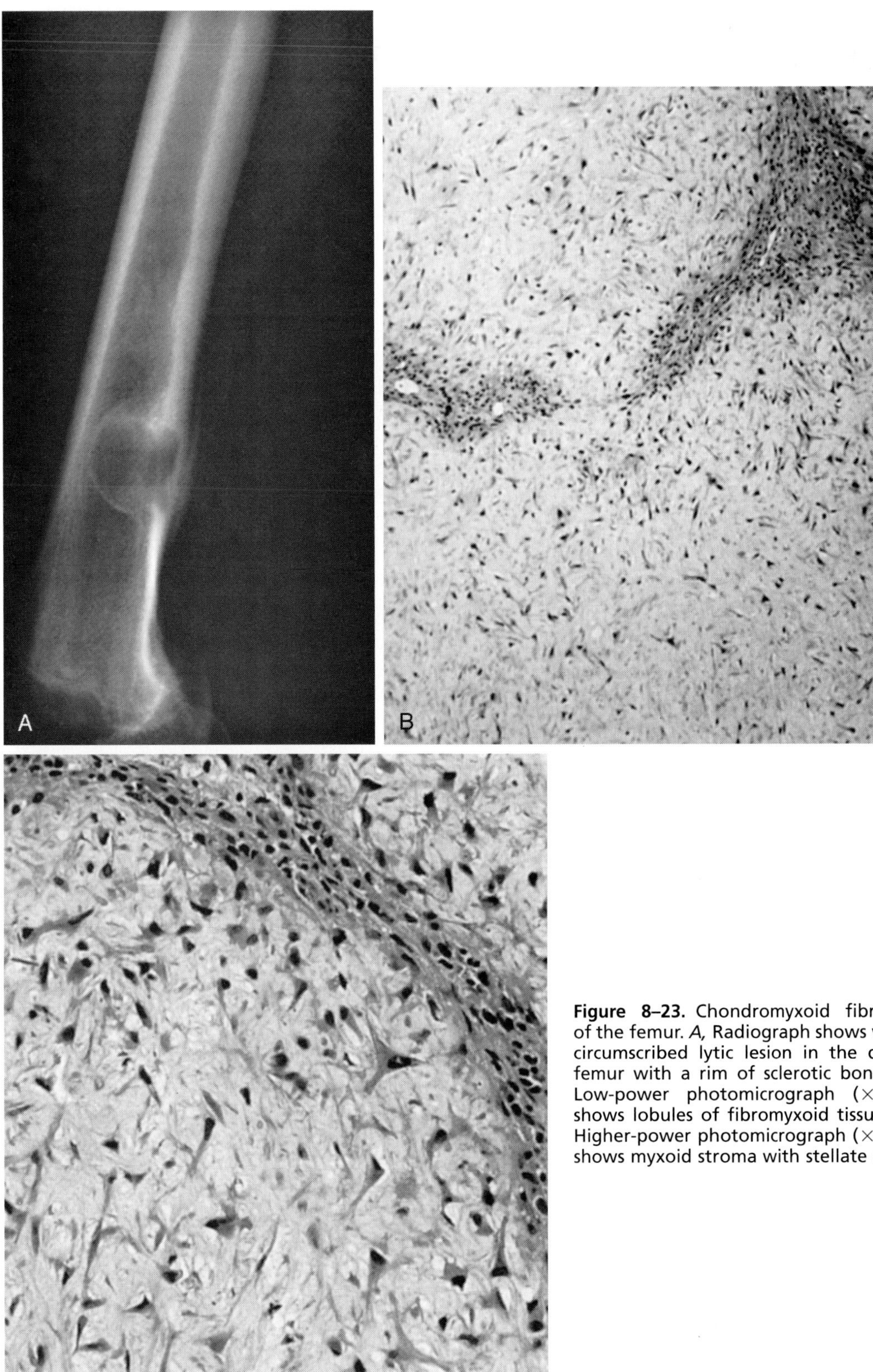

Figure 8–23. Chondromyxoid fibroma of the femur. *A,* Radiograph shows well-circumscribed lytic lesion in the distal femur with a rim of sclerotic bone. *B,* Low-power photomicrograph (×100) shows lobules of fibromyxoid tissue. *C,* Higher-power photomicrograph (×250) shows myxoid stroma with stellate cells.

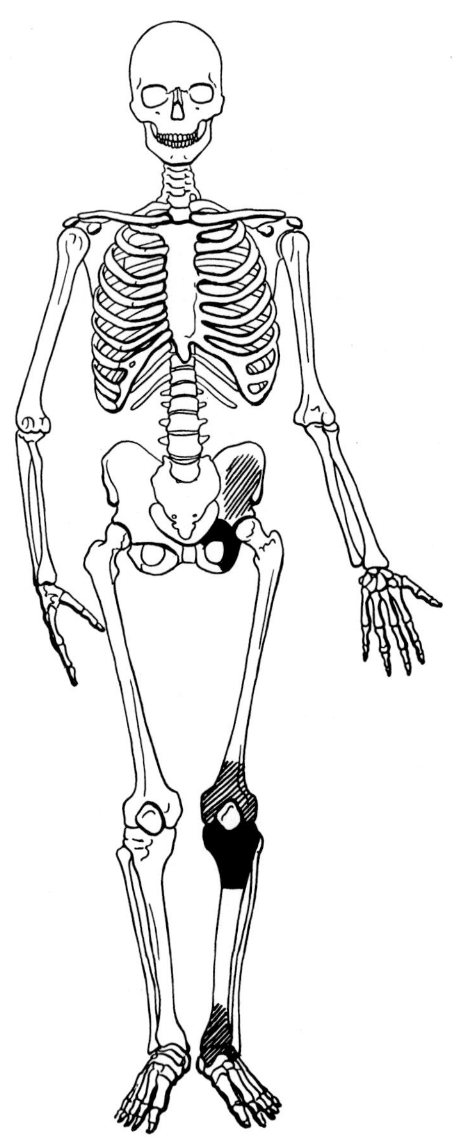

Figure 8–24. Skeletal distribution of the most common sites of chondromyxoid fibroma. The tibia and pelvis are common locations. (From McCarthy, E.F., and Frassica, F.J.: Pathology of Bone and Joint Disorders. Philadelphia, WB Saunders, 1998.)

drosarcoma, including pain and decreased function. The prognosis is poor, and long-term survival is less than 10%. Wide surgical resection and multiagent chemotherapy are the principal methods of treatment.

D. Fibrous Lesions—Truly fibrous neoplasms of bone are not common and number only three: metaphyseal fibrous defect (fibroma), desmoplastic fibroma, and fibrosarcoma.
   1. Metaphyseal Fibrous Defect (Fig. 8–29)—This is a common lesion occurring in young patients. Most of these lesions resolve spontaneously and are probably not true neoplasms. Common names for this lesion include fibroma, myxoma, nonosteogenic fibroma, cortical desmoid, fibromatosis, and xanthoma. Metaphyseal fibrous defect is the most descriptive form. The most common locations are the distal femur, distal tibia, and proximal tibia. Most patients are asymptomatic, and the lesion is discovered incidentally. The radiographic appearance is characteristic, with the lytic lesion that is metaphyseal, eccentric, and surrounded by a sclerotic rim. The cortex may be slightly expanded and thinned. Histologically, there is a cellular, fibroblastic connective tissue background with the cells arranged in whorled bundles (Dahlin). There are numerous giant cells, lipophages, and various amounts of hemosiderin pigmentation. Treatment is observation if the radiographic appearance is characteristic and there is not an excessive risk of pathologic fracture. If more than 75% of the cortex is involved and the patient is symptomatic, curettage and bone grafting are performed.
   2. Desmoplastic Fibroma—This lesion is a rare low-grade malignant fibrous tumor of bone. Radiographically, the lesion is purely lytic. Because the process is low-grade, there will often be residual or reactive trabeculations (or corrugations) of bone. Histologically, this

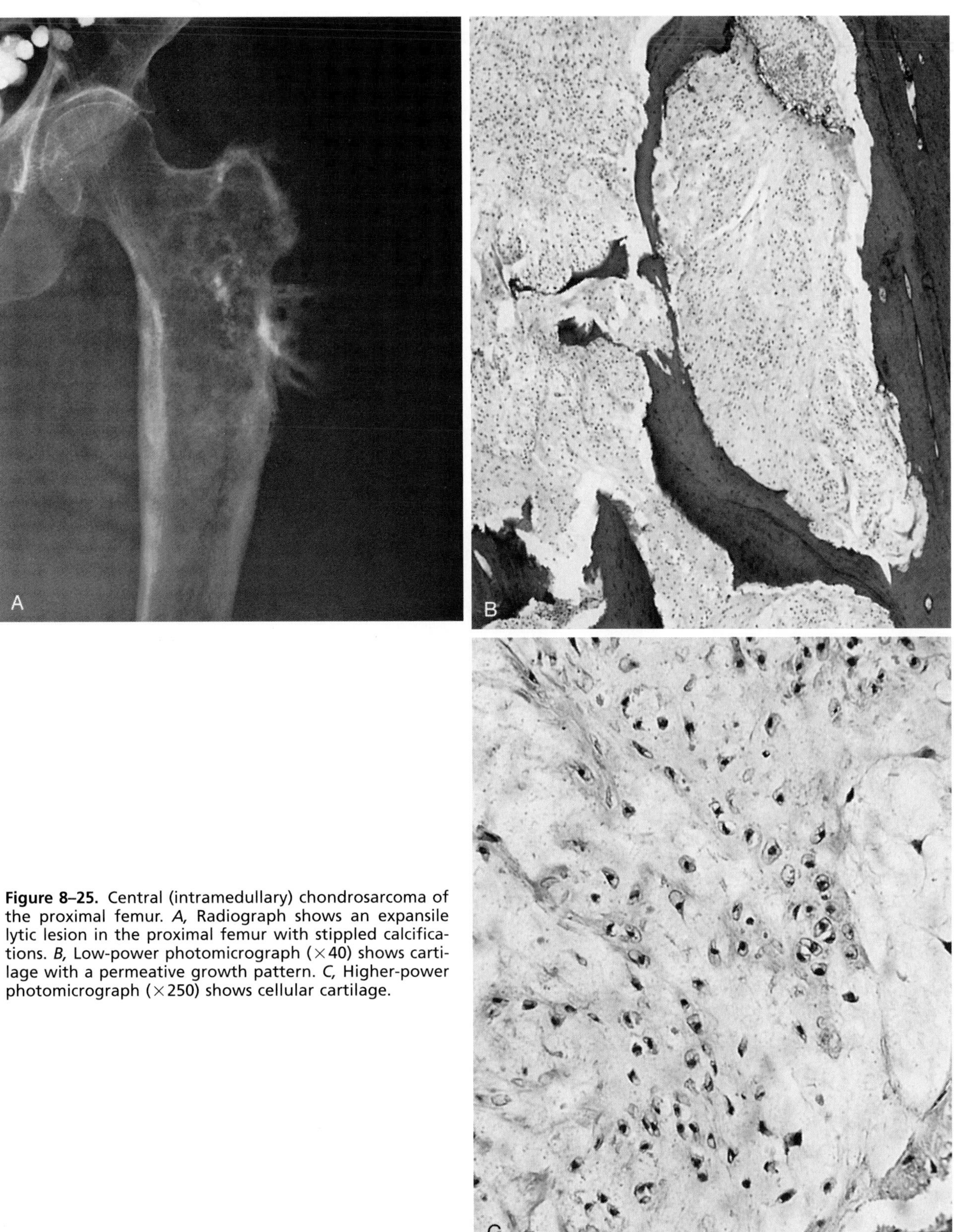

Figure 8–25. Central (intramedullary) chondrosarcoma of the proximal femur. *A,* Radiograph shows an expansile lytic lesion in the proximal femur with stippled calcifications. *B,* Low-power photomicrograph (×40) shows cartilage with a permeative growth pattern. *C,* Higher-power photomicrograph (×250) shows cellular cartilage.

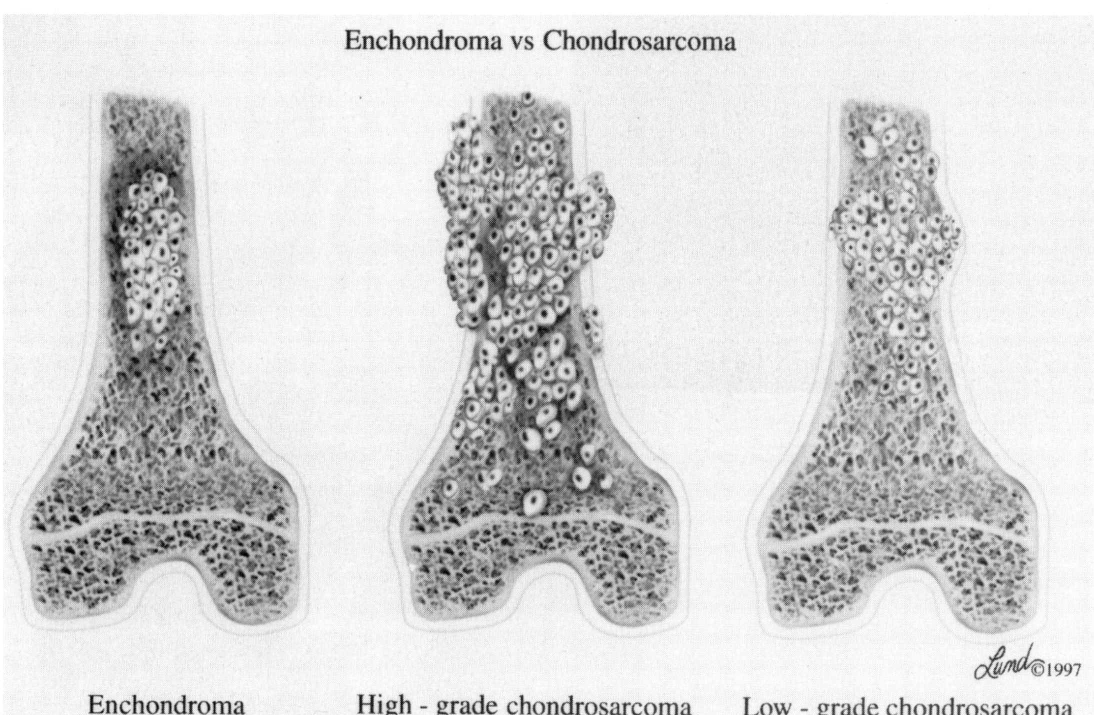

Figure 8–26. Artist's depiction of the three types of intramedullary cartilage tumors: enchondroma, high-grade chondrosarcoma, and low-grade chondrosarcoma. Enchondromas are inactive intramedullary hyaline cartilage tumors. Note that the cortices are not involved. There is no cortical erosion, thickening, expansion, or breakthrough. In contrast, the middle figure shows a high-grade chondrosarcoma with destruction of the cortex and extension into the soft tissues. The figure to the right is a low-grade chondrosarcoma. Note the cortical erosion with expansion of the cortex but no breakthrough. (From McCarthy, E.F., and Frassica, F.J.: Pathology of Bone and Joint Disorders. Philadelphia, WB Saunders, 1998.)

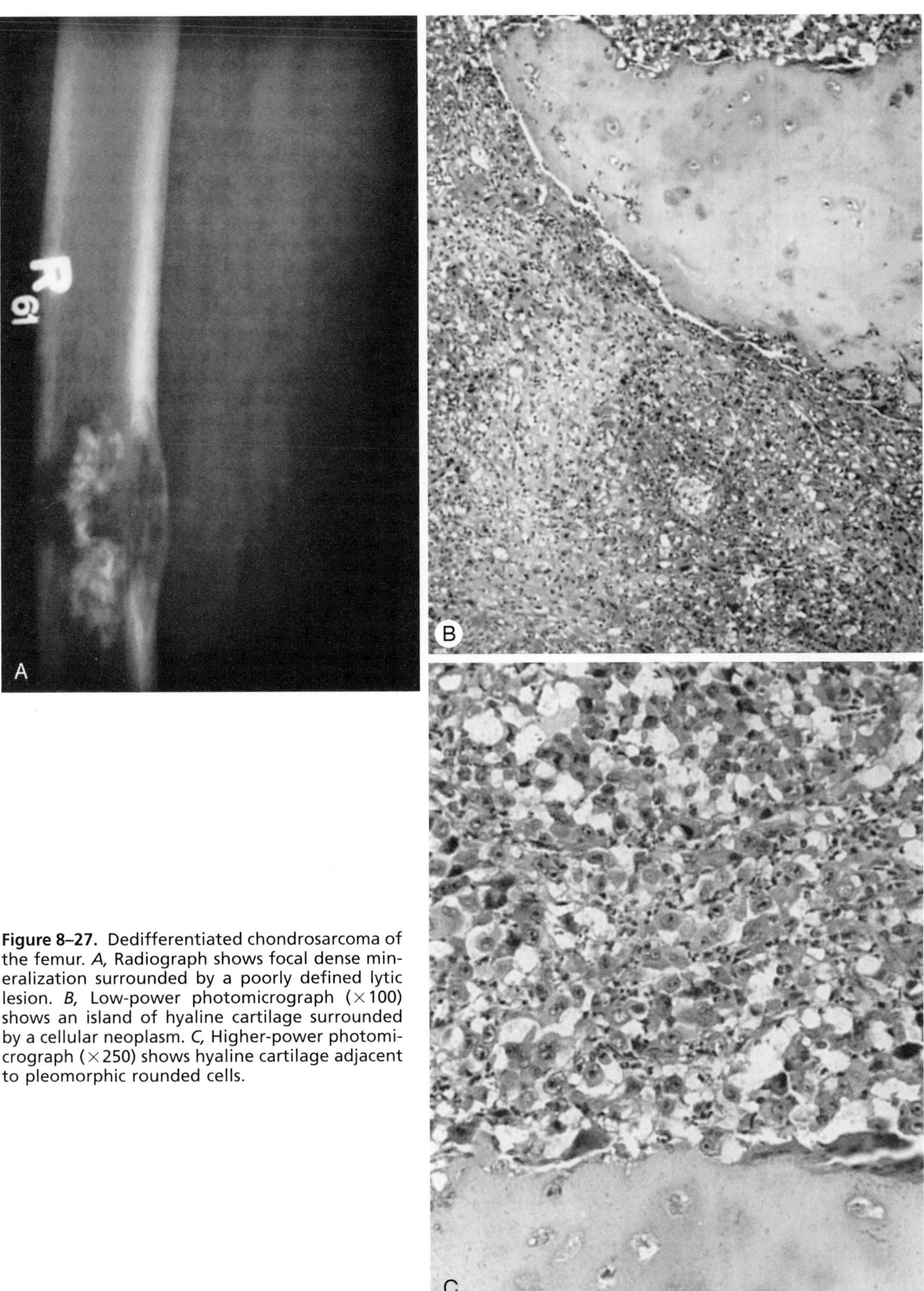

Figure 8–27. Dedifferentiated chondrosarcoma of the femur. *A,* Radiograph shows focal dense mineralization surrounded by a poorly defined lytic lesion. *B,* Low-power photomicrograph (×100) shows an island of hyaline cartilage surrounded by a cellular neoplasm. *C,* Higher-power photomicrograph (×250) shows hyaline cartilage adjacent to pleomorphic rounded cells.

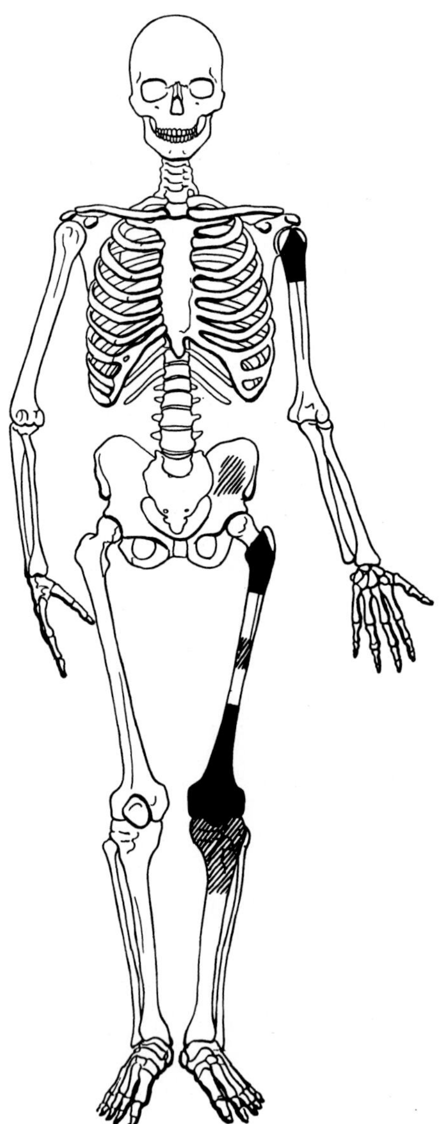

Figure 8–28. Skeletal distribution of the most common sites of dedifferentiated chondrosarcoma. The femur and humerus are the most common sites. (From McCarthy, E.F., and Frassica, F.J.: Pathology of Bone and Joint Disorders. Philadelphia, WB Saunders, 1998.)

lesion is composed of abundant collagen and mature fibroblasts with no cellular atypia. Wide surgical resection is the treatment.

3. Fibrosarcoma (Fig. 8–30)—This malignant tumor of bone has a presentation and localization similar to that of osteosarcoma. The tumor affects primarily an older age group but does occur during all decades of life. Patients present with pain and swelling as with any other malignant bone tumor. Radiographically, there is bone destruction that is typically in a permeative pattern. The histologic features are the same as those of soft tissue fibrosarcoma, with spindle cells, variable collagen production, and a herringbone pattern. Treatment consists in wide surgical resection. Although the prognosis is poor, the role of chemotherapy has not been fully defined; effective regimens for the older patient have not been adequately explored.

E. Histiocytic Lesions—Histiocytic lesions of bone are uncommon. Benign and malignant forms may be encountered.

1. Benign and Atypical Histiocytoma of Bone—These lesions are rare. Patients present with pain, and the radiographs show bone destruction. Histologically, the lesions have nuclei that are indented or grooved, giving a histiocytic appearance. Little is known of the true behavior of these lesions because they are so uncommon. Wide surgical resection is the treatment of choice.
2. Malignant Fibrous Histiocytoma (Fig. 8–31)—These malignant bone tumors have proliferating cells with a histiocytic quality. The nuclei are often indented; the cytoplasm is usually abundant and may be slightly foamy; the nucleoli are often large; and multinucleated giant cells are usually a prominent feature (Dahlin). There may be variable amounts of fibrous tissue found within the lesion, and the fibrogenic areas have a storiform, or cart-

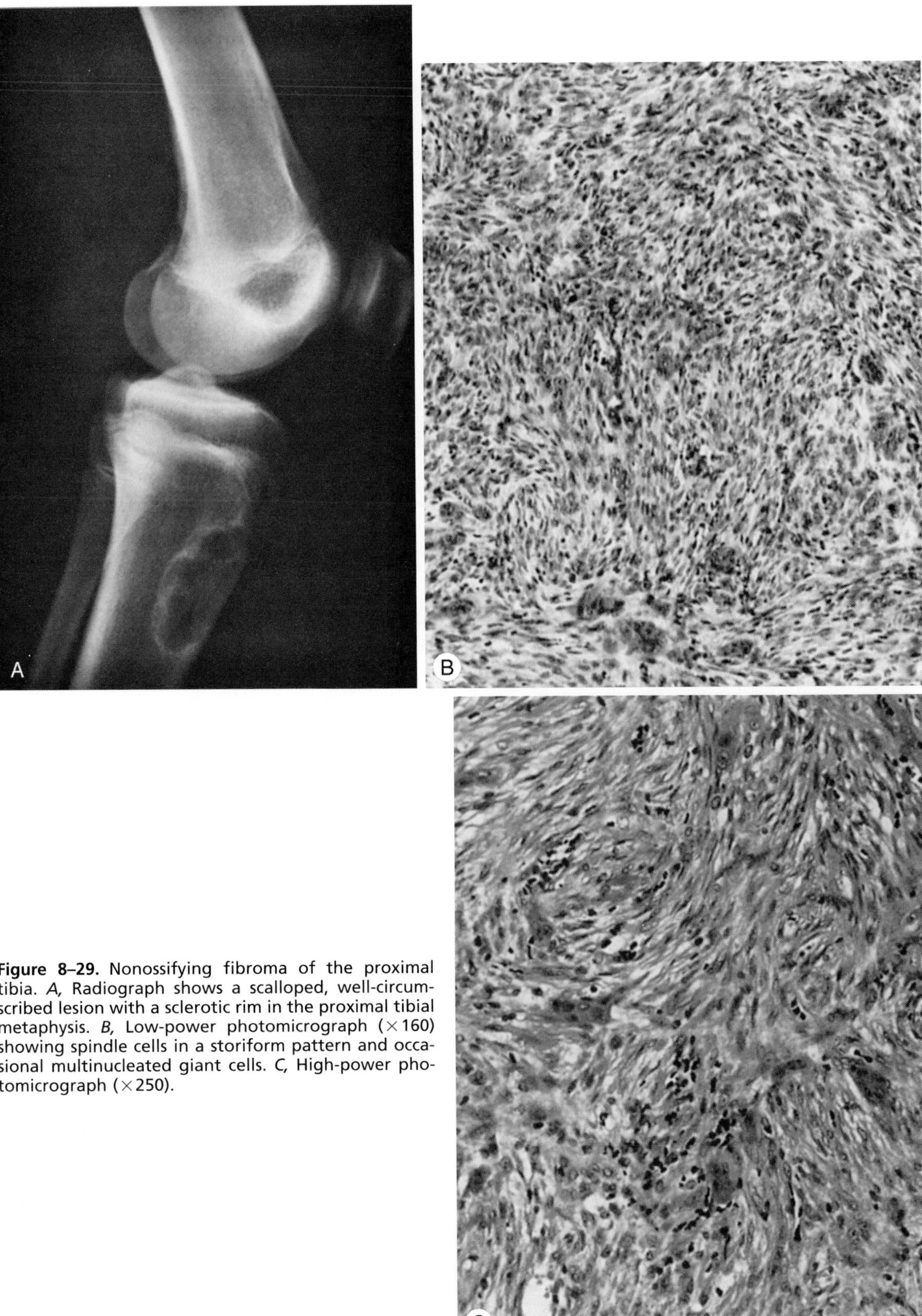

Figure 8–29. Nonossifying fibroma of the proximal tibia. *A,* Radiograph shows a scalloped, well-circumscribed lesion with a sclerotic rim in the proximal tibial metaphysis. *B,* Low-power photomicrograph (×160) showing spindle cells in a storiform pattern and occasional multinucleated giant cells. *C,* High-power photomicrograph (×250).

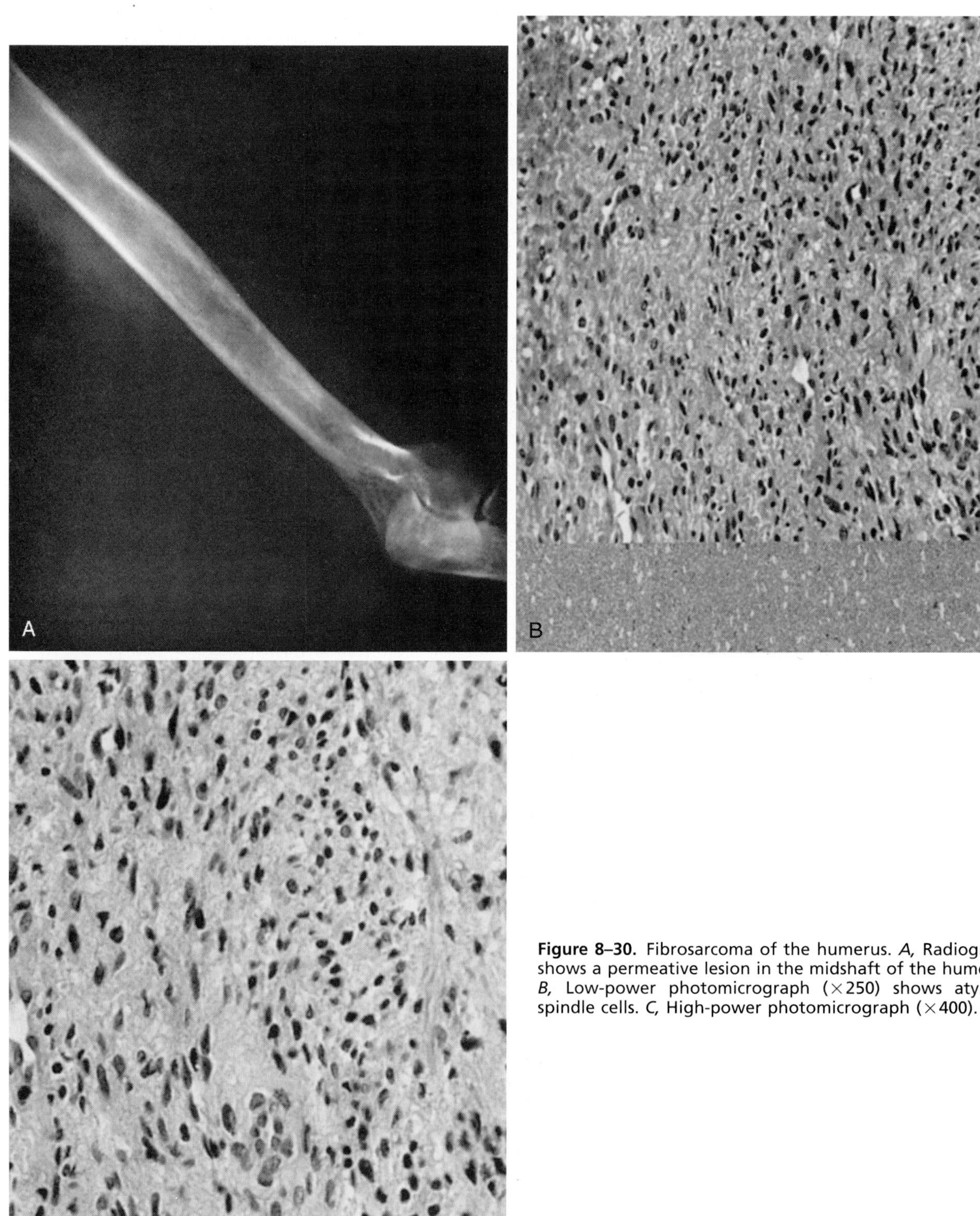

Figure 8–30. Fibrosarcoma of the humerus. *A,* Radiograph shows a permeative lesion in the midshaft of the humerus. *B,* Low-power photomicrograph (×250) shows atypical spindle cells. *C,* High-power photomicrograph (×400).

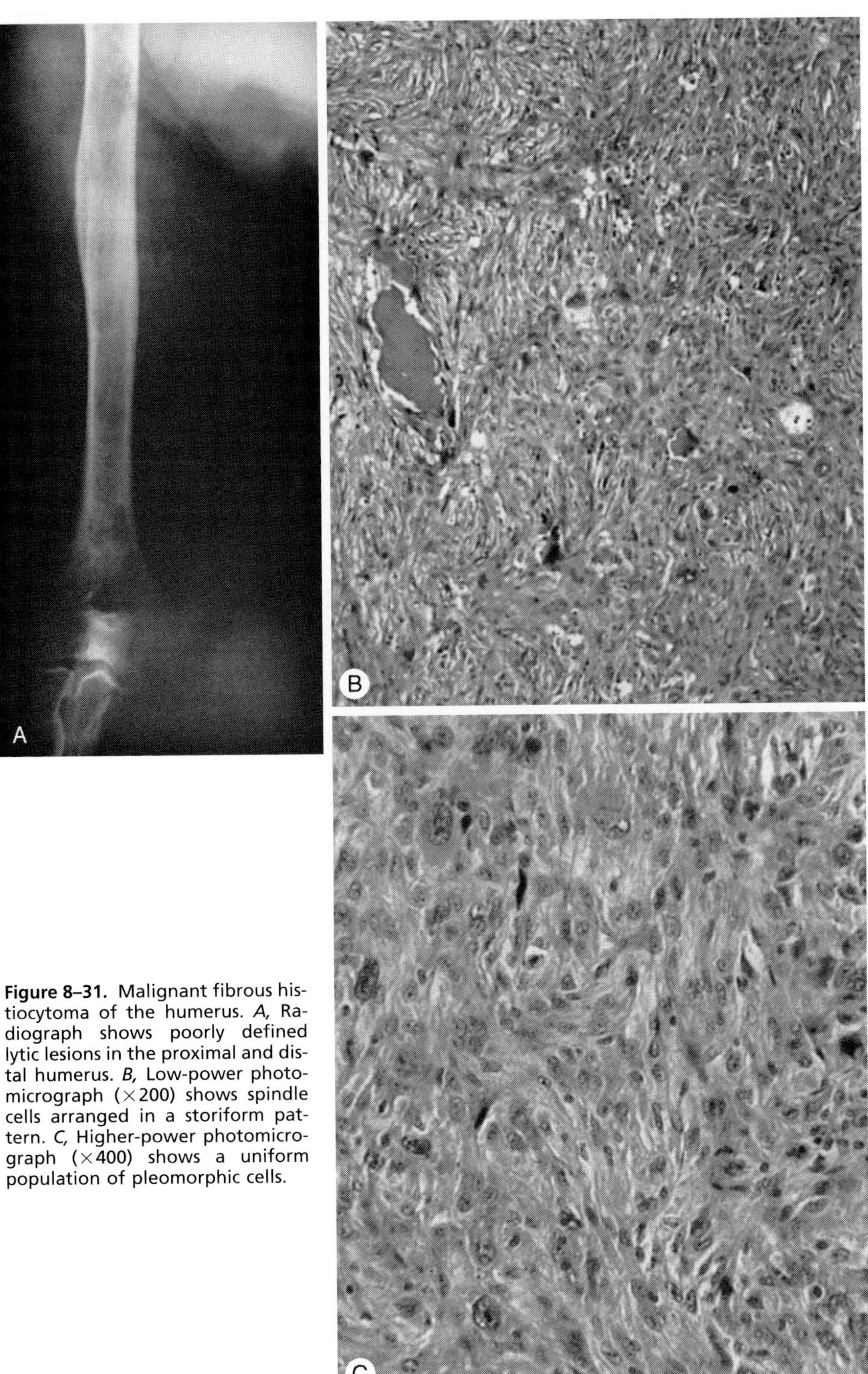

Figure 8–31. Malignant fibrous histiocytoma of the humerus. *A*, Radiograph shows poorly defined lytic lesions in the proximal and distal humerus. *B*, Low-power photomicrograph (×200) shows spindle cells arranged in a storiform pattern. *C*, Higher-power photomicrograph (×400) shows a uniform population of pleomorphic cells.

wheel, appearance. Chronic inflammatory cells are frequently found. Patients present with pain and swelling. The most common locations include the distal femur, proximal tibia, proximal femur, ilium, and proximal humerus (Fig. 8–32). Radiographs usually demonstrate a destructive lesion with either purely lytic bone destruction or a mixed pattern of bone destruction and formation. Treatment is wide surgical excision. Most patients are candidates for multiagent chemotherapy, although few studies have shown chemotherapy to be efficacious for this tumor.

F. Notochordal Tissue (Fig. 8–33)—Chordoma is a malignant neoplasm in which the cell of origin derives from primitive notochordal tissue. This lesion occurs predominantly at the ends of the vertebral column (spheno-occipital region and sacrum) (Fig. 8–34). About 10% of chordomas occur in the vertebral bodies (cervical, thoracic, and lumbar regions). Patients present with an insidious onset of pain. Lesions in the sacrum may present as pelvic pain, low back pain, hip pain, or with primarily gastrointestinal symptomatology (obstipation, constipation, loss of rectal tone). In the vertebral bodies there may be a wide variation in neurologic symptoms due to nerve compression. Patients with a long-standing history of undiagnosed pelvic or low back pain should undergo a rectal examination; more than half of sacral chordomas are palpable with digital examination. Plain radiographs often do not reveal the true extent of sacrococcygeal chordomas. The sacrum is difficult to evaluate on plain radiographs because of overlying bowel gas and fecal material. In addition, the anteroposterior pelvic view reveals bone destruction only at the sacral cortical margins and neural foramina; these areas are not typically involved early. CT scans show midline bone destruction and a soft-tissue mass. The sacrum is often ex-

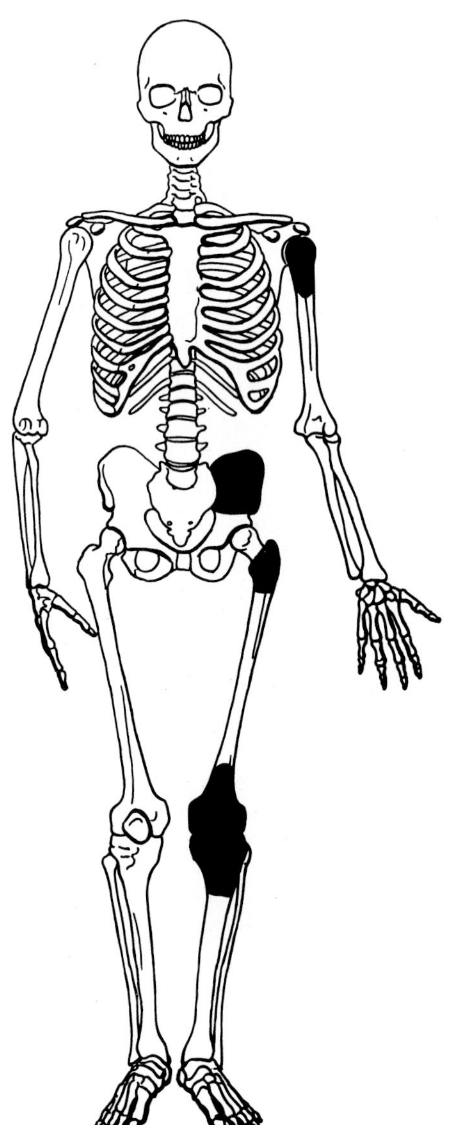

Figure 8–32. Skeletal distribution of the most common sites of malignant fibrous histiocytoma. (From McCarthy, E.F., and Frassica, F.J.: Pathology of Bone and Joint Disorders, Philadelphia, WB Saunders, 1998.)

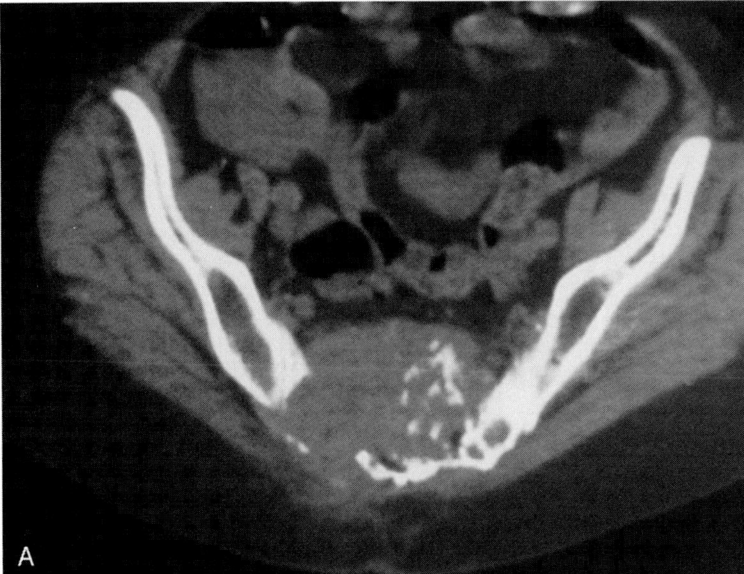

Figure 8–33. Chordoma of the sacrum. *A,* CT scan shows a destructive lesion in the sacrum. *B,* Low-power photomicrograph (×100) shows a lobular arrangement of tissue. *C,* Higher-power photomicrograph (×250) shows nests of physaliferous cells.

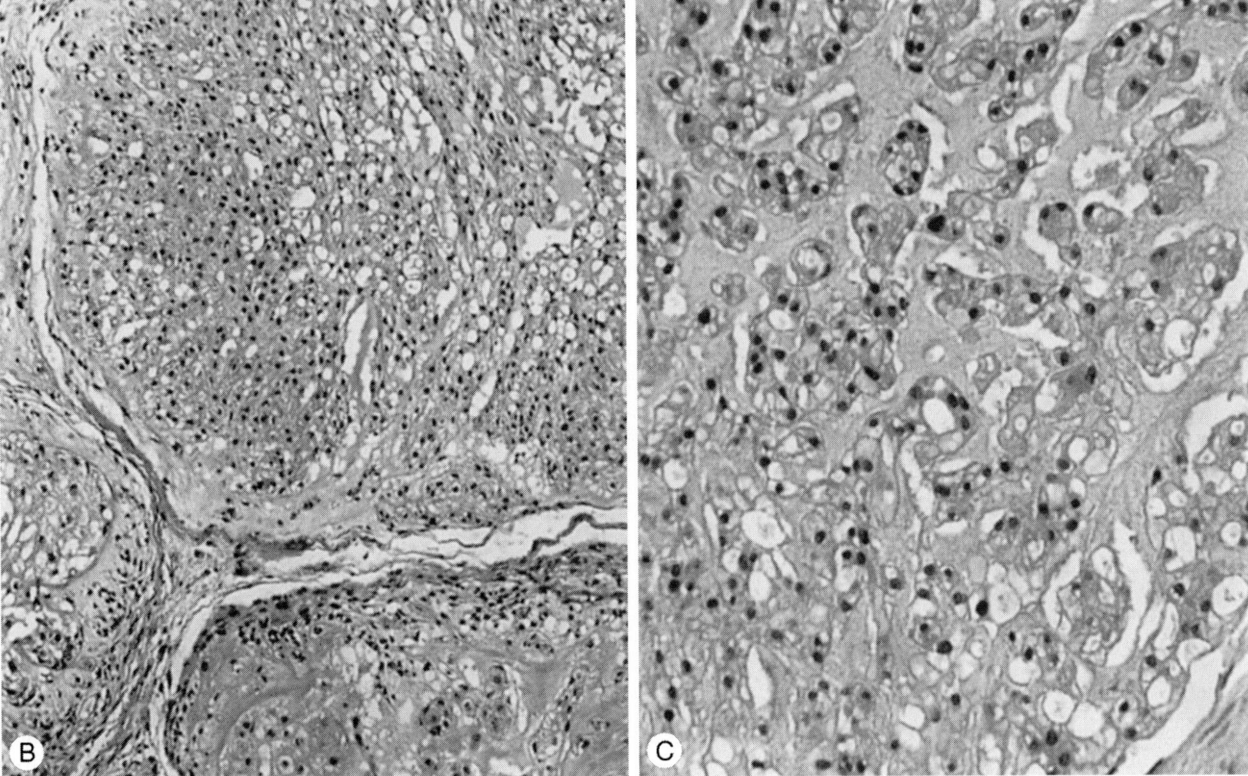

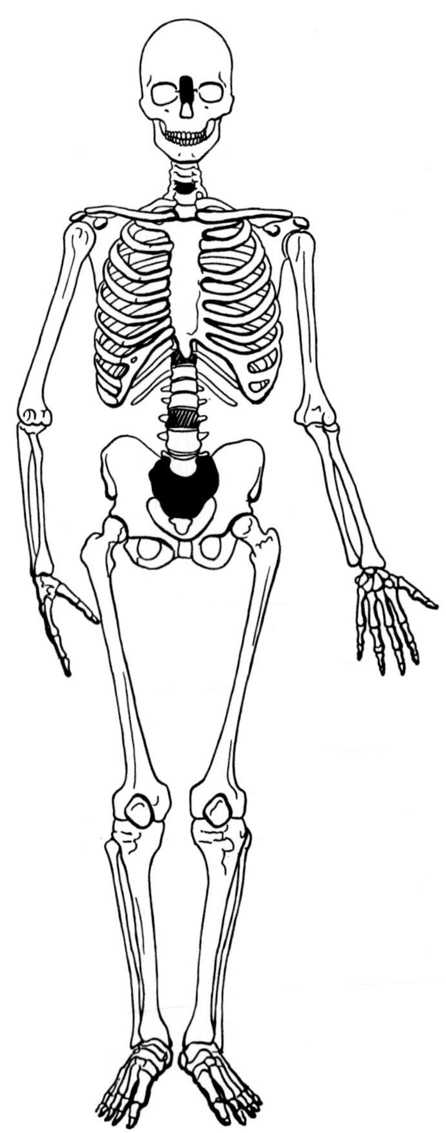

Figure 8–34. Skeletal distribution of the most common sites of chordoma. Chordomas occur exclusively in the spine, with 50% being sacrococcygeal, 40% in the spheno-occipital region, and 10% in the vertebra. (From McCarthy, E.F., and Frassica, F.J.: Pathology of Bone and Joint Disorders. Philadelphia, WB Saunders, 1998.)

panded, and the soft-tissue mass may show irregular mineralization. In the vertebral bodies one often sees areas of both bone formation and bone destruction. The tumor grows in distinct lobules. The chordoma cells sometimes have a vacuolated appearance and are called physaliferous cells. The chordoma cells are often in strands in a mass of mucus. Treatment is resection with a wide surgical margin. Radiation therapy may be added if a wide margin is not achieved. Chordomas may metastasize in about 30–50% of cases, and they often take the patient's life because of local extension.

G. Vascular Tumors—Vascular tumors of bone represent a heterogeneous group of disorders. Benign conditions include hemangioma, lymphangioma, and perhaps vanishing bone disease (Gorham's disease or massive osteolysis). Malignant entities include hemangioendothelioma (hemangiosarcoma) and hemangiopericytoma.

1. Hemangiomas (Fig. 8–35)—These tumors most commonly occur in vertebral bodies. Patients may present with pain or pathologic fracture. Vertebral hemangiomas have a characteristic appearance, with lytic destruction and vertical striations or a coarsened honeycomb appearance (Dahlin). Occasionally, patients have more than one bone involved. Histologically, there are numerous blood channels. Most lesions are cavernous in nature, although some may be a mixture of capillary and cavernous blood spaces.
2. Hemangioendothelioma (Hemangiosarcoma)— Malignant vascular tumors of bone are rare. Patients may be in any age group and present with pain. Approximately one-third of patients have multifocal lesions. Radiographs show a predominantly lytic lesion with no reactive bone formation. The low-grade lesions often have residual trabecular bone. Histologically, the tumor cells form vascular spaces. The lesions range

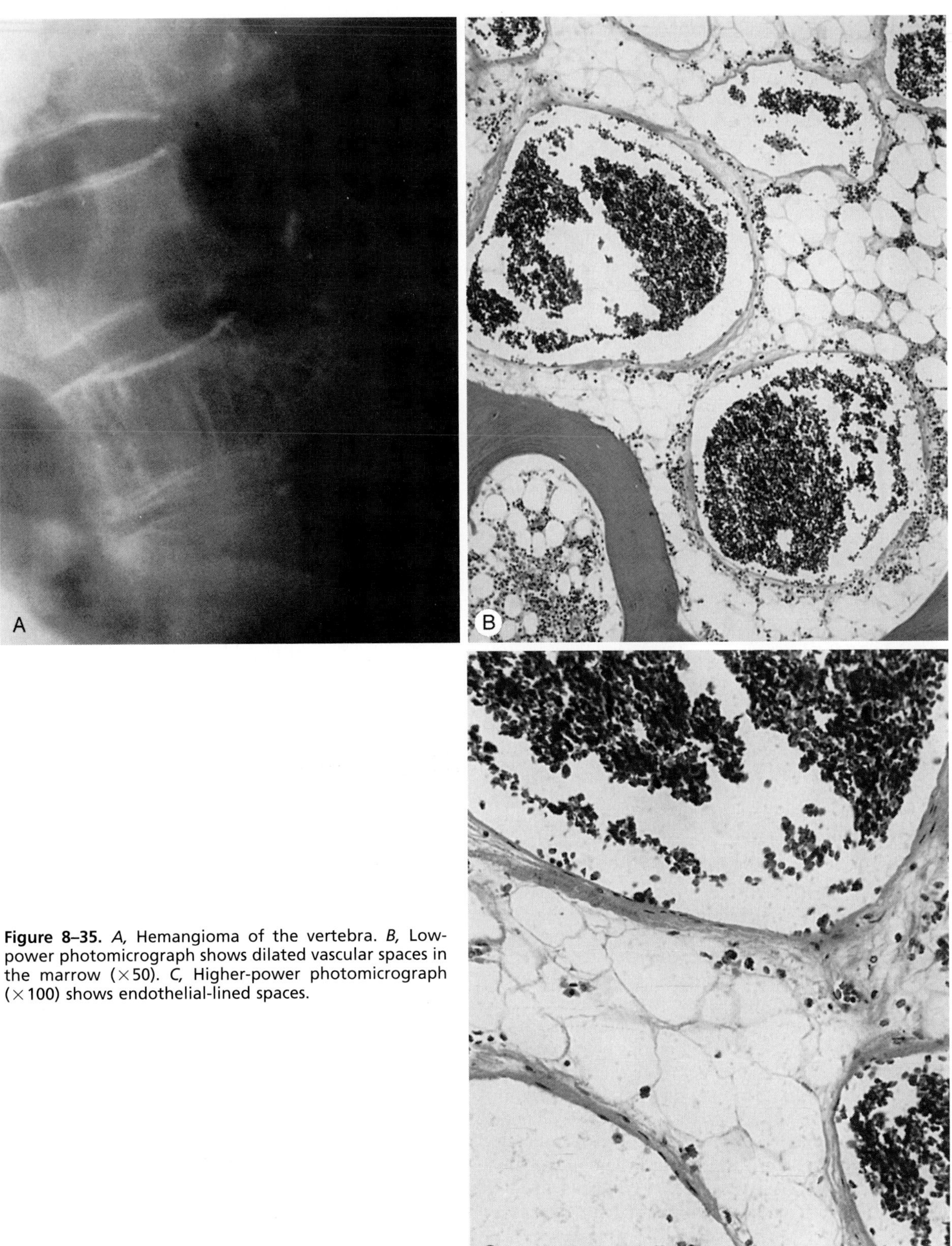

Figure 8–35. *A,* Hemangioma of the vertebra. *B,* Low-power photomicrograph shows dilated vascular spaces in the marrow (×50). *C,* Higher-power photomicrograph (×100) shows endothelial-lined spaces.

from very well-differentiated (easily recognizable vascular spaces) to very undifferentiated tumors (difficult to recognize the vasoformative quality of the tumor). Surgical resection with or without radiotherapy is the treatment. Low-grade multifocal lesions may be treated with radiation alone.

H. Hematopoietic Tumors—Lymphoma and myeloma are the two malignant hematopoietic tumors.

1. Lymphoma (Fig. 8–36)—Lymphoma of bone is common and occurs in three scenarios: (1) as a solitary focus (primary lymphoma of bone), (2) in association with other osseous sites and nonosseous sites (nodal disease and soft-tissue masses), and (3) as metastatic foci (Dahlin). Malignant lymphoma affects individuals at all decades of life. Patients generally present with pain. Large soft-tissue masses may be present. The most common locations include the distal femur, proximal tibia, pelvis, proximal femur, vertebra, and shoulder girdle (Fig. 8–37). The radiographs often show a lesion that involves a large portion of the bone (long lesion). Bone destruction is common and often has a mottled appearance. Reactive bone formation and cortical bone destruction are common. The cortex may be thickened. When lymphoma involves bone, there is a diffuse pattern rather than a nodular pattern (Dahlin). A mixed cell infiltrate is usually present. Treatment centers around multiagent chemotherapy and irradiation. Surgery may be used in selected cases to achieve local control.

2. Myeloma—Plasma cell dyscrasias represent a wide range of conditions, from benign monoclonal gammopathy (Kyle's disease) to multiple myeloma. There are three plasma cell dyscrasias with which the orthopaedist must be familiar: multiple myeloma, solitary myeloma, and osteosclerotic myeloma.

   a. Multiple Myeloma (Fig. 8–38)—This plasma cell disorder commonly occurs in patients between 50 and 80 years of age. Patients usually present with bone pain, most commonly in the spine and ribs, or a pathologic fracture. Fatigue is a common complaint secondary to the associated anemia. Symptoms may be related to complications such as renal insufficiency, hypercalcemia, and the deposition of amyloid. Serum creatinine levels are elevated in about 50% of patients. Hypercalcemia is present in about one-third of patients. The classic radiographic appearance is punched-out lytic lesions. The involved bone may show expansion and a "ballooned" appearance. Osteopenia may be the only finding. Histologically, the classic appearance is sheets of plasma cells. Well-differentiated plasma cells have an eccentric nucleus and a peripherally clumped chromatic "clock face" (Fig. 8–39). There is a perinuclear clear zone (halo) that represents the Golgi apparatus. In contrast, undifferentiated tumors lack some or all of these features, and the cells are anaplastic. The treatment of myeloma is multiagent chemotherapy; surgical stabilization with irradiation is used for impending and complete fractures. Prognosis is related to the stage of disease, with an overall median survival of 18–24 months.

   b. Solitary Myeloma—It is important to differentiate solitary myeloma from multiple myeloma because of the more favorable prognosis in patients with the former. Diagnostic criteria include (1) solitary lesion on skeletal survey, (2) histologic confirmation of plasmacytoma, and (3) bone marrow plasmacytosis of 10% or less. Patients with serum protein abnormalities and Bence-Jones proteinuria of less than 1 g/24 h at presentation are not excluded if they meet the above criteria. The radiographic and histologic features are the same as for multiple myeloma. Treatment is external beam irradiation to the lesion (4500 cGy); when necessary, prophylactic internal fixation is performed.

   c. Osteosclerotic Myeloma—This form is a rare variant in which bone lesions are associated with a chronic inflammatory demyelinating polyneuropathy. Generally, the diagnosis of osteosclerotic myeloma is not made until the polyneuropathy is recognized and evaluated. Sensory symptoms (tingling, pins and needles, coldness) are noted first, followed by motor weakness. Both the sensory and motor changes begin distally, are symmetric, and proceed proximally. Severe weakness is common, but bone pain is not characteristic. Radiographic studies may show a spectrum from purely sclerotic to a mixed pattern of lysis and sclerosis. The lesions usually involve the spine, pelvic bones, and ribs; the extremities are generally spared. Patients may have abnormalities outside the nervous system and have a constellation of findings termed the POEMS syndrome (polyneuropathy, organomegaly, endocrinopathy, M protein, and skin changes). Treatment is difficult, with radiotherapy being the primary modality. The neurologic changes may not improve with treatment.

I. Tumors of Unknown Origin—The three principal tumors of unknown origin are giant cell tumor, Ewing's tumor, and adamantinoma.

1. Giant Cell Tumor (Fig. 8–40)—This distinctive neoplasm has poorly differentiated cells (Dahlin). The lesion is a benign but aggres-

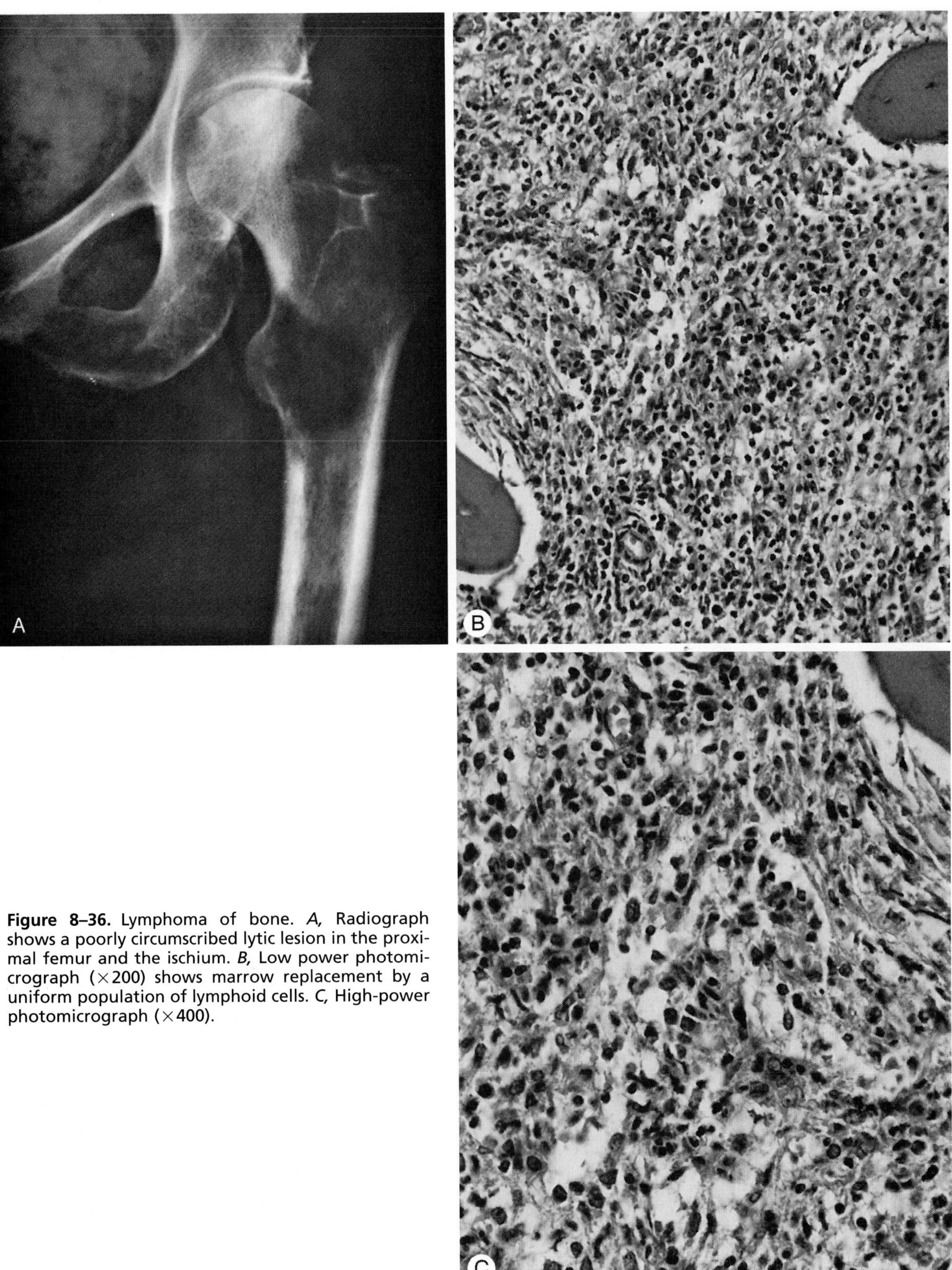

Figure 8–36. Lymphoma of bone. *A,* Radiograph shows a poorly circumscribed lytic lesion in the proximal femur and the ischium. *B,* Low power photomicrograph (×200) shows marrow replacement by a uniform population of lymphoid cells. *C,* High-power photomicrograph (×400).

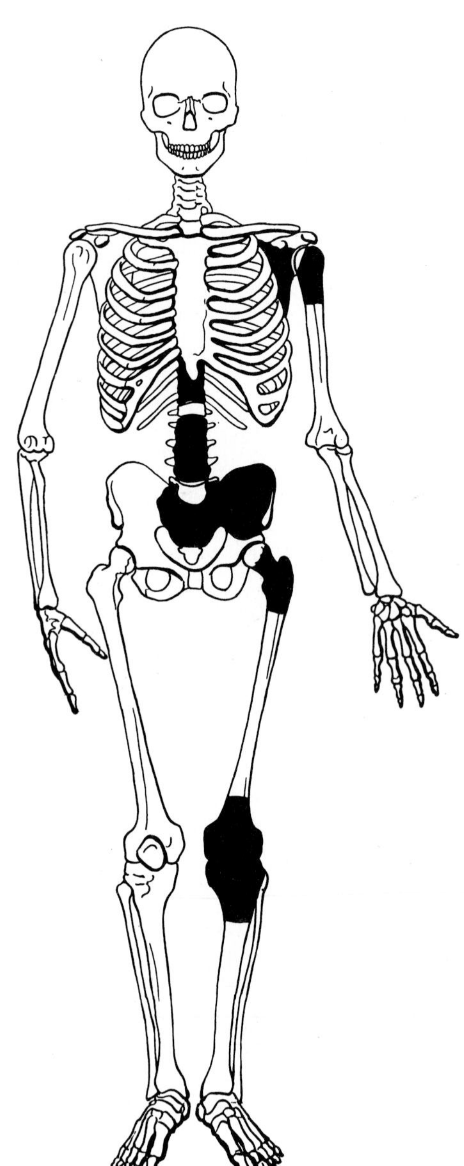

Figure 8–37. Skeletal distribution of the most common sites of lymphoma of bone. The knee, pelvis, and vertebra are common sites. (From McCarthy, E.F., and Frassica, F.J.: Pathology of Bone and Joint Disorders. Philadelphia, WB Saunders, 1998.)

sive process. Further confusion results from the fact that this benign tumor may rarely (<2% of the time) metastasize to the lungs (benign metastasizing giant cell tumor). Unlike most bone tumors, which occur more commonly in males, giant cell tumor is more common in females. The lesion is uncommon in children with open physes. The lesion is most common in the epiphysis of long bones, and about 50% of lesions occur about the knee; the vertebra and sacrum are involved in about 10% of cases (Fig. 8–41). Multicentricity occurs in fewer than 1% of patients; and when multiple lesions occur, hyperparathyroidism should be excluded. Patients present with pain that is usually referable to the joint involved. Radiographs show a purely lytic destructive lesion in the metaphysis; during the early symptomatic phase the radiographs may appear normal; a small lytic focus is difficult to detect. The basic proliferating cell has a round-to-oval or even spindle-shaped nucleus (Dahlin). The giant cells appear to have the same nuclei as the proliferating mononuclear cells. Mitotic figures may be numerous. Giant cell tumors may undergo a number of secondary degenerative changes such as aneurysmal bone cyst formation, necrosis, fibrous repair, foam cell formation, and reactive new bone (Fig. 8–42). Treatment is aimed at removing the lesion with preservation of the involved joint. Extensive exteriorization (removal of a large cortical window over the lesion), curettage with hand and power instruments, and chemical cauterization with phenol are performed. The large resulting defect is usually reconstructed with subchondral bone grafts and methylmethacrylate. Local control using this treatment regimen ranges between 80% and 90%.

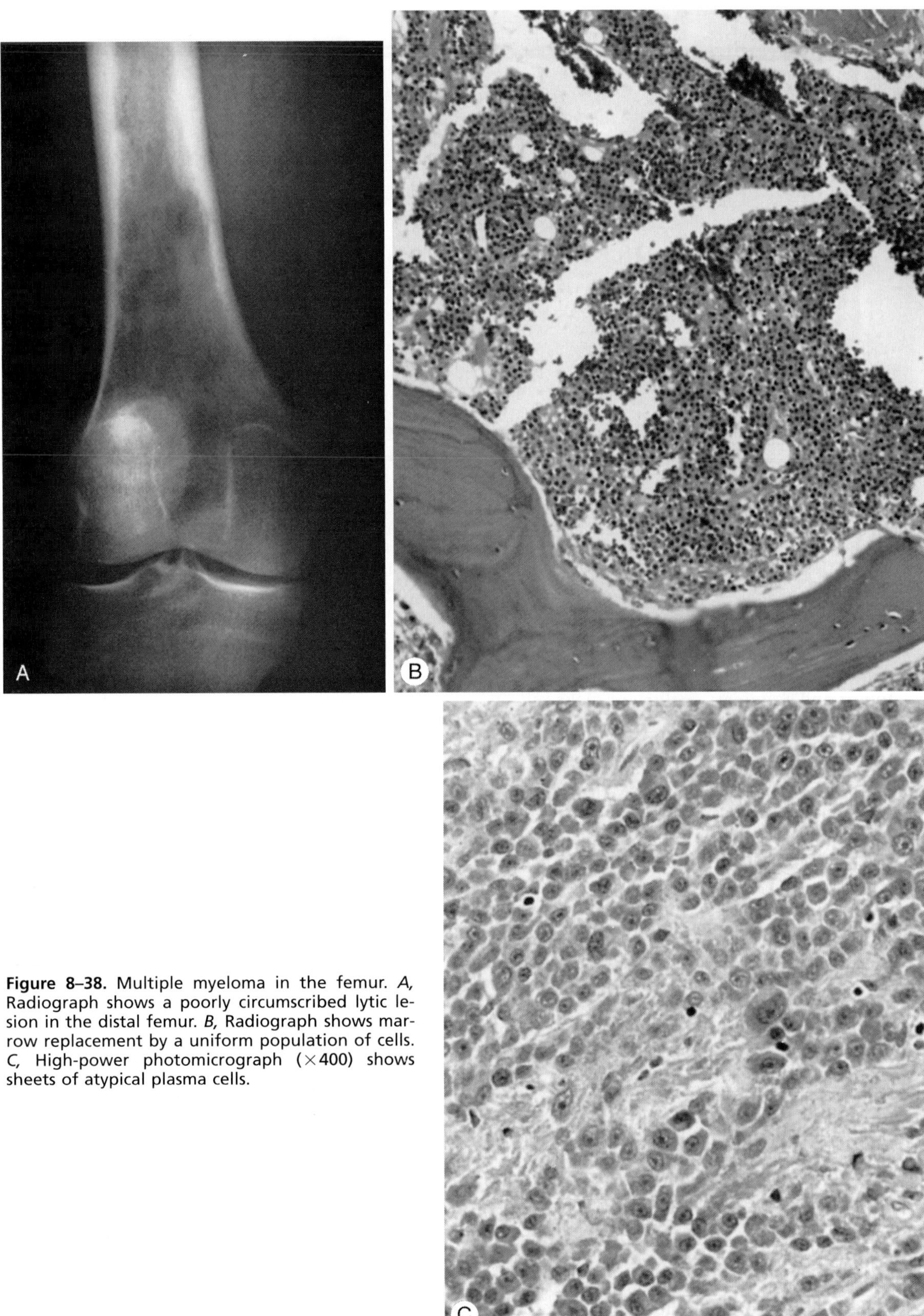

Figure 8–38. Multiple myeloma in the femur. *A,* Radiograph shows a poorly circumscribed lytic lesion in the distal femur. *B,* Radiograph shows marrow replacement by a uniform population of cells. *C,* High-power photomicrograph (×400) shows sheets of atypical plasma cells.

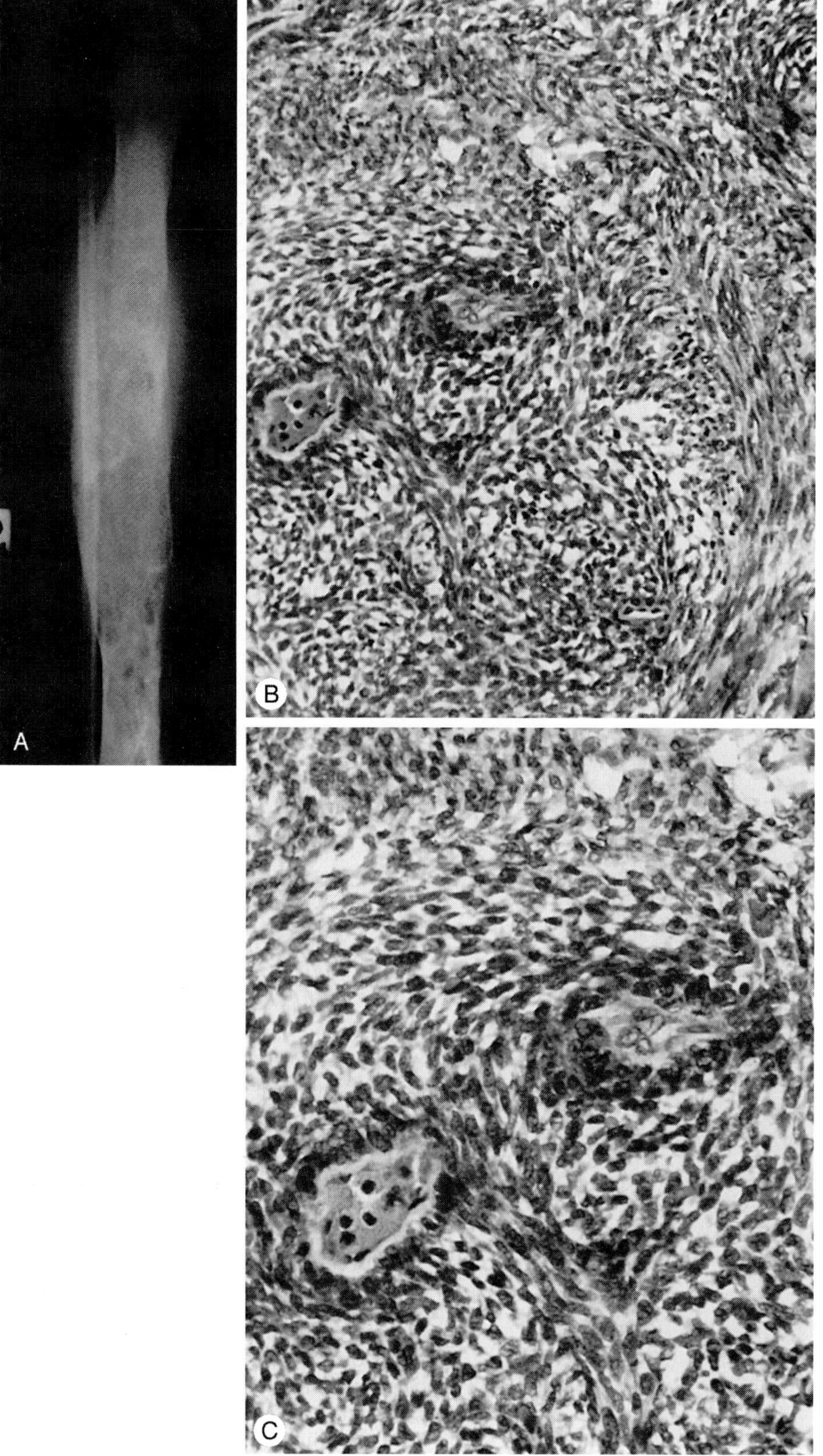

Figure 8–45. Adamantinoma of the tibia. *A,* Radiograph shows a bubbly symmetric lytic lesion in the tibial diaphysis. *B,* Low-power photomicrograph (×250) shows biphasic differentiation with spindle cells and epithelioid cells. *C,* Higher-power photomicrograph (×400).

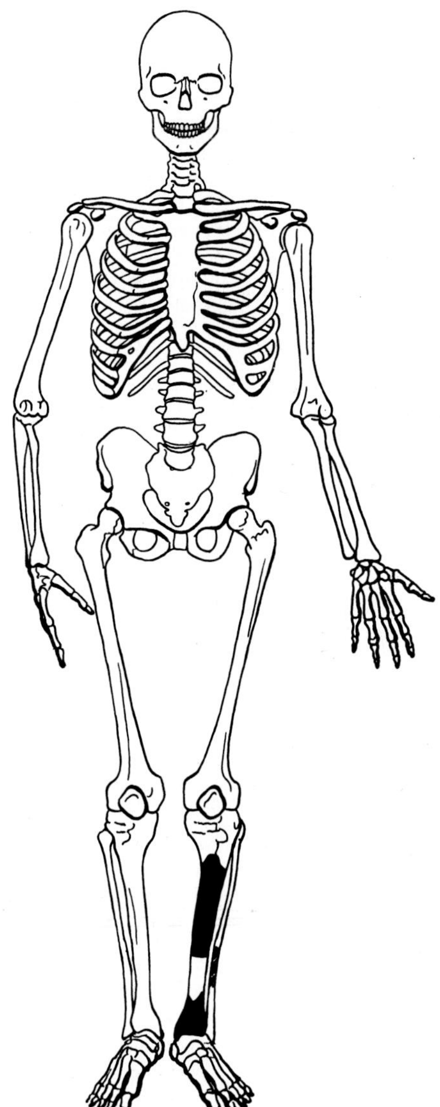

Figure 8–46. Skeletal distribution of the most common sites of adamantinoma. This peculiar tumor most commonly affects the tibia. (From McCarthy, E.F., and Frassica, F.J.: Pathology of Bone and Joint Disorders, Philadelphia, WB Saunders, 1998.)

Treatment of fibrous dysplasia is symptomatic. Internal fixation and bone grafting are used in areas of high stress where nonoperative treatment would not be effective; most patients do not need surgical treatment.

5. Osteofibrous Dysplasia—This rare variant of fibrous dysplasia primarily involves the tibia and is usually confined to the cortices. Bowing is very common, and children may develop pathologic fractures. The lesion typically presents in children younger than age 10. This diagnosis can be made radiographically. In general a biopsy is not necessary. When performed, the biopsy shows fibrous tissue stroma and a background of bone trabeculae with osteoblastic rimming. Nonoperative treatment is preferred until the child reaches maturity.
6. Paget's Disease—This condition is characterized by abnormal bone remodeling. The disease is most commonly diagnosed during the fifth decade of life. The process may be monostotic or polyostotic. Patients usually present with pain. Radiographs demonstrate coarsened trabeculae and remodeled cortices; the coarsened trabeculae give the bone a blastic appearance. Histologically, the characteristic features are irregular broad trabeculae, reversal or cement lines, osteoclastic activity, and fibrous vascular tissue between the trabeculae (Dahlin). Medical treatment of Paget's disease is aimed at retarding the activity of the osteoclasts; agents used include diphosphonates, calcitonin, and methotrexate. The older diphosphonates (e.g., Didronel) stopped both osteoclastic activity and new bone formation; Didronel may cause osteomalacia and cannot be used for more than 6 months. Pamidronate, which can be used only intravenously, does not inhibit bone formation and has become one of the most useful agents in the diphosphonate class of

Table 8–8.

Tumor-like Conditions (Tumor Simulators)

Young Patient
Eosinophilic granuloma
Osteomyelitis
Avulsion fractures
Aneurysmal bone cyst
Fibrous dysplasia
Osteofibrous dysplasia
Heterotopic ossification
Unicameral bone cyst
Giant cell reparative granuloma
Exuberant callus
Adult
Synovial chondromatosis
Pigmented villonodular synovitis
Stress fracture
Heterotopic ossification
Ganglion cyst
Older Adult
Metastatic bone disease
Mastocytosis
Hyperparathyroidism
Paget's disease
Bone infarcts
Bone islands
Ganglion cyst
Cyst secondary to joint disease
Epidermoid cyst

medications. Patients may present with degenerative joint disease, fracture, or neurologic encroachment; joint degeneration is common in the hip and knee. Prior to replacement, arthroplasty patients should be treated in order to decrease bleeding at the time of surgery. Fewer than 1% of patients with Paget's disease develop malignant degeneration with the formation of a sarcoma within a focus of Paget's disease; the symptoms of a Paget's sarcoma are the abrupt onset of pain and swelling. The radiographs usually demonstrate cortical bone destruction and the presence of a soft-tissue mass. Paget's sarcomas are deadly tumors with a poor prognosis (long-term survival is <20%).

7. Metastatic Bone Disease (Fig. 8–51)—This tumor is the most common entity that destroys the skeleton in the older patient. When a destructive bone lesion is found in a patient over age 40, metastases must be considered first; the five carcinomas that are most likely to metastasize to bone are breast, lung, prostate, kidney, and thyroid. The most common locations are the pelvis, vertebral bodies, ribs, and proximal limb girdles. The pathogenesis of skeletal metastases is probably related to Batson's vertebral vein plexus. The venous flow from the breast, lung, prostate, kidney, and thyroid drains into the vertebral vein plexus (Fig. 8–52). The plexus has intimate connections to the vertebral bodies, pelvis, skull, and proximal limb girdles. The radiographs most commonly demonstrate a destructive lesion that may be purely lytic, a mixed pattern of bone destruction and formation, or a purely sclerotic lesion. The histologic hallmark is epithelial cells in a fibrous stroma; the epithelial cells are often arranged in a glandular pattern. Interestingly, the bone destruction is caused not by the tumor cells themselves but rather by activation of osteoclasts (Fig. 8–53). In order to combat the osteoclastic bone destruction many patients are now treated with antiosteoclastic agents such as intravenous pamidronate. Treatment of metastatic bone disease is aimed at controlling pain and maintaining the independence of the patient. Prophylactic internal fixation is performed when impending fracture is present. There are many criteria for fixation. Conditions that put the patient most at risk are the following:
   a. More than 50% destruction of the diaphyseal cortices
   b. Permeative destruction of the subtrochanteric femoral region
   c. More than 50–75% destruction of the metaphysis
   d. Persistent pain following irradiation.

   Patients over age 40 with a single destructive bone lesion without a known primary tumor must still be considered to have metastatic disease. Simon outlined a diagnostic strategy that identifies the primary lesion in up to 80–90% of patients (Table 8–9).

8. Osteomyelitis—Bone infections often simulate primary tumors. Occult infections may occur in all age groups. Patients may present with fever, chills, and bone pain; most commonly, though, patients present with bone pain without systemic symptoms. The radiographs may be nonspecific. Bone destruction and bone formation are usually the characteristic findings of chronic infections; acute infections often produce cortical bone destruction and periosteal elevation. Serpiginous tracts and irregular areas of bone destruction suggest infection rather than neoplasm. Histologically, the lesion is usually apparent with (1) edema of the granulation tissue, (2) numerous new blood vessels, and (3) a mixed cell population of inflammatory cells, plasma cells, polymorphonuclear leukocytes, eosinophils, lymphocytes, and histiocytes. Occasionally, a chronic infection is complicated by a squamous cell carcinoma. One should always biopsy material that has been sent for culture and culture material that has been sent for biopsy. The treatment of osteomyelitis is removal of all dead tissue and appropriate antibiotic therapy.

Text continued on page 440

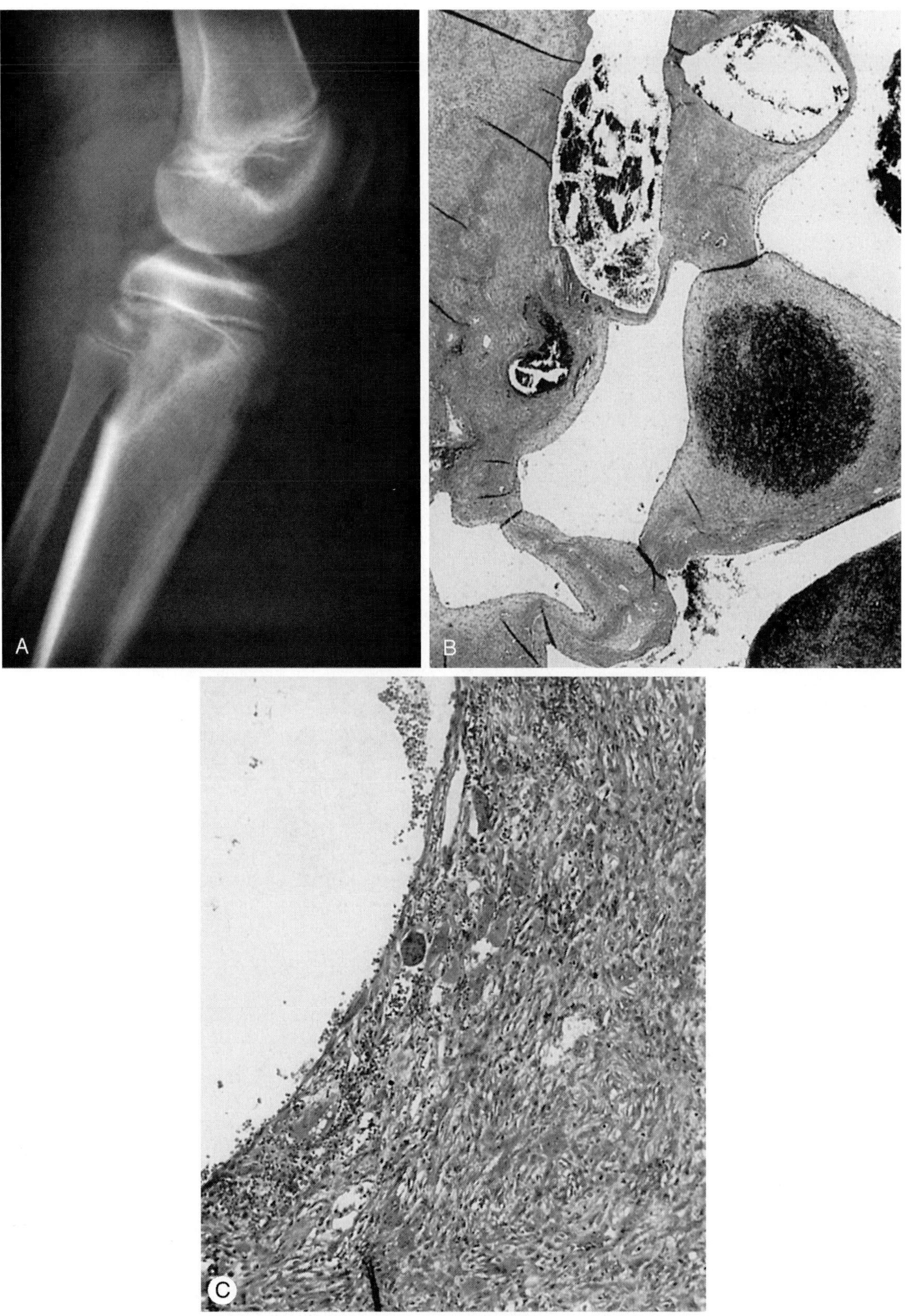

Figure 8–47. Aneurysmal bone cyst of the proximal tibia. *A,* Radiograph shows a well-defined lytic lesion in the posterior tibial metaphysis. *B,* Low-power photomicrograph (×25) shows blood-filled lakes. *C,* Higher-power photomicrograph (×50) shows the wall of the cyst with fibroblasts and occasional multinucleated giant cells.

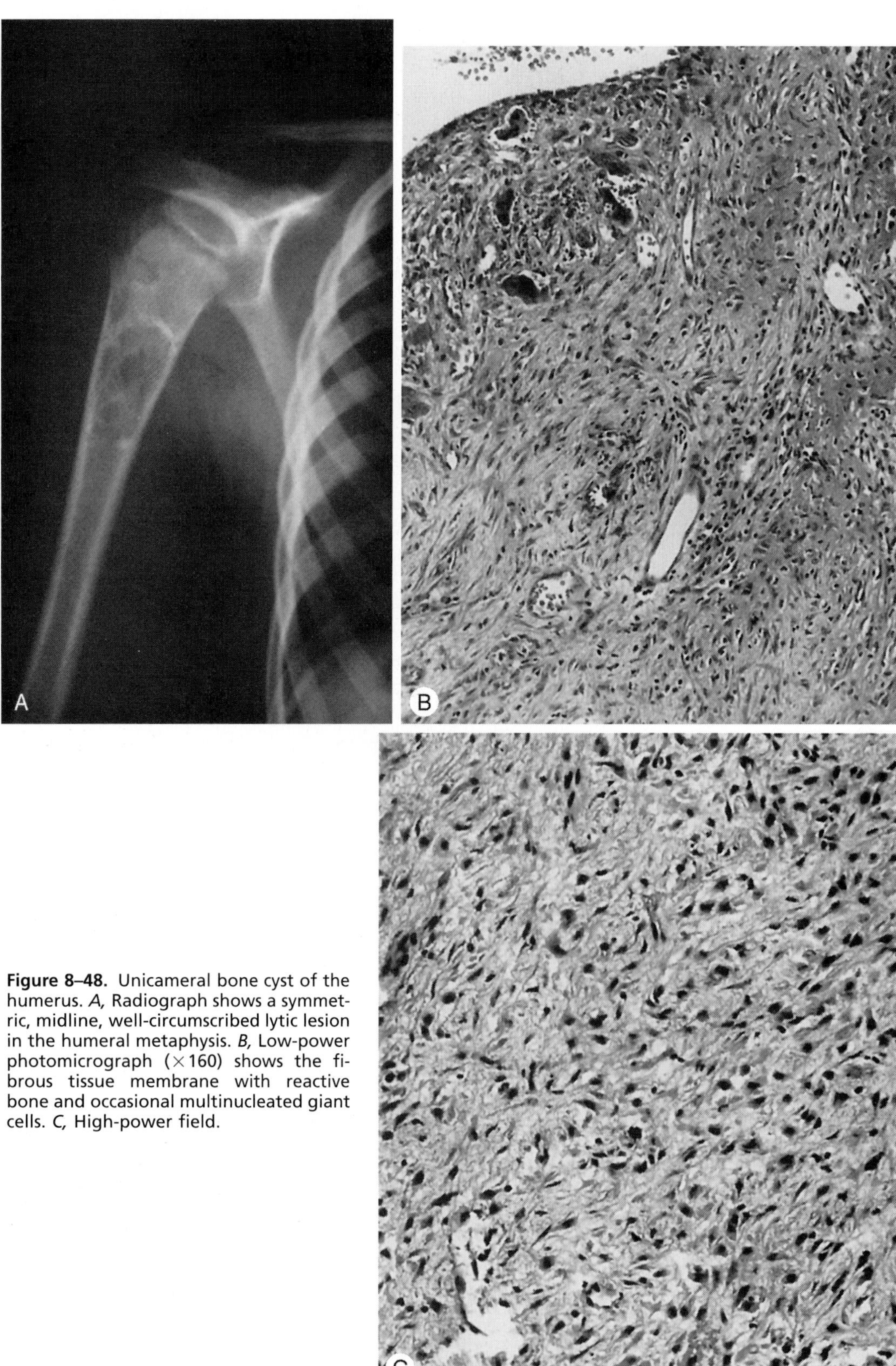

Figure 8–48. Unicameral bone cyst of the humerus. *A,* Radiograph shows a symmetric, midline, well-circumscribed lytic lesion in the humeral metaphysis. *B,* Low-power photomicrograph (×160) shows the fibrous tissue membrane with reactive bone and occasional multinucleated giant cells. *C,* High-power field.

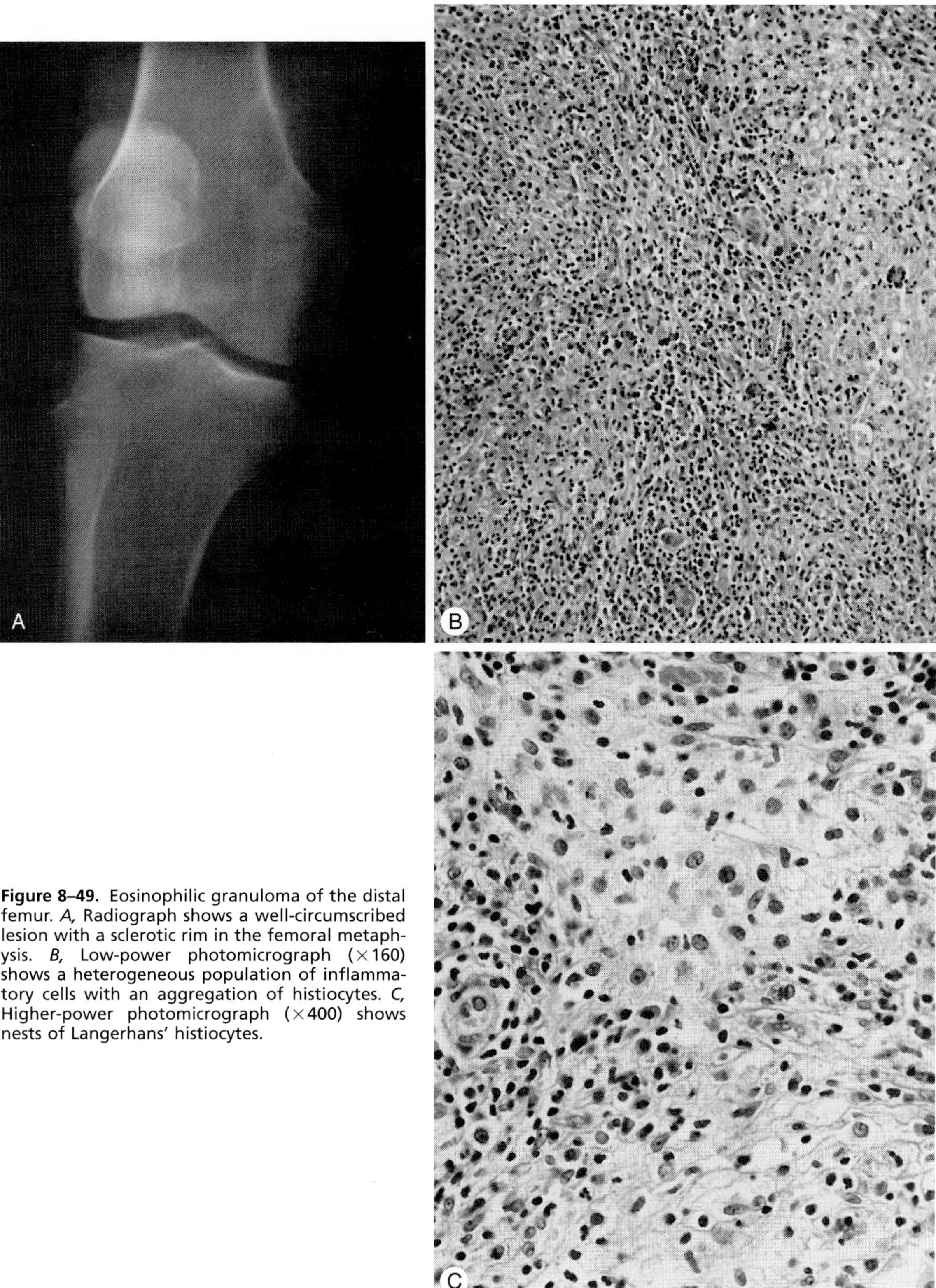

Figure 8–49. Eosinophilic granuloma of the distal femur. *A,* Radiograph shows a well-circumscribed lesion with a sclerotic rim in the femoral metaphysis. *B,* Low-power photomicrograph (×160) shows a heterogeneous population of inflammatory cells with an aggregation of histiocytes. *C,* Higher-power photomicrograph (×400) shows nests of Langerhans' histiocytes.

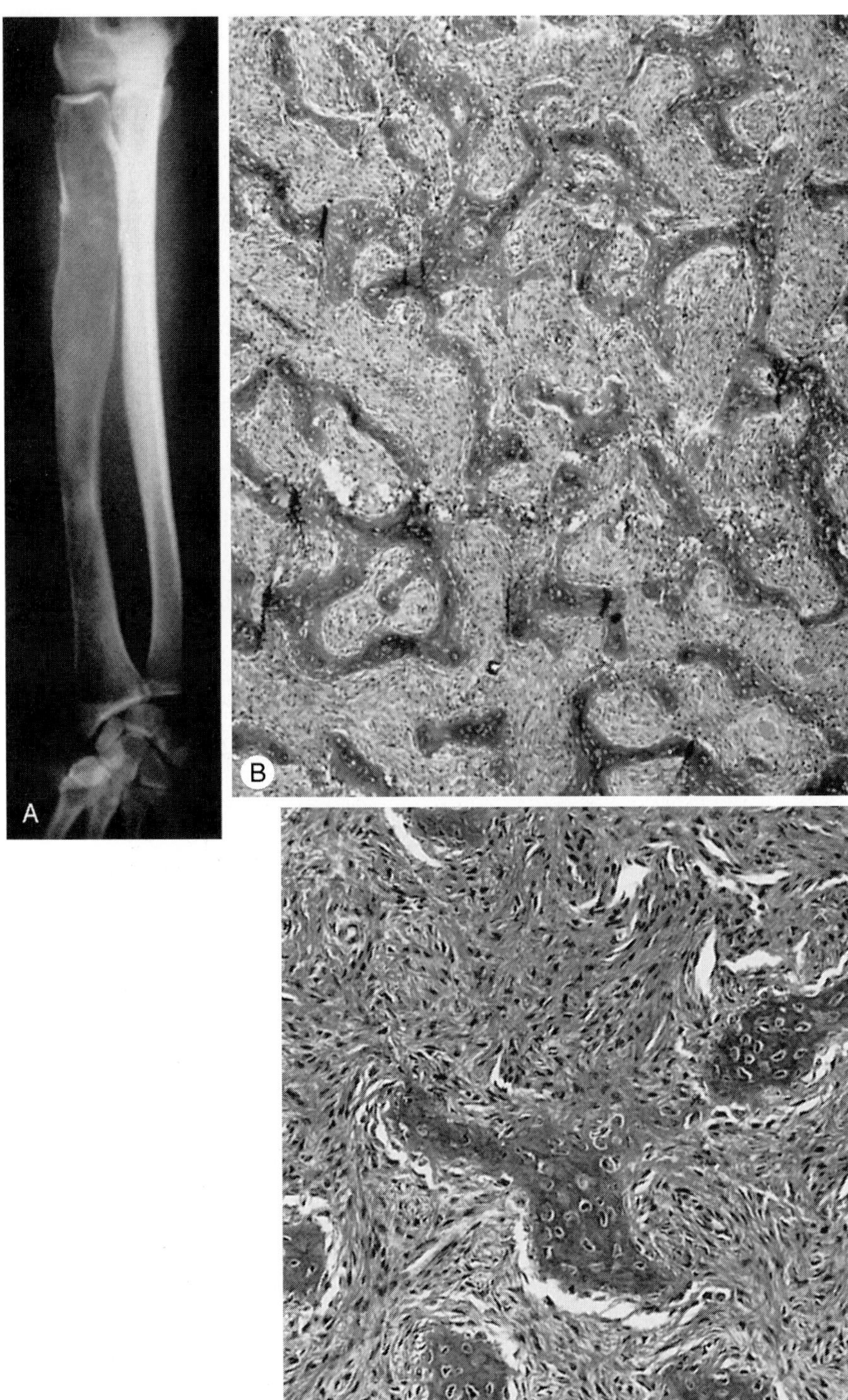

Figure 8–50. Fibrous dysplasia of the radius. *A,* Radiograph shows a long, symmetric, ground-glass lytic lesion of the radius. *B,* Low-power photomicrograph (×50) shows seams of osteoid in a fibrous background. *C,* Higher-power photomicrograph (×160) shows osteoid surrounded by bland fibrous tissue.

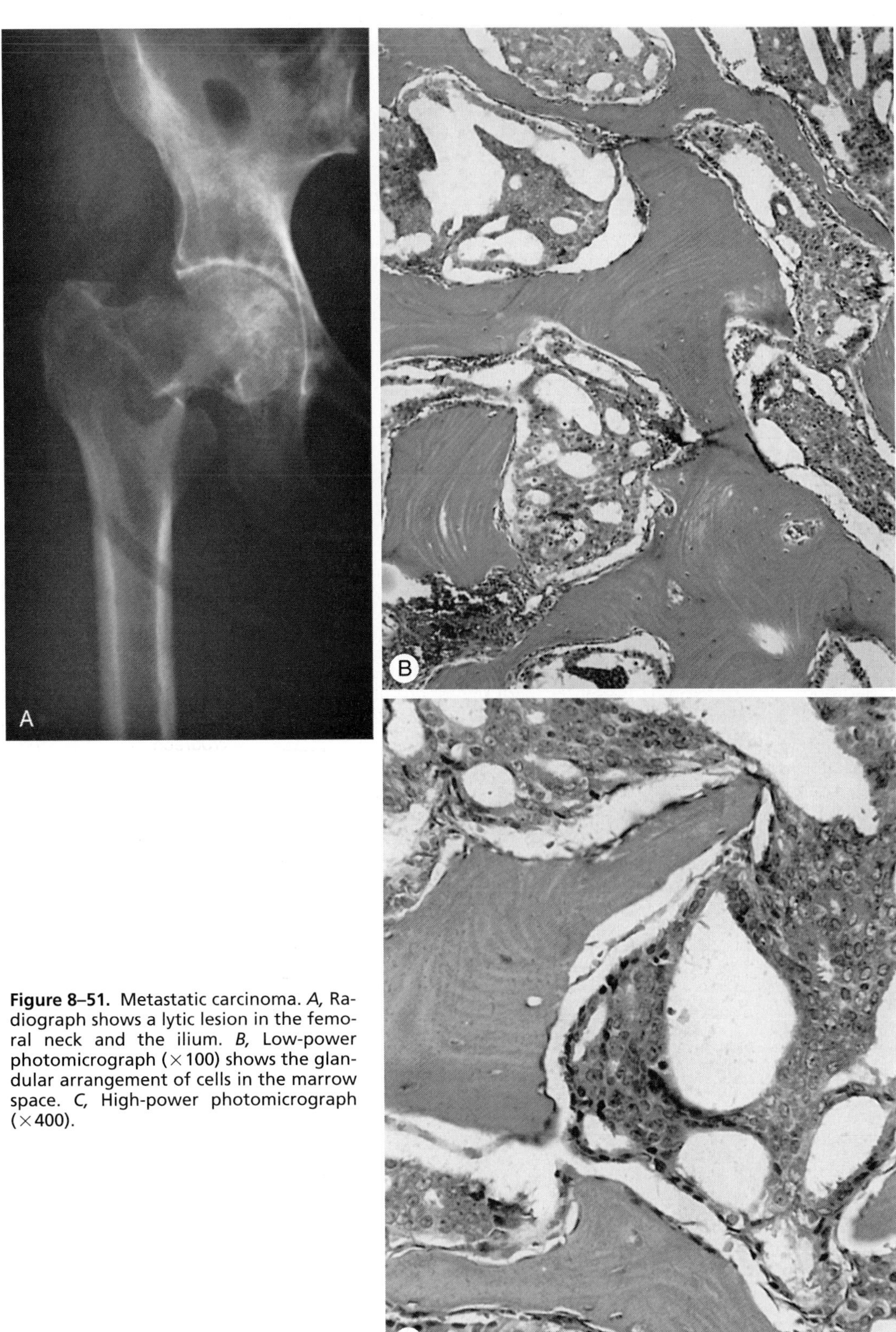

Figure 8–51. Metastatic carcinoma. *A,* Radiograph shows a lytic lesion in the femoral neck and the ilium. *B,* Low-power photomicrograph (×100) shows the glandular arrangement of cells in the marrow space. *C,* High-power photomicrograph (×400).

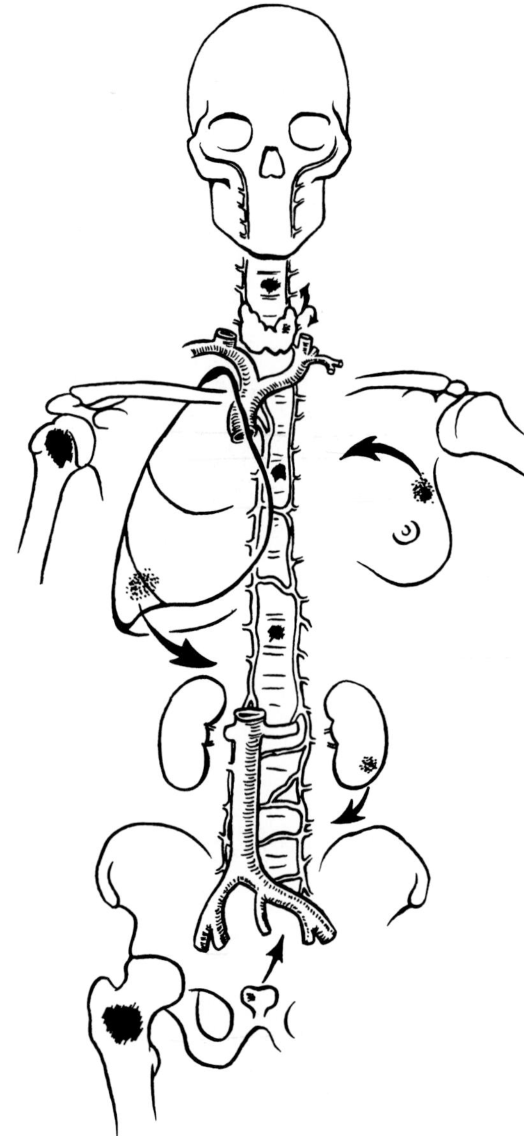

Figure 8–52. Artist's depiction of Batson's venous plexus. This plexus is longitudinal and valveless and extends from the sacrum to the skull. The breast, lung, kidney, prostate, and thyroid glands all connect to this system. Tumor cells can enter this system and spread to the vertebra, ribs, pelvis, and proximal limb girdle. (From McCarthy, E.F., and Frassica, F.J.: Pathology of Bone and Joint Disorders. Philadelphia, WB Saunders, 1998.)

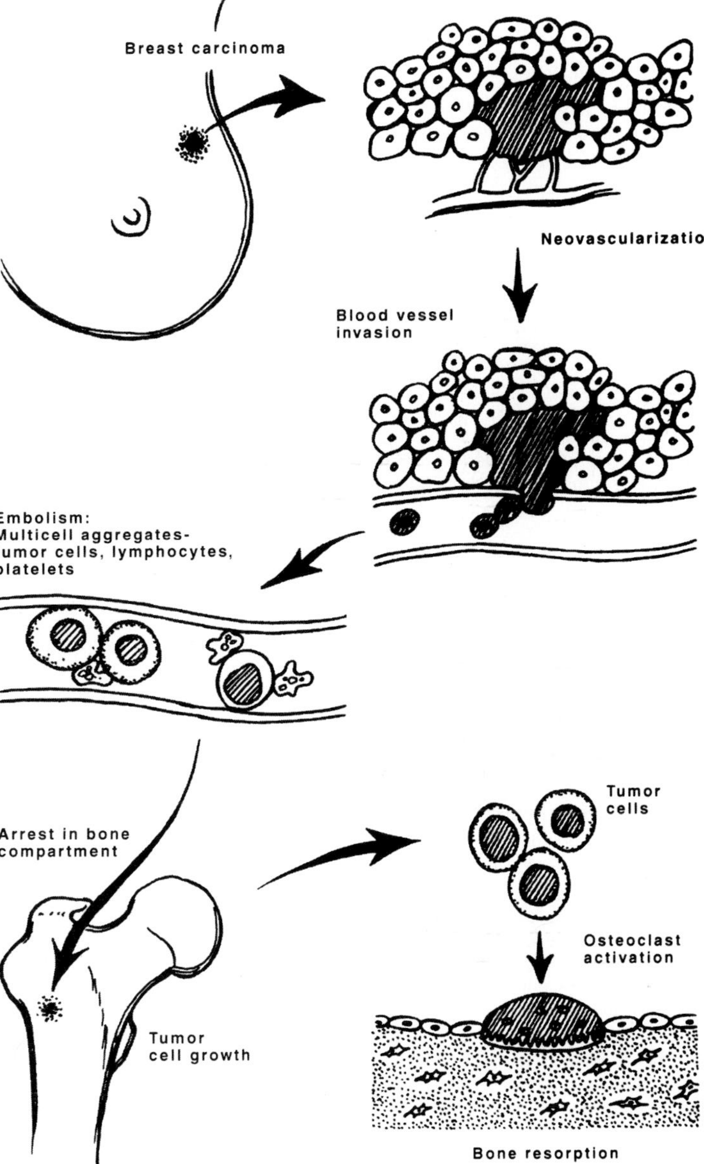

Figure 8–53. The mechanism of bone metastases is complex. Metastatic cells spread into the venous system by vascular invasion and lodge in the medullary cavity. These tumor cells activate osteoclasts, which resorb the host bone. (From McCarthy, E.F., and Frassica, F.J.: Pathology of Bone and Joint Disorders. Philadelphia, WB Saunders, 1998.)

Table 8–9.

Evaluation of the Older Patient with a Single Bone Lesion and Suspected Metastases of Unknown Origin

Plain radiographs in two planes of the affected limb
Technetium bone scan to detect multiple lesions
Radiographic studies to search for occult neoplasms
  Chest radiograph and CT of the chest (to search for occult lung cancer)
  CT of the abdomen or ultrasonography of the abdomen (to detect renal cell cancer *or lymphoma*)
  Skeletal survey (if myeloma is suspected)
Screening laboratory studies
  Complete blood count with differential
  Erythrocyte sedimentation rate
  Chemistry group: liver function test, calcium, phosphorus, alkaline phosphatase
  Serum or urine immunoelectrophoresis

Selected Bibliography

Textbooks

McCarthy, E.F., and Frassica, F.J.: Pathology of Bone and Joint Disorders. Philadelphia, WB Saunders, 1998.
Mirra, J.M.: Bone Tumors: Clinical, Radiologic, and Pathologic Correlations. Philadelphia, Lea and Febiger, 1989.
Sim, F.H.: Diagnosis and Management of Metastatic Bone Disease: A Multidisciplinary Approach. Raven Press, New York, 1988.
Simon, M.A., and Springfield, D.: Surgery for Bone and Soft Tissue Tumors. Lippincott-Raven, Philadelphia, 1998.
Unni, K.K.: Dahlin's Bone Tumors: General Aspects and Data on 11,087 Cases. Lippincott-Raven, Philadelphia, 1996.
Wold, L.E., McLeod, R.A., Sim, F.H., et al.: Atlas of Orthopaedic Pathology. Philadelphia, WB Saunders, 1990.

Reviews

American Joint Committee on Cancer. Soft tissues. In Beahrs, O.H., and Myers, M., eds.: Manual for Staging of Cancer, 3rd ed. Philadelphia, JB Lippincott, 1988.
Enneking, W.F.: Clinical Musculoskeletal Pathology, 3rd ed. Gainesville, University of Florida Press, 1990.
Frassica, F.J., Chang, B.W., Ma, L.D., et al.: Soft tissue sarcomas: General features, evaluation, imaging, biopsy, and treatment. Curr. Orthop. 11:105–113, 1997.
Frassica, F.J., Gitelis, S.G., and Sim, F.H.: Metastatic Bone Disease: General Principles, Pathogenesis, Pathophysiology and Biopsy. Instr. Course Lect. 41:293–300, 1992.
Mindell, E.R.: Chordoma. J. Bone Joint Surg. [Am.] 63:501–505, 1981.
Orthopaedic Knowledge Update Home Study Syllabus I, II, III. Chicago, American Academy of Orthopaedic Surgeons, 1984, 1987, 1990.
Sim, F.H., Frassica, F.J., and Frassica, D.A.: Soft tissue tumors: Evaluation, diagnosis, and management. J. Am. Acad. Orthop. Surg. 2(4):202–211, 1994.
Simon, M.A.: Current concepts review: Biopsy of musculoskeletal tumors. J. Bone Joint Surg. [Am.] 64:1253, 1982.

Recent Articles

Bell, R.S., O'Sullivan, B., Liu, F.F., et al.: The surgical margin in soft tissue sarcoma. J. Bone Joint Surg. [Am.] 71:370, 1989.
Berrey, B.H., Jr., Lord, C.F., Gebhardt, M.C., et al.: Fractures of allografts: Frequency, treatment, and end results. J. Bone Joint Surg. [Am.] 72:825, 1990.
Choong, P.F.M., Pritchard, D.J., Rock, M.G., et al.: Survival after pulmonary metastectomy in soft tissue sarcoma: Prognostic factors in 214 patients. Acta Orthop. Scand. 66:561–568, 1995.
Frassica, F.J., Frassica, D.A., Pritchard, D.J., et al.: Ewing sarcoma of the pelvis: Clinicopathological features and treatment. J. Bone Joint Surg. [Am.] 75:1457–1465, 1993.
Frassica, F.J., Waltrip, R.L., Sponseller, P.D., et al.: Clinicopathologic features and treatment of osteoid osteoma and osteoblastoma in children and adolescents. Orthop. Clin. North Am. 27:559–574, 1996.
O'Connor, M.I., and Sim, F.H.: Salvage of the limb in the treatment of malignant pelvic tumors. J. Bone Joint Surg. [Am.] 71:481, 1989.
Rougraff, B.T., Kneisl, J.S., and Simon, M.A.: Skeletal metastases of unknown origin: A prospective study of a diagnostic strategy. J. Bone Joint Surg. [Am.] 75:1276, 1993.
Peabody, T., Monson, D., Montag, A., et al.: A comparison of the prognoses for deep and subcutaneous sarcomas of the extremities. J. Bone Joint Surg. [Am.] 76:1167, 1994.
Rock, M.G., Sim, F.H., Unni, K.K., et al.: Secondary malignant giant cell tumor of bone: Clinicopathologic assessment of nineteen patients. J. Bone Joint Surg. [Am.] 68:1073, 1986.
Simon, M.A., and Bierman, J.S.: Biopsy of bone and soft tissue lesions. J. Bone Joint Surg. [Am.] 75:616, 1993.
Yaw, K.M., and Wurtz, D.: Resection and reconstruction for bone tumor in the proximal tibia. Orthop. Clin. North Am. 22:133–148, 1991.
Yazawa, Y., Frassica, F.J., Chao, E.Y.S., et al.: Metastatic bone disease: A study of the surgical treatment of 166 pathological humeral and femoral shaft fractures. Clin. Orthop. Rel. Res. 251:213, 1990.

Classic Articles

Bell, R.S., O'Sullivan, B., Liu, F.F., et al.: The surgical margin in soft tissue sarcoma. J. Bone Joint Surg. [Am.] 71:370, 1989.
Berrey, B.H., Jr., Lord, C.F., Gebhardt, M.C., et al.: Fractures of allografts: Frequency, treatment, and end results. J. Bone Joint Surg. [Am.] 72:825, 1990.
Eilber, F.R., Eckhardt, J., and Morton, D.L.: Advances in the treatment of sarcomas of the extremity: Current status of limb salvage. Cancer 54:2695–2701, 1984.
Enneking, W.F., Spanier, S.S., and Goodman, M.A.: A system for the surgical staging of musculoskeletal sarcoma. Clin. Orthop. 153:106–120, 1980.
Enneking, W.F., Spanier, S.S., and Malawer, M.M.: The effect of the anatomic setting on the results of surgical procedures for soft parts sarcoma of the thigh. Cancer 47:1005–1022, 1981.
Heare, T.C., Enneking, W.F., and Heare, M.J.: Staging techniques and biopsy of bone tumors. Orthop. Clin. North Am. 20:273, 1989.
Madewell, J.E., Ragsdale, B.D., and Sweet, D.E.: Radiologic and pathologic analysis of solitary bone lesions. Part I. Internal margins. Radiol. Clin. North Am. 19:715–748, 1981.
Mankin, H.J., Doppelt, S.H., Sullivan, T.R., et al.: Osteoarticular and intercalary allograft transplantation in the management of malignant tumors of bone. Cancer 50:613–630, 1982.
Mankin, H.J., Lange, T.A., and Spanier, S.S.: The hazards of biopsy in patients with malignant primary bone and soft tissue tumors. J. Bone Joint Surg. [Am.] 64:1121–1127, 1982.
Medsger, T.A., Jr.: Twenty-fifth rheumatism review: Paget's disease. Arthritis Rheum. 26:281–283, 1983.
Merkow, R.L., and Lane, J.M.: Current concepts of Paget's disease of bone. Orthop. Clin. North Am. 15:747–764, 1984.
Miller, M.D., Yaw, K.M., and Foley, H.T.: Malpractice maladies in the management of musculoskeletal malignancies. Contemp. Orthop. 23:577–584, 1991.
Pritchard, D.J., Lunke, R.J., Taylor, W.F., et al.: Chondrosarcoma: A clinicopathologic and statistical analysis. Cancer 45:149–157, 1980.
Ragsdale, B.D., Madewell, J.E., and Sweet, D.E.: Radiologic and pathologic analysis of solitary bone lesions. Part II. Periosteal reactions. Radiol. Clin. North Am. 19:749–783, 1981.
Sim, F.H., Beauchamp, C.P., and Chao, E.Y.S.: Reconstruction of musculoskeletal defects about the knee for tumor. Clin. Orthop. 221:188–201, 1987.
Simon, M.A.: Biopsy of musculoskeletal tumors. J. Bone Joint Surg. [Am.] 64:1253–1257, 1982.
Simon, M.A.: Current concepts review: Limb salvage for osteosarcoma. J. Bone Joint Surg. [Am.] 70:307–310, 1988.
Simon, M.A., and Nachman, J.: The clinical utility of pre-operative therapy for sarcomas. J. Bone Joint Surg. [Am.] 68:1458–1463, 1986.

Springfield, D.S., Schmidt, R., Graham-Pole, J., et al.: Surgical treatment for osteosarcoma. J. Bone Joint Surg. [Am.] 70:1124–1130, 1988.

Sweet, D.E., Madewell, J.E., and Ragsdale, B.D.: Radiologic and pathologic analysis of solitary bone lesions. Part III. Matrix patterns. Radiol. Clin. North Am. 19:785–814, 1981.

Wuisman, P., and Enneking, W.F.: Prognosis for patients who have osteosarcoma with skip metastasis. J. Bone Joint Surg. [Am.] 72:60, 1990.

Zimmer, W.D., Berquist, T.H., McLeod, R.A., et al.: Bone tumors: Magnetic resonance imaging versus computerized tomography. Radiology 155:709–718, 1985.

9

Rehabilitation: Gait, Amputations, Prosthetics, Orthotics

Frank Gottschalk

I. **Gait**

A. Human Locomotion—The process of moving from one location to another. Walking is a cyclic, energy-efficient activity for accomplishing that task. Walking requires that one foot be in contact with the ground at all times, with a period when both limbs are in contact with the ground **(double limb support).** Running requires a period when neither limb is in contact with the ground. Prerequisites for normal gait include stance phase stability, swing phase ground clearance, preposition of the foot prior to initial loading (i.e., heel strike), and energy-efficient step length and speed. **Stance phase generally occupies 60%** of the cycle initiated with heel strike and progresses through foot flat, heel off, and toe off. **Swing phase is 40% of the cycle** and starts at toe off and proceeds with limb acceleration to midswing, when the limb decelerates just prior to heel strike of the next cycle.

B. Determinants of Gait—Six determinants of gait contribute to make the process energy-efficient by lessening excursion of the center of body mass from its standing position just anterior to S2. The resultant gait pattern resembles a sinusoidal curve.

1. Pelvic Rotation—The pelvis rotates about a vertical axis alternately to the left and right of the line of progression, lessening the center of mass deviation in the horizontal plane and reducing impact at initial floor contact.
2. Pelvic List—The non–weight-bearing side drops 5 degrees, reducing superior deviation.
3. Knee Flexion at Loading—The stance phase limb is flexed 15 degrees to dampen the impact of initial loading.
4. Foot and Ankle Motion—Through the subtalar joint, damping of the loading response occurs, leading to stability during midstance and efficiency of propulsion at push-off.
5. Knee Motion—Works together with the foot and ankle to decrease necessary limb motion. The knee flexes at heel strike and extends at foot flat.
6. Lateral Pelvic Motion—The motion is 5 cm over the weight-bearing limb, narrowing the base of support and increasing stance phase stability.

C. Muscle Action—Agonist and antagonist muscle groups work in concert during the gait cycle to effectively advance the limb through space. The hip flexors advance the limb forward during swing phase and are opposed during terminal swing prior to heel strike by the decelerating action of the hip extensors. **Most muscle activity is eccentric, which is muscle lengthening while contracting** and allows an antagonist muscle to dampen the activity of an agonist and act as a "shock absorber" (Fig. 9–1). Isocentric contraction defines muscle length, staying constant during contraction (Table 9–1). Some muscle activity can be concentric, in which the muscle shortens to move a joint through space.

D. Gait Nomenclature—The **gait cycle** includes all activity between initial loading (i.e., heel strike) on one limb and the succeeding initial loading on the same limb (Fig. 9–2). The **step** is the distance between toe off and heel strike of the same limb. **Stride** is heel strike to heel strike of the same limb. **Velocity** is a function of cadence (steps per unit time) and stride length. **Stance phase** (60%) of a limb is the period of time when that limb is in contact with the ground. **Swing phase** (40%) is the period when that limb is not in contact with the ground. **Double limb support** is the period of the cycle when both limbs are in contact with the ground. During running there is a period of time when neither limb is in contact with the ground.

E. Pathologic Gait—Abnormal gait patterns can be caused by multiple factors.

1. Muscle weakness or paralysis decreases the ability to normally move a joint through space. A characteristic walking pattern de-

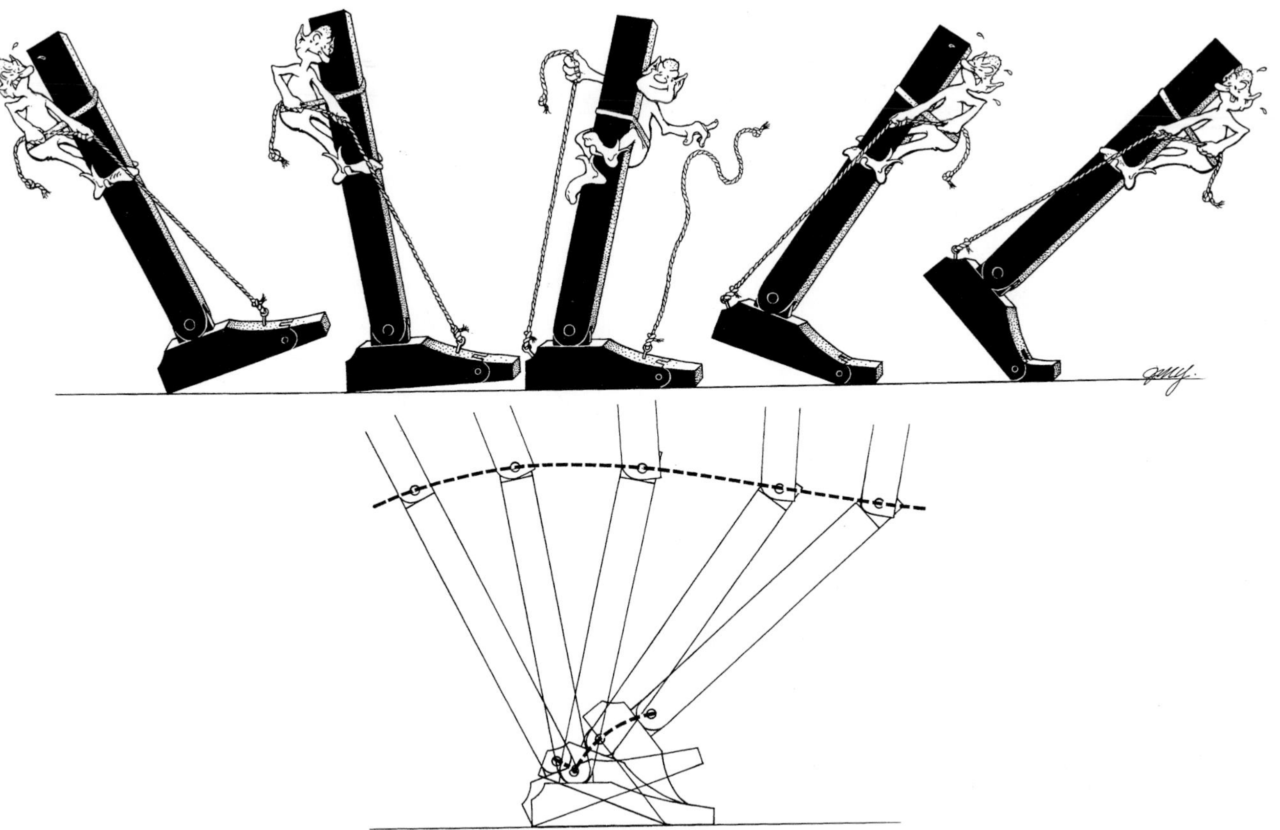

Figure 9–1. Effect of ankle motion, controlled by muscle action, on pathway of knee. The smooth and flattened pathway of the knee during stance phase is achieved by forces acting from the leg on the foot. Foot slap is restrained during initial lowering of the foot; afterward, the plantar flexors raise the heel. (From Inman, V.T., Ralston, H., and Todd, F.: Human Walking, p. 11. Baltimore, Williams & Wilkins, 1981.)

velops based on the specific muscle or muscle group involved and the ability of the individual to achieve a substitution pattern to replace that muscle's action (Table 9–2).

2. Neurologic conditions may alter gait by producing muscle weakness, loss of balance, loss of coordination between agonist and antagonist muscle groups (i.e., spasticity), and late joint contracture. Hip scissoring is associated with overactive adductors, and knee flexion contracture may be caused by hamstring spasticity. **Equinus deformity** of the foot and ankle may result in steppage gait and back setting of the knee.
3. Pain in a limb creates an **antalgic gait** pattern in which the individual has a shortened stance phase to lessen the time that the painful limb is loaded and the swing phase is more rapid.
4. Joint abnormalities alter gait by changing

Table 9–1.

Muscle Action and Function

Muscle	Action	Function
Gluteus medius	Eccentric	Controls pelvic tilt at midstance
Gluteus maximus	Concentric	Powers hip extension
Iliopsoas	Concentric	Powers hip flexion
Hip adductors	Eccentric	Control lateral sway (late stance)
Hip abductors	Eccentric	Control pelvic tilt (midstance)
Quadriceps	Eccentric	Stabilizes knee at heel strike
Hamstrings	Eccentric	Control rate of knee extension (stance)
Tibialis anterior	Concentric	Dorsiflexes ankle at swing
	Eccentric[a]	Slows plantar flexion rate (heel strike)
Gastrocnemius/soleus	Eccentric	Slows dorsiflexion rate (stance)

[a]Predominant role.

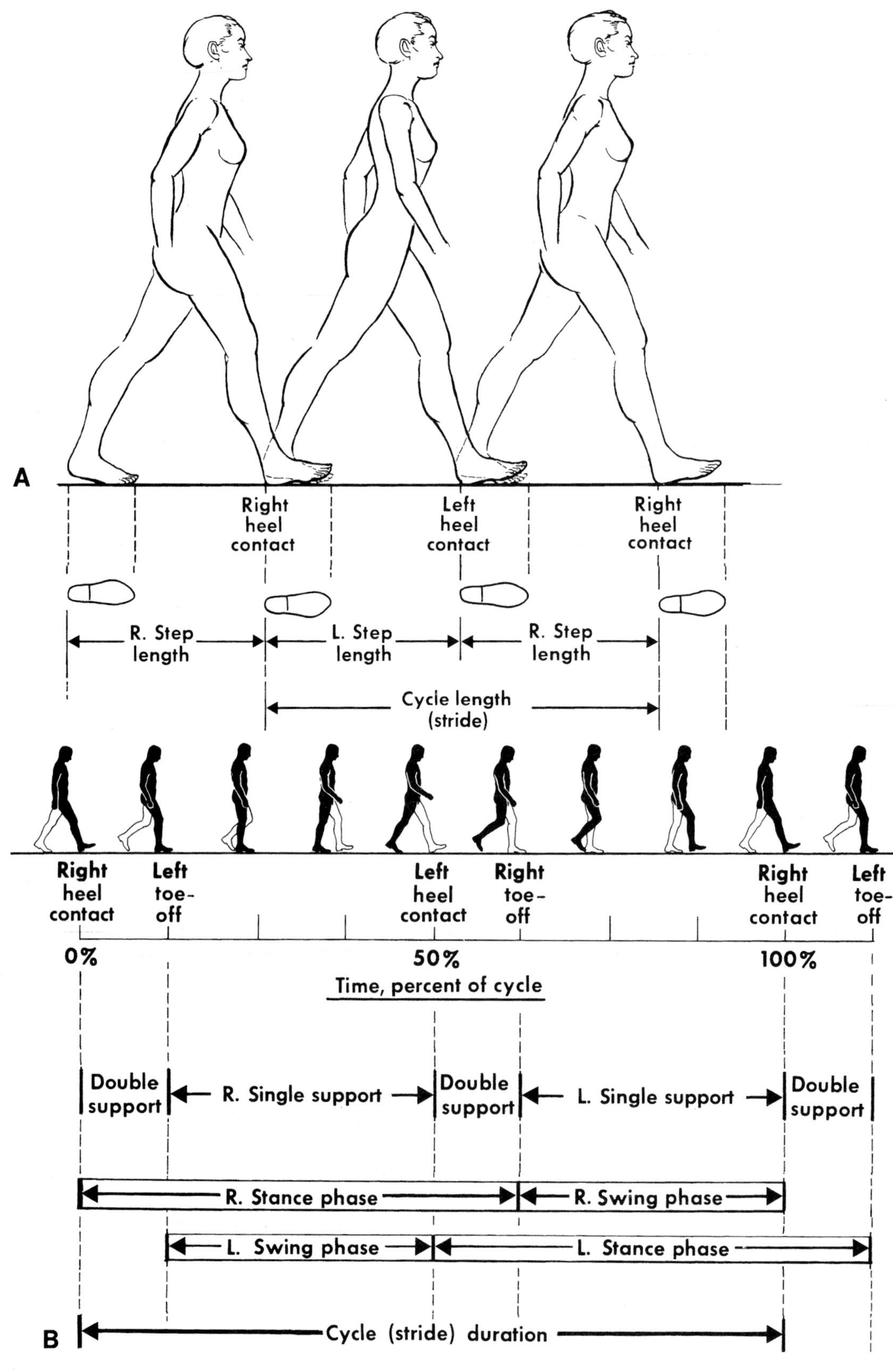

Figure 9–2. Distance and time dimensions of walking cycle. *A,* Distance (length). *B,* Time. (From Inman, V.T., Ralston, H., and Todd, F.: Human Walking, p. 26. Baltimore, Williams & Wilkins, 1981.)

Table 9–2.

Gait Abnormalities Caused by Muscle Weakness

Muscle	Phase	Direction	Type of Gait	Treatment
Gluteus medius	Stance	Lateral	Abductor lurch	Cane
Gluteus maximus	Stance	Backward	Lurch (hip hyperextension)	
Quadriceps	Stance	Forward	Lurch/back knee gait	AFO
	Swing	Forward	Abnormal hip rotation	
Gastrocnemius/soleus	Stance	Forward	Flat foot (calcaneal) gait	±AFO
	Swing	Forward	Delayed heel rise	
Tibialis anterior	Stance	Forward	Foot drop/slap	AFO
	Swing	Forward	Steppage gait	

the motion of that joint or by producing pain.

5. Hemiplegia—Prolongation of stance and double limb support is characteristic. Associated problems are **ankle equinus**, limitation of knee flexion, and increased **hip flexion**. Surgical correction of equinus is 1 year after onset. Gait impairment may be excessive plantar flexion, weakness, and balance problems.
6. Crutches and Canes—Crutches increase stability by providing two additional loading points. **Canes** help shift the center of gravity to the affected side when the cane is used in the opposite hand. This **decreases the joint reaction** forces of the lower limb and reduces pain.

II. **Amputations**—Amputation of all or part of a limb is performed for peripheral vascular disease, trauma, tumor, infection, or congenital anomaly. It is often accomplished as an alternative to limb salvage and should be considered a reconstructive procedure. Because of the psychological implications and the alteration of body self-image, a multidisciplinary team approach should be taken to return the patient to maximum level of independent function. The process should be considered the first step in the rehabilitation of the patient rather than a failure of treatment.

A. Metabolic Cost of Amputation—The metabolic cost of walking is increased with proximal level amputations, being inversely proportional to the length of the residual limb and the number of joints preserved. With more proximal amputation, patients have a decreased self-selected, and maximum, walking speed. **Oxygen consumption is increased** with more proximal level amputation; thus the transfemoral amputee with peripheral vascular disease uses virtually maximum energy expenditure during normal self-selected velocity walking (Table 9–3).

B. Load Transfer—The soft-tissue envelope acts as an interface between the bone of the residual limb and the prosthetic socket. Ideally, it is composed of a mobile, nonadherent muscle mass covering the bone end and full-thickness skin that tolerates the direct pressures and pistoning within the prosthetic socket. It is rare for the prosthetic socket to achieve a perfect intimate fit. A nonadherent soft tissue envelope allows some degree of mobility, or "pistoning," of the bone within the soft-tissue envelope, thus eliminating the shear forces that produce tissue breakdown and ulceration. Load transfer (i.e., weight-bearing) is accomplished by either direct or indirect load transfer. Direct load transfer (i.e., end weight-bearing) is accomplished with knee disarticulation or ankle disarticulation (Syme's amputation). Intimacy of the prosthetic socket is necessary only for suspension. When the amputation is performed through a long bone (i.e., transfemoral or transtibial), the terminal residual limb must be unloaded and the load transferred indirectly by the total contact method. This process requires an intimate prosthetic socket fit and **7–10 de-**

Table 9–3.

Energy Expenditure for Amputation

Amputation Level	% Energy Above Baseline	Speed (m/min)	O_2 Cost (mL/kg/meter)
Long transtibial	10	70	0.17
Average transtibial	25	60	0.20
Short transtibial	40	50	0.20
Bilateral transtibial	41	50	0.20
Transfemoral	65	40	0.28
Wheelchair	0–8	70	0.16

grees of flexion of the knee for transtibial amputation **or 5–10 degrees of adduction of the femur** for transfemoral amputation (Fig. 9–3).

C. Amputation Wound Healing—Depends on several factors, which include vascular inflow, nutrition, and an adequate immune status. Patients with malnutrition or immune deficiency have a high rate of wound failure or infection. **A serum albumin level below 3.5 g/dL** indicates a malnourished patient. **An absolute lymphocyte count below 1500/mm^3** is a sign of immune deficiency. If possible, amputation surgery should be delayed in patients with stable gangrene until these values can be improved by nutritional support, usually in the form of oral hyperalimentation. In severely affected patients, nasogastric or percutaneous gastric feeding tubes are sometimes essential. When infection or severe ischemic pain requires urgent surgery, open amputation at the most distal viable level followed by open wound management can be accomplished until wound healing potential can be optimized. Oxygenated blood is a prerequisite for wound healing and **a hemoglobin of more than 10 g/dL** is necessary. Amputation wounds generally heal by collateral flow, so arteriography is rarely useful for predicting wound healing. Doppler ultrasonography has historically been used as the measure of vascular inflow to predict wound healing in the ischemic limb. An absolute Doppler pressure of 70 mm Hg was originally described as the minimum inflow to support wound healing. The ischemic index is the ratio of the Doppler pressure at the level being tested to the brachial systolic pressure. It is generally accepted that patients require **an ischemic index of 0.5 or greater** at the surgical level to support wound healing. The ischemic index at the ankle (i.e., the ankle-brachial index) has evolved as the gold standard for assessing adequate inflow to the ischemic limb.

Standard Doppler ultrasonography measures arterial pressure. In the normal limb, the **area under the Doppler waveform** tracing is a measure of flow. These values are falsely elevated and nonpredictive in at least 15% of patients with diabetes and peripheral vascular disease because of the **noncompressibility and noncompliance of calcified peripheral arteries.** The **toe pressures (0.5)** are more accurate in these patients. The transcutaneous partial pressure of oxygen ($TcpO_2$) is the present "gold standard" measure of vascular inflow. It records the oxygen-delivering capacity of the vascular system to the level of contemplated surgery. Values **greater than 40 mm Hg** correlate with acceptable wound-healing rates without the false-positive values seen in noncompliant peripheral vascular diseased vessels. **Pressures less than 20 mm Hg** are indicative of poor healing potential.

D. Pediatric Amputation—Pediatric amputations are typically the result of congenital limb deficiencies, trauma, or tumors. The old method for congenital amputations is based on the premise that the limb (or limb segment) was lost before birth, in contrast with the accepted concept of failure of formation. The present system is based on the original work of a 1975 Conference of the International Society for Prosthetics and Orthotics (ISPO) and subsequently an International Organization for Standardization (ISO) standard. Deficiencies are either longitudinal or transverse, with the potential for intercalary deficits. Amputation is rarely indicated in congenital upper limb deficiency; even rudimentary appendages can be functionally useful. In the lower limb, ampu-

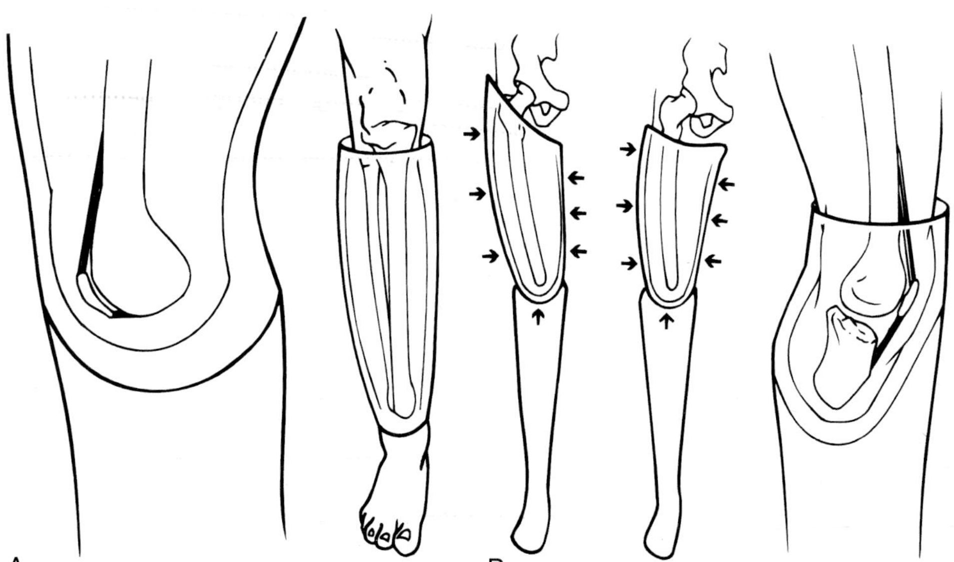

Figure 9–3. *A,* Direct load transfer is accomplished in the (left) through-knee and (right) Syme's ankle disarticulation amputations. *B,* Indirect load transfer is accomplished in above-knee amputations with either (left) a standard quadrilateral socket or (center) an adducted narrow medial-lateral socket. The below-knee amputation (right) transfers weight indirectly with the knee flexed approximately 10 degrees. (From Pinzur, M.: New concepts in lower limb amputation and prosthetic management. Instr. Course Lect. 39:361, 1990.)

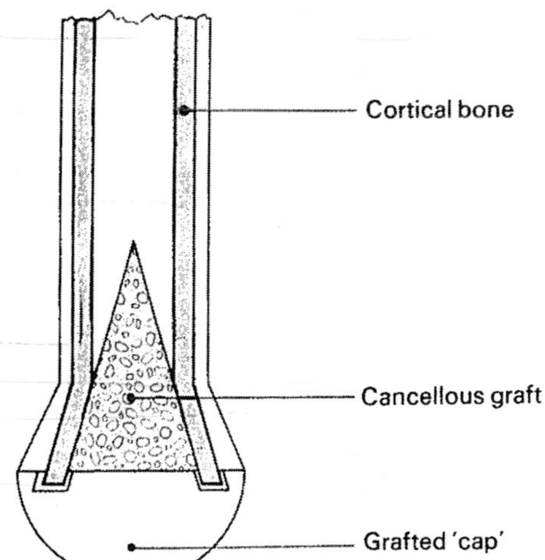

Figure 9–4. Diagram of the stump-capping procedure. The bone end has been split longitudinally. (From Bernd, L., Blasius, K., Lukoschek, M., et al.: The autologous stump plasty: Treatment for bony overgrowth in juvenile amputees. J. Bone Joint Surg. [Br.] 73:203–206, 1991.)

tation of an unstable segment may allow direct load transfer and enhanced walking. In the growing child, disarticulations should be performed only when possible to maintain maximal residual limb length and to prevent terminal bony overgrowth. Such **overgrowth occurs most commonly in the humerus**, fibula, tibia, and femur, in that order; it is most common in diaphyseal amputations. Numerous surgical procedures have been described to resolve this problem, but **the best method is surgical revision** of the residual limb with adequate resection of bone or autogenous osteochondral stump capping (Fig. 9–4).

E. Trauma—The absolute indication for amputation after trauma is an ischemic limb with nonreconstructable vascular injury. Recent studies of severe open tibial fractures reveal that limb salvage is often associated with high mortality and morbidity due to infection, increased energy expenditure for ambulation, and decreased potential to return to work. Early amputation in the appropriate patient may prevent emotional, marital, financial, and addictive problems. Guidelines for immediate or early amputation of mangled limbs differ between upper and lower limbs. When a salvaged upper limb remains sensate and maintains prehensile function, it will often function better than a prosthesis. Sensation is not as crucial in the lower limb, where current prostheses more closely approximate normal function. The salvaged lower extremity with an insensate plantar weight-bearing surface **(loss of tibialis posterior nerve)** is unlikely to provide a durable limb for stable walking and is a potential source of early or late sepsis. The grading scales for evaluating mangled extremities are not absolute predictors but provide reasonable guidelines for determining whether salvage is appropriate.

F. Peripheral Vascular Disease—In order for patients to learn to walk with a prosthesis and care for their residual limb and prosthesis, they must possess certain **cognitive capacities:** (1) memory, (2) attention, (3) concentration, and (4) organization. Patients with cognitive deficits or psychiatric disease have a low likelihood of becoming successful prosthesis users. A majority of patients are diabetic with inherent immune deficiency. Many are malnourished patients with peripheral vascular disease of sufficient magnitude to require amputation and have disease in their coronary and cerebral arteries. Appropriate consultation with physical therapy, social work, and psychology departments is valuable to determine rehabilitation potential. Medical consultation will help determine cardiopulmonary reserve. The vascular surgeon should determine whether vascular reconstruction is feasible or appropriate. The **biologic amputation level** is the most distal functional amputation level with a high probability of supporting wound healing. This level is determined by the presence of adequate viable local tissue to construct a residual limb capable of supporting weight-bearing, an adequate vascular inflow, and serum albumin and total lymphocyte count sufficient to aid surgical wound healing. Amputation level selection is determined by combining the biologic amputation level with the rehabilitation potential to determine the amputation level that maximizes ultimate functional independence.

G. Musculoskeletal Tumors—Advances in chemotherapy and allograft or prosthetic reconstruction have made limb salvage a viable option in extremity sarcomas. The primary goal of musculoskeletal oncologic surgery is to provide adequate surgical margins. If adequate margins can be achieved with limb salvage, the decision can then be based on expected functional outcome. There is still controversy in the literature when limb salvage is compared with amputation regarding energy expenditure to ambulate, quality-of-life measures, and function with activities of daily living. Expected functional outcome should include the psychosocial and body image values associated with limb salvage. These concerns should be balanced with the apparent improved task performance and **reduced concern for late mechanical injury** associated with amputation and prosthetic limb fitting.

H. Technical Considerations—Skin flaps should be full thickness and avoid dissection between tissue planes. Periosteal stripping should be kept to a minimum to allow bone transection; this minimizes regenerative bone overgrowth. Wounds should not be sutured under tension.

Muscles are best secured directly to bone

at resting tension **(myodesis)** rather than to antagonist muscle **(myoplasty)**. Stable residual limb muscle mass can improve function by reducing atrophy and providing a stable soft-tissue envelope over the end of the bone.

All transected nerves form neuromas. The nerve end should come to lie deep in a soft-tissue envelope, away from potential pressure areas. Crushing the nerve may contribute to postoperative phantom or limb pain.

Rigid dressings postoperatively help reduce swelling, decrease pain, and protect the stump from trauma. Early postoperative fitting is done between 5 and 21 days.

I. Complications
   1. **Pain—Phantom limb sensation**, the feeling that all or part of the amputated limb is present, occurs in almost all adults who have undergone amputation. It usually decreases with time. **Phantom pain** is a burning, painful sensation in the amputated part. It is diminished by prosthetic use, physical therapy, compression, and transcutaneous nerve stimulation. A common cause of residual pain is reflex sympathetic dystrophy or causalgia. Amputation should not be performed for this condition.

      Localized stump pain is often related to bony or soft-tissue problems. Referred pain to the limb occurs in a frequent number of cases.
   2. **Edema**—Postoperative edema occurs after amputation. It may impede wound healing and place significant tension on the tissues. Rigid dressings and soft compression help reduce the problem. Swelling occurring after stump maturation is usually caused by poor socket fit, medical problems, or trauma. Persistence of chronic swelling may lead to **verrucous hyperplasia,** which is a wart-like overgrowth of skin with pigmentation and serous discharge. It is treated by a total contact socket, with frequent alterations to accommodate change.
   3. **Joint Contractures**—Usually noted as **hip and knee flexion contractures,** which can be produced at the time of surgery by anchoring the respective muscles with the joints in a flexed position. These can be avoided by ensuring correct positioning of the amputated limb.
   4. **Wound Failure**—May occur in diabetic and vascular patients. If not amenable to local care, **wedge excision** of soft tissue and bone with closure without tension is preferred treatment.

J. Upper Limb Amputations (Fig. 9–5)—Wrist disarticulation has two advantages over transradial amputation:
   1. Preservation of more forearm rotation due to preservation of the distal radioulnar joint; and
   2. Improved prosthetic suspension due to the flare of the distal radius.

   Wrist disarticulation provides challenges to the prosthetist that may outweigh its benefits. Cosmetically, the prosthetic limb is longer than the contralateral limb; and if myoelectric components are used, the motor and battery cannot be hidden within the prosthetic shank. High levels of function can be obtained at this level of amputation. Forearm rotation and strength are directly related to the length of the transradial (below-elbow) residual limb. The optimal length is the junction of the middle and distal thirds of the forearm, where the soft-tissue envelope can be repaired by myodesis and the components of a myoelectric prosthesis can be hidden within the prosthetic shank. Because function at this level is accomplished prosthetically only by opening and closing the terminal device, elbow joint retention is essential. The length and shape of elbow disarticulation provide improved suspension and lever arm capacity. To improve suspension and reduce the need for shoulder harnessing, a 45 to 60 degree distal humeral osteotomy is performed. Patients with **complete brachial plexus** injury and a nonfunctioning hand and forearm may be **best treated** by a **transradial amputation** or elbow disarticulation, which can be fitted with a prosthesis. When not due to Raynaud's or Buerger's diseases, gangrene of the upper limb represents end-stage disease, especially in the diabetic patient. These patients experience a high mortality rate and do not survive beyond 24 months. Localized amputations are unlikely to heal. When surgery becomes necessary, amputation should be performed at the transradial level to achieve wound healing during the final months of the patient's life.

K. Lower Limb Amputations (see Fig. 9–5)—Ischemic patients generally ambulate with a propulsive gait pattern, so they suffer little disability from toe amputation. Traumatic amputees lose some late stance phase stability with toe amputation. The great toe should be amputated distal to the insertion of the flexor hallucis brevis. **Isolated second toe amputation** should be performed just distal to the proximal phalanx metaphyseal flare to act as a buttress, preventing late hallux valgus. Single outer (first or fifth) ray resections function well in standard shoes. Resection of more than one ray leaves a narrow forefoot that is difficult to fit in shoes and often results in a late equinus deformity. Central ray resections are complicated by prolonged wound healing and rarely outperform midfoot amputation.
   1. Transmetatarsal and Lisfranc Tarsal-Metatarsal Amputation—There is little func-

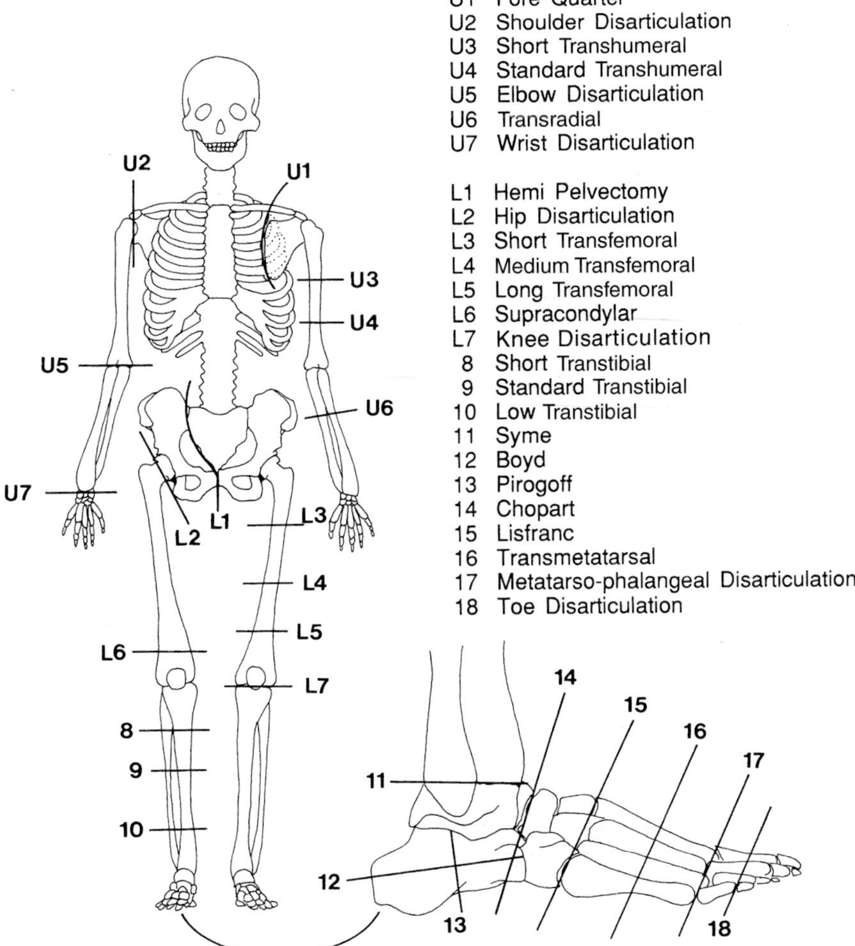

Figure 9–5. Composite illustration of common amputation levels.

tional difference between these two. The long plantar flap acts as a myocutaneous flap and is preferred to fish-mouth dorsal-plantar flaps. Transmetatarsal amputation should be through the proximal metaphyses to prevent late plantar pressure ulcers under the residual bone ends. Percutaneous tendoachilles lengthening should be performed with the Lisfranc amputation to prevent the late development of equinus or equinovarus. Late varus can be corrected with transfer of the tibialis anterior tendon to the neck of the talus. Some authors have reported reasonable functional outcomes with hindfoot amputation (i.e., Chopart's or Boyd's), but most experts recommend avoiding these levels if possible in diabetic and vascular patients. Although children have been reported to function reasonably well, adults retain an **inadequate lever arm** and are prone to experience **fixed equinus** of the heel if tendoachilles lengthening and tibialis anterior tendon transfer are not performed.

2. Ankle Disarticulation (Syme's Amputation)—Allows direct load transfer and is rarely complicated by late residual limb ulcers or tissue breakdown. It provides a stable gait pattern that rarely requires prosthetic gait training after surgery. Surgery should be performed in one stage, even in ischemic limbs with insensate heel pads. A **patent tibialis posterior artery** is necessary to ensure healing. The malleoli and metaphyseal flares should be removed from the tibia and fibula, but the remaining tibial articular surface should be retained to provide a resilient residual limb. The heel pad should be secured to the tibia either anteriorly through drill holes or posteriorly by securing the tendoachilles.
3. Transtibial (Below-Knee) Amputation—Should be performed with a long posterior myocutaneous flap as the preferred method of creating a soft-tissue envelope. Optimal bone length is at least 12–15 cm below the knee joint or longer if adequate gastrocnemius or soleus can be used to construct a durable soft-tissue envelope. Posterior muscle should be secured to the beveled anterior tibia by myodesis. Rigid dressings are preferred during the early postoperative period, and weight-bearing should be initiated 5–21

days after surgery if the residual limb is capable of transferring load.

4. Knee Disarticulation (Through-Knee Amputation)—Presently performed using sagittal skin flaps and covering the end of the femur with gastrocnemius to act as a soft-tissue envelope end pad. The **patella tendon** is sutured to the **cruciate ligaments** in the notch, leaving the patella on the anterior femur. This level is generally used in the nonwalker who can support wound healing at the transtibial or distal level. Knee disarticulation is muscle-balanced, provides an excellent weight-bearing platform for sitting, and provides a lever arm for transfer. When performed in a potential walker, it provides **a direct load transfer** residual limb.
5. Transfemoral (Above-Knee) Amputation—Increases energy cost for walking. Peripheral vascular disease transfemoral amputees are unlikely to become good walkers, so salvaging the limb at the knee disarticulation, or transtibial level, is critical to maintaining functional walking independence. With greater length, the lever arm, suspension, and limb advancement are optimized. The optimal transfemoral bone length is 12 cm above the knee joint to accommodate the prosthetic knee. Adductor myodesis important for maintaining femoral adduction during the stance phase to allow optimal prosthetic function (Fig. 9–6). The major deforming force is into abduction and flexion. Adductor myodesis at normal muscle tension eliminates the problem of **adductor roll** in the groin. Sectioning of **adductor magnus** results in a loss of **70% of adductor pull** (Fig. 9–7). Rigid dressings are difficult to apply and maintain at this level. Elastic compression dressings are used and may be suspended about the opposite iliac crest. Hip disarticulation is infrequently performed, and only an occasional few of these amputees become meaningful prosthetic users because of the high energy requirements. Post-trauma or tumor patients occasionally use the prosthesis for limited activity. These patients sit in their prosthesis and must use their torso to achieve momentum to "throw" the limb forward to advance it.

III. **Prosthetics**

A. Upper Limb—The shoulder provides the center of radius of the functional sphere of the upper limb. The elbow acts as the caliper to position the hand at a workable distance from that center to perform tasks. Multiple joint segment tasks are usually done simultaneously, whereas upper limb prostheses perform these same tasks sequentially; thus joint and residual limb length salvage are directly correlated with functional outcome. Motion at the retained joints is essential to maximize that function. Residual limb length is important for prosthetic socket suspension and providing the lever arm necessary to "drive" the prosthesis through space. Limb salvage is more critical for the upper limb, where sensation is critical to function. An insensate prosthesis provides less function than a partially sensate, partially functional salvaged limb. After amputation, prosthetic fitting should be done as soon as possible, even before complete wound healing has occurred. Outcomes of prosthetic limb use vary from

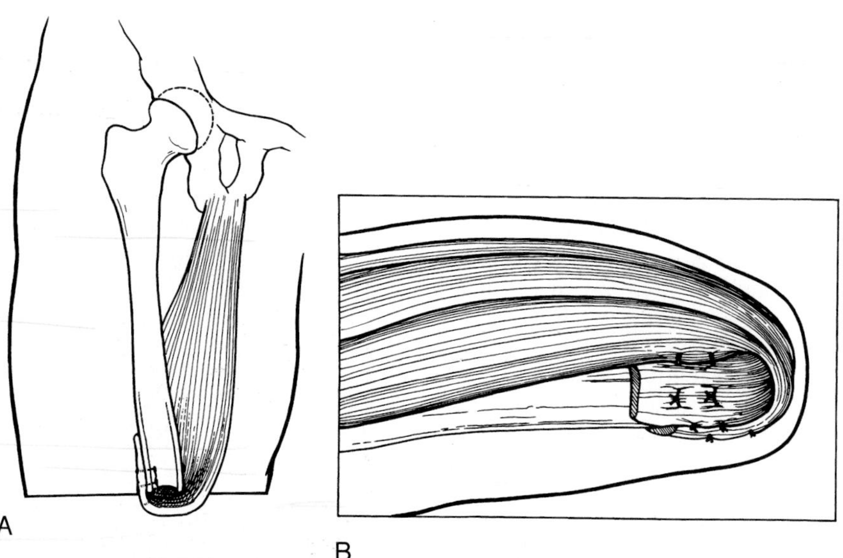

Figure 9–6. *A,* Diagram to show attachment of the adductor magnus to the lateral part of the femur. *B,* Diagram depicting attachment of the quadriceps over the adductor magnus. (From Gottschalk, F.: Transfemoral amputation. In Bowker, J., and Michael, J., eds.: Atlas of Limb Prosthetics, pp. 479–486. St. Louis, Mosby-Year Book, 1992.)

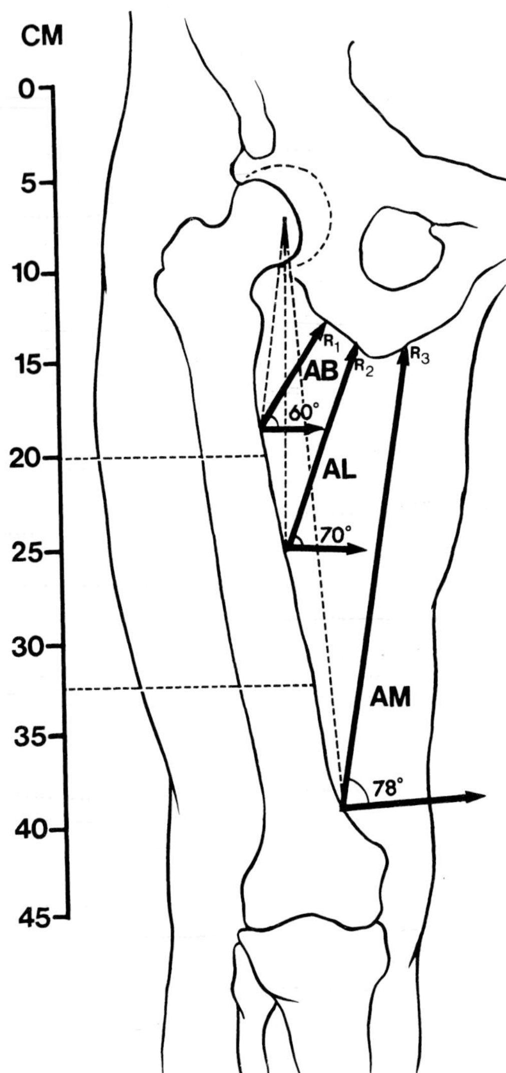

Figure 9–7. Diagram of moment arms of the three adductor muscles. Loss of the distal attachment of adductor magnus will result in a loss of 70% of the adductor pull. (From Gottschalk, F.A., Kourosh, S., Stills, M., et al.: Does socket configuration influence the position of the femur in above-knee amputation? J. Prosthet. Orthot. 1989; 2:94–102.)

70% to 85% when **prosthetic fitting occurs within 30 days** of amputation, in contrast with <30% when started late. **Myoelectric prostheses** provide good cosmesis and are used for **sedentary work**. They can be used in any position including overhead activity. They appear to be most successful in the midlength transradial amputee, where only the terminal device needs to be activated. Body-powered prostheses are used for heavy labor. The **terminal device** is activated by **shoulder flexion and abduction. The elbow is controlled by shoulder extension and depression.** Optimal mechanical efficiency of figure-of-8 harnesses requires the harness ring to be at the spinous process of C7 and slightly to the nonamputated side. When the residual forearm is so short as to preclude an adequate lever arm for driving the prosthesis through space, **supracondylar suspension (Munster socket) and step-up hinges** can be used to augment function. Elbow disarticulation and transhumeral (above-elbow) amputations require two motions to develop prehension, making both levels significantly less efficient and the prosthesis heavier than that for amputation at the transradial level. Prosthetically, the **best function** with the least weight at the lowest cost is provided by **hybrid prosthetic systems** combining myoelectric, traditional body-powered, and body-driven switch components. These levels provide minimal function because the patient must sequentially control two joints and a terminal device. When the lever arm capacity of the humerus is lost in proximal transhumeral or shoulder disarticulation amputations, limited function can be achieved with a manual universal shoulder joint positioned by the opposite hand, combined with lightweight hybrid prosthetic components.

B. Lower Limb
   1. Prosthetic Feet—Several designs are available and are classified into five classes. The single-axis foot is based on an ankle hinge that provides dorsiflexion and plantar flexion. The disadvantages of the single-axis foot include poor durability and cosmesis. The SACH (solid ankle, cushioned heel) foot has been the standard for decades and was appropriate for general use in low-demand patients. It may lead to **overload problems** on the nonamputated foot, and its use is being discontinued. **Articulated dynamic response** feet allow inversion/eversion and rotation of the foot and are useful for activities on uneven surfaces. They may absorb loads and **decrease shear forces** to the residual limb.
   2. Most **dynamic response feet** have a **flexible keel** and are the new standard for general use (Fig. 9–8). Correct **dynamic pros-**

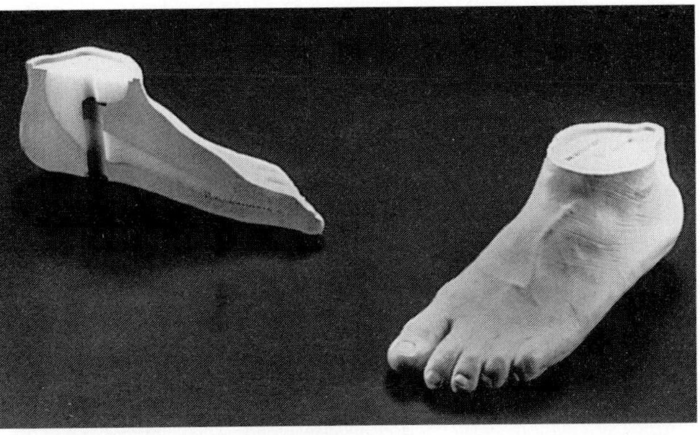

Figure 9–8. Cosmetic appearance of a dynamic response foot (Seattle foot) and cross-section to show internal configuration. (Courtesy of MIND, Seattle, WA.)

thetic foot selection requires information about the patient's height, **weight, activity level**, access for maintenance, cosmesis, and funding. Dynamic response feet may be grouped into articulated and nonarticulated feet, which have short or long keels.

The **keel deforms under load**, becoming a spring and allowing dorsiflexion, thereby decreasing the loading on the sound side and providing a spring-like response for push off. Posterior projection of the keel provides a response at heel strike for smooth transition through stance phase. A saggital split allows for moderate inversion or eversion. **Shortened keels** are not as responsive and are indicated for the moderate activity ambulator, whereas **long keels** are for very high-demand activities. Separate prosthetic feet for running and lower-demand activities may be indicated. The dynamic response feet, including the Seattle foot, Carbon Copy II/III, and the Flex Foot, allow amputees to undertake most normal activities (Fig. 9–9).

3. Prosthetic Shanks—The structural link between prosthetic components. Two varieties exist—endoskeletal, with a soft exterior and load-bearing tubing inside, and exoskeletal, with a hard load-bearing exterior shell. **Rotator units** are sometimes added for patients involved in twisting activities (e.g., golf).
4. Prosthetic Knees—Used in transfemoral and knee disarticulation prostheses and chosen based on patient needs. Prosthetic knees provide controlled knee motion in the prosthesis. **Alignment stability** (the position of the prosthetic knee in relation to the patient's line of weight-bearing) is important in design and fitting of prosthetic knees. Placing the **knee center of rotation posterior** to the weight line allows control in the stance phase but makes flexion difficult. Alternatively, with the knee center of rotation anterior to the weight line, flexion is made easier but at the expense of control. Only the **polycentric knee** takes advantage of both options by having a variable center of rotation. Six basic types of knees are available.
   a. Constant Friction Knee—A hinge that is designed to dampen knee swing via a screw or rubber pad that applies friction to the knee bolt. It is a general utility knee and may be used on uneven terrain. It is the most common knee used in childhood prosthetics. Its major disadvantage is that it allows only single-speed walking and relies solely on alignment for stance phase stability and is therefore not recommended for older, weaker patients.
   b. Variable Friction (Cadence Control) Knee—Allows resistance to knee flexion to increase as the knee extends by employing a number of staggered friction pads. This knee allows walking at different speeds but is not durable and is not available in endoskeletal systems.
   c. **Stance Phase Control** (Weight-Activated, or Safety) Knee—Functions like a constant friction knee during the swing

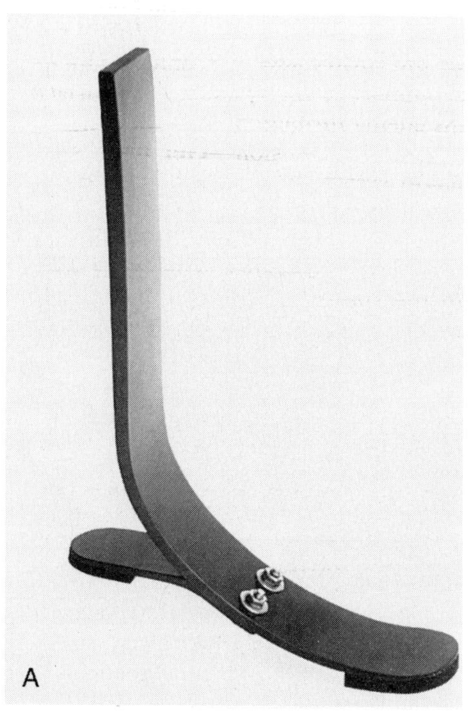

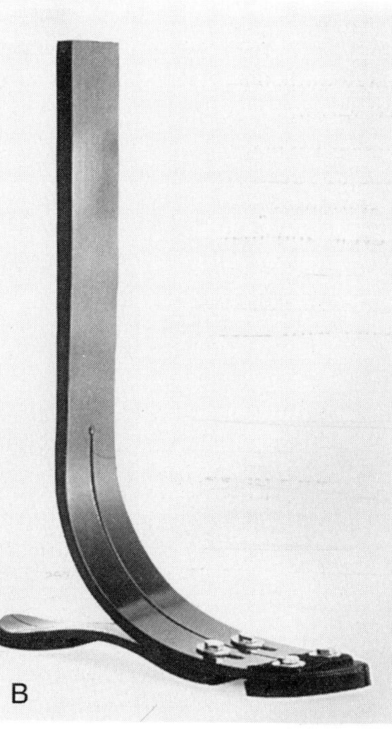

Figure 9–9. *A,* Flex Foot with carbon fiber leaf and posterior projection of keel for heel strike. *B,* Flex Foot with split toe configuration and spring leaf design. (Courtesy of Flex Foot Inc., Aliso Viejo, CA.)

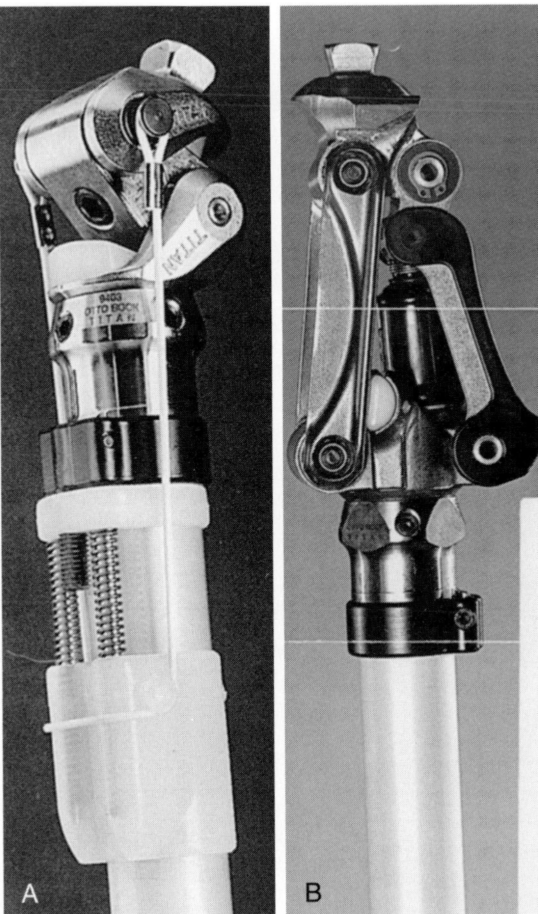

Figure 9–10. *A,* Stance phase control unit for transfemoral prosthesis. *B,* Modular endoskeletal four-bar knee with hydraulic swing-phase control unit. (Courtesy of Otto Bock Orthopaedic Industries, Minneapolis, MN.)

phase but "freezes" by application of a high-friction housing when weight is applied to the limb. Its use is **primarily reserved for older** patients, high-level amputees, or use on uneven terrain.

d. **Polycentric** (Four-Bar Linkage) Knee—has a **moving instant center of rotation** that provides for different stability characteristics during the gait cycle and may allow increased flexion for sitting. It is recommended for patients with transfemoral amputations, patients with knee disarticulations, and bilateral amputees (Fig. 9–10).

e. Manual Locking Knee—Consists of a constant friction knee hinge with a positive lock in extension that can be unlocked to allow function similar to that of a constant friction knee. The knee is often left locked in extension for more stability. The knee has limited indications and is used primarily in weak, unstable patients, those patients just learning to use prostheses, and blind amputees.

f. **Fluid Control** (Hydraulic and Pneumatic) **Knees**—Allows adjustment of cadence response by changing resistance to knee flexion via a piston mechanism. The designing prevents excessive flexion and is extended earlier in the gait cycle, allowing a more fluid gait.

The knee is best used in active patients who prefer greater utility and variability at the expense of more weight.

g. Summary—Information on the various types of prosthetic knees is summarized in Table 9–4.

5. Suspension Systems—Suspension is provided in modern lower extremity prosthetics primarily through socket design and **suspension sleeves**. The use of straps and belts is usually for supplementation. Sockets are prosthetic components designed to provide comfortable functional control and even pressure distribution on the amputated stump. Sockets can be hard (rigid or unlined) or soft (lined with a resilient material and/or flexible shell). In general, suction and socket contour are the primary suspension modalities used. The suction socket provides an airtight seal via a pressure differential between the socket and atmosphere. Total-contact support of the residual limb surface prevents edema formation.

a. Transtibial Suspension—**Gel liner suspension** systems with a locking pin are the preferred method of suspension. Liners are made from silicone, urethane, or thermoplastic elastomer. The sleeve rolls onto the stump, and the locking pin is then locked into the socket (Fig. 9–11).

Table 9–4.

Characteristics of Various Prosthetic Knees

Knee	Action	Advantages	Disadvantages
Constant friction	Limits flexion	Durable, long res	Decreased stability
Variable friction	Varies with flexion	Variable cadence	Durability poor
Stance control	Friction brake	Stability during stance	Durability poor, difficult on stairs
Polycentric	Instant center moves	Stable, increased flexion	Durability poor, heavy
Manual locking	Unlock to sit	Maximum stability	Abnormal gait
Fluid control	Deceleration in swing	Variable cadence	Weight, cost

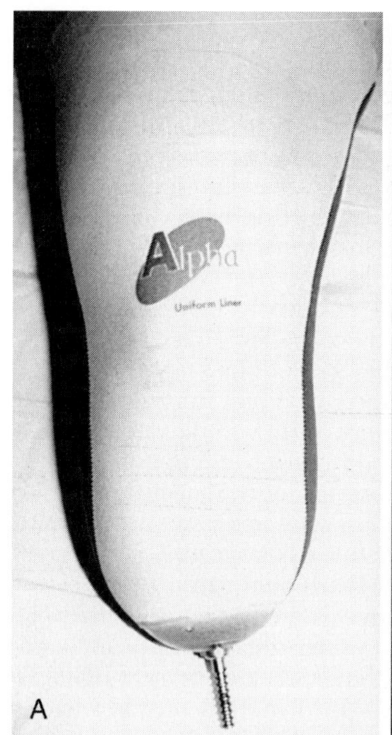

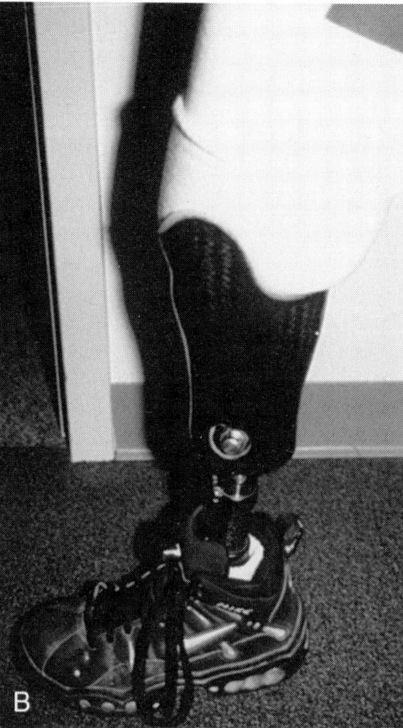

Figure 9–11. *A,* Gel liner suspension with locking pin. *B,* Transtibial prosthesis with liner locked in place.

The liners provide suspension through **suction and friction** and act as the socket interface. Prosthetic socks worn over the liner accommodate volume fluctuation. This suspension allows unrestricted knee flexion and minimal pistoning.

Prosthetic sleeves use friction and negative pressure for suspension. The sleeves fit snugly to the upper third of the tibial prosthesis and are made from neoprene, latex, silicone, or thermoplastic elastomers.

Supracondylar suspension is recommended when the residual limb is less than 5 cm long. The socket is designed to increase the surface area for pressure distribution by raising the medial and lateral socket brim. A wedge may be used in the soft liner.

Supracondylar-suprapatellar suspension encloses the patella in the socket and has a bar proximal to the patella. This design also provides medial-lateral stability, and no additional cuffs or straps are required. Corset-type prostheses can lead to verrucous hyperplasia and thigh atrophy but reduce socket loads, control the direction of swing, and provide some additional weight support.

b. Transfemoral Suspension—Suction suspension is frequently used. This is effected by **surface tension, negative pressure,** and **muscle contraction.** A one-way expulsion valve helps maintain negative pressure and no belts or straps are required. **Stable body weight** is required for this intimate fit. Roll on silicone liners may be used with or without locking pins. The **total elastic suspension** belt, made of neoprene, fastens around the waist and spreads over a larger surface area (Fig. 9–12). It is an excellent auxiliary suspension. **Silesian belts** are used to prevent **socket rotation** in limbs with redundant tissue. Such belts also prevent the socket from slipping off when suction sockets are fitted to short transfemoral stumps and the patient sits.

c. Transfemoral Sockets—Quadrilateral sockets wherein the posterior brim provides a shelf for the ischial tuberosity have been the classic. The design made it difficult to keep the femur in adduction. **Ischial containment** (narrower medial-lateral designs) sockets distribute the proximal and medial concentration of forces more evenly as well as enhance socket rotational control (Fig. 9–13). The ischium and ramus are contained within the socket of these more anatomic, comfortable, and functional designs. Socket design for transfemoral prosthesis allows **for 10 degrees of adduction** of the femur (to stretch the gluteus medius, allowing adequate strength for midstance stability) **and 5 degrees of flexion** (to stretch the gluteus maximus and allow for greater hip extension).

d. Transtibial Sockets—Patella tendon bearing loads all areas of the residual

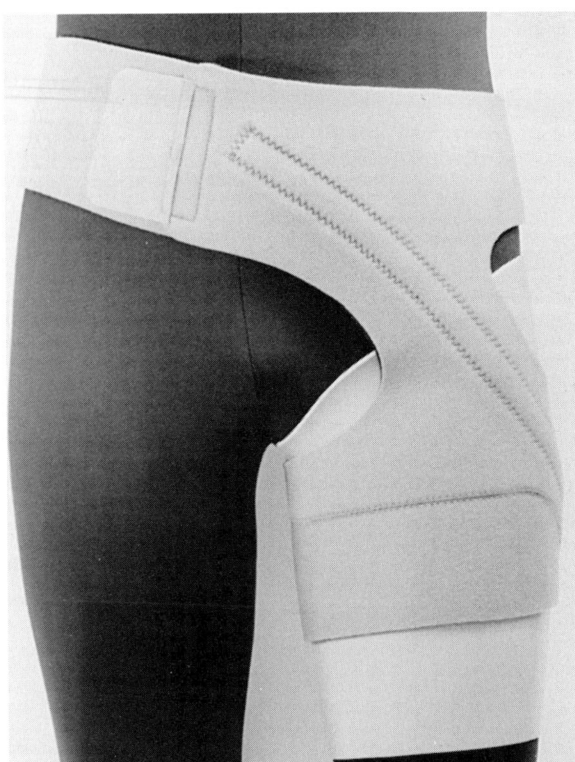

Figure 9–12. Total elastic suspension belt for suspending a transfemoral socket. (Courtesy of Syncor Manufacturers, Green Bay, WI.)

limb that are **weight tolerant** (i.e., patella tendon, medial tibial flare, anterior compartment, gastrocnemius, and fibular shaft). The anterior wedge shape of the socket helps control rotation of the socket on the limb. **Weight intolerant** areas include tibial crest and tubercle, distal fibula and fibular head, peroneal nerve, and hamstring tendons. The patellar tendon bearing supracondylar/suprapatellar socket has proximal extensions over the distal femoral condyles and over the patella.

Total surface bearing is different from total contact, in which different areas have different loads. With total surface bearing, pressure is distributed more equally across the entire surface of the transtibial residual limb and the interface liner material in the socket is important. Urethane liners cope with multidirectional forces by easy material distortion and recovery to original shape. Another liner is made of mineral oil gel with reinforcing fabric. These liners provide good shock-absorbing abilities and reduce skin problems.

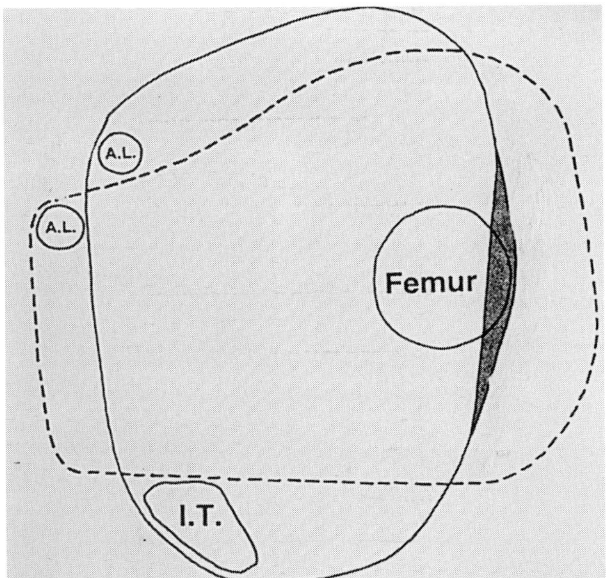

Figure 9–13. Comparison of AKA sockets. Note inclusion of the ischial tuberosity and narrow medial-lateral design of newer CAT-CAM socket shown in solid line. (From Sabolich J.: Contoured adducted trochanteric controlled alignment method. Clin. Prosthet. Orthop. 9:13–17, 1985.)

6. Common Prosthetic Problems
   a. Transtibial—Pistoning during **swing phase** of gait is usually caused by an **ineffective suspension system**. Pistoning in the **stance phase** is due to poor **socket fit** or volume changes in the stump (may require a change in stump sock thickness). Alignment problems are common and are listed in Table 9–5. Pressure-related pain or redness should be corrected with relief of the prosthesis in the affected area. Other problems may be related to the foot—**too soft a foot results in excessive knee extension,** whereas **too hard a foot causes knee flexion and lateral rotation of the toes.**
   b. Transfemoral—Excessive prosthetic length and weak hip abductors or flexors can lead to circumduction, vaulting, and lateral trunk bending. Hip flexion contractures and insufficient anterior socket support can lead to excessive lumbar lordosis (compensatory). Inadequate prosthetic knee flexion can lead to terminal

Table 9–5.

Prosthetic Foot Gait Abnormalities

Foot Position	Gait Abnormality
Inset	Varus strain, pain (proximedial, distolateral), circumduction
Outset	Valgus strain, pain (proxilateral, distomedial), broad-based gait
Forward placement	Increased knee extension (patellar pain) but stable
Posterior placement	Increased knee flexion/instability
Dorsiflexed foot	Increased patellar pressure
Plantar-flexed foot	Drop off, patellar pressure

knee snap. Medial whip (heel in, heel out) can be caused by a varus knee, excessive external rotation of the knee axis, or muscle weakness. Lateral whip (heel out, heel in) is caused by the opposite (valgus knee, internal rotation at knee, and weakness). Table 9–6 summarizes common transfemoral prosthetic gait problems.

c. Stair Climbing—In general, amputees climb stairs by leading with their normal limb and descend by leading with their prosthetic limb ("the good goes up and the bad comes down").

IV. **Orthoses**

A. Introduction—The primary function of an orthosis is control of motion of certain body segments. Orthoses are used to protect long bones or unstable joints, support flexible deformities, and occasionally substitute for a functional task. Orthoses can be static, dynamic, or a combination. **With few exceptions, orthoses are not indicated for correction of fixed deformities or for spastic deformities that cannot be easily controlled manually.** Orthoses are named according to the joint(s) they control and the method used to obtain/maintain that control (e.g., a short-leg, below-the-knee brace is an ankle-foot orthosis, abbreviated AFO).

B. Shoes—Specific shoewear can be used by themselves or in conjunction with foot orthoses. Extra-depth shoes with a high toe box to dissipate local pressures over bony prominences are recommended for diabetic patients. The plantar surface of an insensate foot is protected by use of a pressure-dissipating material. A paralytic or flexible foot deformity can be controlled with more rigid orthotics. SACH heels absorb the shock of initial loading and lessen the transmission of force to the midfoot as the foot passes through the stance phase. A rocker sole can lessen the bending forces on an arthritic or stiff midfoot during midstance as the foot changes from accepting the weight-bearing load to pushing off. It is useful in treating metatarsalgia, hallux rigidus, and other forefoot problems. For the rocker sole to be effective, it must be rigid.

C. **Medial heel outflare** is used to treat severe flat foot of most causes. A foot orthosis is also necessary. Most foot orthoses are used to
1. Align and support the foot,
2. Prevent, correct, or accommodate foot deformities, and
3. Improve foot function.

Three main types of foot orthoses are used: rigid, semi-rigid, and soft. Rigid foot orthoses limit joint motion and stabilize flexible deformities. **Soft orthoses** have best shock-absorbing ability and are used to accommodate fixed deformities of the feet, especially neuropathic, dysvascular, and ulcerative disorders.

D. Ankle-Foot Orthosis (AFO)—This most commonly prescribed lower limb orthosis acts to control the ankle joint. It may be fabricated with metal bars attached to the shoe or thermoplastic elastomer. The orthosis may be rigid, preventing ankle motion, or it can allow free or spring-assisted motion in either plane.

After hindfoot fusions, the primary orthotic goals are absorption of the ground reaction forces, protection of the fusion sites, and protection of the midfoot. The thermoplastic foot section achieves medial-lateral control with high trimlines. When subtalar motion is present, an **articulating AFO** permits motion by a mechanical ankle joint design. Primary factors in **orthotic joint selection** include range of motion, durability, adjustability, and **biomechanical implication** on knee joint. A posterior leaf spring AFO provides stance phase stability for ankle instability in **stance phase.**

E. Knee-Ankle-Foot Orthosis (KAFO)—This orthosis extends from the upper thigh to the foot. It is generally used to control an unstable or paralyzed knee joint. It provides mediolateral stability with prescribed amounts of flexion or extension control. A subset of KAFOs are designated KOs. Knee orthoses can be made of elastic for treatment of patellar pathology or of metal and plastic in the case of anterior cruciate ligament instability.

F. Hip-Knee-Ankle-Foot Orthosis (HKAFO)—This orthosis provides hip and pelvic stability but is rarely used for the adult paraplegic because of the cumbersome nature of the orthosis and the magnitude of effort in achieving minimal gains. Experimentally, it is being used in conjunction with implanted electrodes and computerized functional stimulation of paraplegics. In children with upper-level lumbar myelome-

Table 9–6.

Prosthetic Gait Abnormalities

Gait Abnormality	Prosthetic Problem
Lateral trunk bending	Short prosthesis, weak abductors, poor fit
Abducted gait	Poor socket fit medially
Circumducted gait	Prosthetic too long, excess knee friction
Vaulted gait	Prosthetic too long, poor suspension
Foot rotation at heel strike	Heel too stiff, loose socket
Short stance phase	Painful stump, knee too loose
Knee instability	Knee too anterior, foot too stiff
Medial/lateral whip	Excessive knee rotation, tight socket
Terminal snap	Quadricep weakness, insecure patient
Foot slap, knee hyperextension	Heel too soft
Knee flexion	Heel too hard
Excessive lordosis	Hip flexion contracture, socket problems

ningocele, the reciprocating gait orthoses are modified HKAFOs that can be used for standing and simulated walking.

G. Elbow Orthoses—Hinged elbow orthoses provide minimal stability in the treatment of ligament instabilities. Dynamic spring-loaded orthoses have been successfully used in the treatment of flexion or extension contracture.

H. Wrist and Hand Orthoses (WHO)—The most common use of wrist and hand orthoses today is for postoperative care after injury or reconstructive surgery. These devices are static or dynamic. The opponens splint is successful in pre-positioning the thumb but impairs tactile sensation. Wrist-driven hand orthoses are used in lower cervical quadriplegics. They may be body-powered by tenodesis action or motor-driven. Weight and cumbersomeness are the major limiting factors.

I. Fracture Braces—Fracture bracing remains a valuable treatment option for isolated fractures of the tibia and fibula. Prefabricated fracture orthoses can be used in simple foot and ankle fractures, ankle sprains, and simple hand injuries.

J. Pediatric Orthoses—Many dynamic orthoses are used in children to control motion without total immobilization. The Pavlik harness has become the mainstay for early treatment of developmental dislocation of the hip. Several dynamic orthoses have been used for containment in Perthes' disease.

K. Spine
   1. Cervical Spine—Numerous orthoses are used to immobilize the cervical spine. Effective immobilization ranges from the various types of collars, to posted orthoses that gain purchase about the shoulders and under the chin, to the halo vest, which achieves the most stability by the nature of its fixation into the skull.
   2. Thoracolumbar—Orthoses used for stabilizing mechanical back pain rely on increasing body cavity pressure. Three-point orthoses achieve their control by the length of their lever arm and the subsequent limitation of motion.

V. **Surgery for Stroke and Closed Head Injury**—The orthopaedic surgeon can play a role in the early management of adult-acquired spasticity secondary to stroke or closed head injury when the spasticity interferes with the rehabilitation program. Interventional modalities may include orthotic prescription, serial casting, or motor point nerve blocks with short-acting (bupivacaine HCl) or long-acting (phenol 3–4% in glycerol) agents. Splinting a joint (e.g., the ankle) at neutral is not sufficient to prevent the development of a contracture (e.g., an equinus contracture). When functional joint ranging is insufficient to control deformity, intervention is often indicated. Anesthetic nerve blocks of the posterior tibial or sciatic nerve prior to casting relieves pain and allows for maximum correction of the deformity. Open nerve blocks may be warranted to avoid injecting mixed nerves with large sensory contributions. Surgical intervention in adult-acquired spasticity is delayed until the patient **achieves maximum spontaneous motor recovery (6 months for stroke and 12–18 months for traumatic brain injury).** When patients reach a plateau in functional progress or when their deformity impedes further progress, intervention may be considered. Invasive procedures in this population should be an adjunct to a standard functional rehabilitation program, not an alternative. When surgery is considered for the goal of improving function, patients should be **screened for**

   a. Cognitive deficits,
   b. Motivation, and
   c. Body image awareness.

   Patients should not be confused and must have adequate short-term memory and the capacity for new learning. In addition to specific cognitive strengths, motivation is necessary for patients to utilize functional gains and participate in their rehabilitation program. Body image awareness is essential for surgical intervention to become meaningful and potentially beneficial. Patients who lack the awareness of a limb or its position in space should undergo therapy directed toward improving these deficits before embarking on surgical intervention.

A. Lower Limb—Balance is the best predictor of a patient's ability to ambulate after acquired brain injury. The mainstay of treatment for the dynamic ankle equinus component of this gait deviation is to achieve ankle stability in neutral position during initial floor contact (i.e., heel strike and stance) as well as floor clearance during swing phase. An adjustable AFO with **ankle dorsiflexion and a plantar flexion stop** at neutral is often used during the recovery period, followed by a rigid AFO once the patient has plateaued in recovery. When the dynamic equinus overpowers the holding power of the orthosis and patients "walk out" of their brace, motor balancing surgery is indicated. The **equinus deformity is treated** by percutaneous tendoachilles lengthening. The dynamic varus-producing force in adults is the result of out-of-phase tibialis anterior muscle activity during the stance phase. This dynamic varus deformity is corrected by either **split or complete lateral transfer** of the tibialis anterior muscle.

B. Upper Limb—There is a paucity of literature dealing with acquired spasticity in the upper limb. Invasive intervention can be considered for functional and nonfunctional goals. Surgical release of static contracture is generally performed to assist nursing care or hygiene when the fixed contracture and/or spastic component produces skin maceration or breakdown. A functional use of static contracture release is to improve upper-extremity "tracking" (i.e., arm

10

Adult Trauma

Gregory S. Motley, Tally H. Eddings III,
Richard S. Moore, Jr., and Paul T. Freudigman

I. Introduction—The recent advent of trauma as an orthopaedic subspecialty has brought with it a dramatic increase in our understanding and management of severely injured patients. Advancements have been made in the management of not only the fracture but also the surrounding soft tissues. Controversies surrounding the management of these injuries are noted but not discussed. Every attempt has been made to focus on information relevant to the needs of residents preparing for examinations and the practicing orthopaedist looking for information to add to an already expanding knowledge base.

A. Fracture Description—Fractures are classified according to description or to mechanism of injury. Description of fractures includes location, direction, displacement, and angulation. It also includes the condition of the surrounding soft tissues (open vs. closed) and the involvement of the articular surface. The mechanism of injury is important in the ultimate management of fractures and is commonly used to classify injuries to the ankle, pelvis, and spine.

1. Open Fractures—Open fractures, by definition, communicate through a traumatic wound to the surrounding environment. Therefore, contamination and soft tissue envelope disruption mandate that these injuries be handled with special consideration. Tetanus prophylaxis is routinely administered on presentation. Formal irrigation and débridement within 4 to 8 hours of injury and the administration of appropriate antibiotics are necessary for a successful outcome. A first-generation cephalosporin (low-energy wounds) with an aminoglycoside (high-energy wounds) is the most common regimen. Penicillin is added to "barnyard" injuries and those injuries grossly contaminated with dirt to cover possible *Clostridium* infection. Management also includes stabilization of fractures and soft tissues, prevention of infection, early soft tissue coverage (within 5 days), union of fractures, and return to function. The most important aspect of treatment of open fractures is the emergent débridement in the operating room. Débridement of contaminated, nonviable, necrotic bone and soft tissue is imperative. Stabilization of bone and soft tissues allows maintenance of alignment and length, and reduction of dead space, improves venous and lymphatic return, and thereby provides local host defense against infection. Repeat débridements should be repeated every 48 to 72 hours until definitive skeletal stabilization coincides with adequate soft tissue coverage and closure. Operative cultures of deep tissues taken at the time of débridement provide identification of late infecting organisms up to 60% of the time but usually do not alter the initial clinical management of the injury. Therefore, operative cultures are not mandatory.

2. Classification—Described by Gustilo, this classification is based on the size of the wound and the amount of soft tissue injury present.

Type	Size (cm)	Other Factors
I	<1	Low energy
II	<10	Moderate energy
III	>10	High energy; high-velocity gunshot wounds, close range shotgun wounds, barnyard injuries, segmental fractures, neurovascular injury, open >8 hours

B. Gunshot Wounds (GSWs)—Soft tissue and bony destruction is based on the velocity of the missile (KE = ½ mv). Low-velocity GSWs (<2000 ft/sec—most handguns) cause less soft tissue destruction, and treatment usually consists of entry/exit wound débridement. High-velocity GSWs (>2000 ft/sec—military rifles) can cause massive soft tissue destruction and require two-stage débridement of the entire missile tract. Partially jacketed (dum-dum), unjacketed, and hollow-point bullets cause greater soft tissue destruction. Shotgun wounds, especially at short range, often result in type III wounds because of extensive soft tissue injury. The wadding has a

Subclass	Description
IIIA	Adequate soft tissue coverage
IIIB	Massive soft tissue destruction, bony exposure
IIIC	Fractures associated with repairable vascular injury

high potential for contamination of wounds and must be sought at the time of débridement. Intra-articular missiles should be removed because of the potential for lead intoxication and the certainty of continued articular damage. Nerve injuries associated with GSWs are often temporary (neurapraxia) and are caused by the blast effect of missiles traversing the tissue. Arterial injuries may present as decreased or absent pulses, an expanding hematoma, a thrill, or massive blood loss. Arteriograms should be used liberally if there is any question of an arterial injury.

C. Advanced Trauma Life Support (ATLS)—Protocols should be followed during the evaluation of all major trauma victims with orthopaedic injuries. The treatment of orthopaedic injuries follows adequate stabilization of the patient (life before limb). The trauma score, which is based on respiratory, cardiovascular, and neurologic parameters, is predictive of injury severity and prognosis. The most common abdominal injury is rupture of the spleen, followed by liver injury. Pericardial tamponade should be suspected with a narrow pulse pressure and an elevated diastolic blood pressure. Intravenous pyelography is indicated for gross hematuria only. Head injuries are the most common cause of early death with trauma (Glasgow Coma Scale score < 8). Blood loss of 1500 mL or 30% of blood volume usually results in hypotension and tachycardia with decreased urine output. Treatment includes aggressive fluid administration (crystalloid and blood) as needed. Response to adequate volume replacement is seen with a resumption of adequate urine output. Disseminated intravascular coagulation causes diffuse bleeding and is multifactorial in origin. Treatment consists of identifying and treating all possible causes and replacement of blood factors as needed. The most common thoracic injury is rib fractures. Flail chest is caused by multilevel segmental rib fractures and results in paradoxical chest wall motion. Hemo/pneumothoraces result in an alteration of normal ventilation and perfusion of lung parenchyma and are clinically diagnosed with decreased breath sounds over the affected lung field. Treatment includes immediate chest tube thoracostomy. Pulmonary emboli occur most frequently on the fifth hospital day. Aggressive prophylaxis including pneumatic devices, low molecular weight heparin, and warfarin has decreased the overall incidence of this problem. Umbrella filters are an option in high-risk cases when anticoagulation cannot be done. Fat embolism typically occurs after pelvic or femur fracture, with clinical symptoms 24 to 72 hours after the inciting event. Symptoms include hypoxia, confusion, tachycardia, and petechiae. Treatment consists of supportive pulmonary care and monitoring. In its severe form, it can lead to acute respiratory distress syndrome. This results in significantly decreased lung compliance with poor oxygen and carbon dioxide exchange. Studies suggest that early stabilization of long bone fractures significantly reduces pulmonary complications, intensive care unit stay, and overall hospital stay.

D. General Principles—Reduction of grossly angulated fractures and dislocations is recommended as soon as possible. Immobilization is then employed to prevent displacement of angulation, to decrease movement at the fracture site, and to relieve pain. The goal of all orthopaedic treatment is to restore function. Fracture healing requires an adequate vascular supply, minimal necrosis, anatomic reduction, immobilization, the presence of physiologic stress, and the absence of infection.

E. Complications—Bone healing abnormalities, infection, soft tissue injuries, and bleeding, pulmonary, gastrointestinal, neurologic, and other disorders. Each injury is unique and results in unique complications.

1. Bone Healing Abnormalities—Include delayed union and nonunion, malunion, and avascular necrosis.
   a. Delayed Union—Can be thought of as fractures that still allow free movement of bone ends at 3 to 4 months after injury.
   b. Nonunion—Usually defined as no radiographic evidence of union with clinical motion and pain 6 months after injury. Each fracture has its own expected time to union (femoral neck nonunion defined at 12 months after injury) and therefore a unique time to the definition of nonunion. Too much or too little motion at the fracture site, excessive space between fracture fragments, inadequate fixation, infection, soft tissue interposition, inadequate blood supply, and many other factors can lead to delay in bone healing. Nonunions are classified as hypervascular (hypertrophic) or avascular (atrophic) based on their capability of biologic reaction (vitality of the bone ends) and are classified according to Weber and Chech (Fig. 10–1). Treatment is directed at correction of the cause of the nonunion, if possible, and includes stabilization of bone ends, eradication of infection, restoration of blood supply, surgical excision of interposing tissues, and bone grafting of fracture gaps. Bone grafting is recommended at the time of internal fixation for fractures with comminution in-

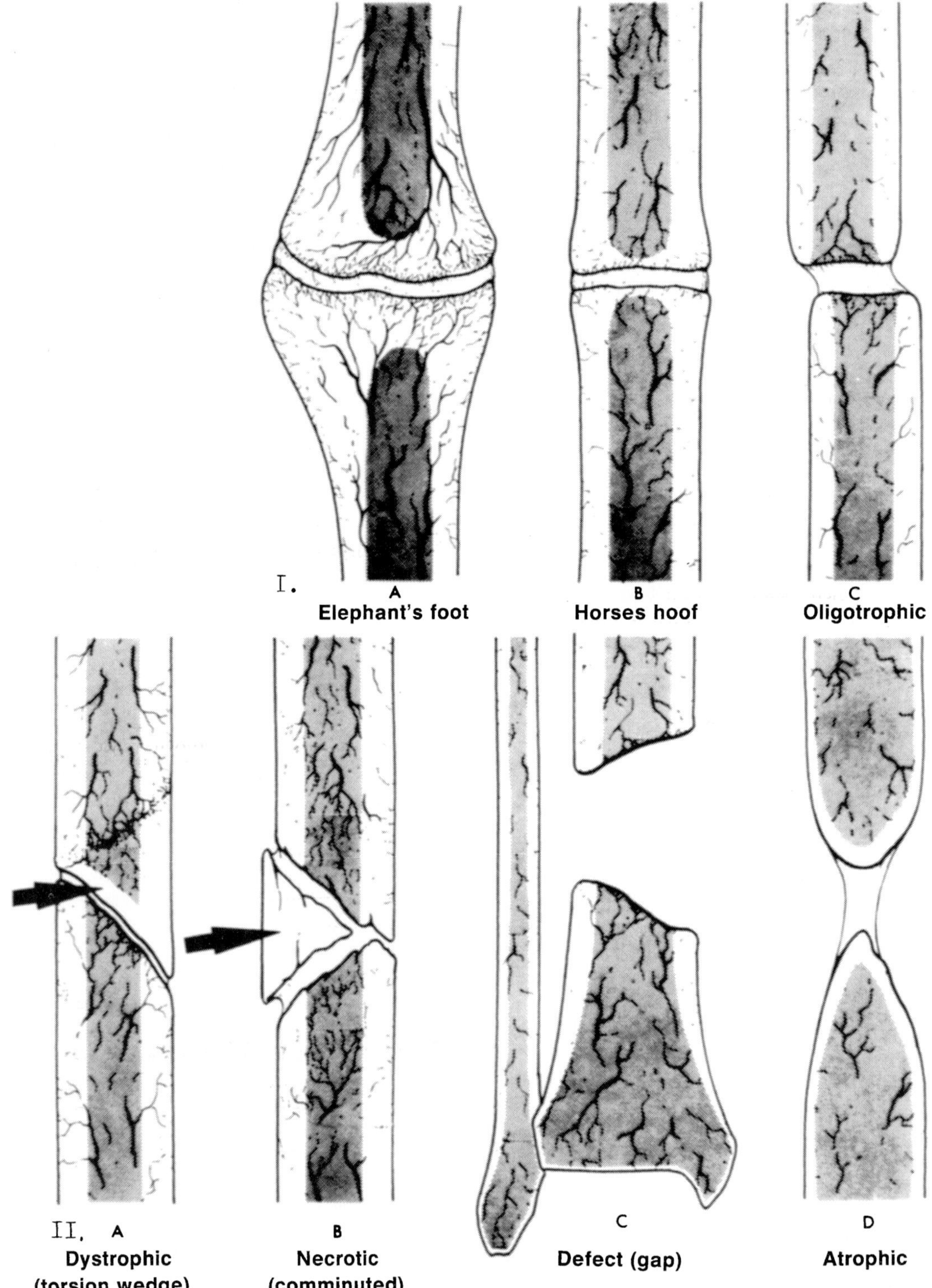

Figure 10–1. Types of nonunion. I—Hypervascular: *A,* Elephant foot. *B,* Horse hoof. *C,* Oligotrophic. II—Avascular: *A,* Torsion wedge. *B,* Comminuted. *C,* Defect. *D,* Atrophic. (From Weber, B.G., and Brunner, C.: The treatment of nonunions without electrical stimulation. Clin. Orthop. 161:25, 1981.)

volving more than one third of the diameter of the bone.

c. Malunion—Bony healing in an unacceptable position in any plane. Initial fracture care is critical in avoidance of this problem. Treatment is directed at correcting the anatomic abnormality.

d. Avascular Necrosis—Caused by the disruption of the blood supply and can lead to nonunion, osteoarthritis, collapse, and other problems. It is more common with intra-articular fractures, especially of the femoral head/neck, femoral condyles, proximal scaphoid, proximal humerus, and talar neck.

2. Infection—A common complication that occurs with the treatment of both open and closed fractures. Infection involving the bone (osteomyelitis) can be acute or chronic. Infected nonunions can be considered chronic, and treatment is based on complete removal of all infected, nonviable bone following the principles of "tumor" surgery with later reconstruction. Acute osteomyelitis is usually hematogenous in origin and occurs in the pediatric population with the greatest frequency.
3. Soft Tissue Injuries—Include direct injuries to vessels, nerves, muscles, and skin envelope.
   a. Arterial Injuries—Require a high index of suspicion for prompt diagnosis and treatment to ensure a successful outcome. Arteriograms should be ordered if any doubt of injury exists. Repair should be performed within 6 hours after injury. Concomitant fasciotomies are usually required.
   b. Compartment Syndrome—Occurs when end-capillary perfusion pressure is less than intracompartmental pressure. Pain is the earliest and most reliable indication of the onset of a compartment syndrome and occurs with passive stretch of muscles traversing the involved compartment. Patients unable to verbalize pain should have compartment pressures measured when appropriate. Pressures greater than 30 mm Hg or within 10 to 30 mm Hg of the diastolic blood pressure require treatment (fasciotomies).
   c. Nerve Injuries—Most often associated with fractures and fortunately are infrequent complications. Examples include sciatic nerve injuries associated with posterior fracture dislocations of the acetabulum and common peroneal injuries associated with proximal fibular fractures, among many others. Most injuries are neurapraxias from stretch, and 70% resolve spontaneously.
4. Pulmonary Complications—Adult respiratory distress syndrome, fat emboli syndrome and pulmonary embolism are discussed in the ATLS section.
5. Bleeding Disorders—Include excessive bleeding, shock, and disseminated intravascular coagulation. Shock is a manifestation of decreased blood flow to the tissues and may present as tachycardia, oliguria, and pale cool extremities. Treatment includes immediate infusion of whole blood, intravenous fluids, and avoidance of albumin. Disseminated intravascular coagulation is caused by microvascular thrombi that consume platelets, initiating a vicious cycle. Laboratory values show decreased antithrombin III and fibrinogen and increased prothrombin and partial thromboplastin times and fibrin split products. Deep muscle hematomas can compress neurovascular structures (iliacus hematoma resulting in femoral nerve compression).
6. Gastrointestinal Complications—Usually the result of blunt abdominal trauma. The most common solid organ injured is the spleen, followed by the liver. Stress ulcers also occur and can be prevented and treated with appropriate H2 blockers. Cast syndrome is a result of compression of the second portion of the duodenum and decreased blood flow through the superior mesenteric artery resulting in bowel ischemia/necrosis. This presents as clinical signs of small bowel obstruction.
7. Other Complications—Included are complex pain syndrome, myositis ossificans, and post-traumatic osteoarthritis. Pain, swelling, discoloration, stiffness, dysesthesias, and temperature abnormalities characterize complex pain syndrome (reflex sympathetic dystrophy). Initial treatment is mobilization of the extremity with organized physical therapy. Other chemotherapeutic regimens are needed if physical therapy fails and include sympathetic blocks. Myositis ossificans can follow injuries with large hematomas and is most common in patients who suffer both elbow fracture/dislocations and traumatic brain injuries (near 100%). It is also seen after extensile exposures to the acetabulum. Post-traumatic arthritis is common after intra-articular fractures if anatomic reductions are not achieved.

F. Soft Tissue Trauma
1. Snake Bites—Can cause extensive soft tissue destruction and may lead to compartment syndrome. Venomous snakes are most commonly pit vipers. These snakes have a triangular head and a pit below their eyes. Elapids are less common, but their venom includes hemotoxins, cytotoxins, and neurotoxins. Systemic symptoms can be severe. Signs include swelling, ecchymosis, and bullae formation.
   a. Treatment—First aid (tourniquet and suction) and hospitalization. Monitoring, use of antibiotics, checking compartment pressures, and administration of antivenin are appropriate. At least five bottles of antivenin are required for a moderate-sized bite, and this treatment can cause serum sickness (sometimes requiring systemic corticosteroids). Fasciotomies are sometimes needed for compartment syndrome.
2. Thermal Injuries—Freezing injuries are the most common cause of bilateral upper- and lower-extremity amputations. Injury may be direct (freezing of tissues with ice crystals in

the extracellular space) or indirect (vascular damage).

   a. Treatment—Based on restoring core body temperature, rapid rewarming of the extremity, débridement, physical therapy, and sometimes anticoagulation and sympathectomy. Psychosocial factors often are important.

3. Heat Injuries—Burns require close management. Treatment is based on burn depth.
   a. Epidermis—Edema, erythema: symptomatic care
   b. Dermis—Blisters, blanching: topical antibiotic, splint, range of motion exercises
   c. Subcutaneous—Waxy, dry: excision, split-thickness skin grafting
   d. Deep—Exposed tissue: amputation, flap, reconstruction
      (1) Burns can also result in compartment syndrome and sometimes require escharotomy/fasciotomy. Contractures are common and often require plasties or releases. Infection is also common.
4. Electrical Injuries—Ignition (burns at site of direct contact), conductant (tunnels along neurovascular structures; number one cause of bilateral high upper-extremity amputations), and arc (high-voltage current jumps across flexor surfaces of joints, leading to late contractures). AC current is more dangerous than DC current. Current density zones resulting from electrical burns are **charred** (unrecognizable tissue), **gray-white** (tissue necrosis), and **red** (thrombosis).
   a. Treatment—Initial débridement of all necrotic muscle and tissue fasciotomy, second-look débridement (at 2 to 3 days), and, finally, definitive flap coverage or amputation. Acute amputation may be required.
5. Chemical Burns—Follow exposure to noxious agents. Severity is based on concentration, duration of contact, penetrability, amount, and mechanism of injury. The mainstay of treatment is copious irrigation. Hydrofluoric acid burns can be successfully treated with calcium gluconate. White phosphorus burns are treated with a 1% copper sulfate solution.
6. Chemotherapeutic Extravasation—Early débridement and secondary coverage is important to reduce the high risk of soft tissue and skin necrosis.
7. High-Pressure Injection Injuries—Occur from accidental injection from paint or grease guns. They usually involve the hand (paint gun injuries are more common and severe because they lead to soft tissue necrosis; grease gun injuries cause fibrosis). A seemingly innocuous entry wound may cover an area of extensive soft tissue destruction. Treatment includes intravenous antibiotics, thorough I&D, and occasionally corticosteroids.

II. Spinal Cord Injuries (SCIs)—Motor vehicle accidents, falls, diving accidents, sports, and GSWs are the usual causes. Young male adults are affected most often. C-spine protection is always needed in the polytrauma patient. Injury level equals the lowest motor and sensory level with normal function. (C6 quad equals normal cervical sixth nerve root function, at least 4/5 motor.) Individual motor and sensory functions must be known at each level. (C7 quad will be able to perform transfers, etc.) SCIs are either **complete**—no function after spinal shock—or **incomplete**—varying patterns with sacral sensory sparing. Spinal shock occurs immediately after SCI, resulting in flaccid paralysis, hypotonia, and areflexia. During this period the bulbocavernosus reflex (BCR) is absent. After BCR returns, spasticity, hyperreflexia, and clonus occur. BCR returns in less than 90% of patients in less than 48 hours and in 100% after 48 hours. If there is no BCR return, then conus medullary injury is ruled out. **Neurogenic** shock results from loss of autonomic reflexes with hypotension and bradycardia and is treated with invasive monitoring, fluids, and vasopressors. Neurogenic shock and hypovolemic shock may coexist, and this possibility must be ruled out. **Autonomic reflexia** presents in SCI patients as headache, sweating, blurred vision, or hypertension and is treated by removing the cause (catheterization of bladder or digital rectal disimpaction). *Initial neurologic examination* is the most sensitive tool in diagnosis, and serial examinations are mandatory to determine treatment plans. The American Spinal Injury Association (ASIA) was formed in 1992 to set standards on systematic neurologic examination.

   A. Frankel Classification—Five broad-based categories have been used in the past 25 years to compare different treatments and are still used by many today.
   B. Syndromes—**Incomplete syndromes** maintain some level of function and potential for partial recovery. See Table 10–1. **Central cord syndrome** is most common and usually occurs from extension in elderly with some pre-existing stenosis. Upper extremities are more affected than lower extremities, and perianal sensation is preserved. **Anterior cord syndrome** is less common and usually occurs from flexion/compression mechanism. Lower extremities are more motor affected than upper extremities, and posterior column sensory pathways are preserved. This syndrome has the worst prognosis. **Brown-Séquard syndrome** is due to ipsilateral penetrating injury and results in ipsilateral motor and contralateral pain and temperature loss. It has the best prognosis for segmental recovery. **Posterior cord syndrome** is rare, with preservation of motor function and loss of sensory function. **Single root injury** is associated with compres-

Table 10–1.

Spinal Cord Injury Syndromes

Syndrome	Pathology	Characteristics	Prognosis
Central	Age >50, extension injuries	Affects upper > lower extremities, motor and sensory loss	Fair
Anterior	Flexion-compression (vertebral A)	Incomplete motor and some sensory loss	Poor
Brown-Séquard	Penetrating trauma	Loss of ipsilateral motor function, contralateral pain and temperature sensation	Best
Root	Foramina compression/herniated nucleus pulposus	Based on level—weakness	Good
Complete	Burst/canal compression	No function below injury level	Poor

sion fracture, burst fracture, or herniated nucleus pulposus.

C. Treatment—Treatment of any spine injury requires C-spine immobilization and good trauma radiologic series (Table 10–2). The C7–T1 junction must be seen (10% of C-spine fractures are at C7–T1). A lateral view will detect 85% of C-spine injuries. Initial skeletal traction is 5 to 10 pounds with follow-up radiograph. Appropriate anatomic pin placement is important to prevent complications to local neurovascular structures. If no overdistraction is present, then additional weight at 5 pounds per level is used for stabilization and reduction. Unstable injuries require operative decompression, reduction, and stabilization. Anterior, posterior, and combined approaches are selected based on the injury pattern, neurologic involvement, and degree of instability. Anterior decompression for incomplete SCI can improve neurologic outcome even as late as 1 year after injury. Acute management also includes methylprednisolone, 30 mg/kg initially within 8 hours and for 23 hours at 5.4 mg/kg, is standard protocol.

Laminectomies are contraindicated unless associated with lamina fracture and dural tear. GSWs to the spinal cord and spine are treated nonoperatively unless there is direct passage through the esophagus or colon or there is progressive neurologic deterioration with proven neurologic compression with either bullet, bony fragments, or hematoma.

III. Spine Fractures

A. Upper Cervical Fractures

1. Occipital Condyle Fracture—Three types occur:

Type I impaction fracture from axial loading
Type II basilar skull fracture from direct blow
Type III avulsion fracture from rotation or lateral bending

Types I and II are usually stable and treated with rigid orthosis. Unstable types I/II and type III injuries are treated with halo or occipitocervical fusion.

2. Atlanto-occipital Dislocation—A rare and usually fatal injury, it occurs by hyperextension, rotation, translation, and/or distraction. Classification is either anterior, posterior, or longitudinal based on lateral radiography. Radiographic evaluation of Wackenheim's line and Power's ratio are used to diagnose and follow treatment. Treatment is with early occipital cervical fusion and fixation and postoperative halo stabilization.

3. C1 Atlas Fracture—Axial load injury creates three injury patterns based on position of head at impact:

Axial + extension = posterior fracture. This is usually stable and is treated with a rigid orthosis.
Axial + flexion = anterior fracture. Treatment is with halo stabilization for 8 weeks and posterior spinal fusion if there is residual atlantoaxial subluxation.
Isolated axial load = Jefferson fracture. This has combined anterior and posterior fractures of the ring and/or lateral mass fractures.

Fracture stability is determined by lateral mass spreading. If this is more than 7 mm, then the transverse ligament is torn, making this an unstable fracture. Treatment is with halo traction for reduction. C1-C2 fusion is used for malunion, nonunion, or atlantoaxial instability greater than 5 mm (Fig. 10–2).

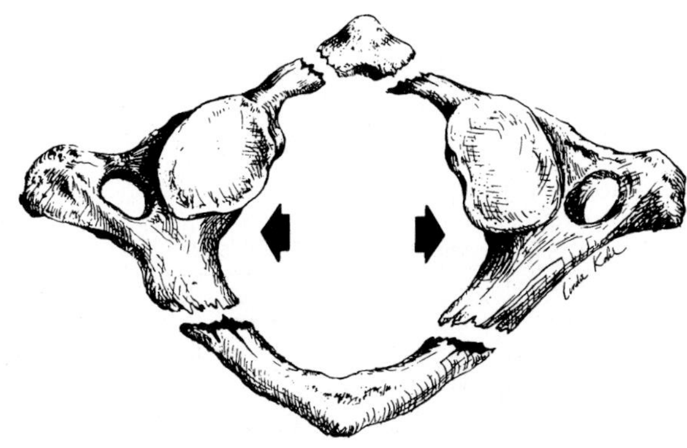

Figure 10–2. Jefferson fracture. (From Urbaniak, J.R.: Fractures of the spine. In Sabiston, D.C., Jr., ed.: Davis-Christopher Textbook of Surgery, p. 1528. Philadelphia, WB Saunders, 1977.)

Table 10–2.

Special Radiographic Views for Specific Injuries

Injury/Location	Eponym/ Description	Technique
Hand and Wrist		
Hand injuries		AP/lateral/oblique, digit: dental film
Fourth and fifth metacarpal	Reverse oblique	Hand placed 45 degrees tilted
Metacarpal head	Brewerton	30 degrees pronated from full supination
Gamekeeper's thumb	Robert	Stress view (with anesthesia); AP hypersupinated (dorsum on cassette)
First metacarpal-trapezium	Burnam	Robert with 15-degree cephalic tilt
Hamate hook/CT	CT view	Tangential through carpal tunnel
Dorsal carpal chip	Dorsal tangential	Tangential of dorsal carpus
Wrist—ulnar variation	Zero rotation	AP, shoulder and elbow at 90 degrees
Carpal instability	Motion	Cineradiography
Radial wrist	Pronation oblique	AP with 45 degrees' pronation
Ulnar wrist	Bura	Superior oblique; AP with 35 degrees' supination
Scaphoid	Series	PA/lateral/oblique fist, PA in ulnar deviation
Forearm and Elbow		
Forearm	Tuberosity	AP elbow with 20 degree tilt to olecranon
Radial head		45 degree lateral of elbow, magnification
Elbow		Check fat pad, anterior humeral line, radius-capitellum
Elbow contracture	AP/lateral	AP humerus, AP forearm
Shoulder		
Shoulder	Trauma	True AP (scapula—45 degrees oblique), scapular lateral (Y)
Shoulder	Axillary lateral	Through axilla with arm abducted
Tuberosities	AP ER/IR	AP with arm in full extension and internal rotation
Impingement	Caudal tilt	AP with 30 degree caudal tilt
Impingement	Supraspinatus outlet	Scapula lateral with 10 degree caudal tilt
Hill-Sachs	Stryker notch	Supine, hand on head, 10 degree cephalic tilt
Bankart	West Point	Prone axillary lateral with 25 degree lateral and posterior tilt
Bankart	Garth	Apical oblique with 45 degree caudal and AP tilt
Acromion injury	Stress	AP both acromions (large cassette) with 10 pounds hanging weight
Acromion injury	Alexander	Scapular lateral with shoulders forward
Acromion arthritis	Zanca	10 degree cephalic tilt of acromion
Spinal cord injury	Hobbs	PA, patient leans over cassette
Spinal cord injury	Serendipity	40 degree cephalic tilt center on manubrium
Clavicle		AP 30 degree cephalic tilt
Spine		
C-spine	Series	AP/lateral/oblique, open-mouth odontoid
C7	Swimmers' view	Lateral through maximally abducted arm
Instability	Flexion/extension	AP with flexion and extension
L-spine	Series	AP/lateral/oblique (foramina), L5/S1 spot lateral
Pelvis and Hip		
Pelvic injury	Inlet	45–50 degrees caudad (assess AP displacement)
Pelvic injury	Outlet	45 degrees cephalad (assess sacroiliac superior displacement)
Pelvic injury—Judet	Iliac oblique	Oblique on ilium (posterior column, anterior acetabulum)
Pelvic injury—Judet	Obturator oblique	Oblique on obturator (anterior column, posterior acetabulum)
Pelvic injury	Push-pull	Outlet view with stress (assess stability)
Sacroiliac injury		Judet views centered on sacroiliac joints
Hip	Surgical lateral	Lateral from opposite side with that hip flexed
Femoral neck		AP with 15 degrees' internal rotation
Knee		
Knee AP & lateral		AP with 5 degrees' flexion, lateral with 30 degrees' flexion
Osteochondral fixation	Notch	Prone 45 degrees from vertical
Knee degenerative joint	Rosenberg	Weight-bearing PA with 45 degrees' flexion
Patella	Merchant	45 degrees' flexion, cassette perpendicular to tibia
Tibial plateau		AP with 10-degree caudal tilt
Tibial plateau		Internal and external oblique views
Foot and Ankle		
Ankle	Mortise	AP with 15 degrees internal rotation
Ankle	Stress	AP with lateral stress, lateral with drawer
Foot	Weight bearing	AP and lateral weight bearing
Midfoot		Include obliques
Talus	Canale	AP with 75 degrees cephalic tilt, pronate 15 degrees
Talar neck		AP with 15 degrees' pronation
Subtalar	Broden	45 degree rotation lateral with varying tilts
Calcaneus	Harris	AP standing, 45-degree tilt
Sesamoid		Tangentials with dorsiflexed toes

AP, anteroposterior; PA, posteroanterior.

4. C1-C2 Subluxation (Atlantoaxial Instability)—Occurs due to transverse ligament rupture. An increased atlantodens interval greater than 5 mm is treated with C1-C2 fusion. Ligament injury without fracture is rare. Anterior subluxation ± fracture is treated with traction reduction and halo. Neurologic injury is more common with this pattern. Posterior subluxation ± fracture is rare and indicates disruption of the apical and alar ligaments and maintenance of the transverse ligament. It requires posterior fusion because of high recurrence. Rotatory subluxation injuries present as head laterally tilted to one side and rotated to the opposite side. Treatment is with traction for reduction, then halo traction or posterior C1-C2 fusion if there is residual atlantoaxial instability (Fig. 10–3).
5. C2 Odontoid Fracture—Flexion (80%) is the most common mechanism. Type I fracture (2–3%) occurs at the upper tip and is usually stable if displacement is less than 2 mm. It is treated with a rigid orthosis for 6 to 8 weeks. Type II fracture (60%) occurs at the junction of the odontoid and C2 body. The nonunion rate is higher and positively related to angulation, displacement, age, and smoking. It is associated with C1 fracture in 16%. Nondisplaced fractures (<5 mm) are treated with halo immobilization for 8 to 12 weeks. Posterior spinal fusion of C1-C2 is done if there is greater than 5 mm displacement, posterior displacement, or imperfect reduction. An anterior odontoid screw may also be used. Type III fractures occur within the superior C2 body and are treated with closed reduction and halo immobilization for 8 to 12 weeks (Fig. 10–4).
6. C2 Isthmus Fracture (Hangman's Fracture)—Injury occurs by hyperextension + axial load + rebound flexion. Neurologic injury is uncommon. Other C-spine injuries are often associated. Type I is a vertical fracture with no angulation treated with a rigid orthosis for 8 to 12 weeks. There is a 30% incidence of degenerative joint disease because of less anterior spontaneous fusion of the anterior annulus/vertebral endplates. In type II injuries, the disc is disrupted and has more than 3 mm of translation, and angulation occurs. Treatment is with closed extension traction if there is more than 6 mm of translation and halo immobilization for 12 weeks. The patient is observed closely, and nonunions are treated with anterior C2-C3 fusion or posterior C1-C3 fusion. Acceptable reduction is less than 4 mm of translation and less than 10 degrees of angulation. A type IIA injury has severe angulation with minimal translation and is treated with extension and compression halo treatment for 6 weeks and fusion as necessary. Type III injury is a vertical fracture with bilateral or unilateral facet dislocation. It has the highest association of neurologic deficits. Treatment is with open reduction, posterior spinal fusion, and halo immobilization (Fig. 10–5).

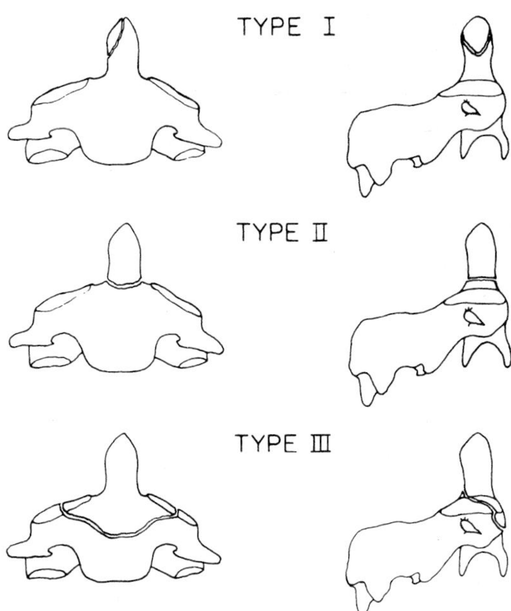

Figure 10–4. Odontoid fracture classification. (From Anderson L.D., and D'Alonzono, R.T.: Fractures of the odontoid process of the axis. J. Bone Joint Surg. [Am.] 56:1664, 1974.)

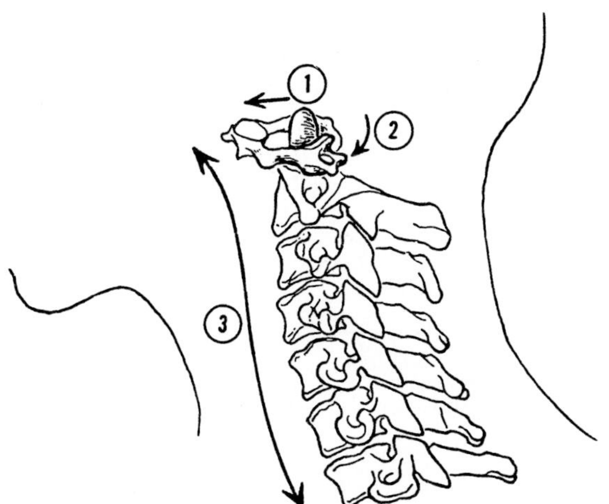

Figure 10–3. Rotatory subluxation of C1–C2. (From Connolly, J.F., ed.: DePalma's The Management of Fractures and Dislocations, an Atlas, 3rd ed., p. 287. Philadelphia, WB Saunders, 1981.)

B. Lower Cervical Fractures
   1. C3-C7 Facet Joint Injuries—These common C-spine injuries occur by flexion or distraction ± rotation. Included are facet subluxations, perched facets, and unilateral or bilateral dislocations ± associated fractures. Unilateral facet dislocations have less than 50% translation. Bilateral facet dislocations have greater than 50% translation, and these

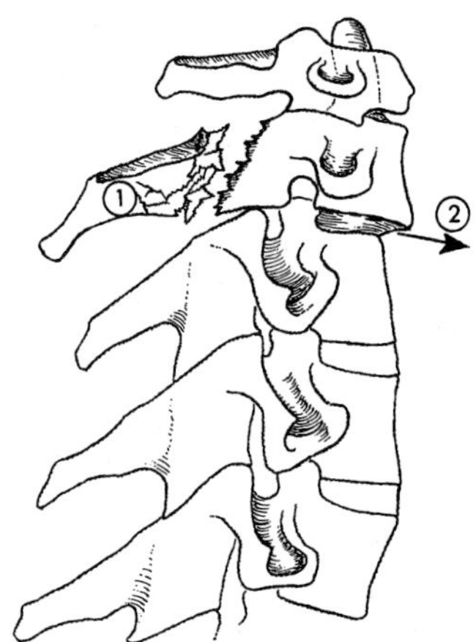

Figure 10–5. Hangman's fracture. (From Connolly, J.F., ed.: DePalma's The Management of Fractures and Dislocations, an Atlas, 3rd ed., p. 312. Philadelphia, WB Saunders, 1981.)

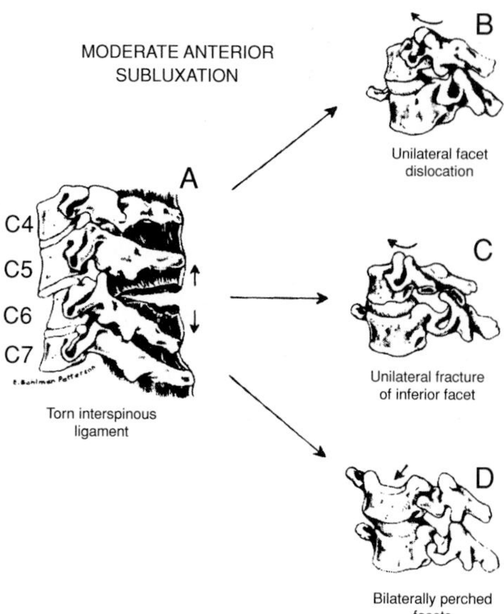

Figure 10–6. Jumped facet. Note 25% displacement with unilateral dislocation and 50% displacement with bilateral dislocation. (From Bohlman, H.H.: Fractures and dislocations of the cervical spine. J. Bone Joint Surg. [Am.] 61:1136, 1979.)

are often associated with nerve root or spinal cord injuries (75%). The most common location for dislocations occurs at C5-C6 and C6-C7 levels. Use of magnetic resonance imaging (MRI) is controversial for closed or operative reductions. Some orthopaedists believe that attempted closed reduction with traction is reasonable in an alert patient with normal results of the neurologic examination. Most believe MRI is warranted before reduction to rule out the possibility of herniated nucleus pulposus (7%). And if herniated nucleus pulposus is present, then anterior open decompression and fusion is suggested. If it is absent, then closed reduction is attempted in the alert, cooperative patient. Open reduction is required if closed reduction has failed or if an unstable fracture pattern is identified followed by posterior spinal fusion. Anterior discectomy should be performed if herniated nucleus pulposus or incomplete injury is present to prevent neurologic injury and decompress spinal canal (Fig. 10–6).

2. C3-C7 Compression Fracture—*Anterior wedge fracture* is due to flexion forces. Injuries occur most often at C4-C5 and C5-C6 levels. Spinal canal compromise is rare. These fractures are stable and treated with a rigid orthosis for 8 to 12 weeks. C-spine instability develops if posterior ligaments are involved. Translation or angular displacement must be ruled out with flexion/extension radiographs. If translation is more than 3.5 mm or angulation is greater than 11 degrees, then it is considered unstable and treated with posterior spinal fusion. If there is an incomplete neurologic injury, then anterior column decompression and fusion is performed (Fig. 10–7).
3. C3-C7 Burst Fractures—These fractures are classified by canal compromise from posterior wall involvement and possible neurologic injury, which is common. They are most often caused by compression-flexion or vertical axial load C5 and C6 vertebral bodies. Posterior ligamentous injury can also occur and needs to be assessed to determine if combined surgical treatment is needed. If there is neurologic involvement, then anterior column decompression and fusion is performed alone only if posterior stability is confirmed. If posterior elements are unstable, then anterior

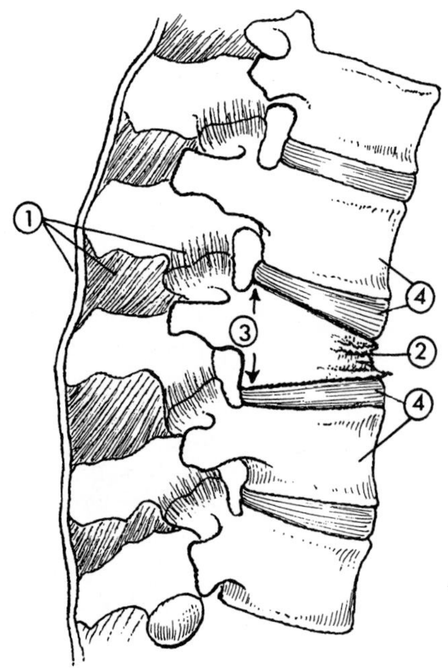

Figure 10–7. Wedge fracture. (From Connolly, J.F., ed.: DePalma's The Management of Fractures and Dislocations, an Atlas, 3rd ed., p. 407. Philadelphia, WB Saunders, 1981.)

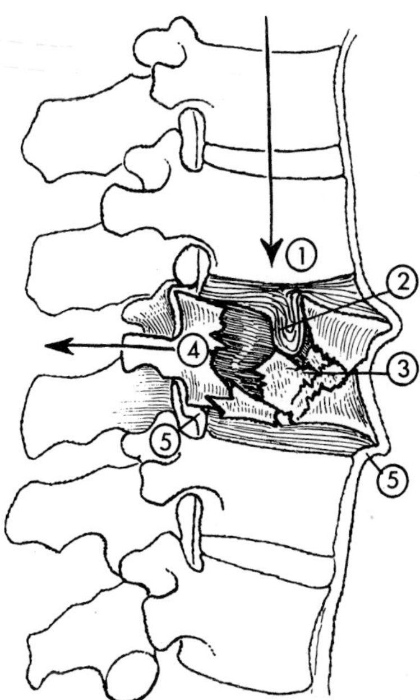

Figure 10–8. Burst fracture. Note retropulsion of bony fragments into spinal canal. (From Connolly, J.F., ed.: DePalma's The Management of Fractures and Dislocations, an Atlas, 3rd ed., p. 409. Philadelphia, WB Saunders, 1981.)

decompression and fusion plus posterior spinal fusion are necessary. If posterior spinal fusion is not combined, then post-traumatic kyphosis is common. Laminectomy is considered only in ankylosing spondylitis (Fig. 10–8).

4. Other C3-C7 Fractures—Lateral mass fractures involve the pedicle and the ipsilateral lamina and can be isolated or associated fractures. If they are stable, then these are treated with a rigid orthosis for 8 to 12 weeks. If they are unstable, then anterior or posterior approaches are indicated, depending on injury. Lamina, pedicle, articular process, or spinous process fractures can be treated with a rigid orthosis or halo immobilization for 8 to 12 weeks if no other instability pattern is identified. Flexion/extension radiographs are checked for ligamentous instabilities.

C. Thoracic and Lumbar Fractures—These affect the spinal transition zone of kyphosis to lordosis. The thoracic T1-T9 levels are usually stable unless there are multiple rib fractures. Most (60%) thoracic and lumbar fractures occur from T11 to the L1 junction, owing to lack of ribs and the facet orientation change from frontal to sagittal. The mechanism of injury is key to the fracture pattern and understanding the classification systems. Motor vehicle collisions with higher energy forces usually experience rotational and distractive forces. Other lower-energy injuries result in compressive and axial forces. Treatment of these fractures is based on the stability of the spine for mobilization, any neurologic injury, and the potential for future compromise. Goals are to maintain neurologic function, minimize further injury, and restore spinal stability and alignment. The Denis three-column anatomic classification is based on anterior, middle, and posterior column anatomy of vertebrae and soft tissues. Fractures are classified according to mechanism of injury and column involvement.

1. Compression Fractures—Occurring in 58% to 89% of all thoracic and lumbar spine fractures, this is the most common fracture pattern. Compression fractures occur by axial load with flexion or lateral bending moment in which the anterior column is disrupted, the middle column remains intact and acts as the fulcrum, and the posterior column is under tensile forces. If compression is greater than 50%, anterior height occurs, or more than 30 degrees of kyphosis is present, then the spine is unstable. Stable fractures are treated with a hyperextension brace or thoracolumbosacral orthosis (TLSO). Stable fractures of the thoracic spine can also be treated with hyperextension exercises. Treatment of unstable fractures is somewhat controversial. Closed reduction and a TLSO may be used and then followed closely for progression of deformity, neurologic deficit, or pain. Otherwise, operative reduction with posterior distraction stabilization and fusion is necessary (Fig. 10–9). Also see Figure 10–7.
2. Burst Fractures—This is a continuum of compression fractures with more axial loading. Burst fractures represent 17% of major spine fractures with five subtypes. Instability and failure occur in the anterior and middle columns. Retropulsion of the superior posterior endplate occur. The posterior column may fail either under compression or tension. Fifty percent of patients with posterior column injuries have a neurologic deficit. Unstable fractures are based on bony instability and neurologic injury. If pedicle or lamina fractures are present, then a three-column injury is defined and one must watch for dural tear and cerebrospinal fluid leak. These fractures are considered unstable if there is more than 50% to 60% anterior compression, 20 to 25 degrees of kyphosis, more than 50% of canal compromise, and a posterior column injury. Incomplete or progressive neurologic deficits require early decompression and stabilization. Treatment of the stable fracture without neurologic deficit is with hyperextension bracing for 3 to 4 months. Complete neurologic injury is treated with indirect stabilization within 72 hours to improve mobilization and decrease complications. Anterior column versus posterior column decompression and fusion is controversial. Posterior pedicle or claw distraction with postoperative computed tomography (CT) to evaluate re-

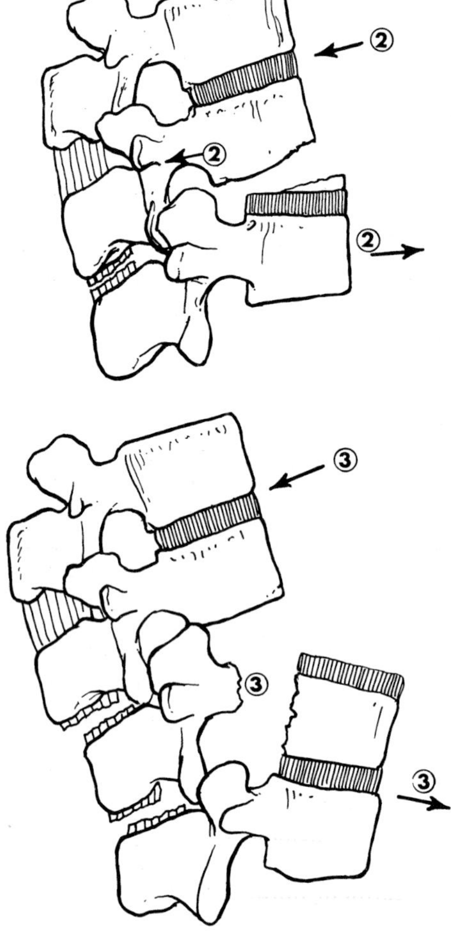

Figure 10–9. Shear fracture. *Top,* Stable. *Bottom,* Unstable. (From Connolly, J.F., ed.: DePalma's The Management of Fractures and Dislocations, an Atlas, 3rd ed., p. 412. Philadelphia, WB Saunders, 1981.)

duction of canal fragments is one option. Posterior bipedicular decompression is another option. Indications for anterior decompression include more than 60% of canal compromise initially or residual after posterior approach, an injury that is more than 7 days old or includes a progressive neurologic deficit initially, and superficial or deep posterior skin wound problems. Newer anterior spine systems have good stability and lower complication rates than previously. Posterior claw systems are excellent for levels above L3. Pedicle screws should be used for fractures at L3 or lower to maintain lordosis and prevent the "flat back" position. L5 burst fractures are usually treated nonoperatively unless there is progressive pain, deformity, or neurologic deficit (see Fig. 10–8).

3. Flexion-Distraction Fractures—Defined by position of fracture fulcrum, these fractures occur either anterior to or within the vertebral body. "Chance fractures" have the fulcrum anteriorly, and distraction occurs through the bone. "Seat-belt fractures" have the fulcrum within the vertebral body, with anterior column compression and distraction through posterior elements. There are various ligamentous, osseoligamentous, or osseous injury patterns that can occur through one or multiple levels. Posterior disruption of interspinous and supraspinous ligaments and ligamentum flavum creates the posterior column instability. The anterior longitudinal ligament is intact in flexion distraction injury versus in fracture/dislocations when it is disrupted. If more than 50% of anterior column height is lost, the injury is posterior, but if the anterior longitudinal ligament is intact, then it is considered a flexion-distraction injury. Treatment depends on location, energy, and fulcrum location. If only osseous injuries occurred with angulation less than 30 degrees, then these are treated with a hypoextension orthosis. Osseous injuries of more than 30 degrees are treated with reduction and posterior spinal fusion. Ligamentous or combination injuries are treated with reduction and posterior spinal fusion. Distraction techniques should **not** be used during reduction. Use decompression techniques as necessary for incomplete injuries. Combined anterior and posterior surgery is done if severe anterior compression exists and there is posterior ligamentous instability (Fig. 10–10).
4. Fracture/Dislocations—These are very unstable fractures with three-column injury. Seventy-five percent of these fractures have neurologic deficits, and 50% of these have complete lesions. Various combinations of rotation, angulation, and translation create mul-

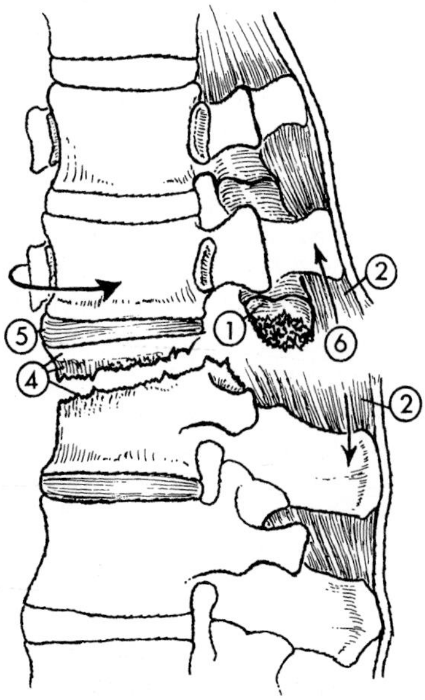

Figure 10–10. Slice fracture. (From Connolly, J.F., ed.: DePalma's The Management of Fractures and Dislocations, an Atlas, 3rd ed., p. 410. Philadelphia, WB Saunders, 1981.)

tiple possibilities. Incomplete lesions need early decompression and fusion. Treatment is early stabilization to prevent further injury. Stabilization is needed for complete neurologic injuries. Anterior column decompression with either anterior or posterior spinal fusion is determined by skin wounds, canal compromise of more than 60 degrees, or significant translation (see Fig. 10–9).

D. Sacral Fractures—The sacrum is a continuum of the lumbar spine and acts as a strut between the two iliac bones through strong ligamentous attachments. The central canal contains the termination of the cauda equina with the respective nerve roots. Most sacral fractures are related to pelvic injury. With the exception of osteoporotic insufficiency fractures, the majority of sacral fractures are from high-energy injuries. This implies a significant number of associated injuries. Bladder and urethral injuries are common. Neurologic injuries may occur in up to 50% of patients with sacral fractures. A careful neurologic evaluation (especially anal sphincter tone, perianal sensation, and bladder function) is imperative. Complete radiographic evaluation includes anteroposterior (AP) pelvis, inlet, and outlet views, in addition to CT. Radiographic signs of pelvic instability include low lumbar transverse process fractures, avulsion fracture of the ischial spine, asymmetry of sacral foramina, and cephalad migration of affected hemipelvis. A bone scan may be useful to identify occult or insufficiency fractures.

1. Patterns
   a. Vertical Fractures—Occur in association with pelvic injuries and can be stable or unstable. Denis describes the fracture in relation to the sacral foramina. A zone 1 injury is lateral and extraforaminal with a low incidence of neurologic and bladder injury. L5 is the most commonly injured nerve root. Zone 2 injuries transverse the foramen with a higher incidence of neurologic injury to L5, S1, and S2 nerve roots. Zone 3 injuries are medial and extraforaminal with central canal involvement. Neurologic injury with bowel and bladder and sexual dysfunction are common.
   b. Transverse Fractures—Commonly occur at S1 to S3. These injuries are usually associated with bladder dysfunction.
   c. H-shaped Fractures—Result of high-energy fractures with two vertical fractures joined together by a transverse component.
2. Treatment—The treatment of sacral fractures is based on the pelvic injury and neurologic deficit. Transverse fractures should be treated with posterior decompression and stabilization. Vertical fractures are treated according to the pelvic injury pattern. If the pelvic ring is stable and there is no neurologic deficit, then treatment consists of short-term protected weight bearing.

IV. Pelvis and Hip Injuries

A. Pelvic Ring Injuries—Pelvic ring injuries are usually the result of high-energy blunt trauma. Patients often have associated serious, life-threatening injuries and should be evaluated following ATLS protocols. Hemorrhage is the leading cause of death with a reported mortality rate of 15%. Other associated serious injuries include urogenital, lumbosacral plexus, and concomitant long bone fractures. Urogenital injuries approach 20%. Lumbosacral plexus injuries approach 8% and occur in up to 50% of patients with "unstable" pelvic ring injuries. Most patients have other extremity fractures, with isolated pelvic ring fractures occurring only 15% of the time. If peritoneal lavage is to be performed, location of catheter insertion should be supraumbilical to avoid penetration of a possible pelvic hematoma and a false-positive result.

1. Relevant Anatomy—The pelvis represents the connection of the lower extremities to the axial skeleton. It is made up of a complementary bony and ligamentous system, which would not withstand physiologic forces one without the other.
2. Stability—*Stability* is described as the ability of the osseoligamentous structures of the pelvis to withstand physiologic stresses without abnormal deformation. Any classification and treatment option should address this concept of stability.
   a. Posterior Stability—The posterior ligamentous complex is the strongest and most important to inherent stability, with the interosseous sacroiliac ligaments the main contributor. The sacroiliac joints and remaining posterior ligaments, including the sacrotuberous, sacrospinous, iliolumbar, and lateral lumbosacral ligaments, all contribute to posterior stability.
   b. Anterior Stability—Anterior stability is achieved with the rami and symphysis pubis, which is composed of a bony articulation covered in hyaline cartilage. The ligamentous union between the articular surfaces is composed of fibrocartilage and collagen. The arcuate ligament or the inferior pubic ligament supports the inferior portion of the symphysis.
3. Imaging—A standard AP pelvis view following ATLS guidelines is an adequate screening tool looking for pelvic ring injuries (see Table 10–2). If any lesion of the anterior or posterior pelvis is suspected, inlet and outlet views of the pelvis are indicated. The inlet view is obtained with the patient supine and the beam tilted 60 degrees cephalad. The outlet view is then obtained with the beam tilted 45 degrees caudad. Signs indicating occult or frank instability of the pelvis are seen on

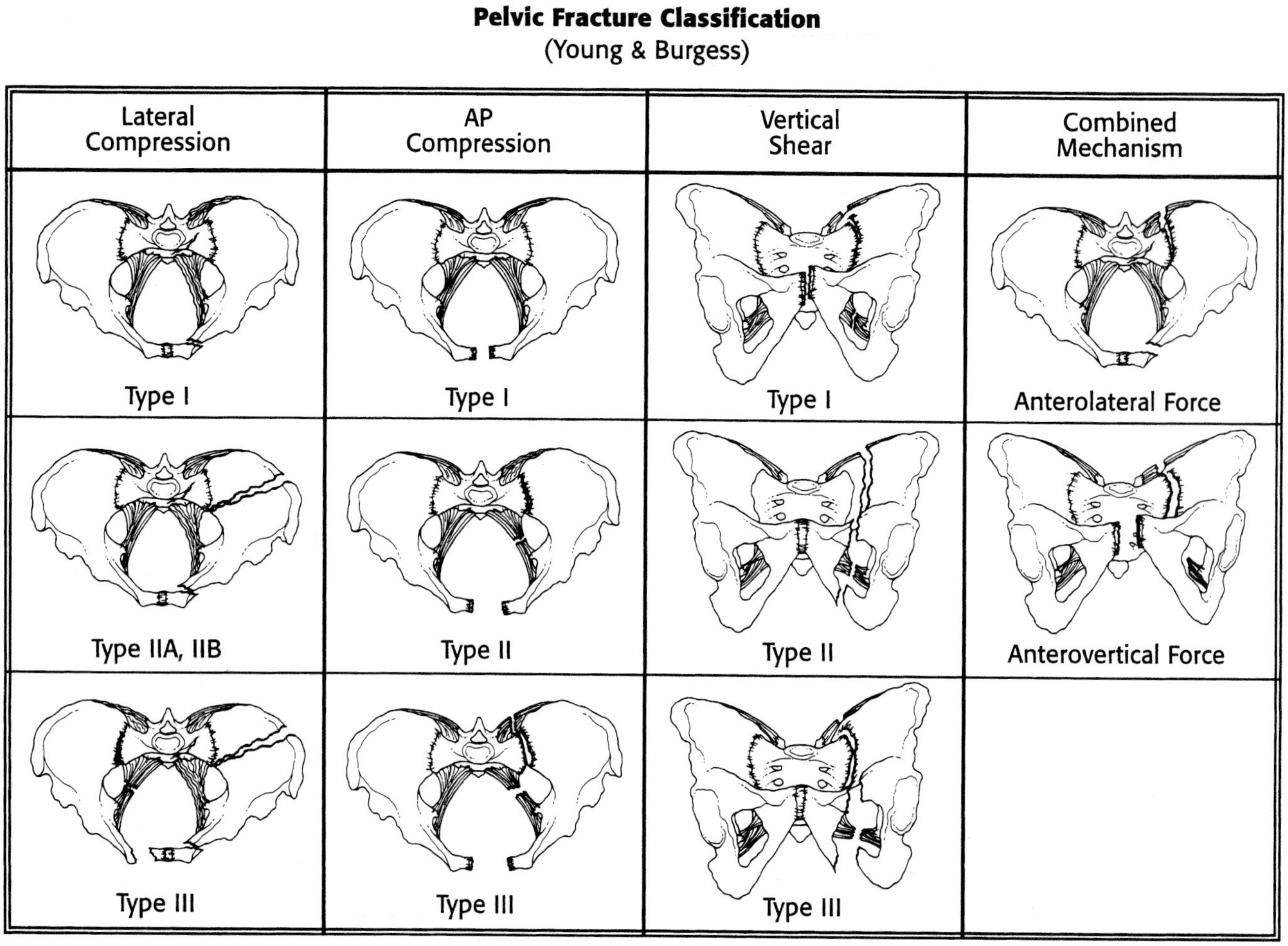

Pelvic Fracture Classification
(Young & Burgess)

Lateral Compression	AP Compression	Vertical Shear	Combined Mechanism
Type I	Type I	Type I	Anterolateral Force
Type IIA, IIB	Type II	Type II	Anterovertical Force
Type III	Type III	Type III	

Figure 10–11. Modified Pennal classification system. (From Orthopaedic Knowledge Update. Chicago, American Academy of Orthopaedic Surgeons.)

all projections. A fracture of the L5 spinous process on the AP view is almost always associated with instability. An avulsion fracture of the sacrospinous ligament from the ischial spine or the adjacent sacrum is also suspicious. The inlet view is valuable in determining the displacement of the pelvis in the AP plane. The outlet view is most helpful in evaluating superior displacements of the posterior half of the pelvis and rotational deformities of the hemipelvis. CT is a necessity in evaluation of pelvic ring disruptions. The images obtained reveal posterior pathology in detail and are required to determine stability.

4. Classification—Classification of pelvic ring fractures has been described by Tile and by Young and Burgess. Stable fracture patterns do not disrupt the ligamentous structures of the pelvic ring (Fig. 10–11).
   a. Stable Fractures—Avulsion fractures, iliac wing fractures, nondisplaced fractures, and transverse fractures of the sacrum.
   b. Unstable Fractures—Injuries that demonstrate both radiographic and clinical findings. Radiographic findings include displacement of the posterior sacroiliac complex of greater than 1 cm, the presence of a fracture gap versus impaction, avulsion fractures, and fractures of the transverse process of L5. Clinical findings consistent with instability include leg-length discrepancy, an obvious rotational deformity of one hemipelvis, marked posterior displacement, gross instability demonstrated with palpation, internal visceral injuries, scrotal or labial swelling/ecchymosis, and open wounds.
5. Treatment—Treatment is directed at restoring the stability of the pelvis to facilitate mobilization and healing (Chart 10–1). The most important factor affecting morbidity and mortality is posterior displacement. Obviously, stable fracture patterns may be treated with early mobilization and weight bearing with an expected good result. It is accepted that isolated fractures of the rami are stable and do not require fixation. Pubic symphysis disruptions of less than 2.5 cm may

Chart 10–1. Management Protocol for Pelvic Ring Disruption

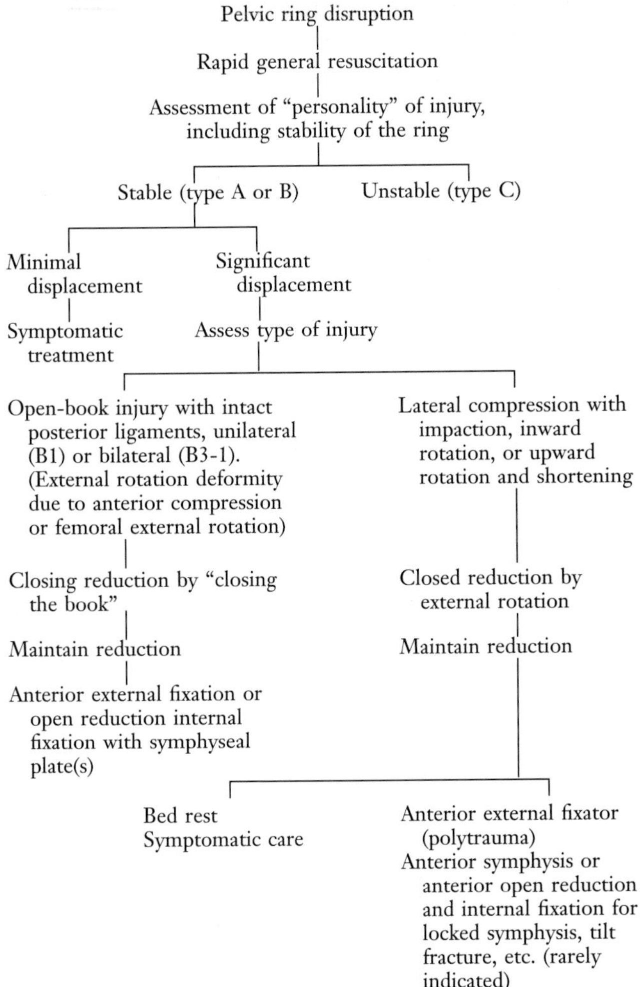

Tile, M.: Fractures of the Pelvis and Acetabulum. Williams & Wilkins, 1995.

be observed if the fracture is clinically stable. Unstable fracture patterns require fixation based on the personality of the injury and associated injuries. Other fractures that require fixation include the "locked symphysis" and the "tilt fracture." The tilt fracture is a displaced superior rami fracture that projects posteriorly into the perineum and is associated with dyspareunia in females.

Methods of achieving stability include external fixation, internal fixation, and percutaneous fixation. Percutaneous intramedullary screw fixation is as strong as plate and screw fixation biomechanically for displaced rami fractures. Acute management of the hemodynamically unstable patient with a pelvic ring injury centers around identifying the source of bleeding, concomitant fluid resuscitation, decreasing the pelvic volume, and obtaining stability. If after these goals have been achieved and the patient remains unstable, then angiography is indicated.

a. Open Pelvic Fractures—Open pelvic fractures deserve emergent attention. Open iliac wing fractures should be treated with internal fixation after irrigation and débridement. Vaginal lacerations should alert the treating surgeon to the possibility of an open fracture. Speculum examination is recommended with emergent irrigation and débridement and fixation of the pelvis. Fractures that communicate with the rectum, perineum, or colon require a diverting colostomy early in the management.

6. Complications—Pain is the most common reason for a poor outcome. Malunion or residual displacements of greater than 1 cm are associated with pain (75%). Other factors that are associated with a poor outcome include leg-length discrepancy of 2 cm, nonunion, permanent nerve injury, and urethral injury. Deep vein thrombosis occurs in approximately 60% of patients with pelvic fractures. The rate of pulmonary embolism is 10 times more frequent in this patient population as well, with rates approaching 2%.

   Retroperitoneal hematoma is seen most frequently with a lateral compression type 3 injury pattern (60%). This pattern also demonstrates the highest frequency of pelvic vascular injury (23%). However, embolization of pelvic vascular injuries is rarely required in lateral compression patterns (1.7%) when compared with all other patterns (20%). Mortality for open pelvic fractures approaches 30% and increases with the patient's physiologic age at time of injury (Fig. 10–12; see Fig. 10–11 and Chart 10–1).

B. Acetabular Fractures—Acetabular fractures are usually the result of high-energy blunt trauma. The fracture pattern that results is related to the position of the femoral head at the time of impact, the resulting force vector, and the quality of the underlying bone. Patients often have associated injuries and should be evaluated according to ATLS protocols. Associated injuries include bowel, bladder, and sciatic nerve injuries and (most common) other long bone fractures. Open acetabular fractures have a high mortality and require urgent stabilization. In patients who have both unstable pelvic ring injuries and acetabular fractures, the priority is given to fixation of the pelvic ring first.

1. Imaging—Radiographic evaluation includes the AP pelvis and oblique views of the affected hip (Judet views) (see Table 10–2). The AP pelvis view is included in the evaluation of all trauma patients and serves as a screening tool for acetabular fractures. Once identified, an acetabular fracture can be further investigated with oblique views. The obturator oblique view shows in profile the anterior

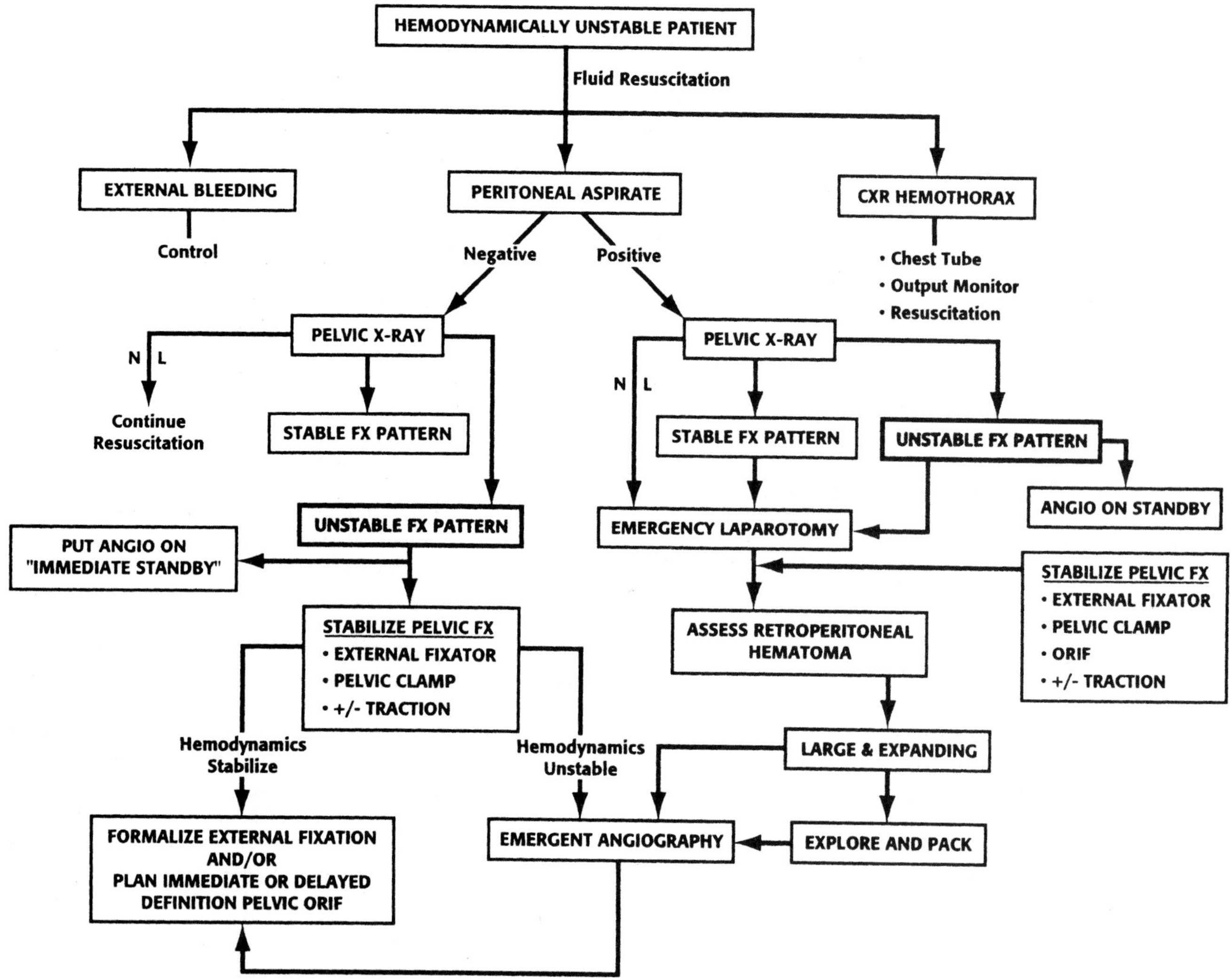

Figure 10–12. Suggested management guidelines in the hemodynamically unstable patient. (From Orthopaedic Knowledge Update. Chicago, American Academy of Orthopaedic Surgeons.)

column and the posterior wall and is characterized by the obturator foramen seen in its entirety. The iliac oblique view shows in profile the posterior column and the anterior wall and is characterized by the ilium seen in its entirety. The iliopectineal line represents the anterior column. The ilioischial line represents the posterior column.

CT evaluation is of absolute necessity in evaluation of these injuries. It allows the treating surgeon to evaluate the extent of the articular involvement, to identify marginal impaction injuries, to identify intra-articular debris and joint incongruency, and to further evaluate the fracture pattern for preoperative planning. Surgical indications are also based partially on radiographic criteria. Roof arc angles of less than 45 degrees on plain radiographs indicate dome articular displacement and are an indication for open reduction and internal fixation (ORIF). (Both column fractures and posterior wall fractures cannot be evaluated by roof arc measurements.) CT evaluation of the posterior wall fragment allows determination of hip stability based on degree of posterior wall involvement. Fragments less than or equal to 20% of the posterior wall are considered stable and do not require ORIF. Fragments that are greater than or equal to 40% of the posterior wall are considered unstable and require ORIF. Twenty to 40% is a gray zone, and clinical assessment of stability of the hip is required for correlation. CT can also identify the marginal impaction fracture, which is considered operative. Intra-articular debris needs to be removed but can be done on an elective basis. Operative fractures include joint debris removal as part of the procedure.

2. Classification—Described by Letournel and Judet, the classification is based on anatomical description of fracture patterns. Ten patterns have been described with five basic patterns and five associated patterns. The five

basic patterns include the posterior wall, the posterior column, the anterior wall, the anterior column, and the transverse. The five complex fracture patterns include combinations of the simple patterns, and all have at least two fracture planes. These include the posterior wall with an associated posterior column fracture, the transverse fracture with associated posterior wall, the anterior column fracture with a posterior hemitransverse component, the "T" fracture, and the both-column fracture. Posterior column fractures and T-shaped fractures have a fracture that extends into the obturator foramen. The both-column fracture is characterized by disassociation of the articular surface of the acetabulum from the ilium. The transverse fracture will have some articular surface attached to the ilium and is divided into three subtypes based on the location of the fracture in relation to the cotyloid fossa (Fig. 10–13).

3. Treatment
   a. Nonoperative Treatment—Options include longitudinal skeletal traction, which is indicated when there is severe osteoporosis, sepsis, and systemic illness that prevents operative treatment. Secondary congruency can be seen in some both-column acetabular fractures, and these can be treated by closed means as well. Observation is indicated for nondisplaced fractures. Trochanteric traction is never indicated.
   b. Operative Treatment—Indications include when there is greater than 3 mm of articular stepoff, posterior wall fractures of greater than 40%, marginal impaction fractures, loss of acetabular congruency, intra-articular debris, irreducible fracture/dislocations (an orthopaedic emergency), and fractures whose roof arc measurements are less than 45 degrees. External fixation has no role in the treatment of acetabular fractures.
   c. Surgical Approaches—Surgical approaches to the acetabulum are directed at addressing the displaced fracture fragments and can be simple or extensile. The *Kocher-Langenbeck approach* is the workhorse of most acetabular surgery and gives access to the posterior wall and the posterior column below the greater sciatic notch. The *ilioinguinal approach* gives access to the interior of the ilium, the anterior column including the quadrilateral plate, and the superior pubic ramus to the symphysis. It is the workhorse for both-column fractures. Extensile approaches (including triradiate, extended iliofemoral, and the combined) provide access to both columns simultaneously. Each approach has its own associated complications. The posterior approach may damage the blood supply to the femoral head at the level of the medial femoral circumflex artery, which lies just under the superior border

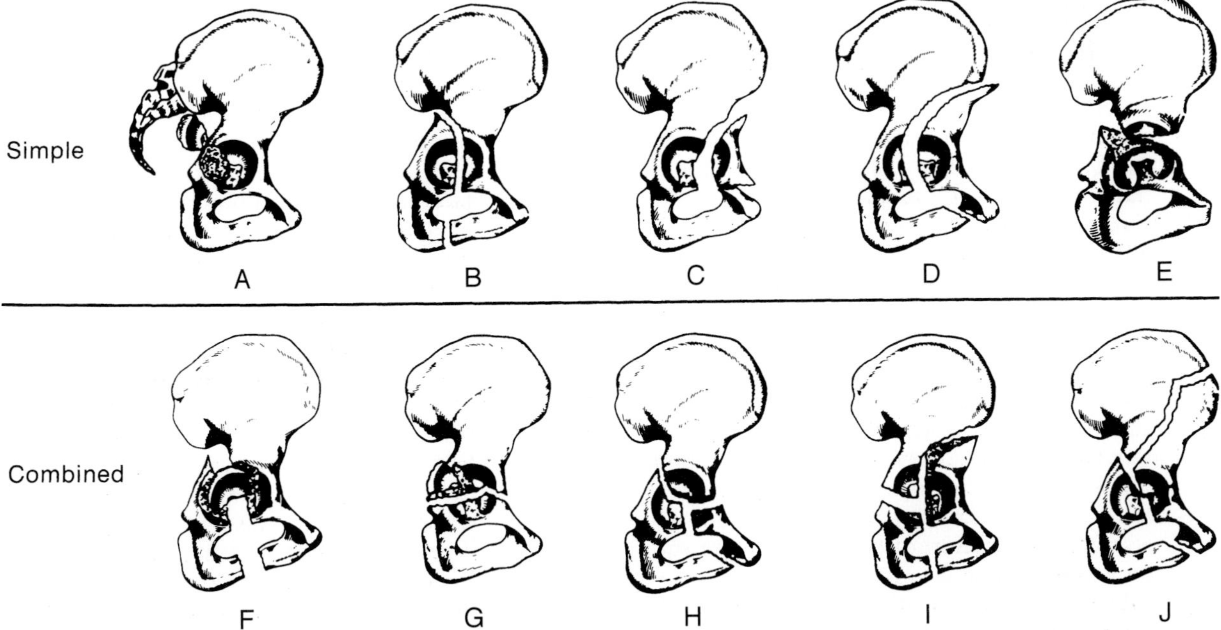

Figure 10–13. Letournel classification of acetabular fractures. *A,* Posterior wall. *B,* Posterior column. *C,* Anterior wall. *D,* Anterior column. *E,* Transverse. *F,* Posterior column and posterior wall. *G,* Transverse and posterior wall. *H,* T fracture. *I,* Anterior column and posterior hemitransverse. *J,* Both columns. (From Matta, J.M.: Trauma: Pelvis and acetabulum. In Orthopaedic Knowledge Update II, p. 348. Chicago, American Academy of Orthopaedic Surgeons, 1987.)

of the quadratus femoris muscle. The sciatic nerve is at risk with the posterior approach as well. This is minimized by maintaining hip extension and knee flexion to decrease tension on the nerve and by careful retraction of the nerve under the protection of the external rotators. The ilioinguinal approach is associated with thrombosis of the femoral artery/vein, injury to the femoral nerve, and injury to the lateral femoral cutaneous nerve. Severe bleeding from laceration of the corona mortis branch of the obturator artery is a potential complication of this approach. The extended iliofemoral approach has the highest incidence of heterotopic ossification and is associated with posterior gluteal muscle death if the superior gluteal artery is not patent preoperatively (requires preoperative arteriogram for evaluation). Combined anterior and posterior approaches have the disadvantage of incomplete simultaneous fracture visualization.

4. Complications—Infection, bleeding, thromboembolism, neurovascular injury, heterotopic ossification, post-traumatic arthritis, and decreased hip strength are just a few of the numerous complications that may occur. *Infection* is increased with the presence of overlying abrasions, which compromise the surgical approach. Closed degloving injuries or fat shear injuries (Morel-Lavalle) are associated with increased infection rates and must be débrided at the time of surgery. *Prior incisions* (antegrade femoral nailing) must be irrigated and débrided during the acetabular approach and are associated with a higher incidence of infection. Thromboembolism is common and approaches 60% or more of patients with pelvic trauma. Heterotopic ossification occurs 20% to 100% of the time in patients undergoing acetabular surgery. Indomethacin has been shown to reduce the overall incidence, especially in patients with head trauma and those undergoing extensile approaches. Low-dose irradiation has also been proven effective in reducing heterotopic ossification. Hip fusion or total hip arthroplasty can address post-traumatic arthritis. Total hip arthroplasty has a worse outcome after acetabular fracture when compared with total hip arthroplasty for osteoarthritis. Intraoperative use of fluoroscopy aids in avoiding intra-articular penetration of hardware during surgical stabilization (see Fig. 10–13).

C. Hip Dislocations—Hip dislocations are usually the result of a high-energy mechanism through a direct axial blow to the femur. The position of the leg at the time of impact influences the direction of dislocation. A limb that is adducted, flexed, and internally rotated at the time of impact results in a posterior dislocation. A limb that is abducted and flexed at the time of impact will result in an anterior dislocation. External rotation results in a dislocation above the superior ramus, and internal rotation results in a dislocation within the obturator foramen. The hip joint is an inherently stable construct, with approximately 70% of the femoral head covered at any position by the acetabular articular cartilage and labrum. The iliofemoral ligament anteriorly and the ischiofemoral ligament posteriorly combine with the capsule to aid in stability and prevent pathologic motion. The blood supply to the femoral head has been well described. Please see discussion under Femoral Neck Fractures. Avascular necrosis is a complication of hip dislocations and occurs approximately 15% of the time, and the incidence increases with the time to relocation (reduction before 6-hour mark imperative). The sciatic nerve is in close proximity to the posterior capsule and is at risk for injury in posterior dislocations with the peroneal division most vulnerable. This injury is seen with a frequency of up to 20% of the time and has a poor prognosis. A nerve that was intact before relocation and subsequently is lost requires surgical exploration.

1. Imaging—Radiographic evaluation of hip dislocations includes the standard AP pelvis view (see Table 10–4). This view allows comparison of the medial clear space to the normal side. Dislocations, associated acetabular fractures, and femoral head fractures are usually identified from this view. Judet views of the pelvis are useful in further evaluation of the direction of dislocation and associated injuries of the acetabulum. Cross-table lateral films confirm the direction of dislocation. Post-reduction AP pelvis views may reveal subtle differences in the medial clear space distance alluding to incarcerated fragments. CT after reduction is required for any fracture/dislocation but may not be necessary in simple dislocations with normal post-reduction radiographs. MRI is useful in evaluation of the viability of the femoral head in suspect osteonecrosis and in evaluation of the labrum.
2. Classification—Posterior and anterior hip dislocations are further classified by the comprehensive description. Under the comprehensive description, type 1 represents a pure dislocation without associated fractures and demonstrates no instability post reduction. Type 2 represents an irreducible dislocation without associated fractures. Type 3 dislocation represents an unstable hip post reduction or has incarcerated fragments. Type 4 dislocation has an associated operative acetabular fracture. Type 5 dislocation has an associated femoral head or neck fracture.
3. Treatment—Treatment of these injuries is

directed by prompt reduction of the femoral head into the acetabulum. Type 2 dislocations must be openly reduced. Type 3 dislocations must undergo removal of incarcerated fragments. Avulsions of the ligamentum teres, which reduce into the cotyloid fossa, require no further treatment if the post-reduction CT demonstrates a concentric reduction. Type 3 dislocations without incarcerated fragments but demonstrating instability after reduction should have capsular/labral repairs within the first week. Type 4 dislocations require reconstruction of the acetabulum for maintenance of stability. Type 5 dislocations require emergent reduction and stabilization as well.

4. Complications—Osteonecrosis of the femoral head, traumatic arthritis (most common), sciatic nerve injury, and rarely recurrent dislocations.

V. Lower Extremity Fractions and Dislocations

A. Femoral Head Fractures—Femoral head fractures are associated with hip dislocations and pelvic/acetabular fractures. Seventy percent of the articular surface is responsible for load transfer through the hip. A spectrum of injury includes articular depression or impaction, osteochondral fractures, or large articular fracture segments with a 10% to 68% incidence. Femoral head fractures are associated most often with anterior hip dislocations. Posterior hip dislocations have a 7% incidence. Clinically, the same mechanism and physical findings are found as in hip dislocations.

1. Imaging—The same radiographic views used in hip dislocations are used. Judet views may help diagnose a femoral head fracture not seen on AP views. After hip reduction, AP radiographs are used to determine concentricity of the joint. CT is required for more precise evaluation of femoral head fracture and treatment planning.

2. Classification—Pipkin's classification is the most commonly used format and is based on dividing the femoral head at the fovea. Type I fracture occurs below the fovea; type II fracture occurs above the fovea; type III fracture is associated with femoral neck fracture; and type IV fracture is associated with an acetabular fracture. Type II fracture keeps the foveal artery intact to the fracture segment and has a better prognosis but does involve the weight-bearing dome surface. Brumback's classification includes the associated spectrum of fractures, including shear osteochondral fractures.

3. Treatment—After gentle hip reduction, description and size of the fracture determine treatment. A type I fracture with less than 1 mm of stepoff is treated with 4 weeks of traction and then touchdown weight bearing for 4 weeks. Larger stepoff requires an anterior approach for either excision of small fragments or ORIF with buried screws for a large-enough fragment. All type II fractures require CT-confirmed anatomic reduction; and if reduction is not obtained through closed reduction, then ORIF through the anterior approach is performed. If small fragments are present, then the approach is determined by CT. The same holds true for irreducible hip dislocations: if anterior, then an anterior approach is used. In femoral head fractures requiring ORIF, this rule is not standard and extensile or combined approaches may be necessary. An anterior approach does not increase the risk of osteonecrosis but does increase heterotopic ossification.

B. Femoral Neck Fractures—An increasing aging population has led to an increase in overall fractures of the proximal femur. In young patients this fracture is a result of high-energy trauma. Older patients suffer this fracture from low-energy falls. Hip fractures can be classified into intracapsular and extracapsular. Intracapsular hip fractures can be divided into displaced and nondisplaced. Intracapsular fractures of the proximal femur occur more frequently in women, whites, and patients with pre-existing medical problems, including disturbances of vision, balance, and neurologic disorders.

1. Imaging—Imaging of acute fractures requires an AP pelvis, cross-table lateral hip, and views of the ipsilateral femoral shaft for completeness. Normal trabecular patterns crossing from acetabulum to head, neck, and trochanteric regions are followed to look for subtle changes (see Fig. 10–17). CT is useful for assessing comminution. MRI is useful in assessing femoral head viability and occult femoral neck fractures. When used for diagnosis of occult femoral neck fractures, MRI has proven the most cost-effective method.

2. Classification—*Garden's classification* of intracapsular fractures includes nondisplaced fractures (types I and II) and displaced fractures (types III and IV). *Pauwels' classification* of intracapsular fractures stresses the orientation of the fracture, with vertical orientation having the worst prognosis and highest incidence of osteonecrosis (Figs. 10–14, 10–15).

a. Nondisplaced Fractures—May result from a traumatic event, in young patients from a high-energy mechanism and in older patients from a low-energy mechanism. This results in the truly nondisplaced fracture or the valgus impaction type.

b. Displaced Fractures—Have a worse prognosis and a higher rate of osteonecrosis and nonunion than nondisplaced fractures. The blood supply may be disrupted in this pattern.

c. Fatigue Fractures—Can be classified into

fracture is considered a surgical emergency. Every attempt is made to obtain an anatomic reduction first by closed means and then by open reduction if necessary. Fixation is best with cannulated screws placed in parallel with the starting points at or above the lesser trochanter for the inferior screws. Screws placed below the lesser trochanter are associated with a higher subtrochanteric fracture rate. The most important factor in fixation is the density of bone. There is no mechanical advantage to more than three screws placed in a triangular pattern. Older patients with displaced femoral neck fractures benefit from primary hemiarthroplasty. Indications include low demand patients and those with chronic medical problems. Physiologically younger patients with active lifestyles whose likelihood of success with internal fixation is low may benefit from primary total hip arthroplasty. Posterior approach is not associated with a higher dislocation rate in patients with Parkinson's disease.

Patients with rheumatoid arthritis and osteoarthritis may benefit from primary total hip arthroplasty. Results of primary total hip arthroplasty after femoral neck fracture have not been as good as those of primary total hip arthroplasty for rheumatoid arthritis and osteoarthritis. Patients with metabolic bone disease, including those with chronic renal failure or hyperparathyroidism, are at increased risk for complications associated with internal fixation. In these patients primary cemented prosthetic replacement is the treatment of choice. Patients unable to comply with limited weight-bearing status postoperatively may benefit from compression screw and side plate construct with a derotational screw placed proximal and center. This is associated with an increased risk for osteonecrosis. Osteoporosis is not more common in patients with hip fracture than in age-matched patients without hip fracture. Osteoarthritis is not associated with femoral neck fractures.

5. Complications—Young adults are at increased risk for development of nonunion and osteonecrosis. Overall rates of osteonecrosis approach 10% for nondisplaced fractures and up to 40% in displaced fractures. Nonunion rates are higher in displaced fractures and range from 10% to 30%. *Nonunion* can be defined as no healing at 12 months after injury. MRI is the study of choice to look at viability of the femoral head. A patient with a viable femoral head and a nonunion of a femoral neck fracture is a candidate for removal of the hardware and an intertrochanteric valgus osteotomy with fixation of the femoral neck (80% success reported). Osteotomy is also indicated for young patients with osteonecrosis and less than 50% femoral head involvement. The goal of osteotomy is to bring a viable portion of the femoral head under the weight-bearing portion of the acetabulum. A free vascularized fibular graft is also a possible alternative in the treatment of a young person with a nonunion with or without osteonecrosis. Malunion of 20 degrees varus/valgus is associated with increased rates of osteonecrosis.

   Ipsilateral femoral neck fractures in conjunction with femoral shaft fractures occur 3% of the time. Neck fracture takes priority and is missed up to 30% of the time. Fixation is dependent on the surgeon, who may use cannulated screws with antegrade/retrograde plating of the shaft fracture or second-generation intramedullary nailing.
6. Treatment Algorithm
   a. Young Patient—closed reduction and internal fixation (CRIF) versus ORIF
   b. Old Patient

      Activity level high, bone stock good: CRIF versus ORIF
      Sedentary, medical problems, and poor bone stock: Bipolar hemiarthroplasty versus primary total hip arthroplasty
      Multiple medical problems with low life expectancy and poor bone stock: Unipolar hemiarthroplasty

   c. Nonambulatory Patient—Trial of conservative treatment. Failure warrants resection arthroplasty versus hemiarthroplasty for comfort and hygiene (Fig. 10–17).

C. **Intertrochanteric Femur Fractures**—This region is best defined from the base of the femoral

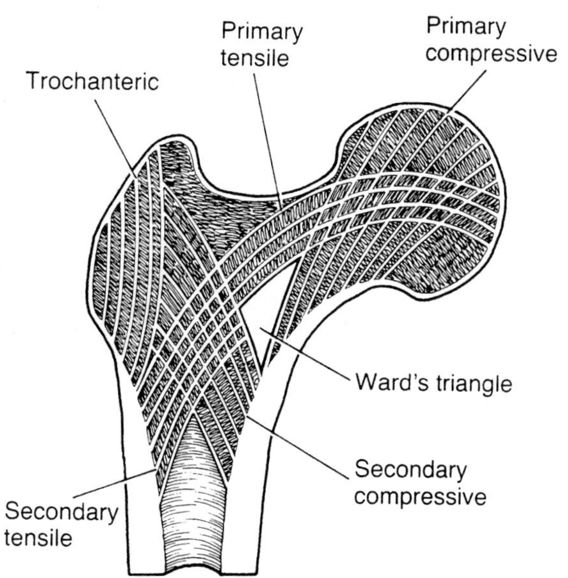

Figure 10–17. Bony trabecular groups as seen in the proximal femur. (From Evarts, C.M., ed.: Surgery of the Musculoskeletal System, 2nd. ed., p. 2552. Churchill Livingstone, 1990.)

neck to the distal portion of the lesser trochanter. These fractures occur in young patients from high-energy trauma and in older patients from low-energy trauma. They are associated with a high mortality rate in the elderly.

1. Risk Factors—Risk factors include a positive maternal history of hip fracture (doubles risk) and physiologic co-morbidities such as impaired vision and balance. Hospitalized patients demonstrate this injury pattern at 11 times the frequency of age-matched controls living at home.
2. Classification—The classification described by Jensen and Evans stresses the anatomic reducibility and postfixation stability for a given fracture.
   a. Stable Fractures—Avulsion fractures of the greater and lesser trochanters. The degree of displacement determines treatment. Fractures with more than 1 cm of displacement require surgical intervention.
   b. Unstable Fractures—Three-part and four-part patterns that usually demonstrate posteromedial comminution. Included is the reverse obliquity pattern.
3. Treatment—Treatment for unstable patterns is operative. A successful outcome depends on bone quality, stability of postoperative construct, and overall alignment. The reduced fracture position, after fixation, determines the rate of secondary displacement. Timing of open reduction remains controversial. Patients with severe comminution (basilar neck and intertrochanteric extension) may benefit from calcar-replacing hemiarthroplasty. The sliding hip screw is the implant of choice. The center/center location of the compression screw within 1 cm of subchondral bone is ideal. The angle of implant is not as critical. Medial displacement osteotomies are of no advantage over anatomic reductions and cause increased limb shortening. Stable constructs often collapse to a stable medial displacement. The larger the posterior medial fragment is, the greater its contribution to postoperative stability. The reverse obliquity pattern requires a fixed-angle device, either 95-degree blade or compression screw and side plate. Gamma nails provide some advantages. The intramedullary location shifts the moment of inertia medially, allowing greater calcar load sharing. A short lever arm decreases the bending moment. A sliding screw allows for compression of the fracture in controlled manner. Decreased fracture exposure may contribute to healing when this device is used. Secondary fracture at the distal end of nail is the most common complication of gamma nail use.
4. Complications—The most common complication is implant failure, with rates approaching 16%. Placing a compression screw in a posterior position has a higher failure rate, with cutout approaching 30%. Patients with rheumatoid arthritis have higher complication rates with osteonecrosis approaching 10%, infection approaching 10%, and revision to total hip arthroplasty at 30% (Fig. 10–18).

D. **Subtrochanteric Femur Fractures**—The subtrochanteric region starts at the lesser trochanter and extends 5 cm distally. This proximal portion of the femur is composed primarily of cortical bone and is slower to heal than the metaphyseal bone of the intertrochanteric region. It is also subject to strong muscular pull from the iliopsoas, short external rotators, and hip abductors. Fractures in this region are subject to long lever arms and increased bending moments leading to implant failure before union.
   1. Classification—Classification has been described by Russell-Taylor and allows implant choice based on fracture type. Type 1 fractures do not have extension into the piriformis fossa, and therefore closed intramedullary nailing techniques are possible. Type 1A fractures do not include the lesser trochanter, whereas type 1B fractures do. Type 1B fractures require cephalomedullary interlocking. Type 2 fractures extend into the greater trochanter and involve the piriformis fossa.

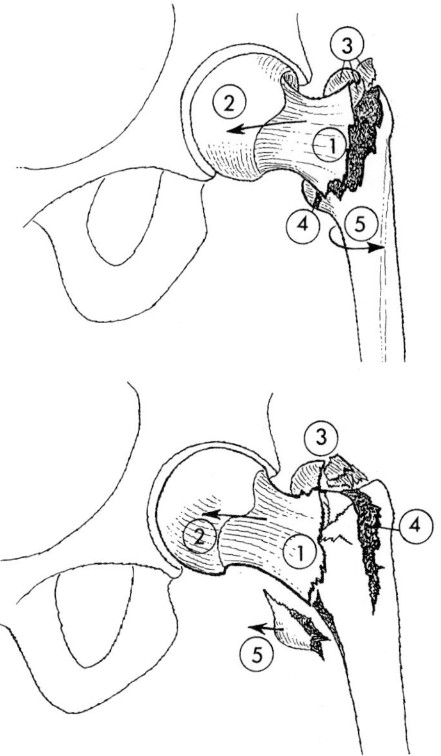

Figure 10–18. Intertrochanteric hip fracture classification. *Top,* Stable. *Bottom,* Unstable. (From Connolly, J.F., ed.: DePalma's The Management of Fractures and Dislocations, an Atlas, 3rd ed., p. 1372. Philadelphia, WB Saunders, 1981.)

Again, type 2A fractures do not involve the lesser trochanter, whereas type 2B fractures do.

2. Treatment—Treatment of these fractures is operative. First-generation intramedullary nails are usually not sufficient. Second-generation nails with fixation into the femoral head and neck are the implant of choice. An alternative is a fixed-angle device with a long side plate again gaining purchase in the head and neck region that should be used whenever there is extension into the piriformis fossa. Extensive comminution of the medial cortex (involvement of the lesser trochanter) requires bone grafting. Any fracture that has extension into the piriformis fossa cannot be treated with intramedullary techniques (type 2 fractures). These require a hip compression screw with or without bone grafting depending on the degree of medial comminution (involvement of the lesser trochanter requires addition of bone graft, type 2B).
3. Complications—Complications include loss of fixation and implant failure, nonunion, malunion, and infection. Compression screw fixation most often fails in osteopenic bone where the screw cuts out of the femoral head. *Intramedullary nails* fail when they are not statically interlocked, there was unrecognized extension into the piriformis fossa resulting in proximal cutout, and there was failure of the device due to insufficient strength. Length and rotational differences are the most common types of malunion. Nonunion can be defined as persistent pain after 6 months with no radiographic evidence of healing. It is best treated with a reamed intramedullary nail statically locked (Fig. 10–19).

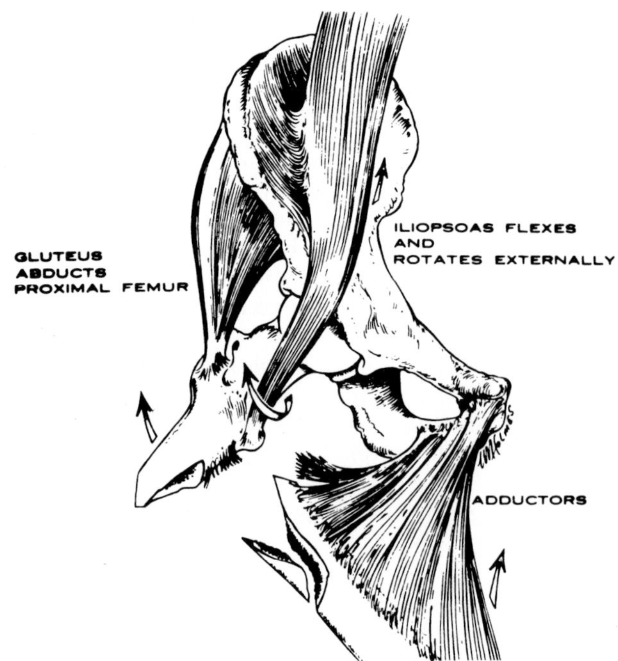

Figure 10–19. The muscle forces acting on a Type II subtrochanteric fracture. (From Froimson, A.L.: Treatment of comminuted subtrochanteric fractures of the femur. Surg. Gynecol. Obstet. 131:460, 1970.)

E. **Femoral Diaphyseal Fractures**—ATLS protocols apply during evaluation. Associated injuries are serious and common in this patient population.
   1. Imaging—Imaging should include AP and lateral views of femur, knee, and hip and an AP pelvis view.
   2. Classification—Classification by Winquist and Hansen describes the degree of comminution. This is useful in determination of stability of postoperative construct. The Orthopaedic Trauma Association classification describes the location and geometry of the fracture, the degree of comminution, and the severity of the soft tissue injury.
   3. Treatment—Treatment of these fractures is operative, and options include external fixation, intramedullary nailing, and plating. External fixation is used for severe soft tissue injuries requiring multiple débridements, unstable patients, and arterial injuries before repair. Conversion to intramedullary nailing is possible after external fixation up to 3 weeks after surgery without increased infection rates. Plating is reserved for treatment of the shaft fracture in ipsilateral neck-shaft injuries. Plating has higher associated complications when compared with intramedullary nailing, including a higher infection rate (6%), higher delayed union (9%), and loss of fixation (9%). *Intramedullary nailing* is the standard of care and has the advantages of near-percutaneous fracture treatment, relative stability, and proven results. Complications include infection (1%), shortening (2%), and malrotation (3%). The successful union in acceptable alignment occurs 99% of the time.
      a. Timing—Early stabilization (within 24 hours) of shaft fractures has been proven to decrease pulmonary complications, hospitalization, and overall costs in the multiply-injured patient. This also facilitates early mobilization.
      b. Reaming—There are no randomized prospective studies that prove the benefit of unreamed technique in patients with coexisting pulmonary injury. Deep flutes and small shafts decrease intramedullary pressures when compared with reamers of other designs.
      c. Locking—Static interlocking does not inhibit fracture healing, and routine dynamization is unnecessary.
      d. Biomechanics—Bending stiffness is related to diameter (radius to the fourth power). Slotted nails have decreased torsional stiffness (40 times).

e. Implant Failure—Failure occurs at the fracture site in subtrochanteric fractures. It will occur at the interlocking site if a screw is within 5 cm of fracture location.
f. GSW Femur Fractures—Treatment is with local wound care and reamed intramedullary nailing for low-velocity injuries. Shotgun and high-velocity injuries should be managed as Gustilo grade III open femur fractures.
g. Open Fractures—Adequate débridement, irrigation, antibiotics, and delayed closure with reamed intramedullary nailing is recommended. Severely contaminated wounds or wounds that have had delayed treatment are contraindications to immediate intramedullary nailing.
h. Infection—Débridement with removal of infected tissue and dead bone and antibiotics are necessary with retention of the intramedullary nail until union is achieved. Eradication of infection may require removal of the nail after union.
i. Nonunion—Exchanged nailing with reaming is successful 50% of the time. Extensive comminution may require bone grafting. Infected nonunion after initial intramedullary nailing is best treated with organism-specific intravenous antibiotics and exchange nailing with reaming.
j. Nerve Injury—Pudendal (most common) and sciatic nerve injuries are usually the result of traction and represent a neurapraxia that usually spontaneously resolves. Pudendal nerve injury in males is suggested when complaints include impotence and penile numbness after intramedullary nailing of the femur.
k. Heterotopic Ossification—This is the most frequent complication after reamed intramedullary nailing, approaching 25%. Fortunately, it is rarely clinically important. Pulsatile lavage does not appear to lower the incidence of ossification.
l. Malunion—Immediate recognition of malrotation can be treated with correction and replacement of interlocking screws. Malunion is most common in distal third fractures. Rotational malunion of up to 15 degrees is well tolerated.
m. Ipsilateral Femoral and Tibial Shaft Fractures—Urgent fixation of both is required if the patient's condition permits, with priority given to fixation of the femur (Fig. 10–20).

F. **Supracondylar Femur Fractures**—Result from high-energy mechanisms in young patients and low-energy falls in the elderly. Fractures in this region represent 4% to 7% of all femur fractures; and if hip fractures are excluded, they represent 31% of all femur fractures. The supracondylar region extends to 5 cm above the metaphyseal flare to the articular surfaces. The lateral condyle is larger in the AP dimension than the medial condyle. The condyles together form a trapezoid.
1. Imaging—Radiographic evaluation includes AP and oblique views of the knee and radiographs of the femoral and tibial shafts (see Table 10–4). CT evaluation has not been proven to change the classification or treatment of this injury. Angiography is indicated in a pulseless extremity after gross skeletal alignment has been achieved.
2. Classification—Classification as by the AO group includes extra-articular, unicondylar, and bicondylar fractures.
3. Treatment—Nondisplaced fractures of the condyles can be treated with cast bracing, non–weight bearing, and early motion. All

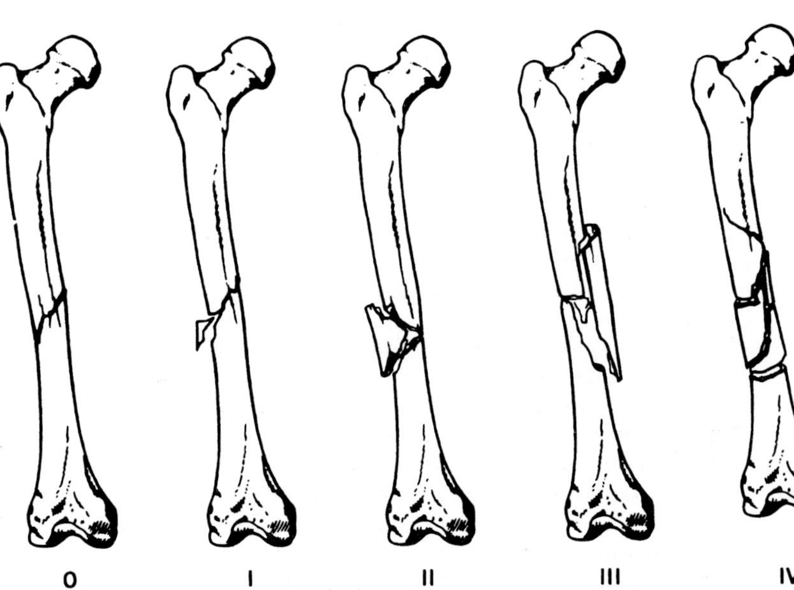

Figure 10–20. Winquist and Hanson classification of femoral shaft fractures. (*Note:* Type V [not shown] has segmental bone loss.) (From Johnson, K.D.: Femur: Trauma. In Orthopaedic Knowledge Update III, p. 514. Chicago, American Academy of Orthopaedic Surgeons, 1990.)

displaced fractures should be treated operatively. Articular fractures should be reduced anatomically and fixed rigidly. Fixation options include ORIF, intramedullary nailing, and CRIF. With ORIF the lateral approach is the most common. The articular surface is reduced anatomically and fixed with lag screws. The articular construct is then fixed to the diaphysis with a fixed-angle device restoring the axial alignment, rotation, and length. The 95-degree condylar screw and side plate can be used if the fracture does not extend to within 4 cm of the articular surface. The 95-degree fixed angle condylar bladeplate can be used if the fracture does not extend to within 2 cm of the articular surface and has one less degree of freedom than the screw. Condylar buttress plates are used in severely comminuted articular fractures. Medial endosteal substitution plates (intramedullary plates) can be used for restoration of the medial column and do not require periosteal or soft tissue stripping. Bone grafting of osseous defects and early range of motion are important adjuvants to rigid internal fixation. *Intramedullary nailing* can be used for supracondylar fractures as well. Surgical techniques are the same as ORIF, with fixation of the articular surface anatomically first, either by closed or open means, and then fixation of this construct to the diaphysis. Nails can be inserted antegrade or retrograde and can be rigid or flexible. The presence of a coronal fracture is a relative contraindication to intramedullary nailing. Nails are at an increased risk of failure, especially when interlocking screws are placed within 5 cm of the fracture. Antegrade nailing of these fractures is associated with a higher angular malunion rate than other treatment options. External fixation is reserved for unstable patients unable to undergo long surgical procedures, open fractures with severe soft tissue injury requiring multiple débridements, and as a temporizing measure in fractures with an associated vascular injury during arterial repair (Fig. 10–21).

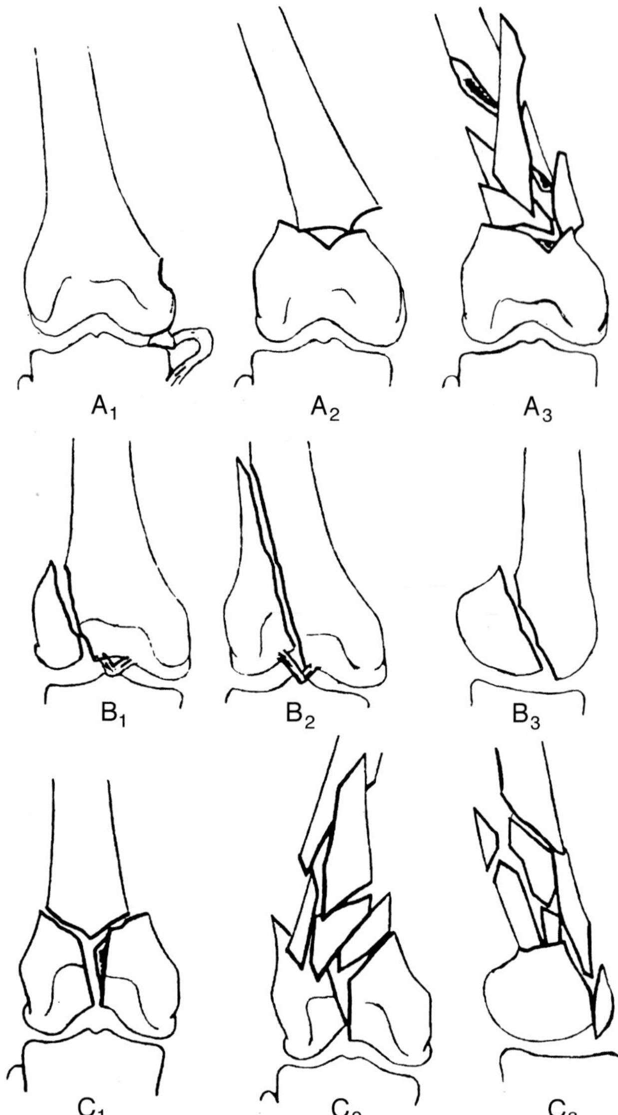

Figure 10–21. AO/ASIF classification of supracondylar fractures. *A,* Extra-articular. *B,* Unicondylar. *C,* Bicondylar. (From Johnson, K.D.: Femur: Trauma. In Orthopaedic Knowledge Update III, p. 521. Chicago, American Academy of Orthopaedic Surgeons, 1990.)

G. Knee Dislocations—Traumatic dislocations of the knee are probably underdiagnosed. The capsular destruction allows spontaneous reductions to occur and prevents a tense hemarthrosis from accumulating. This injury is the result of a high-energy mechanism, and associated injuries are common. Patients presenting with an acute knee dislocation require careful examination to rule out neurovascular injuries. The treatment of this injury strives for a painless, stable knee with a normal range of motion and strength. Complications are common. Knee dislocations should be considered an orthopaedic emergency and often require a multidisciplinary approach to their management.

1. Imaging—Radiographic evaluation includes AP and lateral views of the knee (see Table 10–4). Oblique views of the knee are helpful in evaluating associated fractures. Arteriograms are often required to rule out associated popliteal artery injuries. In dislocations with an absent pulse and obvious ischemia after reduction require an intraoperative arteriogram. In dislocations in which there are diminished pulses on post-reduction examination, arteriograms are required if close observation is not possible and before any use of a tourniquet. MRI is valuable in evaluation of soft tissue injuries associated with dislocations.
2. Classification—Classification of knee dislocations is based on the direction and mechanism of injury. Anterior, posterior, medial,

lateral, and rotational represent the five major types of knee dislocation. The anterior and posterior are the most common. The posterolateral is the most common rotational dislocation. Many dislocations cannot be classified, and the direction (type) remains unknown and includes global instability (Fig. 10–22).

3. Treatment—Treatment is aimed at restoring normal function. Prompt evaluation is required, noting in detail the neurovascular examination before and after reduction. A vascular injury is present when there is no pulse, active bleeding, expanding hematoma, and/or a bruit-thrill. This requires an intraoperative arteriogram and a vascular surgery consultation. Repair is best accomplished with a reverse saphenous vein graft. Amputation rates approach 30% if repair is not accomplished within the first 7 to 12 hours and approach 0% if done within the first 6 hours. Clinical signs that are associated with suspected vascular injuries after knee dislocations include diminished pulse or capillary refill, neurologic deficit, hypotension, decreased temperature, nonexpansile hematoma, or decreased arterial systolic pulse pressures. Pulse differential is the most sensitive clinical sign of arterial injury (85% sensitive). These patients require arteriography if vascular injury is suspected. Patients who have obvious clinical signs of vascular injury after knee dislocations, including absent pulses, active bleeding, expanding hematoma, bruits or thrill, and ischemia, require intraoperative arteriograms. Ligamentous lesions can be approached nonsurgically, acutely, or on a delayed basis. Nonsurgical management requires a period of immobilization and is associated with stiffness. Acute reconstruction centers on the posterior cruciate ligament and is done within the first 3 weeks. The posterior cruciate ligament is reconstructed first to avoid the development of a flexion contracture. Delayed reconstruction emphasizes regaining motion and then treating instabilities later. Posterolateral and lateral collateral ligamentous injuries benefit from early repair versus delayed reconstruction. The medial collateral ligament can be treated nonoperatively after cruciate ligament reconstruction.

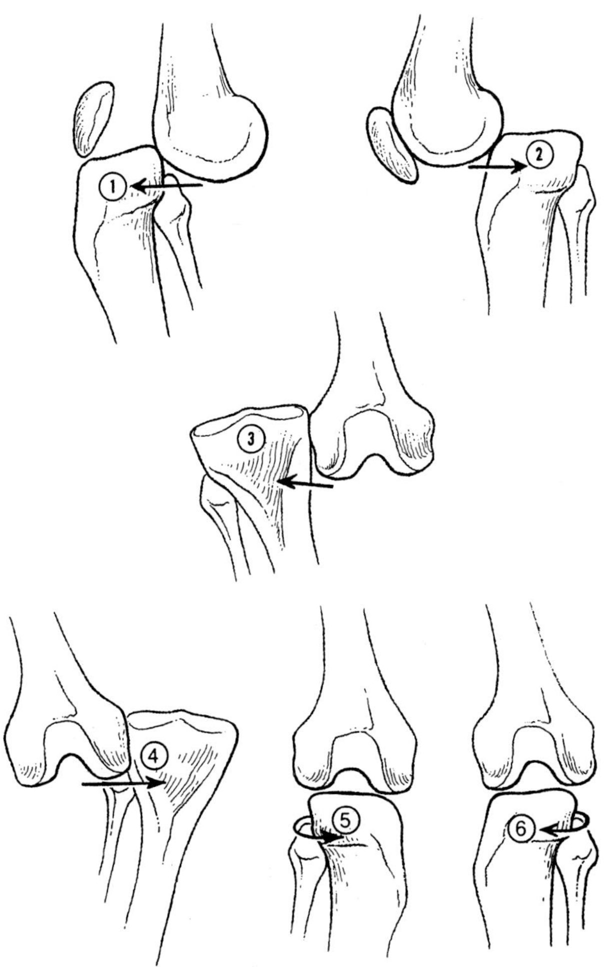

Figure 10–22. Dislocations of the knee. 1, Anterior. 2, Posterior. 3, Lateral. 4, Medial. 5, Anteromedial. 6, Anterolateral. (From Connolly, J.F., ed.: DePalma's The Management of Fractures and Dislocations, an Atlas, 3rd ed., p. 1621. Philadelphia, WB Saunders, 1981.)

4. Complications—Complications include stiffness (most common), vascular injury (40%; most common with anteroposterior dislocations), peroneal nerve injury (10–40%; incomplete lesions have better prognosis), compartment syndrome (associated with reperfusion after long ischemic times), and pain. Stiffness after 3 months of aggressive physical therapy requires manipulation with use of general anesthesia. See Figure 10–22.

H. **Extensor Mechanism Injuries**—Patellar fractures and disruption of the patellar tendon and quadriceps tendon are rare injuries. Mechanisms vary from a direct blow to quadriceps contraction. Examination often reveals extensor disruption with a patient unable to perform an active straight-leg raise. Palpable defects in the region of the patellar/quadriceps tendon with an extensor lag are indicative of an injury to that tendon. Hemarthrosis is often seen with patellar fractures.

1. **Patellar Fractures**—Most fractures are transverse in orientation and are best seen radiographically on lateral projection (see Table 10–2). Vertical fractures are rare and are best seen on sunrise projection. Nondisplaced fractures of the patella are treated nonsurgically with 6 weeks of casting in extension followed by progressive range-of-motion exercises. Displaced fractures have 3 mm of cortical separation or 2 mm of articular stepoff and should be openly reduced and fixed surgically. Inferior pole fractures of the pa-

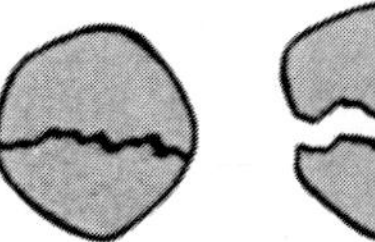
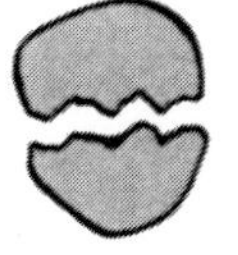
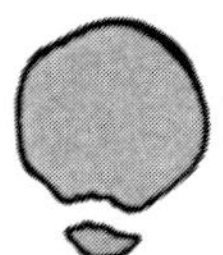
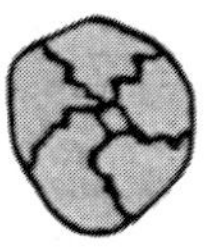
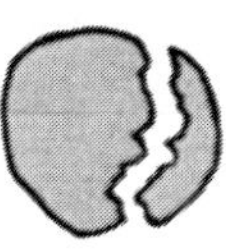

Figure 10–23. Types of patellar fractures. (From Weissman, B.N.W., and Sledge, C.B.: Orthopedic Radiology, p. 553. Philadelphia, WB Saunders, 1986.)

tella are extra-articular. Fractures of the inferior pole with an intact extensor mechanism can be treated with casting and progressive range-of-motion exercises. When extensor lag is present, treatment is as for patellar tendon rupture with advancement with an attempt at retention of pole fragments and ORIF. Comminuted or stellate fractures are difficult to manage. Every attempt at anatomic reduction and fixation of the largest fragments with retention of the construct should be made. Patellectomy is reserved for fractures in which no portion can be anatomically reduced (within 2 mm) and fixed to another. Retention of the largest articular fragment is also indicated.

Complications associated with patellar fractures include infection, hardware failure, delayed union, malunion, and loss of knee motion. Loss of fixation can occur after ORIF and with early motion. Fragments that displace more than 3 mm require repeat ORIF if there is no improvement in fracture position on a full-extension radiograph. Delayed union is initially treated with a decrease in range-of-motion exercises. Widely separated fragments should be approximated, restoring the extensor mechanism. If patellofemoral arthrosis is present at the time of repair, consideration of total patellectomy is made. Loss of knee motion is common. Physical therapy is beneficial. Manipulation under anesthesia can be performed if physical therapy fails to improve overall motion. Arthroscopic lysis of adhesions can be performed after 12 months of conservative treatment.

2. Patellar Dislocations—Acute traumatic lateral patellar dislocations should be reduced with the knee in full extension. The patellar-femoral ligament has been disrupted. Treatment consists of 6 weeks of cylinder casting followed by progressive range of motion exercises with attention to vastus medialis obliquus strengthening.
3. Patellar Tendon Rupture—Injury usually occurs in patients who are younger than 40 years old and athletically active. Repair is accomplished with heavy permanent suture through drill holes in the patella. Approach is through the midline. The tendon end should be freshened, and attention to the length of the repair should be determined to avoid patellofemoral articular incongruence. Augmentation with an 18-gauge wire is recommended to relieve stress on the repair. The retinaculum should also be repaired if possible. Range of motion should be assessed in the operating room and stability of the repair noted. Late repairs are associated with poor results. The patella is brought into position through preoperative skeletal traction to stretch the contracted quadriceps tendon. The repair is performed and augmented using the semitendinosus and gracilis tendons (after Ecker). Tibial tubercle avulsions should be repaired with a lage screw and washer construct after open reduction. The addition of a small plate adds to the strength of the construct.
4. Quadriceps Tendon Ruptures—This injury usually occurs in patients who are older than age 40 years and sedentary. The diagnosis is frequently missed on initial examination. Having a high index of suspicion in a patient who reports loss of terminal knee extension, weakness, and swelling leads to proper diag-

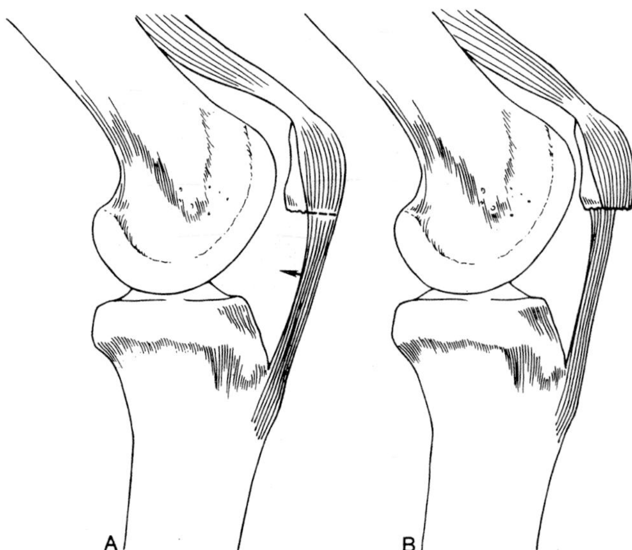

Figure 10–24. Proper and improper techniques for partial patellectomy. *A,* Patellar ligament sutured too far anteriorly, resulting in a tilted patella. *B,* Proper position of patellar ligament. (From Evarts, C.M., ed.: Surgery of the Musculoskeletal System, 2nd ed., p. 3465. Churchill Livingstone, 1990.)

nosis. Patients often have a palpable defect at the superior pole of the patella. Nonoperative treatment is preferred in patients with a defect but an intact extensor mechanism and a partial tear. Operative repair is indicated in a patient who cannot demonstrate extension against gravity. The most common site of rupture is 0 to 2 cm above the superior pole. Surgical repair is performed through a midline incision, with end-to-end primary repair having the best outcome. Most surgeons recommend augmentation with a partial-thickness turndown of the quadriceps tendon over the primary repair (after Scuderi). In chronic ruptures of the tendon, of greater than 2 weeks' duration, the quadriceps tendon is retracted and scarred to the anterior femur. A Codivilla V-Y lengthening is indicated to restore length and patellofemoral articulation. All late repairs are associated with a poor outcome when compared with early repair (Figs. 10–23 to 10–25).

I. Tibial Plateau Fractures—These fractures involve the articular surface of the proximal tibia usually resulting from a combination of axial loading and varus/valgus stress. This injury demonstrates a bimodal pattern involving men in their 40s and women in their 70s, reflecting high- and low-energy mechanisms, respectively.

1. Evaluation—Evaluation of the patient in the emergency department adheres to the principles of ATLS. Secondary survey of the involved extremity includes evaluation of the overlying skin envelope looking for areas of ecchymosis, abrasion, contusion, and laceration that can affect surgical timing and approach. Careful evaluation of the limb above and below the fracture is necessary. Detailed neurovascular examination should be documented before and after gross skeletal alignment is achieved if the patient's overall condition permits.
2. Imaging—Radiographs should include AP, lateral, and oblique views of the knee (see Table 10–2). The femur and tibia should also be included, as should comparison views of the uninvolved knee. If possible, traction views aid in preoperative planning and identi-

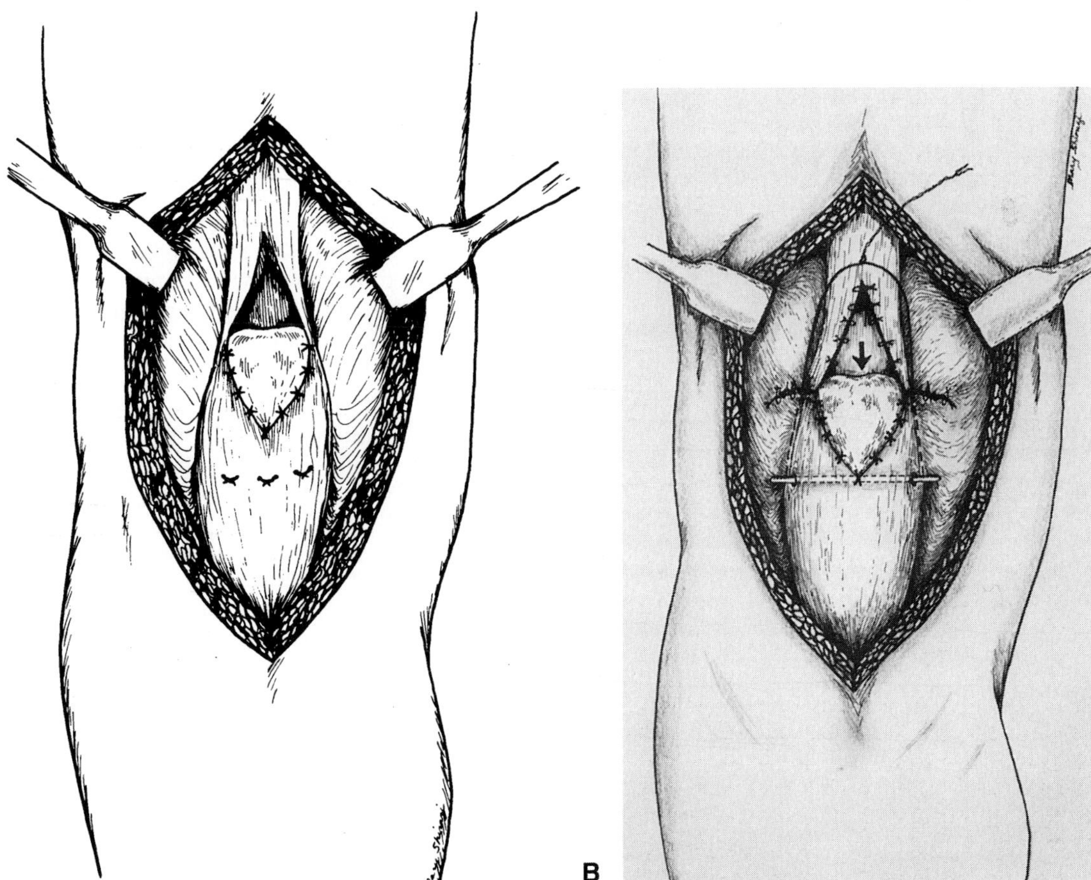

Figure 10–25. *A,* Scuderi's flap reinforcement. This triangular flap is based 2 cm above the site of the rupture. It is 5 cm wide at its base and approximately 6–8 cm long. The flap should be approximately 3 mm thick. *B,* If approximation of the rupture edges proves difficult, a Bennett-type quadriceps tendon lengthening is performed by completing the Scuderi flap incision down through the full thickness of the tendon. A retention suture, with a pull-out wire is fastened to a Steinmann pin in the patella. (From Evarts, C.M., ed.: Surgery of the Musculoskeletal System, 2nd ed., p. 3514. Churchill Livingstone, 1990.)

fication of major fracture fragments. CT has been proven to change the classification and surgical approach 10% to 15% of the time and is helpful in delineating the borders of depressed segments. MRI has recently proven accurate in evaluation of associated soft tissue injuries, adding information that previously was unavailable preoperatively. MRI is not as accurate as CT in showing bone detail.

3. Associated Injuries—Associated soft tissue injuries include the medial collateral ligament tears as the most common ligamentous injury, followed by the anterior cruciate ligament tears. Injuries to the medial cruciate ligament occur most frequently with Schatzker I and II fracture patterns. Anterior cruciate ligament injuries occur most frequently with Schatzker II and VI injuries. Approximately 50% of all tibial plateau fractures have associated meniscal tears, which are reparable.
4. Classification—Classification of tibial plateau fractures has been described by Schatzker, the AO group, and bicondylar fractures subclassified by Honkonen and associates. Schatzker described six basic patterns of injury, starting with the lateral condyle and moving medially:

   Type I: Lateral split
   Type II: Split-depression
   Type III: Pure depression type fracture of the lateral condyle
   Type IV: Medial condylar fracture that may involve the tibial spine
   Type V: Bicondylar fracture with an intact metaphysis
   Type VI: Bicondylar fracture with metaphyseal diaphyseal disassociation.

   The AO classification system describes extra-articular fractures as A, intra-articular fractures as B, and complex intra-articular fractures as C, with subdivisions in each category. This classification system is more descriptive but does not include associated soft tissue injuries. Bicondylar fractures are divided into laterally tilted, medially tilted, and symmetric axial displacement.
5. Treatment—Treatment of tibial plateau fractures is based on stability and fracture pattern. Stability is described as having less than 10 degrees of laxity in full extension to varus/valgus stress regardless of fracture pattern. Patients demonstrating "stability" can be treated nonsurgically with cast bracing, early range-of-motion exercises, and delayed weight bearing.

   Surgical indications are continuing to change and remain controversial. It is generally accepted that all displaced fractures of the medial plateau be reduced and fixed. Any varus tilting should be corrected. Lateral tilt of up to 5 degrees is tolerated. Separation in the lateral condyle of 5 mm or more or articular stepoff of 3 mm or more requires reduction and fixation. Similarly, all medial bicondylar and axial bicondylar tibial plateau fractures should be fixed. Laterally tilted bicondylar tibial plateau fractures follow the criteria of the lateral (3 mm stepoff and 5 mm displacement) and medial (any displacement or stepoff) condyles. Surgical treatment options include ORIF, CRIF, arthroscopy assisted, and external fixation. ORIF should be done through full-thickness flaps, avoiding overlying abrasions usually through a midline approach. Minimal periosteal stripping is recommended, as is bone grafting of metaphyseal defects and preservation of the meniscus. Repair of associated injuries to cruciate and collateral ligaments also appears to improve long-term results.

   Surgical approaches are varied and include the limited medial or lateral inverted "L", the longitudinal midline, and extensile. Additional incisions are used, if needed, including the posteromedial and posterolateral. Osteotomy of the tibial tubercle and Z plasty of the patellar tendon have also been described but have limited indications. The Y incision is associated with unacceptable wound complications and is contraindicated. Arthrotomy is followed by release of the coronary ligaments of the meniscus or sectioning of the anteromedial horn to facilitate articular visualization and reduction. These are then repaired at closure. External fixation can be used in conjunction with limited ORIF and CRIF to stabilize severely comminuted high-energy injuries, limiting the amount of iatrogenic soft tissue insult. External fixators can be placed medially to prevent late varus deformity in bicondylar fracture patterns. They can be placed spanning the knee in conjunction with limited ORIF. Hybrid ring fixators can also be used for fixation, allowing early knee motion. It is important to keep fine wires at least 15 mm away from the joint surface to prevent infection.
6. Complications—Complications include infection, malunion, nonunion, peroneal nerve palsy, post-traumatic arthritis, and compartment syndrome. Infection rates increase with severity of the fracture pattern, the surgical approach (most important factor), and the surgical time. Extensive soft tissue stripping with devascularization of the fracture fragments increases infection rates. Malunion rates are higher with closed versus open treatment of these injuries. Peroneal nerve injuries are seen with equal frequency in both closed and open management. Post-traumatic arthritis occurs with both open and closed

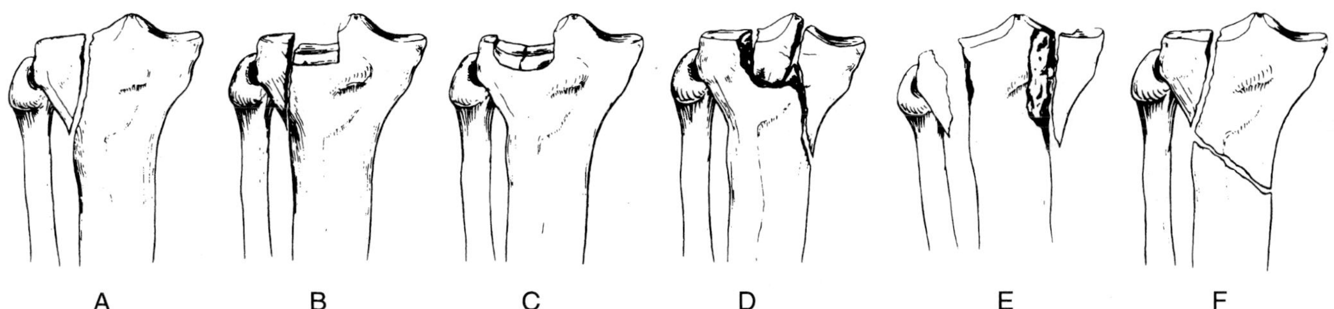

Figure 10–26. Diagram of the Schatzker classification of tibial plateau fractures. *A,* Type I, cleavage of wedge fracture of the lateral tibial plateau. *B,* Type II, lateral split/depression fracture. *C,* Type III, pure central depression. *D,* Type IV, medial condyle fracture (may involve tibial spine). *E,* Type V, bicondylar fracture. *F,* Type VI, metaphyseal/diaphyseal disassociation. (From Schatzker, J., McBroom, R., and Bruce, D.: The tibial plateau fracture: The Toronto experience 1968–1975. Clin. Orthop. 138:94–104, 1979.)

treatment. Compartment syndrome is rarely seen with this injury (Figs. 10–27 and 10–28).

J. Tibial Shaft Fractures—These are the most common long bone fractures. ATLS protocol is required if the mechanism is high energy and associated injuries are suggested. Location of the fracture and its "personality" determine the appropriate fixation. Soft tissue management is paramount for successful treatment with aggressive débridements and early coverage for open fractures.

1. Imaging—AP and lateral radiographs of the tibia are sufficient for diagnosis (see Table 10–2). Radiographs should include the knee and the ankle following the rule of "a joint above and a joint below the fracture."
2. Treatment—Relies on mechanism of injury, associated injuries, condition of the soft tissue envelope, and location of the fracture.
   a. Closed Treatment—Isolated closed tibial shaft fractures with low-energy mechanism should be treated initially closed with long-leg casting. Early conversion to functional bracing and weight bearing avoids joint stiffness and promotes healing. Acceptable alignment has been described. The usual accepted criteria are varus/valgus angulation to 5 to 7 degrees; AP angulation to 10 degrees, with shortening to 1 cm; cortical apposition of 50%; and rotational alignment within 10 degrees. External rotation is better tolerated than internal rotation. Complications of closed treatment include a delayed union rate of 19%, nonunion rate of 4%, AP malunion of 13%, varus/valgus malunion rate of 21%, and significant length deformity of 5%. The most common complication of closed treatment is loss of ankle range of motion.
   b. Operative Treatment—Operative treatment is indicated in any patient who fails closed treatment, has multiple injuries, has an ipsilateral femoral shaft fracture, has an open or segmental fracture, and has fractures associated with compartment syndrome or vascular injury. A relative indication for operative treatment includes morbid obesity, which precludes long-leg casting. Options include external fixation, intramedullary nailing, plating, and hybrid ring fixation.

   External fixation should be used in patients with open fractures for management of severe soft tissue injuries including burns, compartment syndrome, and multitrauma patients unable to undergo prolonged periods of anesthesia. When used to treat diaphyseal fractures the union rate approaches 95% with a 20% malunion rate. The most common complication with external fixation is pin tract infection (50%), and it is associated with thermal necrosis during pin insertion. All pin sites should be predrilled before insertion to help avoid this complication. Pin diameter is proportional to its bending rigidity by the fourth power. Thus, small increases in pin diameter dramatically affect its bending rigidity. End-to-end bone contact, if

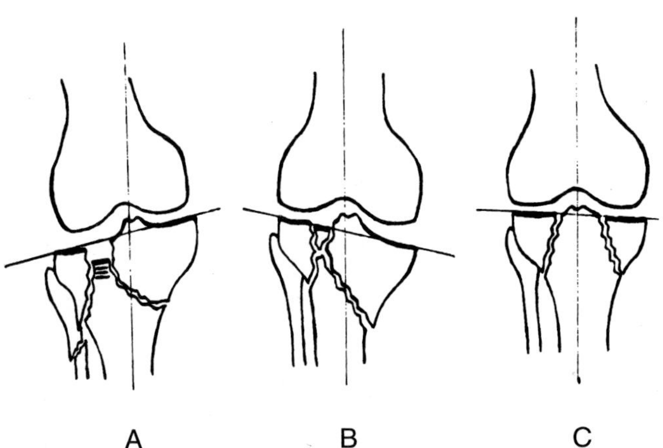

Figure 10–27. Subtypes of bicondylar fractures. *A,* Laterally tilted. *B,* Medially tilted. *C,* Symmetric axial displacement. (From Honkonen, S.E., and Jarvinen, M.J.: Classification of fractures of the tibial condyles. J. Bone Joint Surg. [Br.] 74:840–847, 1992.)

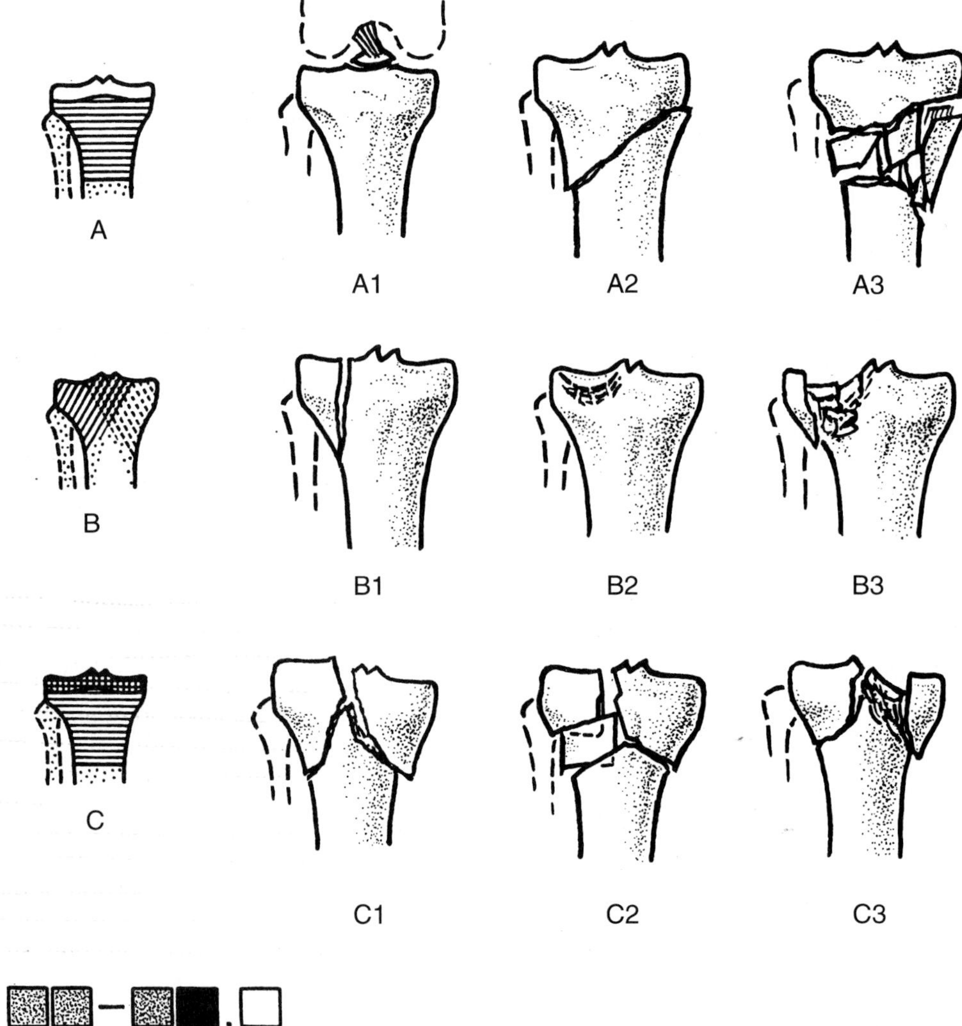

Figure 10–28. AO/ASIF universal classification system for tibial plateau fractures (see text). (From Müller, M.E., Nazarian, S., Koch, P., et al., eds.: The Comprehensive Classification of Fractures of Long Bones. Berlin, Germany, Springer-Verlag, 1990.)

possible, has the greatest influence on fixator stability. Construct is improved with pins in close location to the fracture, the bar lowered close to the axis of the tibia (cube of the side bar to bone distance—affects pin rigidity proportionally), placement of the fixator in the sagittal plane, placing the pins as far apart as possible in each fragment, adding another fixator in a perpendicular plane and connecting it to the first, and the number of pins used.

Intramedullary nailing is the gold standard of operative treatment with the lowest complication rate. Reaming is used for closed fractures and is controversial in open fractures. Interlocking is used routinely for rotational stability. Extending the use of intramedullary nailing to proximal and distal metaphyseal fractures has led to complications. A higher incidence of malunion exists in the AP plane for proximal fractures and in the varus/valgus plane for distal fractures. Hardware failure occurs more frequently in this subset as well, which reflects the higher malunion rate. The most common complication of intramedullary nailing of the tibia is anterior knee pain.

Hybrid ring fixation can be used to treat fractures of the proximal and distal metaphysis.

3. Complications—Nonunion and delayed union rates are increased with increasing fracture displacement, bone loss, associated fibular fractures, comminution, and infection. The incidence of nonunion increases also with the severity of open fractures. Distribution of nonunion is equal when comparing proximal, middle, and distal thirds. Infection is a common complication encountered in the treatment of tibial shaft fractures. The incidence of infection increases with the se-

verity of the soft tissue injury. The white blood cell count, sedimentation rate, and C-reactive protein level will be elevated. Radiographs will show an involucrum, sequestra, decreased mineralization, and/or periosteal reaction. Bone and indium scans are usually nondiagnostic. Aspiration can be helpful, but negative aspiration does not exclude infection. Bone grafting for treatment of grade 3A/3B open tibial fractures is safe after 3 months if the soft tissue envelope has shown no evidence of infection. The posterolateral approach is preferred with an autogenous iliac crest graft.

K. Tibial Plafond Fractures—Tibial plafond fractures can be described as an injury to the articular surface of the distal tibia, which differs from ankle fractures in the degree of articular surface involved and the mechanism of injury. Ankle fractures are usually the result of a rotational force.

1. Classification—These fractures are classified according to the direction and degree of rotation by Lauge-Hanson. Tibial plafond fractures are the result of axial loading and are classified based on the degree of articular involvement by Reudi (Fig. 10–26).
2. Patterns—Fracture patterns reflect the position of the foot at loading, with dorsiflexion resulting in anterior tibial articular fractures and plantarflexion resulting in posterior tibial articular fractures. The cartilage injury is more severe than the common ankle fracture and therefore carries a worse prognosis. The surrounding soft tissues are involved as well in this high-energy injury and often dictate treatment options and timing.
3. Imaging—Radiographic evaluation includes an ankle series, tibia view, comparison views, and traction views (see Table 10–2). CT is useful in identification of major fracture fragments, planning surgical approaches, and evaluation of the articular involvement.
4. Treatment—Treatment options are limited to operative methods because all nonoperative measures have been abandoned. Optimum timing for operative treatment is within the first 8 to 12 hours. The soft tissues are not excessively swollen, and full-thickness flaps placed more than 7 cm apart are readily closed without undue tension. After this initial window, operative intervention should be delayed for 7 to 10 days to allow the soft tissues to "calm down." The skin envelope should "wrinkle" to pinch. Axial alignment can be maintained during this time with calcaneal traction or an external fixator placed across the joint with pins in the calcaneus and in the first metatarsal. Major fracture fragments are reduced by ligamentotaxis and allow plain film evaluation in traction.

   Principles of operative intervention include

   1. Restoration of fibular length with or without fixation
   2. Reconstruction of the articular surface through "fracture windows" with minimal periosteal stripping
   3. Full-thickness flaps centered over the major fragments with at least 7 cm of separation
   4. Bone grafting of metaphyseal deficits
   5. Medial stabilization with plating or external fixation

5. Complications—Complications associated with this injury are high. Unacceptable infection rates associated with ORIF have led surgeons to search for alternatives. One method that has gained support is ORIF of the fibula, limited ORIF of the articular surface, and medial external fixation. This approach respects the severity of the soft tissue injury and allows the goals of operative intervention to be achieved. Articulated external fixators across the ankle joint allow early motion but are associated with a higher incidence of pin-track infections. Wound complications should be aggressively addressed with judicious use of free tissue transfers. Deep infections may require removal of devascularized bone, which includes a portion of the articular surface. Even though this is not ideal, to eradicate the source of infection, all devascularized bone should be removed. Hardware should be retained until union is achieved.

   Early arthrodesis is a salvage for severely comminuted fractures. Soft tissues should be allowed to heal 6 to 12 weeks before arthrodesis and should be limited to "unreconstructable" fractures. Gross alignment of fracture fragments may facilitate delayed arthrodesis should this be required later. This goal may be achieved with ligamentotaxis alone or in combination with limited ORIF.

   Medial wounds during closure should take priority. This allows coverage of neurovascular structures, hardware, and the tibiotalar joint. The lateral wound is easily skin grafted for closure and avoids undue tension and its associated problems (Fig. 10–29).

L. Talar Body Fractures—Relatively uncommon fractures with high rate of complications including osteonecrosis, ankle or subtalar degenerative joint disease, and disabling pain. It is a high-energy injury classified by location (anterior, middle, posterior body, processes) and fracture pattern (coronal, sagittal). Treatment requires open anatomic reduction and rigid fixation or excision of a fragment if it is too small for fixation. Mid-body fractures are best approached with medial malleolar osteotomy and posterior fractures are best approached posterolaterally.

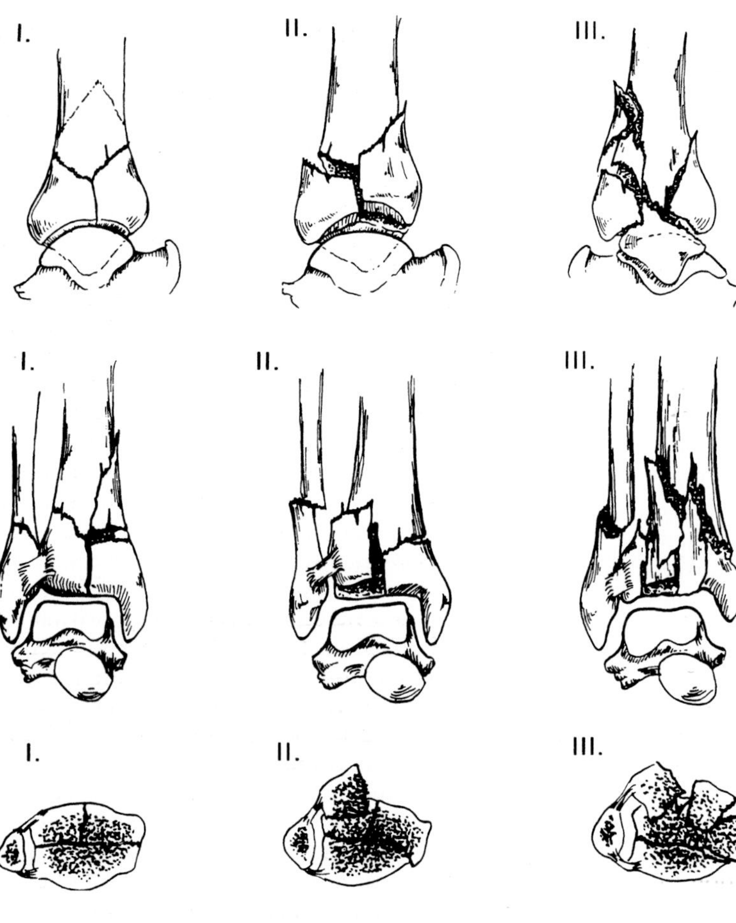

Figure 10–29. Tibial pilon fractures. I, Minimally displaced. II, Incongruous. III, Comminuted. (From Kozin, S.H., and Berlet, A.C.: Handbook of Common Orthopaedic Fractures, p. 131. Medical Surveillance, West Chester, PA, 1989.)

Postoperative management is with non–weight bearing, the duration of which is controversial. There is a relatively high incidence of osteonecrosis, delayed union, or nonunion. Late postoperative arthrosis is managed with fusion.

M. Talar Neck Fractures—The most common fracture of the talus, its mechanism is hyperdorsiflexion. Because no tendons or muscles attach to the talus, the blood supply is limited and there is a high incidence of avascular necrosis.

1. Classification—The classification of Hawkins and Canale is based on displacement of fracture.

   Type I: Nondisplaced vertical fracture (risk of avascular necrosis [AVN] less than 10%)
   Type II: Displaced with subtalar dislocation/subluxation (AVN risk greater than 40%)
   Type III: Displaced with talar body dislocation (AVN risk greater than 90%)
   Type IV: Displaced with talar head subluxation and body extrusion (AVN risk 100%).

2. Treatment—Type I fractures can be treated with non–weight bearing and a cast in slight plantarflexion for 4 to 6 weeks. Types II, III, and IV require ORIF with lag screw technique. There is a recent trend to use titanium screws to allow better visualization with MRI to evaluate vascularity of the dome. Postoperative treatment is controversial. Initial treatment is with a non–weight-bearing cast. Patients are followed radiographically for development of Hawkins' sign (subchondral lucency in the dome at 6 weeks), which indicates revascularization. Osteonecrosis is managed with delayed weight bearing or patella tendon bearing cast and arthrosis with delayed fusion.

3. Complications—Complications include osteonecrosis, delayed union, malunion, and nonunion.

N. Talar Head Fractures—Least common of talus fractures, these injuries occur with high-energy axial loading and usually part of a more complex fracture or ligamentous injury. Treatment is similar to that for other talar fractures with anatomic reduction and stable fixation. Small fragments that will not accept fixation should be excised. Healing usually occurs at 6 weeks in a partial or full weight-bearing cast. Talonavicular arthritis may occur and require fusion.

O. Talar Process Fractures—Lateral process fractures are the most common injury. These are often missed, and symptoms are attributed to "ankle sprain."

1. Classification—Hawkins' classification:

   Type I: Nondisplaced
   Type II: Large into talofibular and talocalcaneal joints
   Type III: Comminuted

2. Treatment—Treatment is based on size of fragment and degree of displacement. Nondisplaced fractures are treated in a cast for 6 weeks with 4 weeks non–weight bearing. Displaced fractures require ORIF or excision of small fragments.

P. Posterior Process Fracture—Rule out the trigonum. Twenty-five percent affect the posterior facet articular cartilage. The flexor hallucis longus runs between the medial and lateral tubercles. The posterior talofibular ligament inserts on the lateral tubercle, and the posterior third of the deltoid inserts on the medial tubercle. Hyperplantarflexion or inversion is the mechanism of injury. Treatment is with a short-leg cast for 6 weeks. If the fracture is displaced and fragments are large, then ORIF is used. Small fragments are excised.

Q. Subtalar Dislocation—A high-energy injury, there is simultaneous talocalcaneal and talonavicular dislocation. There is a significant incidence of open dislocation due to tenuous soft tissues and high energy. Eighty-five percent are medial dislocations. Associated fractures occur in 50%. Treatment is with closed reduction with traction under sedation or general anesthesia and a short-leg cast for 4 weeks. Irreducible dislocations must be opened. Medial dislocation is usually obstructed by the capsule or extensor brevis muscle in the talonavicular joint. Obstruction to lateral dislocation is if the posterior tibial tendon is greater than 2 mm and there is comminution.

R. Calcaneus Fractures

1. Classification—Based on facet displacement and posterior facet comminution seen with CT.

   Type I: Nondisplaced posterior facet
   Type II: Single fracture line posterior facet
   Type III: Secondary fracture line with three main posterior fragments
   Type IV: Three fracture lines with 4+ fragments

2. Evaluation—Radiographic evaluation involves a lateral view for Gusiane angle and Broden's view for subtalar joint congruency (see Table 10–2). CT should be oriented 90 degrees to the posterior facet. Extra-articular fractures make up 25% of calcaneal fractures. These include anterior process, posterosuperior tuberosity body, and medial or lateral process fracture.

3. Treatment—Nondisplaced or extra-articular fractures are placed in a cast with early range-of-motion exercises. ORIF is used for large fragments and small fragments are excised. Treatment of intra-articular fractures remains controversial. Many surgeons still favor closed treatment with or without manipulation. Poor results have been found with displacement. Most authors recommend ORIF for a displaced fracture with reduction of calcaneal width, correction of varus hindfoot, and restoration of articular height and congruity. The lateral approach is most common. Fixation is with low profile plates. Consider primary subtalar fusion in type IV injuries.

4. Complications—Complications include compartment syndrome in 10%, difficulty with shoewear due to heel widening, peroneal impingement, sural nerve injury, post-traumatic arthritis, malunion, and skin problems. There is a high incidence of tarsal tunnel syndrome.

S. Tarsometatarsal Fracture/Dislocation (Lisfranc)—This complex injury is often unrecognized. The second and third metatarsals are the keystones for tarsometatarsal stability. Plantar ligaments are much stronger and, therefore, dorsal dislocations are more common. Lisfranc's ligament extends from the second metatarsal to the medial cuneiform, bypassing the first metatarsal. The plantar branch of the anterior tibial artery and the deep peroneal nerve emerge from between the first and second metatarsals. Radiographic evaluation is important. There is a high index of suspicion with small fractures of the first or second metatarsal base on the AP view or with dorsal displacement of the second or third metatarsals on the lateral view, avulsion fractures of the medial pole of the navicular, and crush injuries of the cuboid. Stress views taken with regional anesthesia are helpful if there is no radiographic evidence of injury but pain and swelling over the tarsometatarsal joints.

1. Classification—Classification is homolateral, isolated with medial or lateral displacement of a portion of the tarsometatarsal complex, or divergent.

2. Treatment—Treatment requires anatomic reduction for best results. Some authors recommend open management of all fractures; however, if fracture is anatomically reduced, then use percutaneous pin fixation for 6 weeks with cast immobilization for 3 months. If fracture is displaced, then use ORIF and removal of osteochondral fragments. Screws remain in for at least 6 months with weight bearing begun at 3 months.

T. Midtarsal Fractures

1. Classification—Classified as five injuries to the region: medial, longitudinal, lateral, plantar stress, and crush. The classification is based on direction of force and resulting deformity. Any combination of injuries can occur. The medial fracture is most common owing to inversion injury dislocating the talonavicular joint. The longitudinal high-energy fracture has higher associated injuries and a poor prognosis. Lateral injury has a "nutcracker" effect on the cuboid with navicular tuberosity fracture. Plantar injury occurs after dorsal lip fractures of the navicular, talus, and anterior process. Crush injuries are often open, with numerous patterns.

2. Treatment—Treatment is early anatomic reduction and realignment of the midtarsal area. Nondisplaced fractures may be treated with cast immobilization, but displacement occurs frequently because of unrecognized instability. Percutaneous pin fixation for 6 weeks is preferred with ORIF of large fragments.

U. Navicular Fractures—Included are cortical avulsion fractures (47%), tuberosity fractures (24%), and body fractures (29%). Treatment requires restoration of anatomic joint surface while maintaining mobility of the talonavicular joint. ORIF fragments of the navicular are stabilized to the cuneiform with a temporary smooth Kirschner wire through the talonavicular joint for additional stabilization. The stress fracture is managed with non–weight bearing in a cast for 6 to 8 weeks.

V. Cuboid Fracture—This avulsion or compression fracture ("nutcracker") occurs between the calcaneus and metatarsal. Minimal impaction is treated with a non–weight bearing cast for 6 to 8 weeks. Large fragments are stabilized with ORIF, non–weight bearing for 6 to 8 weeks.

W. Metatarsal Fractures—The first metatarsal is the most mobile of the metatarsals. It bears one third of the body weight through two sesamoid bones. The anterior tibial tendon elevates the metatarsal and supinates the forefoot. The peroneal longus plantarflexes the metatarsal and pronates the forefoot. Nondisplaced fractures are treated in a short-leg cast for 2 to 3 weeks. Displaced fractures require anatomic ORIF.

Metatarsal shaft fractures and neck fractures when nondisplaced can be treated with partial weight bearing in a short-leg walking cast or padded cast shoe for 2 to 3 weeks. Displaced fractures require reduction and pinning or ORIF. Intra-articular fracture with displacement requires anatomic reduction with ORIF. Stress fractures usually involve the second metatarsal. Nondisplaced stress fractures can be treated with activity restriction and a short-leg walking cast or orthosis. Complete or displaced stress fractures are treated as acute fractures. The fifth metatarsal fracture is a metadiaphyseal fracture ("Jones fracture"). A unique blood supply is provided by the medial nutrient artery feeding proximally. A watershed area may explain the high nonunion rate. There is also a high ratio of cortical to cancellous bone. It is characterized as acute, stress fracture, or chronic nonunion.

Treatment is controversial. Acute nondisplaced fractures can be treated with a non–weight-bearing short-leg cast for 6 weeks and then partial weight bearing for 2 weeks. In an elite athlete a cannulated screw is used with return to full activity at 8 weeks. Stress fractures require activity restriction and non–weight bearing in a cast for 6 to 8 weeks. Predisposing factors such as genu varum or heel varus should be corrected. High-performance athletes warrant a surgical approach. Chronic nonunion or a delayed-healing stress fracture requires ORIF, bone graft, and a short-leg weight-bearing cast.

Metaphyseal fractures typically of the base of the fifth metatarsal can usually be managed with weight bearing in a short-leg cast or orthosis. Avulsion fractures of the base of the fifth metatarsal occur with acute inversion in plantarflexion and are caused by the lateral plantar aponeurosis and if nondisplaced or minimally displaced can be managed similarly. Intra-articular fractures should be managed with ORIF if there is more than 2 mm of displacement.

X. Phalangeal Fractures of Foot—Lesser phalangeal and interphalangeal joint fractures can usually be treated with reduction and buddy splinting. Surgery is reserved for markedly displaced fractures or open fractures. Great toe proximal phalanx fractures are treated more aggressively with pinning or ORIF. The first interphalangeal joint is more forgiving; its fracture requires closed reduction and immobilization. Sesamoid fractures are treated conservatively in a cast shoe for 4 to 8 weeks. If there is nonunion, bone graft is done; if this is persistent, then meticulous excision should be done.

VI. Upper Extremity Fractures and Dislocations

A. Sternoclavicular Joint Dislocation—The sternoclavicular joint is incongruent, and its stability is primarily due to its ligamentous structures. It is supported by the costoclavicular ligament, interclavicular ligaments, intra-articular disc ligament, and the anterior, superior, and posterior capsular ligaments (strongest). Injuries usually manifest as dislocations (either anterior or posterior). In patients younger than 25 years of age these usually represent physeal injuries of the medial clavicle: SH type I or II (Fig. 10–30).

1. Diagnosis—Diagnosis is usually evident on physical examination. Foreshortening is evident of the affected side, and there is a tender prominence at the sternoclavicular joint in anterior dislocations. Posterior dislocations are often associated with symptoms of dyspnea or dysphagia owing to compression of the trachea and esophagus. The "Serendipity" view (40 degree cephalic tilt; see Table 10–2) and CT are often necessary to determine the direction of dislocation.
2. Treatment—Treatment of acute anterior dislocations consists of closed reduction with the patient supine with a bump between the shoulders. Abduction and posterior pressure is placed on the medial end of the clavicle. Frequently unstable, the dislocation is immobilized in a figure-of-eight brace with hand and elbow range of motion. Irreducible or recurrent dislocations can be managed nonoperatively with an excellent functional result.

Treatment of acute posterior dislocations

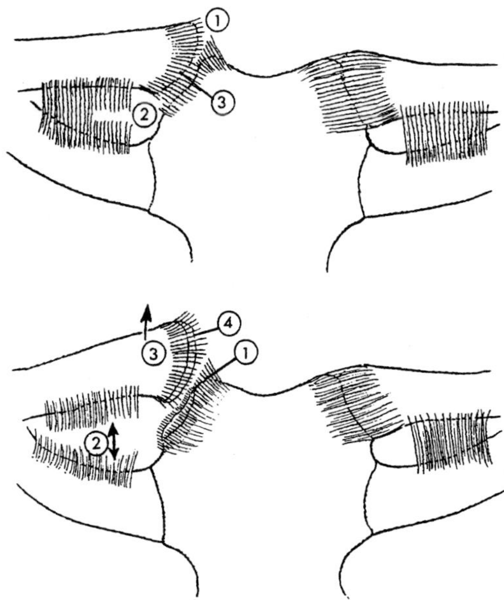

Figure 10–30. Sternoclavicular dislocations. *Top,* Partial injury. *Bottom,* Complete sternoclavicular dislocation. (From Connolly, J.F., ed.: DePalma's The Management of Fractures and Dislocations, an Atlas, 3rd ed., p. 560. Philadelphia, WB Saunders, 1981.)

is complicated by the proximity of neurovascular structures. Closed reduction in the operating room is recommended with thoracic surgery backup. Shoulder abduction is done with a percutaneous towel clip. If the dislocation is irreducible, open reduction and ligamentous reconstruction is done. A figure-of-eight brace is used for 6 weeks.

3. Complications—Complications are related to injuries to the associated structures. Chronic symptomatic dislocations can be managed by resection of the medial 1 to 1.5 cm of the clavicle.

B. ***Clavicle Fractures***

1. Classification

Group I: Fractures of the middle third (85%)
Group II: Fractures of the distal third (10%)
  Type I: Nondisplaced interligamentous fracture
  Type II: Fracture medial to coracoclavicular ligaments with displacement of medial fragment
  Type IIA: Conoid and trapezoid ligaments intact and attached to distal fragment
  Type IIB: Conoid disrupted but trapezoid intact and attached to distal fragment
  Type III: Fracture extends into acromioclavicular joint
  Type IV: Periosteal sleeve fracture with ligaments attached to periosteum
  Type V: Comminuted fracture with ligaments attached to an inferior fragment
Group III: Fractures of the medial third (5%)

2. Treatment—The majority of group I and III fractures heal uneventfully with sling or figure-of-eight immobilization for 6 to 8 weeks. Shortening and deformity are common but are not usually a problem. Indications for acute operative management include open fractures, displaced fractures with compromise of skin, and associated vascular injuries requiring repair. Methods of fixation include modified Hagie intramedullary pin, AO 3.5 plate, and external fixation. Management of group II injuries varies. ORIF is recommended for type II injuries. Type I and minimally displaced type III, IV, and V fractures can be managed nonoperatively with a sling or figure-of-eight.

3. Complications—These are uncommon. Nonunion occurs in 1% to 5%, although this is likely underestimated. The majority of nonunions occur in the middle third, but lateral third fractures are more prone to develop nonunions. Nonunion is more common in open, displaced, or high-energy fractures or with inadequate immobilization or poor patient compliance. Hypertrophic nonunions may result in neurologic or vascular compression. Symptomatic nonunions of the middle third are managed with ORIF using a modified Hagie pin or AO 3.5 plate with bone grafting. Symptomatic distal third nonunions are managed with excision ± ligamentous reconstruction.

C. Acromioclavicular Joint—This joint is extremely stable from strong static and dynamic stabilizers. Horizontal stability is primarily provided by the acromioclavicular ligaments and vertical stability by the coracoclavicular ligaments. With greater displacement, the conoid ligament provides primary restraint to superior translation and the trapezoid provides restraint to acromioclavicular joint compression. The trapezius and deltoid provide dynamic support.

1. Classification (Fig. 10–31)

Type I: Sprain
Type II: Acromioclavicular ligament disruption/preservation of coracoclavicular ligaments
Type III: Disruption of acromioclavicular and coracoclavicular ligaments with 25% to 100% subluxation
Type IV: Posterior dislocation of clavicle
Type V: Detachment of deltoid and trapezius muscles with 100% to 300% subluxation
Type VI: Inferior dislocation of clavicle

2. Treatment—Type I and II injuries are treated with rest, sling, and early range-of-motion exercises. Return to activity is allowed at 3 months. Treatment of type III injuries is controversial. The majority of type III injuries are managed nonoperatively with rehabilitation for 3 to 6 months. Operative repair may be considered in heavy laborers and high-performance athletes. Types IV, V, and VI are

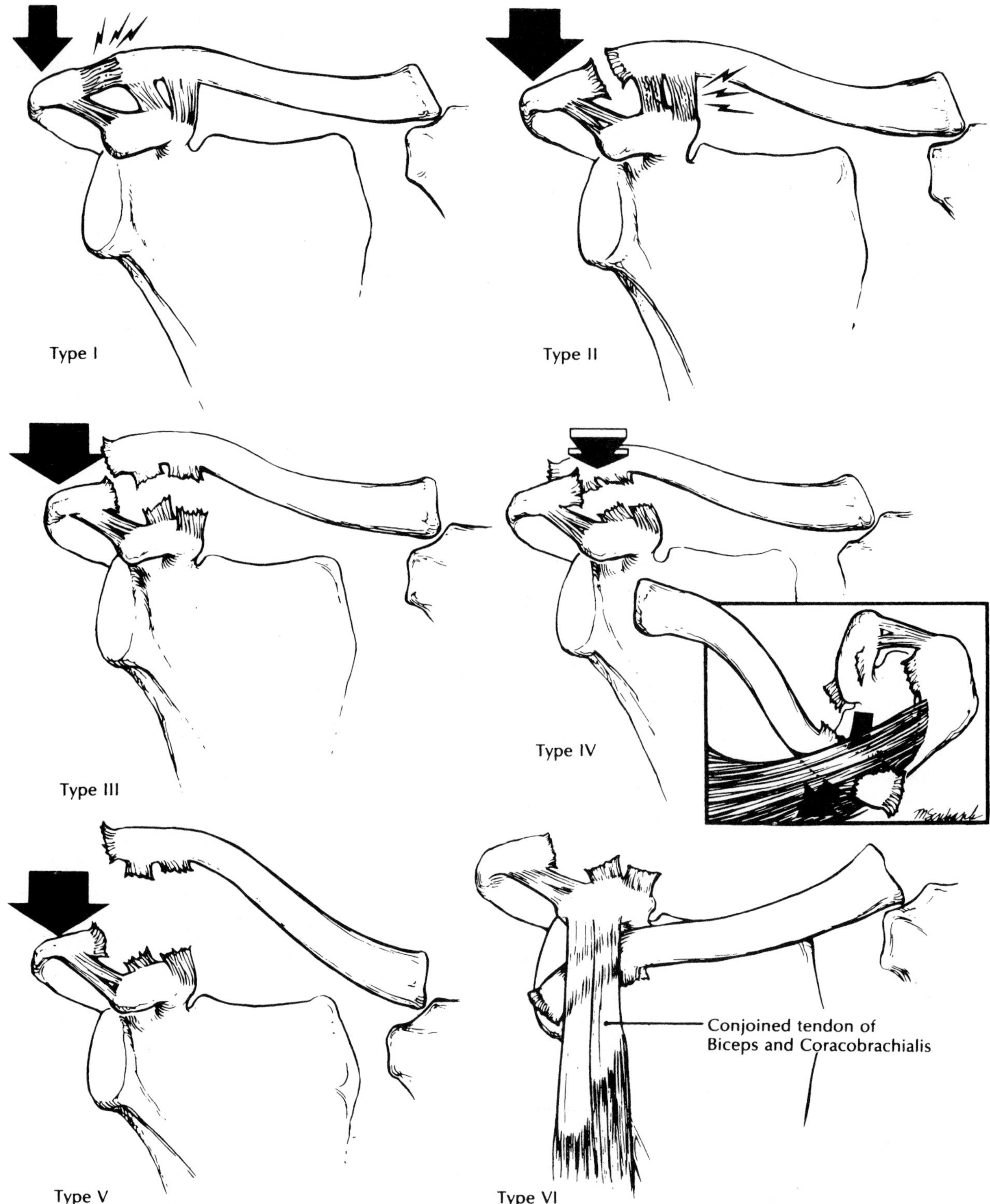

Figure 10–31. Classification of acromioclavicular injuries. (From Neer, C.S., and Rockwood, C.A.: Fractures and dislocations of the shoulder. In Rockwood, C.A., and Green, D.P., eds.: Fractures in Adults, 2nd ed., p. 871. Philadelphia, JB Lippincott, 1984.)

treated with open reduction and repair with acromioclavicular joint fixation versus coracoclavicular repair ± distal clavicle excision. Late symptomatic injuries can be managed with distal clavicle excision.

D. Scapular Fractures—Uncommon fractures make up less than 1% of all fractures. Fifty percent involve the scapular body and spine. High-energy fractures have a high incidence of associated injuries. Radiographic studies including AP, scapular Y, and axillary views and CT are useful for evaluating fracture pattern (see Table 10–2).

1. Classification
   Multiple classification systems are based anatomically.
   a. Zdravkovic 1974

      Type I: Scapular body fractures
      Type II: Apophyseal fractures including the coracoid and acromion
      Type III: Fractures of the superlateral angle including the neck and glenoid

      This system was devised to separate the type III fractures, which are generally considered most difficult to treat.
   b. Thompson 1985

      Class I: Coracoid, acromion, and small body fractures
      Class II: Glenoid and neck fractures
      Class III: Major scapular body fractures

      This system was devised to separate class II and III fractures, which are more likely to have associated injuries.
   c. Idberg Classification of Glenoid Fractures

      Type I: Anterior avulsion fracture
      Type II: Transverse/oblique fracture—inferior glenoid free
      Type III: Upper third glenoid and coracoid
      Type IV: Horizontal glenoid fracture through body
      Type V: Combination of II to IV
2. Treatment—Ninety percent of scapular fractures can be treated nonoperatively. Short-term immobilization is followed by progressive range of motion. Most fractures heal in 6 weeks with little or no functional deficit. Surgical management is aimed at restoring rotator cuff function and stability of the glenohumeral joint. Indications for surgery include involvement of more than 25% of the glenoid fossa with associated humeral subluxation, intra-articular stepoff of more than 5 mm, more than 40 degrees of angulation of a neck fracture. Seventy percent have good to excellent results with ORIF using appropriate indications. The approach (anterior vs. posterior) is based on the position of major fracture fragments.
3. Associated Injuries—These high-energy fractures have a high incidence of associated injuries: rib fractures with pneumo/hemothorax, pulmonary contusion, closed-head injuries, brachial plexus, and vascular injuries. Scapulothoracic dissociation is a rare separation of the scapulothoracic articulation. Intrathoracic dislocation is treated with closed reduction, management of pulmonary injury, and immobilization for 3 to 6 weeks. Lateral dissociation ("closed forequarter amputation") is associated with a high incidence of vascular injury (subclavian most common). Partial or complete plexus injury is treated with stabilization of dissociation with ORIF of clavicle and acromioclavicular and sternoclavicular joints and vascular repair as indicated. Prognosis is poor.

E. Proximal Humeral Fractures—Represent 5% to 7% of all fractures and 76% of all humeral fractures in patients older than age 40 years. Falls are the most common mechanism in elderly persons with osteoporotic bone. Treatment requires accurate assessment of fracture pattern, bone quality, individual functional requirements of patient, compliance, and rehabilitation potential.
   1. Classification (Fig. 10–32)—The proximal humerus consists of four parts: greater tuberosity, lesser tuberosity, head, and shaft. Fracture classification is based on displacement of the four fragments. Fragments are considered displaced if separated by 1 cm or angulated more than 45 degrees from anatomic position. Displacement is due to deforming forces of cuff, pectoralis muscles, and deltoid muscles. Careful radiographic evaluation is necessary to accurately assess fracture pattern and displacement. CT is often helpful.
   2. Treatment—One-part fractures are treated with sling immobilization, early range of motion (1–2 weeks), and isometric exercises. Close radiographic follow-up is required to evaluate displacement.
      a. Two-Part Fractures—In these surgical neck fractures both tuberosities remain on the humeral head and the cuff is intact. The shaft is displaced medially by pull of the pectoralis major. Closed reduction is attempted. If fracture is stable, early progressive range-of-motion exercises are begun. If the fracture is unstable, percutaneous pinning versus ORIF is done.
      b. Greater Tuberosity Fractures—Often associated with anterior dislocation. The tuberosity is retracted posteriorly by pull of

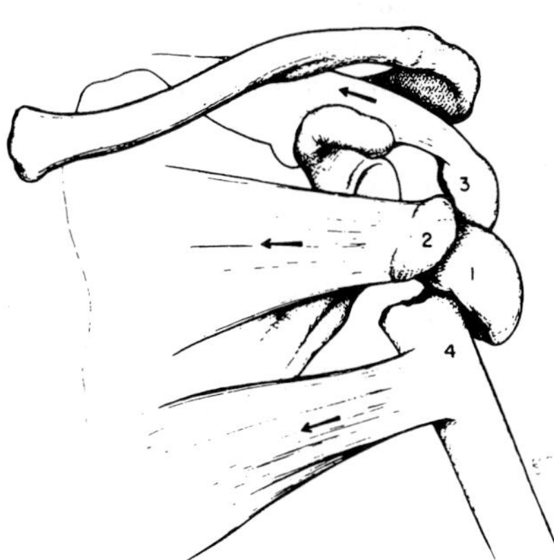

Figure 10–32. Proximal humeral fracture. Four parts: 1, head; 2, lesser tuberosity; 3, greater tuberosity; 4, humeral shaft. (From Neer, C.S., and Rockwood, C.A.: Fractures and dislocations of the shoulder. In Rockwood, C.A., and Green, D.P., eds.: Fractures in Adults, 2nd ed., p. 696. Philadelphia, JB Lippincott, 1984.)

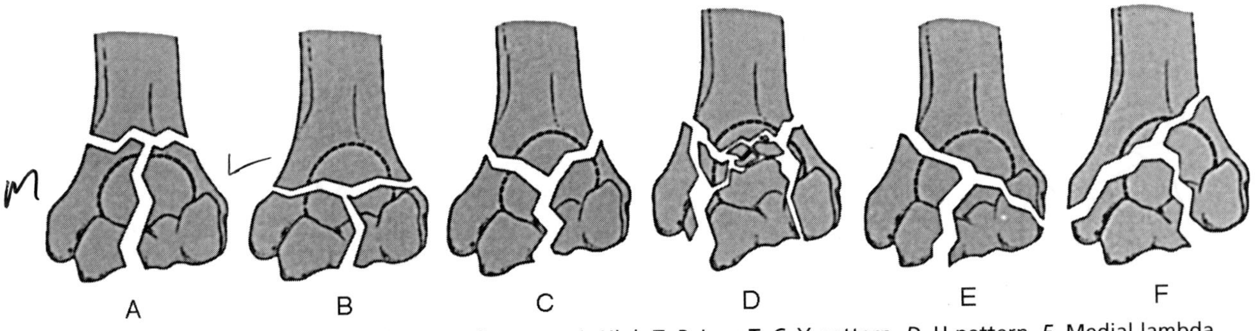

Figure 10–36. Bicolumn distal humerus fractures. *A,* High T. *B,* Low T. *C,* Y pattern. *D,* H pattern. *E,* Medial lambda. *F,* Lateral lambda. (From Browner, B.: Skeletal Trauma, vol. 2, pp. 1159–1163. Philadelphia, WB Saunders, 1992.)

severe soft tissue injury or bone loss, an unreliable patient, and an inability to obtain or maintain reduction.

Indications for ORIF include open fractures, vascular injuries, floating elbow, polytrauma with multiple extremities, closed-head injury, and pathologic fracture. Fixation options include intramedullary nailing antegrade or retrograde or ORIF with AO 4.5 compression plate. A minimum of six cortices and preferably eight cortices should be above and below the fracture.

1. Humeral Fractures and Associated Radial Nerve Palsy—Neurologic status must be documented before reduction. Incidence is 5% to 10%, and most represent traction injuries. There is a high incidence of spontaneous recovery even with a Holstein-Lewis fracture. Exploration is mandatory in open fractures with palsy, intact function before reduction with deficit after reduction, deficit after ORIF unless nerve isolated and protected intraoperatively, or persistent deficit 3 to 4 months after injury with no electromyographic evidence of recovery. Exploration of Holstein-Lewis fractures (long spiral oblique fracture in distal third) is controversial.
2. Humeral Shaft Nonunion—Higher rate of nonunion occurs in operatively treated fractures than in nonoperatively treated fractures unless they have been optimally stabilized. Management of nonunion is ORIF with stable plate fixation. A minimum of six cortices above and below is preferable. Supplemental autogenous bone graft should be used. Persistent nonunion occurs despite adequate stabilization and bone grafting; free vascularized fibular graft may be required. Infection should be ruled out.

H. Distal Humerus Fractures

1. Anatomy—Bony anatomy consists of diverging medial and lateral columns supporting the trochlea, creating a triangular construct of two functionally independent joints. The lateral column diverges 20 degrees anteriorly to end in the capitellum. The medial column diverges 45 degrees and ends proximal to the trochlear articular surface. The distal humerus tilts forward 30 degrees; the trochlea has 3 to 8 degrees of internal rotation and a valgus inclination of 2 to 6 degrees.
2. Classification—There are multiple classification systems based on the condylar concept. No single system is comprehensive. Extra-articular fractures are either supracondylar or transcondylar. Most adult distal humeral fractures involve the articular surface. Lateral condylar fractures are much more common than medial fractures. Jupiter has classified bicolumn fractures based on orientation of major fracture lines (Fig. 10–36). The AO/ASIS classification is being used more frequently:

   Type A: Periarticular/extra-articular distal humerus fractures: A1, avulsion fracture; A2, metaphyseal; A3, metaphyseal with comminution.

   Type B: Partial intra-articular fracture with or without column involvement: B1, lateral condylar; B2, medial condylar; B3, articular fracture without column.

   Type C: Entire articular fracture with both-column disruption: C1, no significant articular or metaphyseal comminution; C2, no articular comminution but significant metaphyseal comminution; C3, both articular and metaphyseal comminution.

3. Treatment—Treatment is based on stable anatomic reduction and early active range of motion. Only nondisplaced fractures with enough innate stability to allow early range of motion should be treated nonoperatively.
   a. Type A—Extra-articular fracture. Most avulsion fractures are medial and if there is more than 1 cm of displacement or medial instability, then ORIF is recommended.
   Type A2—Type A2 and A3 extra-articular fractures disrupt the medial and lateral columns and require ORIF. Posterior triceps splitting or sparing approach is most commonly used. Distal diaphyseal fractures can often be managed with 4.5 dynamic compression plates (DCPs). Dual-plate fixation provides more rigid stability

with distal metaphyseal fracture. The plate should be placed at 90 degrees, with a posterolateral and medial position providing the best mechanical rigidity. The 3.5 Recon or DCPs are preferred.

b. Type B—Partial articular fracture. The Milch Classification is used primarily to determine potential stability.
Medial and lateral humeral condylar fracture (Fig. 10–37).

Milch I: Lateral trochlear ridge intact
Milch II: Fracture through lateral trochlear ridge

Milch type I fractures are less common. Nondisplaced fractures can be treated with a period of 2 to 3 weeks of splinting followed by range-of-motion exercises. A displaced fracture should undergo ORIF. Milch type II fractures are unstable and require ORIF. In children, Milch type I fractures are true Salter-Harris type IV physeal injuries. Milch type II fractures are type II Salter-Harris physeal injuries.

c. Type C—Unstable patterns that require articular reconstruction and both-column stabilization.

I. Capitellum Fracture (Fig. 10–38)
   1. Classification

   Type I: Hahn-Steinthal: Fracture in the coronal plane
   Type II: Kocher-Lorenz: Sleeve fracture of the articular surface with little osseous bone
   Type III: Comminuted

   2. Treatment—Nondisplaced fractures can typically be treated with 2 to 3 weeks of splinting with progressive range-of-motion exercises. If fragments are displaced more than 2 mm and large enough to accept fixation, ORIF is recommended. If fragments are too small, excision is advised.
      a. Intra-articular Fracture with Both-Column Disruption—Treatment of these fractures is technically demanding and almost always operative: posterior exposure with intra-articular Chevron osteotomy versus subperiosteal reflection of the triceps. The ulnar nerve is isolated and protected. The goal is anatomic reduction of the articular surface with transcondylar screws. The trochlea is then fixed to the shaft by dual plating technique. Posterolateral and medial plates provide the greatest rigidity. Postoperatively, there is a short period of immobilization followed by early range-of-motion exercises.
   3. Complications—Nonunion after ORIF ranges from 1% to 11% and is usually associated with inadequate fixation. Olecranon osteotomy nonunion has also been reported, particularly after transverse intra-articular osteotomies. Nonunions are managed by revision ORIF with bone grafting. Nonunions can occur and require complex reconstructive osteotomies. Ulnar neuropathy is also common, especially with valgus deformities or nonunions. Routine ulnar nerve transposition is recommended during the initial procedure. Late neuropathies usually respond well to stabilization of the fracture and transposition of the nerve. Heterotopic ossification after ORIF of distal humerus fractures has been estimated at approximately 4% (much higher with traumatic brain injury). Prophylaxis with indomethacin and, rarely, radiation has been recommended. Treatment is late excision after maturity.

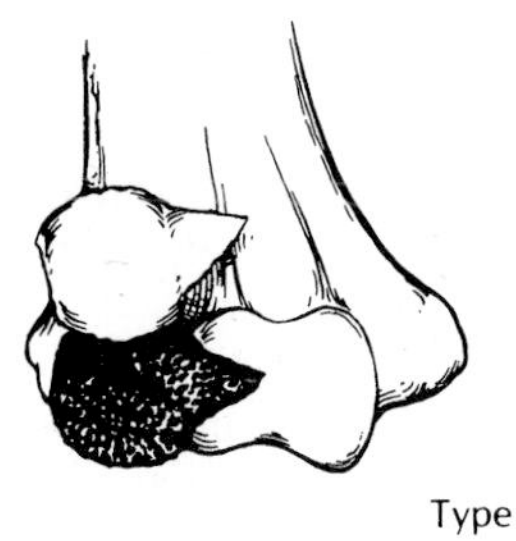
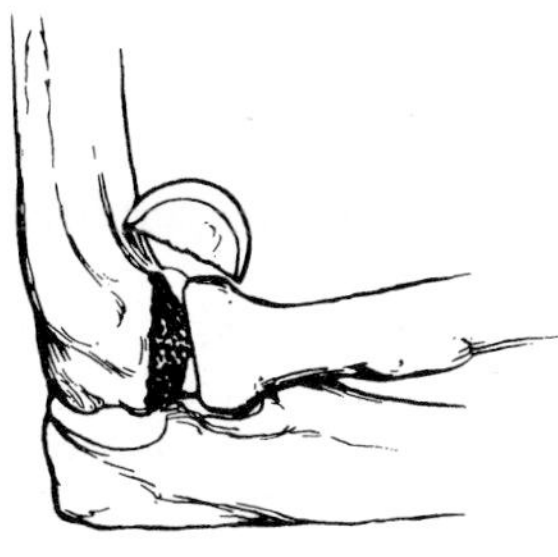

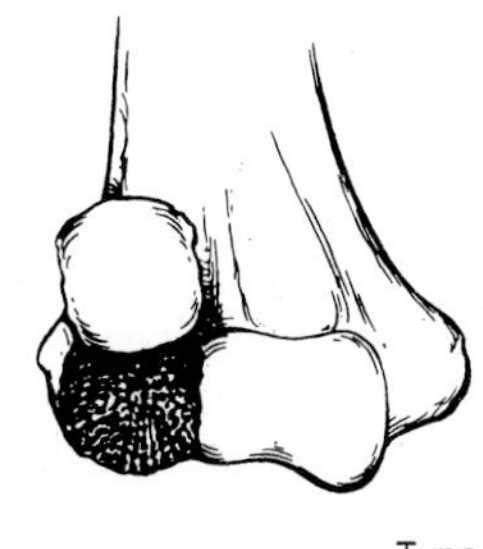
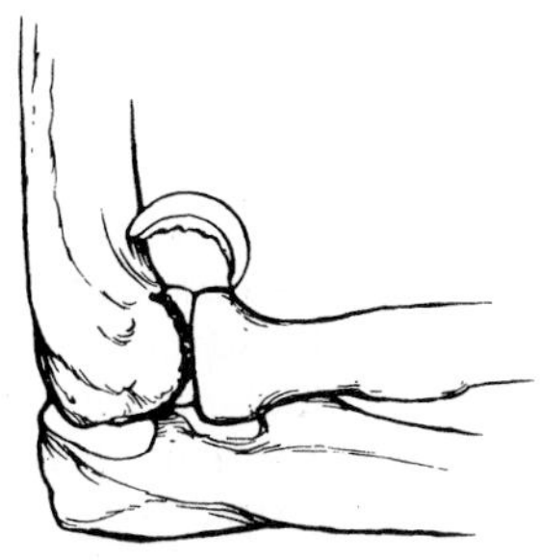

Figure 10–38. Capitellar fractures. Note presence of subchondral bone in type I fracture. (From DeLee, J.C., Green, D.P., and Wilkins, K.E.: Fractures and dislocations of the elbow. In Rockwood, C.A., and Green, D.P., eds.: Fractures in Adults, 2nd ed., p. 591. Philadelphia, JB Lippincott, 1984.)

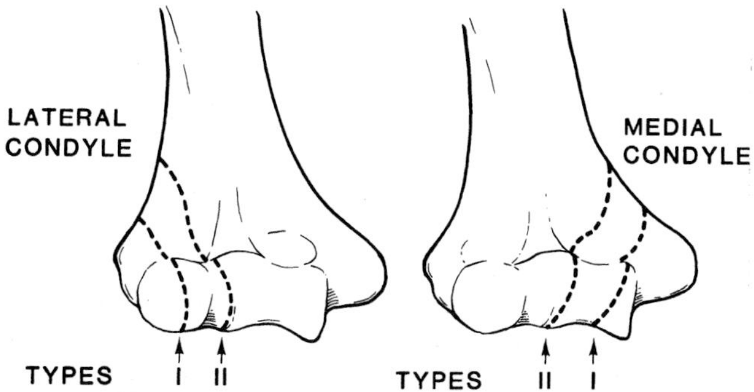

Figure 10–37. Humeral condyle fractures. (From Gelman, M.I.: Radiology of Orthopedic Procedures, Problems and Complications, vol. 24, p. 56. Philadelphia, WB Saunders, 1984.)

J. Olecranon Fractures
   1. Classification—Olecranon fractures are common with varied mechanisms of injury and fracture patterns. Multiple classification patterns have been developed; however, no single system is widely accepted.
   2. Treatment—Nondisplaced fractures are uncommon. Criteria are less than 2 mm of displacement and no increase with 90 degrees of flexion or active extension. The elbow should be splinted in 30 to 45 degrees of flexion with close radiographic follow-up. Nondisplaced and simple avulsion fractures can be associated with triceps rupture. Displaced fractures require ORIF to restore the extensor mechanism. Transverse fractures can be treated with tension band technique supplemented with Kirschner wires or an intramedullary screw. Oblique fractures are more amenable to management with a bicortical interfragmentary screw, supplemental plate, or tension band. Comminuted fractures are best managed with plate fixation placed on the dorsal (tension) surface. In severely comminuted fractures, excision of the fragment and reattachment of the triceps can provide results equivalent to ORIF. Excision of greater than 50% of the olecranon can result in instability.

K. Coronoid Fractures—The coronoid process is important for anterior stability. It functions as an anterior buttress of the greater sigmoid fossa and is the attachment site for the anterior bundle of the medial collateral ligament and anterior capsule. Coronoid fractures are common and are associated with 10% of elbow dislocation and with recurrent instability after dislocation.
   1. Classification

      Type I: Avulsion of the tip
      Type II: Less than 50% fracture (stable)
      Type III: Greater than 50% fracture (unstable)

   2. Treatment—Type I and II fractures can usually be managed with closed reduction and early mobilization if stable. Type III fractures require ORIF to restore stability.

L. Radial Head Fractures—These common injuries account for 33% of elbow fractures and are associated with 20% of elbow trauma cases. Head and neck fractures occur in 50% to 60% of elbow dislocations. The mechanism of injury is usually an axial load on a pronated forearm. Fracture most commonly occurs in the anterolateral portion of the radial head in the area without articular cartilage and with less tensile strength of the subchondral bone.
   1. Classification (Mason) (Fig. 10–39)

      Type I: Undisplaced
      Type II: Displaced single fracture
      Type III: Comminuted
      Type IV: Radial head fracture with associated dislocation (Johnson modification)

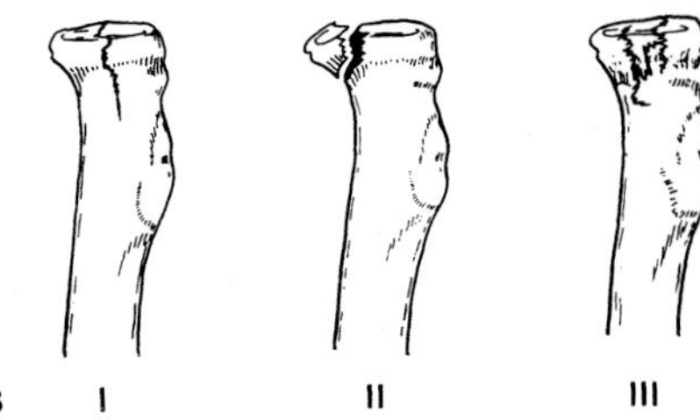

Figure 10–39. Anterior shoulder dislocation. *Top,* Subglenoid. *Middle,* Subcoracoid. *Bottom,* Subclavicular. (From Connolly, J.F., ed.: DePalma's The Management of Fractures and Dislocations, an Atlas, 3rd ed., p. 617. Philadelphia, WB Saunders, 1981.)

   2. Treatment
      a. Type I—Fractures without other soft tissue injuries can usually be treated nonoperatively with good results. Early mobilization reduces disability time and enhances elbow motion. If greater than one third of the radial head is involved, displacement can occur and close radiographic follow-up is necessary.
      b. Type II—Type II fractures treated surgically result in less pain and improved function and grip strength. ORIF is the preferred treatment with 1.5- to 2.7-mm screws, and with plate if humeral neck is involved. Hardware should be placed in the "safe zone" of approximately 100 degrees, found by bisecting midline of the radial neck in neutral forearm rotation. Small fragments can be excised.
      c. Types III and IV—Treatment of type III and IV fractures is operative. Timing of surgery and management of associated injuries are controversial. ORIF and salvage of the radial head are recommended, if possible. If resection of a fragment of the radial head is necessary, the elbow should be tested in 30 degrees of flexion to valgus stress to determine the status of the medial collateral ligament. If unstable, primary repair of this ligament should be performed. A radial head spacer can be placed in conjunction with lateral capsular and ligamentous repair. If associated with interosseous membrane and distal radioulnar joint disruption (Essex-Lopresti), realignment and stabilization of the disruption is done for 4 to 6 weeks with primary fixation of the radial head or temporary use of radial head implant until the soft tissues have healed.

M. Elbow Dislocations
   1. Anatomy—The elbow is the second most commonly dislocated joint in the body. This dislocation accounts for 20% of all dislocations and is second only to dislocation of the shoulder. Stability of the elbow is provided by highly congruent bony anatomy and strong ligamentous supports. The medial collateral ligament is the primary stabilizer and is com-

posed of the anterior oblique ligament, posterior oblique ligament, and small transverse ligament. The anterior oblique is the strongest and most well defined and is the main stabilizer to valgus stress. The lateral collateral ligament is primarily a thickening of the capsule consisting of the radial collateral ligament, lateral ulnar collateral ligament, and accessory collateral ligament. It is the main stabilizer with posterolateral stress.

2. Classification—Classified by direction of dislocation. Posterolateral dislocation is most common (more than 80% of all dislocations). Anterior, medial, lateral, and diversion dislocations occur.
3. Treatment—The initial treatment of all dislocations is nonsurgical. Closed reduction is done using gentle traction under anesthesia. Check range of motion and stability after reduction. Full flexion and extension should be present with no subluxation. Post-reduction radiographs should be obtained to confirm reduction and rule out fracture. Stable reduction can be splinted in 90 degrees of flexion for 7 to 10 days, followed by progressive range-of-motion exercises.

   Unstable reductions without fracture can be immobilized for 2 to 3 weeks, followed by range-of-motion exercises. Greater than 3 weeks' immobilization has been shown to be detrimental to elbow motion. Open treatment is indicated for persistent instability, intra-articular fragments, medial epicondylar fractures with displacement greater than 5 mm, and type III coronoid process fractures.
   a. Associated Injuries—Radial head and neck fractures occur in 50% to 60% of elbow dislocations. Medial and lateral epicondylar fractures occur in 10%. Associated coronoid fractures occur in 10%.
   b. Elbow Instability—Elbow dislocation can lead to a spectrum of instability described as circular that results from lateral to medial capsular and ligamentous disruption occurring in three stages. Stage I is posterolateral rotatory subluxation with tear of the lateral ulnar collateral ligament, posterolateral capsule, and radial collateral ligament. Stage II is subluxation or incomplete dislocation with the above involved structures plus an anterior capsule tear.

      Stage III is a result of either partial or complete medial collateral ligament tear. Posterolateral instability is present in 1% to 2% of simple dislocations. In patients younger than 16 years old this is usually related to the radial collateral ligament. In older patients it is due to an ulnar portion of the lateral collateral ligament. Diagnosis is made by the pivot shift test, which is subluxation associated with extension, valgus, and supination. With flexion beyond 30 to 60 degrees in pronation, reduction or a "clunk" is felt. This is treated with reconstruction of the lateral ulnar collateral ligament.

N. Forearm Fracture—Fractures of the forearm commonly result from high-energy trauma and are associated with systemic and musculoskeletal injuries. Examination of the injured extremity as well as the whole patient is essential. A detailed neurologic and vascular examination is critical. Radiographic evaluation should include AP and lateral views of the forearm, wrist, and elbow x-ray to rule out other associated injuries (see Table 10–2).
   1. Classification—Forearm fractures are most often characterized by description of fracture location, fracture configuration, presence of any radial ulnar or radial humeral articular involvement, and associated soft tissue injuries.
      a. Monteggia Fractures—Dislocation of radial head and ulnar fracture (Fig. 10–40).

         Type I (60%): Anterior radial head dislocation and apex anterior proximal third ulnar fracture
         Type II (15%): Posterior radial head dislocation and apex posterior proximal third ulnar fracture
         Type III: Lateral radial head dislocation and proximal ulnar metaphyseal fracture
         Type IV: Anterior dislocation of the radial head associated with proximal third radius and ulnar fractures

      b. Galeazzi Fractures—Fracture of distal third of the radius with associated distal radioulnar joint injury. Radiographic signs of distal radioulnar joint injury include ulnar styloid fracture, widened distal radioulnar joint on AP view, dislocation of the distal radioulnar joint on lateral view, and 5 mm of radial shortening.
   2. Treatment—Nonoperative treatment is limited to nondisplaced isolated ulnar fracture in the distal two thirds with less than 50% displacement and less than 10 degrees of angulation. These fractures can usually be managed with a functional fracture brace with good interosseous mold after 7 to 10 days of long-arm cast immobilization. The proximal third of the ulna or a more displaced fracture requires ORIF.

      Operative management is the favored treatment option for forearm fractures. Shaft fractures should be treated with anatomic reduction with stabile fixation and early range-of-motion exercises. Separate approaches to the ulna and radius decrease the synostosis rate. The volar (Henry) approach is optimal for distal third shaft fractures, and the dorsal (Thompson) approach is best for middle third

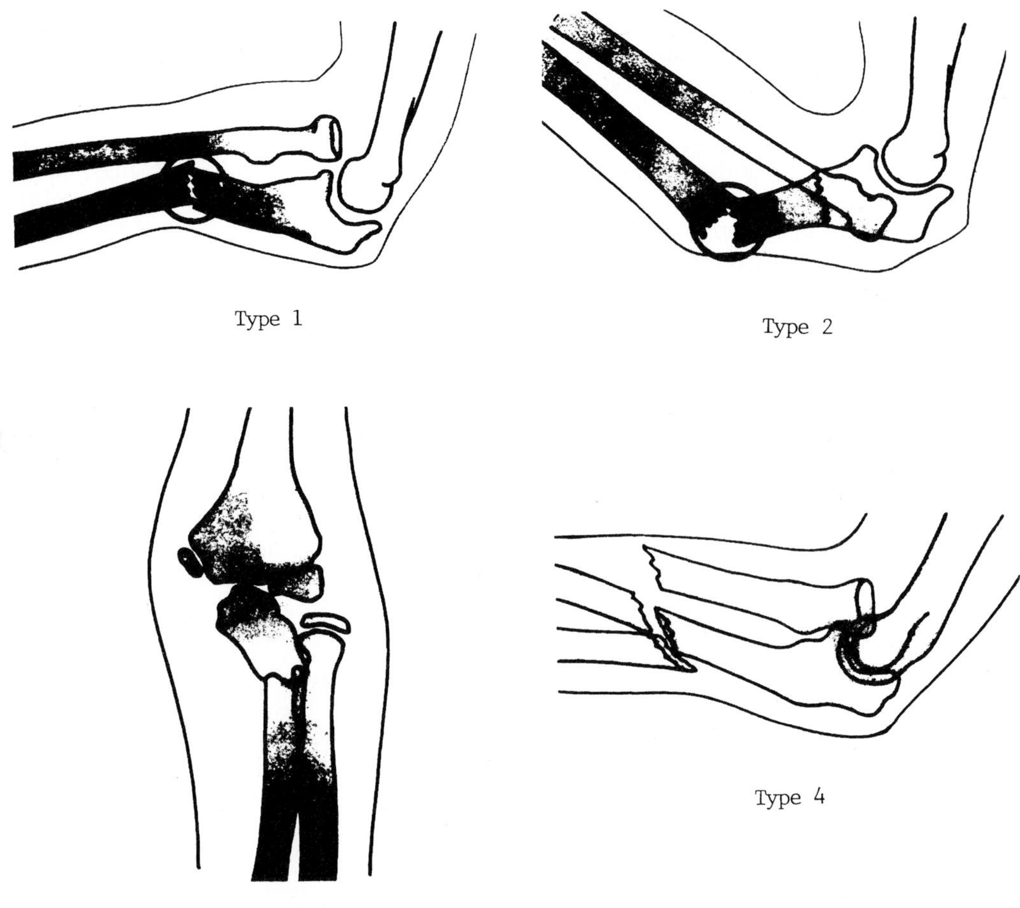

Figure 10–40. Classification of Monteggia's fractures. (From Reckling, F.W., and Cordell, L.D.: Unstable fracture-dislocations of the forearm. Arch. Surg. 96:1004, 1968. Copyright 1968 American Medical Association.)

shaft fractures. The proximal third fractures can be approached through a volar extensile approach or a dorsal approach. With a dorsal approach the posterior interosseous nerve is at risk. A direct subcutaneous approach is used for the ulna. Fixation is with three 3.5-mm DCPs with seven cortices of each main fragment including the interfrag screw; eight cortices are recommended if there is significant comminution. Primary bone grafting should be considered if there is more than one third comminution. A short course of postoperative splinting is followed by early range-of-motion exercises unless proximal or distal injuries prohibit mobilization. Intramedullary fixation has become more common; however, this technique is associated with a high rate of nonunion, especially in both-bone forearm fracture.

a. Monteggia Fracture—Requires early accurate diagnosis, anatomic reduction, and ORIF of ulna. The radial head typically relocates with reduction of the ulna. Irreducible radial head dislocations are associated with posterior interosseous nerve entrapment and postoperative cast or splint immobilization in 90 degrees with early (less than 3 weeks) progressive range-of-motion exercises.
b. Galeazzi Fracture—Treatment is ORIF of radius fracture with stabilization of the distal radioulnar joint either in supination or with reduction and percutaneous pinning for 4 to 6 weeks.

3. Complications—Forearm fractures are at risk for compartment syndrome especially in open fractures, low-velocity gunshot wounds, vascular injury, and coagulopathies. Diagnosis of compartment syndrome is clinical, with pain with passive stretch as the primary symptom, confirmed with compartment pressures. Neurologic injury is uncommon in closed fractures with the exception of injury to the posterior interosseous nerve with Monteggia fractures.

Hardware removal is controversial and is associated with fractures after plate removal in 4% to 20%. The radial refracture is decreased if hardware is left in for 15 to 24 months. Increased refracture rates are also associated with large 4.5-mm plates. After hardware removal splint protection is warranted for 6 to 8 weeks.

Synostosis occurs in an average of 3% of fractures. A higher risk of synostosis is associated with fixation beyond 2 weeks, both-bone forearm fractures at the same level, high-energy injuries, closed-head injuries, infections, single incision approach to both fractures, and bone graft placed along the interosseous membrane.

O. Distal Radius Fractures—Distal radius fractures are the most common of all orthopaedic injuries. They account for 74% of all forearm fractures and one sixth of all fractures seen in emergency departments; 50% involve the radiocarpal or radioulnar joints. They occur in bimodal distribution: younger patients have high-energy injuries, and older patients have injuries associated with falls.

1. Classification—Several classification systems have been described based on mechanism and anatomic description. **Frykman** describes **types I to VIII** (Fig. 10–41). Melone describes intra-articular fractures based on four parts—shaft, radial styloid, dorsomedial, and palmar medial fragment (Fig. 10–42): **type I** is minimally displaced; **type II** is carpus displacement; **type III** is volar spike; and **type IV** is volar fragment rotated.
2. Eponyms

Colles': Dorsal displacement
Smith's: Volar displacement
Dorsal Barton: Dorsal radial rim (Fig. 10–43)
Chauffeur's: Radial styloid (Fig. 10–44)
Volar Barton's: Volar radial rim

3. Evaluation—Thorough neurovascular examination should be carried out. The median nerve is the most commonly injured and primarily neurapraxic. Check the forearm compartment and evaluate the shoulder and elbow, especially in an elderly patient or with high-energy injuries. Distal radioulnar joint injury with an irreducible joint is usually due to extensor carpi ulnaris tendon entrapment.
   a. Radiographic Evaluation—Lateral view is normal volar tilt of 11 degrees. Posteroanterior (PA) view is normal radial length of 12 mm. Inclination is 23 degrees.
   b. Criteria for Acceptable Reduction—Change in palmar tilt less than 10 degrees, radial shortening less than 2 mm; change in radial angle less than 5 degrees, less than 1 to 2 mm; articular stepoff.
4. Treatment—The principle of treatment is to restore articular congruity, distal radial anatomy, and radial ulnar relationship; maintain reduction; obtain union; and restore functional range of motion. Certainly, instability of the fracture and reduction are keys to management. The pre-reduction films are the most important for determining fracture stability. Instability criteria include widely displaced intra-articular fractures, volar or dorsal comminution, dorsal angulation (apex volar) greater than 20 degrees or significant osteoporosis, initial fracture displacement or shortening greater than 5 mm, or dorsal comminution, articular margin fracture, and pal-

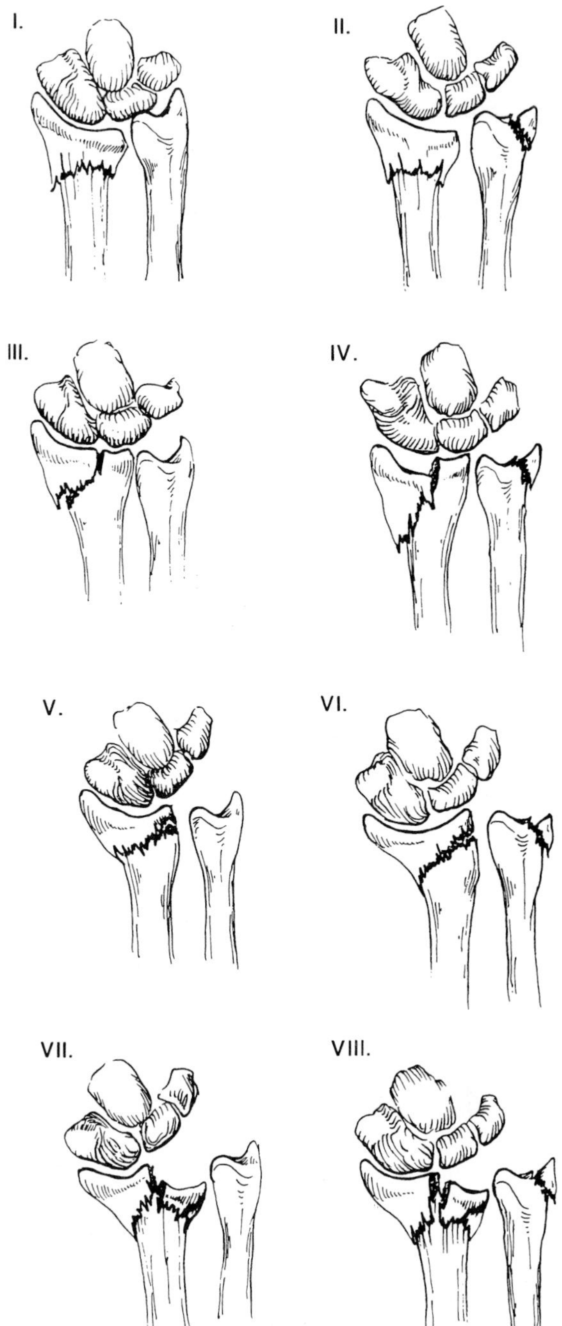

Figure 10–41. Frykman's classification of distal radius fractures. Note even numbers with ulnar styloid involvement. (From Kozin, S.H., and Berlet, A.C.: Handbook of Common Orthopaedic Fractures, pp. 17, 19. West Chester, PA, Medical Surveillance, 1989.)

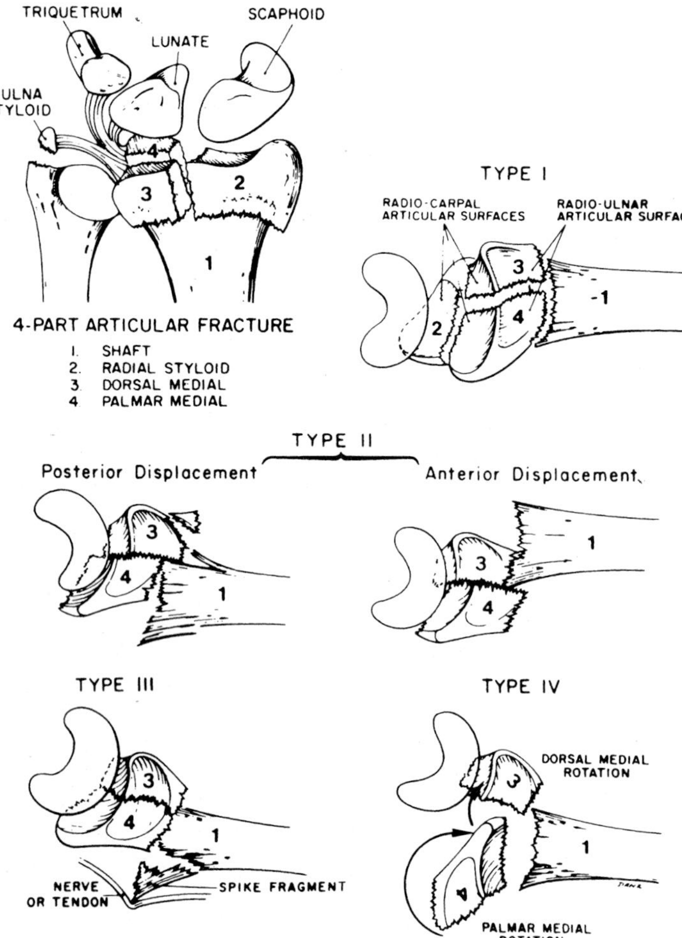

Figure 10–42. Melone classification of distal radius fractures. (From Melone, C.P., Jr.: Open treatment for displaced articular fractures of the distal radius. Clin. Orthop. 202:104, 1986.)

marly displaced and comminuted extra-articular fractures.

Treatment options include closed reduction with casting versus percutaneous pins, external fixation, or ORIF. Closed reduction and casting require close follow-up for redisplacement over a 2- to 3-week period. Repeat reduction attempts are associated with less than 50% satisfactory result. Percutaneous pinning is done to maintain sagittal alignment in unstable extra-articular fracture. Percutaneous pins do not maintain length when volar or bicortical comminution is present. External fixation is the treatment of choice for unstable extra-articular fractures with comminution and with unstable comminuted in-

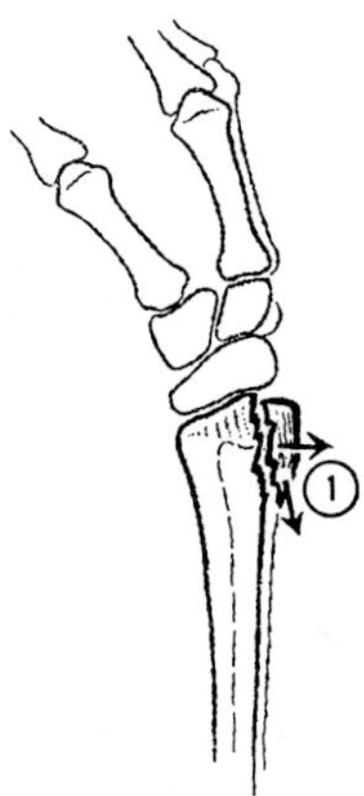

Figure 10–43. Dorsal Barton's fracture. (From Connolly, J.F., ed.: DePalma's The Management of Fractures and Dislocations, an Atlas, 3rd ed., p. 1032. Philadelphia, WB Saunders, 1981.)

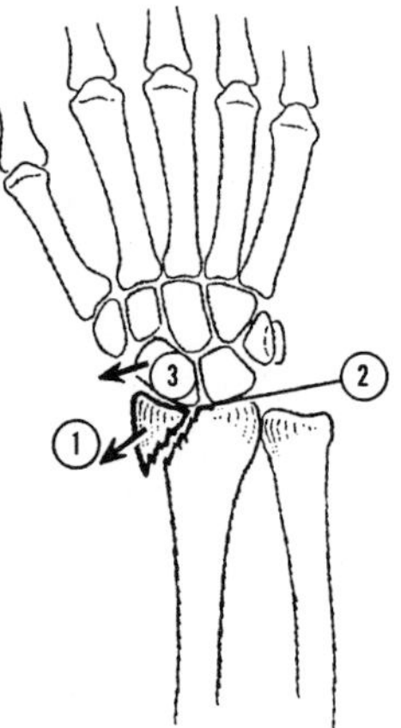

Figure 10–44. Radial styloid fractures. (From Connolly, J.F., ed.: DePalma's The Management of Fractures and Dislocations, an Atlas, 3rd ed., p. 1033. Philadelphia, WB Saunders, 1981.)

tra-articular fractures. External fixation does not reliably restore the 10-degree palmar tilt because the stronger volar ligaments become taut before the dorsal ligaments are restored to length. Complication rates of 15% to 60% have been reported associated with external fixation, with complications including pin tract infection, pin loosening, fracture complications, radial sensory iatrogenic nerve injury, and stiffness of the wrist and hand. Limiting duration of external fixation, carpal distraction of less than 5 mm, and neutral wrist position provide the best result. ORIF is done for articular marginal fractures and complex comminuted intra-articular fracture. Complex fractures may require a combination of external fixation, pin fixation, and ORIF. The approach is directed by the major articular fragment and the direction of displacement.

5. Complications
   a. Neurologic Injury—The median nerve is the most commonly involved; usually there is neurapraxia associated with traction due to fracture displacement or hematoma. Ulnar neuropathies are associated with distal radioulnar joint injuries.
   b. Tendon Injury—Distal radioulnar joint injuries may entrap the extensor carpi ulnaris or extensor digiti minimi. Late attritional ruptures can also occur, with the extensor pollicis longus most common.
   c. Distal Radioulnar Joint Injury—Fractures of the base of the ulnar styloid are associated with TFC injury. Treatment is with anatomic reduction of the ulnar styloid and immobilization in supination to stabilize the joint. Late joint complications include arthrosis, instability, weak grip, and limited forearm rotation. Restoring radial length is the key to avoiding these problems. Late management of chronic instability and pain is associated with distal ulnar excision (Darrach) or distal radioulnar joint fusion and creation of proximal ulnar pseudarthrosis.
   d. Radial Carpal Arthrosis—Stepoff of more than 1 to 2 mm leads to radiographic arthrosis. Greater than 90%, given the results of these findings, are symptomatic. This emphasizes the importance of an anatomic reduction. Extra-articular malunion or nonunion requires opening wedge osteotomy, ORIF, and bone grafting. Ulnar shortening should be added if radial length is not restored.
   e. Carpal Injury—Scaphoid fracture is most common in young adults and in high-energy fractures. In unstable distal radius fractures, ORIF is done of the scaphoid. The scapholunate ligament is the most commonly injured. Extra-articular nonunion can result in carpal instability.

P. Scaphoid Fractures—Scaphoid fractures often have subtle presentations characterized by pain and tenderness in the snuffbox. A high level of suspicion is necessary to avoid complications that would delay recognition and treatment. Thorough x-ray evaluation includes PA, lateral, and PA with ulnar deviation views (see Table 10–2). Initial x-ray sensitivity is 64%. If x-ray evaluation is normal but there is a high index of suspicion, a thumb spica cast is used for immobilization and radiography is repeated in 10 to 14 days. If x-ray films remain negative, then bone scan, CT, tomogram, or MRI is done. A delay in diagnosis of more than 28 days is associated with 45% nonunion. Early diagnosis and treatment in less than 28 days is associated with only 5% nonunion.
   1. Classification (Fig. 10–45)—Scaphoid fractures are classified by level, direction, stability, and chronicity; neck fractures, waist-horizontal fractures, waist-transverse fractures, and proximal pole fractures. Proximal pole fractures have higher rates of nonunion and osteonecrosis from the unique blood supply of the scaphoid: dorsal and distal supply resulting in high incidence of proximal pole necrosis. Type A fractures are acute-stable; type B are acute-unstable; type C are delayed union, and type D are nonunion. Criteria for fracture instability include displacement greater than 1 mm, any angulation, a scapholunate angle greater than 45 degrees, and a capitolunate angle greater than 15 degrees.

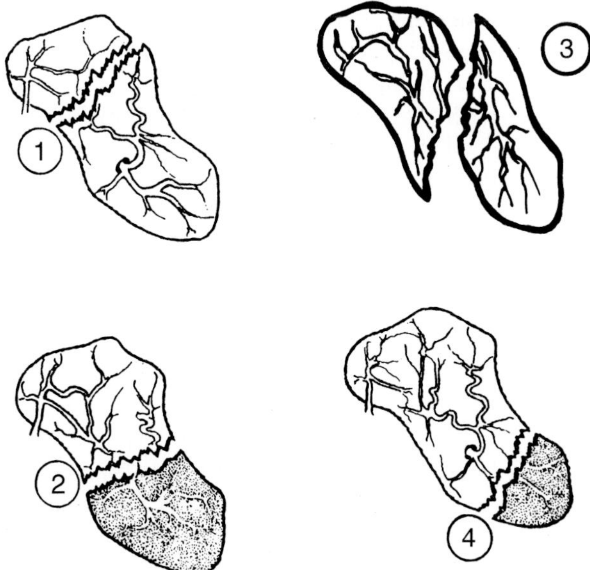

Figure 10–45. Classification of scaphoid fractures. *1,* Neck. *2,* Waist. *3,* Body. *4,* Proximal pole. Note progressive risk of avascular necrosis with proximal transverse fractures. (From Weissman, B.N., and Sledge, C.B.: Orthopedic Radiology, p. 1060. Philadelphia, WB Saunders, 1986.)

2. Treatment—Nondisplaced distal fractures can be managed with immobilization in a short-arm thumb spica cast for 8 to 12 weeks. Nondisplaced proximal and mid-body or waist fractures are managed with 6 weeks of immobilization in a long-arm thumb spica cast followed by a short-arm thumb spica cast until union. Displaced fractures require stable ORIF. Volar comminuted fractures require a volar approach; however, minimally displaced waist and proximal pole fractures can be managed through a dorsal approach.

   Nondisplaced, nonunion, or delayed union fractures can be managed with corticocancellous bone grafting. Displaced nonunions require ORIF with trapezoid or wedge grafting. Salvage procedures include scaphoid excision with four-corner fusion, proximal row carpectomy, and wrist arthrodesis.

Q. Carpal Fractures and Ligamentous Injuries

1. Capitate Fracture—These fractures occur rarely in isolation but are commonly associated with perilunate dislocations. Osteonecrosis is not uncommon, owing to a predominant palmar retrograde blood supply. Scaphoid fractures are commonly associated. This results from hyperdorsiflexion of the wrist with fracture through the waist of the scaphoid and neck of the capitate. Treatment is reduction and immobilization and requires ORIF. The proximal pole of the capitate can rotate 180 degrees. If nonunion of the proximal pole occurs, treatment is fusion of the capitate of the scaphoid and lunate. Capitate fractures can also be associated with carpometacarpal fracture/dislocations. This usually results in a coronal split-type fracture of the fourth and fifth metacarpals and requires ORIF for stabilization.
2. Hamate Fractures—Hamate body fractures are uncommon and are usually associated with fourth and fifth carpometacarpal fracture/dislocations. If they are nondisplaced, closed treatment with a cast is usually satisfactory. If they are displaced or unstable, then closed reduction with percutaneous pinning or ORIF is indicated. Fractures of the hook of the hamate are more common and often a source of chronic pain when unrecognized. They are common in golfers, baseball players, and racquet sport players. Clinically there is ill-defined pain, tenderness over the hamate, ulnar nerve symptoms, and flexor tendon symptoms or attritional rupture. Radiographic evaluation includes the carpal tunnel view and a 45-degree supination oblique view. CT is also useful. An acute injury of less than 7 to 10 days can be treated with 6 weeks of immobilization, often with good result. If nonunion is chronic, management is with excision of the small fragment or ORIF if the fragment is large enough.
3. Triquetral Fractures—Triquetral fractures represent the third most common carpal fracture behind the scaphoid and lunate fracture. Typically, these fractures are asymptomatic. The most common types are shear caused by impingement of the ulnar styloid with dorsiflexion and ulnar deviation. This is typically a flake seen on the lateral x-ray film and can be managed with 4 to 6 weeks of cast immobilization. If the patient remains symptomatic with impingement symptoms, the fragment can be excised. Body fractures are rare. If the fractures are nondisplaced, management is with cast immobilization. If they are displaced, these fractures require ORIF.
4. Trapezial Fractures—Isolated fractures are uncommon and account for only 5% of all carpal fractures. Usually associated are carpometacarpal dislocations or Bennett fractures. Fractures are most easily visualized on anterior oblique projection with ulnar deviation.
   a. Body Fracture—There are six patterns with various mechanisms. Intra-articular displaced fractures require ORIF.
   b. Trapezial Ridge Fracture—From direct blow or fall on the palm of the hand. Type I is a base of ridge fracture, and type II is a tip of ridge fracture. A high index of suspicion for the injury leads to a carpal tunnel view or CT. Type II tip fractures are treated with immobilization in a cast for 6 weeks with molded abduction of the first ray. Type I base fracture often requires early excision because nonunion is usually common. Chronic pain associated with either type usually responds to excision.
5. Pisiform Fractures—Relatively uncommon, accounting for only 1% to 3% of all carpal fractures. Fifty percent are associated with distal radius, hamate, or triquetrum fractures. Local pain and tenderness and a history of a direct blow to this area are suggestive of fracture. Thirty-degree supination oblique x-ray films, tomograms, or CT is helpful. Treatment is with a short-arm cast in 30 degrees of wrist flexion and ulnar deviation for 6 weeks. If painful nonunion develops, excision is done.
6. Carpal Ligamentous Injuries—The complex wrist anatomy allows wide range of motion and force transmission from the arm to the hand. The extrinsic (radius to carpus) and intrinsic (carpal bone to carpal bone) ligaments maintain the overall alignment. The obliquely oriented major extrinsic ligaments (radioscapholunate and radioulnar triquetral and the dorsoradial triquetral ligament) resist the tendency of the carpus to migrate ulnarly and palmarly. The intrinsics, scapholunate, and lunotriquetral ligaments support the lunate in its balanced anatomic position. Disruption of the scapholunate ligament allows

the lunate to follow the triquetrum's position of extension, which results in radiographic dorsal intercalated segmental instability (Fig. 10–46). Lunate triquetral ligament disruption allows the lunate to follow the scaphoid into a position of flexion and a volar intercalated segmental instability pattern.

a. Classification—Mayfield has defined a reproducible pattern of progressive perilunate instability. With hyperextension, ulnar deviation, and intercarpal supination, ligamentous disruption progresses from scapholunate to capitolunate to lunate triquetral and finally to dislocation of the lunate. These are classified as stages I to IV (Fig. 10–47).
b. Radiographic Evaluation—Carpal instability manifests as malalignment of the carpal bones. The PA x-ray view allows evaluation of the scapholunate interval as well as the carpal height index (.54). If there is scapholunate disruption there will also be foreshortening of the scaphoid and the "ring sign" (cortical silhouette of the tuberosity). The scapholunate gap should be less than 2 mm. This may be accentuated with a closed-fist view. The lateral x-ray view allows measurement of the scapholunate angle, defined by the long axis of the scaphoid in relation to the long axis of the lunate. The average is 47 degrees (range: 30–60 degrees). The capitolunate angle range is 0 to 15 degrees; that of the radiolunate angle is −25 to +10 degrees.

   The final pathway of these injuries results in either a dorsal perilunate injury with the carpus dorsal and the lunate remaining seated within the lunate fossa or a palmar lunate dislocation with the capitate residing in the lunate fossa. This injury pattern is purely ligamentous and is referred to as a lesser arc injury. Dislocations involving fractures including the radial styloid, scaphoid, capitate, and triquetrum are termed greater arc injuries. Combinations of both may occur, with the most common being the transscaphoid perilunate dorsal fracture/dislocation.

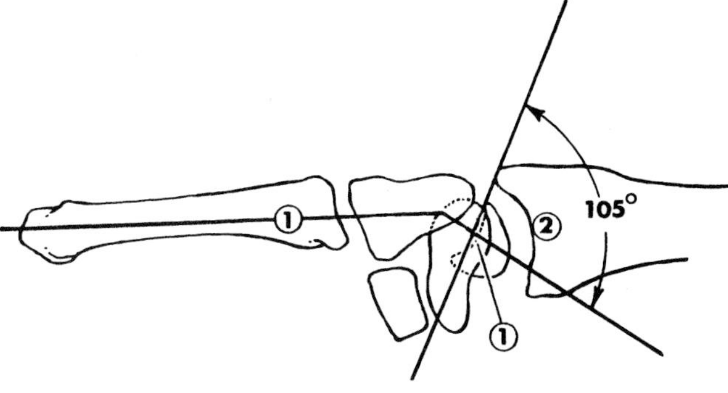

Figure 10–46. Dorsal intercalary segmental instability (DISI). Note scapholunate angle >70 degrees, consistent with a DISI pattern. (From Connolly, J.F., ed.: DePalma's The Management of Fractures and Dislocations, an Atlas, 3rd ed., p. 1085. Philadelphia, WB Saunders, 1981.)

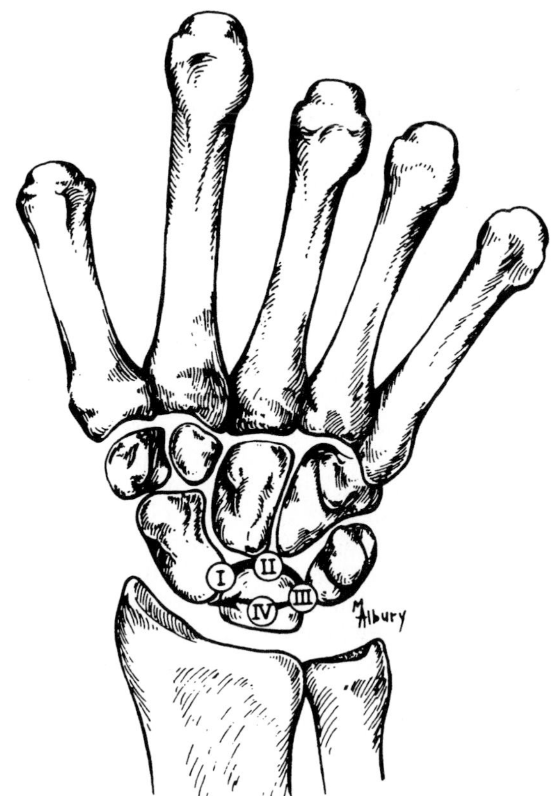

Figure 10–47. Perilunar instability—stages. I, Scapholunate. II, Capitolunate. III, Triquetrolunate. IV, Dorsal radiocarpal (leading to lunate dislocation). (From Mayfield, J.K.: Mechanism of carpal injuries. Clin. Orthop. 149:50, 1980.)

c. Treatment—Treatment is based on the degree of injury and includes closed reduction with immobilization, closed reduction with percutaneous pinning, ORIF, and external fixation. Closed reduction alone is associated with a high failure rate; 60% have loss of reduction. ORIF maintains reduction in 75% of cases. Surgical approach depends on the direction and type of dislocation. Pure dorsal ligamentous dislocation can be managed with a palmar approach to repair the palmar capsular rent and a dorsal approach to repair scapholunate and lunotriquetral ligaments. Kirschner wire stabilization is required after reduction. Fracture/dislocations may be approached in various directions.
d. Complications—In 50% of cases, even with early treatment and satisfactory results, patients still develop stiffness and degenerative joint disease. Associated neurologic injuries are major factors in determining outcome. Decreased range of motion, pinch, and grip strength often prevent a return to a previous occupation.

e. Axial Injuries—Longitudinal axial carpus dislocations are also possible without perilunate injury. Axial-radial or axial-ulnar longitudinal disruption may occur with or without fractures. These are often a high-energy injury and can be associated with significant skin and soft tissue injury. Neurovascular injury (ulnar nerve most common) and intrinsic muscle injury are common. Treatment involves management of the soft tissue injury, neurovascular injuries, and ORIF of the bony disruptions.

R. Dislocations in the Hand

1. Hamatometacarpal Fracture/Dislocation—The ulnar carpometacarpal joint consists of an articulation with the fourth and fifth metacarpal bases with the hamate. The hamate has two distinct facets and a bony ridge, producing a saddle joint similar to the trapezium. This allows significant mobility with a flexion extension arc of 20 degrees and rotational motion for thumb opposition. This is the most commonly recognized carpometacarpal injury in fracture/dislocations. Dislocation is associated with high energy and produces significant pain and swelling. Evaluation requires a minimum of three views of the hand, including pronation oblique films. CT is helpful to define the degree of displacement and intra-articular components. Dislocations can be treated with closed reduction and stable casting; however, most authors recommend percutaneous pinning, owing to late subluxation and symptoms. Fracture/dislocations can be treated with closed reduction and pinning. A patient with significant articular stepoff should undergo ORIF.

2. First Carpometacarpal Dislocation—The thumb carpometacarpal ligaments are strong but lax enough to allow freedom of motion. The anterior oblique ligament and the intermetacarpal ligament are the primary stabilizers. There are lesser contributions from the dorsoradial ligament and the posterior oblique ligament. True dislocations without fracture are uncommon. Evaluation requires true AP radiography of the ray with the hand and thumb maximally pronated. Treatment is with closed reduction with traction and pronation and percutaneous pinning. Postoperatively, a thumb spica cast is used for 4 weeks, followed by a course of therapy with protective splinting for an additional 4 to 6 weeks. Chronic instability can be a significant problem.

3. First Metacarpophalangeal Dislocation (Fig. 10–48)—The metacarpophalangeal joint of the thumb is a multiaxial diarthrodial joint that primarily allows flexion and extension with some variable degrees of adduction, abduction, and rotation. Stability is crucial for the thumb to properly function in its role of grip and pinch. Ulnar and radial collateral ligaments extend from the condyles and metacarpal to the volar portion of the proximal phalanx and volar plate in a primary stabilizer. These are supplemented by accessory collateral ligaments and the ulnar musculature volarly. Treatment consists of closed reduction and splinting.

a. **Ulnar Collateral Ligament Injuries** (Gamekeeper's or Skier's Thumb; Fig. 10–49)—Forceful radial deviation of the thumb results in injuries to the ulnar collateral ligament complex. These are painful and debilitating in the acute phase and can lead to chronic instability if not recognized and appropriately treated. Examina-

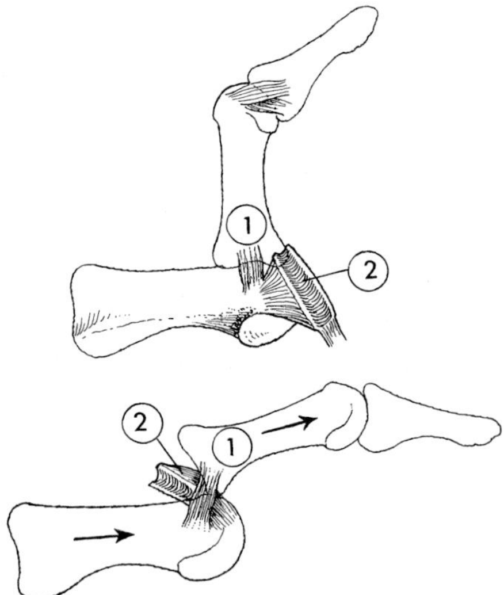

Figure 10–48. Thumb metacarpophalangeal dislocation. *Top,* Simple. *Bottom,* Complex; note interposition of volar plate. (From Connolly, J.F., ed.: DePalma's The Management of Fractures and Dislocations, an Atlas, 3rd ed., p. 1152. Philadelphia, WB Saunders, 1981.)

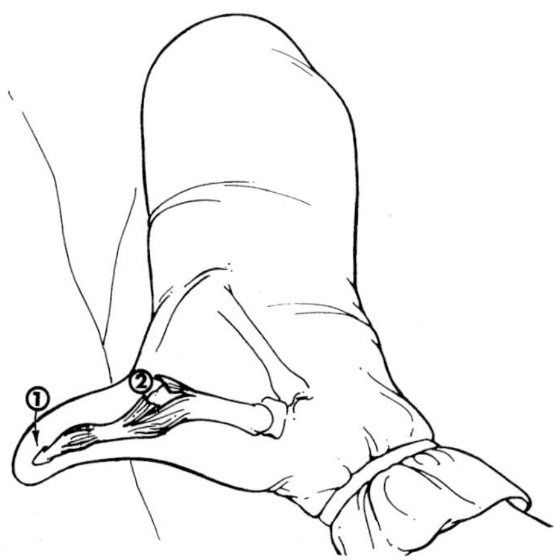

Figure 10–49. Gamekeeper's thumb (ulnar collateral ligament injury). (From Connolly, J.F., ed.: DePalma's The Management of Fractures and Dislocations, an Atlas, 3rd ed., p. 1151. Philadelphia, WB Saunders, 1981.)

tion reveals tenderness over the ulnar collateral ligament and often over the volar plate. Static radiographs are initially obtained to rule out avulsion fracture off the proximal phalanx. Dynamic radiographs are often useful to rule out subluxation with stress. Partial tears will not open up greater than 35 to 45 degrees on stress testing and can advance with thumb spica casting for 4 to 6 weeks, followed by progressive protected range-of-motion exercises. Complete rupture, opened up greater than 30 to 45 degrees, can be associated with a Stener lesion. This is an interposition of the adductor hood between the ruptured ligament and its insertion on the proximal phalanx. These injuries will not heal without open reduction and repair of the ligament to its bed. Postoperatively, a thumb spica cast is maintained for 4 to 6 weeks, followed by progressive protective range-of-motion exercises.

b. **Radial Collateral Ligamentous Injuries**—These injuries are rare and not as debilitating as the ulnar collateral ligament injuries. They occur secondary to forced ulnar deviation. The majority can be treated nonoperatively with splinting and late reconstruction as needed.

4. Dislocations of the Thumb—Simple dorsal dislocations can be managed with closed reduction and immobilization for 3 weeks in a thumb spica cast. Complex irreducible dislocations often occur secondary to interposition of the volar plate and flexor pollicis longus (see Fig. 10–45). These require open reduction, reapproximation of soft tissues, and thumb spica immobilization postoperatively.
5. Metacarpophalangeal Dislocations in the Fingers—Metacarpophalangeal dislocations are much less common in proximal interphalangeal injury; however, loss of motion at the metacarpophalangeal joint can have a profound effect on hand function and is very disabling. Radiographs can be difficult to interpret on the lateral view, and oblique views are necessary for complete assessment. A Brewerton view is helpful with collateral injuries, and skyline views are of benefit for impaction injuries. Collateral ligament injuries at the metacarpophalangeal joint are uncommon and usually occur in the ulnar three digits. Treatment is with a splint in 50 degrees of metacarpophalangeal flexion for 3 weeks and then buddy tape with progressive mobilization over 3 weeks. If associated with an avulsion fracture and if there is more than 2 to 3 mm of displacement or more than 20% of the joint surface, ORIF is recommended. Simple dorsal dislocations can be managed with closed reduction and 7 to 10 days of immobilization, followed by buddy taping. Complex irreducible dislocations often have interposition of the volar plate and a "buttonhole effect." The index finger metacarpal head can also be entrapped between the lumbricals radially and the flexor tendons ulnarly. Clinically, this is suggested by puckering of the volar skin, an intra-articular sesamoid on x-ray films, and parallelism of the joints. Open reduction is recommended through a volar or dorsal approach, followed by mobilization in 30 degrees for 1 week and progressive extension-block splinting. Volar dislocations are rare but require open reduction.
6. Proximal Interphalangeal Dislocations
   a. Anatomy—The proximal interphalangeal joint is a hinged joint with significant stability primarily derived from strong volar plate and ligaments that were reinforced by the adjacent tendon and retinacular structures. A proximal phalanx articular surface consists of two concentric condyles on the intercondylar notch that articulate intermittently with two depressions and a flap based in the middle phalanx. This high degree of articular congruency provides additional stability. The collateral ligaments at the proximal interphalangeal are 2 to 3 mm thick and insert distally and volarly on the volar third of the middle phalanx to the volar plate. This conjoined attachment of the collateral ligaments in the volar plate is a crucial element for proximal interphalangeal joint stability.
   b. Classification—Despite the stability of the proximal interphalangeal joint, pure dislocation is prominent. Dislocations are the most common articular injury in the hand. They can be classified as dorsal, volar, or lateral. The collateral ligaments are partially entered, and the volar plate is avulsed from the middle phalanx. Interposition of the volar plate may necessitate open reduction.
   c. Treatment
      (1) Dorsal Dislocation
         (a) Type I—Hyperextension, volar plate avulsion. These injuries can be treated with reduction followed by buddy taping or extension block splinting for 2 weeks.
         (b) Type II—Dorsal complete dislocation with volar plate avulsion and bilateral collateral ligament injury. Treatment is with reduction and extension block splinting in 20 degrees for 3 weeks.
         (c) Type III—Fracture/dislocation. Stable fractures are treated with extension block splinting for 2 to 3 weeks, followed by progressive

mobilization. An unstable fracture involving more than 40% of the articular surface or with subluxation requires ORIF. Severely comminuted fractures require volar plate arthroplasty.

(2) Volar Dislocation—Although these dislocations are not as common as dorsal dislocations, they herald a much more significant injury pattern. The mechanism of injury is typically an axial load on a partially flexed joint with some rotational component. The condyles of the proximal phalanx buttonhole through the extensor mechanism, and with pure volar dislocation this often results in avulsion of the central slip, resulting in a boutonnière deformity. If a rotatory component is involved, a single condyle of the middle phalanx often buttonholes between the central slip and lateral band. As the dislocation completes, the lateral band subluxes into the joint, becoming entrapped between the dorsal aspect of the middle phalanx and the volar aspect of the proximal phalanx. Flexion and longitudinal traction are necessary for reduction of the majority of this dislocation; however, it is often irreducible and requires open reduction. In treatment of these injuries it is crucial to confirm the integrity of the central slip (Fig. 10–50). If there is evidence of injury, treatment is as for a boutonnière deformity with proximal interphalangeal extension splinting and active distal interphalangeal motion followed by progressive protected range-of-motion exercises. With the central slip intact and stable concentric reduction, protective range-of-motion exercises are done with buddy taping.

7. Distal Interproximal Dislocations—These dislocations are uncommon. Dorsal dislocations are more common than palmar ones, and these injuries often involve disruption of both collateral ligaments and the palmar plate. They can be managed with closed reduction and immobilization for 1 to 2 weeks. Palmar disruption is important to document the integrity of the terminal extensor tendon. If there is extensor lag, treatment is with a minimum 8-week course of splinting as for a mallet injury.

S. Metacarpal Fractures

1. Thumb Metacarpal Fractures—Thumb metacarpal base fractures are the second most common of all metacarpal fractures, constituting 25%; and they make up 80% of all thumb fractures. They more commonly occur in the dominant hand. Half occur in patients younger than 30, and they are found more often in males than females. The injury is caused by an axial force directed through a partially flexed thumb. Three major types (Fig. 10–51) include (1) Bennett's intra-articular fracture with small volar ulnar fragment, which remains attached to the anterior oblique fracture; (2) Rolando's intra-articular fracture, either T or Y or comminuted, with a volar fragment remaining attached to the anterior oblique ligament; and (3) extra-articular fracture, both transverse and oblique.

a. Evaluation—Requires a true AP view with maximal forearm pronation and the thumb on the cassette (Robert's) and a true lateral view with the forearm flat and the hand pronated 20 degrees and the x-ray tube angled at 10 degrees (see Table 10–2).

b. Treatment—Epibasal transverse fractures can usually be managed with closed reduction and thumb spica casting for 4 to 6 weeks. Supplemental pinning is recommended for displacement of more than 30 degrees. Oblique fractures usually require pinning due to innate instability. An attempt should be made at closed reduction and percutaneous pinning to the trapezium in the index metacarpal for Bennett's fractures. ORIF is done if the fracture is

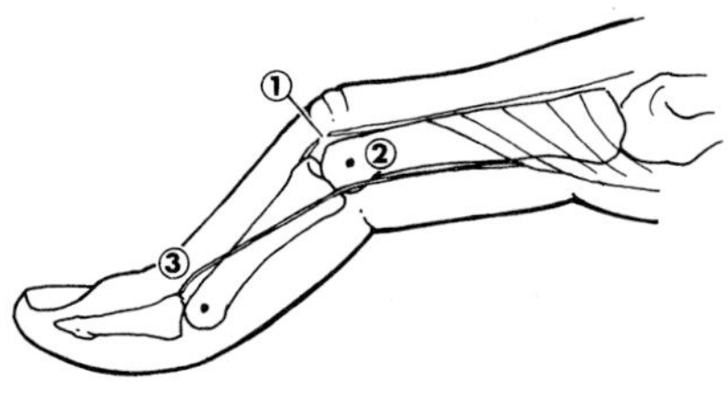

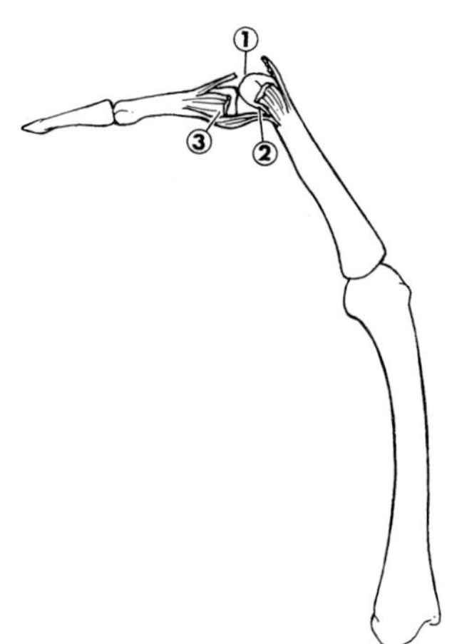

Figure 10–50. Boutonnière deformity, an injury to the central slip with volar subluxation of lateral bonds. (From Connolly, J.F., ed.: DePalma's The Management of Fractures and Dislocations, an Atlas, 3rd ed., p. 1149. Philadelphia, WB Saunders, 1981.)

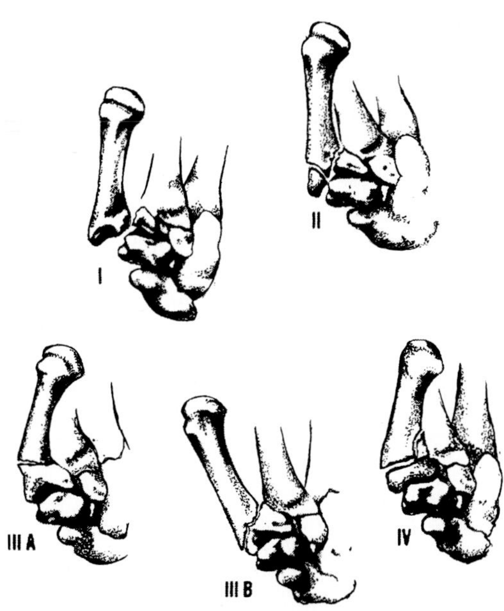

Figure 10–51. Classification of first metacarpal base fractures. *I,* Bennett's fracture. *II,* Rolando's fracture. *IIIA,* Transverse extra-articular fracture. *IIIB,* Oblique extra-articular fracture. *IV,* SH II epiphyseal fracture (pediatric). (From Green, D.P., and O'Brien, E.T.: Fractures of the thumb metacarpal. South. Med. J. 65:807, 1972.)

irreducible, is unstable, or has a noncongruent articular surface. The Rolando T or Y fracture is best managed with ORIF if the fragment is large enough. If there is significant comminution, external fixation is combined with percutaneous pinning and bone grafting.

2. Small Metacarpal Base Fracture—Fractures of the base of the fifth metacarpal are known as reverse Bennett's fractures. Four fracture patterns have been described: epibasal, two-part, three-part, and comminuted. Treatment of epibasal and two-part fractures is closed reduction with percutaneous pinning and casting for 6 weeks. ORIF is done for inadequate articular reduction. Treatment of three-part or comminuted fractures is reduction with ligamentotaxis and supplemental percutaneous pinning or ORIF.
3. Metacarpal Shaft Fractures—The metacarpals are stabilized by the intrinsic muscles, the lumbricals, and the strong intermetacarpal ligaments. The central two metacarpals are more stable because of border stability. The index and long fingers have less motion and are less tolerant of angulation than the more mobile fourth and fifth metacarpals. Transverse fractures tend to angulate apex dorsal owing to the palmar pole of the interosseous muscles. Ten degrees of angulation is acceptable in the second and third metacarpals whereas the fourth and fifth will tolerate 20 to 30 degrees. Oblique fractures tend to shorten, and spiral fractures tend to rotate. Rotation is very poorly tolerated and results in digital overlap with flexion.

   The transverse nondisplaced fractures can be treated in a three-point cast for 3 to 4 weeks with the metacarpophalangeal joint at 70 degrees of flexion. Displaced transverse fractures are treated with closed reduction and casting if stable; otherwise, percutaneous pinning or ORIF is used. Oblique or spiral fractures require reduction and fixation with percutaneous pinning or ORIF.
4. Metacarpal Neck Fractures—These fractures usually result from an axial load to a closed fist and most commonly involve the ring and small fingers. Rotational deformity or lateral deviation should be corrected. Ten to 15 degrees of angulation can be accepted in the index and long fingers, and the ring and small fingers can tolerate 35 to 45 degrees. Too much flexion results in loss of knuckle prominence, a prominent metacarpal head in the palm, and "pseudo clawing." If rotational alignment is acceptable, immobilization with a splint or cast is done for 2 to 3 weeks. A displaced or open fracture is treated with open reduction with percutaneous pinning to an adjacent metacarpal or with ORIF.
5. Metacarpal Head Fractures—Intra-articular fractures of the metacarpal head are uncommon and are usually open. Patterns of injury include vertical, horizontal, oblique, and comminuted. The third metacarpal is the most common metacarpal involved. Radiographic findings can be subtle; a skyline view is helpful: the dorsal surface of the hand is flat on the cassette with the metacarpophalangeal joint flexed 70 degrees and the x-ray tube angled 15 degrees radial and ulnar to the metacarpal. Treatment is anatomic restoration with ORIF of large fragments. Comminuted fractures may best be treated with traction and external fixation followed by early motion. Loss of range of motion of the metacarpophalangeal joint is very debilitating to hand function.

T. Phalangeal Fractures and Tendinous Injuries—Phalangeal fractures are described as extra-articular base, intra-articular base, diaphyseal, phalangeal neck fractures, phalangeal condylar fractures, and unicondylar/bicondylar fractures.
1. Proximal Phalanx Extra-Articular Base Fractures—May angulate less than a midshaft fracture but is more disabling in loss of function. Treatment is with initial reduction and cast treatment with metacarpophalangeal joints in 70 degrees. If the fracture is unstable or fails to reduce, percutaneous pinning or ORIF is done.
2. Intra-Articular Base Fractures—Three types include collateral ligament avulsion, compression, and vertical shear. Nondisplaced ligament avulsion fractures can be treated with

buddy taping and early range-of-motion exercise. Displaced and unstable fractures need reduction, tension banding, or ORIF. Proximal and middle phalanx intra-articular vertical base fractures require reduction with pinning or ORIF with lag screw. Intra-articular compression fractures do not predictably reduce with longitudinal traction and require elevation of the articular surface, bone grafting, and ORIF.

3. Proximal and Middle Phalanx Diaphyseal Fractures—Middle phalanx fractures displace owing to forces of the central slip attached dorsally and proximally, extensor tendon insertion dorsally and distally, and the flexor superficialis insertion volarly and distally. Proximal to the flexor digitorum superficialis insertion they angulate dorsally; distal to this insertion they angulate volarly. Proximal phalanx fractures angulate volarly owing to the interosseous muscles. Stable nondisplaced or impacted fractures can be treated with buddy taping and progressive range of motion. Displaced fractures require closed reduction and immobilization with a short-arm cast and dorsal block component. Fractures that are irreducible or unstable will require internal fixation.
4. Proximal and Middle Phalangeal Neck Fractures—Extremely uncommon in the adult, these fractures are easily reduced with traction but difficult to control. Treatment is percutaneous pinning for 4 weeks with cast protection for an additional 3 weeks.
5. Proximal and Middle Phalangeal Condylar Fractures—Intra-articular fractures demand anatomic reduction, rigid fixation, and early motion. Nondisplaced fractures may be treated with digital splint for 7 to 10 days, followed by buddy taping and range-of-motion exercises with close radiographic follow-up. Displaced fractures require ORIF through a dorsal approach with stable fixation and early range-of-motion exercises.
6. Distal Phalanx Fractures—The distal phalanx is the most common bone fractured in the hand (50%). The long finger and thumb are usually involved. Because of the unique soft tissue anatomy, this fracture is usually stable and reduction is not necessary unless the articular surface is involved. Splinting is for comfort and can usually be discontinued by 4 weeks. Radiographic union may take up to 6 months but is usually asymptomatic. Shaft fractures are usually nondisplaced and can be treated with splinting for 3 to 4 weeks until nontender. Displaced fractures can undergo closed reduction. If instability is persistent, percutaneous pinning is done. Shaft fractures are often associated with nail matrix injuries and a subungual hematoma. One should carry a high suspicion of an underlying matrix injury.
7. Tendinous Injuries—Avulsion injury of the extensor digitorum longus (mallet finger). There is disruption of the insertion of the tendon into the distal phalanx.
   a. Classification

      Type I: Extensor tendon stretch with 15 to 30 degree extensor lag
      Type II: Extensor tendon torn with 30 to 60 degree extensor lag
      Type III: Extensor tendon avulsion flake
      Type IV: Extensor tendon avulsion fragment or "bony mallet"

   b. Treatment—Treatment of types I through III is extension immobilization: type I, 6 weeks followed by night-time splinting for 3 to 4 weeks; types II and III, 8 weeks continuous splinting and 3 to 4 weeks of night splinting. A Kirschner wire is used only if the patient's occupation precludes splinting. Most bony mallet injuries can be managed with extension splinting for 8 weeks; however, a volar displacement or involvement of more than 50% of the articular surface should be treated with ORIF.
8. Flexor Digitorum Profundus Avulsion Injury (Jersey Finger)—Avulsion from insertion of the tendon to the distal phalanx. The ring finger is most commonly affected. Patients present with inability to flex the distal interproximal joint, tenderness, and a prominence in the digit or palm.
   a. Classification

      Type I: Tendon retraction to palm rupturing vincula
      Type II: Tendon retracts to proximal interphalangeal joint held by vinculum
      Type III: Large bony fragment catches on A4 pulley at middle phalanx
      Type IV: Bony avulsion with tendon avulsed from fragment

   b. Treatment and Timing—Type I tendon is dysvascular; therefore, repair should be done within 7 to 10 days at the insertion site using a pullout suture over a button. Type II repair is possible for up to 6 weeks. In type III ORIF of the fragment to the distal phalanx is done. Type IIIa repair is of the articular fragment with secondary repair of the distal phalanx. Postoperative dynamic tendon rehabilitation is done with a dorsal block splint, passive flexion, and active extension exercises.

Selected Bibliography

General

Amadio, P.C.: Current concepts review: Pain dysfunction syndromes. J. Bone Joint Surg. [Am.] 70:944–949, 1988.

Amato, J.J., Rhinelander, H.F., and Cleveland, R.J.: Post-traumatic adult respiratory distress syndrome. Orthop. Clin. North Am. 9:693–713, 1978.

Barach, E., Tomlanovich, M., and Nowak, R.: Ballistics: A pathophysiologic examination of the wounding mechanisms of firearms: I and II. J. Trauma 26:225–235, 374–383, 1986.

Berquist, T.H., ed.: Imaging of Orthopedic Trauma and Surgery, Philadelphia, WB Saunders, 1986.

Blick, S.S., Brumback, R.J., Poka, A., et al.: Compartment syndrome in open tibia fractures. J. Bone Joint Surg. [Am.] 68:1348–1353, 1986.

Bone, L.B.: Emergency treatment of an injured patient. In Browner, B., Jupiter, J.B., Levine, A.M., et al., eds.: Skeletal Trauma, vol. 1. Philadelphia, WB Saunders, 1992, pp. 127–136.

Border, J.R., Allgower, M., Hansen, S.T., Jr., et al., eds.: Blunt Multiple Trauma. New York, Marcel Dekker, 1990.

Brighton, C.T.: Current concepts review: The treatment of nonunions with electricity. J. Bone Joint Surg. [Am.] 63:847–851, 1981.

Chapman, M.W., ed.: Operative Orthopaedics. Philadelphia, JB Lippincott, 1988.

Connolly, J.F., ed.: DePalma's The Management of Fractures and Dislocations, an Atlas, 3rd ed. Philadelphia, WB Saunders, 1981.

Fry, D.E.: Multiple System Organ Failure. St. Louis, Mosby–Year Book, 1992.

Gelman, M.I.: Radiology of Orthopedic Procedures, Problems and Complications, vol. 24. Philadelphia, WB Saunders, 1984.

Godina, M.: Early microsurgical reconstruction of complex trauma of the extremities. Plast. Reconstr. Surg. 78:285–292, 1986.

Gossling, H.R., and Pellegrini, V.D., Jr.: Fat embolism syndrome: A review of the pathophysiology and physiological basis of treatment. Clin. Orthop. 165:68–82, 1982.

Gustilo, R.B., Merkow, R.B., and Templeman, D.: Current concepts review: The management of open fractures. J. Bone Joint Surg. [Am.] 72:299–303, 1990.

Heinrich, S.D., Gallagher, D., Harris, M., and Nadell, J.M.: Undiagnosed fractures in severely injured children and young adults. J. Bone Joint Surg. [Am.] 76:561–572, 1994.

Johansen, K., Danines, M., Howey, T., et al.: Objective criteria accurately predict amputation following lower extremity trauma. J. Trauma 30:508–572, 1990.

Johnson, K.D., Cadambi, A., and Seibert, G.B.: Incidence of adult respiratory distress syndrome in patients with multiple musculoskeletal injuries: Effect of early operative stabilization of fractures. J. Trauma 25:375–383, 1985.

Kozin, S.H., and Berlet, A.C.: Handbook of Common Orthopaedic Fractures. West Chester, PA, Medical Surveillance, 1990.

MacKenzie, E.J., Burgess, A.R., McAndrew, M.P., et al.: Patient oriented functional outcome after unilateral lower extremity fracture. J. Orthop. Trauma 7:393–401, 1993.

Matsen, F.A., III, Winquist, R.A., and Krugmire, R.B., Jr.: Diagnosis and management of compartmental syndromes. J. Bone Joint Surg. [Am.] 62:286–291, 1980.

May, J.W., Jr., Jupiter, J.B., Weiland, A.J., et al.: Current concepts review: Clinical classification of post-traumatic osteomyelitis. J. Bone Joint Surg. [Am.] 71:1422, 1989.

Muller, M.E., Allgower, M., Schneider, R., et al.: Manual of Internal Fixation, 3rd ed. Berlin, Springer-Verlag, 1991.

Orthopaedic Knowledge Update Home Study Syllabus I, II, III, and IV. Chicago, American Academy of Orthopaedic Surgeons, 1984, 1987, 1990, 1993.

Pape, H.C., Dwenger, A., Grotz, et al.: Does the reamer type influence the degree of lung dysfunction after femoral nailing following severe trauma? An animal study. J. Orthop. Trauma 7:300–309, 1994.

Phillips, T.F., and Contreras, D.M.: Current concepts review: Timing of operative treatment of fractures in patients who have multiple injuries. J. Bone Joint Surg. [Am.] 72:784, 1990.

Pollak, R., and Myers, R.A.M.: Early diagnosis of the fat embolism syndrome. J. Trauma 18:121–123, 1978.

Rockwood, C.A., Jr., and Green, D.P., eds.: Fractures in Adults, 3rd ed. Philadelphia, JB Lippincott, 1991.

Steinberg, M.E.: Blood supply to the femoral head and avascular neurosis. Op. Tech. Orthop. 4:94–103, 1994.

Ward, W.G., and Nunley, J.A.: Occult orthopaedic trauma in the multiply injured patient. J. Orthop. Trauma 5:308–312, 1991.

Weber, B.G., and Chech, O.: Pseudoanthrosen. Bern, Huber, 1973.

Spine

Allen, B.L., Jr., Ferguson, R.L., Lehmann, T.R., and O'Brien, R.P.: A mechanistic classification of closed, indirect fractures and dislocations of the lower cervical spine. Spine 7:1–27, 1982.

Bohler, J.: Anterior stabilization for acute fractures and non-unions of the dens. J. Bone Joint Surg. [Am.] 64:18–27, 1982.

Bohlman, H.H.: Acute fractures and dislocations of the cervical spine: An analysis of three hundred hospitalized patients and review of the literature. J. Bone Joint Surg. [Am.] 61:1119–1142, 1979.

Bohlman, H.H.: Treatment of fractures and dislocations of the thoracic and lumbar spine. J. Bone Joint Surg. [Am.] 67:165–169, 1985.

Bradford, D.S., and McBride, G.G.: Surgical management of thoracolumbar spine fractures in incomplete neurologic deficits. Clin. Orthop. 218:201–216, 1987.

Denis, F.: The three column spine and its significance in the classification of acute thoracolumbar spinal injuries. Spine 8:817–831, 1983.

Denis, F.: Updated classification of thoracolumbar fractures. Orthop. Trans. 6:8, 1982.

Drummond, D., Guadagni, J., Keene, J.S., et al.: Interspinous process segmental spinal instrumentation. J. Pediatr. Orthop. 4:397–404, 1984.

Jacobs, R.R., and Casey, M.P.: Surgical management of thoracolumbar injuries: General principles and controversial considerations. Clin. Orthop. 189:22–35, 1984.

Kramer, K.M., and Levine, A.M.: Unilateral facet dislocation of the lumbosacral junction: A case report and review of the literature. J. Bone Joint Surg. [Am.] 71:1258, 1989.

Rizzolo, S.J., and Cotler, J.M.: Unstable cervical spine injuries—specific treatment approaches. J. Am. Acad. Orthop. Surg. 1:57–66, 1993.

Schatzker, J., Rorabeck, C.H., and Waddell, J.P.: Fractures of the dens (odontoid process): An analysis of thirty-seven cases. J. Bone Joint Surg. [Br.] 53:392–405, 1971.

Southwick, W.O.: Current concepts review: Management of fractures of the dens (odontoid process). J. Bone Joint Surg. [Am.] 62:482–486, 1980.

White, A.A., Southwick, W.O., and Panjabi, M.M.: Clinical instability in the lower cervical spine: A review of past and current concepts. Spine 1:15–27, 1976.

Pelvis and Hip

Bosse, M.J., Poka, A., Reinert, C.M., et al.: Heterotopic ossification as a complication of acetabular fracture: Prophylaxis with low-dose irradiation. J. Bone Joint Surg. [Am.] 70:1231–1237, 1988.

Bucholz, R.W.: The pathologic anatomy of Malgaigne fracture-dislocations of the pelvis. J. Bone Joint Surg. [Am.] 63:400–404, 1981.

Dalal, S.A., Burgess, A.R., Siegal, J.H., et al.: Pelvic fracture and multiple trauma: Classification by mechanism is key to pattern of organ injury, resuscitative requirements and outcome. J. Trauma 29:981–1000, 1989.

Denis, F., Davis, S., and Comfort, T.: Sacral fractures: An important problem: Retrospective analysis of 236 cases. Clin. Orthop. 227:67–81, 1988.

Dreinhofer, K.E., Schwarzkopf, S.R., Haas, N.P., et al.: Isolated dislocation of the hip: Long term results in 50 patients. J. Bone Joint Surg. [Br.] 76:6–12, 1994.

Epstein, H.C.: Traumatic Dislocation of the Hip. Baltimore, Williams & Wilkins, 1980.

Epstein, H.C., Wiss, D.A., and Cozen, L.: Posterior fracture dislocation of the hip with fractures of the femoral head. Clin. Orthop. 201:9–17, 1985.

Fassler, P.R., Swiontkowski, M.F., Kilrow, A.W., and Routt, M.L.: Injury of the sciatic nerve associated with acetabular fracture. J. Bone Joint Surg. [Am.] 75:1157–1166, 1993.

Hanson, P.B., Milne, J.C., and Chapman, M.W.: Open fractures of the pelvis—review of 43 cases. J. Bone Joint Surg. [Br.] 73:325–329, 1991.

Horwitz, S.M.: The management of pathological hip fractures. Op. Tech. Orthop. 4:122–129, 1994.

Judet, R., Judet, J., and Letournel, E.: Fractures of the acetabulum: Classification and surgical approaches for open reduction. J. Bone Joint Surg. [Am.] 46:1615–1646, 1964.

Juliano, P.J., Bosse, M.J., and Edwards, K.J.: The superior gluteal artery and complex acetabular procedures: A cadaveric angiographic study. J. Bone Joint Surg. [Am.] 76:244–248, 1994.

Koval, K.J., and Zuckerman, J.D.: Current concepts review: Functional recovery after fracture of the hip. J. Bone Joint Surg. [Am.] 76:751–758, 1994.
Koval, K.J., and Zuckerman, J.D.: Hip fractures: I. Evaluation and treatment of femoral neck fractures. II. Hip fractures: Evaluation and treatment of intertrochanteric fractures. J. Am. Acad. Orthop. Surg. I: 2:141–149, 1994; II: 2:150–156, 1994.
Kyle, R.F.: Fractures of the proximal part of the femur. J. Bone Joint Surg. [Am.] 76:924–950, 1994.
Kyle, R.F., Wright, T.M., and Burstein, A.H.: Biomechanical analysis of the sliding characteristics of compression hip screw. J. Bone Joint Surg. [Am.] 62:1308–1314, 1980.
Lange, R.H., and Hansen, S.T., Jr.: Pelvic ring disruptions with symphysis pubis diastasis: Indications, technique, and limitations of anterior internal fixation. Clin. Orthop. 201:130–137, 1985.
Latenser, B.A., Gentilello, L.M., Tarver, A.A., et al.: Improved outcome with early fixation of skeletally unstable pelvic fractures. J. Trauma, 31:28–31, 1991.
Letournel, E., and Judet, R.: Fractures of the Acetabulum. Elson, R.A., transl., ed. New York, Springer-Verlag, 1981.
Lu-Yao, G.L., Keller, R.B., Littenberg, B., and Wennberg, J.E.: Outcomes after displaced fractures of the femoral neck—meta analysis of 106 published reports. J. Bone Joint Surg. [Am.] 76:15–25, 1994.
Matta, J., Anderson, L., Epstein, H., and Henricks, P.: Fractures of the acetabulum: A retrospective analysis. Clin. Orthop. 205:230–240, 1986.
Matta, J.M., and Saucedo, T.: Internal fixation of pelvic ring fractures. Clin. Orthop. 242:83–97, 1989.
Matta, J.M., Mehne, D.K., and Roffi, R.: Fractures of the acetabulum: Early results of a prospective study. Clin. Orthop. 205:241–250, 1986.
McMurtry, R., Walton, D., Dickinson, D., et al.: Pelvic disruption in the polytraumatized patient: A management protocol. Clin. Orthop. 151:22–30, 1980.
Mears, D.C., and Rubash, H.: Pelvic and acetabular fractures. Thorofare, NJ, Slack, 1986.
Mears, D.C., Capito, C.P., and Deleeuw, H.: Posterior pelvic disruptions managed by the use of the double cobra plate. Instr. Course Lect. 37:143–150, 1988.
Naam, N.H., Brown, W.M., Hurd, R., et al.: Major pelvic fractures. Arch. Surg. 118:610–616, 1983.
Riemer, B.L., Butterfield, S.L., Ray, R.L., and Daffner, R.H.: Clandestine femoral neck fractures with ipsilateral diaphyseal fractures. J. Orthop. Trauma 7:443–449, 1993.
Rizzo, P.F., Gould, E.S., Lyden, J.P., et al.: Diagnosis of occult fractures about the hip: Magnetic resonance imaging compared with bone-scanning. J. Bone Joint Surg [Am.] 75:395–401, 1993.
Routt, M.L.C., Jr., and Swiontkowski, M.F.: Operative treatment of complex acetabular fractures: Combined anterior and posterior exposures during the same procedure. J. Bone Joint Surg. [Am.] 72:897, 1990.
Stahaeli, J.W., Frassica, F.J., and Sim, F.H.: Prosthetic replacement of the femoral head for fracture of the femoral neck in patients who have Parkinson disease. J. Bone Joint Surg. [Am.] 70:565–568, 1988.
Swiontkowski, M.F.: Current concepts review: Intracapsular fractures of the hip. J. Bone Joint Surg. [Am.] 76:129–138, 1994.
Tile, M.: Fractures of the Pelvis and Acetabulum. Baltimore, Williams & Wilkins, 1984.
Tile, M.: Pelvic ring fractures: Should they be fixed? J. Bone Joint Surg. [Br.] 70:1–12, 1988.
Young, J.W.R., and Burgess A.R.: Radiographic Management of Pelvic Ring Fractures: Systematic Radiographic Diagnosis. Baltimore: Urban & Schwarzenberg, 1987.

Thigh and Leg

Arneson, T.J., Melton, L.J., III, Lewallen, D.G., et al.: Epidemiology of diaphyseal and distal femoral fractures in Rochester, Minnesota, 1965–1984. Clin. Orthop. 234:188–194, 1988.
Behrens, F., and Searls, K.: External fixation of the tibia: Basic concepts and prospective evaluation. J. Bone Joint Surg. [Br.] 68:246–254, 1986.
Blair, B., Koval, K.J., Kummer, F., et al.: Basicervical fractures of the proximal femur: A biomechanical study of 3 internal fixation techniques. Clin. Orthop. 306:256–263, 1994.
Bonar, S.K., and Marsh, J.L.: Unilateral external fixation for severe pilon fractures. Foot Ankle 14:57–64, 1993.
Bone, L., and Bucholz, R: The management of fractures in the patient with multiple trauma. J. Bone Joint Surg. [Am.] 68:945–949, 1986.
Bone, L.B., Cassman, S., Stegemann, P., and France, J.: Prospective study of union rate of open tibial fractures treated with locked unreamed intramedullary nails. J. Orthop. Trauma 8:45–49, 1994.
Bone, L.B., Johnson, K.D., Weigelt, J., et al.: Early versus delayed stabilization of femoral fractures: A prospective randomized study. J. Bone Joint Surg. [Am.] 71:336, 1989.
Boynton, M.D., and Schmeling, G.J.: Nonreamed intramedullary nailing of open tibial fractures. J. Am. Acad. Orthop. Surg. 2: 107–114, 1994.
Brumback, R.J., Ellison, T.S., Molligan, H., et al.: Pudendal nerve palsy complicating intramedullary nailing of the femur. J. Bone Joint Surg. [Am.] 74:1450–1455, 1992.
Brumback, R.J., Reilly, J.P., Poka, A., et al.: Intramedullary nailing of femoral shaft fractures. J. Bone Joint Surg. [Am.] 70:1441–1462, 1988.
Caudle, R.J., and Stern, P.J.: Severe open fractures of the tibia. J. Bone Joint Surg. [Am.] 69:801–807, 1987.
Cierny, G., III, Byrd, H.S., and Jones, R.E.: Primary versus delayed soft tissue coverage for severe open tibial fractures: A comparison of results. Clin. Orthop. 178:54–63, 1983.
Delamarter, R.B., Hohl, M.E., Jr.: Ligament injuries associated with tibial plateau fractures. Clin. Orthop. 250:226–233, 1990.
DeLee, J.C., and Stiehl, J.B.: Open tibia fracture with compartment syndrome. Clin. Orthop. 160:175–184, 1981.
Den Hartog, B.D., Bartal, E., and Dooke, F.: Treatment of the unstable intertrochanteric fracture: Effect of the placement of the screw, its angle of insertion, and osteotomy. J. Bone Joint Surg. [Am.] 73:726–733, 1991.
Desjardins, A.L., Roy, A., Paiement, G., et al.: Unstable intertrochanteric fracture of the femur: A prospective randomised study comparing anatomical reduction and medial displacement osteotomy. J. Bone Joint Surg. [Br.] 75:445–447, 1993.
Gustilo, R.B., Mendoza, R.M., and Williams, D.N.: Problems in the management of type III (severe) open fractures: A new classification of type III open fractures. J. Trauma 24:742–746, 1984.
Gustilo, R.B., Merkow, R.L., and Templeman, D.: Current concepts review: The management of open fractures. J. Bone Joint Surg. [Am.] 72:299, 1990.
Hack, D.J., and Johnson, E.E.: The use of the unreamed nail and tibial fractures with concomitant preoperative or intraoperative elevated compartment pressure or compartment syndrome. J. Orthop. Trauma 8:203–211, 1994.
Hansen, S.T., and Winquist, R.A.: Closed intramedullary nailing of the femur: Kuntscher technique with reaming. Clin. Orthop. 138:56–61, 1979.
Holbrook, J.L., Swiontkowski, M.F., and Sanders, R.: Treatment of open fractures of the tibial shaft: Ender nailing versus external fixation: A randomized, prospective comparison. J. Bone Joint Surg. [Am.] 71:1231, 1989.
Hume, E., and Catalano, J.B., Ipsilateral neck and shaft fractures of the femur. Op. Tech. Orthop. 4:111–115, 1994.
Lachiewicz, P.F., and Funcik, T.: Factors influencing the results of open reduction and internal fixation of tibial plateau fractures. Clin. Orthop. 259:210–215, 1990.
Lhowe, D.W., and Hansen, S.T.: Immediate nailing of open fractures of the femoral shaft. J. Bone Joint Surg. [Am.] 70:812–820, 1988.
Mast, J.W., Spiegel, F.G., and Pappas, J.N.: Fractures of the tibial pilon. Clin. Orthop. 230:68–82, 1988.
Mawhinney, I.N., Maginn, P., and McCoy, G.F.: Tibial compartment syndromes after tibial nailing. J. Orthop. Trauma 8:212–214, 1994.
Nowotarski, P., and Brumback, R.J.: Immediate interlocking nailing of fractures of the femur caused by low to mid velocity gunshots. J. Orthop. Trauma. 8:134–141, 1994.
Pritchett, J.W.: Supracondylar fractures of the femur. Clin. Orthop. 184:173–177, 1984.
Richards, R.R., Waddell, J.P., Sullivan, T.R., et al.: Infra-isthmal fractures of the femur: A review of 82 cases. J. Trauma 24:735–741, 1984.
Riemer, B.L., Butterfield, S.L., Ray, R.L., et al.: Clandestine femoral neck fractures with ipsilateral diaphyseal fractures. J Orthop. Trauma 7:443–449, 1993.

Schatzker, J., and Lambert, D.C.: Supracondylar fractures of the femur. Clin. Orthop. 138:77–83, 1979.

Suedkamp, N.P., Barbey, N., Vueskens, A., et al.: The incidence of osteitis in open fractures: An analysis of 948 open fractures (a review of the Hanover experience). J. Orthop. Trauma 7:473–482, 1993.

Swiontkowski, M.F., Hansen, S.T., Jr., and Kellam, J.: Ipsilateral fractures of the femoral neck and shaft: A treatment protocol. J. Bone Joint Surg. [Am.] 66:260–268, 1984.

Talucci, R.C., Manning, J., Lampard, S., et al.: Early intramedullary nailing of femoral shaft fractures: A cause of fat embolism syndrome. Am. J. Surg. 146:107–110, 1983.

Tornetta, P., Bergman, M., Watnik, N., et al.: Treatment of grade III B open tibial fractures—a prospective randomized comparison of external fixation in non-reamed locked nailing. J. Bone Joint Surg. [Br.] 76:13–19, 1994.

Webb, L.X., Winquist, R.A., and Hansen, S.T.: Intramedullary nailing and reaming for delayed union or nonunion of the femoral shaft: A report of 105 consecutive cases. Clin. Orthop. 212:133–141, 1986.

Whittle, A.P., Russell, T.A., Taylor, J.C., and Lavelle, D.G.: Treatment of open fractures of the tibial shaft with the use of interlocking nailing without reaming. J. Bone Joint Surg. [Am.] 74:1162–1171, 1992.

Winquist, R.A., Hansen, S.T., Jr., and Clawson, D.K.: Closed intramedullary nailing of femoral fractures: A report of five hundred and twenty cases. J Bone Joint Surg. 66A:529–539, 1984.

Wiss, D.A., and Brien, W.W.: Subtrochanteric fractures of the femur: Results of treatment by interlocking nailing. Clin. Orthop. 283:231–236, 1992.

Zickel, R.E.: Subtrochanteric femoral fractures. Orthop. Clin. North Am. 11:555–568, 1980.

Knee

Benirschke, S.K., Agnew, S.G., Mayo, K.A., et al.: Immediate internal fixation of open, complex tibial plateau fractures: Treatment by standard protocol. J. Orthop. Trauma 6:76–86, 1992.

Carpenter, J.E., Kasman, R., and Matthews, L.S.: Fractures of the patella. J. Bone Joint Surg. [Am.] 75:1550–1561, 1993.

Fernandez, D.L.: Anterior approach to the knee with osteotomy of the tibial tubercle for bicondylar tibial fractures. J. Bone Joint Surg. [Am.] 70:208–219, 1988.

Georgiadis, G.M.: Combined anterior and posterior approaches for complex tibial plateau fractures. J. Bone Joint Surg. [Br.] 76:285–289, 1994.

Haas, S.B., and Callaway, H.: Disruptions of the extensor mechanism. Orthop. Clin. North Am. 23:687–695, 1992.

Iannacone, W.M., Bennett, F.S., DeLong, W.G., et al.: Initial experience with the treatment of supracondylar femoral fractures using the supracondylar intramedullary nail: A preliminary report. J. Orthop. Trauma 8:322–327, 1994.

Jensen, D.B., Rude, C., Duus, B., and Bjerg-Nielsen, A.: Tibial plateau fractures; A comparison of conservative and surgical treatment. J. Bone Joint Surg. [Br.] 72:49–52, 1990.

Koval, K., Sanders, R., Borrelli, J., et al.: Indirect reduction and percutaneous screw fixation of displaced tibial plateau fractures. J. Orthop. Trauma 6:340–346, 1992.

Moore, T.M.: Fracture-dislocation of the knee. Clin. Orthop. 156:128–140, 1981.

Saltzman, C.L., Goulet, J.A., McClellan, R.T., et al.: Results of treatment of displaced patellar fractures by partial patellectomy. J. Bone Joint Surg. [Am.] 72:1279, 1990.

Sanders, R.: Patella fractures and extensor mechanism injuries. In Browner, B.D., Jupiter, J.B., Levine, A.M., et al. (eds.): Skeletal Trauma: Fractures, Dislocations, Ligamentous Injuries, vol. 2. Philadelphia, WB Saunders, 1992, pp. 1685–1716.

Schatzker, J., McBroom, R., and Bruce, D.: The tibial plateau fracture: The Toronto experience, 1968–1975. Clin. Orthop. 138:94–104, 1979.

Siliski, J.M., Mahring, M., and Hofer, H.P.: Supracondylar-intercondylar fractures of the femur: Treatment by internal fixation. J. Bone Joint Surg. [Am.] 71:95–104, 1989.

Weber, M.J., Janecki, C.J., McLeod, P., et al.: Efficacy of various forms of fixation of transverse fractures of the patella. J. Bone Joint Surg. [Am.] 62:215–220, 1980.

Ankle and Foot

Canale, S.T., and Kelly, F.B.: Fractures of the neck of the talus. J. Bone Joint Surg. [Am.] 60:143–156, 1978.

DeCoster, T.A., and Miller, R.A.: Management of traumatic foot wounds. J. Am. Acad. Orthop. Surg. 2:226–230, 1994.

DeLee, J.C., and Curtis, R.: Subtalar dislocation of the foot. J. Bone Joint Surg. [Am.] 64:433–437, 1982.

Faciszewski, T., Burks, R.T., and Manaster, B.J.: Subtle injuries of the Lisfranc joint. J. Bone Joint Surg. [Am.] 72:1519, 1990.

Giachino, A.A., and Uhthoff, H.K.: Current concepts review: Intraarticular fractures of the calcaneus. J. Bone Joint Surg. [Am.] 71:784–787, 1989.

Goossens, M., and De Stoop, N.: Lisfranc's fracture-dislocations: Etiology, radiology, and results of treatment: A review of 20 cases. Clin. Orthop. 176:154–162, 1983.

Harper, M.C., and Hardin, G.: Posterior malleolar fractures of the ankle associated with external rotation-abduction injuries: Results with and without internal fixation. J. Bone Joint Surg. [Am.] 70:1348–1356, 1988.

Lindsay, W.R.N., and Dewar, R.P.: Fractures of the os calcis. Am. J. Surg. 95:555–576, 1958.

Macey, L.R., Benirschke, S.K., Sangeorzan, B.J., and Hansen, S.T.: Acute calcaneal fractures: Treatment, options, and results. J. Am. Acad. Orthop. Surg. 2:36–43, 1994.

Marti, R.K., Raaymakers, E.L., and Nolte, P.A.: Malunited ankle fractures—the late results of reconstruction. J. Bone Joint Surg. [Br.] 72:709–713, 1990.

McReynolds, I.S.: The Case for Operative Treatment of Fractures of the Os Calcis. Philadelphia, WB Saunders, 1982.

Ovadia, D.N., and Beals, R.K.: Fractures of the tibial plafond. J. Bone Joint Surg. [Am.] 68:543–551, 1986.

Sangeorzan, B.J., Benirschke, S.K., Mosca, V., et al.: Displaced intraarticular fractures of the tarsal navicular. J. Bone Joint Surg. [Am.] 71:1504, 1989.

Segal, D.: Displaced Ankle Fractures Treated Surgically and Postoperative Management. St. Louis, CV Mosby, 1979.

Stephenson, J.R.: Treatment of displaced intra-articular fractures of the calcaneus using medial and lateral approaches, internal fixation, and early motion. J. Bone Joint Surg. [Am.] 69:115–130, 1987.

Swanson, T.V., Bray, T.J., and Holmes, G.B.: Fractures of the talar neck: A mechanical study of fixation. J. Bone Joint Surg. [Am.] 74:544–551, 1992.

Shoulder

Flatow, E.L., Pollock, R.G., and Bigliani, L.U.: Operative treatment of two part, displaced surgical neck fractures of the proximal humerus. Op. Tech. Orthop. 4:2–8, 1994.

Goss, T.P.: Current concepts review: Fractures of the glenoid cavity. J. Bone Joint Surg. [Am.] 74:299–305, 1992.

Goss, T.P.: Double disruptions of the superior shoulder suspensory complex. J. Orthop. Trauma 7:99–106, 1993.

Green, A., and Norris, T.R.: Humeral head replacement for four part fractures and fracture dislocations. Op. Tech. Orthop. 4:13–20, 1994.

Herscovici, D., Jr., Fiennes, A.G., Allgower, M., et al.: The floating shoulder-ipsilateral, clavical and scapular neck fractures. J. Bone Joint Surg. [Br.] 74:362–366, 1992.

Jaberg, H., Warner, J.P., and Jakob, R.P.: Percutaneous stabilization of unstable fractures of the humerus. J. Bone Joint Surg. [Am.] 74:508–515, 1992.

Klassen, J.F., and Cofield, R.H.: Surgical management of scapular fractures, Op. Tech. Orthop. 4:58–63, 1994.

Schlegel, T.F., and Hawkins, R.J.: Displaced proximal humeral fractures: Evaluation and treatment. J. Am. Acad. Orthop. Surg. 2:54–66, 1994.

Schlegel, T.F., and Hawkins, R.J.: Hemiarthroplasty for the treatment of proximal humeral fractures. Op. Tech. Orthop. 4:21–25, 1994.

Schlegel, T.F., and Hawkins, R.J.: Internal fixation of three part proximal humeral fractures. Op. Tech. Orthop. 4:9–12, 1994.

Sidor, M.L., Zuckerman, J.D., Lyon, T., and Koval, K.: The Neer classification system for proximal humeral fractures—an assessment of interobserver reliability and intraobserver reproducibility. J. Bone Joint Surg. [Am.] 75:1745–1750, 1993.

Siebenrock, K.A., and Gerber, C.: The reproducibility of classification

Table 11–4.

Muscles of the Shoulder

Muscle	Origin	Insertion	Action	Innervation
Trapezius	Spin. proc. C7–T12	Clavicle, scapula (AC, SP)	Rotate scapula	CN XI
Lat. dorsii	Spin. proc. T6–S5, ilium	Humerus (ITG)	Ex., add., IR humerus	Thoracodorsal
Rhomboid maj.	Spin. proc. T2–T5	Scapula (med. border)	Adduct scapula	Dorsal scapular
Rhomboid min.	Spin. proc. C7–T1	Scapula (med. spine)	Adduct scapula	Dorsal scapular
Lev. scapulae	T. proc. C1–C4	Scapula (sup. med.)	Elevate, rotate scapula	C3, C4
Pectoralis maj.	Sternum, ribs, clavicle	Humerus (L-ITG)	Add., IR arm	M and L PN
Pectoralis min.	Ribs 3–5	Scapula (coracoid)	Protract scapula	MPN
Subclavius	Rib 1	Inf. clavicle	Depress clavicle	U trunk
Serratus ant.	Ribs 1–9	Scapula (vent. med.)	Prevent winging	Long thoracic
Deltoid	Lateral clavicle, scapula	Humerus (deltoid tub.)	Abduct arm (2)	Axillary
Teres major	Inf. scapula	Humerus (M-ITG)	Add., IR, ext.	L subscapular
Subscapularis	Ventral scapula	Humerus (LT)	IR arm, ant. stability	U and L subscapular
Supraspinatus	Sup. scapula	Humerus (GT)	Abd. (1), ER arm stability	Suprascapular
Infraspinatus	Dorsal scapula	Humerus (GT)	Stability, ER arm	Suprascapular
Teres minor	Scapula (dorsolateral)	Humerus (GT)	Stability, ER arm	Axillary

ITG, intertubercular groove; AC, acromion; SP, spinous process; LT, lesser tuberosity; GT, greater tuberosity.

against the glenoid. Table 11–4 presents specifics on these muscles. The shoulder has been described as having four supporting layers (Fig. 11–4).

Layer	Structure
I	Deltoid Pectoralis major
II	Clavipectoral fascia Conjoined tendon, short head biceps and coracobrachialis Coracoacromial ligament
III	Deep layer of subdeltoid bursa Rotator cuff muscle (subscapularis, supraspinatus, infraspinatus, teres minor)
IV	Glenohumeral joint capsule Coracohumeral ligament

D. Nerves—Peripheral nerves that innervate muscles about the upper extremity derive from the brachial plexus. This plexus, formed from the ventral primary rami of C5–T1, lies under the clavicle, extending from the scalenus (between scalenus medius and scalenus anterior) anterior to the axilla. The brachial plexus is organized into five components: *r*oots, *t*runks, *d*ivisions, *c*ords, and *b*ranches (remember the mnemonic *R*ob *T*aylor *d*rinks *c*old *b*eer). There are five roots (C5–T1, although C4 and T2 can have small contributions), three trunks (upper, middle, lower), six divisions (two from each trunk), three cords (posterior, lateral, medial), and multiple branches, as illustrated in Figure 11–5. Note that there are four preclavicular branches (from roots and upper trunk): dorsal scapular nerve, long thoracic nerve, suprascapular nerve, and **nerve to subclavius.**

E. Vessels (Fig. 11–6)—The subclavian artery arises either directly from the aorta (left subclavian) or from the brachiocephalic trunk (right subclavian). It then emerges between the scalenus anterior and medius muscles and becomes the axillary artery at the outer border of the first rib. The axillary artery is divided into three portions based on its relationship to the pectoralis minor (the first is medial to it, the second is under it, and the third is lateral to it). Each part of the artery has as many branches as the number of that portion (e.g., the second part has two branches).

Part	Branch	Course
1	Supreme thoracic	Medial—to serratus anterior and pecs
2	Thoracoacromial	Four branches (deltoid, acromial, pectoralis, clavicular)
	Lateral thoracic	Descends to serratus anterior
3	Subscapular	Two branches (thoracodorsal and circumflex scapular → triangular space)
	Ant. circumflex humeral	Circles humerus anteriorly, blood supply to humeral head
	Post. circumflex humeral	Post. humerus → quadrangular space

F. Surgical Approaches to the Shoulder—Include the anterior approach (reconstructions and arthroplasties), lateral approach (acromioplasty and cuff repair), and posterior approach (posterior reconstruction).

1. Anterior Approach (Henry) (Fig. 11–7)—Explores the interval between the deltoid (axillary n.) and the pectoralis major (medial and lateral pectoral n.). The cephalic vein is dissected and retracted laterally with

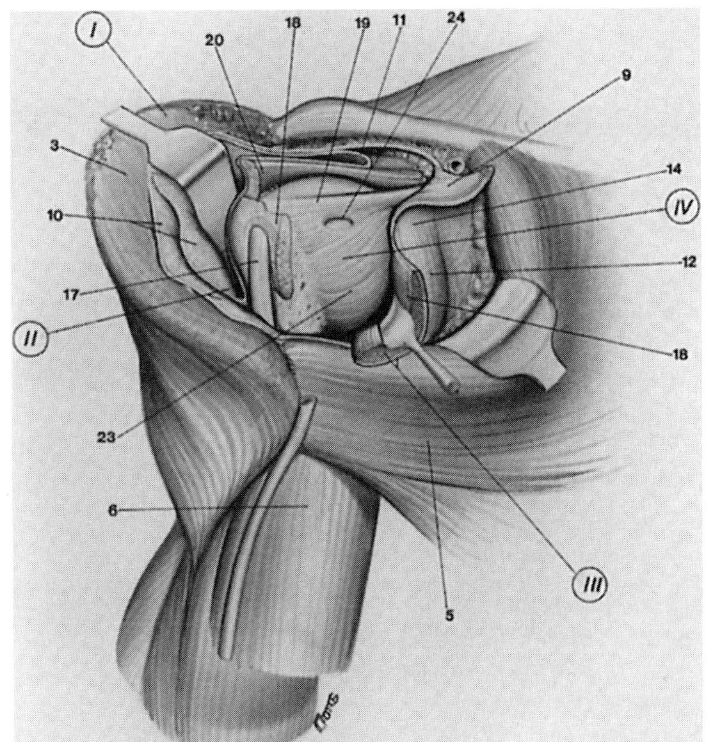

Figure 11–4. Anterior aspect of the right shoulder depicting the four layers *(encircled Roman numerals)*. The lateral retractor is placed deep to layer 2, demonstrating the ease of dissection in the plane of the bursa around the lateral aspect of the proximal humerus. The subscapularis and supraspinatus (layer 3) have been reflected, disclosing layer 4 (capsule and coracohumeral ligament). The usual shape and position of the defect in the rotator interval (if present) is depicted; it is variable (3 = deltoid; **5 = pectoralis major**; 6 = biceps; 9 = C-A ligament; 10 = fasci (II); 11 = deep layer of subacromial tendon b, and subscapular; 12 = conjoined tendon; 14 = tip of coracoid process; 17 = biceps long hd.; 18 = deep layer subacromial b, and subscapular; 19 = coracohumeral ligament; 20 = supraspinatus under deep bursa layer; 23 = joint capsule; 24 = hiatus in capsule. (From Cooper, D.E., O'Brien, S.J., and Warren, R.F.: Supporting layers of glenohumeral joint. Clin. Orthop. 289:151, 1993.)

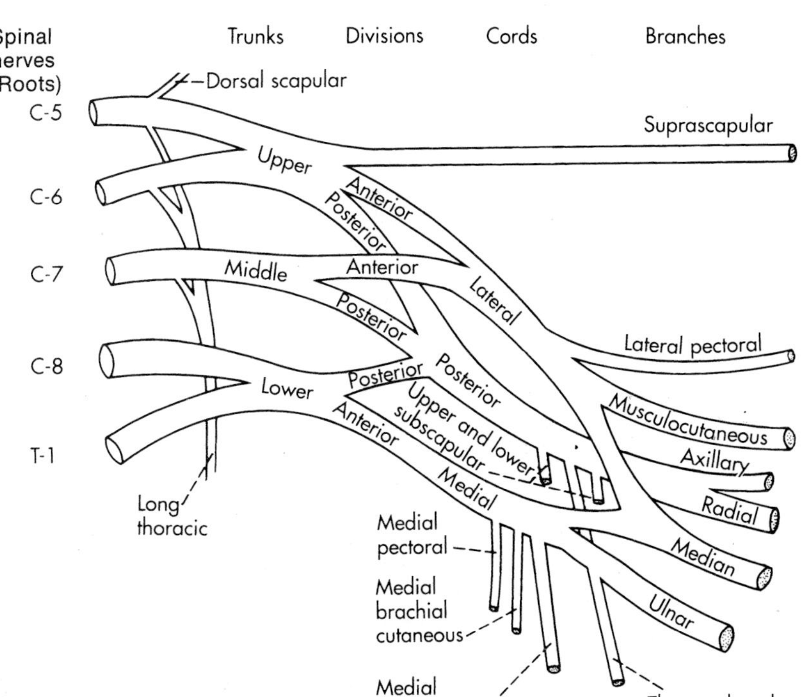

Figure 11–5. Brachial plexus. (From Jenkins, D.B.: Hollinshead's Functional Anatomy of the Limbs and Back, 6th ed., Fig. 5–7. Philadelphia, W.B. Saunders, 1991.)

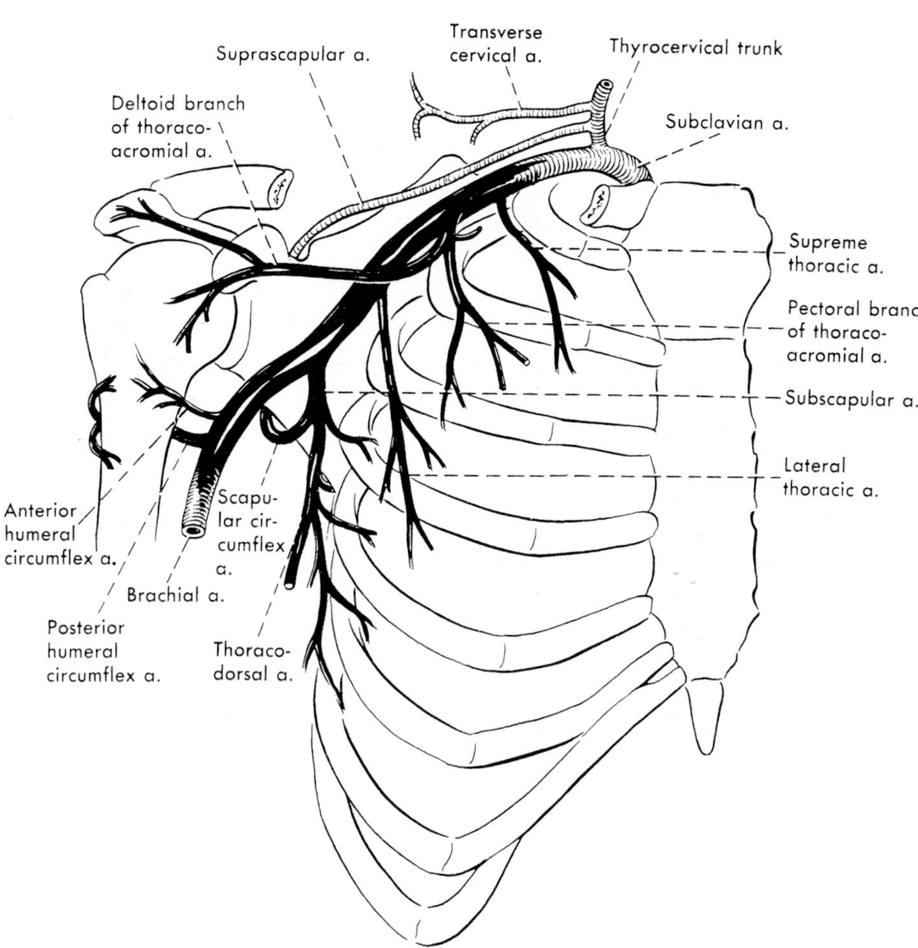

Figure 11–6. Branches of the axillary artery. (From Jenkins, D.B.: Hollinshead's Functional Anatomy of the Limbs and Back, 6th ed., p. 77. Philadelphia, W.B. Saunders, 1991.)

the deltoid, and the underlying subscapularis is exposed. The latter is then divided (preserving the most inferior fibers to protect the axillary n.), and the shoulder capsule is encountered. The **musculocutaneous nerve** should be protected by avoiding dissection medial to the coracobrachialis. This nerve usually penetrates the biceps/coracobrachialis 5–8 cm below the coracoid, but it enters these muscles proximal to this 5-cm "safe zone" almost 30% of the time. The **axillary nerve,** which is **just inferior** to the shoulder **capsule,** must be protected during procedures in this area. Abduction and external rotation of the arm will help displace the nerve from the surgical field.

2. Lateral Approach—Involves splitting the deltoid muscle or subperiosteal dissection of the muscle from the acromion. This maneuver exposes the supraspinatus tendon well and allows for repairs of the rotator cuff. The deltoid should not be split more than **5 cm below the acromion** to avoid injury to the **axillary nerve.**
3. Posterior Approach (Fig. 11–8)—Uses the internervous plane between the infraspinatus (suprascapular nerve) and teres minor (axillary nerve). This plane can be approached by detaching the deltoid from the scapular spine or by splitting the deltoid (Rockwood's). After this interval is found, the posterior capsule lies immediately below it. The axillary nerve and the posterior circumflex humeral artery both run in the **quadrangular space** below the teres minor, so it is important to stay above this muscle. **Excessive medial retraction of the infraspinatus can injure the suprascapular nerve.**

G. Arthroscopy—Portals for arthroscopy (discussed in Chapter 3, Sports Medicine) include the anterior superior (musculocutaneous nerve at risk with portals medial), the anterior inferior (must be above the subscapularis and lateral to the conjoint tendon), and the posterior (inferior portals may risk the axillary nerve).

III. Arm

A. Osteology—The humerus is the only bone of the arm and the largest and longest bone of the upper extremity. It is composed of a shaft and two articular extremities. The hemispherical head, directed superiorly, medially, and slightly dorsally, articulates with the much smaller scapular glenoid cavity. The *anatomic neck,* directly below the head, serves as an

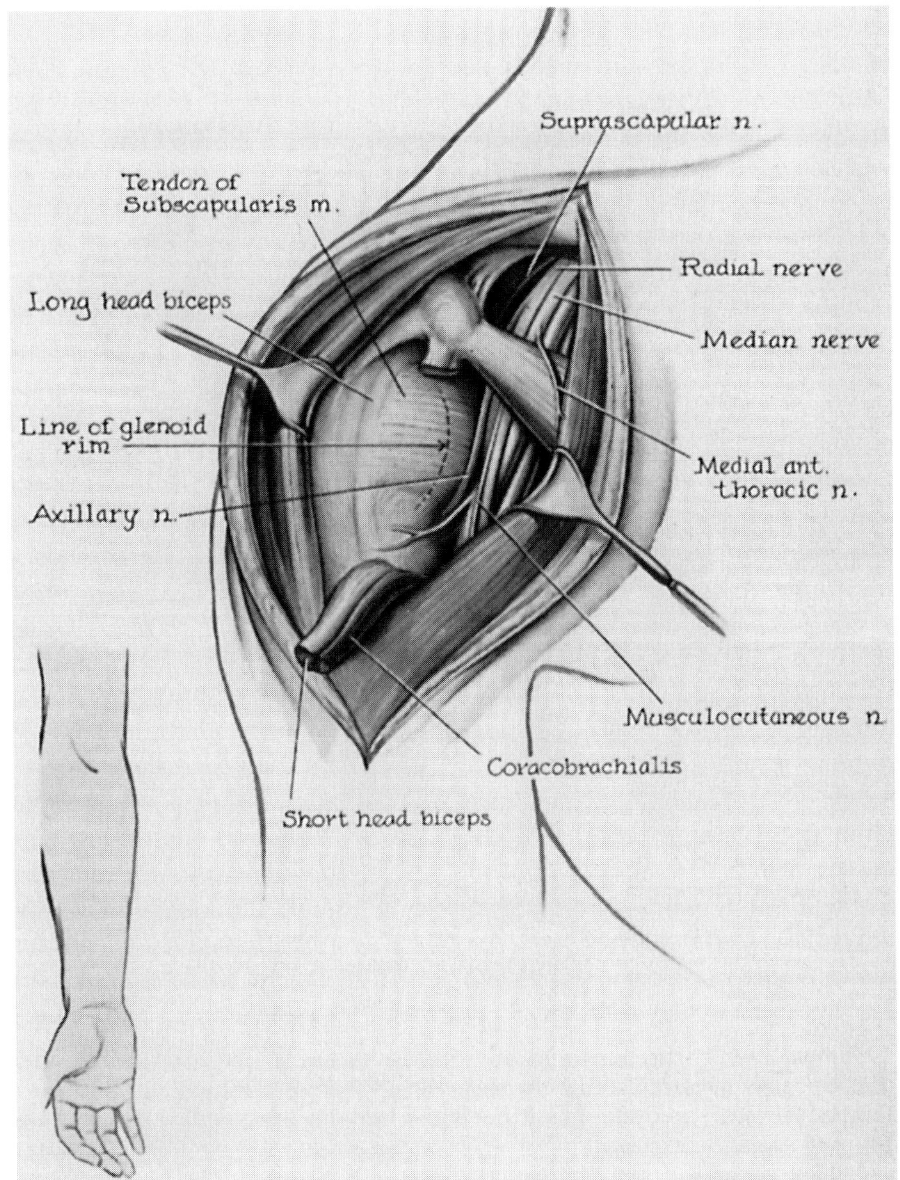

Figure 11–7. Anterior approach to the shoulder through the deltopectoral interval. (From Kaplan, E.B.: Surgical Approaches to the Neck, Cervical Spine, and Upper Extremity, p. 57. Philadelphia, W.B. Saunders, 1966.)

attachment for the shoulder capsule. The *surgical neck* is lower and is more often involved in fractures. The greater tuberosity, lateral to the head, serves as the attachment for the supraspinatus, infraspinatus, and teres minor muscles (anterior to posterior, respectively). The lesser tuberosity, located anteriorly, has only one muscular insertion: the last rotator cuff muscle, the subscapularis. The bicipital groove (for the tendon of the long head of the biceps) is situated between the two tuberosities. The shaft of the humerus has a notable groove for the radial nerve posteriorly in its midportion, adjacent to the deltoid tuberosity. Distally, the humerus flares into medial and lateral epicondyles and forms half of the elbow joint with a medial spool-shaped trochlea (articulates with the olecranon of the ulna) and a globular capitulum (which opposes the radial head). The normal articular alignment of the distal humerus has a 7 degree valgus tilt (carrying angle). The humerus has one primary and seven secondary ossification centers.

Ossification Center	Age at Appearance	Age at Fusion
Body (primary)	8 weeks (fetal)	Blend at 6 years, unites at 20 years
Head	1 year	
Greater tuberosity	3 years	
Lesser tuberosity	5 years	
Capitulum	2 years	Blend and unites with body at 16–18 years
Medial epicondyle	5 years	
Trochlea	9 years	
Lateral epicondyle	13 years	

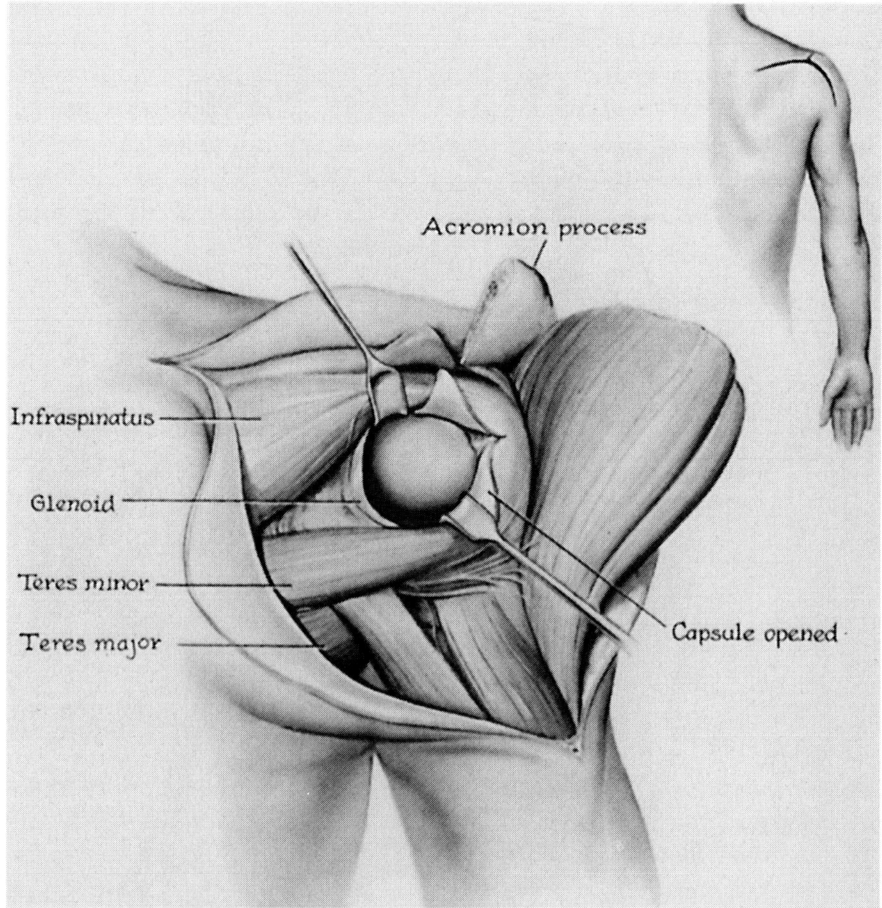

Figure 11–8. Posterior approach to the shoulder through the infraspinatus—teres minor interval. (From Kaplan, E.B.: Surgical Approaches to the Neck, Cervical Spine, and Upper Extremity, p. 61. Philadelphia, W.B. Saunders, 1966.)

B. Arthrology—The humerus articulates with the scapula on its upper end, forming the glenohumeral joint (discussed earlier), and with the radius and ulna on its lower end, forming the elbow joint. The elbow is composed of a compound ginglymus (hinge) joint (humeroulnar) and a trochoid (pivot) joint (humeroradial).

Articulation	Components
Humeroulnar	Trochlea and trochlear notch
Humeroradial	Capitulum and radial head
Proximal R-U	Radial notch and radial head

The ligaments of the elbow joint include a relatively weak capsule and the following ligaments (Fig. 11–9).

Ligament	Components	Comments
Ulnar collateral	Anterior and posterior	Ant. fibers key
Radial collateral	Triangular	Weaker, less distinct
Annular	Osseofibrous ring	
Quadrate	Annular lig. → radial neck	Rotatory movements
Oblique cord	Coronoid base → radius	

C. Muscles of the Arm—There are four muscles of the arm (Table 11–5). The triceps muscle helps form borders for two important spaces (Fig. 11–10). The **triangular space** is bordered by the teres minor (superiorly), teres major (inferiorly), and long head of the triceps (laterally); it contains the circumflex scapular vessels. The **quadrangular, or quadrilateral, space** is also bordered by the teres minor (superiorly) and the teres major (inferiorly), with the long head of the triceps forming its medial border and the humerus forming the lateral border. The quadrangular space **transmits the posterior humeral circumflex vessels and the axillary nerve.** The **triangular interval** is immediately inferior to the quadrangular space and is bordered by the teres major (superiorly), long head of the triceps (medially), and lateral head of the triceps or the humerus (laterally). Through this interval the profunda brachii artery and **radial nerve can be seen.**

D. Nerves—Four major nerves traverse the arm, two giving off branches to arm musculature and two that innervate distal musculature (Fig. 11–11). Most of the cutaneous innervation of the arm arises directly from the brachial plexus.

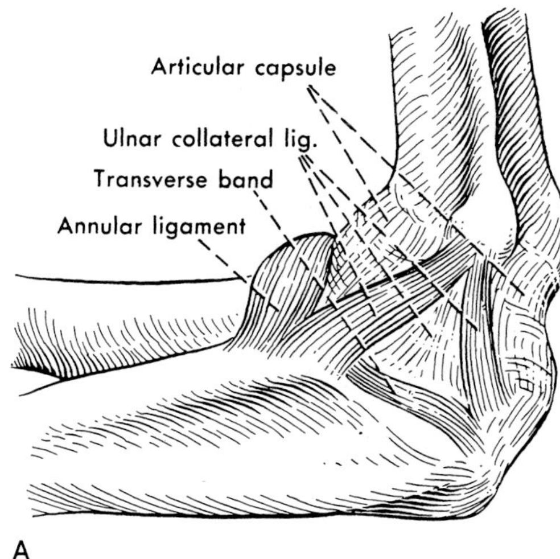

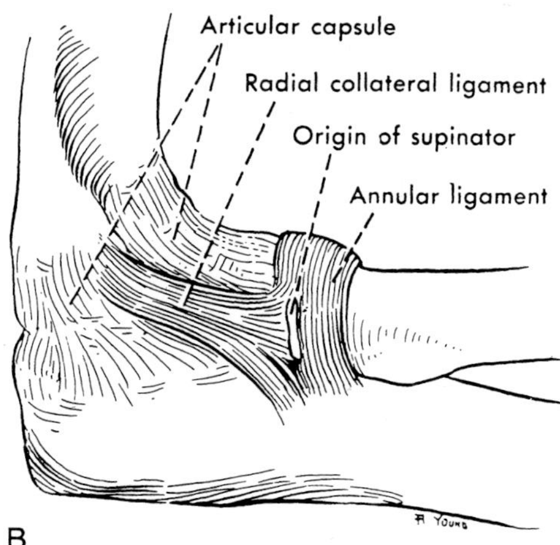

Figure 11–9. Elbow ligaments. *A,* Medial view. *B,* Lateral view. (From Jenkins, D.B.: Hollinshead's Functional Anatomy of the Limbs and Back, 6th ed., p. 108. Philadelphia, W.B. Saunders, 1991.)

1. Musculocutaneous Nerve—Formed from the lateral cord of the brachial plexus, this nerve pierces the coracobrachialis 5–8 cm distal to the coracoid and then branches to supply this muscle, the biceps, and the brachialis. It also gives off a branch to the elbow joint before it **becomes the lateral antebrachial cutaneous nerve of the forearm.**
2. Radial Nerve—Formed from the posterior cord of the brachial plexus, this nerve spirals around the humerus (medial lateral), supplying the triceps muscles. It emerges on the lateral side of the arm between the brachialis and brachioradialis anterior to the lateral epicondyle (where it supplies the anconeus muscle).
3. Median Nerve—From the medial and lateral cords of the brachial plexus, this nerve accompanies the brachial artery along the arm, crossing it during its course (lateral medial). It supplies some branches to the elbow joint but has no branches in the arm itself.
4. Ulnar Nerve—The continuation of the medial cord of the brachial plexus, this nerve remains medial to the brachial artery in the arm and then runs behind the medial epicondyle of the humerus, where it is quite superficial. It also has branches to the elbow but not arm branches.
5. Cutaneous Nerves—The supraclavicular nerve (C3, C4) supplies the upper shoulder. The axillary nerve supplies the shoulder joint and the overlying skin (in accordance with Hilton's law). The medial, lateral, and dorsal brachial cutaneous nerves supply the balance of the cutaneous innervation of the arm.

E. Vessels—The brachial artery originates at the lower border of the tendon of the teres major and continues to the elbow, where it bifurcates into the radial and ulnar arteries (see Fig. 11–11). Lying medial in the arm, the brachial artery curves laterally to enter the cubital fossa (formed by the distal humerus proximally, the brachioradialis laterally, and the pronator teres medially). Its principal branches include the deep brachial (also known as the profunda, this artery accompanies the radial nerve posteriorly), the superior and inferior ulnar collaterals, and nutrient and muscular branches.

Table 11–5.

Muscles of the Arm

Muscle	Origin	Insertion	Action	Innervation
Coracobrachialis	Coracoid	Mid. humerus medial	Flexion, adduction	Musculocutaneous
Biceps	Coracoid (SH) Supraglenoid (LH)	Radial tuberosity	Supination, flexion	Musculocutaneous
Brachialis	Ant. humerus	Ulnar tuberosity (ant.)	Flexes forearm	Musculocut., radial
Triceps	Infraglenoid (LH) Post. humerus (lat H) Post. humerus (MH)	Olecranon	Extends forearm	Radial

SH, short head; LH, long head; lat H, lateral head; MH, medial head.

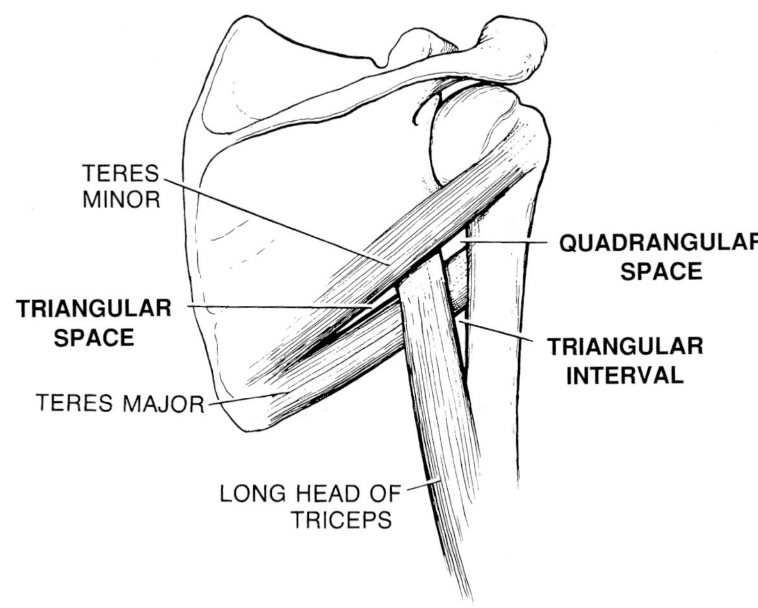

Figure 11–10. Quadrangular space. (From Kaplan, E.B.: Surgical Approaches to the Neck, Cervical Spine, and Upper Extremity, p. 53. Philadelphia, W.B. Saunders, 1966.)

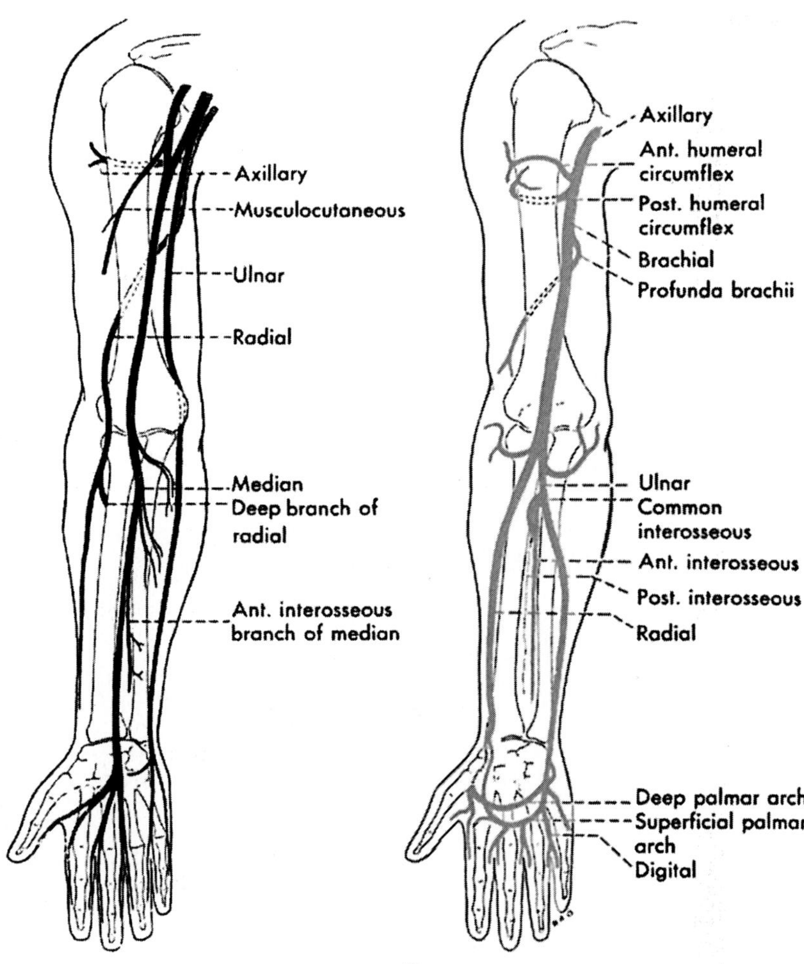

Figure 11–11. Nerves and vessels of the upper extremity. *A,* Principal nerves. *B,* Chief arteries. (From Jenkins, D.B.: Hollinshead's Functional Anatomy of the Limbs and Back, 6th ed., p. 62. Philadelphia, W.B. Saunders, 1991.)

The supratrochlear artery is the least flexible branch; these collateral vessels can bind up the brachial artery with distal humerus fractures. Anastomoses around the elbow (medial to lateral) are as follows.

Superior Branch	Inferior Branch
Superior ulnar collateral	Posterior ulnar recurrent
Inferior ulnar collateral	Anterior ulnar recurrent
Mid. collateral branch of deep brachial	Interosseous recurrent
Rad. collateral branch of deep brachial	Radial recurrent

F. Surgical Approaches to the Arm and Elbow—Proximally include the anterior and posterior approaches and distally include anterolateral and lateral approaches to the humerus and numerous approaches to the elbow.

1. Anterolateral Approach to the Humerus (Fig. 11–12)—Depends on the internervous plane between the deltoid (axillary nerve) and the pectoralis major (medial and lateral pectoral nerves) proximally and between the fibers of the brachialis (radial nerve and musculocutaneous nerve) distally. The radial and axillary nerves are at risk mainly for forceful retraction. The anterior circumflex humeral vessels may need to be ligated with a proximal approach.
2. Posterior Approach to the Humerus (Fig. 11–13)—Utilizes the interval between the lateral and long heads of the triceps superficially and a **muscle-splitting approach for the medial (deep) head.** The radial nerve (which limits proximal extension of this approach) and deep brachial artery must be identified and protected, and the ulnar nerve is jeopardized unless subperiosteal dissection of the humerus is meticulous.
3. Anterolateral Approach to the Distal Humerus (Fig. 11–14)—Uses the interval between the brachialis (musculocutaneous and radial nerves) and the brachioradialis (radial nerve). The radial nerve again must be identified and protected.
4. Lateral Approach to the Distal Humerus—Exploits the interval between the triceps and the brachioradialis by elevating a portion of the common extensor origin from the lateral epicondyle. Proximal extension jeopardizes the radial nerve.
5. Posterior Approach to the Elbow (Fig. 11–15)—Detachment of the extensor mechanism of the elbow gives excellent exposure for many elbow fractures. The olecranon osteotomy (best done with a chevron cut 2 cm distal to the tip) should be predrilled and the ulnar nerve protected. An alternative approach splits the triceps and leaves the olecranon intact.

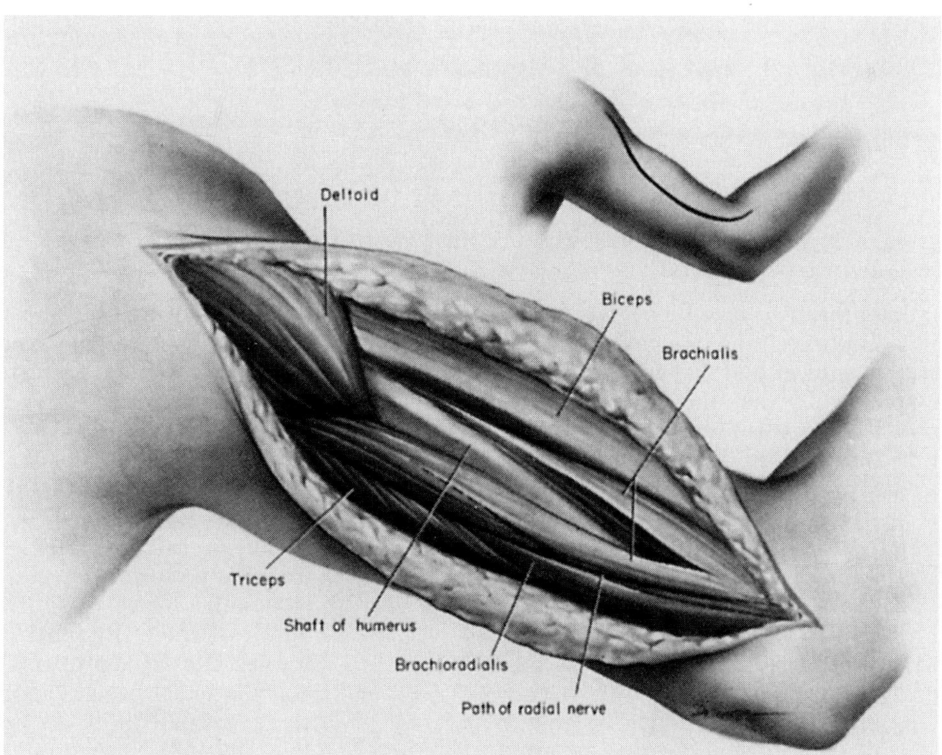

Figure 11–12. Lateral approach to the arm. (From Kaplan, E.B.: Surgical Approaches to the Neck, Cervical Spine, and Upper Extremity, p. 74. Philadelphia, W.B. Saunders, 1966.)

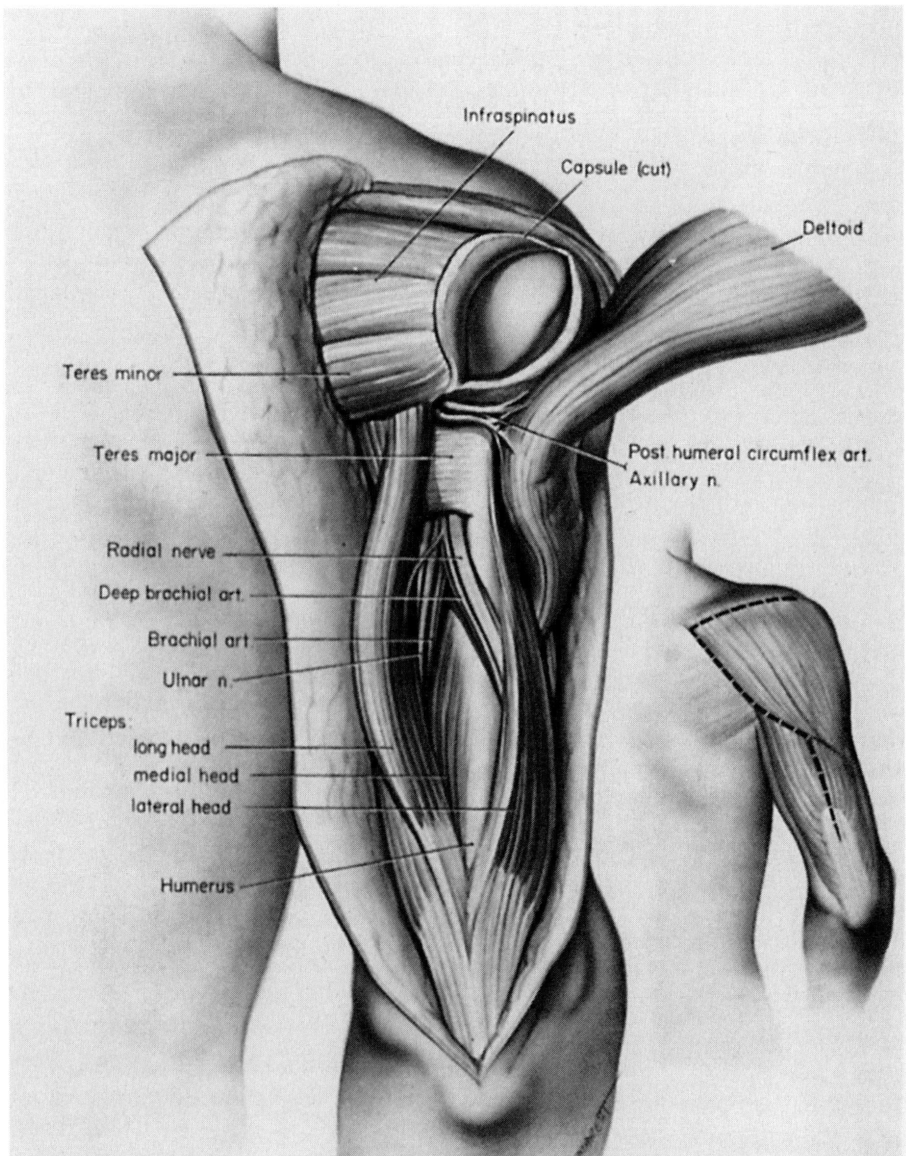

Figure 11–13. Posterior approach to the arm. (From Kaplan, E.B.: Surgical Approaches to the Neck, Cervical Spine, and Upper Extremity, p. 73. Philadelphia, W.B. Saunders, 1966.)

6. Medial Approach to the Elbow—Exploits the interval between the brachialis (musculocutaneous nerve) and the triceps (radial nerve) proximally and the brachialis and pronator teres (median nerve) distally. The ulnar and medial antebrachial cutaneous nerves are in the field and must be protected.
7. Anterolateral Approach to the Elbow (Henry's)—An extension of the same approach to the distal humerus, this approach is a brachialis (musculocutaneous nerve) splitting approach proximally and is between the pronator teres (median nerve) and the brachioradialis distally. The lateral antebrachial cutaneous nerve must be protected superficially and the radial nerve (and its branches) deep (supinate the forearm). Additionally, the brachial artery (which lies under the biceps aponeurosis) must be carefully protected. Branches of the radial recurrent artery must be ligated with this approach.
8. (Postero)Lateral (Kocher's) Approach to the Elbow (Fig. 11–16)—Uses the interval between the anconeus (radial nerve) and the main extensor origin (extensor carpi ulnaris—posterior interosseous branch of the radial nerve [posterior interosseous nerve—PIN]). **Pronation of the arm moves the PIN anteriorly and radially,** and the radial head is approached through the proximal supinator fibers. Extending this approach distal to the annular ligament increases the risk to the PIN.

G. Arthroscopy—Portals for elbow arthroscopy

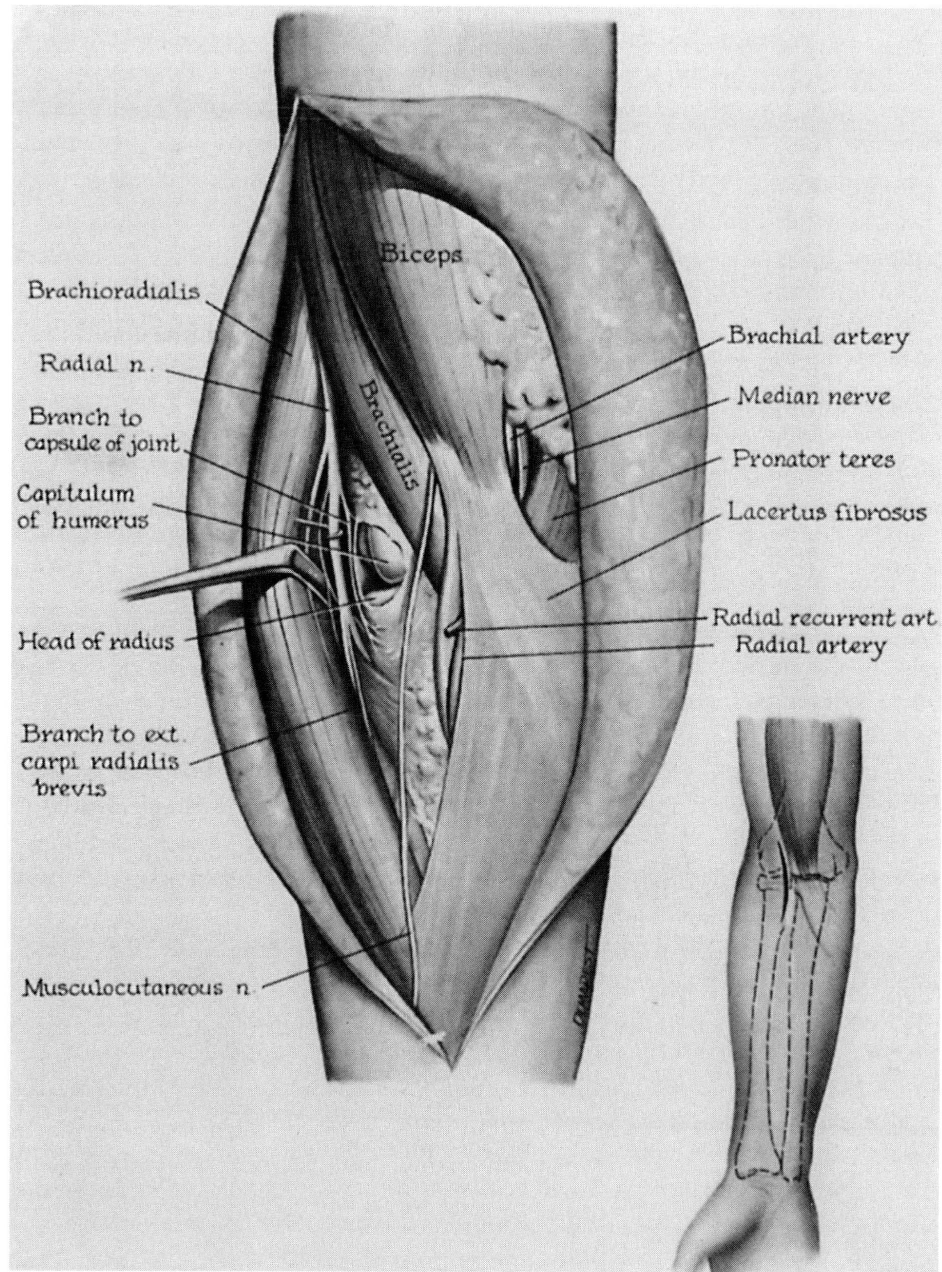

Figure 11–14. Anterior approach to the elbow. (From Kaplan, E.B.: Surgical Approaches to the Neck, Cervical Spine, and Upper Extremity, p. 77. Philadelphia, W.B. Saunders, 1966.)

include the anterolateral portal (radial nerve risk), the anteromedial portal (risks the medial antebrachial cutaneous and median nerves), and posterolateral portals.

IV. Forearm

A. Osteology—The forearm includes two long bones—the ulna and radius, which articulate with the humerus (principally the ulna)—and the carpi (principally the radius).

1. Ulna—A long prismatic bone occupying the medial forearm and consisting of a body and two extremities. Proximally, the ulna is composed of two curved processes, the olecranon and the coronoid processes, with an intervening trochlear notch. Distally, the ulna tapers and ends in a lateral head and a medial styloid process. The ulna has one primary and two secondary ossification centers.

Ossification Center	Age at Appearance	Age at Fusion
Body (primary)	8 weeks (fetal)	
Distal ulna	5 years	20 years
Olecranon	10 years	16 years

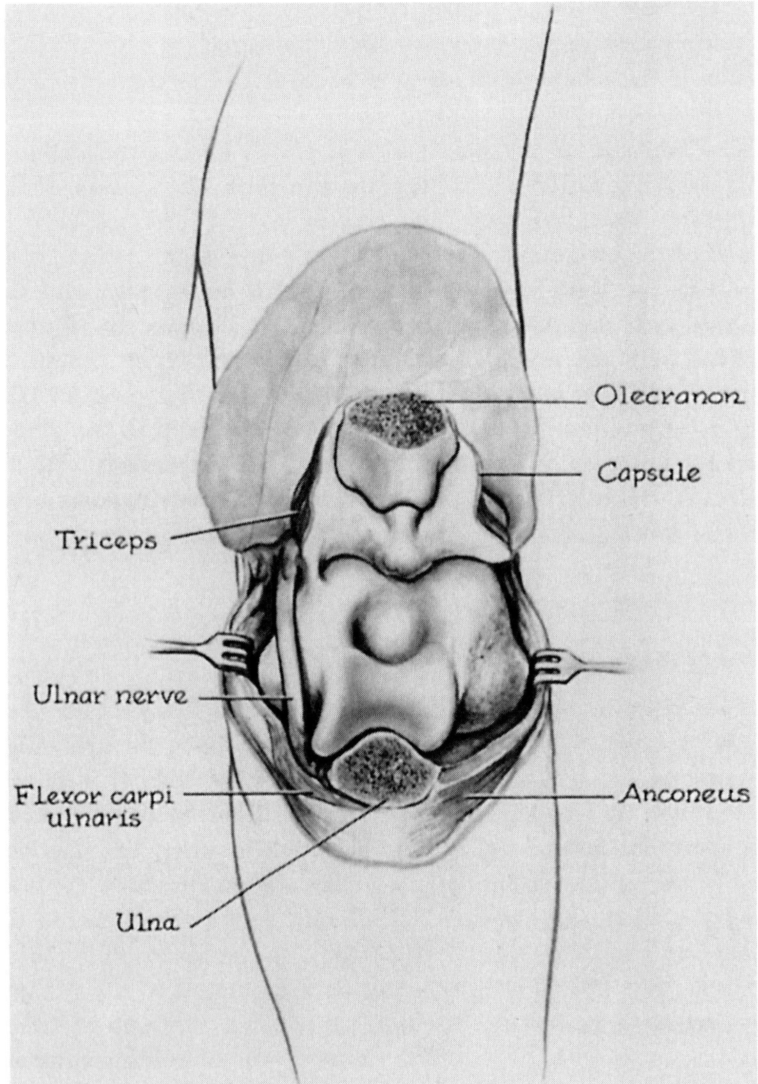

Figure 11–15. Posterior approach to the elbow. (From Kaplan, E.B.: Surgical Approaches to the Neck, Cervical Spine, and Upper Extremity, p. 82. Philadelphia, W.B. Saunders, 1966.)

2. Radius—Like the ulna, the radius has a body and two extremities. The proximal radius is composed of a head with a central fovea, a neck, and a proximal medial radial tuberosity (for insertion of the biceps tendon). The radius has a gradual bend (convex laterally) and gradually increases in size distally. The distal extremity of the radius is composed of the carpal articular surface, an ulnar notch, a dorsal tubercle (Lister's tubercle, which is at the level of the scapholunate joint), and a lateral styloid process. The radius is also ossified via three centers.

Ossification Center	Age at Appearance	Age at Fusion
Body (primary)	8 weeks (fetal)	
Distal radius	2 years	17–20 years
Proximal radius	5 years	15–18 years

B. Arthrology—The radius and ulna articulate proximally at the elbow joint (discussed earlier) and distally at the wrist. The wrist consists primarily of the radiocarpal joint but also includes the distal radioulnar articulation with its triangular fibrocartilage complex.
   1. Radiocarpal Joint—An ellipsoid joint involving the distal radius and the scaphoid, lunate, and triquetrum. This joint is usually located at the level of the proximal wrist flexion crease. Covered by a loose capsule, the wrist relies heavily on ligaments, especially volar ligaments, for stability. They include the volar and dorsal radiocarpal ligaments and the ulnar and radial collateral ligaments.
   2. Triangular Fibrocartilage Complex (Fig. 11–17)—Originates from the most ulnar portion of the radius and extends into the caput ulna and the ulnar wrist to the base of the fifth metacarpal. It includes the following components.

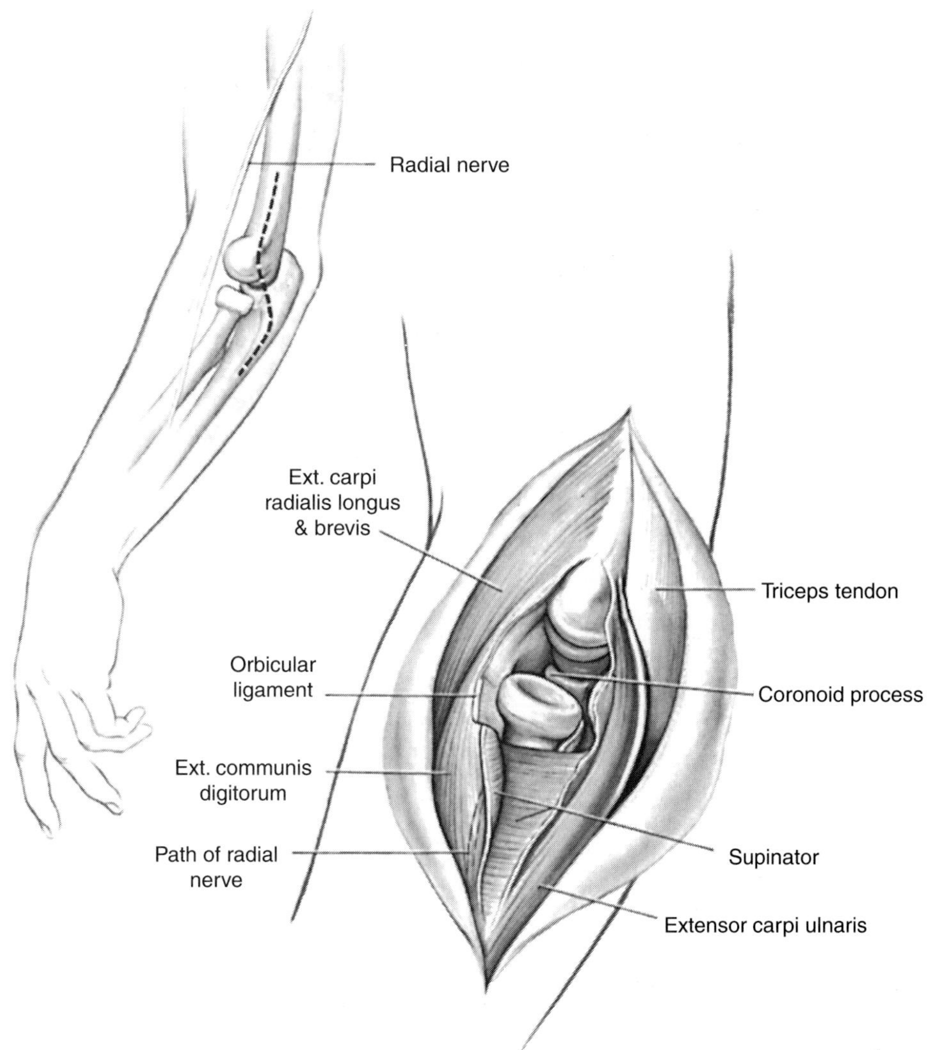

Figure 11–16. Lateral approach to the elbow. (From Kaplan, E.B.: Surgical Approaches to the Neck, Cervical Spine, and Upper Extremity, p. 83. Philadelphia, W.B. Saunders, 1966.)

Component	Origin	Insertion
Dorsal and volar radioulnar ligament (RUL)	Ulnar radius	Capnut ulna
Articular disc	Radius/ulna	Triquetrum
Prestyloid recess	Disc	Meniscus homologue
Meniscus homologue	Ulna/disc	Triquetrum/UCL
Ulnar collateral ligament	Ulna	Fifth metacarpal

C. Muscles of the Forearm (Fig. 11–18)— Arrangement based on both location and function into volar flexors (superficial and deep) and dorsal extensors (superficial and deep) (Table 11–6).

D. Nerves—The nerves of the upper arm continue into the forearm (Fig. 11–19).

1. Radial Nerve—Anterior to the lateral epicondyle, the radial nerve runs between the brachialis and brachioradialis and divides into anterior and deep (PIN) branches. The PIN splits the supinator and supplies all of the extensor muscles (except the mobile wad [brachioradialis, extensor carpi radialis brevis, extensor carpi radialis longus]). The superficial branch of the radial nerve passes to the dorsal radial surface of the hand in the distal third of the forearm by passing between the brachioradialis and extensor carpi radialis longus.
2. Median Nerve—Lies medial to the brachial artery at the elbow, superficial to the brachialis muscle. In the forearm the median nerve **splits** the two heads of the **pronator teres** and then **runs between the flexor digitorum superficialis (FDS) and flexor digitorum profundus (FDP),** becoming more superficial at the flexor retinaculum, where it continues into the hand. It has branches to all the superficial flexor muscles of the forearm except the flexor carpi ulnaris (FCU). Its anterior interosseous

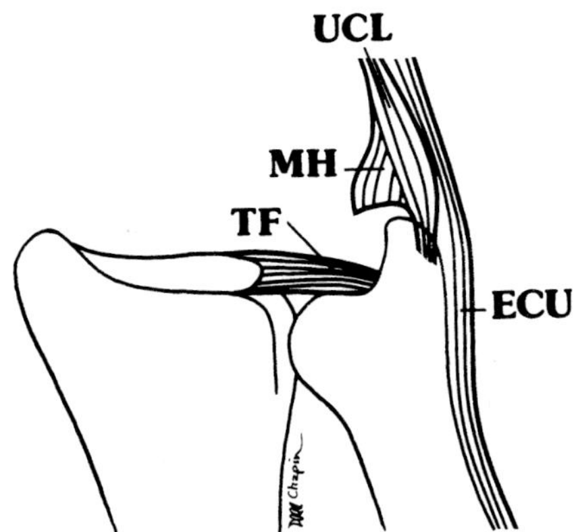

Figure 11–17. Triangular fibrocartilage complex (TFCC). UCL, ulnar collateral ligament; MH, meniscal homologue; TF, transverse fibers (radioulnar ligament); ECU, extensor carpi ulnaris. (From Weissman, B.N., and Sledge, C.B.: Orthopedic Radiology, p. 115. Philadelphia, W.B. Saunders, 1986.)

branch, which runs between the flexor pollicis longus (FPL) and FDP, supplies all the deep flexors except the ulnar half of the FDP.

3. Ulnar Nerve—Enters the forearm between the two heads of the FCU, which it supplies, and then **runs between the FCU and FDP** (and **innervates the ulnar half of this muscle**). It lies more superficial at the wrist and enters the hand through Guyon's canal.
4. Cutaneous Nerves—In the forearm are the **lateral antebrachial cutaneous nerve** (the continuation of the musculocutaneous nerve **that passes lateral to the cephalic vein** after emerging laterally from between the biceps and brachialis at the elbow), the medial antebrachial cutaneous nerve (a

Table 11–6.

Muscles of the Forearm

Muscle	Origin	Insertion	Action	Innervation
Superficial Flexors				
Pronator teres (PT)	Med. epicondyle and coronoid	Mid. lat. radius	Pronate, flex forearm	Median
Flexor carpi radialis (FCR)	Med. epicondyle	2nd and 3rd Metacarpal bases	Flex wrist	Median
Palmaris longus (PL)	Med. epicondyle	Palmar aponeurosis	Flex wrist	Median
Flexor carpi ulnaris (FCU)	Med. epicondyle and post. ulna	Pisiform	Flex wrist	**Ulnar**
Flexor digitorum superficialis (FDS)	Med. epicondyle and ant. radius	Base of middle phalanges	Flex PIP	Median
Deep Flexors				
Flexor digitorum profundus (FDP)	Ant. and med. ulna	Base of distal phalanges	Flex DIP	**Median-ant. interosseous/and ulnar**
Flexor pollicis longus (FPL)	Ant. and lat. radius	Base of distal phalanges	Flex IP, thumb	Median-ant. interosseous
Pronator quadratus (PQ)	Distal ulna	Volar radius	Pronate hand	Median-ant. interosseous
Superficial Extensors				
Brachioradialis (BR)	Lat. supracondylar humerus	Lat. distal radius	Flex forearm	Radial
Ext. carpi radialis longus (ECRL)	Lat. supracondylar humerus	2nd Metacarpal base	Extend wrist	Radial
Ext. carpi radialis brevis (ECRB)	Lat. epicondyle of humerus	3rd Metacarpal base	Extend wrist	Radial
Anconeus	Lat. epicondyle of humerus	Proximal dorsal ulna	Extend forearm	Radial
Extensor digitorum (ED)	Lat. epicondyle of humerus	Extensor aponeurosis	Extend digits	Radial-post. interosseous
Extensor digiti minimi	Common extensor tendon	Small finger extensor carpi ulnaris	Extend small finger	Radial-post. interosseous
Ext. carpi ulnaris (ECU)	Lat. epicondyle of humerus	5th Metacarpal base	Extend/adduct hand	Radial-post. interosseous
Deep Extensors				
Supinator	Lat. epicondyle of humerus, ulna	Dorsolateral radius	Supinate forearm	Radial-post. interosseous
Abductor pollicis longus (APL)	Dorsal ulna/radius	1st Metacarpal base	Abduct thumb, extend	Radial-post. interosseous
Extensor pollicis brevis (EPB)	Dorsal radius	Thumb proximal phalanx base	Extend thumb MCP	Radial-post. interosseous
Extensor pollicis longus (EPL)	Dorsolateral ulna	Thumb dorsal phalanx base	Extend thumb IP	Radial-post. interosseous
Extensor indicis proprius (EIP)	Dorsolateral ulna	Index finger extensor apparatus (ulnarly)	Extend index finger	Radial-post. interosseous

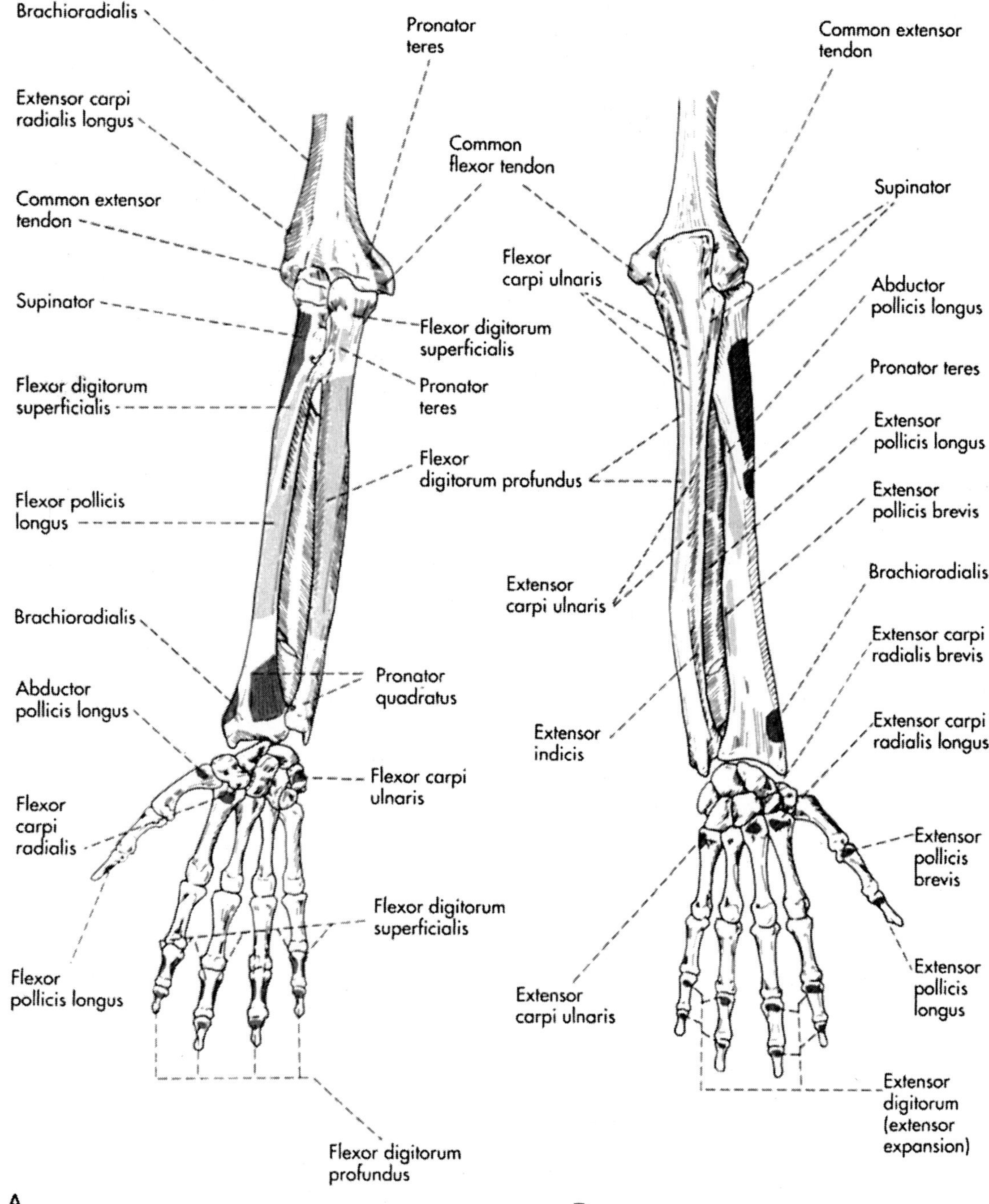

Figure 11–18. Origins and insertions of muscles of the forearm. (From Jenkins, D.B.: Hollinshead's Functional Anatomy of the Limbs and Back, 6th ed., Fig. 8–4. Philadelphia, W.B. Saunders, 1991.)

branch from the medial cord of the brachial plexus), and the posterior antebrachial cutaneous nerve (a branch of the radial nerve given off in the arm).

E. Vessels (see Fig. 11–19)—At the elbow the brachial artery enters the cubital fossa (bordered by the two epicondyles, the brachioradialis, and the pronator teres and overlying the brachialis and supinator). It then divides at the level of the radial neck into the radial and ulnar arteries.

1. Radial Artery—Runs initially on the pronator teres, deep to the brachioradialis, and continues to the wrist between this muscle and the flexor carpi radialis (FCR). Forearm branches include the radial recurrent (see earlier) and muscular branches.
2. Ulnar Artery—The larger of the two branches, it is covered by the superficial flexors proximally (between the FDS and FDP). Distally, the artery lies on the FDP, between the tendons of the FCU and FDS.

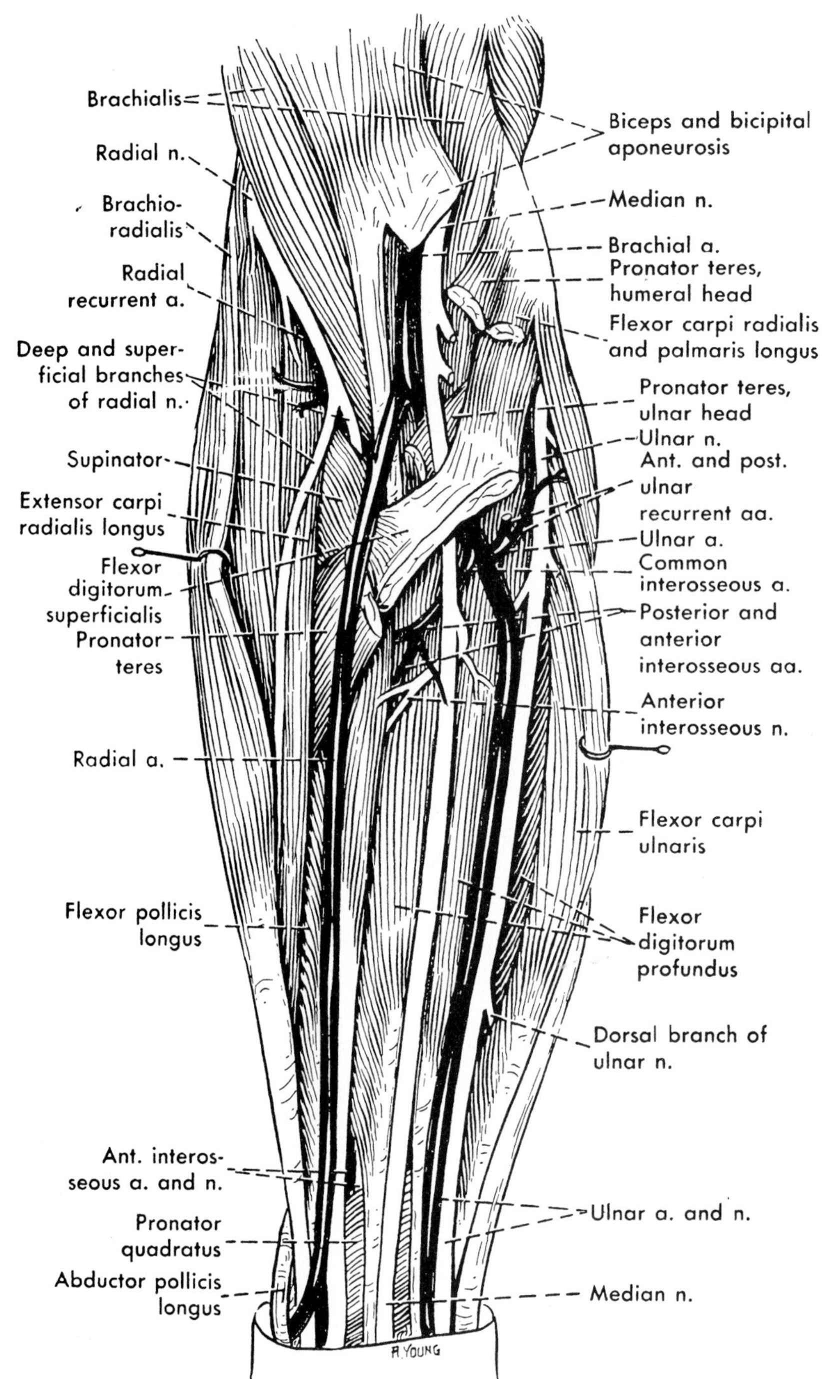

Figure 11–19. Arteries (*black*) and nerves (*white*) of the forearm. (From Jenkins, D.B.: Hollinshead's Functional Anatomy of the Limbs and Back, 6th ed., p. 131. Philadelphia, W.B. Saunders, 1991.)

Forearm branches include the anterior and posterior ulnar recurrent (discussed earlier), the common interosseous (with anterior and posterior branches), and several muscular and nutrient arteries.

F. Surgical Approaches to the Forearm

1. Anterior Approach (Henry's) (Fig. 11–20)—Utilizes the interval between the brachioradialis (radial n.) and the pronator teres (or FCR distally) (median n.). Proximally it is necessary to isolate and ligate the **leash of Henry** (radial artery branches) and subperiosteally to strip the supinator from its insertion. It is essential to protect the superficial branch of the radial nerve (retract laterally) and the brachioradialis. Distally, it is necessary to dissect off the FPL and pronator quadratus. Supination of the forearm displaces the PIN ulnarly.
2. Dorsal (Posterior) Approach (Thompson) (Fig. 11–21)—Utilizes the interval between the extensor carpi radialis brevis (radial n.)

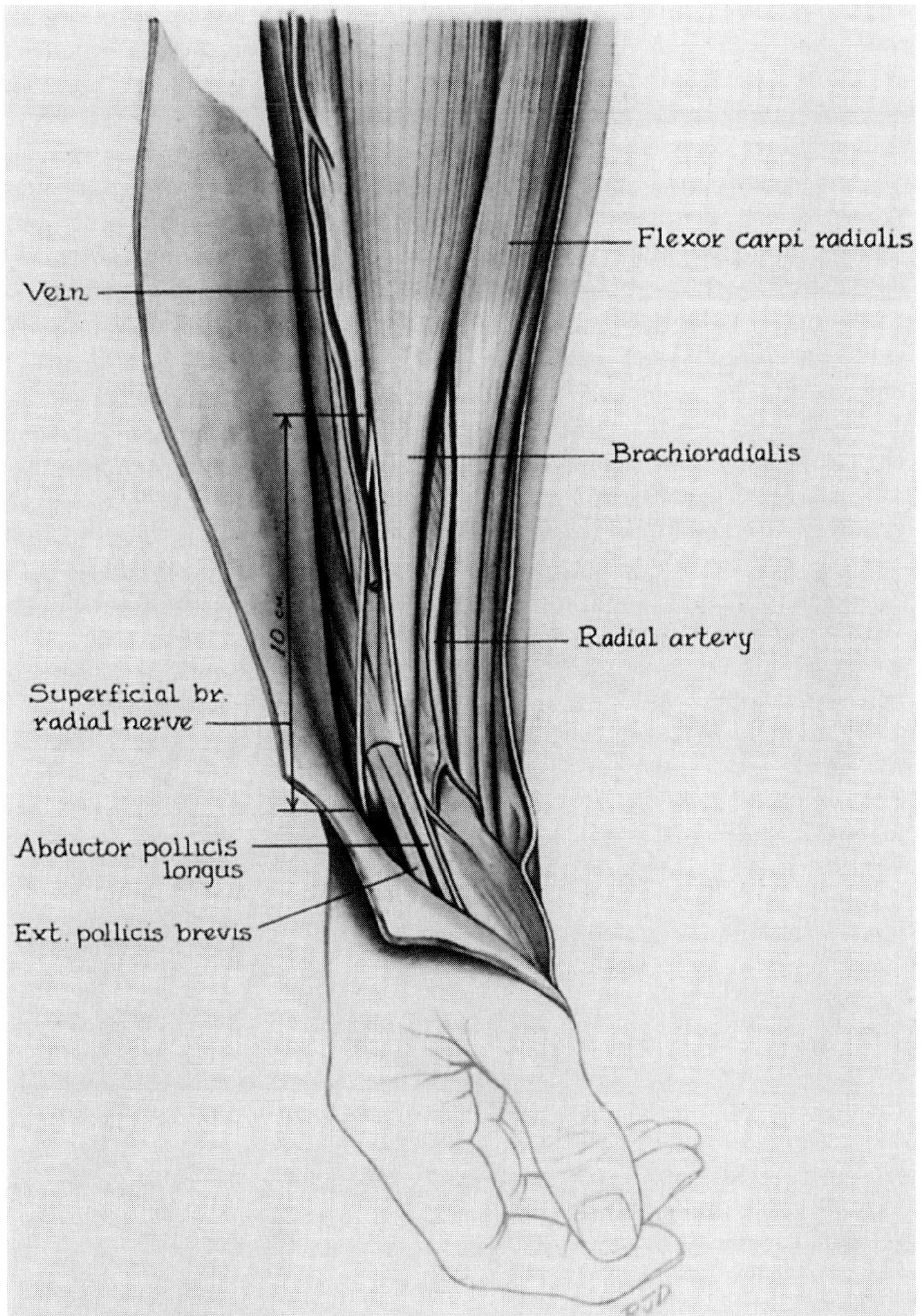

Figure 11–20. Anterior (Henry) approach to the forearm. (From Kaplan, E.B.: Surgical Approaches to the Neck, Cervical Spine, and Upper Extremity, p. 92. Philadelphia, W.B. Saunders, 1966.)

and extensor digitorum communis (EDC) (or extensor pollicis longus distally) (PIN). The PIN must be identified and protected when using this surgical approach. **Excessive retraction of the supinator can injure the posterior interosseous nerve.**

3. Exposure of the Ulna—Via the interval between the extensor carpi ulnaris (PIN) and the FCU (ulnar n.).
4. Cross-sectional diagrams of middle and distal forearm are available (Figs. 11–22, 11–23).

V. Wrist and Hand

A. Osteology

1. Carpal Bones—Each carpal bone has six surfaces, with proximal, distal, medial, and lateral surfaces for articulation and palmar and dorsal surfaces for ligamentous insertion. Ossification begins at the capitate (usually present at 1 year of age) and proceeds in a counterclockwise direction. Therefore the hamate is the second carpus to ossify (1–2 years), followed by the triquetrum (3 years), lunate (4–5 years),

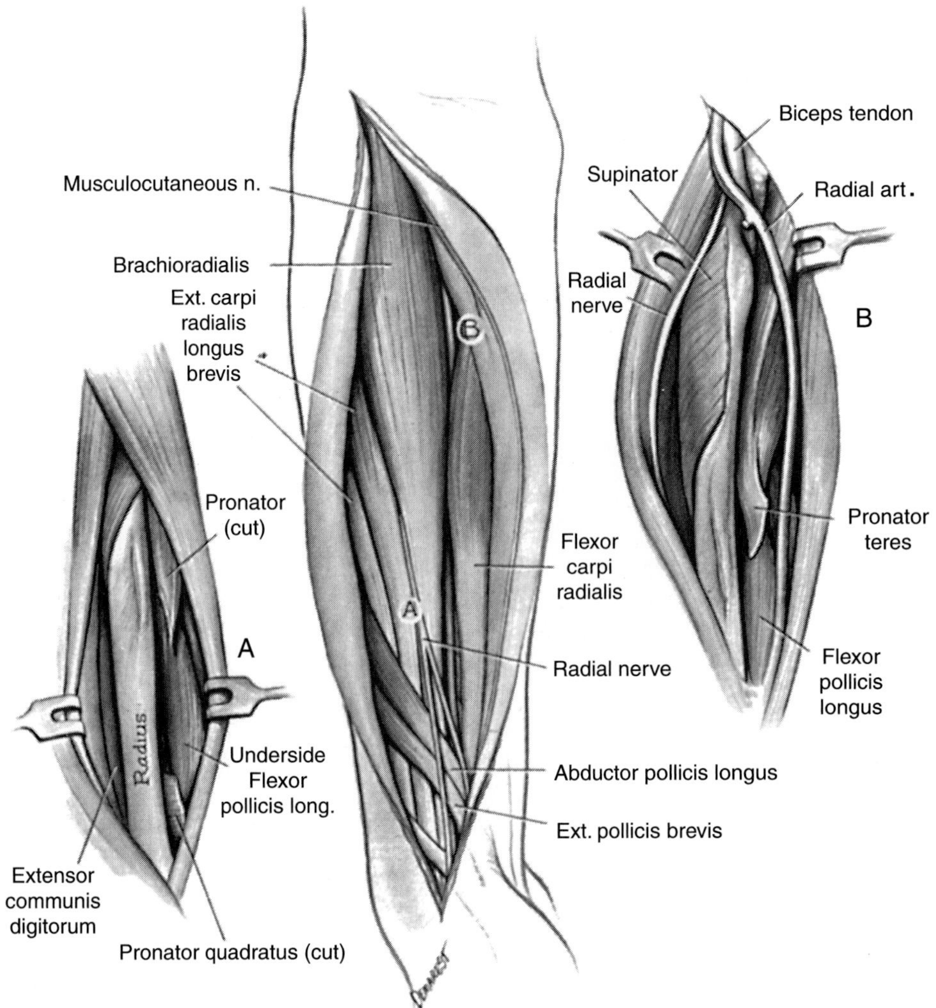

Figure 11–21. Dorsal (Thompson) approach to the forearm. (From Kaplan, E.B.: Surgical Approaches to the Neck, Cervical Spine, and Upper Extremity, p. 90. Philadelphia, W.B. Saunders, 1966.)

scaphoid (5 years), trapezium (6 years), and trapezoid (7 years). The pisiform, which is a large sesamoid bone, is the last to ossify (9 years). Several key features are important to recognize in the individual carpal bones.

Bone	Important Features	No. of Articulations
Scaphoid	Tubercle (TCL, APB), distal vascular supply	5
Lunate	Lunar shape	5
Triquetrum	Pyramid shape	3
Pisiform	Spheroidal (TCL, FCR)	1
Trapezium	FCR groove, tubercle (opponens, APB, FPB, TCL)	4
Trapezoid	Wedge shape	4
Capitate	Largest bone, central location	7
Hamate	Hook (TCL)	5

TCL, transverse carpal ligament.

2. Metacarpals—Have two ossification centers: one for the body (primary center of ossification), which ossifies at 8 weeks of fetal life (like most long bones), and one at the neck, which usually appears before age 3. The first metacarpal is a primordial phalanx and has its secondary ossification center located at the base (like the phalanges). Several characteristics allow identification of the individual metacarpals.

Metacarpal	Distinctive Features
I (thumb)	Short, stout, base is saddle-shaped
II (index)	Longest, largest base, medial at base
III (middle)	Styloid process
IV (ring)	Small quadrilateral base, narrow shaft
V (small)	Tubercle at base (ECU)

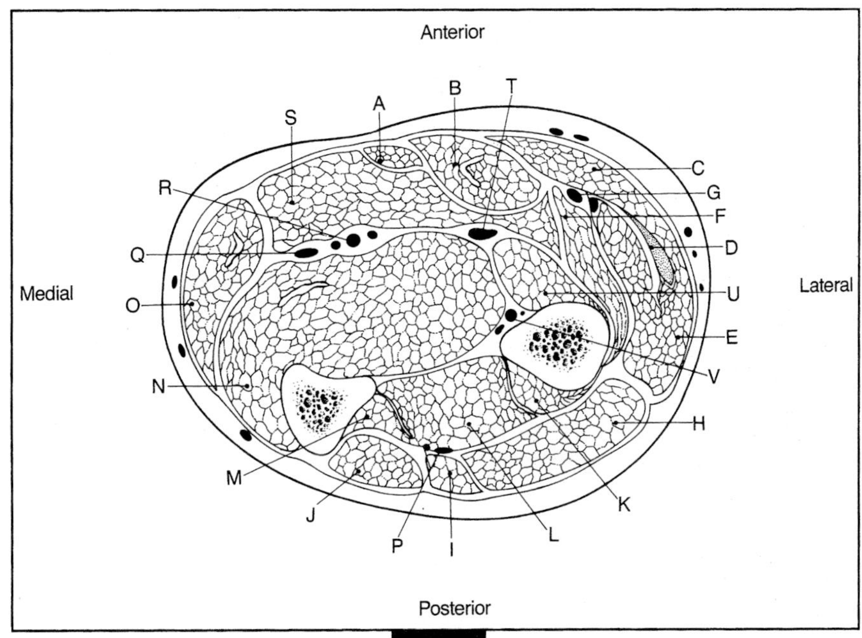

Figure 11–22. Cross-section of the mid-forearm. (From Callaghan JJ., ed.: Anatomy Self-Assessment Examination, Fig. 39. Park Ridge, IL, American Academy of Orthopaedic Surgeons, 1991.)

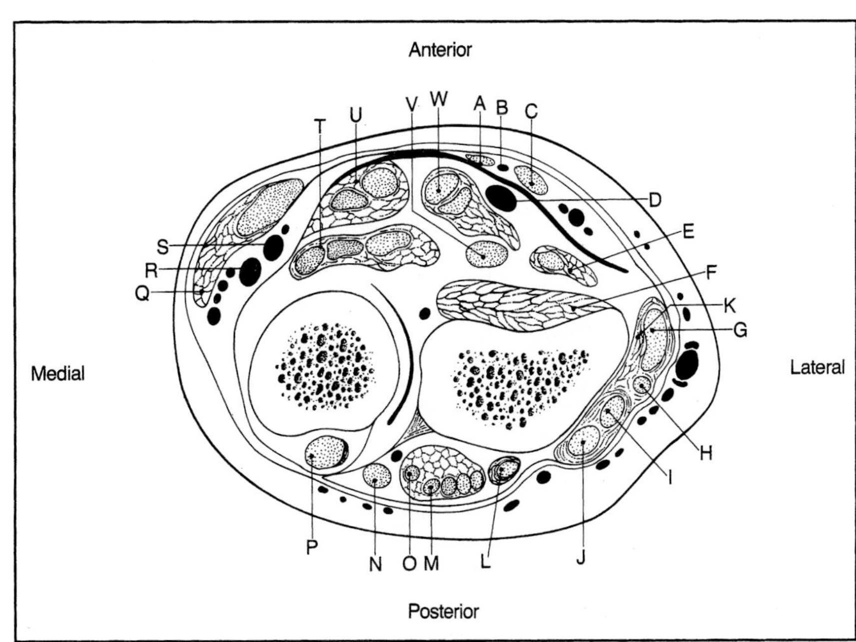

Figure 11–23. Cross-section of the distal forearm proximal to the distal radioulnar joint. (From Callaghan, JJ., ed.: Anatomy Self-Assessment Examination, Fig. 38. Park Ridge, IL, American Society of Orthopaedic Surgeons, 1991.)

3. Phalanges—The 14 phalanges (three for each finger and two for the thumb) are similar. They all have secondary ossification centers at their bases that appear at ages 3 (proximal), 4 (middle), and 5 (distal). The bases of the proximal phalanges are oval and concave, with smaller heads ending in two condyles. The middle phalanges have two concave facets at their bases and pulley-shaped heads. The distal phalanges are smaller and have palmar ungual tuberosities distally.

B. Arthrology

1. Radiocarpal (Wrist) Joint—Ellipsoid joint made up of the distal radius, scaphoid, lunate, triquetrum, and the following ligamentous structures.

Structure	Attachments	Distinctive Features
Articular capsule	Surrounds joint	Reinforced by volar and dorsal RCL
Volar radiocarpal ligament (RCL)	Radius, ulna, scaphoid, lunate, triquetrum, capitate	Oblique ulnar, strong
Dorsal radiocarpal ligament	Radius, scaphoid, lunate, triquetrum	Oblique radial, weak

Structure	Attachments	Distinctive Features
Ulnar collateral ligament	Ulna, triquetrum, pisiform, TCL	Fan-shaped, two fascicles
Radial collateral ligament	Radius, scaphoid, trapezium, TCL	Radial artery adjacent

TCL, transverse carpal ligament.

The palmar radiocarpal ligament is the strongest supporting structure, although it has a weak area on the radial side (the space of Poirier) that lends less support to the scaphoid, lunate, and trapezoid. It may be related to wrist instability with injury.

2. Intercarpal Joints
   a. Proximal Row—Scaphoid, lunate, and triquetral are gliding joints. Two dorsal intercarpal ligaments connect the scaphoid and lunate and the lunate and triquetral bones. Two palmar intercarpal ligaments connect the scaphoid and lunate and the lunate and triquetral bones. The dorsal intercarpal ligaments are stronger. Interosseous ligaments are narrow bundles connecting the lunate and scaphoid and the lunate and triquetral bones (Fig. 11–24).
   b. Pisiform Articulation—The pisotriquetral joint has a thin articular capsule. The pisiform is also connected proximally by the ulnar collateral and palmar radiocarpal ligaments. The pisohamate ligament and pisometacarpal ligaments help extend the pull of the FCU.
   c. Distal Row—Trapezium, trapezoid, capitate, and hamate gliding joints. The dorsal intercarpal ligaments connect the trapezium with the trapezoid, the trapezoid with the capitate, and the capitate with the hamate. The palmar ligaments do the same. The interosseous ligaments are much thicker in the distal row, connecting the capitate and hamate (strongest), the capitate and trapezoid, and the trapezium and trapezoid (weakest).
   d. Midcarpal Joint—Transverse articula-

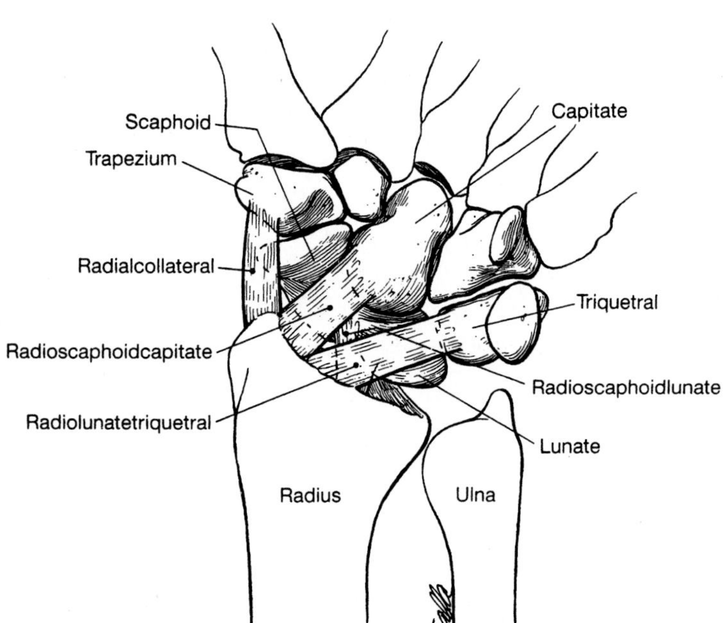

Figure 11–24. Extrinsic radiocarpal ligaments. (From Mooney, J.F., Siegel, D.B., and Koman, L.A.: Ligamentous injuries of the wrists in athletes. Clin. Sports Med., 11:129–139, 1992.)

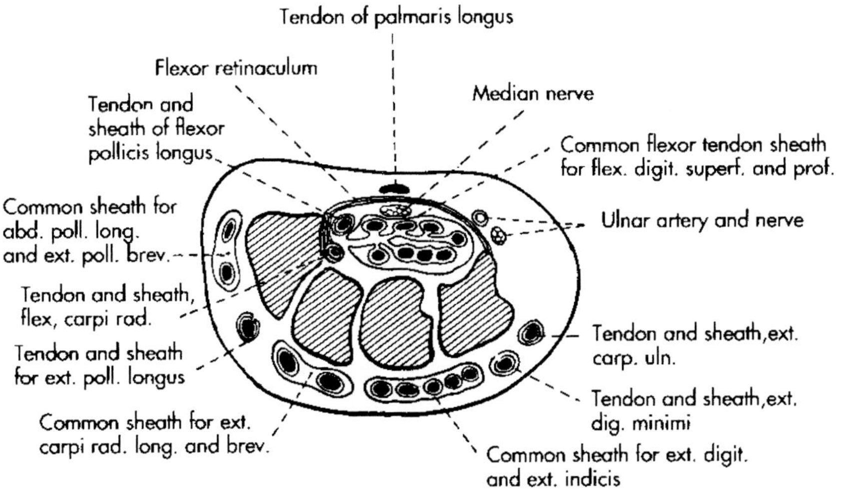

Figure 11–25. Components of the carpal tunnel. (From Jenkins, D.B.: Hollinshead's Functional Anatomy of the Limbs and Back, 6th ed., p. 162. Philadelphia, W.B. Saunders, 1991.)

tions between the proximal and distal rows are reinforced by palmar and dorsal intercarpal ligaments and carpal collateral ligaments (radial is stronger).

3. Carpometacarpal (CMC) Joints
   a. Thumb CMC Joint—A highly mobile saddle joint. It is supported by a capsule and radial, palmar, and dorsal CMC ligaments.
   b. Finger CMC Joints—Gliding joints with capsules, dorsal CMC ligaments (strongest), palmar CMC ligaments, and interosseous CMC ligaments.
4. Metacarpophalangeal Joints—Ellipsoid joints covered by palmar (volar plate), collateral, and deep transverse metacarpal ligaments.
5. Interphalangeal Joints—Hinge joints with capsules and obliquely oriented collateral ligaments.
6. Other Important Structures
   a. Extensor Retinaculum—Covers the dorsum of the wrist and contains six synovial sheaths (Figs. 11–25, 11–26).

Compartment	Contents	Pathologic Condition Involving Tendons
1	APL, EPB	de Quervain's tenosynovitis
2	ECRL, ECRB	Tennis elbow/extensor tendonitis
3	EPL	Rupture at Lister's tubercle (after wrist fractures)
4	EDC, EIP	Extensor tenosynovitis
5	EDM	Rupture (rheumatoid)
6	ECU	Snapping at ulnar styloid

Lister's tubercle separates the second and third compartments.

   b. Transverse Carpal Ligament ([TCL]; Flexor Retinaculum)—Forms the roof of the carpal tunnel (see Fig. 11–25), which contains the long flexor tendons and the median nerve. FDS tendons of the long and ring finger are volar to the tendons of the index and small fingers in the tunnel. The retinaculum is attached medially to the pisiform and the hook of the hamate and laterally to the tuberosity of the scaphoid and the ridge of the trapezium. It also forms the floor of Guyon's canal, which is bordered as well by the hook of the hamate and the pisiform and is covered by the volar carpal ligament. Entrapment of the ulnar nerve in this canal is possible (Fig. 11–27).
   c. Triangular Fibrocartilage Complex—Formed by the triangular fibrocartilage, ulnocarpal ligaments (volar ulnolunate and ulnotriquetral ligaments), and a meniscal homologue. Injuries to this structure are a common cause of ulnar wrist pain (see Fig. 11–17).
   d. Intrinsic Apparatus—Complex arrangement of structures that surround the digits (Fig. 11–28). The following structures are important.

Structure	Attachments	Significance
Sagittal bands	Covers MCP	Allows MCP extension
Transverse (sagittal) fibers	Volar plate	Allows MCP flexion (interossea)
Lateral bands	Covers PIP	Allows PIP extension (lumbricals)
Oblique retinacular ligament (Landsmeer's ligament)	A4 pulley, terminal tendon	Allows DIP extension (passive)

   e. Flexor Sheath (Fig. 11–29)—Covers the flexor tendons in the finger, protecting

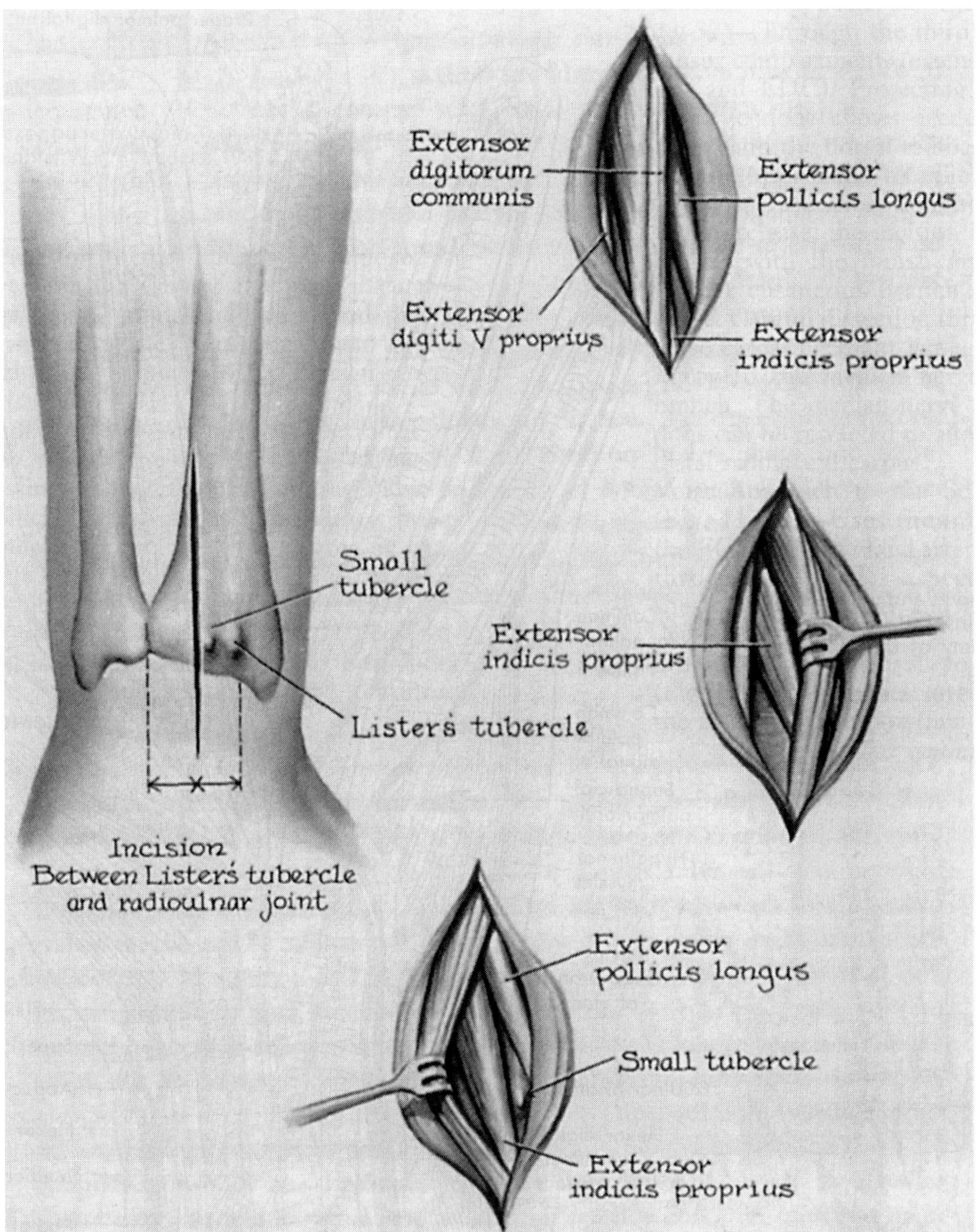

Figure 11–32. Dorsal wrist approach. (From Kaplan, E.B.: Surgical Approaches to the Neck, Cervical Spine, and Upper Extremity, p. 112. Philadelphia, W.B. Saunders, 1966.)

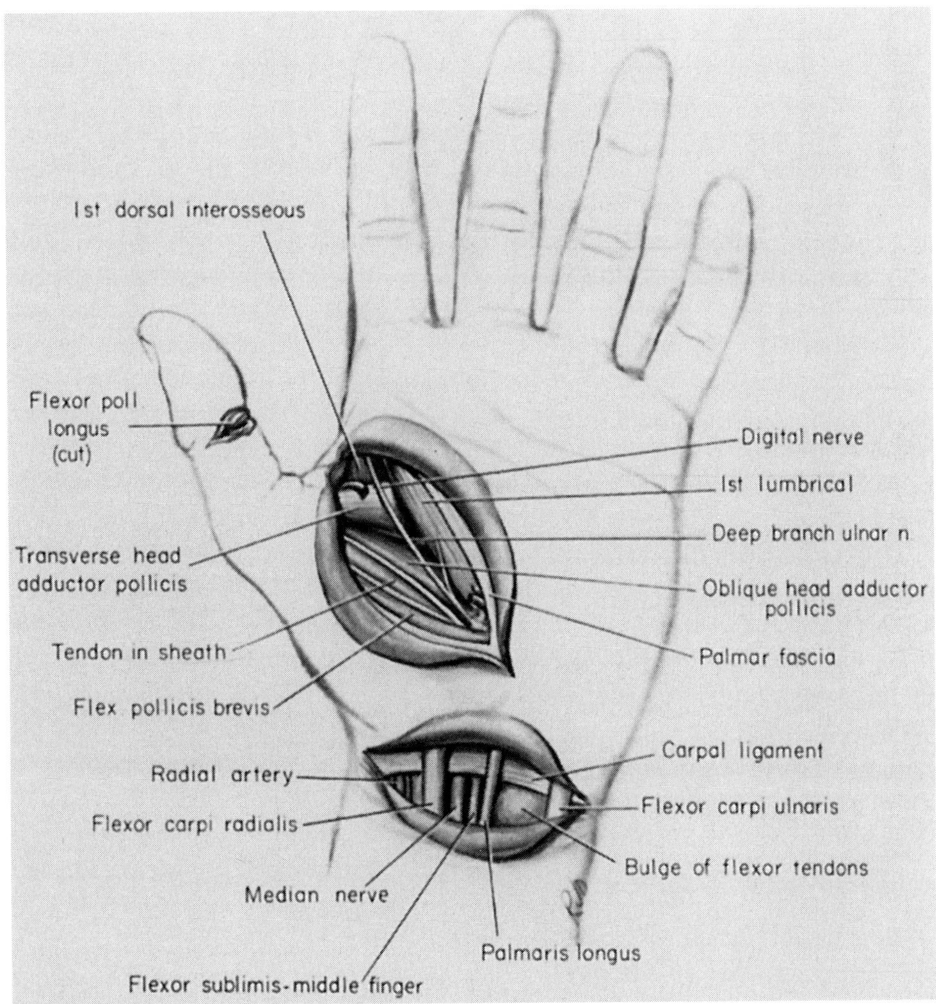

Figure 11–33. Approach to the carpal tunnel and thenar muscles. (From Kaplan, E.B.: Surgical Approaches to the Neck, Cervical Spine, and Upper Extremity, p. 97. Philadelphia, W.B. Saunders, 1966.)

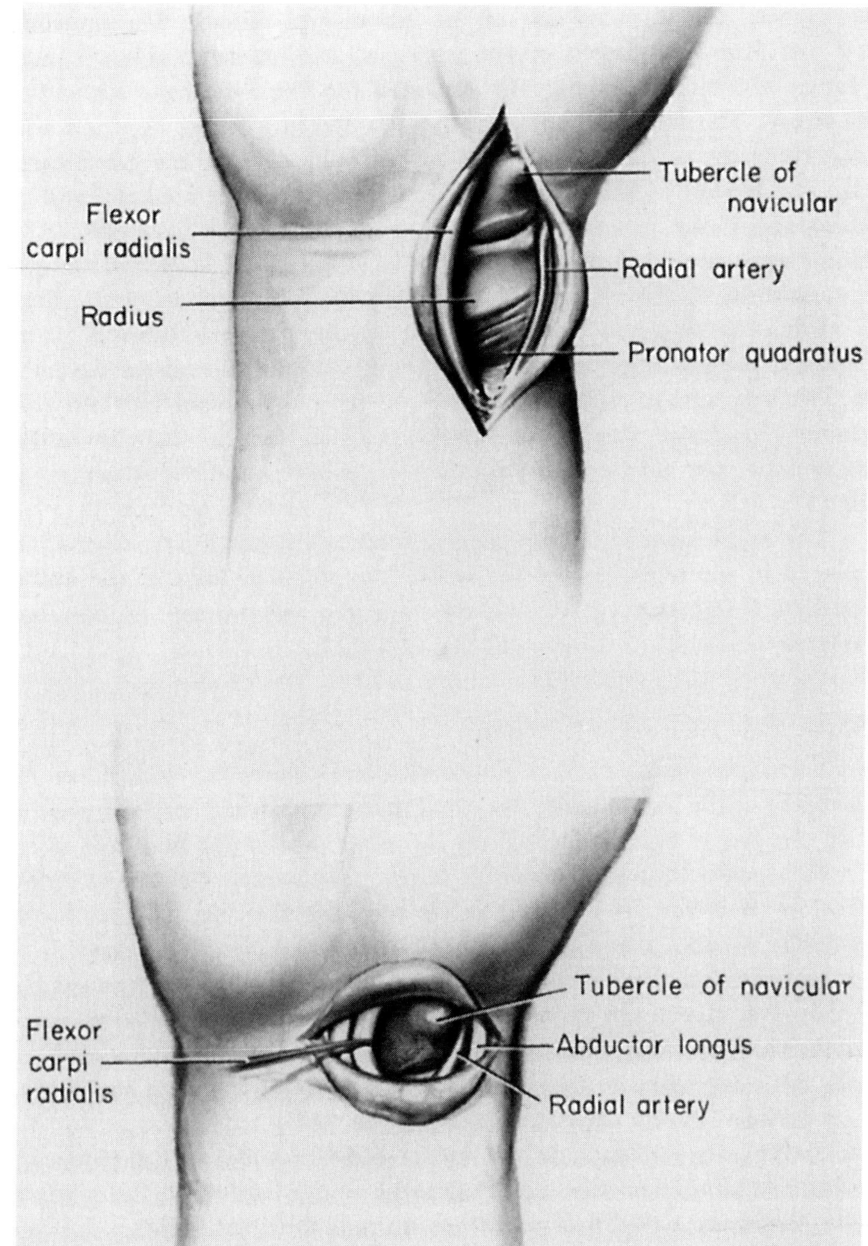

Figure 11–34. Russé's approach to the scaphoid. (From Kaplan, E.B.: Surgical Approaches to the Neck, Cervical Spine, and Upper Extremity, p. 101. Philadelphia, W.B. Saunders, 1966.)

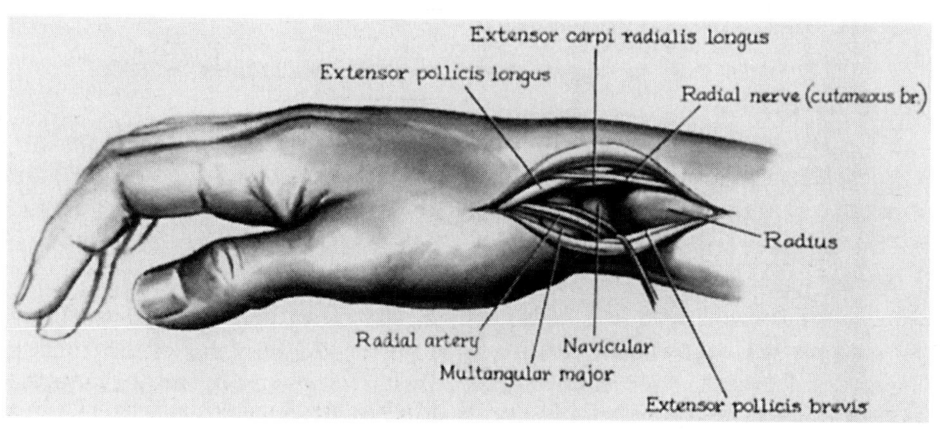

Figure 11–35. Dorsal approaches to the scaphoid. (From Kaplan, E.B.: Surgical Approaches to the Neck, Cervical Spine, and Upper Extremity, p. 107. Philadelphia, W.B. Saunders, 1966.)

sal wrist compartment), protecting the superficial radial nerve and radial artery (deep).

5. Volar Approach to the Flexor Tendons (Bunnell's)—Zigzag incisions across the flexor creases help to expose the flexor sheaths. The digital sheaths should be avoided.
6. Midlateral Approach to the Digits—Good for stabilization of fractures and neurovascular exposure, this approach uses a laterally placed incision at the dorsal extent of the interphalangeal (IP) creases. Exposure of the digital neurovascular bundle is carried out volar to the incision.

G. Arthroscopy—Portals used for wrist arthroscopy are based on the dorsal compartments. The 1-2 portal (risks the radial artery), 6-R and 6-U portals (radial and ulnar to the sixth compartment—risks the ulnar nerve and artery) are the most dangerous. The commonly used 3-4 and 4-5 portals are safer.

VI. Spine

A. Osteology

1. Introduction—The spine contains 33 vertebrae. There are 7 cervical, 12 thoracic, 5 lumbar, 5 sacral, and 4 coccygeal vertebrae. The total length of the spine averages about 71 cm. Normal curves include cervical lordosis, thoracic kyphosis, and lumbosacral lordosis. The vertebral bodies generally increase in width craniocaudally with the exception of T1–T3. Important topographic landmarks include the mandible (C2–C3), **hyoid cartilage (C3)**, thyroid cartilage (C4/C5), **cricoid cartilage (C6)**, vertebra prominens (C7), spine of scapula (T3), tip of scapula (T7), and iliac crest (L4–L5).
2. Cervical Spine—Unique features include foramina in each transverse process. The spinous processes are bifid, and the vertebral foramina are triangular. The atlas (C1) is unique in that it contains no vertebral body and no spinous process. It does contain two lateral masses. The axis (C2) has a vertical projection called the dens, or odontoid process, that articulates with the atlas. It also possesses superior and inferior facets. The seventh cervical vertebra is unique because it has a prominent nonbifid posterior spinous process and no anterior tubercle.
3. Thoracic Spine—Unique features include costal facets (present on all 12 vertebral bodies and the transverse processes of T1–T9) and a rounded vertebral foramen. The first thoracic vertebra contains a large, prominent spinous process.
4. Lumbar Spine—These vertebrae are the largest. They contain short laminae and pedicles and massive vertebral bodies. They also have mammillary processes that project posteriorly from the superior articular facet. The transverse processes are thin and long (with the exception of the fifth lumbar vertebra).
5. Sacrum—Fusion of five spinal elements. The promontory is the anterosuperior portion that projects into the pelvis. There are usually four pairs of pelvic sacral foramina located both anteriorly and posteriorly that transmit respective branches of the upper four sacral nerves. There is also a sacral canal, which opens caudally into the sacral hiatus.
6. Coccyx—Fusion of the lowest four spinal elements; it attaches dorsally to the gluteus maximus, the external anal sphincter, and the coccygeal muscles.
7. Ossification—There are three primary ossification centers for each vertebra: two ossification centers in the centrum and one cartilaginous center for each arch. The arches unite dorsally at the third month of fetal life. Five secondary ossification centers (two transverse processes, one spinous process, and two body end plates) do not appear until after puberty. Ossification of the atlas, axis, sacral, and coccygeal vertebrae are unique. The axis (C2) ossifies from five primary and two secondary centers. Of note, the dens is formed from two primary growth centers that originate from the "centrum," or body of the atlas (C1). Mammillary processes arise from additional ossification centers in the lumbar vertebrae. The arches fuse with the centrum during the seventh year of life in the following order: thoracic, cervical, lumbar, and finally sacral. Failure of arch formation results in spina bifida.

B. Arthrology

1. Ligaments

a. General Arrangement—The vertebral bodies are bound together by the strong anterior longitudinal ligament (ALL) and the weaker posterior longitudinal ligament (**PLL**). The ALL is usually thickest at the center of the vertebral body and thins at the periphery. Separate fibers extend from one to five levels. The PLL extends from the occiput to the posterior sacrum. It is separated from the center of the vertebral body by a space that allows passage of the dorsal branches of the spinal artery. The PLL is hourglass-shaped, with the wider (yet thinner) sections located over the discs. Ruptured discs tend to occur lateral to these expansions. Ligamentous capsules overlying the zygapophyseal joints and the intertransverse ligaments contribute little to interspinous stability. The **liga-**

mentum flavum is a strong, yellow, elastic ligament connecting the laminae. It runs from the anterior surface of the superior lamina to the posterior surface of the inferior lamina and is constantly in tension. Hypertrophy of the ligamentum flavum is said to contribute to nerve root compression. The **supraspinous** and **interspinous** ligaments lie dorsal to and between the spinous processes, respectively. The supraspinous ligament begins at C7 and is in continuity with the ligamentum nuchae (which runs from C7 to the occiput). Their relative contribution to interspinous stability is unknown.

b. Specialized Ligaments
   1. Atlanto-occipital Joint—Consists of two articular capsules (anterior and posterior) and the **tectoral membrane** (a cephalad extension of the PLL). It is further stabilized by the ligamentous attachments to the dens.
   2. Atlantoaxial Joint—The **transverse ligament** is the major stabilizer of the median atlantoaxial joint. This articulation is further stabilized by the apical ligament (longitudinal), which together with the transverse ligament composes the **cruciate** ligament. Additionally, a pair of **alar, or "check," ligaments** run obliquely from the tip of the dens to the occiput (Fig. 11–36).
   3. Iliolumbar Ligament—This stout ligament connects the transverse process of L5 with the ilium. Tension on this ligament in patients with unstable vertical shear pelvic fractures can lead to avulsion fractures of the transverse process.

2. Facet (Apophyseal) Joints—The orientation of the facets of the spine dictates the plane of motion at each relative level. The facet orientation varies with spinal level. In the sagittal plane, the orientation is 45 degrees in the cervical spine, 60 degrees in the thoracic spine, and 90 degrees in the lumbar spine. In the coronal plane, the orientation is 0 degrees (neutral) in the cervical spine, 20 degrees posterior in the thoracic spine, and 45 degrees anterior in the lumbar spine. **In the cervical spine the superior articular facet is anterior and inferior to the inferior articular process of the vertebra above**. Nerve roots exit near the superior articulating process. In the lumbar spine the superior articular facet is anterior and lateral to the inferior articular facet.
3. Discs—The intervertebral discs are fibrocartilaginous, with an obliquely oriented

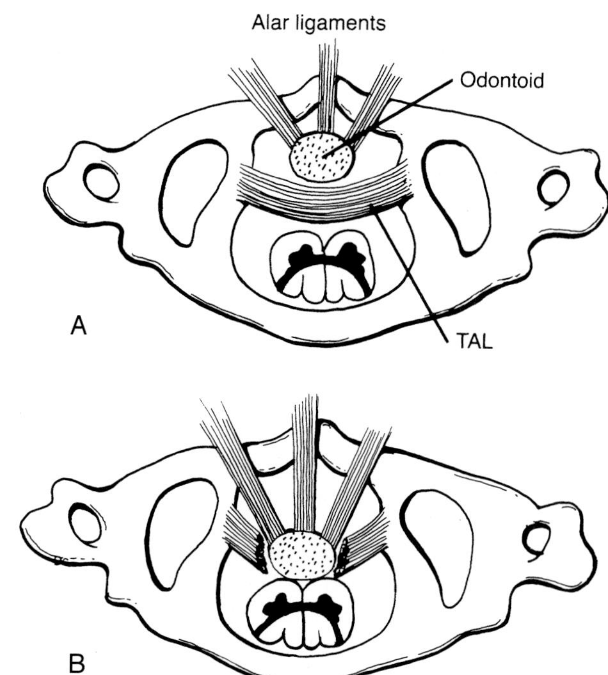

Figure 11–36. The atlanto-axial complex as seen from above *(A)*. The disruption of the transverse ligament (TAL) with intact alar ligaments results in C1–C2 instability without cord compression *(B)*. (From DeLee, J.C., and Drez, D., Jr.: Orthopaedic Sports Medicine, Principles and Practices, vol. 1, p. 432. Philadelphia, W.B. Saunders, 1994; *B* redrawn from Hensinger, R.N.: Congenital anomalies of the atlantoaxial joint. The Cervical Spine Research Society Editorial Committee. The Cervical Spine, 2nd ed., p. 242. Philadelphia, J.B. Lippincott, 1989.)

annulus fibrosus composed of **type I collagen** and a softer central **nucleus pulposus** made of **type II collagen.** The discs account for 25% of the total spinal columnar height. They are attached to the vertebral bodies by hyaline cartilage, which is responsible for the vertical growth of the column. The distinction between the nucleus and annulus becomes less apparent as one ages.

C. Spinal Musculature
   1. Neck—The neck is divided, for functional purposes, into the anterior and posterior regions.
      a. Anterior—The anterior neck muscles include the superficial platysma muscle (CN VII innervated), stylohyoid and digastric muscles (CN XII) above the hyoid, and "strap" muscles below the hyoid. Important strap muscles include the sternohyoid and omohyoid in the superficial layer and the thyrohyoid and sternothyroid in the deep layer; all are innervated by the ansa cervicalis. Laterally, the sternocleidomastoid (CN XI and ansa) runs obliquely across the neck and inserts into the ipsilateral side; it rotates the head to the contralateral side. Three triangles are formed by

these muscles. The anterior triangle (borders: sternocleidomastoid, midline of the neck, and the lower border of the mandible) is the largest area. Three smaller triangles include the submandibular, carotid (bordered by the posterior aspect of the digastric and the omohyoid, and used for the anterior approach to C5), and posterior (bordered by the trapezius, sternocleidomastoid, and clavicle).

b. Posterior—The posterior neck muscles form the borders of the **suboccipital triangle.** This triangle is formed by the superior and inferior heads of the obliquus capitis muscle and the rectus capitis posterior major muscle. The vertebral artery and the first cervical nerve are within this triangle, and the greater occipital nerve (C2) is superficial.

2. Back—The back is blanketed by the trapezius (superiorly) and the latissimus dorsi (inferiorly). The rhomboids and levator scapulae are deep to this layer. Refer to Table 11–4 for specifics on these muscles. The deep muscles of the back are arranged into two groups: erector spinae and transversospinalis group. The erector spinae run from the transverse and spinous processes of the inferior vertebrae to the spinous processes of the superior vertebrae. They stabilize and extend the back. All of the deep back musculature is innervated by dorsal primary rami of spinal nerves.

D. Nerves

1. Spinal Cord—The cord extends from the brain stem to L1, where it terminates as the conus medullaris. It is enclosed within the bony spinal canal with variable amounts of space (greatest in the upper cervical spine). The cord also varies in diameter (widest at the origin of plexi). In cross-section, the cord has both geographic and functional boundaries (Fig. 11–37). It is divided in the midline anteriorly by a fissure and posteriorly by the sulcus. The posterior funiculi (**dorsal columns**) are located dorsally and receive ascending fibers, which deliver deep touch, proprioception, and vibratory sensation. The **lateral spinothalamic tract** transmits pain and temperature (it is the site for chordotomy for intractable pain). Descending in the **lateral corticospinal tract** are fibers that transmit instructions for voluntary muscle contraction. The ventral spinothalamic tract transmits light touch sensation, and the **ventral corticospinal tract** delivers cortical messages of voluntary contraction. Pathways to the hand and upper extremity are usually localized centrally within this area (hence the clinical findings of anterior cord syndrome). The **spinal cord tapers at L1 (conus medullaris)**, and a small filum terminale continues with surrounding nerve roots contained within a common dural sac (cauda equina) to its termination in the coccyx.

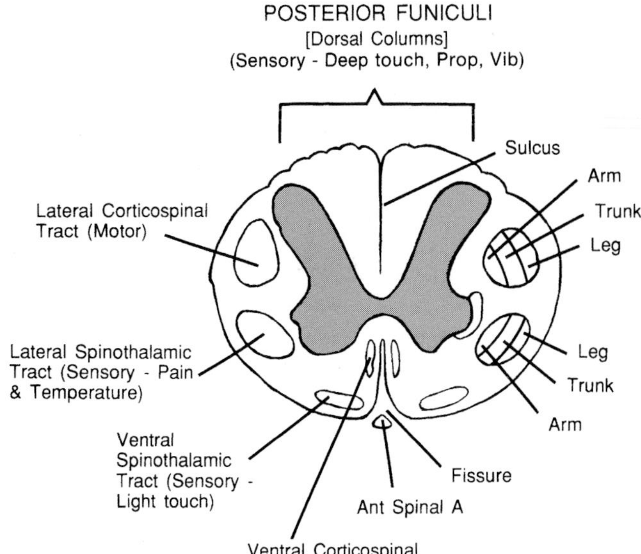

Figure 11–37. Cross-section of the spinal cord.

2. Nerve Roots (Fig. 11–38)—Within the subarachnoid space the dorsal root (and ganglia) and ventral roots converge to form the spinal nerve. The nerve becomes "extradural" as it approaches the intervertebral foramen (dura becomes epineurium) at all levels above L1. Below this level, the nerves are contained within the cauda equina. In the **cervical spine the numbered nerve exists at a level *above* the pedicle of corresponding vertebral level (e.g., C2 exists at C1–C2)**. In the lumbar spine the nerve root transverses the respective disc space above the named vertebral body and exits the respective foramen under the pedicle (Fig. 11–39). Herniated discs usually impinge on the traversing nerve root and the facet joint. After exiting the foramen the spinal nerve delivers dorsal primary rami, which supply the muscles and skin of the neck and back regions. The ventral rami supply the anteromedial trunk and the limbs. With exception of the thoracic nerves, ventral rami are grouped in plexuses before delivering sensorimotor functions to a general region.

3. Sympathetic Chain—The cervical sympathetic chain is a deep structure closely associated with the longus capitis and colli muscles, **posterior to the carotid sheath**. The chain is anterior to the longus capitis muscle and the transverse processes of the vertebrae. The sympathetic chain has three

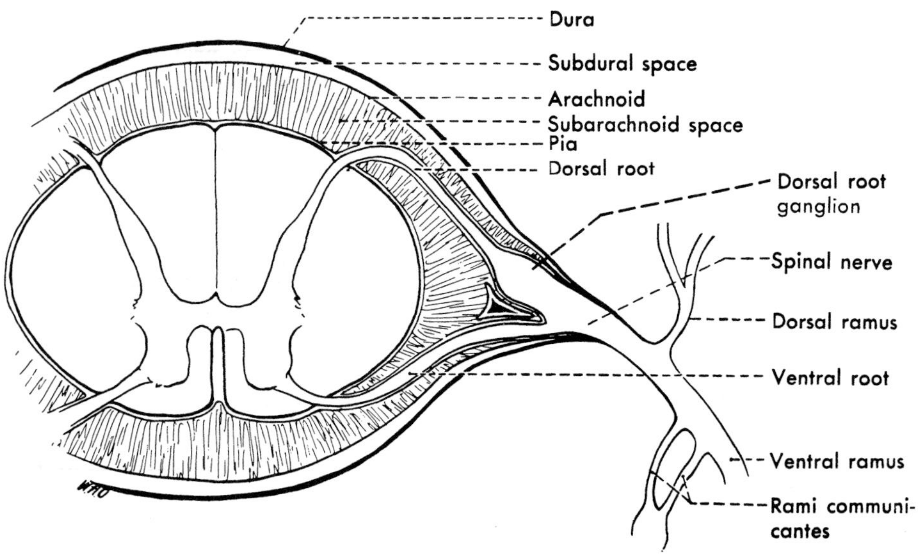

Figure 11–38. Spinal nerves. (From Jenkins, D.B.: Hollinshead's Functional Anatomy of the Limbs and Back, 6th ed., p. 205. Philadelphia, W.B. Saunders, 1991.)

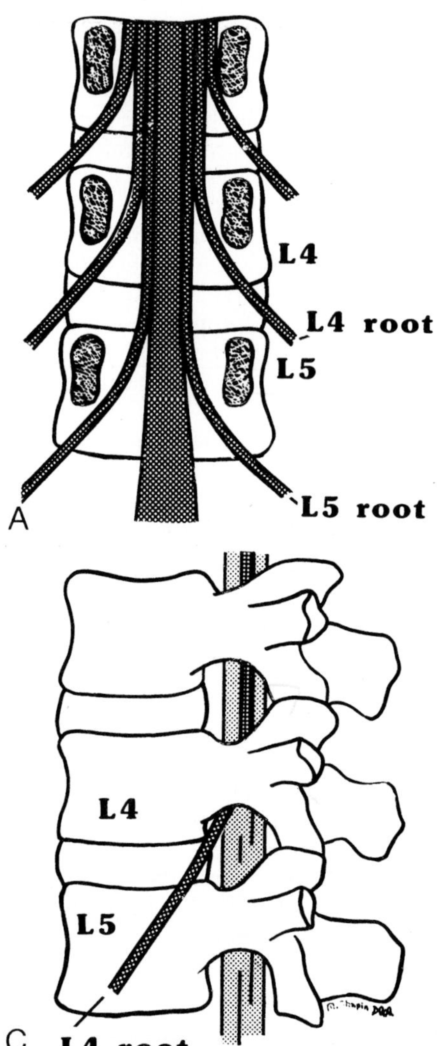

Figure 11–39. Nerve root locations in relation to vertebral landmarks. (From Weissman, B.N., and Sledge, C.B.: Orthopedic Radiology, p. 283. Philadelphia, W.B. Saunders, 1986.)

ganglia: superior, middle, and inferior. **Disruption of the inferior ganglia can lead to Horner's syndrome.**

Ganglia	Location	Other
Superior	C2–C3	Largest
Middle	C6	Variable
Inferior	C7–T1	"Stellate"

E. Vascular Supply to the Spine—Spinal blood supply is usually derived from the segmental arteries via the **aorta (which lies on the left side of the vertebral column with the inferior vena cava and azygos vein on the right).** The primary supply to the dura and posterior elements is from the dorsal branches. The ventral branches supply the vertebral bodies via ascending and descending branches, which are delivered underneath the PLL in four separate ostia. **The vertebral artery** (a branch of the subclavian) ascends through the transverse foramina of C1–C6 (anterior to and not through C7), **posterior to the longus colli muscle,** then posterior to the lateral masses, along the cephalad surface of the posterior arch of C1 (atlas), passes ventromedially around the spinal cord and through the foramen magnum before uniting at the midline basilar artery. The artery of **Adamkiewicz** (great anterior medullary artery) enters through the left intervertebral foramen in the lower thoracic spine. It should be preserved during dissections at this level. Arterial supply to the spinal cord is from anterior and posterior spinal arteries and segmental branches of the vertebral artery and dorsal arteries, which travel via the dorsal and ventral rootlets to the respective dorsal and anterolateral portions of the cord. The venous drainage of the vertebral bodies is primarily via the central sinusoid located on the dorsum of each vertebral body.

F. Surgical Approaches to the Spine

1. Anterior Approach to the Cervical Spine (Fig. 11–40)—A transverse incision is based on the desired level (e.g., for C5 one should enter the carotid triangle). The platysma is retracted with the skin. The pretracheal fascia is exposed to explore the interval between the **carotid sheath (contains the internal and common carotid arteries, the internal jugular vein, and the vagus nerve [CN X])** and the trachea. The prevertebral fascia is sharply incised and the longus colli muscle gently retracted (protecting the recurrent laryngeal nerve [a branch of the vagus nerve that lies outside the sheath]) to expose the vertebral body. The right recurrent laryngeal nerve can lie outside the carotid sheath and must be identified. By dissecting the longus muscles subperiosteally, one also protects the stellate ganglion (avoiding Horner's syndrome). Occasionally it is necessary to split the fibers of the omohyoid.
2. Posterior Approach to the Cervical Spine—After a midline approach through the ligamentum nuchae, the superficial layer (trapezius) and intermediate layer (splenius, semispinalis, longissimus capitis) are reflected laterally, and the vertebrae are exposed. The vertebral artery is especially vulnerable as it leaves the foramen transversarium and travels above and medially to pierce the atlanto-occipital membrane at its lateral angle. The greater occipital nerve (C2) and the third occipital nerve C3) should also be protected in the suboccipital region. Access to the spinal canal is via laminectomy or facetectomy (Fig. 11–41).
3. Anterior Approach to the Thoracic Spine—A transverse incision is made approximately two ribs above the level of interest. Dissection over the top of the rib is

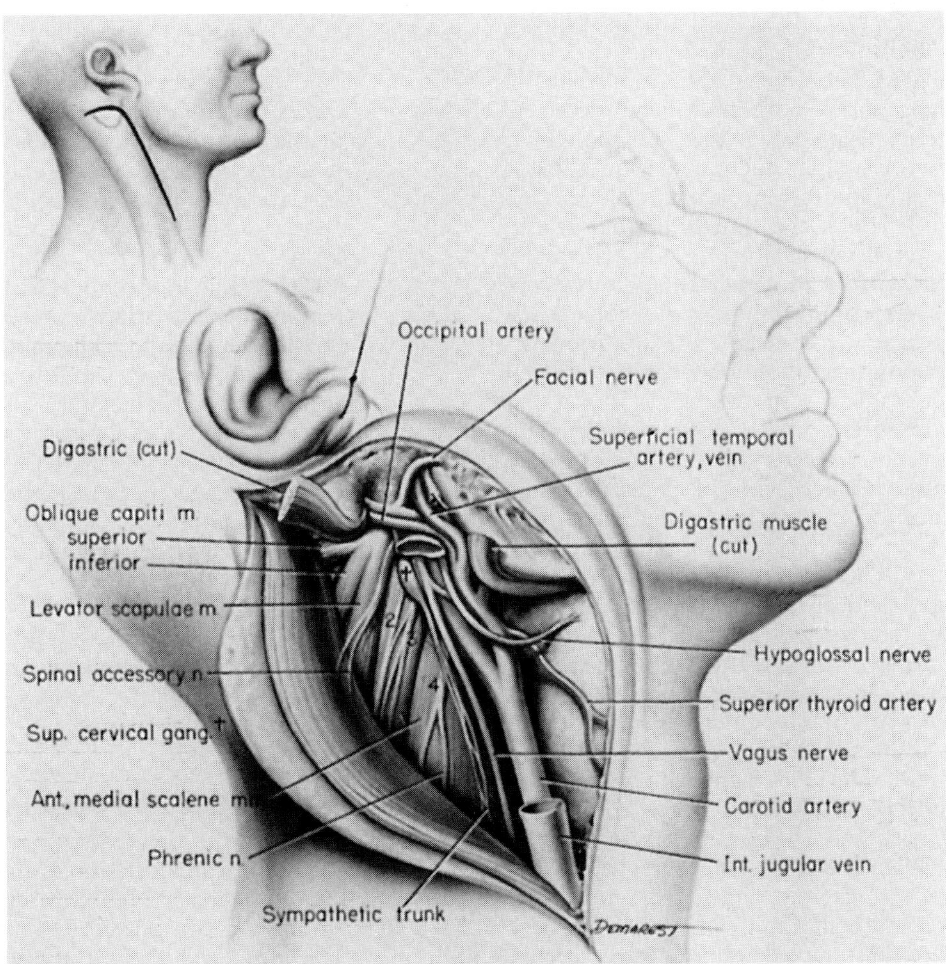

Figure 11–40. Approach to the anterior neck. (From Kaplan, E.B.: Surgical Approaches to the Neck, Cervical Spine, and Upper Extremity, p. 23. Philadelphia, W.B. Saunders, 1966.)

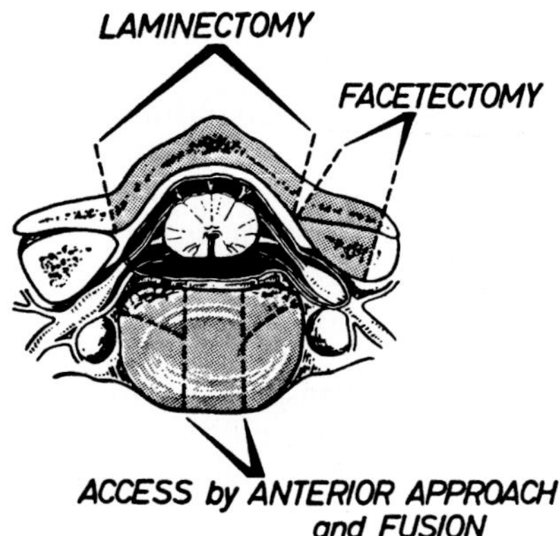

Figure 11–41. Approach to the cervical spine. (From Rothman, R.H., and Simeon, F.A.: The Spine, 2nd ed., p. 484. Philadelphia, W.B. Saunders, 1982.)

carried out to avoid injuring the intercostal neurovascular bundle (which lies on the inferior internal surface of the rib). The rib is further dissected and removed from the field. **The right-sided approach is favored to avoid the aorta, segmental arteries, artery of Adamkiewicz (T9–T11), and thoracic duct (in the upper thoracic spine on the left side of the esophagus and behind the carotid sheath).** The esophagus, aorta, vena cava, and pleura of the lungs should be identified and protected.

4. Posterior Approach to the Thoracolumbar Spine—A straight midline incision is made over the spinous processes and carried down through the thoracolumbar fascia. Paraspinal musculature is subperiosteally dissected from the attached spinous processes, exposing the posterior elements. Structures at risk include the posterior primary rami (near facet joints) and segmental vessels (anterior to the plane connecting the transverse processes). Partial laminectomy allows greater exposure of the cord and discs. Pedicle screw placement is at the junction of the lateral border of the superior facet and the middle of the transverse process. These screws should be angled 15 degrees medially and in line with the slope of the vertebra as seen on lateral radiographs.
5. Anterior Approach to the Thoracolumbar Spine—An oblique incision is centered over the tenth rib, which is exposed and removed. The diaphragm is incised near its periphery, and dissection is carried into the retroperitoneum. The peritoneum is swept away from the psoas and vertebral bodies. Segmental arteries (which cross anteriorly at the mid-body level) are ligated. Risks of this approach include injuries to the ureter, internal iliac vessels, and **lumbar plexus nerves (including the superior hypogastric; injury to this plexus can cause sexual dysfunction and retrograde ejaculation).**

VII. Pelvis and Hip

A. Osteology—The pelvic girdle is composed of two innominate (coxal) bones that articulate with the sacrum. Each innominate bone, in turn, is composed of three united bones: the ilium, ischium, and pubis. Distinctive parts of each innominate bone include the acetabulum (vinegar cup) and the obturator foramen. The acetabulum is anteverted and obliquely oriented. The posterosuperior articular surface is thickened to accommodate weight-bearing. The inferior surface is deficient and contains the acetabular, or cotyloid, notch. This notch is bound by the transverse acetabular ligament. The greater sciatic notch is located posterior and superior to the acetabulum, between the posteroinferior iliac spine and the ischial spine. The anterior superior iliac spine is prominent and palpable at the lateral edge of the inguinal ligament. It is the origin for the sartorius muscle and the transverse and internal abdominal muscles. The posterior superior iliac spine is usually located 4–5 cm lateral to the S2 spinous process. It may be marked topographically by a dimple and is an excellent source for bone graft. The anterior inferior iliac spine is less prominent and provides the origin of the direct head of the rectus femoris. The arcuate line delineates a thick column of bone that extends from the auricular process of the ilium to the pectineal line and represents the weight-bearing column. The outer surface of the iliac wing contains the anterior, posterior, and inferior gluteal lines, which form borders for the origins of the gluteal muscles. The iliopectineal eminence is a raised region anteriorly that represents the union of the ilium and pubis. The iliopsoas muscle traverses a groove between this eminence and the anteroinferior iliac spine. Ossification centers of the pelvis are as follows.

Center	Type	Age at Appearance	Age at Fusion
Ilium	Primary	2 months	15 years
Ischium	Primary	4 months	15 years
Pubis	Primary	6 months	15 years
Acetabulum	Secondary	12 years	15 years
Iliac crest	Secondary	16 years	25 years
Ant. inf. iliac spine	Secondary	16 years	25 years
Ischial tuberosity	Secondary	16 years	25 years
Pubis	Secondary	16 years	30 years

The proximal femur is composed of the femoral head (articulates with the acetabulum), neck, and greater and lesser trochanters. The inner architecture of the proximal femur includes an intricate arrangement of primary and secondary trabeculae (Fig. 11–42).

B. Arthrology

1. Hip—The hip joint is a spheroidal, or ball-

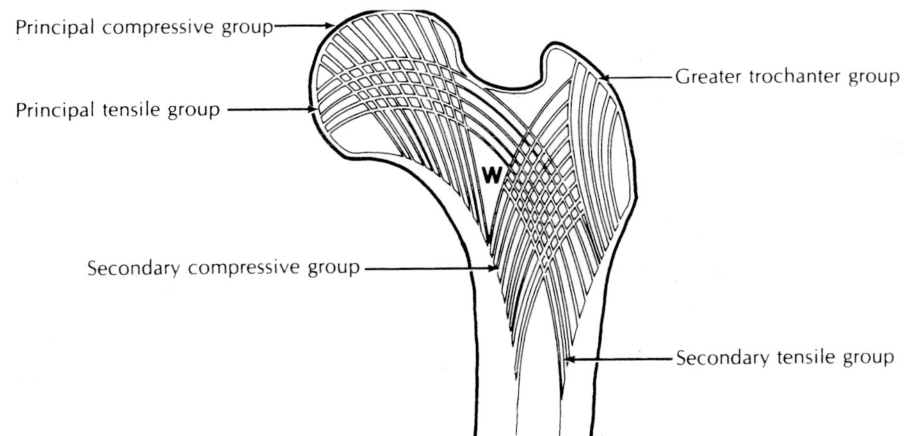

Figure 11–42. Hip trabeculae. (From DeLee, J.C.: Fractures and dislocations of the hip. In Rockwood, C.A., Jr., Green, D.P., and Buchholz, R.W., eds.: Fractures in Adults, 3rd ed., p. 1488. Philadelphia, J.B. Lippincott, 1991.)

and-socket, type of diarthrodial joint. Its stability is based primarily on the bony architecture, which also allows good motion. The acetabulum is deepened by the fibrocartilaginous rim, called the labrum. The joint capsule extends anteriorly across the femoral neck to the trochanteric crest; however, posteriorly it extends only partially across the femoral neck (Fig. 11–43). The fibrous capsule that encloses the joint contains circular fibers that can be recognized better posteriorly as the zona orbicularis. A series of three ligaments compose the capsule anteriorly. The *iliofemoral*, or Y, ligament of Bigelow is the strongest ligament in the body and attaches the anterior inferior iliac spine to the intertrochanteric line in an inverted Y fashion. The remaining anterior ligaments, the *ischiofemoral* and *pubofemoral* ligaments, are weaker but lend additional stability. Inside the joint, the ligament of teres arises from the apex of the cotyloid notch and attaches to the fovea of the femoral head. It transmits an arterial branch of the posterior division of the **obturator artery** to the femoral head (less significant in adults).

2. Sacroiliac (SI) Joint—A true diarthrodial gliding joint supported by three groups of ligaments: posterior SI ligaments, anterior SI ligaments, and interosseous ligaments. Of these structures, the posterior ligaments, which have been compared to the trusses of a suspension bridge (Tile), provide the most stability and strength to the joint.
3. Symphysis Pubis—Connects the two hemipelvii anteriorly and is united with a fibrocartilaginous disc and supported by the superior pubic ligament and the arcuate pubic ligament.
4. Other ligaments include the sacrospinous and sacrotuberous ligaments, which outline the boundaries for the greater and lesser sciatic foramina. The **sacrospinous ligament** (anterior sacrum ischial spine) is the inferior border of the **greater** sciatic foramen and the superior border of the **lesser** sciatic foramen. The lesser sciatic foramen is bordered inferiorly by the **sacrotuberous ligament** (anterior sacrum ischial tuberosity). The piriformis, sciatic nerve, and other important structures exit the greater sciatic foramen. The short external rotators of the hip exit the lesser sciatic foramen.

C. Muscles of the Pelvis and Hip (Table 11–8; Fig. 11–44)

Pubofemoral ligament
Ant. inf. iliac spine
Iliofemoral ligament
Ischiofemoral ligament
Greater trochanter
Lesser trochanter
A
B

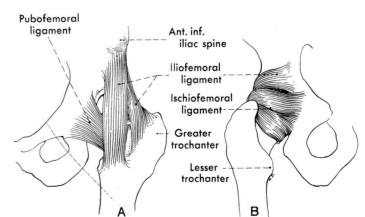

Figure 11–43. Hip capsule. *A,* Anterior view. *B,* Posterior view. (From Jenkins, D.B.: Hollinshead's Functional Anatomy of the Limbs and Back, 6th ed., p. 230. Philadelphia, W.B. Saunders, 1991.)

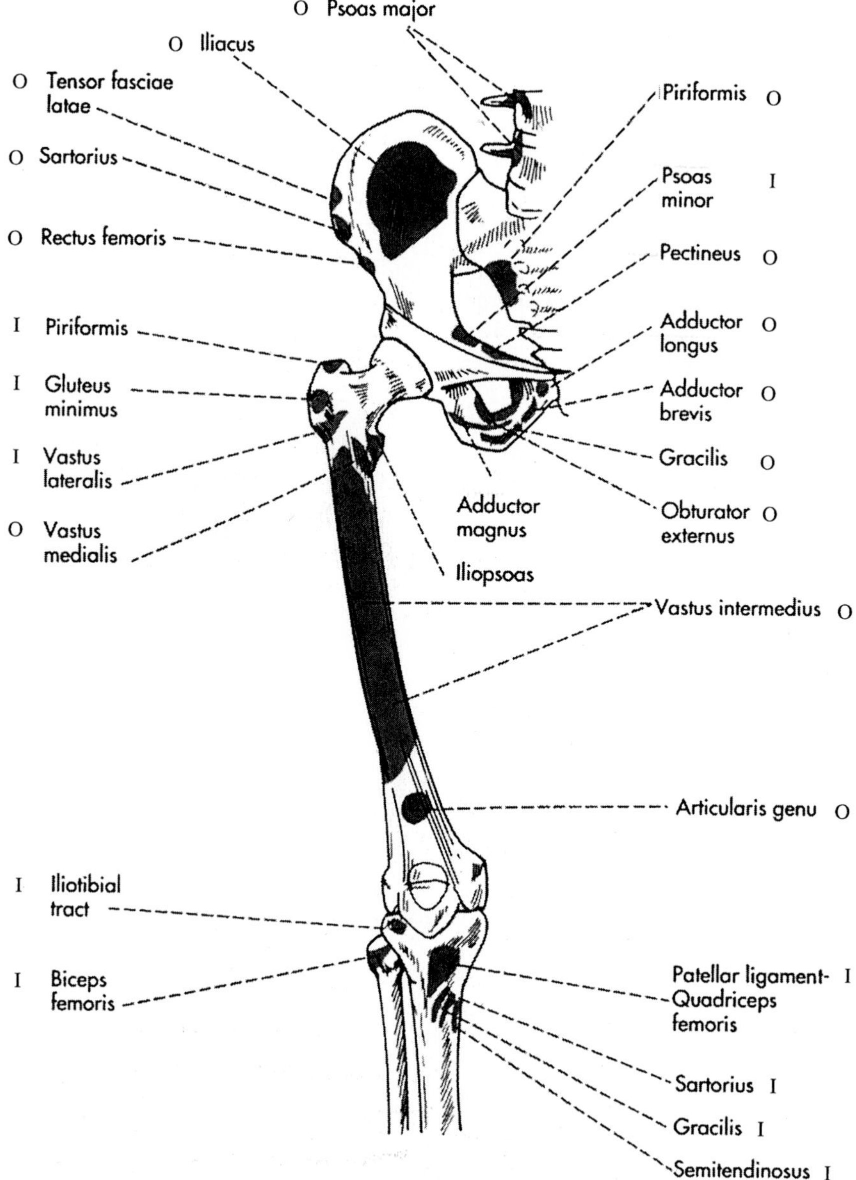
O Psoas major
O Iliacus
O Tensor fasciae latae
O Sartorius
O Rectus femoris
I Piriformis
I Gluteus minimus
I Vastus lateralis
O Vastus medialis
Piriformis O
Psoas minor I
Pectineus O
Adductor longus O
Adductor brevis O
Gracilis O
Obturator externus O
Adductor magnus
Iliopsoas
Vastus intermedius O
Articularis genu O
I Iliotibial tract
I Biceps femoris
Patellar ligament-Quadriceps femoris I
Sartorius I
Gracilis I
Semitendinosus I

Figure 11–44 *See legend on opposite page*

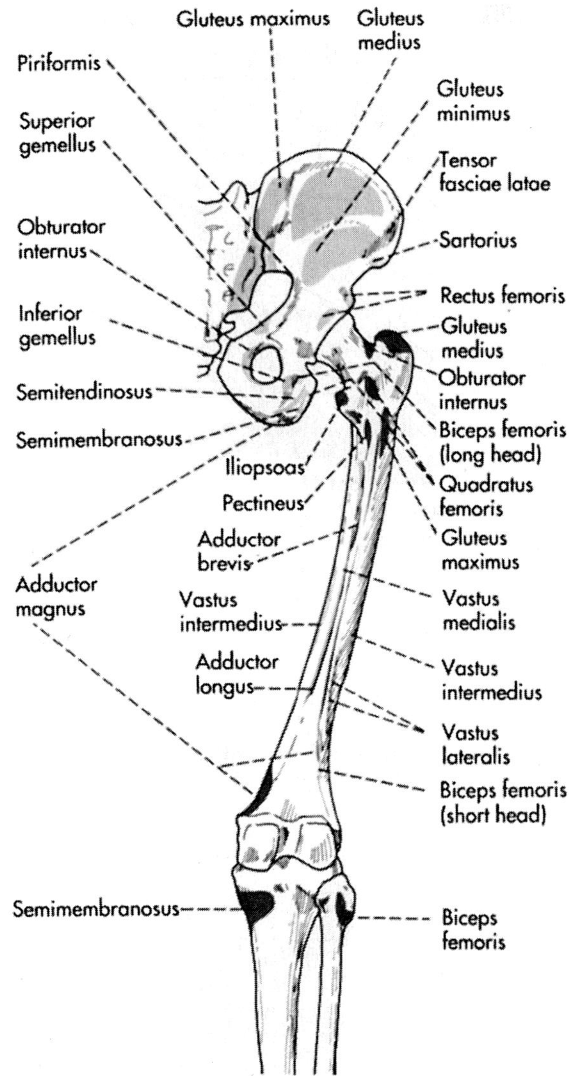

Figure 11–44. Origins and insertions of muscles of the hip and leg. O, origin; I, insertion. Origins = light areas; insertions = dark areas. (Adapted from Jenkins, D.B.: Hollinshead's Functional Anatomy of the Limbs and Back, 6th ed., Figs. 16–7, 17–3. Philadelphia, W.B. Saunders, 1991.)

Table 11–8.

Muscles of the Pelvis and Hip

Muscle	Origin	Insertion	Nerve	Segment
Flexors				
Iliacus	Iliac fossa	Lesser trochanter	Femoral	L234 (P)
Psoas	Transverse processes of L1–L5	Lesser trochanter	Femoral	L234 (P)
Pectineus	Pectineal line of pubis	Pectineal line of femur	Femoral	L234 (P)
Rectus femoris	AIIS, acetabular rim	Patella → tibial tubercle	Femoral	L234 (P)
Sartorius	ASIS	Proximal medial tibia	Femoral	L234 (P)
Adductors				
Post. adductor magnus	Inferior pubic ramus/ischial tuberosity	Linea aspera/adductor tubercle	Obturator (P) and Sciatic (tibial)	L234 (A)
Adductor brevis	Inferior pubic ramus	Linea aspera/pectineal line	Obturator (P)	L234 (A)
Adductor longus	Anterior pubic ramus	Linea aspera	Obturator (A)	L234 (A)
Gracilis	Inf. symphysis/pubic arch	Proximal medial tibia	Obturator (A)	L234 (A)
External Rotators				
Gluteus maximus	Ilium post to post gluteal line	Iliotibial band/gluteal sling (femur)	Inf. gluteal	L5–S2 (P)
Piriformis	Ant. sacrum/sciatic notch	Proximal greater trochanter	Piriformis	S12 (P)
Obturator externus	Ischiopubic rami/obturator membrane	Trochlear fossa	Obturator	L234 (A)
Obturator internus	Ischiopubic rami/obturator membrane	Medial greater trochanter (MGT)	Obturator internus	L5–S2 (A)
Superior gemellus	Outer ischial spine	MGT	Obturator internus	L5–S2 (A)
Inferior gemellus	Ischial tuberosity	MGT	Quadratus femoris	L4–S1 (A)
Quadratus femoris	Ischial tuberosity	Quadrate line of femur	Quadratus femoris	L4–S1 (A)
Abductors				
Gluteus medius	Ilium between post. and ant. gluteal lines	Greater trochanter	Superior gluteal	L4–S1 (P)
Gluteus minimus	Ilium between ant. and inf. gluteal lines	Ant. border of greater trochanter	Superior gluteal	L4–S1 (P)
Tensor fasciae latae (TFL) [tensor fascia femoris (TFF)]	Anterior iliac crest	Iliotibial band	Superior gluteal	L4–S1 (P)

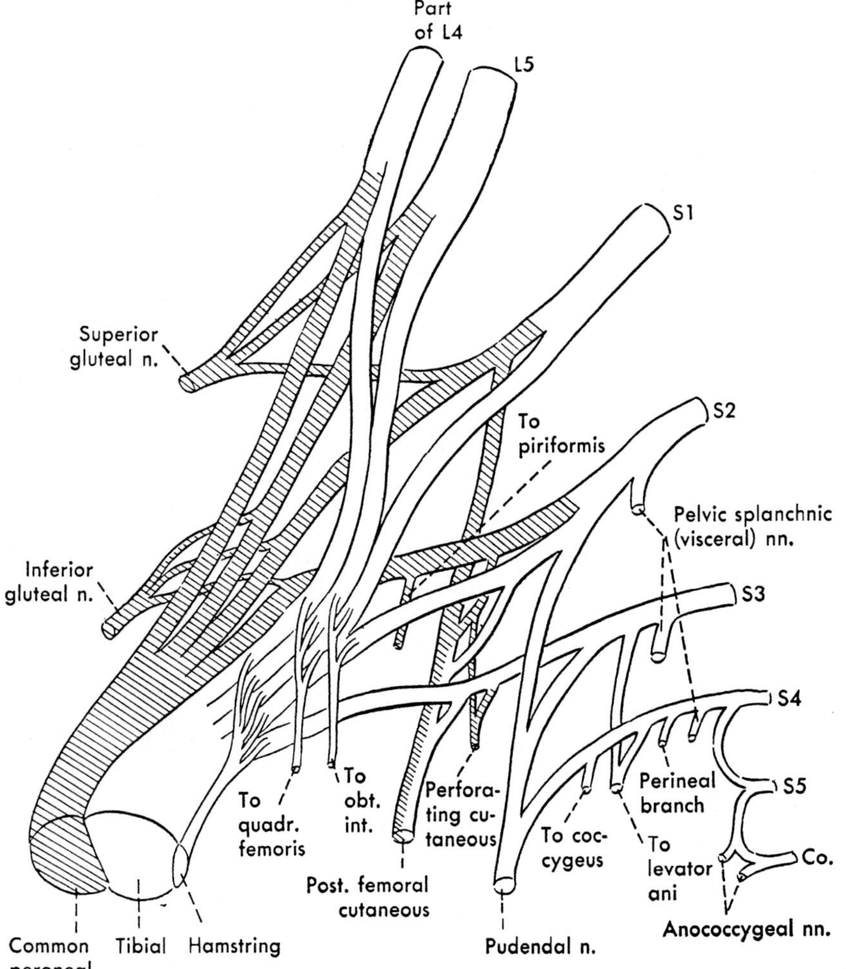

Figure 11–45. Sacral plexus. Anterior division *(unshaded)* and posterior division *(shaded)*. (From Jenkins, D.B.: Hollinshead's Functional Anatomy of the Limbs and Back, 6th ed., p. 256. Philadelphia, W.B. Saunders, 1991.)

Nerves	Level	Innervation
Anterior Division		
Subcostal	T12	Sensory: subxiphoid region
Iliohypogastric	L1	Sensory: posterolat. buttock/above pubis Motor: transversus abdominis/Int. oblique
Ilioinguinal	L1	Sensory: inguinal area
Genitofemoral	L1–L2	Sensory: Proximal anteromed. thigh, scrotum/mons Motor: cremaster
Obturator	L2–L4	Motor: Ext. oblique/adductor longus/adductor magnus (ant.)/gracilis
Posterior Division		
Lateral femoral cutaneous (LFCN)	L2–L3	Sensory: Lateral thigh
Femoral	L2–L4	Motor: Psoas/iliacus/quadratus/sartorius/pectineus/articularis genu
Accessory obturator	L2–L4	Motor: Psoas

D. Nerves

1. Lumbosacral Plexus

a. Lumbar Plexus—The lumbar plexus involves the ventral primary rami for T12–L4 but may display the usual prefixed (T11–L3) and postfixed (L1–L5) variations (see chart as shown at the top of this page).

b. Sacral Plexus (Fig. 11–45)—The sacral plexus typically involves the ventral primary rami of L4–S3. It is formed in the pelvis anterior and lateral to the sacrum. It provides a significant amount of innervation to the limb.

Nerves	Level	Innervation
Anterior Division		
Tibial	L4–S3	Semimembranosus/semitendinosus/biceps (long head)/adductor magnus/sup. gemellus/soleus/plantaris/popliteus/tibialis posterior/flexor digitorum longus/flexor hallucis longus
Quadratus femoris	L4–S1	Quadratus femoris/inf. gemellus
Obturator internus	L5–S2	Obturatorius internus/sup. gemellus
Pudendal	S2–S4	Sensory: perineal Motor: bulbocavernosus/urethra/urogenital diaphragm
Coccygeus	S4	Coccygeus
Levator ani	S3–S4	Levator ani
Posterior Division		
Peroneal	L4–S2	Biceps (short head)/tibialis anterior/extensor digitorum longus/peroneus tertius/extensor hallucis longus Peroneus longus and brevis/extensor hallucis brevis/extensor digitorum brevis

Nerves	Level	Innervation
Sup. gluteal	L4–S1	Gluteus medius and minimus/TFL
Inf. gluteal	L5–S2	Gluteus maximus
Piriformis	S2	Piriformis
Post. femoral cutaneous (PFCN)	S1–S3	Sensory: posterior thigh

2. Relationships—The lumbar plexus is found on the surface of the quadratus lumborum under (and within) the substance of the psoas major muscle. The genitofemoral nerve pierces the psoas and then lies on the anteromedial surface of the psoas. The femoral nerve lies between the iliacus and the psoas. The lateral femoral cutaneous nerve lies on the surface of the iliacus muscle and exits the pelvis under the lateral attachment of the inguinal ligament. Virtually all important nerves about the hip leave the pelvis by way of the sciatic foramen. The major reference point for the greater sciatic nerve and related structures in the hip is the piriformis muscle ("key" to the sciatic foramen). The **superior gluteal nerve and artery lie above the piriformis,** and virtually everything else leaves below the muscle (remember POP'S IQ [lateral to medial nerves]: *p*udendal, *o*bturator internus, *p*ostfemoral cutaneous, *s*ciatic, *i*nferior gluteal, *q*uadratus femoris). Two nerves leave the greater sciatic foramen and reenter the pelvis via the lesser foramen (pudendal and nerve to obturator internus). In addition to the peripheral nerves, a plexus of parasympathetic nerves cover the lower aorta and the anterior sacrum. These nerves should be protected to prevent sexual dysfunction. Anteriorly, the great nerves and vessels enter the thigh (and into the **femoral triangle**) under the inguinal ligament (Fig. 11–46). The borders of this tri-

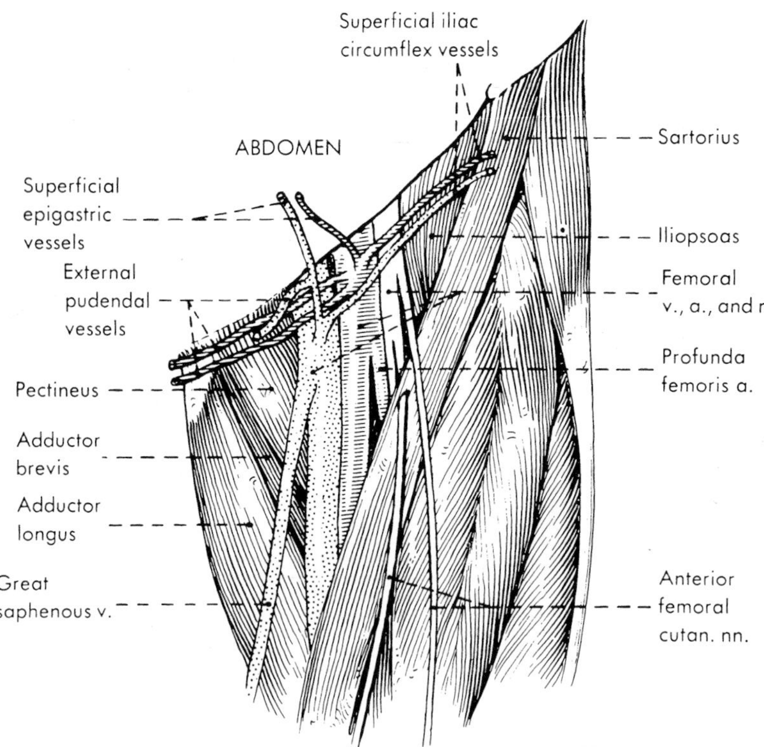

Figure 11–46. Femoral triangle. (From Jenkins, D.B.: Hollinshead's Functional Anatomy of the Limbs and Back, 6th ed., p. 243. Philadelphia, W.B. Saunders, 1991.)

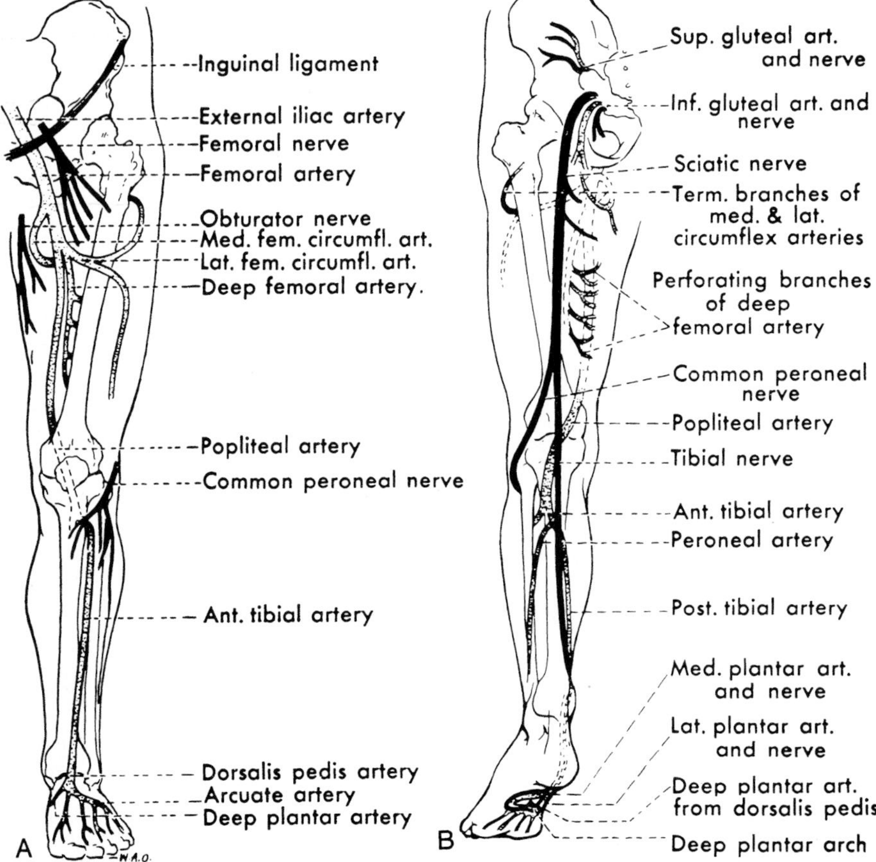

Figure 11–47. Nerves and vessels of the lower extremity. *A,* Anterior view. *B,* Posterior view. (From Jenkins, D.B.: Hollinshead's Functional Anatomy of the Limbs and Back, 6th ed., p. 221. Philadelphia, W.B. Saunders, 1991.)

angle include the sartorius laterally, the pectineus medially, and the inguinal ligament superiorly. Within the triangle, from lateral to medial, are the femoral *n*erve, *a*rtery, and *v*ein *a*nd the *l*ymphatic vessels (remember NAVAL). The **floor of the femoral triangle** (again, lateral to medial) is made up of the **iliacus,** psoas, pectineus, and the adductor longus. The femoral nerve descends between the iliacus and psoas and delivers numerous branches to muscle, overlying skin, and the hip joint (in accordance with Hilton's law). A spontaneous **iliacus hematoma may irritate the femoral nerve** owing to its proximity. At the apex of the triangle the saphenous nerve branches off and travels under the sartorius muscle. The obturator nerve exits the pelvis via the obturator canal. It splits into anterior and posterior divisions within the canal. The anterior division proceeds anteriorly to the obturator externus and posteriorly to the pectineus, supplying the adductor longus and brevis and the gracilis; it then delivers cutaneous branches to the medial thigh. The posterior division supplies the obturator externus, adductor brevis, and upper part of the adductor magnus, and it delivers other branches to the knee joint. Referred pain from the hip to the knee can be from the continuation of the branch to the adductor magnus. **The obturator nerve can be injured by retractors placed behind the transverse acetabular ligament.**

E. Vessels (Fig. 11–47)—The aorta branches into the common iliac arteries anterior to the L4 vertebral body. The common iliac vessels, in turn, divide into the internal (or *hypogastric;* medial) and external (lateral) iliacs at the S1 level. Important internal iliac branches include the **obturator** (the posterior branch **supplies the transverse acetabular ligament**), **superior gluteal (can be injured in the sciatic notch)**, and inferior gluteal (supplies the gluteus maximus and the short external rotators) (Fig. 11–48). The superficial circumflex iliac

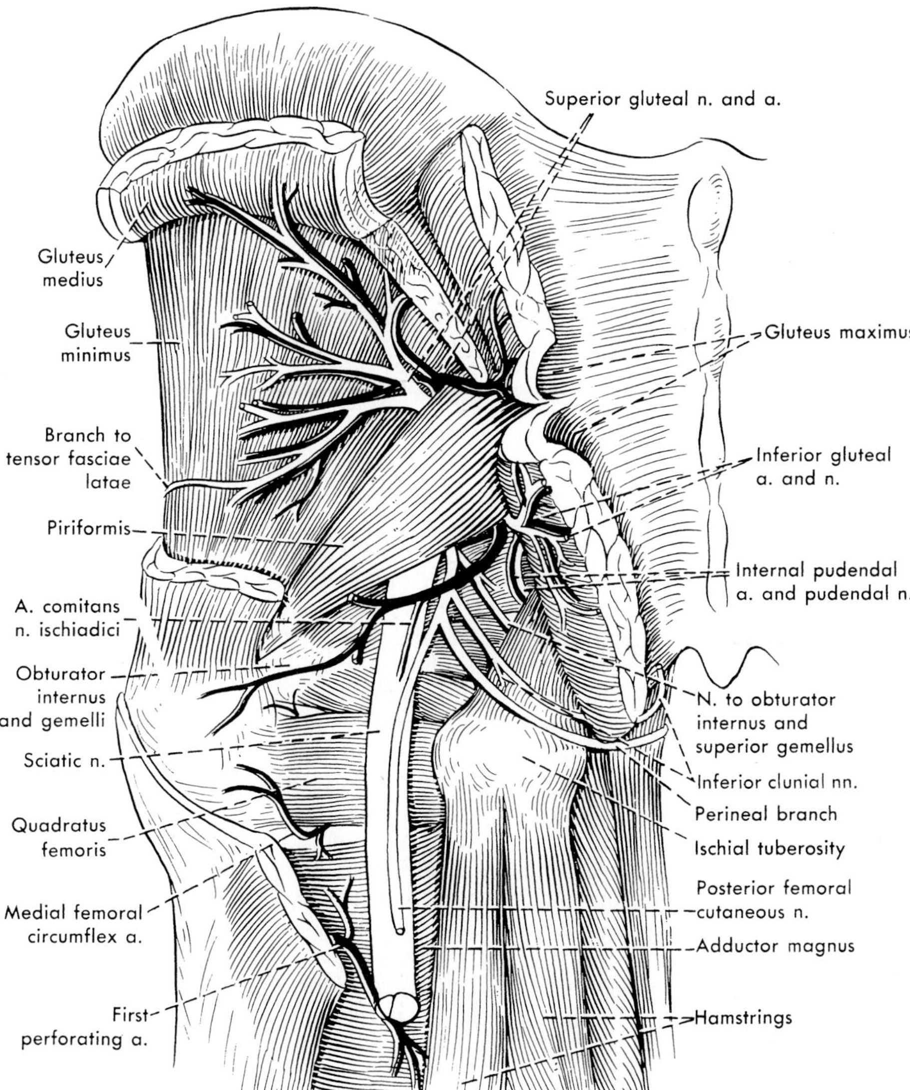

Figure 11–48. Posterior hip anatomy. Note relationship of structures to the piriformis muscle. (From Jenkins, D.B.: Hollinshead's Functional Anatomy of the Limbs and Back, 6th ed., p. 260. Philadelphia, W.B. Saunders, 1991.)

artery lies adjacent to the lateral femoral cutaneous nerve. The **external iliac artery** continues under the inguinal ligament to become the femoral artery. It **can be injured by anterosuperior quadrant acetabular screw placement** during total hip arthroplasty, and the **obturator artery and vein are jeopardized by anteroinferior screws and acetabular retractors.** The femoral artery enters the femoral triangle and delivers the profunda femoris, which supplies the anteromedial portion of the thigh and the perforators, which pierce the lateral intermuscular septum to supply the vastus lateralis muscle. The profunda has two other important branches: the medial and lateral femoral circumflex arteries. The lateral femoral circumflex travels obliquely and deep to the sartorius and rectus femoris. It delivers an ascending branch (at risk during anterolateral approaches) that proceeds to the greater trochanteric region and a descending branch that travels laterally under the rectus femoris. The **medial femoral circumflex,** which supplies most of the blood to the **femoral head,** runs between the pectineus and the iliopsoas and then in the interval between the obturator externus and adductor brevis muscles and in the **interval between the adductor magnus and brevis.** It proceeds distally anterior to the quadratus femoris. The cruciate anastomosis is the confluence of the ascending branch of the first perforating artery, the descending branch of the inferior gluteal artery, and the transverse branches of the medial and lateral femoral circumflex arteries. It lies at the inferior margin of the quadratus femoris muscle. The superficial femoral artery continues on the medial side of the thigh (between the vastus medialis and adductor longus) toward the adductor (Hunter's) canal. In the posteromedial thigh it becomes the popliteal artery in the popliteal fossa.

F. Approaches to the Pelvis and Hip
1. Posterior Approach to the Iliac Crest—A curvilinear incision is made just inferior to the crest beginning at the posterior superior iliac spine. After identifying the iliac crest, the gluteus maximus fibers are subperiosteally dissected from the outer table. Risks of this approach include the greater sciatic notch (superior gluteal artery and sciatic nerve) and the **cluneal nerves (8 cm anterolateral to the posterior superior iliac spine).**
2. Anterior Approach to the Iliac Crest—An oblique incision is made lateral to the anterior superior iliac spine, and the crest is exposed through the interval between the external oblique and the gluteus medius. Risks are to the greater sciatic notch, the inguinal ligament, and the lateral femoral cutaneous nerve.
3. Anterior (Smith-Peterson) Approach to the Hip (Fig. 11–49)—Takes advantage of the internervous plane between the sartorius (**femoral nerve**) and the tensor fascia femoris (**superior gluteal nerve**). It is useful for hemiarthroplasty and open reduction of the congenitally dislocated hip. Retract the lateral femoral cutaneous nerve anteriorly and ligate the **ascending branch of lateral femoral circumflex artery (which lies superficial to the rectus).** For deeper dissection, approach the interval between the gluteus medius and rectus femoris. Detach the origin of both heads of the rectus femoris. Retract the rectus medially and the gluteus medius laterally. Dissect any attachments of the iliopsoas to the inferior capsule and perform a capsulotomy. Dangers are to **the lateral femoral cutaneous nerve**, which is located anterior or medial to the sartorius about 6–8 cm below the anterior superior iliac spine. The femoral nerve and vessels can sometimes be injured with aggressive medial retraction of the sartorius.
4. Anterolateral (Watson-Jones) Approach to the Hip (Fig. 11–50)—This approach can be used for total hip arthroplasty as popularized by Watson-Jones. There is no true internervous plane, but it utilizes the **intermuscular plane between the tensor fascia femoris and gluteus medius**. After the incision and superficial dissection, the fascia lata is split to expose the vastus lateralis. Detach the anterior third of the gluteus medius from the greater trochanter and the entire gluteus minimus. Dissect the reflected head of the rectus femoris (and capsular attachment of the iliopsoas if necessary) and retract medially. Perform a capsulotomy. Dangers of this approach include damage to the femoral nerve by ex-

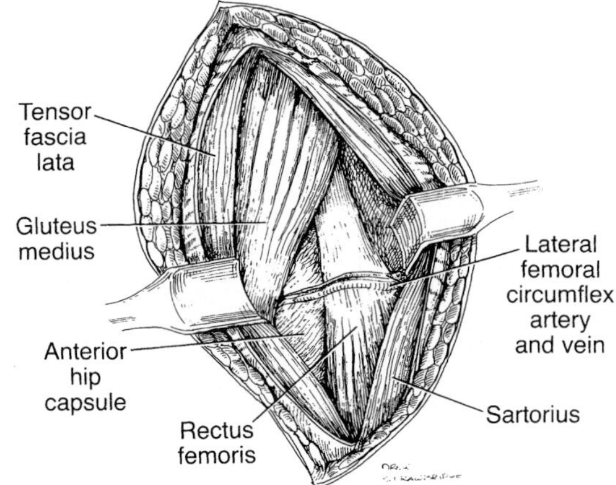

Figure 11–49. Anterior approach to the hip. (From Steinberg, M.E.: The Hip and Its Disorders, p. 92. Philadelphia, W.B. Saunders, 1991.)

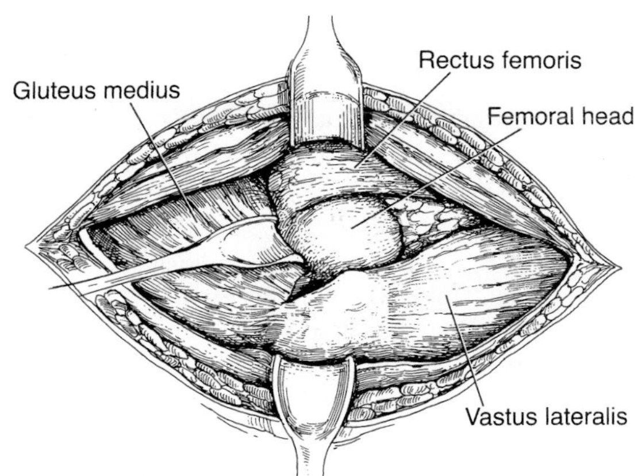

Figure 11–50. Anterolateral approach to the hip. (From Steinberg, M.E.: The Hip and Its Disorders, p. 93. Philadelphia, W.B. Saunders, 1991.)

cessive medial retraction, denervation of the tensor fascia femoris if the intermuscular interval is exploited too superiorly (the superior gluteal nerve lies about 5 cm above the acetabular rim), and injury to the descending branch of the **lateral femoral circumflex artery** with anterior and inferior dissection.

5. Lateral (Hardinge's) Approach to the Hip (Fig. 11–51)—Useful for total hip arthroplasty bipolar hemiarthroplasty and revision work, this approach utilizes an incision that splits both the gluteus medius and the vastus lateralis in tandem. Incise the skin and the fascia lata to expose the gluteus medius and the vastus. Incise the gluteus medius from the greater trochanter, leaving a cuff of tissue and the posterior one-half to two-thirds attached. Extend this incision to split the gluteus medius proximally. Distally, split the vastus along its anterior one-fourth down to the femoral shaft. Detach the gluteus minimus from its insertion. The hip capsule is exposed for further dissection. Dangers include injury to the femoral nerve and possible denervation of the gluteus medius **(superior gluteal nerve) if the split is too proximal (more than 5 cm proximal to the greater trochanter).**
6. Posterior (Moore or Southern) Approach to the Hip (Fig. 11–52)—The internervous plane in one version is between the gluteus maximus (inferior gluteal nerve) and the gluteus medius and the tensor fascia femoris (superior gluteal nerve). Most surgeons, however, approach the hip by splitting the fibers of the gluteus maximus. Incise the skin and the fascia lata along the posterior border of the femur, and then split the fibers of the gluteus maximus bluntly. Next, expose the short external rotators close to their insertion into the greater trochanter. Reflect them laterally to protect the sciatic nerve and expose the posterior hip capsule. A portion of the quadratus femoris may be taken down with the short external rotators, but one must be aware of the significant bleeding that can come from the inferior portion of this muscle (ascending branches of medial femoral circumflex artery). Dangers include sciatic neurapraxia if the sciatic nerve is not properly protected by the short external rotators. Additional trouble may be encountered if the inferior gluteal artery is damaged during the splitting of the gluteus maximus.
7. Medial (Ludloff) Approach to the Hip (Fig. 11–53)—Used occasionally for pediatric adductor releases and open reductions, this approach uses the interval between the adductor longus and gracilis. Deep, the interval is between the adductor brevis and magnus. Structures at risk include the anterior division of the **obturator nerve and medial femoral circumflex artery** (between the adductor brevis and the adductor mag-

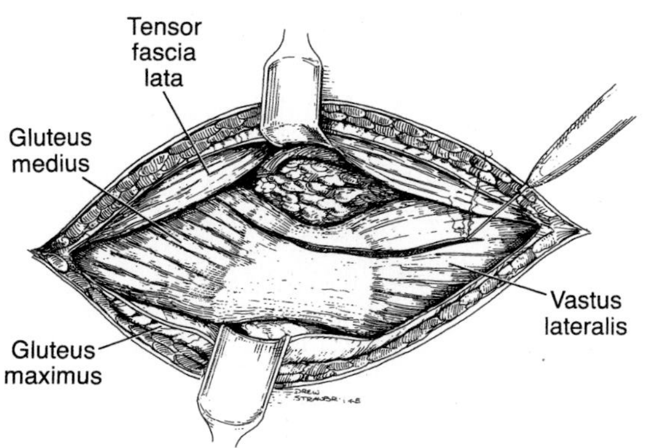

Figure 11–51. Lateral approach to the hip. (From Steinberg, M.E.: The Hip and Its Disorders, p. 95. Philadelphia, W.B. Saunders, 1991.)

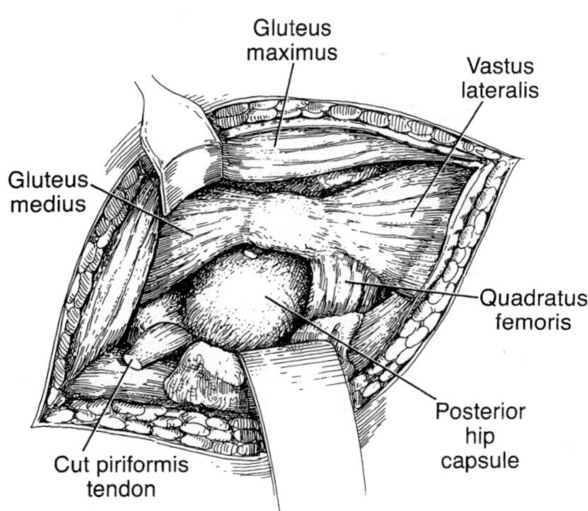

Figure 11–52. Posterior approach to the hip. (From Steinberg, M.E.: The Hip and Its Disorders, p. 98. Philadelphia, W.B. Saunders, 1991.)

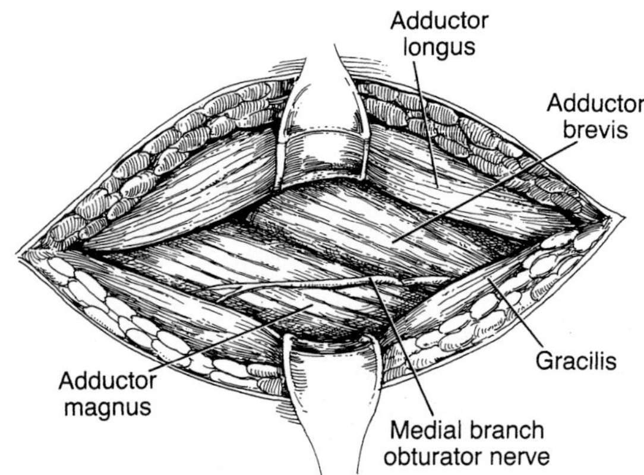

Figure 11–53. Medial approach to the hip. (From Steinberg, M.E.: The Hip and Its Disorders, p. 99. Philadelphia, W.B. Saunders, 1991.)

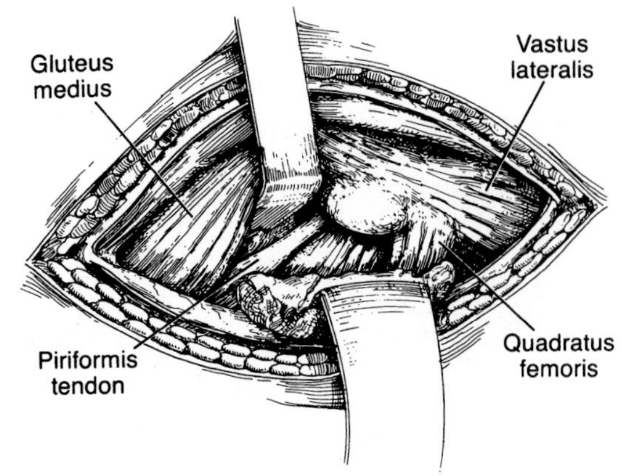

Figure 11–54. Posterolateral approach to the hip. (From Steinberg, M.E.: The Hip and Its Disorders, p. 96. Philadelphia, W.B. Saunders, 1991.)

nus/pectineus). **The deep external pudendal artery (anterior to the pectineus near the adductor longus origin) is also at risk proximally.**

8. Acetabular Approaches—Used primarily for open reduction and internal fixation (ORIF) of pelvic fractures, these approaches are basically extensions of incisions for exposure of the hip discussed earlier. The Kocher-Langenbeck incision is a posterolateral approach that provides access to the posterior column/acetabulum (Fig. 11–54). The ilioinguinal incision relies on mobilization of the rectus abdominis and iliacus, exposing the anterior column. Three windows are available with this approach. The first window gives access to the internal iliac fossa and the anterior sacro-iliac joint. The second window (between the iliopectineal fascia and the external iliac vessels) gives access to the pelvic brim and part of the superior pubic ramus. The third window (below the vessels and the spermatic cord) provides access to the quadrilateral plate and retropubic space (Fig. 11–55). The extended iliofemoral incision allows access to both columns by reflecting the gluteal muscles and tensor posteriorly and dividing the obturator internus and piriformis.

G. Arthroscopy—Hip arthroscopy portals include the anterolateral and posterolateral portals (adjacent to the superior border of the greater trochanter) and the anterior portal (femoral nerve and lateral femoral cutaneous nerve risk).

VIII. Thigh

A. Osteology of the Femur

1. Introduction—The femur is the largest bone of the body. The upper portion contains a head, neck, and two trochanters connected posteriorly by a crest. The neck-shaft angle averages about 127 degrees, although it begins at 141 degrees in the fetus. The anteversion varies from 1 to 40 degrees but averages 14 degrees. Below the lesser trochanter is a ridge known as the pectineal line, which continues as the linea aspera with medial and lateral ridges that diverge at the lower end to meet the medial and lateral supracondylar ridges. There are two femoral condyles; the medial condyle is larger. The more prominent medial epicondyle supports the adductor tubercle.
2. Ossification—The ossification center of the body of the femur appears at the seventh fetal week. The femoral head is usually not present at birth but appears as one large physis that includes both trochanters at about 11 months and fusing at 18 years. The greater trochanter becomes distinct at 5 years and the lesser at 9 years; both fuse at 16 years. The distal femoral physis appears at birth and fuses at 19 years.

B. Muscles of the Thigh

1. Anterior Thigh (Table 11–9)—See Table 11–8 for rectus femoris, sartorius.

Table 11–9.

Muscles of the Anterior Thigh

Muscle	Origin	Insertion	Innervation
Vastus lateralis	Iliotibial line/greater trochanter/lateral linea aspera	Lateral patella	Femoral
Vastus medialis	Iliotibial line/medial linea aspera/supracondylar line	Medial patella	Femoral
Vastus intermedius	Proximal anterior femoral shaft	Patella	Femoral

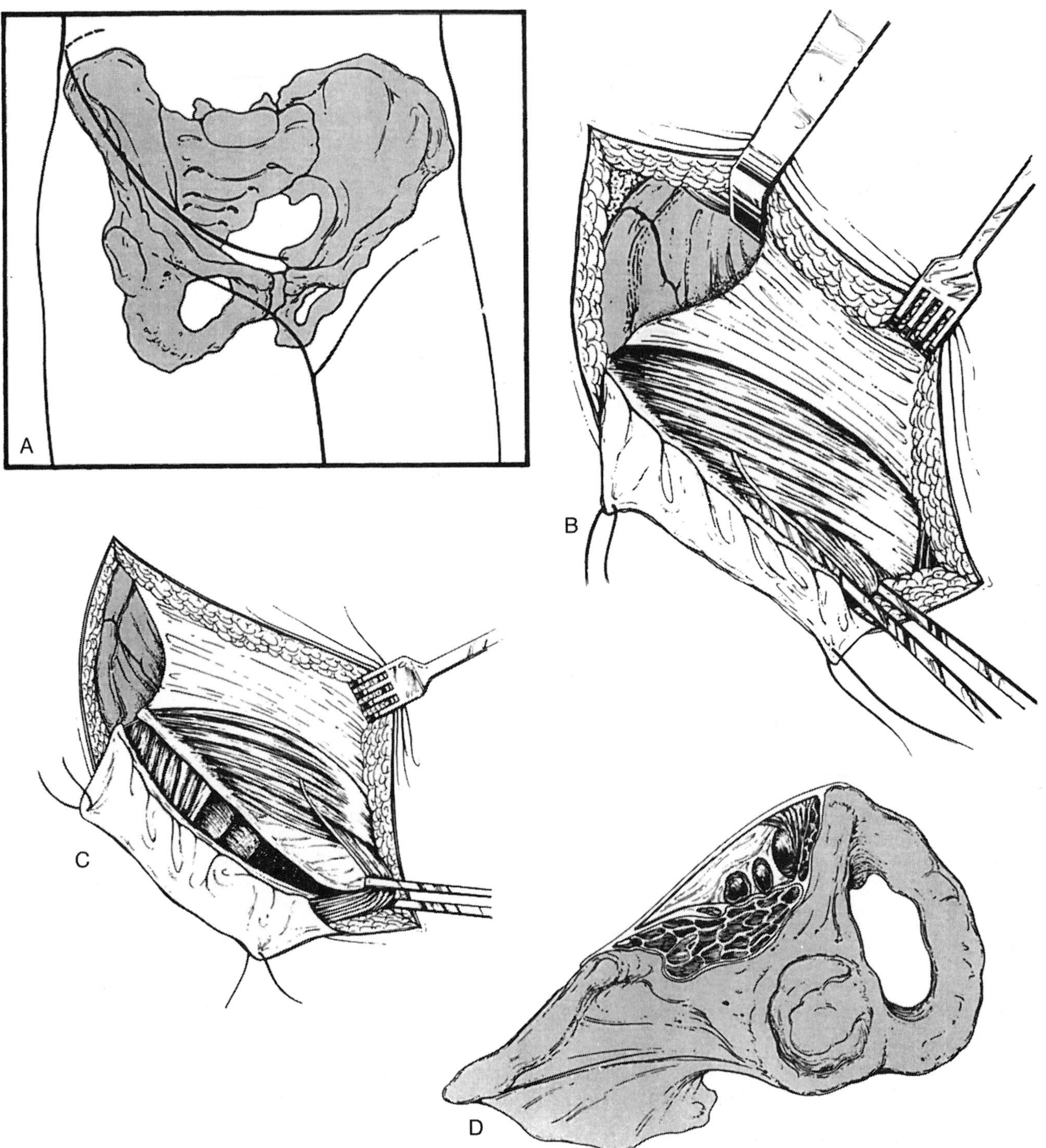

Figure 11–55. The ilioinguinal approach. *A,* The skin incision. *B,* The internal iliac fossa has been exposed, and the inguinal canal has been unroofed by distal reflection of the external oblique aponeurosis. *C,* An incision along the inguinal ligament detaches the abdominal muscles and transversalis fascia, giving access to the psoas sheath, the iliopectineal fascia, the external aspect of the femoral vessels, and the retropubic space of Retzius. *D,* An oblique section through the lacuna musculorum and lacuna vascularum at the level of the inguinal ligament.

Illustration continued on following page

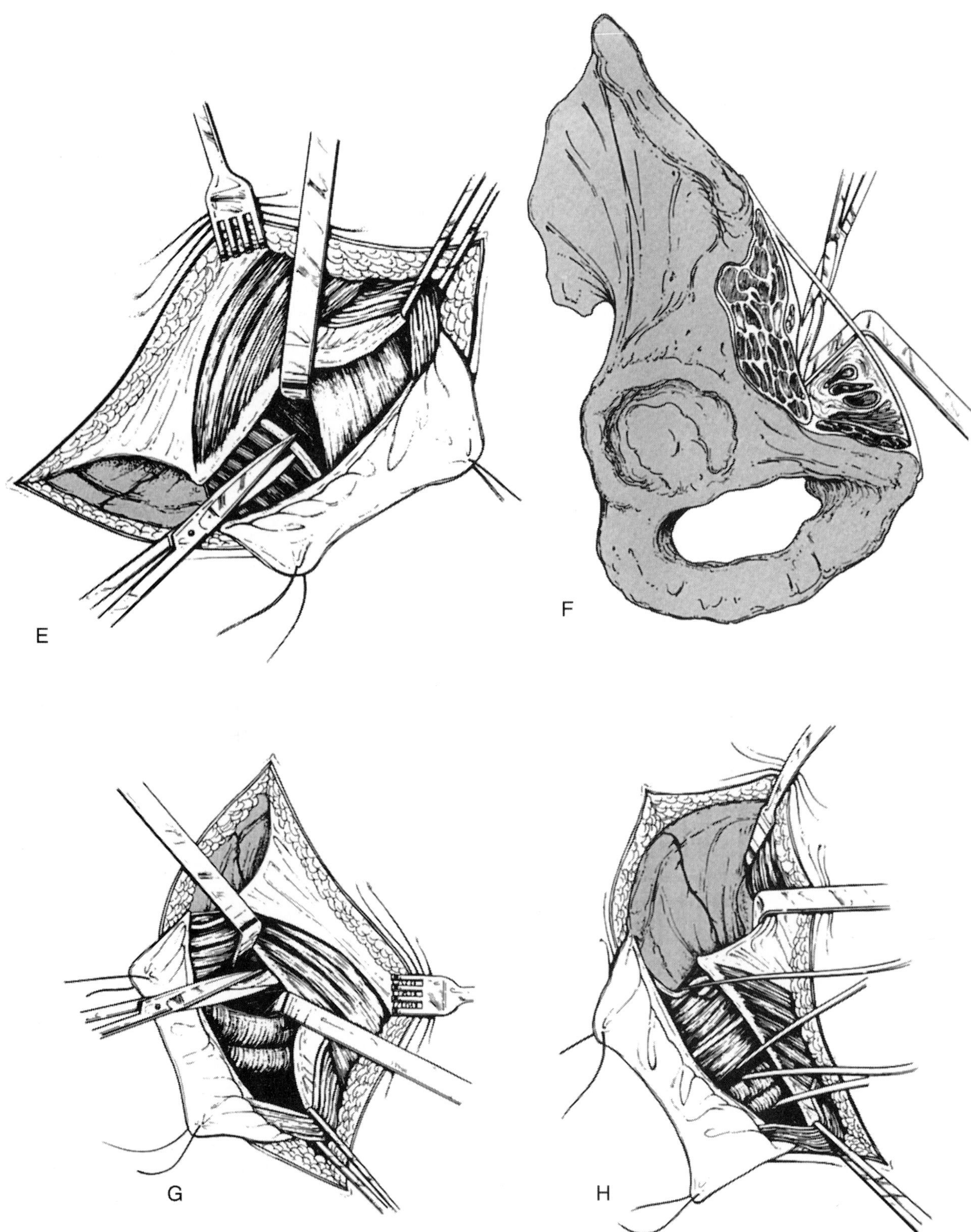

Figure 11–55 *Continued. E,* Division of the iliopectineal fascia to the pectineal eminence. *F,* An oblique section that demonstrates division of the iliopectineal fascia. *G,* Proximal division of the iliopectineal fascia from the pelvic brim to allow access to the true pelvis. *H,* The first window of the ilioinguinal approach, which gives access to the internal iliac fossa, the anterior sacroiliac joint, and upper portion of the anterior column.

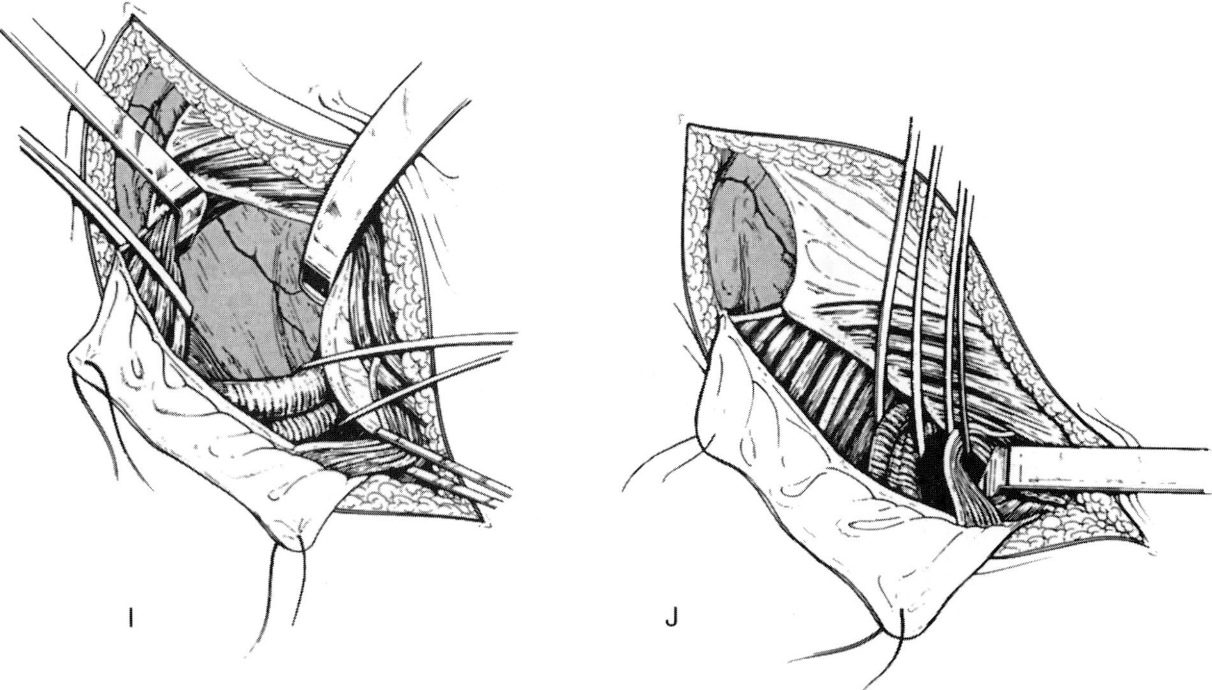

Figure 11–55 *Continued. I,* The second window of the ilioinguinal approach, giving access to the pelvic brim from the anterior sacroiliac joint to the lateral extremity of the superior pubic ramus. The quadrilateral surface and posterior column are accessible beyond the pelvic brim. *J,* Access to the symphysis pubis and retropubic space of Retzius, medial to the spermatic cord and femoral vessels. (From Browner B.D., Jupiter J.B., Levine, A.M., and Trafton, P.G.: Skeletal Trauma: Fractures, Dislocations, Ligamentous Injuries, pp. 907–909, Fig. 32–5*A–J*. Philadelphia, W.B. Saunders, 1992.)

2. Medial Thigh—See Adductors in Table 11–8.
3. Posterior Thigh (Table 11–10)
4. Cross-Sectional Diagram (Fig. 11–56)

C. Nerves and Vessels (see also VII, Pelvis and Hip, and IX, Knee and Leg)—The sciatic nerve emerges from its foramen below the piriformis muscle and lies posterior to the other short external rotators. It descends below the gluteus maximus and proceeds posteriorly to the adductor magnus and between the long head of the biceps and the semimembranosus. Before it emerges from the popliteal fossa, it divides into the common peroneal nerve and the tibial nerve. The common peroneal nerve diverges laterally and traverses the lateral knee region under cover of the biceps femoris. The tibial nerve emerges into the popliteal fossa lateral, proceeds posteriorly to the vessel, then descends between the heads of the gastrocnemius. After supplying the profundus (described earlier), the superficial femoral artery descends under cover of the sartorius muscle and proceeds between the adductor group and the vastus medialis into the adductor canal. At the level above the medial epicondyle, the artery supplies a supreme geniculate branch, then passes through

Table 11–10.

Muscles of the Posterior Thigh

Muscle	Origin	Insertion	Innervation
Biceps (long head)	Medial ischial tuberosity	Fibular head/lateral tibia	Tibial
Biceps (short head)	Lat. linea aspera/lat. intermuscular septum	Lateral tibial condyle	Peroneal
Semitendinosus	Distal med. ischial tuberosity	Anterior tibial crest	Tibial
Semimembranosus	Proximal lat. ischial tuberosity	Oblique popliteal ligament Posterior capsule Posterior/medial tibia Popliteus Medial meniscus	Tibial

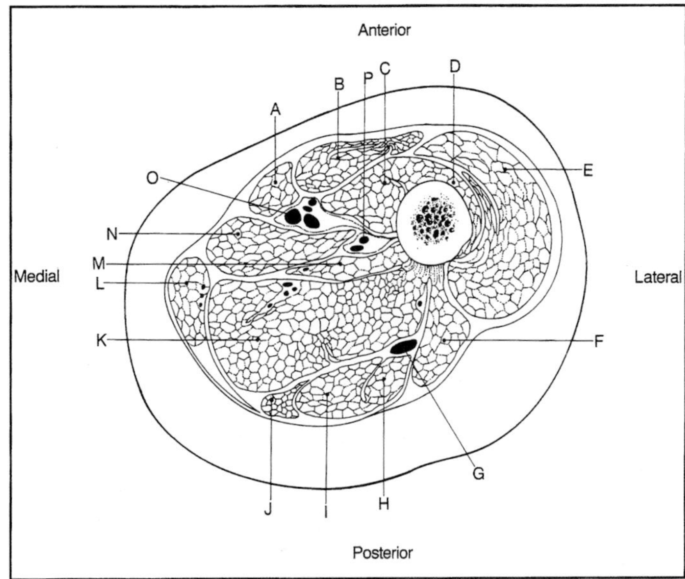

Figure 11–56. Cross-section of the proximal thigh. (From Callaghan, J.J., ed.: Anatomy Self-Assessment Examination, Fig. 53. Park Ridge, IL, American Academy of Orthopaedic Surgeons, 1991.)

a defect in the adductor magnus (adductor hiatus) and emerges in the popliteal fossa. The vein is usually posterior to the artery.

D. Approaches to the Thigh
   1. Lateral Approach to the Thigh—The lateral approach is used for ORIF of intertrochanteric and femoral neck fractures. This approach can be extended for access to shaft and supracondylar fractures. There is no true internervous plane. Split the fascia lata in line with the femoral shaft. Include part of the tensor fascia femoris if necessary. Then bluntly dissect the vastus lateralis in line with its fibers or dissect the fibers of the intermuscular septum. Identify and coagulate the various perforators from the profunda femoris.
   2. Posterolateral Approach to the Thigh—This approach may be used for exposure of the entire length of the femur through an internervous plane. It exploits the interval between the vastus lateralis (femoral nerve) and the hamstrings (sciatic nerve). Incise the fascia under the iliotibial band and retract the vastus superiorly. Continue anteriorly to the lateral intermuscular septum with blunt dissection until the periosteum over the linea aspera is reached. The danger of this dissection lies in the series of perforating vessels from the profundus that pierce the lateral intermuscular septum to reach the vastus. If approached without care, these vessels can retract and bleed underneath the septum.
   3. Anteromedial Approach to the Distal Femur—This approach may be used for ORIF of distal femoral and femoral shaft fractures. Explore the interval between the rectus femoris and vastus medialis and extend to a point medial to the patella. Retract the rectus laterally. Explore the interval to reveal the vastus intermedius. It may be necessary to open the knee joint. If so, incise the medial patellar retinaculum and split a portion of the quadriceps tendon just lateral to the medial border. After identifying the vastus intermedius, split it along its fibers to expose the femur. Dangers include injury to the medial superior geniculate artery and the infrapatellar branch of the saphenous nerve because both cross the site of exposure. Additionally, one must leave an adequate cuff of tissue for a strong patellar retinacular repair or risk lateral subluxation of the patella.
   4. Posterior Approach to the Thigh—This rare approach may be used for exploration of the sciatic nerve. It makes use of the internervous interval between the sciatic nerve (biceps femoris) and the femoral nerve (vastus lateralis). Identify and protect the posterior femoral cutaneous nerve (between the biceps and the semitendinosus). Next, explore the interval between the biceps and the lateral intermuscular septum. Detach the origin of the short head of the biceps from the linea aspera. This maneuver allows exposure of the femur at the midshaft level. In the lower thigh, retract the long head of the biceps laterally to expose the sciatic nerve. It lies on the surface of the adductor magnus and may be retracted laterally to expose this portion of the femur.

IX. Knee and Leg
   A. Osteology
      1. Patella—Commonly known as the kneecap, the patella is the largest sesamoid bone (about 5 cm in diameter). It serves three functions: It is a fulcrum for the quadriceps;

it protects the knee joint; and it enhances lubrication and nutrition of the knee. The patella is said to have the thickest articular surface in the body, probably because of the loads it must transmit. Although sometimes subdivided, the articular surface of the patella has two facets, medial and lateral, separated by a vertical ridge. The lateral facet is broader and deeper than the medial facet. Somewhat triangular in shape, the apex of the patella gives rise to the patella, and they fuse sometime between the second and sixth year of life. An accessory or "bipartite" patella may represent failure of fusion of the superolateral corner of the patella and is commonly confused with patellar fractures.

2. Tibia—The tibia is the second longest bone in the body (behind the femur). It consists of a proximal extremity with medial (oval and concave) and lateral (circular and convex) facets. The intercondylar eminence separates the medial and lateral facets and the anterior and posterior cruciate ligaments. The tibial tubercle is an oblong elevation on the anterior surface of the tibia where the patella tendon inserts. Gerdy's tubercle lies on the lateral side of the proximal tibia and is the insertion of the iliotibial tract. The tibial shaft is triangular in cross-section and tapers to its thinnest point at the junction of the middle and distal thirds and then again widens to form the tibial plafond. Distally, the tibia forms an inferior quadrilateral surface for articulation with the talus and the pyramid-shaped medial malleolus. Laterally, the fibular notch forms an articulation with the fibula. The tibia is formed from three ossification centers.

Ossification Center	Age at Appearance	Age at Fusion
Body (primary)	7 weeks (fetal)	
Proximal (secondary)	Birth	20 years
Distal (secondary)	Second year	18 years

3. Fibula—This long slender bone is composed of a head, a shaft, and a distal lateral malleolus. The styloid process of the head serves as the attachment for the fibular collateral ligament and the biceps tendon. Lying just below the head, the neck of the fibula is grooved by the common peroneal nerve. The expanded distal fibula is known as the lateral malleolus and extends beyond the distal margin of the medial malleolus. Together with the inferior distal surface of the tibia, these structures make up the ankle mortise. Like the tibia, the fibula is also formed from three ossification centers.

Ossification Center	Age at Appearance	Age at Fusion
Body (primary)	8 weeks (fetal)	
Proximal (secondary)	Third year	25 years
Distal (secondary)	Second year	20 years

B. Arthrology

1. Knee—Much more than a simple ginglymus or hinge-type of joint, the knee is a compound joint consisting of two condyloid joints and one sellar joint (patellofemoral articulation). The medial and lateral femoral condyles articulate with the corresponding tibial facets. Intervening menisci serve to deepen the concavity of the facets, help protect the articular surface, and assist in rotation of the knee (Fig. 11–57). The peripheral one-third of the menisci are vascular (and can be repaired); the inner two-thirds are nourished by synovial fluid. Stability of the knee is enhanced by a complex arrangement of ligaments (Table 11–11; Fig. 11–58). The cruciate ligaments are crucial to anteroposterior stability, and the collateral ligaments provide varus/valgus stability. Each cruciate ligament is made up of two portions, or bundles. **The anterior cruciate ligament is composed of an anteromedial portion that is tight in flexion and a posterolateral portion that is tight in extension. The posterior cruciate ligament has an anterolateral portion that is tight in flexion and a posteromedial portion that is tight in extension.** In addition, several muscles and tendons traverse the knee, giving it dynamic stability.

Location	Muscles
Anterior	Quadriceps
Lateral	Biceps and popliteus
Medial	Pes anserinus (sartorius, gracilis, semitendinosus), semimembranosus (with five attachments)
Posterior	Medial and lateral heads of the gastrocnemius, plantaris

2. Superior Tibiofibular Joint—A plane or gliding joint that is strengthened by the anterior and posterior ligaments of the head of the fibula.

C. Muscles of the Leg—Commonly divided into groups based on compartments (anterior, lateral, superficial posterior, and deep posterior) (Table 11–12). Origins and insertions are noted in Figure 11–59. **The popliteal fossa**

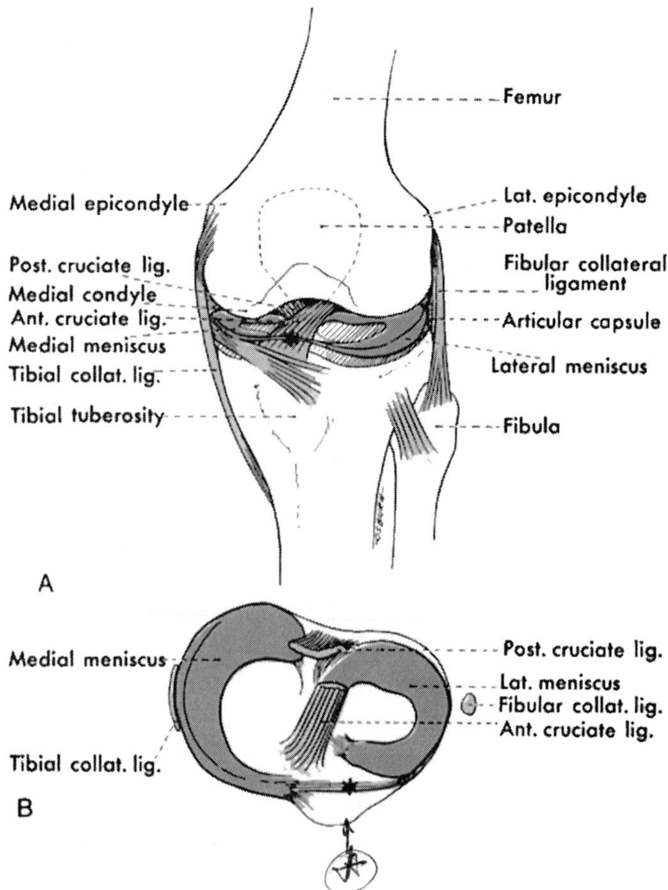

Figure 11–57. Ligaments of the knee. (From Jenkins, D.B.: Hollinshead's Functional Anatomy of the Limbs and Back, 6th ed., Fig. 16–1. Philadelphia, W.B. Saunders, 1991.)

Table 11–11.

Ligaments of the Knee

Ligament	Origin	Insertion	Function
Retinacular	Vastus medialis and lateralis	Tibial condyles	Forms anterior capsule
Posterior fibers	Femoral condyles	Tibial condyles	Forms posterior capsule
Oblique popliteal	Semimembranosus tendon	Lateral femoral condyle/ posterior capsule	Strengthens capsule
Deep medial collateral (MCL)	Medial epicondyle	Medial meniscus	Holds med. meniscus to femur
Superficial MCL	Medial epicondyle	Medial condyle of tibia	Resists valgus force
Arcuate	Lat. femoral condyle, over popliteus	Post. tibia/fibular head	Posterior support
Lateral collateral (LCL)	Lateral epicondyle	Lateral fibular head	Resists varus force
Anterior cruciate (ACL)	Anterior intercondylar tibia	Posteromed. lat. femoral condyle	Limits hyperextension/sliding
Posterior cruciate (PCL)	Posterior sulcus tibia	Anteromed. femoral condyle	Prevents hyperflexion/sliding
Coronary	Meniscus	Tibial periphery	Meniscal attachment
Wrisberg	Posterolateral meniscus	Med. femoral condyle (behind PCL)	Stabilizes lat. meniscus
Humphrey	Posterolateral meniscus	Med. femoral condyle (in front)	Stabilizes lat. meniscus
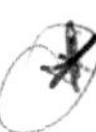 Transverse meniscal	Anterolateral meniscus	Anteromedial meniscus	Stabilizes menisci

Table 11–12.

Muscles of the Leg

Muscle	Origin	Insertion	Action	Innervation
Anterior Compartment				
Tibialis anterior	Lateral tibia	Med. cuneiform, 1st metatarsal	Dorsiflex, invert foot	Deep peroneal (L4)
Extensor hallucis longus (EHL)	Mid. fibula	Great toe distal phalanx	Dorsiflex, extend toe	Deep peroneal (L5)
Extensor digitorum longus (EDL)	Tibial condyle/fibula	Toe middle and distal phalanges	Dorsiflex, extend toes	Deep peroneal (L5)
Peroneus tertius	Fibula and EDL tendon	5th Metatarsal	Evert, plantar flex, abduct foot	Deep peroneal (S1)
Lateral Compartment				
Peroneus longus	Proximal fibula	Med. cuneiform, 1st metatarsal	Evert, plantar flex, abduct foot	Superficial peroneal (S1)
Peroneus brevis	Distal fibula	Tuberosity of 5th metatarsal	Evert foot	Superficial peroneal (S1)
Superficial Posterior Compartment				
Gastrocnemius	Post. med. and lat. femoral condyles	Calcaneus	Plantar flex foot	Tibial (S1)
Soleus	Fibula/tibia	Calcaneus	Plantar flex foot	Tibial (S1)
Plantaris	Lat. femoral condyle	Calcaneus	Plantar flex foot	Tibial (S1)
Deep Posterior Compartment				
Popliteus	Lat. femoral condyle, fibular head	Proximal tibia	Flex, IR knee	Tibial (L5S1)
Flexor hallucis longus (FHL)	Fibula	Great toe distal phalanx	Plantar flex great toe	Tibial (S1)
Flexor digitorum longus (FDL)	Tibia	2nd–5th Toe distal phalanges	Plantar flex toes, foot	Tibial (S1S2)
Tibialis posterior	Tibia, fibula, interosseous membrane	Navicular, med. cuneiform	Invert/plantar flex foot	Tibial (L4L5)

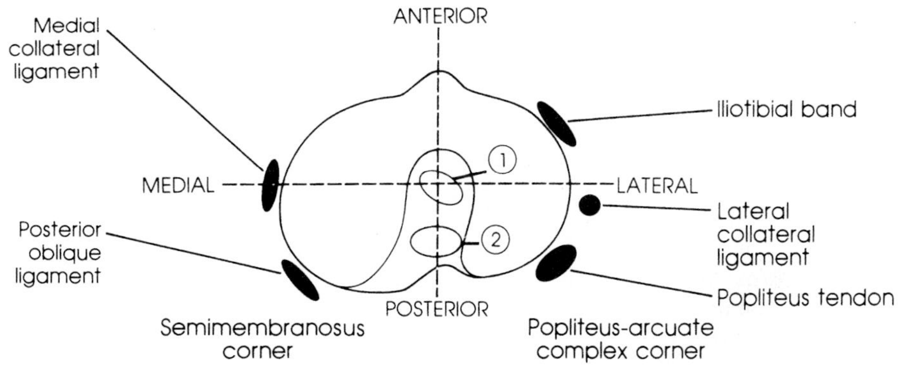

Figure 11–58. Ligaments of the knee. 1, Anterior cruciate ligament; 2, posterior cruciate ligament. (From Magee, D.J.: Orthopedic Physical Assessment, p. 285. Philadelphia, W.B. Saunders, 1987.)

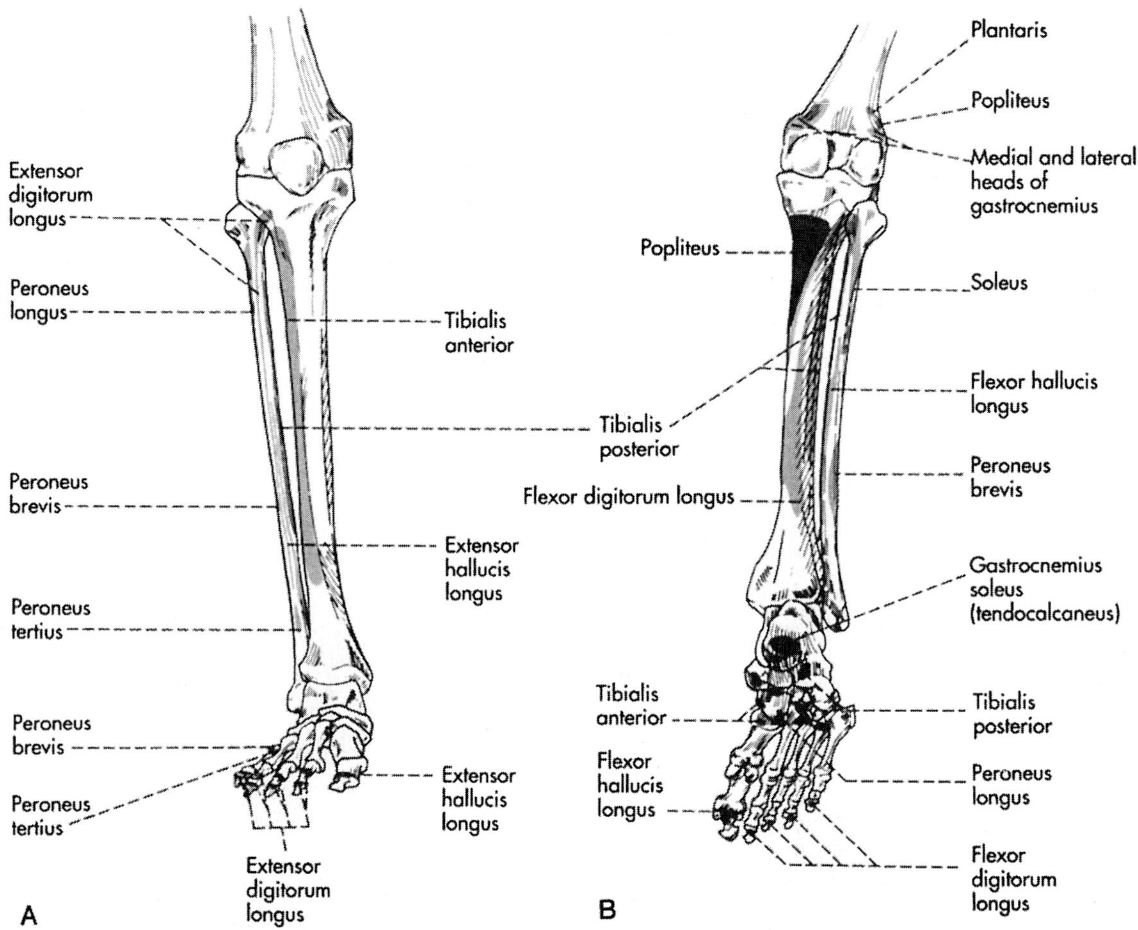

Figure 11–59. Origins and insertions of leg and foot muscles. (From Jenkins, D.B.: Hollinshead's Functional Anatomy of the Limbs and Back, 6th ed., Fig. 19–3. Philadelphia, W.B. Saunders, 1991.)

is bordered by the gastrocnemius muscles, semimembranosus, and biceps. The plantaris muscle makes up the floor of the fossa.

D. Nerves (Fig. 11–60)—Motor branches to the muscles of the leg are from terminal divisions of the sciatic nerve (in the distal thigh) and the tibial and common peroneal nerves and their branches.

1. Tibial Nerve—Continues in the thigh deep to the long head of the biceps and enters the popliteal fossa. It then crosses over the popliteus muscle and splits the two heads of the gastrocnemius, passing deep to the soleus on its course to the posterior aspect of the medial malleolus. It terminates as the medial and lateral plantar nerves. Muscular branches supply the posterior leg along its course.
2. Common Peroneal Nerve—The smaller terminal division of the sciatic, this nerve runs laterally in the popliteal fossa in the interval between the medial border of the biceps and the lateral head of the gastrocnemius. Then it winds around the neck of the fibula, deep to the peroneus longus, where it divides into superficial and deep branches. **This nerve can be injured with traction and with lateral meniscal repair.**
   a. Superficial Peroneal Nerve—Runs along the border between the lateral and anterior compartments in the leg, supplying muscular branches to the peroneus longus and brevis. It terminates in two cutaneous branches supplying the dorsal foot.
   b. Deep Peroneal Nerve—Sometimes known as the anterior tibial nerve, this nerve runs along the anterior surface of the interosseous membrane, supplying the musculature of the anterior compartment.
3. Cutaneous Nerves—Important cutaneous nerves include the saphenous nerve and the sural nerve. The saphenous nerve is the continuation of the femoral nerve of the thigh, and it becomes subcutaneous on the medial aspect of the knee between the sartorius and gracilis (where it is sometimes injured during procedures about the knee, e.g., meniscal repair). The saphenous nerve supplies sensation to the medial aspect of the leg and foot. The sural nerve, which is

often used for nerve grafting and which can cause painful neuromas when inadvertently cut, is formed by cutaneous branches of both the tibial (medial sural cutaneous) and common peroneal (lateral sural cutaneous) nerves. It lies on the lateral aspect of the leg and foot.

E. Vessels (see Fig. 11–60)—Branches of the popliteal artery, the continuation of the femoral artery, supply the leg. The artery enters the popliteal fossa between the biceps and semimembranosus and descends underneath the tibial nerve and terminates between the medial and lateral heads of the gastrocnemius, dividing into the anterior and posterior tibial arteries. Several genicular branches are given off in the popliteal fossa, including the medial and lateral geniculates (which supply the menisci) and the middle geniculate (which supplies the cruciate ligaments). **The superior lateral geniculate can be injured during lateral release procedures. The descending geniculate artery (a branch of the femoral artery proximal to Hunter's canal) supplies the**

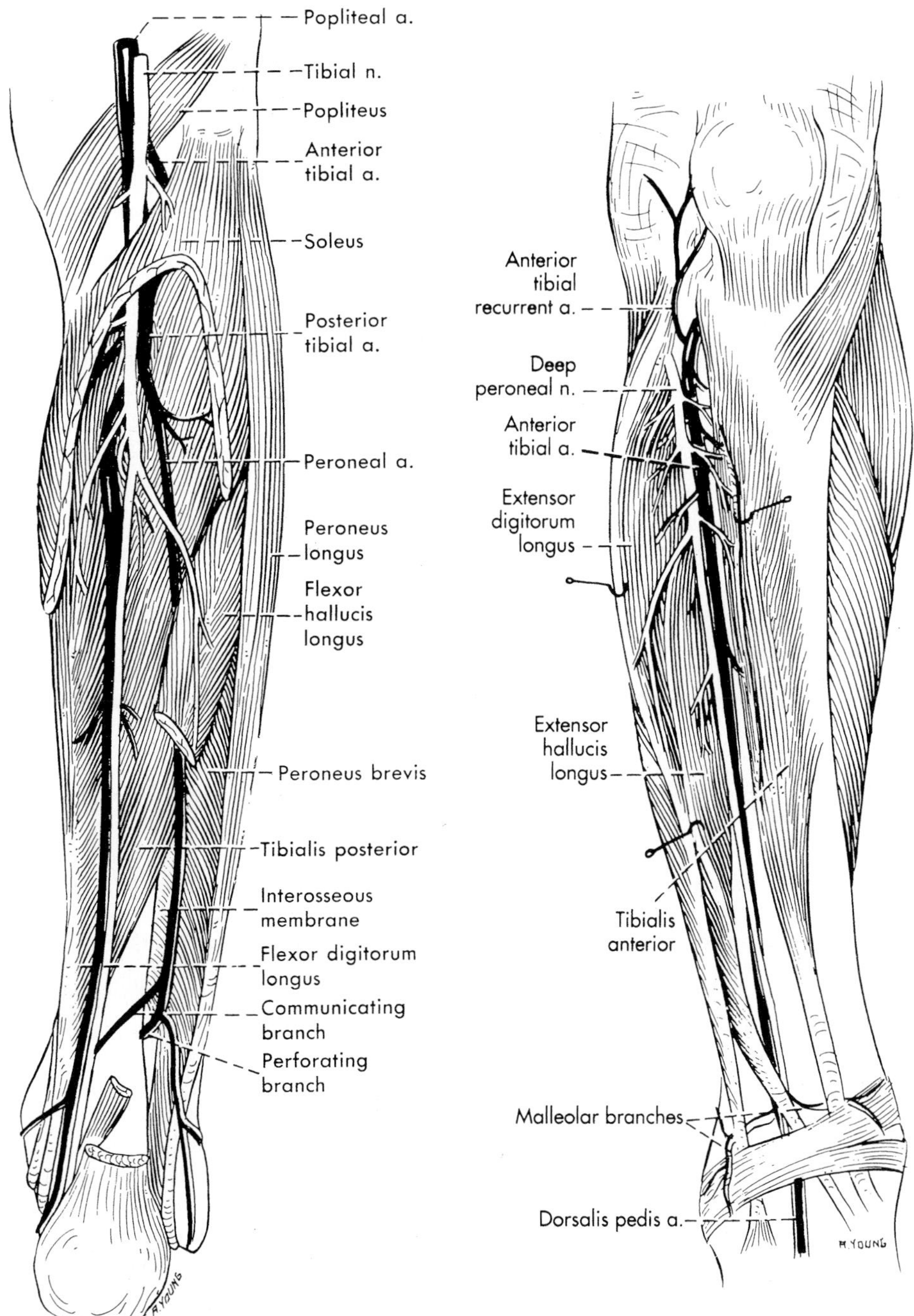

Figure 11–60. Nerves and vessels of the leg. *Left,* Posterior. *Right,* Anterior. (From Jenkins, D.B.: Hollinshead's Functional Anatomy of the Limbs and Back, 6th ed., pp. 292, 296. Philadelphia, W.B. Saunders, 1991.)

vastus medialis at the anterior border of the intermuscular septum.

1. Anterior Tibial Artery—The first branch of the popliteal artery, this vessel passes between the two heads of the tibialis posterior and the interosseous membrane to lie on the anterior surface of that membrane between the tibialis anterior and extensor hallucis longus until it terminates as the dorsalis pedis artery.
2. Posterior Tibial Artery—Continues in the deep posterior compartment of the leg, coursing obliquely to pass behind the medial malleolus, where it terminates by dividing into medial and lateral plantar arteries. Its main branch, the peroneal artery, is given off 2.5 cm distal to the popliteal fossa and continues in the deep posterior compartment, lateral to its parent artery, between the tibialis posterior and flexor hallucis longus (FHL), eventually terminating in calcaneal branches.

F. Surgical Approaches to the Knee and Leg

1. Medial Parapatellar Approach to the Knee—Used most commonly for total knee arthroplasty, this approach utilizes a midline incision and a medial parapatellar capsular incision. The infrapatellar branch of the saphenous nerve is sometimes cut with incisions that stray too far medially, leading to a painful neuroma.
2. Medial Approach to the Knee (Fig. 11–61) —Used for repair of the medial collateral ligament and capsule, this approach is in the interval between the sartorius and medial patellar retinaculum. Three layers are commonly recognized (from superficial to deep).

   The saphenous nerve and vein must be identified and protected.

Layer	Components
1	Pes anserinus tendons
2	Superficial MCL
3	Deep MCL, capsule, POL

3. Lateral Approach to the Knee (Fig. 11–62) —Used primarily for exploring and repairing damaged ligaments, this approach utilizes the plane between the iliotibial band (superior gluteal nerve) and the biceps (sciatic nerve). The common peroneal nerve, located near the posterior border of the biceps, must be isolated and retracted. The popliteus tendon is also at risk and should be identified. **The lateral inferior geniculate artery is posterior to the lateral collateral ligament between the lateral head of the gastrocnemius and the posterolateral capsule; it must also be identified and coagulated. The superior**

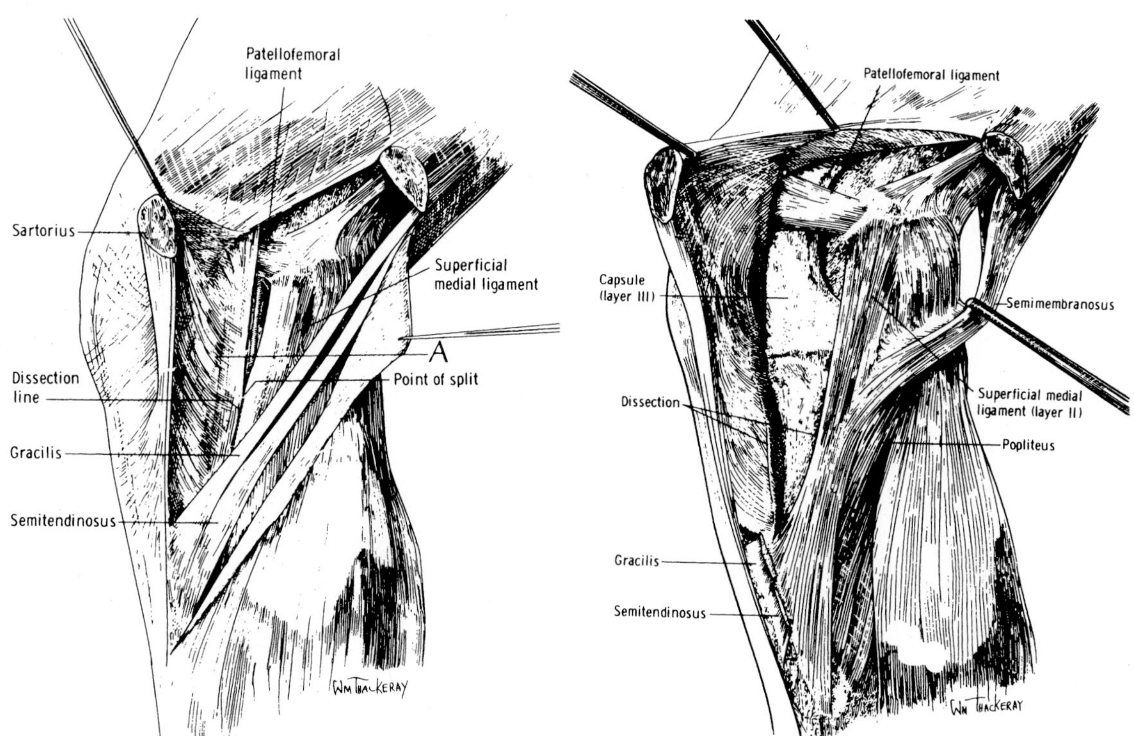

Figure 11–61. Medial structures of the knee. (Warren, L.F., and Marshall, J.L.: The supporting structures and layers of the medial side of the knee. J. Bone Joint Surg. [Am.] 61:58, 1979.)

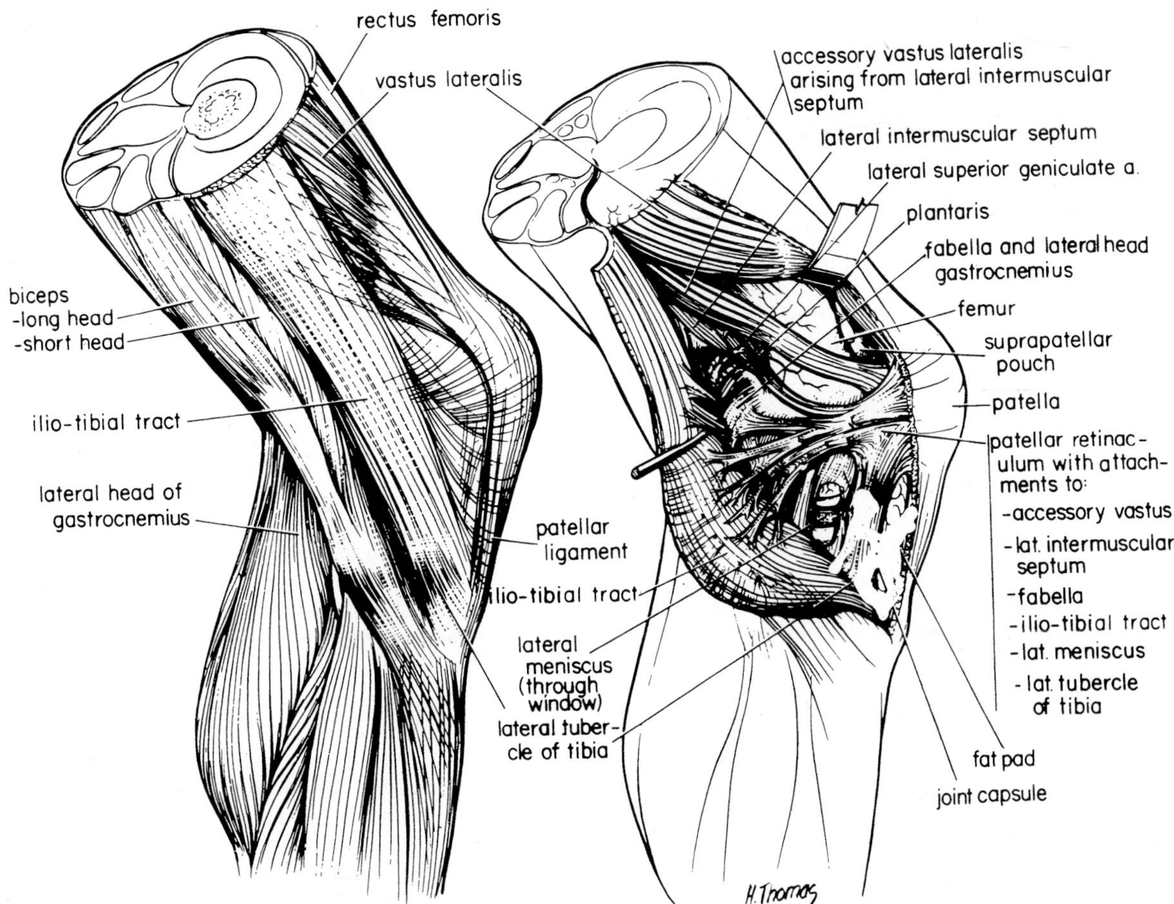

Figure 11–62. Lateral structures of the knee. (From Seebacher, J.R., Inglis, A.E., Marshall, J.L., and Warren R.F.: The structure of the posterolateral aspect of the knee. J. Bone Joint Surg. [Am.] 64:533, 1982.)

lateral geniculate is located between the femur and vastus lateralis.

4. Posterior Approach to the Knee—Occasionally required to address posterior capsular pathology, this approach uses an S-shaped incision beginning laterally and ending medially (distally). The popliteal fossa is exposed using the small saphenous vein and medial sural cutaneous nerves as landmarks. The two heads of the gastrocnemius can be detached if greater exposure is necessary. An alternative approach is to mobilize the medial head of the gastrocnemius (lateral to the semimembranosus) and retract it laterally, using its muscle belly to protect the neurovascular structures.
5. Anterior Approach to the Tibia—May be used for ORIF of fractures and bone grafting; it relies on subperiosteal elevation of the tibialis anterior.
6. Posterolateral Approach to the Tibia—Used typically for bone grafting of tibial nonunions, this approach utilizes the internervous plane between the soleus and the FHL (tibial nerve) and the peroneal muscles (superficial peroneal nerve). The FHL is detached from its origin on the fibula, and the tibialis posterior is detached from its origin along the interosseous membrane to reach the tibia. Neurovascular structures in the posterior compartment (including the peroneal artery) are protected by the muscle bellies of the FHL and tibialis posterior.
7. Approach to the Fibula—Through the same interval as the posterolateral approach to the tibia but stays more anterior and relies on isolation and protection of the common peroneal nerve in the proximal dissection.

G. Arthroscopy—Arthroscopic portals for knee arthroscopy commonly include the inferomedial and inferolateral portals and a proximal (medial or lateral) portal. Posterior portals can place certain neurovascular structures at risk (lateral—common peroneal nerve; medial—saphenous nerve and vein).

X. Ankle and Foot

A. Osteology—The 26 bones of the foot include 7 tarsal bones, 5 metatarsals, and 14 phalanges.

1. Tarsus—Includes the talus, calcaneus, cuboid, navicular, and three cuneiforms.

a. Talus—Articulates with the tibia and fibula in the ankle mortise and with the calcaneus and navicular distally. It is made up of a body with three articular surfaces (the trochlea, including surfaces for the malleoli articulations, and the posterior and middle calcaneal facets) and a posterior process (for the posterior talofibular ligament). The neck of the talus connects with the head, which in turn articulates with the navicular distally and the calcaneus inferiorly.

b. Calcaneus—Largest and strongest bone in the foot. It has three surfaces that articulate with the talus: a large posterior surface, an anterior surface, and a middle surface. Distally, there is an articular surface that receives the cuboid bone. The **sustentaculum tali is an overhanging horizontal eminence on the anteromedial surface of the calcaneus**. It supports the middle articular surface above it and allows plantar vessels and nerves to pass below it. The calcaneal tuberosity posteriorly is bounded by medial and lateral processes.

c. Cuboid—Lies on the lateral aspect of the foot, is grooved by the peroneus longus, and has four facets for articulation with the calcaneus, the lateral cuneiform, and the fourth and fifth metatarsals.

d. Navicular—The most medial tarsal bone; lies between the talus and the cuneiforms. Proximally, the surface is oval and concave for its articulation with the head of the talus. Distally, the navicular has three articular surfaces, one for each of the cuneiforms.

e. Cuneiforms—Medial, intermediate, and lateral, these three bones articulate with the navicular and posterior cuboid (lateral cuneiform) and the first three metatarsals. The intermediate cuneiform does not extend as far distally as the medial cuneiform, allowing the second metatarsal to "key" into place.

2. Metatarsals—Five bones, numbered from medial to lateral, span the distance between the tarsals and the phalanges. In general, their shape and function are similar to those of the metacarpals of the hand.
3. Phalanges—Also similar to the hand. The great toe has two phalanges, and the remaining digits have three.
4. Ossification—Each tarsus has a single ossification center, except the calcaneus, which has a second center posteriorly. The calcaneus, talus, and usually the cuboid are present at birth. The lateral cuneiform appears during the first year, the medial cuneiform

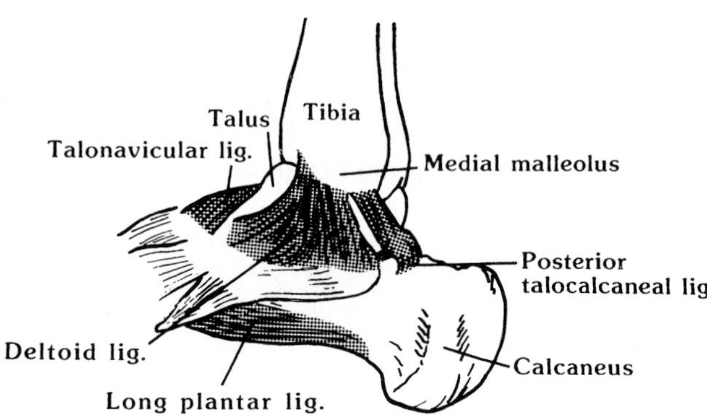

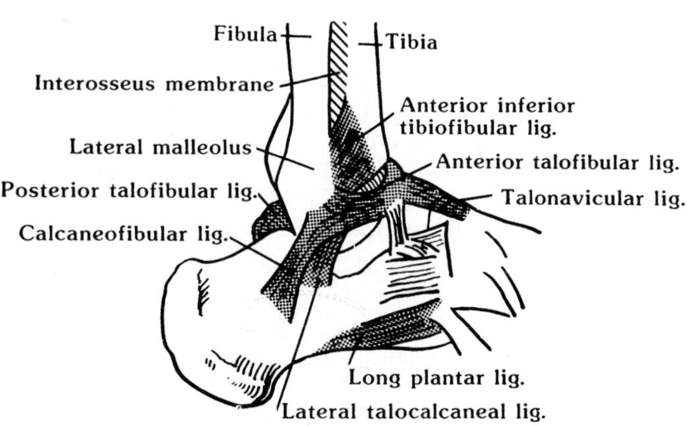

Figure 11–63. Ankle ligaments. *Top,* Medial. *Bottom,* Lateral. (From Weissman, B.N., and Sledge, C.B.: Orthopedic Radiology, pp. 593, 594. Philadelphia, W.B. Saunders, 1986.)

Table 11–13.

Ligaments of the Intertarsal Joints

Ligament	Common Name	Origin	Insertion
Interosseous talocalcaneal	Cervical	Talus	Calcaneus
Calcaneocuboid/calcaneonavicular	Bifurcate	Calcaneus	Cuboid and navicular
Calcaneocuboid-metatarsal	Long plantar	Calcaneus	Cuboid and 1st–5th metatarsals
Plantar calcaneocuboid	Short plantar	Calcaneus	Cuboid
Plantar calcaneonavicular	Spring	Sustentaculum tali	Navicular
Tarsometatarsal	Lisfranc	Med. cuneiform	2nd Metatarsal base

during the second year, and the intermediate cuneiform and navicular during the third year. The posterior center for the calcaneus usually appears at the eighth year. The second through fifth metatarsals have two ossification centers: a primary center in the shaft and a secondary center for the head that appears at age 5–8. The phalanges and first metatarsal have secondary centers at their bases that appear during the third or fourth year proximally and the sixth to seventh year distally.

B. Arthrology

1. Inferior Tibiofibular Joint—Formed by the medial distal fibula and the notched lateral distal tibia, this joint is supported by four ligaments. **The anteroinferior tibiofibular ligament is an oblique band that connects the bones anteriorly. Avulsion of this ligament may result in a Tillaux fracture.** The posterior tibiofibular ligament is smaller but serves a similar function posteriorly. The inferior transverse ligament lies just below the posterior tibiofibular ligament and provides additional posterior support for the mortise. Finally, an interosseous ligament also connects the two bones.
2. Ankle Joint (Fig. 11–63)—A ginglymus, or hinge, joint is formed by the malleoli and the talus. It is supported by the following ligaments.

Ligament	Origin	Insertion
Capsule	Tibia	Talus
Deltoid		
Tibionavicular	Med. malleolus	Navicular tuberosity
Tibiocalcaneal	Med. malleolus	Sustentaculum tali
Post. tibiotalar	Med. malleolus	Inner side of talus
Deep	Med. malleolus	Medial surface of talus
ATFL	Lat. malleolus	Transversely to talus anteriorly
PTFL	Lat. malleolus	Transversely to talus posteriorly
Calcaneofibular (CFL)	Lat. malleolus	Obliquely posteriorly to calcaneus

The posterior tibiofibular ligament is strong, and the anteroinferior tibiofibular ligament is weak; therefore the anteroinferior tibiofibular ligament is most commonly injured in ankle sprains.

3. Intertarsal Joints (Fig. 11–64)—Relatively self-explanatory, but there are several ligamentous structures that deserve highlighting (Table 11–13).
4. Other Joints—Tarsometatarsal joints are gliding joints supported by dorsal, plantar, and interosseous ligaments. The intermetatarsal joints are supported by similar ligaments, and the deep transverse metatarsal ligaments interconnect the metatarsal heads. The metatarsophalangeal joints are supported by plantar and collateral ligaments, and IP joints are supported mainly by their capsules.

C. Muscles (Fig. 11–65)—The arrangement of muscles and tendons in the foot is best considered in layers (Table 11–14). On the plantar surface intrinsic muscles dominate the first and third layers, and extrinsic tendons are more important in the second and fourth layers. Tendons are arranged about the toe as shown in Figure 11–66. Tendons about the foot and ankle are shown in Figure 11–67.

D. Nerves (see Fig. 11–61)—Nerves of the ankle and foot are branches of proximal nerves discussed earlier.

1. Tibial Nerve—Splits into two branches under the flexor retinaculum: medial and lateral plantar nerves. Both of these nerves run in the second layer of the foot. The medial plantar nerve runs deep to the abductor hallucis, and the lateral plantar nerve runs obliquely under the cover of the quadratus plantae. **The distribution of the sensory and motor branches of the plantar nerves is similar to that in the hand.** The medial plantar nerve (like the median nerve of the hand) supplies plantar sensation to the medial 3½ digits and motor to only a few plantar muscles (flexor hallucis brevis, abductor hallucis, flexor digitorum brevis, and first lumbrical). The lateral plantar nerve (like the ulnar nerve in the hand) supplies plantar sensation to the lat-

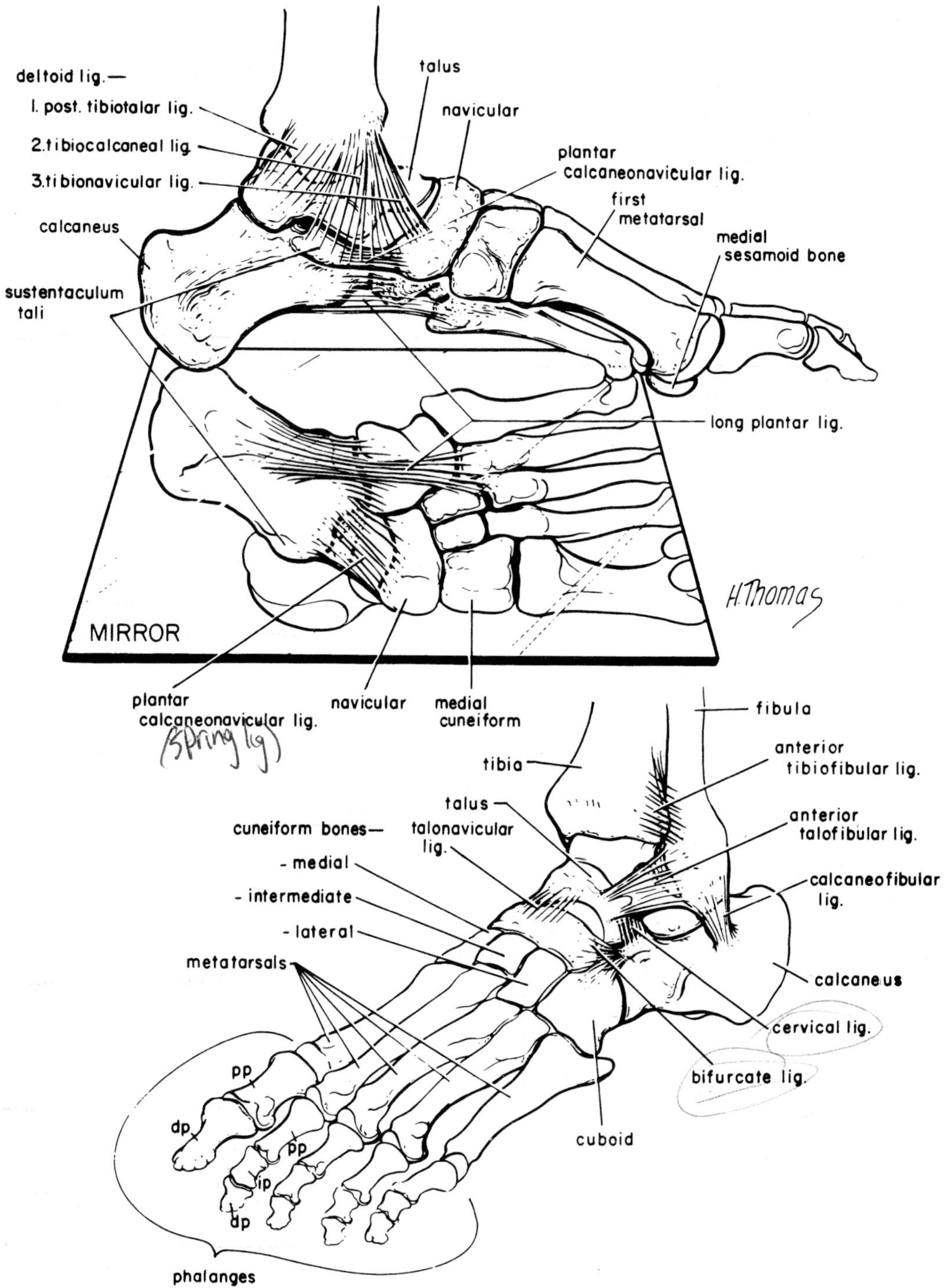

Figure 11–64. Ligaments of the foot. (From Jahss, M.H.: Disorders of the Foot, p. 14. Philadelphia, W.B. Saunders, 1982.)

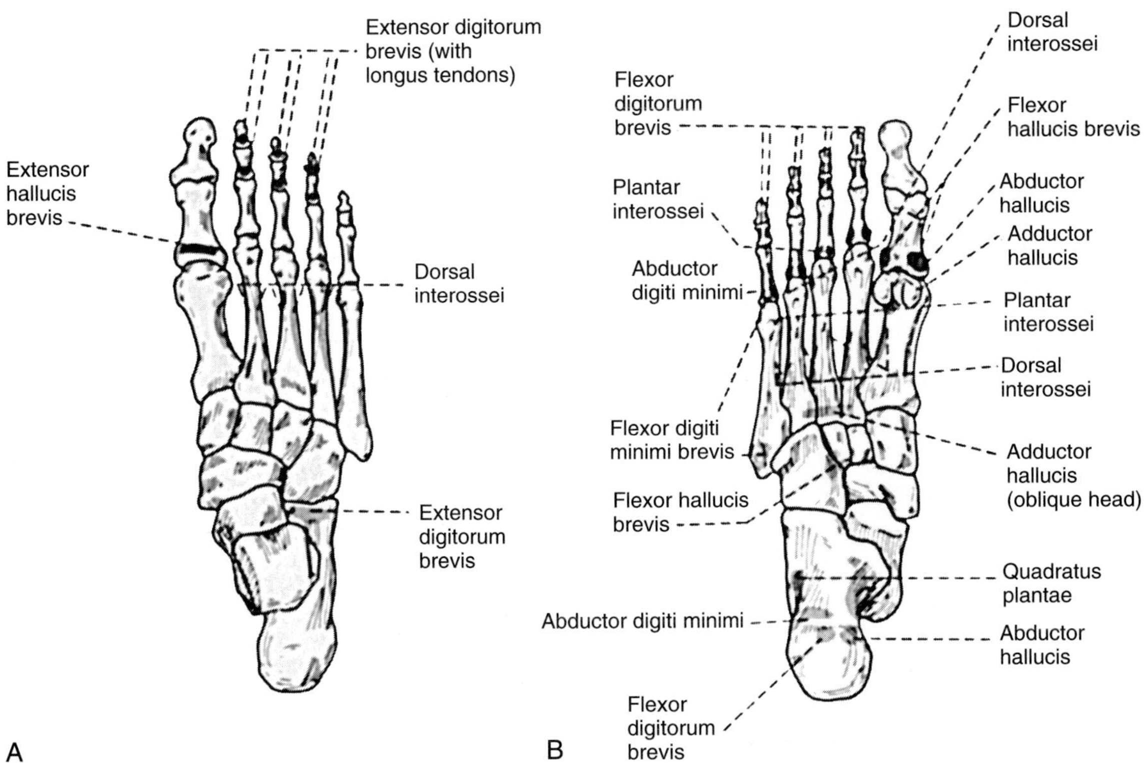

Figure 11–65. Origins and insertions of muscles of the foot. *A,* Dorsal view. *B,* Plantar view. (From Jenkins, D.B.: Hollinshead's Functional Anatomy of the Limbs and Back, 6th ed., Fig. 20–7. Philadelphia, W.B. Saunders, 1991.)

Table 11–14.

Muscles of the Ankle and Foot

Muscle	Origin	Insertion	Action	Innervation
Dorsal Layer				
Extensor digitorum brevis (EDB)	Superolateral calcaneus	Base of proximal phalanges	Extend	Deep peroneal
First Plantar Layer				
Abductor hallucis	Calcaneal tuberosity	Base of great toe proximal phalanx	Abduct great toe	Med. plantar
Flexor digitorum brevis (FDB)	Calcaneal tuberosity	Distal phalanges of 2nd–5th toes	Flex toes	Med. plantar
Abductor digiti minimi	Calcaneal tuberosity	Base of 5th toe	Abduct small toe	Lat. plantar
Second Plantar Layer				
Quadratus plantae	Med. and lat. calcaneus	FDL tendon	Helps flex distal phalanges	Lat. plantar
Lumbricals	FDL tendon	EDL tendons	Flex MTP, extend IP	Med. and lat. plantar
FDL and FHL	Tibia/fibula	Distal phalanges of digits	Flex toes/invert foot	Tibial
Third Plantar Layer				
Flexor hallucis brevis (FHB)	Cuboid/lat. cuneiform	Proximal phalanx of great toe	Flex great toe	Med. plantar
Adductor hallucis	Oblique: 2nd–4th metatarsals Transverse: MTP	Proximal phalanx of great toe lat.	Adduct great toe	Lat. plantar
Flexor digiti minimi brevis (FDMB)	Base of 5th metatarsal head	Proximal phalanx of small toe	Flex small toe	Lat. plantar
Fourth Plantar Layer				
Dorsal interosseous	Metatarsal	Dorsal extensors	Abduct	Lat. plantar
Plantar interosseous	3rd–5th Metatarsals	Proximal phalanges medially	Adduct toes	Lat. plantar
(Peroneus longus and tibialis posterior)	Fibula/tibia	Med. cuneiform/ navicular	Evert/invert foot	Superficial peroneal/ tibial

Note: For abduction and adduction in the foot, the second toe serves as the reference.

tib post. inserts: tuberosity of navicular, medial & middle cuneiform bases # 2,3,4 MT

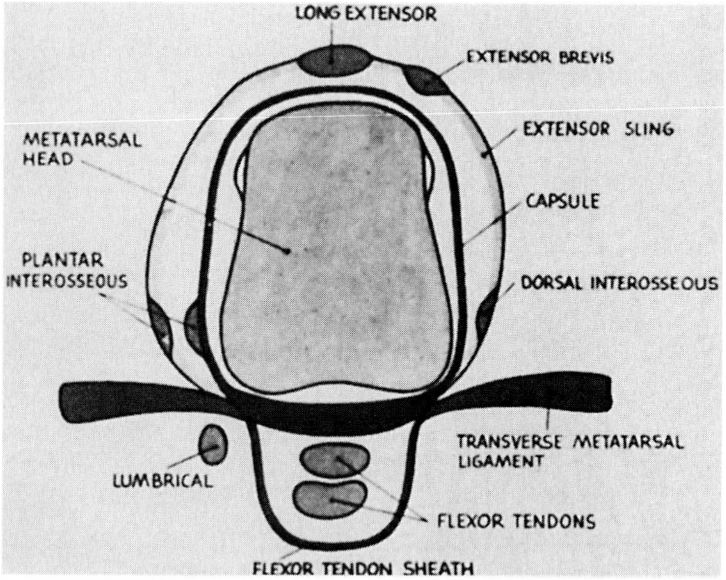

Figure 11–66. Cross-section of the toe at the metatarsal base. (From Jahss, M.H.: Disorders of the Foot, p. 623. Philadelphia, W.B. Saunders, 1982.)

eral 1½ digits and the remaining intrinsic muscles of the foot.

2. Common Peroneal Nerve—Splits into superficial and deep branches in the leg and has terminal branches in the foot as well. The lateral terminal branch of the deep peroneal nerve ends in the proximal dorsal foot by supplying the extensor digitorum brevis (EDB) muscle. The medial terminal branch of the deep peroneal nerve supplies sensation to the first web space. The **bulk of the remaining sensation to the dorsal foot is supplied by the medial and intermediate dorsal cutaneous nerves of the superficial peroneal nerve.**

E. Vessels—Like the nerves that run with them, there are two main arteries that supply the ankle and foot.
   1. Dorsalis Pedis Artery—Continuation of the anterior artery of the leg, it provides the blood supply to the dorsum of the foot via its lateral tarsal, medial tarsal, arcuate, and first dorsal metatarsal branches. Its largest branch, the deep plantar artery, runs between the first and second metatarsals and contributes to the plantar arch (see Fig. 11–67*A*).
   2. Posterior Tibial Artery—Divides into medial and lateral plantar branches under the abductor hallucis muscle. The larger lateral branch receives the deep plantar artery and forms the plantar arch in the fourth layer of the plantar foot.

F. Important Neurovascular Relationships—May be seen in a coronal section (Fig. 11–68).

G. Surgical Approaches
   1. Anterior Approach to the Ankle—Used primarily for ankle fusion, this approach utilizes the interval between the extensor hallucis longus and extensor digitorum longus. Before incising the extensor retinaculum, care must be taken to protect the superficial peroneal nerve. The deep peroneal nerve and anterior tibial artery, which lie directly in this interval, must be retracted medially with the extensor hallucis longus.
   2. Approach to the Medial Malleolus—This approach is commonly used for ORIF of ankle fractures. It is superficial and can be approached anteriorly or posteriorly. The anterior approach jeopardizes the saphenous nerve and the long saphenous vein; the posterior approach places the structures running behind the medial malleolus (posterior tibial artery; FDL; posterior tibial artery, vein, and nerve; and FHL) at risk. A posteromedial approach, behind the medial malleolus, can be made through the tendon sheath of the posterior tibialis.
   3. Posteromedial Approach to the Ankle/Foot—Used for clubfoot release in children, this approach begins medial to the Achilles tendon and curves distally along the medial border of the foot. Care must be taken to protect the posterior tibial nerve/artery and their branches. The posterior tibialis tendon is a landmark for the location of the subluxated navicular in the clubfoot.
   4. Lateral Approach to the Ankle—Used for ORIF of distal fibula fractures, this approach is subcutaneous. The sural nerve (posterolateral) and the superficial peroneal nerve (anterior) must be avoided.
   5. Lateral Approach to the Hindfoot—Used for triple arthrodesis, this approach uses the internervous plane between the peroneus tertius (deep peroneal nerve) and peroneal tendons (superficial peroneal nerve). The fat pad covering the sinus tarsi is re-

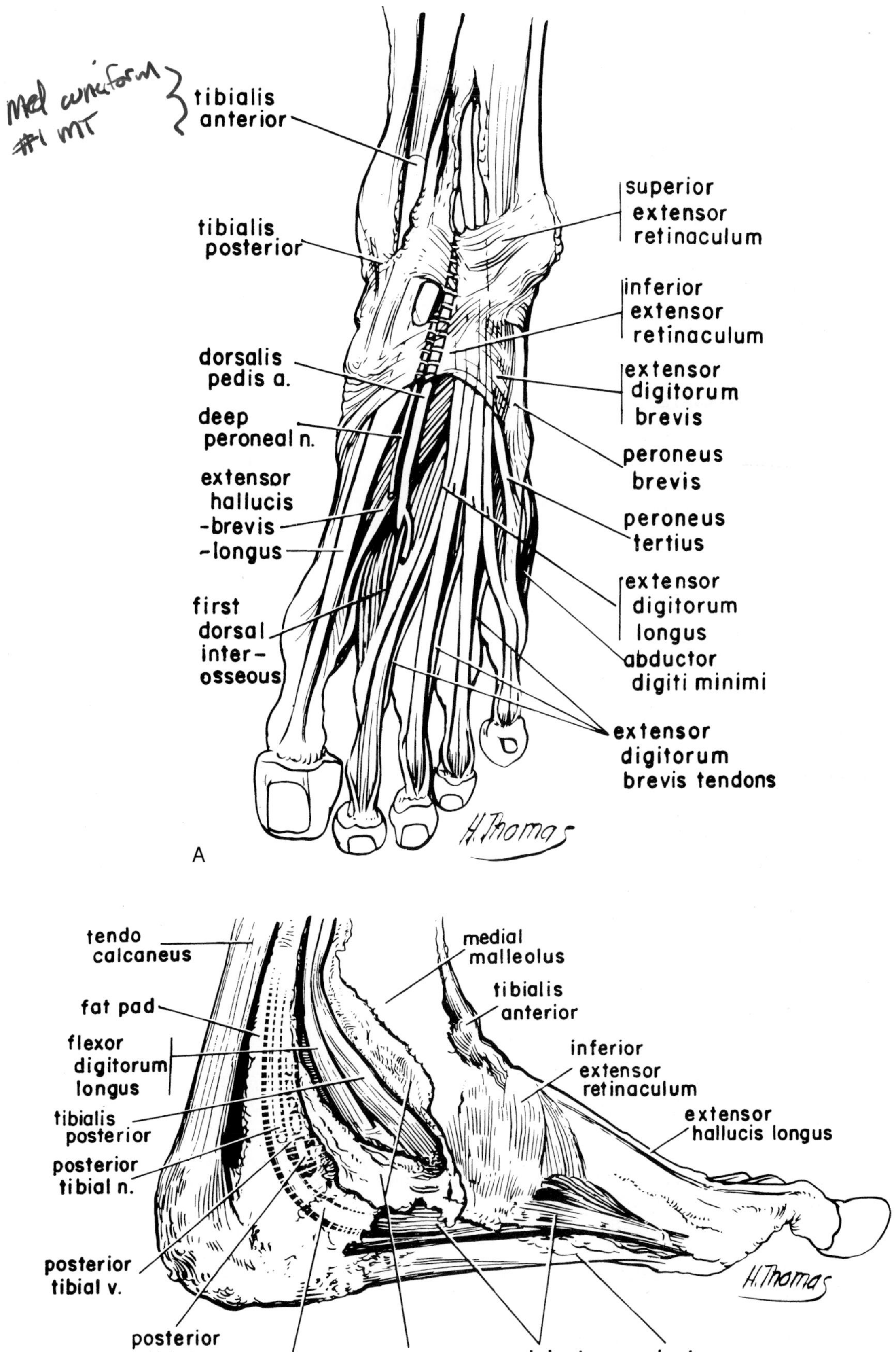
tibialis anterior
tibialis posterior
dorsalis pedis a.
deep peroneal n.
extensor hallucis
-brevis
-longus
first dorsal inter-osseous
superior extensor retinaculum
inferior extensor retinaculum
extensor digitorum brevis
peroneus brevis
peroneus tertius
extensor digitorum longus
abductor digiti minimi
extensor digitorum brevis tendons
H. Thomas
A
tendo calcaneus
fat pad
flexor digitorum longus
tibialis posterior
posterior tibial n.
posterior tibial v.
posterior tibial a.
flexor hallucis longus
flexor retinaculum (reflected)
abductor hallucis
plantar aponeurosis
medial malleolus
tibialis anterior
inferior extensor retinaculum
extensor hallucis longus
H. Thomas
B

Figure 11–67 *See legend on following page*

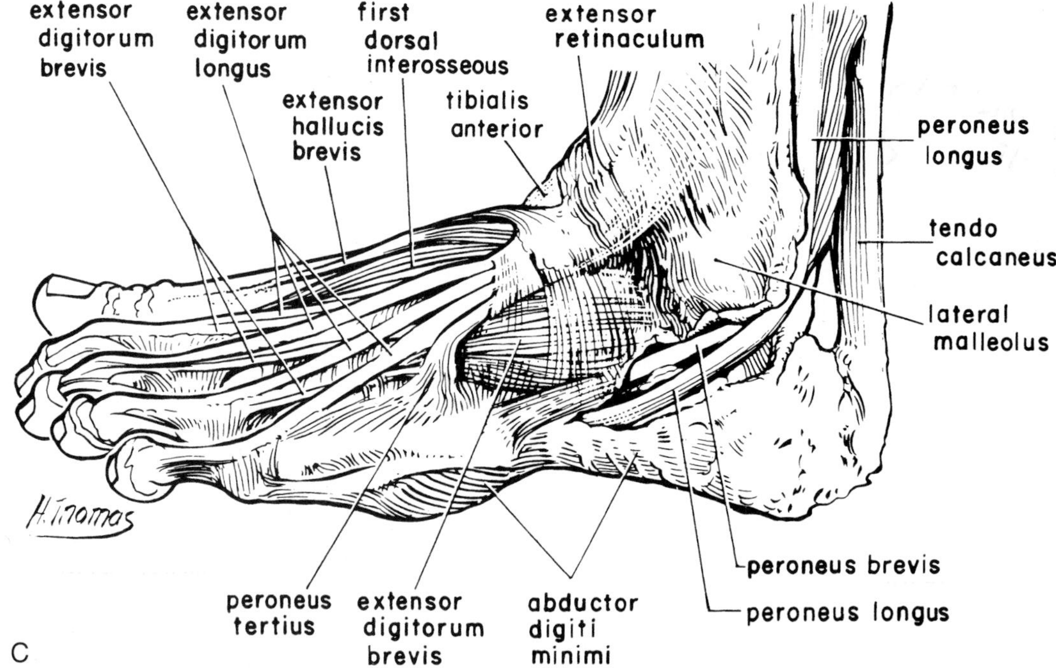

Figure 11–67. Muscles and tendons of the foot. *A*, Dorsal view. *B*, Medial view. *C*, Lateral view. (From Jahss, M.H.: Disorders of the Foot, pp. 18–20. Philadelphia, W.B. Saunders, 1982.)

moved, and the EDB is reflected from its origin to expose the joints. The lateral branch of the deep peroneal nerve (which supplies the EDB) must be protected with this approach. Deep penetration with an instrument from this approach can injure the FHL.

6. Anterolateral Approach to the Midfoot—Requires release of the EDB. The risk of this approach, commonly used for excision

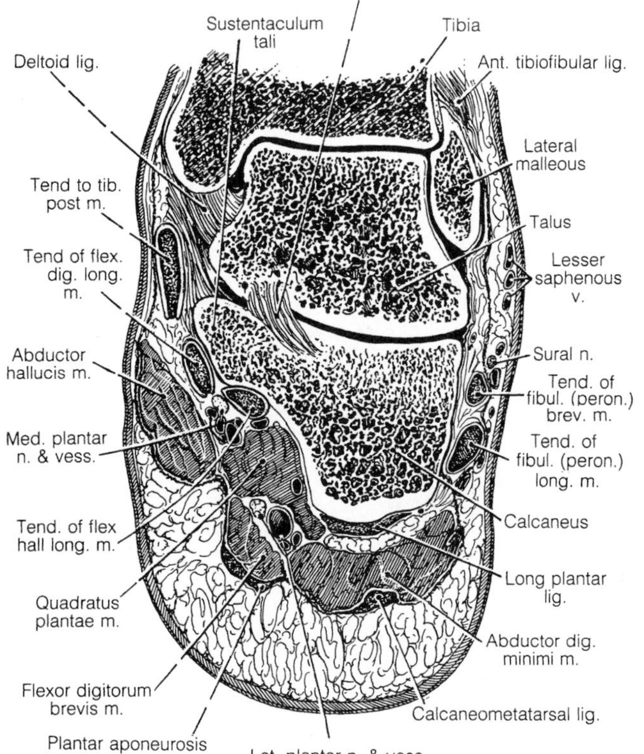

Figure 11–68. Vertical section of the ankle. (From Essentials of Human Anatomy, 9th ed., by Russell T. Woodburne and Willima E. Burkel. Copyright 1957, 1994 by Oxford University Press, Inc. Used by permission of Oxford University Press, Inc.)

of a calcaneonavicular bar, is to the calcaneal navicular (Spring) ligament.

7. Approach to the midfoot and digits is direct and is not discussed in detail. In general, care must be taken to protect digital nerves/arteries.

H. Arthroscopy—Portals used in ankle arthroscopy can put important structures at risk. The anterolateral portal can jeopardize the dorsal lateral cutaneous branch of the superficial peroneal nerve. The anteromedial portal can damage the greater saphenous vein. Anterior central portals are no longer recommended because of risk to the dorsalis pedis artery. Posteromedial portals can injure the posterior tibial artery (and are not recommended), and the posterior lateral portal can injure the sural nerve.

XI. Summary

A. Important anatomic landmarks are summarized in Table 11–1.

B. Surgical Approaches—Key internervous intervals are summarized in Tables 11–2 and 11–3.

Selected Bibliography

Arnoczky, S.P., and Warren, R.F.: Microvasculature of the human meniscus. Am. J. Sports Med. 10(2):90–95, 1982.

Bohlman, H.H.: The Neck. In D'Ambrosia, R., ed.: Muskuloskeletal Disorders. Philadelphia, J.B. Lippincott, 1977.

Bora, F.W.: The Pediatric Upper Extremity. Philadelphia, W.B. Saunders, 1986.

Browner, B.D., Jupiter, J.B., Levine, A.M., et al.: Skeletal Trauma. Philadelphia, W.B. Saunders, 1992.

Callaghan, J.J., ed.: Anatomy Self-Assessment Examination. Park Ridge, IL, American Academy of Orthopaedic Surgeons, 1991.

Cervical Spine Research Education Committee: The Cervical Spine, 2nd ed. Philadelphia, J.B. Lippincott, 1989.

Chapman, M.W., ed.: Operative Orthopaedics. Philadelphia, J.B. Lippincott, 1988.

Chapman, M.W., ed.: Gray's Anatomy, 30th American ed. Philadelphia, Lea & Febiger, 1985.

Cooper, D.E., O'Brien, S.J., and Warren, R.F.: Supporting layers of the glenohumeral joint. Clin. Orthop. 289:144–155, 1993.

Crock, H.V.: An atlas of the arterial supply of the head and neck of the femur in man. Clin. Orthop. 152:17, 1980.

DeLee, J.C., and Drez, D., Jr.: Orthopaedic Sports Medicine: Principles and Practice. Philadelphia, W.B. Saunders, 1994.

Doyle, J.R.: Anatomy of the finger flexor tendon sheath and pulley system. J. Hand Surg. [Am.] 13:473–484, 1988.

Girgis, F.G., Marshall, J.L., and Monajem, A.R.S.: The cruciate ligaments of the knee joint: Anatomical, functional, and experimental analysis. Clin. Orthop. 106:216–231, 1975.

Harding, K.: The direct lateral approach to the hip. J. Bone Joint Surg. [Br.] 64:17–19, 1982.

Henry, A.K.: Extensive Exposure, 2nd ed. New York, Churchill Livingstone, 1973.

Hollinshead, W.H.: Anatomy for Surgeons, vol. 3, 2nd ed. New York, Harper & Row, 1969.

Hoppenfield, S., and DeBoer, P.: Orthopaedics: The Anatomic Approach. Philadelphia, J.B. Lippincott, 1984.

Jahss, M.H.: Disorders of the Foot. Philadelphia, W.B. Saunders, 1987.

Jenkins, D.B.: Hollinshead's Functional Anatomy of the Limbs and Back, 6th ed. Philadelphia, W.B. Saunders, 1991.

Kaplan, E.B.: Surgical Approaches to the Neck, Cervical Spine, and Upper Extremity. Philadelphia, W.B. Saunders, 1966.

Ludloff, K.: The open reduction of the congenital hip dislocation by an anterior incision. Am. J. Orthop. Surg. 10:438, 1913.

Magee, D.J.: Orthopaedic Physical Assessment. Philadelphia, W.B. Saunders, 1987.

Mooney, J.F., Siegel, D.B., and Koman, L.A.: Ligamentous injuries of the wrist in athletes. Clin. Sports Med. 11(1):129–139, 1992.

Morrey, B.F., and An, K.N.: Articular and ligamentous contributions to the stability of the elbow joint. J. Sports Med. 11:315–319, 1983.

Morrey, B.F., and An, K.: Functional anatomy of the ligaments of the elbow. Clin. Orthop. 210:84–90, 1985.

Netter, F.H.: The CIBA Collection of Medical Illustrations, vol. 8: Musculoskeletal System, Part I. Summit, NJ, Ciba-Geigy, 1987.

Orthopaedic Knowledge Update Home Study Syllabus I, II, and III. Chicago, American Academy of Orthopaedic Surgeons, 1984, 1987, 1990.

Rockwood, C.A., Jr., and Green, D.P., eds.: Fractures in Adults, 3rd ed. Philadelphia, J.B. Lippincott, 1991.

Rothman, R.H., and Simeon, F.A.: The Spine, 2nd ed. Philadelphia, W.B. Saunders, 1982.

Ruge, D., and Wiltse, L.L., eds.: Spinal Disorders: Diagnosis and Treatment. Philadelphia, Lea & Febiger, 1977.

Sarrafian, S.K.: Anatomy of the Foot and Ankle. Philadelphia, J.B. Lippincott, 1983.

Seebacher, J.R., Inglis, A.E., Marshall, J.L., et al.: The structure of the posterolateral aspect of the knee. J. Bone Joint Surg. [Am.] 64:536–541, 1982.

Steinberg, M.E.: The Hip and Its Disorders. Philadelphia, W.B. Saunders, 1991.

Tubiana, R.: The Hand. Philadelphia, W.B. Saunders, 1985.

Turkel, S.J., Panio, M.W., Marshall, J.L., and Girgis, F.G.: Stabilizing mechanisms preventing anterior dislocation of the gleno-humeral joint. J. Bone Joint Surg. [Am.] 63:1208–1217, 1981.

Verbiest, H.A.: Lateral approach to the cervical spine: Technique and indications. J. Neurosurg. 28:191–203, 1968.

Warren, I.F., and Marshall, J.L.: The supporting structures and layers on the medial side of the knee. J. Bone Joint Surg. [Am.] 61:56–62, 1979.

Watkins, R.G.: Surgical Approaches to the Spine. New York, Springer-Verlag, 1983.

Weissman, B.N., and Sledge C.B.: Orthopedic Radiology. Philadelphia, W.B. Saunders, 1986.

Woodburne, R.T., and Burkel, W.E.: Essentials of Human Anatomy, 9th ed. New York, Oxford Unversity Press, 1994.

12

Principles of Practice and Statistics

Damian M. Rispoli, Kerry G. Jepsen, and Kevin D. Plancher

I. Impairment, Disability, Handicap
  A. Definitions
    1. Impairments are defined as conditions that interfere with an individual's activities of daily living. Impairment is the loss of use of or derangement of any body part, system, or function. Impairment is what the physician determines based on the objective results of a physical examination.
    2. Disability may be defined as an alteration of an individual's capacity to meet personal, social, or occupational demands or statutory or regulatory requirements because of impairment.
    3. Handicap is related to, but different from the concepts of disability and impairment. Under federal law an individual is handicapped if he or she has an impairment that substantially limits one or more of life's activities, has a record of such impairment, or is regarded as having such impairment. This definition is so broad that almost any person may be considered to be handicapped.
  B. Impairment
    1. An impaired individual is not necessarily disabled. For example, a surgeon who loses a hand will be disabled in terms of the ability to operate; the surgeon may be fully capable of being the chief of a hospital medical staff and may not be at all disabled with respect to that occupation.
    2. Permanent impairment is impairment that has become static or well-stabilized with or without medical treatment and is not likely to remit despite maximal medical treatment.
  C. Disability
    1. Disability may be thought of as the gap between what a person can do and what the person needs or wants to do.
    2. Permanent disability occurs when the degree of capacity becomes static or well-established and is not likely to increase despite continuing use of medical or rehabilitative measures.
    3. To meet the definition of disability, an individual's impairment or combination of impairments must be of such severity that he or she is not only unable to do the work previously done but also cannot perform any other kind of substantial gainful work, considering the individual's age, education, and work experience.
    4. Provisions of the Americans with Disabilities Act (ADA).
      a. Effective July 22, 1992, for private-sector organizations that employ 25 or more employees.
      b. Accommodation refers to modifications of a job or workplace that enables a disabled employee to meet the same job demands and conditions required of any other employee in the same or similar job.
      c. Under the ADA, identification of an individual as having a disability does not depend on the results of a medical examination.
      d. An individual may be identified as having a disability if there is a record of an impairment that has substantially limited one or more major life activities.
    5. Disability causes additional illness.
      a. Feelings of displacement, depression, and suicide increase as disabilities protract.
      b. There is a higher incidence of drug and alcohol abuse, family disruption, and divorce among disabled workers.
      c. Return to employment must be the goal of treatment.
    6. Cost of disability.
      a. The workers' compensation system experienced double-digit increases in cost during the 1970s and 1990s.
      b. Total cost of workers' compensation was approximately $5.2 billion in 1971 and $57.3 billion dollars in 1993.

c. Back injuries were the leading force in driving up medical indemnity expenses.

II. Informed Consent
 A. Decision-making capacity.
  1. A patient must be able to understand the clinical circumstances and the indications for a procedure.
  2. A patient must be able to understand the alternative approaches to the procedure.
  3. A patient must be able to weigh among the alternative approaches and be able and willing to express in an understandable fashion his or her choices.
 B. The level of capacity required of a patient is related to the risks of a procedure and the risk:benefit ratio.
  1. In circumstances when a patient lacks the ability for decision-making, informed consent may be obtained by a legal guardian or in situations deemed medically necessary by a physician.
  2. Special informed consent rules apply to emergencies and minors.
   a. A medical emergency is an unconscious or incapacitated person with a life- or limb-threatening condition requiring immediate medical attention, and treatment can proceed without informed consent.
   b. Consent rules for minors vary greatly from state to state. The surgeon must be aware of those that apply locally. Generally, consent for treatment of minors is obtained from the parent or guardian for all but emergency conditions.
 C. Informed consent as a tool for communication.
  1. Informed consent is a means to facilitate clear communication between the physician and the patient or guardian.
  2. This form should include diagnosis, indications for treatment and treatment proposed, expected outcomes, risks and complications of the proposed approach, and the alternatives with their risks and complications.
  3. An entry should be also be made in the permanent record creating the so-called double consent.
  4. Some states have specific guidelines on the disclosure of risks and complications. However, the majority of the states use the **professional or reasonable physician standard.** Another standard that may be used is the **patient viewpoint standard,** which is based on what a reasonable person would want to know if faced with a similar medical decision.
  5. Most litigation results from unexpected consequences of a procedure. Properly informed patients will be aware of and have decided to accept both benefits and risks.

III. Elements of Malpractice
 A. Malpractice is defined as negligence by a health-care provider that results in injury to a patient. A malpractice suit is a civil action filed by a patient alleging that a physician's negligence resulted in an injury for which the patient desires compensation.
  1. Negligence is the result of failure to exercise the degree of diligence and care that a reasonable and prudent person would exercise under the same or similar conditions.
  2. Medical negligence is composed of four elements: duty, **breach of duty, causation,** and **damages.**
   a. The duty of the physician is to provide care equal to the local standard.
    i. Standard of care is not universal and is established by local expert opinion.
    ii. **Residents and fellows are held to the same standard of care as board-certified orthopaedists.**
   b. **Breach of duty** occurs when action or failure to act deviates from the standard of care.
   c. **Causation** must demonstrate that failure to meet the standard of care was the direct cause of the patient's injuries.
   d. **Damages** are monies awarded as compensation for injuries sustained as the result of medical negligence.
    i. **Special damages** are actual expenses such as medical/rehabilitative expenses and lost wages.
    ii. **General damages** or "noneconomic losses" are awards for pain and suffering, disfigurement, etc.
    iii. **Punitive damages** serve as a penalty for blatant disregard or incompetence. These are seldom awarded.
    iv. **Ad damnum clause** is the portion of a plaintiff's complaint that specifies the amount of money sought for damages in a suit. Some states do not allow this clause to be included as part of a lawsuit.
  3. The **comparative negligence doctrine** awards damages based on the percentage of responsibility for the result by each party.
  4. **Contributory negligence** bars recovery of damages if there was negligence on the part of the plaintiff.
  5. **Modified comparative fault** bars recovery of damages if the plaintiff's percentage of negligence exceeds 50%.

B. Bad Faith Action—The filing of a claim and pursuit of action regardless of the lack of reasonable grounds for filing the claim. In these circumstances the physician may countersue for damages.

C. Expert testimony.
1. Expert testimony is used to determine the standard of care and whether a breach of conduct has occurred.
2. The American Academy of Orthopaedic Surgeons (AAOS) definition of expert testimony.
   a. A physician with an unrestricted license to practice medicine.
   b. Satisfactory completion of the educational requirements of the American Board of Orthopaedic Surgery or a recognized specialty board.
   c. Be qualified by experience or have demonstrated competence in the subject of the case.
   d. Be familiar with clinical practice and applicable standard of care in orthopaedic surgery at the time of the incident.
3. The expert should ensure the testimony is nonpartisan, scientifically correct, and clinically accurate. The expert should testify only to the facts.
4. It is unethical to accept compensation based on the outcome of the litigation; however, reasonable compensation commensurate with time and expertise is acceptable.

D. Res ipsa loquitor.
1. Certain cases do not require expert testimony.
2. This is the legal doctrine of **res ipsa loquitor** ("the thing speaks for itself"). Examples of this are wrong-site surgery, surgical equipment inadvertently left in the patient, and failure of a physician to attend to a persistently complaining patient in distress.

E. Statute of limitations.
1. A plaintiff must file the malpractice suit within the statute of limitations.
   a. Commonly, the **statute of limitations is 2 years.** However, this may vary by state.
   b. The statute of limitations for **minors** may also vary by state; it is generally considered to be **2 years from the time of the incident or until the individual's 18th birthday to file a claim.**

F. Discovery.
1. Discovery is the process by which both parties find out about each other's cases and is a period of information-gathering.
2. Discovery is formed by several techniques of fact-gathering.
   a. **Interrogatories**—Written questions answered in writing under oath.
   b. **Deposition**—Pretrial oral testimony given under oath.
   c. **Production Request**—Producing documents regarding a claim.
   d. **Request for Admission**—Admitting or denying factual statements under oath.

IV. Medical Records

A. Medical records represent the best defense in a malpractice lawsuit.
1. Medical records must be maintained for 7 years after the last date of treatment.
2. Records are confidential and can be released only to the patient, the attorney, or an authorized representative on receipt of a signed request.
3. **The physician must never forget that risk management begins the moment a patient is engaged in a physician-patient relationship.**

B. Accurate and complete medical records protect both the patient and physician from errors and misinterpretations. Records should be:
1. Well documented, detailing the history, observations, and reasons for treatment provided.
2. Legible and clear.
3. Accurate and properly identify the appropriate patient.
4. A logical sequence of the events and factors affecting treatment decisions.
5. An outline of the treatment plan, including risks, benefits, and alternatives.
6. Free from editorial comments or casual criticism of the patient or other health-care providers.

C. Medical records should never be altered.
1. All corrections should be made by amendments. Amendments should accurately reflect the reason for correction and be placed following the last entry.
2. Any errant entry should be lined through so that it remains legible. The reason for the correction, the date, time, and the physician's initials must be included.
3. Removing or obscuring an entry shatters credibility and is indefensible.
4. Attempts to supplement or clarify entries after notification of a lawsuit constitutes tampering.

D. On notification of a lawsuit, the medical records should be secured, inventoried, and copied. Copies of the medical record must be made available to the patient or the attorney in a reasonable amount of time. **The medical record must not be withheld to ransom payment of outstanding bills.**

V. Physician-Patient Relationship

A. The physician-patient relationship is a consensual relationship.
   1. The relationship is established by a telephone call, a visit, or by the choice of a consultant from a provider list.
   2. Rights and responsibilities related to the relationship.
      a. The patient has a right to courteous, confidential, and prompt treatment.
      b. The patient has the responsibility to be compliant with the treatment plan.
      c. Physicians have the responsibility to request appropriate consultation and to relinquish responsibility when the care of the patient reaches outside their scope of practice.
      d. Physicians must read their managed care contract before committing to the relationship. They must understand their legal responsibilities before executing an agreement to be supervising physicians for an allied health-care company.
   3. Physicians who utilized empathy in their day-to-day interactions with patients increase the perception that they are caring and enhance their day-to-day enjoyment of medical practice.
   4. Effective communication enhances patient compliance and increases quality of outcome.
   5. Office staff interactions with the patient may have a direct effect on the physician-patient relationship.
      a. Having established policies and procedures to guide the patient through the system will foster a positive relationship.
      b. As an employer, hire wisely, supervise diligently, and weigh carefully the needs of your practice and your patients when hiring employees.

B. The difficult patient.
   1. Each patient's individual needs should be identified and focused on by the physician rather than responded to generally.
      a. Characterization of patients in terms such as "loser," "addict," "druggie," "troll," or "gomer" is stereotyping. Such terms divert the physician's attention from the issue that must be tackled with each individual.
      b. It is helpful to attempt to understand difficult patients by exploring the individual circumstances from the patient's perspective.
      c. Try to attempt to evaluate goals for care in terms that the patient would both agree with and understand.
      d. The physician may need to modify the aim. This may include the need at times to reformulate the focus from cure to incremental improvement or palliation.
   2. Ending the physician-patient relationship.
      a. Physicians must always provide emergent treatment to continuity patients.
      b. For patients with whom an insolvable conflict occurs or for patients who can no longer pay for their services, the physician may sever the physician-patient relationship so long as an alternative source of care can be identified.
      c. This is best accomplished in writing and should provide the patient with ample time to establish care with the new provider.
      d. Medical records should be forwarded to the accepting physician, including a medical history and a summary of treatments rendered. Date of shipping and receipt of records should be documented.

C. Abandonment.
   1. Wrongful termination of the physician-patient relationship consists of four basic elements.
      a. There must be an established physician-patient relationship.
      b. The patient must have a reasonable expectation that care will be provided.
      c. The patient must have a medical need that requires medical attention, the absence of which will result in harm or injury.
      d. Causation must be established. The failure to provide care must produce injury or harm.
   2. Abandonment may take many forms.
      a. It may be alleged that the patient's follow-up is inadequate to recognize common complications.
      b. Failure to provide an appointment to an established patient even if the patient has not paid previous bills, missed other appointments, has been noncompliant, or has sought interim care from another provider.
      c. Premature discharge from an inpatient setting.
      d. If illness, personal conflict, or vacation prevents the physician from attending to patient care, immediate notice must be issued to allow the patient the opportunity to seek care elsewhere.
      e. If a patient does not appear for important follow-up appointments, a certified letter should be sent instructing the patient to follow-up.

D. Medical referrals.
   1. A medical referral aims to obtain services that the referring physician is unable to render to the patient.

a. Selection of a consultant should be based primarily on the consultant's ability to handle the patient's clinical care.
b. Choice of a consultant involves not only consideration of technical skill but also the elements of the physician-patient relationship, insurance type accepted by the consultant, and perhaps even factors such as gender or ethnicity.
c. Under no circumstances should consideration be influenced by factors such as kickback.
d. Monetary compensation in exchange for referrals is illegal.
e. It is also unacceptable for the primary care physician to choose a consultant incapable of providing the necessary care just because that consultant was picked by a health plan.
f. It is the physician's responsibility to ensure that health plans to which they subscribe permit adequate access to qualified specialists. If not, the physicians must lobby for referral outside their panel.

VI. Malpractice Insurance

A. There are two basic types of malpractice insurance: occurrence and claims-made.
1. **Occurrence coverage** covers the insured for all claims resulting from action during the period of employment covered by the policy regardless of when the claim is filed. It continues to cover the physician for occurrences during a specific time period even after the physician has ceased working at that particular job/location.
2. **Claims-made coverage** covers the insured during a particular period of employment covered by the policy. Claims filed after the expiration of the policy (usually when the physician leaves a particular job/employer) are not covered even if the events occurred during the period of coverage.
a. **Tail coverage** is a separate policy that covers the physician for all claims made for actions occurring during the period of coverage; this essentially makes an occurrence policy.
b. **Prior acts coverage** protects the insured from claims resulting from events for which claims have yet to be filed.
3. **Locum tenens coverage** is coverage that is extended to a physician temporarily replacing the policyholder.
4. **Slot coverage** covers duties encountered while practicing in a specific position through which several physicians may rotate.

B. Policies may have specific restrictions or exclusions.
1. Some policies cover only direct patient care.
2. Activities such as peer review, quality assurance, and utilization review may be covered by the insurance policy or by a health-care contract.
3. **Hold Harmless Clause**—This contractual statement attempts to shift liability from the employer to the physician. Insurance carriers do not generally cover this contractual obligation.

C. **Surcharging or Experience Rating**—Insurance plans may assess points against a physician based on the number of claims filed and dollar amounts awarded on behalf of the insured.

D. **The Good Samaritan Act**—This act grants immunity for good faith acts performed by persons at the scene of an emergency. Immunity is not given if the act constitutes gross, willful, or wanton neglect. This does not extend to care given in expectation of payment by persons who routinely render care in an emergency room or by the patient's admitting, attending, or treating physician.

VII. Special Liability Status of Residents and Fellows—The status of residents and fellows as licensed physicians who are functioning as employees while in a training/educational program creates a special relationship between them and their patients and supervisors.

A. Failure to inform a patient of residency/fellow status may result in claims of fraud, deceit, misrepresentation, assault, battery, and lack of informed consent.

B. Residents and fellows are responsible for their own actions. In addition, their supervisors may also be held accountable for the actions of their residents and fellows. This is known as **vicarious liability.**

C. **Respondeat superior**—An agency relationship is established from the fact that the resident has been authorized to act for or represent the supervising physician. As an agent for the supervisor, all acts of the relationship are considered to be under the direction of the supervisor. This term means "let the master answer." This doctrine is also known as "borrowed servant" or the "captain of the ship." This relationship is independent of the specific employer of the trainee.

D. **Residents and fellows are held to the same standard of care as a fully trained practicing orthopaedist, regardless of their level of training.** Residents should not attempt to perform procedures that are beyond their level of training. Appropriate consultation with their supervisor is imperative in any situation. Lack of appropriate consultation puts the resident at risk of acting independent of the supervisor.

VIII. Ethical Practice of Orthopaedic Surgery

A. Physician-patient contract.

1. An orthopaedic surgeon may choose whom he or she will treat. The surgeon may not discriminate based solely on race, color, gender, sexual orientation, religion, or national origin.
2. After engaging the patient, the surgeon may not neglect the care of the patient.
3. The patient may enter into or withdraw from the physician-patient contract at any time without penalty.

B. HIV testing and treatment of the HIV-infected patient.

1. Explicit informed consent is required for HIV testing.
2. The implications of HIV testing may have substantial social and economic consequences for the individual testing positive.
   a. Future life, disability, and health insurance may be difficult to obtain if medical records contain a positive HIV result.
   b. HIV positivity may compromise the ability to obtain housing and employment and cause social injuries.
   c. Many states have statutes requiring that explicit consent be documented in the medical record or that written consent be provided before HIV testing is performed.
   d. The orthopaedic surgeon should know the law in his or her particular state.
3. Reasons why an orthopaedist may order an HIV test.
   a. The HIV status of an individual might affect the physician's consideration of diagnosis and of therapeutic alternative.
   b. Knowledge of a positive HIV test result may lead the physician and operating room team to uphold infection precautions more strongly, thus reducing the risk of HIV transmission from the patient.
   c. To avoid performing procedures on patients who are HIV-infected.
      i. This would diminish a patient's access to necessary medical care and in almost all cases is ethically unacceptable.
      ii. The physician has a fiduciary responsibility to act in the best interest of his or her patient, but this does not include actions that place the physician at substantial risk.
      iii. It has been shown that many physicians overestimate their risk of HIV transmission from a patient.
      iv. Deciding whether a particular surgical procedure places an undue risk on the surgeon and the operative team, that surgeon must attempt to accurately gauge the actual risk associated with the patient.

C. Industry and the orthopaedic surgeon.

1. Medicine and industry work together in improving the treatment of patients. This relationship is even more pronounced in orthopaedics because of the required implants, materials, and techniques.
2. Ethical conduct demands that the educational support of the orthopaedist by industry is not excessive, does not profit the company directly, and has the purpose of improving patient care through education.
3. Personal gifts should not exceed $100 dollars in value and should have educational benefit. Cash or direct payments should never be accepted.
4. Subsidies for conferences or professional meetings are acceptable as they represent an opportunity for continuing medical education. Any subsidy should be paid directly to the conference sponsor. **Educational subsidies should not be applied to personal expenses (travel, lodging) for attendees.**
5. It is acceptable for faculty to receive honoraria and reimbursement for travel, lodging, and meals in return for their participation.

D. Loyalties and conflicts of interest.

1. The physician's role is to use his or her expertise to select the best possible orthopaedic hardware, medication, or treatment for a particular patient's needs. Decisions should be based on:
   a. Clinical trials in the published medical literature.
   b. The clinician's expertise.
   c. The clinician's perspective of the patient's preference.
   d. Monetary issues should enter into the decision process in the realm of cost-effectiveness.
      i. Monetary considerations may include limitations of the patient's resources or needs.
      ii. There is no role in this decision for consideration of factors that benefit the physician. This is particularly true for financial compensation.
2. Compensation may potentially affect a physician's decision-making concerning

the choice of a particular hardware, medication, or treatment.

a. **In this circumstance, the physician must disclose to the patient that he or she receives this financial compensation.**

3. In circumstances in which a physician has developed a novel therapeutic modality that is clearly superior to anything else available, the clinician might state to the patient, "I participated in development of this product and received compensation for its use. Based on published clinical trials and in my opinion, it is the best product for your use."

E. Advertising.
   1. Federal and state antitrust laws protect truthful advertising.
   2. Truthful advertising must not contain any overtly false claim nor imply a false claim that would affect a reasonably prudent person. It should only include claims that can be substantiated by the physician and not omit any fact that would influence a reasonably prudent person.
   3. Claims should be representative of expected results for the average patient.
   4. Care should be exercised when using terms like "safe and effective," because the lay person equates these terms with no risk and a guarantee of a good result.
   5. Advertising of physicians' qualifications should reflect the amount of formal training and degree of expertise and competence.

F. Royalties.
   1. Similar to financial interests, any items of money, including royalties received from a manufacturer, must be disclosed to the patient.
   2. It is unethical to receive any payment (excluding royalties) from the manufacturer for the use of its product.
   3. It is unethical for the physician to agree to **exclusively use** a product for which the physician receives royalties.

G. Patents—The nature of medical practice builds on innovations and ideas and to claim exclusive rights to a procedure denies all former individual contributions. The additional fallout from such patents would limit medical education, increase the cost of delivered services, and jeopardize the quality of patient care. The AAOS states that procedure patents are unethical.

H. Second Opinions—Definition of specific relationships between physicians and their responsibilities to their colleagues and patients can avoid inappropriate actions. Clear and direct communication between parties involved can eliminate most problems.
   1. **Consultation** implies that the treating physician retains care for the patient but is requesting additional diagnostic or treatment expertise from the consultant. **It is unethical for the consulting physician to solicit care of a patient** or to proffer slanderous accusations about the referring physician.
   2. **Referral** implies the treating physician desires to share care of the patient for a specific service. This request may be temporary or permanent and should be made clear at the outset by the physicians involved.
   3. **Transfer** by the treating physician implies complete transfer of care to the accepting physician. All transfers must be made with the consent of the patient.
   4. Second opinions secured by third party payers prior to authorizing procedures are usually governed by contractual agreements. The physician must be aware of provisions in the contract regarding assumption of care.

IX. Research—Clinical and basic research provides a tremendous opportunity for improvement of the diagnosis and treatment of orthopaedic disease.

A. Ethical research is conducted when the primary goal is to improve methods of detection or treatment of illness. It should be designed to produce useful, reproducible information and should not be redundant or serve to further individuals or institutions financially or professionally.

B. Results should be reported honestly, accurately, and in a timely fashion. Misrepresentation or falsifying data is unethical.

C. Withholding critical information to protect financial interest may create an ethical conflict and jeopardize patient care.

D. Sponsorship by industry has represented a potential conflict of interest or bias; however, significant developments have been made possible by their involvement, and this form of cooperative effort is gaining acceptance. Specific ethical problems arise with this type of research funding.
   1. Financial interests of the researcher through stock holdings, stock options, or profit-sharing agreements with the funding corporation may introduce bias or jeopardize objectivity in reporting results.
   2. It is unethical once a researcher is involved in a project funded by a corporation to buy or sell the corporation's stock until the project is complete or results are made a matter of public record.
   3. All areas of corporate involvement including resources, materials, and sponsorship must be disclosed as part of reporting results.

E. **Human research subjects require a vol-**

untary informed consent before participating in any research protocol. Their medical care must not be contingent on their participation, and they must be allowed to withdraw from the study at any time without penalty. Each subject must be able to demonstrate understanding of the information and the ability to make a responsible decision. The decision must be voluntary and not the result of undue pressure or influence. A voluntary informed consent must include the following:

1. An explanation of the proposed procedure.
2. Likely effects and risks of the procedure.
3. Possible side effects in a language easily understood by the patient.
4. Methods and conditions of participation.

F. Responsibilities of the principal investigator (PI) and the coauthors.

1. The PI remains responsible for all aspects of the research project, even when duties have been delegated to others.
2. The PI is also responsible for accurately representing efforts of individuals or agencies involved in the research and citing contributions from other researchers or publications.
3. Coauthors must have made a significant contribution to the design of, collection of data for, and forming of the document.
4. Each coauthor should sign an affidavit stating that he or she has reviewed the manuscript and agrees with all results and conclusions presented therein prior to publication.
5. Resident research should be conducted under the supervision of an attending surgeon. However, the attending surgeon must contribute to the work in actual fact or in a consultative capacity.

G. Scientific publications—Scientific publications create information that impacts other research and direct care of patients. If error in scientific method or failure to replicate results is found, the PI is responsible to accurately report them.

X. The Impaired Physician

A. A surgeon (resident, fellow, or attending) who discovers chemical impairment, dependence, or incompetence in a colleague or supervisor has the responsibility to ensure the problem is identified and treated.

B. Mechanisms exist for the proper identification and treatment of the impaired physician.

1. Misconduct can be reported to state and local agencies. One must be sure to act in "good faith" with reasonable evidence when reporting such incidences.
2. If a patient is at risk for immediate harm or injury by an impaired physician, one should assert authority and relieve the physician of the patient care and then address the problem with the senior hospital staff as soon as possible.

XI. Sexual Misconduct—Sexual misconduct in a physician's relationships with patients, coworkers, staff, or colleagues cannot be tolerated. Sexual relationships between individuals while maintaining a professional supervisor/trainee relationship, even if consensual, create the potential for sexual exploitation and the loss of objectivity. Supervisors may need to be reassigned or responsibilities may need to be modified to avoid potential conflict.

A. Sexual harassment can be characterized as:

1. Quid Pro Quo—Harassment is directly linked to employment or advancement.
2. Hostile Environment Harassment—Verbal or physical conduct (gestures, innuendo, humor, pictures, etc.) promotes a hostile environment in the workplace.

B. The adopted standard for offensive behavior is the "reasonable woman" test. If a reasonable woman would have found the behavior objectionable, then harassment may have occurred.

C. Individuals in medical training programs are considered employees of the school that is training them. This status allows them to pursue harassment claims under the Civil Rights Act.

D. Sexual misconduct with patients.

1. This is simply a form of sexual exploitation.
2. Such misconduct is unethical and may represent malpractice or even criminal acts of assault. Courts have maintained that a patient is unable to give meaningful consent to sexual or romantic advances.
3. Many states have laws prohibiting physicians from pursuing relationships with current or former patients.
   a. These laws protect the patient from exploitation.
   b. They help the physician to maintain objectivity in diagnosis and treatment.
   c. The physician-patient relationship must be terminated before pursuing any romantic interest. Even then, it may still be unethical if the physician exploits certain confidences, trust, or emotions learned while serving as the patient's physician.

XII. Violence—Each year intentional violence claims 20,000 lives, is responsible for over 300,000 hospitalizations, and causes millions of injuries. It is estimated that 1.4 million children in the United States suffer some form of maltreatment each year. As many as 2000 children die each year from abuse. **The U.S. Child Abuse Prevention and Treatment Act of 1974 requires orthopaedic surgeons to report all suspected cases**

of child abuse to local authorities. Failure to report suspected child abuse might result in state disciplinary actions.

A. Physicians have a specific legal duty to identify and report violence against children.
B. Child protective services and social workers should be alerted and the events and home circumstances should be investigated.
C. These statutes provide immunity for physicians when reporting such cases provided they act in good faith, even if the information is protected by the physician-patient privilege.
D. Elderly abuse has been estimated to affect 2 million older Americans each year. Many states have provided legislation to protect physicians who report elderly abuse from liability.
E. Reporting of spousal abuse is not protected. A physician may encourage a patient to pursue such measures. If the physician believes that an individual is truly incapable of self-protection, then a court order may be obtained to permit reporting.

XIII. Managed Care—Health maintenance organizations (HMOs) have become increasingly prevalent. Currently one in five persons with health insurance is enrolled in an HMO. This shift has necessitated physician groups to contract with HMOs. HMOs are shifting to create direct access to certain specialties. Orthopaedics is a specialty that lends itself to direct contracting with managed care groups. In order to re-establish both economic control and clinical autonomy, many physicians are forming alliances to compete for and negotiate contracts with HMOs. It is essential to understand the basic principles of each form of organization.

A. Health Maintenance Organization (HMO)—Any organization that arranges or provides a health-care plan to enrollees on a prepaid basis.
B. Preferred Provider Organization (PPO)—A group of health-care providers, including hospitals, who agree to provide health-care services on a fee-for-service basis to a group of insured patients.
C. Physician Practice Management (PPM) Company—This is currently the most popular concept emerging in the United States. The PPM company represents large physician groups and acts as an intermediary between the physicians and the HMOs. PPMs are usually created by purchasing physician-owned practices and their hard assets. Physicians retain control by serving on a governing board.
D. Independent Practice Association (IPA)—IPAs contract directly with physicians for provision of services to HMO members. Physicians maintain their independence, and the IPA has no ownership role in the practices, but it allows physicians to contract collectively.
E. Management Service Organization (MSO)—MSOs provide various administrative services for either a set fee or a percentage of revenues. They are not involved with contract negotiations or other aspects of delivering care.
F. Physician Hospital Organization (PHO)—PHOs form to market physician and hospital services for volume contracts to HMOs. They have generally performed poorly.
G. Physician-Sponsored Organization (PSO)—These networks provide services identical to those of an HMO except they are owned and operated by physician members. Antitrust laws have been amended to allow physician ownership of HMOs. This organization eliminates the HMO intermediary and associated expenses.

XIV. Physician Statements by the AAOS

A. Regarding reimbursement of the first assistant at surgery.
   1. No national standard exists.
   2. Quality of care must be maintained, and the ultimate decision remains for the operating surgeon.
B. Regarding the scope of orthopaedic practice and the managed care arrangement.
   1. The AAOS opposes any arrangement in which orthopaedic surgeons are excluded from the provision of musculoskeletal care.
   2. The AAOS approves immediate performance and interpretation of diagnostic imaging and studies.
   3. The AAOS opposes any policy that prohibits orthopaedists from performing x-ray studies. Orthopaedists are entitled to adequate compensation for their interpretation of diagnostic imaging studies.
C. Regarding second opinions.
   1. Both the patient and the orthopaedist are free to enter or discontinue the relationship with any existing contract with a third party.
D. Regarding discovery after surgery.
   1. If after the surgical procedure it is determined that the surgery was performed at the wrong site, as soon as reasonably possible the surgeon should discuss the mistake with the patient and, if appropriate, with the patient's family and recommend an immediate plan to rectify the mistake unless there is a medical reason not to proceed.

XV. Introduction to Statistics—As a consumer of medical research, the orthopaedic surgeon needs to have a firm grasp of statistical concepts. The ability to discern superior from inferior research allows the surgeon to make sound clinical decisions and enhance surgical outcomes. An ability to understand statistics allows a surgeon to generalize with confidence about a given population based on the study of a small subset of that population. It enables critical evaluation of large chunks of data by reducing them to understandable indices. Relationships can be identified, outcomes can be measured and predicted, and practice can be based on proven fact in place of chance occurrence.

XVI. Basic Terminology

A. Basic terminology in design.

1. **Hypothesis**—A supposition or unproven theory. The research hypothesis is the theory believed to be true. The null hypothesis is the opposite of the research hypothesis.
2. **Theory**—A hypothesis with proof; a grouping of relationships based on scientific proof.
3. **Natural Law**—A collection of proven theories; an event or occurrence that has been proved to occur in a specific manner in a given set of circumstances.
4. **Population**—A collection of all possible measurements that could be used to address a hypothesis.
5. **Sample**—A subset of the population. Samples should be random; that is, all members of the population should have an equal chance of being selected to ensure the sample is representative of the population as a whole. Nonrandom samples introduce bias into the study.
6. **Bias**—A flaw in impartiality that alters the manner in which measurement, analysis, or assessment is recorded, conducted, or interpreted. Two forms of bias are selection and observation/information.
   a. Selection bias is introduced by a nonrandom selection of a sample from a given population.
   b. Observational or informational bias is when a measurement/outcome is affected by the characteristics of the study group itself.
   c. Lost to follow-up. This is a potential bias for a study outcome. The question remains: are these patients better or worse from the study population or sample?
   d. Ways to minimize the introduction of bias into a study include randomization, masking (formerly referred to as blinding), and meticulous attention to the study protocol.
7. **Confounding Factors**—Variables that can interfere with the researcher's ability to draw statistically valid conclusions. Matching is a strategy utilized to minimize the effect of confounding factors. Always try to minimize bias and confounding factors to increase the strength of a study.
8. **Efficacy**—A term important in outcomes research that refers to a treatment working under ideal conditions.
9. **Effectiveness**—Another term important in outcomes research that refers to how a treatment works in real-world conditions.
10. **Inclusion/Exclusion criteria**—Criteria determined during experimental design that define the study population.
11. **Randomization**—Minimizes confounding variables to equalize them in all small groups.
12. **Accuracy**—This tests the issue of data differentiation. The ideal test should always be accurate.
13. **Precision**—The ability to repeat measurements accurately.
14. **Matching**—Matching controls decrease confounding variables. Example: All people with the same age are put together in a study.
15. **Instrument**—A measurement tool.

B. Basic terminology in assessment.

1. Once a study has been evaluated or designed using the preceding principles, then the manner in which the data are subsequently collected or interpreted must be designed or assessed. This leads to the principle of accuracy: specifically, the ability to correctly identify data collected or evaluated by a study. The concept of precision is slightly different; it is the ability to arrive at the same data point with repeated testing. Other critical concepts in assessment of tests are sensitivity, specificity, positive predictive value, and negative predictive value.
   a. **Sensitivity** is the ability of a test to detect that which is truly positive.
   b. **Specificity** is the ability to detect that which is truly negative.
   c. Positive predictive value is the chance that a condition is present if identified by a positive test.
   d. Negative predictive value is the opposite, the chance that a condition is not present as identified by a negative test result.

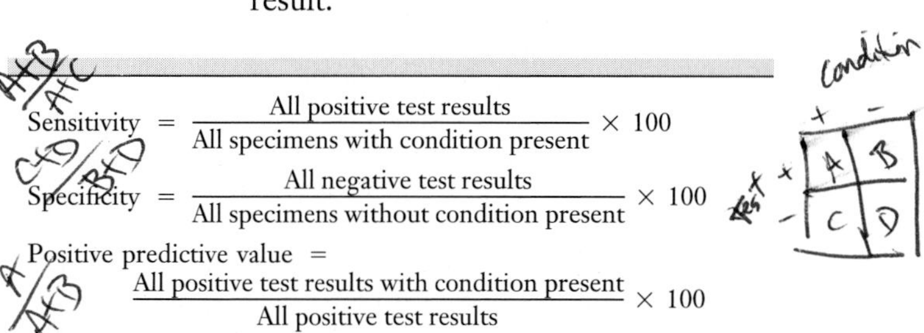

$$\text{Sensitivity} = \frac{\text{All positive test results}}{\text{All specimens with condition present}} \times 100$$

$$\text{Specificity} = \frac{\text{All negative test results}}{\text{All specimens without condition present}} \times 100$$

$$\text{Positive predictive value} = \frac{\text{All positive test results with condition present}}{\text{All positive test results}} \times 100$$

$$\text{Negative predictive value} = \frac{\text{All negative test results without condition present}}{\text{All negative test results}} \times 100$$

2. When dealing with a clinical condition, it is important to remember that these concepts are intimately intertwined. As the sensitivity of a test increases, the negative predictive value increases, a desirable trait for a screening test for an uncommon condition. If a condition is common, then a test with higher specificity and subsequently a higher positive predictive value is more desirable.
3. Prevalence is the total occurrence of a condition in a population whether diagnosed or not. Incidence refers to those conditions identified/diagnosed in a population during a specific time interval. These concepts are critical in designing or evaluating a study to determine whether the study will accurately answer the hypothesis it proposes without under- or overestimation.

XVII. Statistical Power/Power Analysis—Accepting or rejecting the null hypothesis is the basic thrust of all scientific studies. The research hypothesis becomes that which the scientist theorizes to be true. The null hypothesis is the antithesis; it is that which the scientist hopes to statistically reject. The scientist may be correct or incorrect. **Rejecting a true null hypothesis is referred to as a type I or alpha error.** In this case, the scientist's research hypothesis was falsely accepted as positive; hence, this is a false-positive result. The probability of committing a type I error is the P-value. **Accepting a false null hypothesis is a type II or beta error.** The scientist has falsely accepted a negative null hypothesis; hence, this is a false-negative result. Beta is used to signify the frequency of a type II error occurring. Alpha is the frequency of a type I error occurring. Alpha and beta are inversely related.

Power is akin to a type II error or the probability of rejecting the null hypothesis when it is actually false. Power is the likelihood that a statistically significant difference would be found between two groups given that a difference truly did exist. Increasing sample size and improving experimental design can maximize power. Sample size is the number of subjects in a study population. A **power analysis** is a statistical process that allows experimenters to determine the sample size that allows them to make statistically valid conclusions based on a study design. A simple estimate of sample size can be determined using the Rule of Three. The Rule of Three is that if a condition has an occurrence of 1 in 10, then the researcher needs a population three times this number (30) for a statistically significant study.

Probability mathematics allows one to quantify uncertainty and randomness. There are many different statistical tests that can be utilized to arrive at a probability statement, or P-value, for a given study design. The P-value is defined as the probability that the null hypothesis is false; thus, it is the probability of the researcher committing a type I error. The stated P-value in a study alerts the reader of the magnitude of chance that the study arrived at the conclusion serendipitously. It is imperative to note that in a multiple comparison study, the chance of making a conclusion by chance alone increases, and the P-value should be adjusted downward (Fig. 12–1).

Type I error = Alpha, false-positive (Protect against with significance levels.)
Type II error = Beta, false-negative (Protect against with statistical power.)

XVIII. Hypothesis Testing—P-values less than 0.05 are generally accepted as statistically significant. A P-value less than a given number assigns statistical significance to a finding. This, however, does not immediately assign clinical significance to a finding. This is where the idea of confidence intervals assists critical evaluation of a study. Based on a normal distribution, the 95% confidence interval means all values falling within $\pm \sim 2$ standard deviations from the mean. A confidence interval is the range of values that includes the true value within a given probability (usually 95%).

XIX. Statistical Tests

A. Discrete data are also known as noncontinuous, categorical, or qualitative. This type of

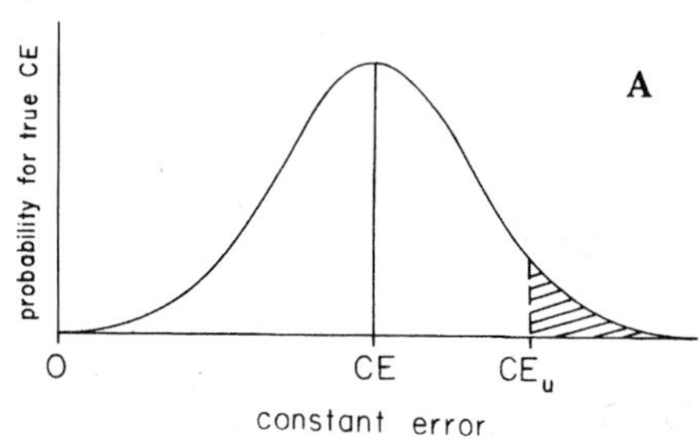

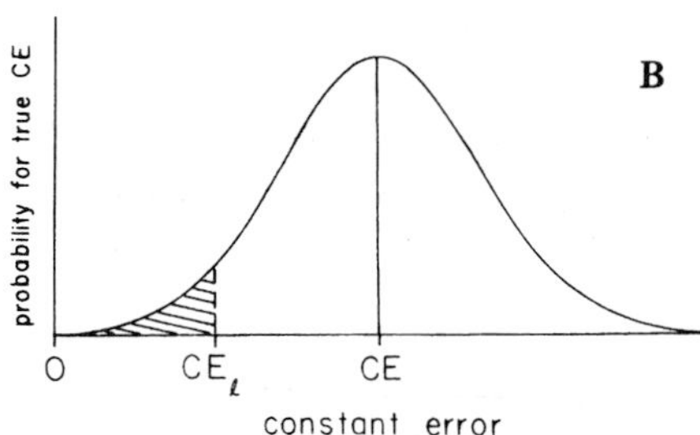

Figure 12–1. *A,* One-sided 95% upper limit of constant error, CE_u. *B,* One-sided 95% lower limit of constant error, CE_L. (From Kaplan, L.A., and Pesce, A.J.: Clinical Chemistry: Theory, Analysis and Correlation, 3rd ed. St. Louis, Mosby, 1996.)

data is defined by its ability to be placed into specific categories. This type of data is statistically evaluated using P-values, the chi-square test, and Fisher's exact test. The chi-square test concerns the frequency with which an observation occurs and is used to evaluate discrete data to generate a P-value. Fisher's exact test generates a more conservative estimate of the P-value and is used when the study numbers are small.

B. Continuous data vary over a continuous range. Continuous data are evaluated using these statistical measures: central tendency, variation, and distribution of the data. Tests for continuous data include the one-sample t-test, the independent two-sample t-test, the paired t-test, and the analysis of variance (ANOVA) test.

1. One-sample t-test—Compares the sample mean value to a known mean of a standard variable. This test calculates a t-value that is used to obtain a P-value from a statistics chart.
2. Two-sample t-test—Compares the mean values between two independent groups. The paired t-test allows comparison between two dependent samples.
3. ANOVA—Simply an extension of the t-test and allows determination of a statistically significant difference in the mean values when more than two independent groups are being compared. It relies on two sources of variation: between group and within group.
4. These statistical tests represent only the most basic of statistical procedures; the quality investigator will enlist the aid of a trained statistician to assist in data analysis.

C. The normal distribution is the key concept to understand. Normal is a statistical concept; it is not related to an anatomic condition or disease state. Some refer to the normal distribution as the "gaussian distribution" to avoid such confusion (Fig. 12–2). The normal distribution is a theoretical probability distribution determined by two quantities, the mean and standard deviation (SD). The mean is the total numeric sum of all the values divided by the number of values. The SD is simply the square root of the variance, where variance is the mean of the squared deviations about the mean of the data. Changing the mean shifts the entire curve along the X axis (abscissa), whereas changing the SD changes the "width" of the curve along the X axis. The normal distribution is unimodal, bell-shaped, and symmetrical at a horizontal line equal to the mean value. Virtually all observations in a normal distribution occur within mean ± 3 SD, 95% within mean ± 2 SD, and 2/3 within mean ± 1 SD. The mean is a measure of central tendency. Other terms include:

1. Median—The middlemost observation.
2. Mode—The most frequently occurring observation.
3. Standard Deviation—A measure of spread or variation.
4. Range—The highest minus lowest value.
5. Mean Deviation—The average value of all deviation from the mean.
6. Variance—The average of the squares of each observation's deviation from the mean.
7. Standard Error of the Mean—When comparing different samples with different means, the standard error of the mean

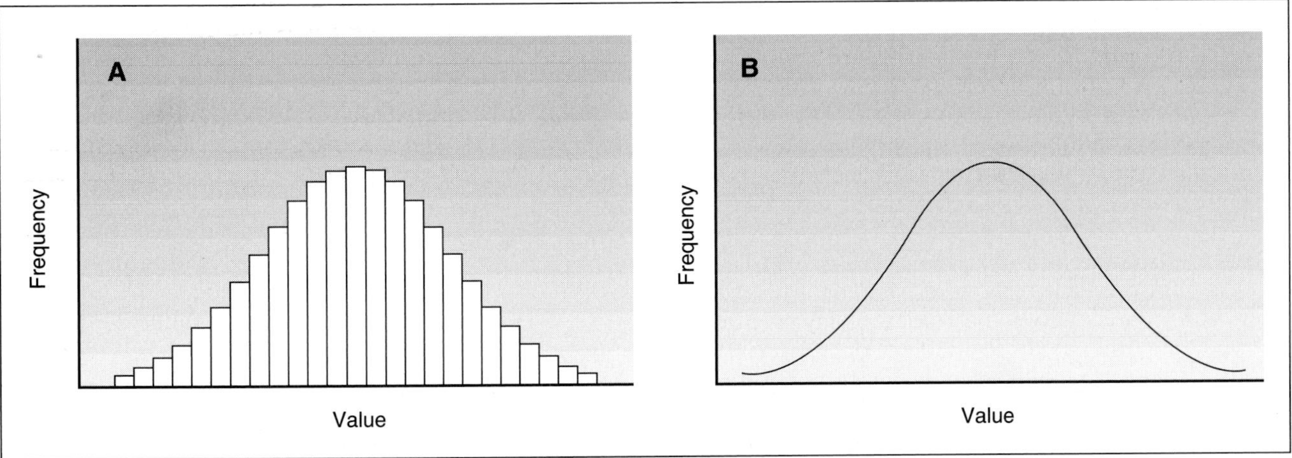

Figure 12–2. Illustration of the normal (gaussian) distribution. Diagram A shows a probability distribution of actual data, plotted as a histogram with very narrow ranges, and diagram B shows the way this idea is represented, for simplicity, in textbooks, articles, and tests. (From Jekel, J. F., Elmore, J. G., and Katz, D. L.: Epidemiology, Biostatistics, and Preventive Medicine. Philadelphia, WB Saunders, 1996.)

must be used, which is the standard deviation of the distribution of sample means.

D. Correlation analysis and regression analysis refer to methods by which two variables are shown to be related.
   1. Correlation analysis gives a value that allows for the assessment of the extent to which two sets of data or variables are related.
   2. Regression analysis utilizes a mathematic equation to calculate approximate values of a variable from known values of another variable.

E. Validity and reliability.
   1. Reliability refers to the ability to repeat the same results/measurements.
      a. Intra- and interobserver error can affect reliability and must be adequately accounted for and controlled within the experimental design.
   2. Validity refers to the extent to which an experimental value represents a true value.
      a. The study of biologic systems introduces biologic variability into an investigation.
      b. The method of distinguishing biologic variability from measurement error is the ANOVA test, from which a reliability coefficient/interclass correlation coefficient can be derived.

XX. Types of Studies

A. Descriptive—Descriptive studies take available data and arrange and present them to highlight or demonstrate differences or significant findings. Case reports, case series, correlational studies, and cross-sectional studies are examples of descriptive studies. These studies cannot show cause-and-effect relationships, but they are highly useful in showing associations that may be studied further.
   1. Case Reports and Case Series—A presentation/description of a disease or condition that occurred in one patient. Case series present information from multiple patients with a similar disease or condition. These generate speculative associations, which can be further tested by analytical studies.
   2. Correlational Studies—Studies that use very large sample sizes to identify associations between a disease or injury and another studied variable. Correlational studies are best used to generate a research hypothesis and a worthy study, but no conclusions can be drawn.
   3. Cross-Sectional Studies—This type of study evaluates a group at one point in time. Often described as a "snapshot" of a population or sample. Causal links between diagnosis and variables are found, but no conclusions are assumed.

B. Analytic—Analytic studies are designed to compare exposures to risk factors and disease states. They allow for hypothesis testing and statistical analysis. The two major types of analytic studies are cohort and experimental. Cohort studies are those in which the researcher does not influence or alter the conditions of the group being studied. The researcher is an observer who records occurrences as they happen. In experimental studies, the researcher is actively involved in controlling and altering the conditions of the group as a part of the experimental design or protocol.
   1. Case Control—Subjects in the study group are chosen for the presence of an injury or the presence of a disease. The group is then analyzed to identify associated, clinically relevant information. Case control studies by definition begin with a population and its disease and cannot be evaluated prospectively to determine exposure.
   2. **Prospective Cohort Study**—A study in which a group of disease-free subjects is followed over time to identify onset of disease or injury. This type of study identifies incidence. Cohort studies are useful for establishing relative risk.
   3. **Meta-analysis**—The combining of several smaller cohort studies into one larger cohort to examine treatment and outcome variables.
   4. Outcomes Research—A branch of clinical epidemiology that makes a scientific measurement of the effect of a condition on the life of a patient. The data are reported in a way that allows comparison to the work of other investigators. The rising cost of health care, varying regional practice patterns, and poor methods of clinical research in the past have spawned the recent interest in outcomes research. The only validated research instruments are the General Health Assessment (SF36) and the Sickness Impact Profile. Others, such as the Harris Hip Score, Hospital for Special Surgery Knee rating, and the International Knee Documentation Committee, have not been validated or tested for reliability.
   5. Interventional Study—Also known as a clinical trial and involves the testing of an intervention. The gold standard of studies is the randomized, blinded clinical trial. This type of study is usually designed to minimize the impact of bias and confounding factors.

XXI. Epidemiology

A. Epidemiology is the study of the frequency and cause of disease in human populations. The terminology of this field permeates the medical literature and therefore an understanding of these terms is critical in the evaluation and design of experiments. Concepts such as prevalence and incidence measure the frequency of disease within a given population.

1. Prevalence is defined as the total number of affected individuals at a single point in time divided by the total number of individuals at risk for the disease or condition in a population.

$$\text{Incidence} = \text{New cases developing over a period of time}$$

$$\text{Cumulative incidence} = \frac{\text{New cases developing over a period of time}}{\text{Total cases without the disease at the start of the time period}}$$

$$\text{Incidence rate} = \frac{\text{New cases developing over a period of time}}{\text{Total person-time of observation}}$$

$$\text{Relative risk} = \frac{\text{Incidence of condition in population exposed}}{\text{Incidence of condition in population not exposed}}$$

2. Incidence is defined as the number of new cases of the disease or condition that arise during a specified time interval.
3. Cumulative incidence is the incidence divided by the total number of individuals at risk for the disease or condition in a population. Unfortunately, cumulative incidence does not account for varying time periods.
4. The incidence rate is the number of new cases in a specified time interval divided by the population at risk but without disease. It gives a far better estimation of the significance of exposure.

B. Measures of disease association allow definition of the relationship between exposure to a risk factor and the disease or condition studied.

1. Relative risk is the estimation of this association. It is defined as the incidence in the exposed group divided by the incidence in the unexposed group.
2. As the relative risk approaches 1, the incidence rates of both groups reach equality. Above 1, a positive correlation between the risk and the condition being studied exists. Below 1, the exposure is exerting a protective effect on the population being exposed.
3. Relative risk can be approximated retrospectively by calculating the odds ratio.
4. The odds ratio is the odds of exposure in those with the condition/disease compared with the odds in those without disease.

Selected Bibliography

Brickmeyer, N.J., Weinstein, J.N.: Clinical epidemiology. In Beaty, J.H., ed.: Orthopaedic Knowledge Update 6. Am. Acad. Orthop. Surg. 89–95, 1999.

Colton, T.: Statistics in Medicine. Boston, Little Brown & Co., 1974.

Committee on Professional Liability: Guide to the Ethical Practice of Orthopaedic Surgery, 3rd ed. Illinois, AAOS, 1998.

Committee on Professional Liability: Managing Orthopaedic Malpractice Risk. Illinois, AAOS, 1996.

Committee on Professional Liability: Medical Malpractice: A Primer for Orthopaedic Residents and Fellows. Illinois, AAOS, 1993.

Dawson-Saunders, B., Trapp, R.G., eds.: Basic and Clinical Biostatistics. Norwalk, CT, Appleton & Lange, 1990.

Elam, K., Taylor, V., Ciol, M.A., et al.: Impact of a workers' compensation practice guideline on lumbar spine fusion in Washington state. Med. Care 35:417–424, 1997.

Ellrodt, G., Cook, D.J., Lee, J., et al.: Evidence-based disease management. JAMA 278:1687–1692, 1997.

Ellwood, P.M.: Shattuck lecture: Outcomes management, a technique of patient experience. N. Engl. J. Med. 318:1549–1556, 1988.

Epstein, A.M.: The outcomes movement: Will it get us where we want to go? N. Engl. J. Med. 323:266–270, 1990.

Feinstein, A.R., ed.: Clinical Epidemiology: The Architecture of Clinical Research. Philadelphia, W.B. Saunders, 1985.

Ficarra, B.: Medicolegal Examination, Evaluation, and Report. Florida, CRC Press Inc., 1987.

Fletcher, R.H., Fletcher, S.W., Wagner, E.H., eds.: Clinical Epidemiology: The Essentials, 2nd ed. Baltimore, Williams & Wilkins, 1988.

Gartland, J.J.: Orthopaedic clinical research: Deficiencies in experimental design and determinations of outcome. J. Bone Joint Surg. 70A:1357–1364, 1988.

Gottlieb, S., Einhorn, T.: Beyond HMOs: Understanding the next wave of changes in health-care organization. J. Am. Assoc. Orthop. Surg. 6:75–83, 1998.

Greenfield, M.V., Kuhn, J.E., Wojyts, E.M.: Current concepts: A statistical primer. Am. J. Surg. Med. 24:3–6; 25:1–6; 26:1–3.

Hennekens, C.H., Buring, J.E., Mayrent, S.L., eds.: Epidemiology in Medicine. Boston, Little Brown & Co., 1987.

Hinkle, D.E., Jurs, S.G., Wiersma, W.: Applied Statistics for the Behavioral Sciences. Boston, Houghton-Mifflin, 1979.

Hulley, S.R., Cumings, S.R., eds.: Designing Clinical Research. Baltimore, Williams & Wilkins, 1988.

Ingelfinger, J.A., Mosteller, F., Thibodeau, L.A., et al., eds.: Biostatistics in Clinical Medicine, 3rd ed. New York, McGraw-Hill, 1994.

Int J Technol Assess Health Care 13(2), 1997.

Kelsey, J.L., ed.: Epidemiology of Musculoskeletal Disorders. New York, Oxford University Press, 1982.

Kreder, H.J., Wright, J.G., McLeod, R.: Outcome studies in surgical research. Surgery 121:223–225, 1997.

Laupacis, A., Sekar, N., Stiell, G.: Clinical prediction rules: A review and suggested modifications of methodological standards. JAMA 277:488–494, 1997.

Lieber, R.L.: Experimental design and statistical analysis. In Simon, S.R., ed.: Orthopaedic Basic Science. Chicago, AAOS, 1994.

Martin, D.P., Engelberg, R., Agel, J., et al.: Development of a musculoskeletal extremity health status instrument: The Musculoskeletal Function Assessment Instrument. J. Orthop. Res. 14:173–181, 1996.

Mozena, J.P., Emerick, C.E., Black, S.C., eds.: Clinical Guideline Development: An Algorithm Approach. Gaithersburg, MD, Aspen Publishers, 1996.

National Health Lawyers Association: Colloquium report on legal issues related to clinical practice issues. Washington, DC, 1995.

Petitti, D.B., ed.: Meta-Analysis, Decision Analysis, and Cost-Effectiveness Analysis: Methods for Quantitative Synthesis in Medicine. New York, Oxford University Press, 1994.

Rosenberg, A.G.: Practice guidelines. In Beaty, J.H., ed.: Orthopaedic Knowledge Update 6. Am. Acad. Orthop. Surg. 97–102, 1999.

Schootman, M., Powell, J.W., Albright, J.P.: Statistics in sports injury research. In DeLee, J.C., Drez, D., Jr.: Orthopaedics Sports Medicine: Principles of Practice. Philadelphia, WB Saunders, 1994.

Szabo, R.M.: Statistical analysis as related to hand surgery. J. Hand Surg. 22A:376–384, 1997.

Szklo, M.: Design and conduct of epidemiological studies. Prev. Med. 16:142–149, 1987.

Whimster, W.F.: Biomedical Research. New York, Springer-Verlag, 1997.

Winslade, W.J.: The Texas Medical Jurisprudence Examination: A Self-Study Guide. Texas: University of Texas Medical Branch, 1997.

Wright, J.G.: Outcomes Assessment. In Beaty, J.H., ed.: Orthopaedic Knowledge Update 6. Am. Acad. Orthop. Surg. 103–106, 1999.

Wright, J.G., McLeod, R.S., Lossing, A.: Measurement in surgical clinical research. Surgery 119:241–244, 1996.

Index

Note: Page numbers in *italics* indicate illustrations; those followed by t indicate tables.

— B —

— D —

— E —

— G —

— H —

— I —

— N —

— O —

— P —

— Q —

— R —

— S —

— T —

— U —

— V —

— W —

— X —

— Y —

— Z —

Spinal dysplasias

SED
MED
psadoAchadr
Kneists
drastroph dwarf

Marf fibrillin
Achadropl FGFR3
OI col 1A1 1A2

Genes SED/Kneist col2A1
MED col9A2